Musculoskeletal Injuries and Conditions

Musculoskeletal Injuries and Conditions

Assessment and Management

Se Won Lee, MD
Associate Professor
Department of Clinical Physical Medicine and Rehabilitation
Albert Einstein College of Medicine
Fellowship Director, Sports Medicine
Director
Electrodiagnostic Laboratory
Department of Rehabilitation Medicine
Montefiore Medical Center
Bronx, New York

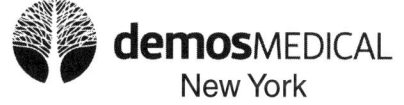

Visit our website at www.demosmedical.com

ISBN: 9781620700983
e-book ISBN: 9781617052750

Acquisitions Editor: Beth Barry
Compositor: Newgen KnowledgeWorks

Copyright © 2017 Springer Publishing Company.
Demos Medical Publishing is an imprint of Springer Publishing Company, LLC.

All rights reserved. This book is protected by copyright. No part of it may be reproduced, stored in a retrieval system, or transmitted in any form or by any means, electronic, mechanical, photocopying, recording, or otherwise, without the prior written permission of the publisher.

Medicine is an ever-changing science. Research and clinical experience are continually expanding our knowledge, in particular our understanding of proper treatment and drug therapy. The authors, editors, and publisher have made every effort to ensure that all information in this book is in accordance with the state of knowledge at the time of production of the book. Nevertheless, the authors, editors, and publisher are not responsible for errors or omissions or for any consequences from application of the information in this book and make no warranty, expressed or implied, with respect to the contents of the publication. Every reader should examine carefully the package inserts accompanying each drug and should carefully check whether the dosage schedules mentioned therein or the contraindications stated by the manufacturer differ from the statements made in this book. Such examination is particularly important with drugs that are either rarely used or have been newly released on the market.

Library of Congress Cataloging-in-Publication Data
Names: Lee, Se Won, author.
Title: Musculoskeletal injuries and conditions: assessment and management / Se Won Lee.
Description: New York: Demos Medical Publishing, [2017] | Includes bibliographical references.
Identifiers: LCCN 2016025422| ISBN 9781620700983 | ISBN 9781617052750 (e-book)
Subjects: | MESH: Musculoskeletal Diseases—diagnosis | Musculoskeletal Diseases—therapy | Musculoskeletal System—injuries | Physical Examination | Handbooks | Outlines
Classification: LCC RC925.5 | NLM WE 39 | DDC 617.4/7044—dc23
LC record available at https://lccn.loc.gov/2016025422

Special discounts on bulk quantities of Demos Medical Publishing books are available to corporations, professional associations, pharmaceutical companies, health care organizations, and other qualifying groups. For details, please contact:

Special Sales Department
Demos Medical Publishing
11 West 42nd Street, 15th Floor, New York, NY 10036
Phone: 800–532-8663 or 212–683-0072; Fax: 212–941-7842
E-mail: specialsales@demosmedical.com

Printed in the United States of America by Bradford & Bigelow.
16 17 18 19 20 / 5 4 3 2 1

This book is dedicated to my wife (Hyunjoo), my daughter (Jane), and my mentors (Dr. Dennis D. J. Kim and Dr. Mooyeon Oh-Park). It is also dedicated to the Physical Medicine and Rehabilitation faculty at Montefiore Medical Center (Dr. Matthew Bartels, Dr. Mark Thomas, Dr. Stanley Wainapel, Dr. Sikha Guha, Dr. Eathar Saad, Dr. Yuxi Chen, Dr. Yumei Wang, Dr. Karen Morice, Dr. Andrew Gitkind, Dr. Emal Wahezi, Dr. Sooyeon Kim, Dr. Olivera Pekovic, Dr. Jeffrey Nissinoff, Dr. Gary Inwald, Dr. Maria Castro, Dr. Meg Krilov, Dr. David Prince, Dr. Anna Lasak, Dr. Rani Kathirithamby, Dr. David Cancel, Dr. Grigory Syrkin, Dr. Huma Naqvi, and Dr. Maria Reyes), and past, present, and future fellows and residents.

Contents

Abbreviations xv
Preface xvii
Acknowledgments xix

1. APPROACH TO THE PATIENT WITH A MUSCULOSKELETAL PROBLEM 1

History and Physical Examination 1
  Chief Complaint 1
  Neurological Impairment 4
  Other History 6
  Past Medical History (Limited to MSK Problems) 8
  Review of Systems 8
  Other MSK Symptoms 9
  Physical Examination 9
  Provocative Test 11

Clinically Oriented Anatomy 12
  Tendon and Ligament 12
  Muscle and Fascia 16
  Bursa 20
  Bone and Joint 20
  Nervous System 26

Biomechanics 28
  Introduction 28
  Clinical Application 29
  Gait Cycle 29
  Gait Dysfunction 31

Workup 33
  MSK Imaging 33
  Radiographs 33
  Advanced Imaging 36
  Scanning Protocol Modified From AIUM Protocol 45
  Other Workup: Laboratory Investigation 56

Treatment 57
  Patient Education 57
  Pharmacologic Management 57
  Local Intervention 64
  Physical and Occupational Therapy 69
  Orthoses 75
  Treatment Based on Different Anatomical Pathologies 76

References 78

2. NECK 83

Epidemiology of Neck Pain 83
  Neck Pain in the General Population 83
  Neck Pain in Athletes 83
  Neck Pain at Work 83

Differential Diagnosis 83
  Unusual Causes of Neck Pain 84
  Neurological Symptoms Associated With Neck Pain 85

Anatomy 87
  Regional Anatomy 87
  Spine Complex (Bone and Joint) 87
  Ligament 90
  Nerve: Root and Plexus 90
  Muscle 92
  Fascia 95
  Blood Supply 95

Biomechanics 96

Physical Examination 97
  Inspection 97
  Palpation 97
  Neurologic Examination and Special Examination 97

Diagnostic Studies 99
  Plain Radiographs 99
  MRI 100
  Point-of-Care Ultrasonagraphy 100
  CT Scan 101
  Electromyography (EMG) 101

Treatment 101
  Nonoperative Management 101
  Surgery 102

Nerve and Spinal Cord Pathology 103
  Cervical Radiculopathy 103
  Noncompressive Radiculopathy 104
  C5 (Nerve Root) Palsy 104
  Greater Occipital Neuralgia 105
  Supraclavicular Nerve Entrapment Syndrome 106

Cervical Myelopathy 106
Cervical Cord Neurapraxia 107
Ossification of Posterior Longitudinal Ligament (OPLL) 107
Syringomyelia 108
Chiari Malformation 108
Drop Head Syndrome 109

Bone and Joint Pathology 109
Cervical Facet Pathology 109
Whiplash-Associated Injury 110
Degenerative Disc Disease 110
Rheumatoid Arthritis 111
Cervical Spine Disorder in Down Syndrome 111
Klippel–Feil Anomaly 112
Fracture 112
Metastatic Cervical Spine Tumor 114

Muscle and Ligament Pathology 114
Cervical Strain/Sprain 114
Myofascial Pain Syndrome 115

References 115

3. SHOULDER 119

Epidemiology of Shoulder Pain 119
Shoulder Pain in the General Population 119
Shoulder Pain in Athletes 119
Shoulder Pain at Work 119

Differential Diagnosis 119
Musculoskeletal (MSK) Causes of Shoulder Pain Based on Location 119
Neuropathic Causes of Shoulder Pain 122
Extrinsic Causes of Shoulder Pain 122
Neurological Symptoms 122
Snapping Shoulder 123
Shoulder Instability 123

Anatomy 124
Bone, Joint, and Ligament 124
Nerve 126
Bursa 126
Muscle 127

Biomechanics 129
Shoulder Movement 129
Subacromial Impingement 130
Subcoracoid Impingement: Roller Wringer Effect 130
Suprascapular Nerve Traction With Scapula Position 130
Biomechanics of Throwing 131
Shoulder Stability 131

Physical Examination 132
Inspection 132
Palpation 132
Range of Motion 132
Strength of Rotator Cuff Muscles 133
Special Tests 133

Diagnostic Studies 135
Plain Radiographs 135
Point-of-Care Ultrasonography 136
MRI/MRA 136
CT Scan 137

Treatment 137
Nonoperative Management 137
Surgery 138

Tendon and Bursa Pathology 139
Impingement Syndrome 139
Rotator Cuff Tendinopathy and Tear 142
Calcific Tendinopathy 143
Biceps Long-Head Tendon Pathologies 144
Pectoralis Muscle Strain and Tear 146

Joint and Bone Pathology 146
AC Joint Sprain and Injury 146
AC Osteoarthritis 147
Distal Clavicle Osteolysis 148
Glenohumeral Joint Pathologies 148
Shoulder Osteoarthritis 149
Shoulder Instability 150
Multidirectional Instability 151
SLAP (Superior Labral Anteroposterior) Lesion 151
Bennett Lesion 152
Rheumatologic Disease 152
Infectious Pathology 154
Osteonecrosis of the Humeral Head 155
Little League Shoulder 155
Sternoclavicular (SC) Sprain/Injury 156
SC Osteoarthritis 156
Fracture 156

Neuropathy and Vascular Dysfunction 158
Brachial Amyotrophy (Parsonage Turner Syndrome) 158
Cervical Radiculopathy 159
Stinger Syndrome (Burner) 159
Thoracic Outlet Syndrome (TOS) 159
Effort Thrombosis (Paget–Schroetter Syndrome) 160
Axillary Artery Occlusion 161
Suprascapular Neuropathy 161
Quadrilateral Space Syndrome 162

References 162

4. ELBOW 167

Epidemiology of Elbow Pain 167
Elbow Pain in the General Population 167
Elbow Pain in Athletes 167
Elbow Pain at Work 167

Differential Diagnosis 167
Elbow Instability 169
Snapping Elbow 169
Stiffness 169

Anatomy   170
   Bone and Joint   170
   Ligament   171
   Nerve   171
   Muscle   172

Biomechanics   174
   Kinetic and Kinematics   174
   Elbow Stability   174
   Elbow Function in ADL   174

Physical Examination   175
   Inspection   175
   Palpation   175
   Range of Motion   175
   Special Tests   176

Diagnostic Studies   177
   Plain Radiographs   177
   Point-of-Care Ultrasonography   177
   MRI/MRA   178
   CT Scan   178

Treatment   178
   Nonoperative Management   178
   Surgery   179

Tendon, Ligament, and Bursa Pathology   179
   Lateral Epicondylitis   179
   Lateral Collateral Ligament Sprain   180
   Medial Epicondylitis   180
   Little League Elbow   181
   Ulnar Collateral Ligament (UCL) Injury   181
   Valgus Extension Overload Syndrome
     (Posteromedial Impingement)   182
   Distal Biceps Tendinopathy/Tear   182
   Bicipitoradial Bursitis   183
   Triceps Tendinopathy and Tear   183
   Olecranon Bursitis   183

Bone and Joint Pathology   184
   Osteoarthritis   184
   Osteochondritis Dissecans
     of the Elbow (Capitellum)   184
   Posterior Impingement of the Elbow   185
   Rheumatoid Arthritis   185
   Myositis Ossificans   186
   Fracture   186
   Elbow Dislocation   189

Neuropathy   189
   Ulnar Neuropathy   189
   Radial Tunnel Syndrome   192
   Posterior Antebrachial Cutaneous
     Neuropathy   193
   Median Neuropathy at Elbow   193
   Other Nerves   194
References   194

5. WRIST AND HAND   197

Epidemiology of Wrist and Hand Pain   197
   Wrist and Hand Pain in the General
     Population   197
   Wrist and Hand Pain in Athletes   197
   Wrist and Hand Pain at Work   197

Differential Diagnosis   197
   MSK Causes of Wrist and Hand Pain
     Based on Location   197
   Neuropathic Causes of Wrist
     and Hand Pain   199
   Differential Diagnosis of
     Finger/Wrist Drop   200
   Snapping   200

Anatomy   200
   Bone, Joint, and Ligament   200
   Nerve   204
   Muscle   206
   No Man's Land   208

Biomechanics   208
   Forearm Movement and RU Joint   208
   ROM of Wrist and Hand   208
   Proximal Carpal Movements   208
   Wrist Stability   209
   Biomechanics of Hand   209

Physical Examination   209
   Inspection   209
   Palpation   210
   Special Tests of Wrist and Hand   211
   Special Examination of Hand (Finger)   213

Diagnostic Studies   214
   Plain Radiographs   214
   Point-of-Care Ultrasonography   214
   MRI/MRA   215
   CT Scan   215
   Electromyography (EMG)   215

Treatment   216
   Nonoperative Management   216
   Surgery   217

Tendon and Ligament Pathology   218
   Wrist Extensor Tendon Disorders   218
   Wrist Flexor Tendon Disorders   220
   Trigger Fingers   221
   Retinacular Cyst   221
   Dupuytren's Disease   222
   Gamekeeper's (Skier's) Thumb
     and Stener's Lesion   222
   Finger Sprain and Strain   223
   Volar Plate Injury   224
   Central Slip Extensor Injury   224

Nerve Entrapment Syndrome   224
  Carpal Tunnel Syndrome (CTS)   224
  Anterior Interosseous Neuropathy   225
  Ulnar Neuropathy at Wrist   225
  Superficial Radial Neuropathy   226

Bone and Joint Pathology   227
  First Carpometacarpal (CMC) Osteoarthritis
    (Trapeziometacarpal)   227
  Osteoarthritis of the Wrist   227
  Pisotriquetral (PT) Arthritis/Instability   228
  Rheumatoid Arthritis of the Wrist
    and Hand   228
  Ligament Sprain and Instability   230
  Ganglion Cyst   232
  Carpal Boss   233
  Tumor   233
  Fracture   234

Other Pathology   237
  Hypothenar Hammer Syndrome   237
References   238

6. BACK   241

Epidemiology of Back Pain   241
  Back Pain in the General Population   241
  Back Pain in Children   241
  Back Pain in Athletes   241
  Back Pain at Work   241

Differential Diagnosis   242
  Working Definition of Low Back   242
  Differential Diagnosis Based on
    Mode of Onset   243
  Classification and Differential Diagnosis
    of Spine Deformity   244
  Differential Diagnosis of Severe
    Back Spasm   244
  Differential Diagnoses of Bowel and
    Bladder Dysfunction Related to Spine
    Pathologies   244
  Differential Diagnosis of Chest
    Wall Pain   244
  Differential Diagnosis of Buttock Pain   246

Anatomy   247
  Bone and Joint   247
  Nerve   250
  Artery   252
  Muscle   252

Biomechanics   253
  Lumbar Spine Biomechanics   254

Physical Examination   256
  Inspection   256
  Palpation   256
  Neurological and Other Examination   256
  Red Flags   258

Diagnostic Studies   259
  Plain Radiographs   259
  CT Scan   260
  MRI   260
  Serologic Tests   262
  Electromyography (EMG)   262

Treatment   263
  Nonoperative Management   263
  Surgery   264

Back Pain   265
  Nerve and Spinal Cord Pathology   265
  Bone and Joint Pathology   270
  Muscle and Ligament Pathology   280

Chest Wall Pain   281
  Bone and Joint Pathology   281
  Nerve Pathologies   283
  Muscle Strain   283

Buttock Pain   284
  Bone and Joint Pathology   284
  Tendon and Bursa Pathology   286
  Ischiogluteal Bursitis   288
  Neuropathy   288
  Miscellaneous Pathology   289
References   290

7. HIP AND THIGH   295

Epidemiology of Hip Pain   295
  Hip Pain in the General Population   295
  Hip Pain in Children   295
  Hip Pain in Athletes   295
  Hip Pain at Work   295

Differential Diagnosis   295
  Differential Diagnosis of Hip Pain
    Based on Location   295
  Snapping Hip (Coxa Saltans)   299
  Differential Diagnosis of Groin Mass   300
  Differential Diagnosis of Hip Instability   300

Anatomy   300
  Bone and Joint   300
  Ligament   301
  Nerve   302
  Muscle   302

Biomechanics   303
  Kinematic and Kinetic   303
  Hip Stability   304

Physical Examination   304
  Inspection   304
  Palpation   305
  Range of Motion   305
  Special Examination   305

Diagnostic Studies   306
  Plain Radiographs   307

Point-of-Care Ultrasonography   307
MRI/MRA   308

Treatment   *308*
Nonoperative Management   308
Surgery   308

Joint and Bone Pathology   *309*
OA of Hip   309
Labral Tear   310
Femoroacetabular Impingement   311
Avascular Necrosis of Hip   312
Stress Fracture   312
Osteitis Pubis   313
Avulsion Fracture and Apophyseal Injuries   314
Hip Pointer   314
Hip Dislocation   315
Tumor or Tumorlike Lesion   315

Bursitis and Tendinopathy   *315*
Lateral Hip   315
Groin   317

Neuropathy   *319*
Lateral Femoral Cutaneous Nerve   319
Anterior Femoral Cutaneous Neuralgia   320
Obturator Neuropathy   320
Border Nerve Syndrome (Ilioinguinal, Iliohypogastric, and Genitofemoral Nerves)   320
Posterior Femoral Cutaneous Neuropathy   321

Other Pathology   *321*
Myositis Ossificans   321
Transient Osteoporosis   321

Pediatric Hip Pathology   *322*
Individual Conditions   323
Transient Synovitis or Irritable Hip   323

References   *323*

8. KNEE   327

Epidemiology of Knee Pain   *327*
Knee Pain in the General Population   327
Knee Pain in Athletes   327
Knee Pain at Work   327

Differential Diagnosis   *327*
MSK (Musculoskeletal) Causes of Knee Pain Based on Location   327
Neuropathic Causes of Knee and Leg Pain   330
Differential Diagnosis of Knee Swelling   331
Differential Diagnosis of Subjective Knee Instability   331
Differential Diagnosis of Painful Knee Snapping   331

Anatomy   *331*
Bone and Joint   331
Ligament and Meniscus   332
Nerve   334

Biomechanics   *334*
Kinematic and Kinetic   334
Knee Stability   336

Physical Examination   *337*
Inspection   337
Palpation   337
Range of Motion   337
Special Examination   338

Diagnostic Studies   *340*
Plain Radiographs   340
Point-of-Care Ultrasonography   341
MRI   341
MR and CT Arthrography   342

Management   *342*
Nonoperative Management   342
Surgery   343

Intra-Articular Structures   *344*
Bone and Joint Pathology   344
Inflammatory Arthropathy   347
Osteochondritis Dissecans   348
Spontaneous Osteonecrosis of the Knee   349
Proximal Tibiofibular Sprain and Instability   349
Meniscus Pathology   350
Ligament Injury   351
Plica Syndrome   353

Extra-Articular Structures (Bursa, Tendon, Ligament Pathology)   *354*
Medial Knee Pathology   354
Lateral Knee Pathology   356
Anterior Knee Pathology   356
Posterior Knee Pathology   359

Neuropathy   *360*
Saphenous Neuropathy; Gonalgia Paresthetica   360
Peroneal Neuropathy   361

References   *362*

9. LEG   367

Epidemiology of Leg Pain   *367*
Leg Pain in the General Population   367
Leg Pain in Athletes   367

Differential Diagnosis   *367*
Differential Diagnoses Based on Location of Pain   368
Differential Diagnosis of Calf Pain and Cramps   368
Differential Diagnosis of Leg Swelling   368
Differential Diagnosis of Atrophy and Pseudohypertrophy   369
Differential Diagnosis of Common Tibial Deformity   369
Other History to Ask   369

Anatomy   *369*
Cross-Sectional Anatomy   369
Bones   369
Muscles   370

Physical Examination 371
　Inspection 371
　Palpation 371
　Neurological Examination 371
　Evaluation of Foot for Pes Planus (Overpronation)
　　and Pes Cavus (With Supination) 371

Diagnostic Studies 371
　Plain Radiographs 371
　MRI 371
　Point-of-Care Ultrasonography (US) 372
　CT Scan 372
　Vascular Study and Other Tests 372

Treatment 372
　Nonoperative Management 372

Musculoskeletal Pathology 373
　Medial Tibial Stress Syndrome 373
　Chronic Exertional Compartment
　　Syndrome (CECS) 373
　Stress Fracture (of Tibia) 374
　Medial Gastrocnemius Tear 375
　Plantaris Tendon and Soleus Muscle Tear 375

Neuropathy 376
　Superficial Peroneal Neuropathy 376
　Tibial Neuropathy—Soleal Sling Syndrome 376
　Saphenous Neuritis 376
　Lateral Sural Cutaneous Neuropathy 376

Vascular Pathology 377
　Arterial Disease 377
　Venous Disease 378

Other Pathology 380
　Restless Legs Syndrome 380
　Statin Myopathy 380

References 380

10. ANKLE AND FOOT 383

Epidemiology of Ankle and Foot Pain 383
　Foot and Ankle Pain in the General
　　Population 383
　Foot and Ankle Pain in Athletes 383
　Foot and Ankle Pain at Work 383

Differential Diagnosis 383
　Musculoskeletal (MSK) Causes of Foot
　　and Ankle Pain Based on Location 383
　Differential Diagnosis of MSK Hindfoot
　　and Ankle Pain 385
　Differential Diagnosis of MSK Midfoot Pain 386
　Differential Diagnosis of MSK Forefoot Pain 386
　Neuropathic Causes of Foot and Ankle Pain
　　Based on Location 386
　Other Causes of Severe (Disabling)
　　Foot Pain 387
　Common Causes of Pes Cavus
　　(High Arch Foot) 387
　Differential Diagnosis of Pes Planus
　　(Flat Foot, Normal up to 6 Years) 387
　Differential Diagnosis of Ankle Equinus 387
　Differential Diagnosis of Ankle Instability 388
　Differential Diagnosis of Snapping Ankle 388
　Lateralization of Pain 388
　Differential Diagnosis of Neuropathic
　　Ankle and Foot Pain 388

Anatomy 388
　Bone and Joint 388
　Ligament 390
　Retinaculum 390
　Nerve 391
　Muscle 392

Biomechanics 394
　Kinetic and Kinematic 394
　Ankle and Foot in Gait 394
　Foot Alignment and Deformity 394

Physical Examination 395
　Inspection 395
　Palpation 396
　Range of Motion 396
　Special Tests 397

Diagnostic Studies 399
　Plain Radiographs 399
　Point-of-Care Ultrasonography 400
　MRI 401
　CT Scan 401

Treatment 401
　Nonoperative Management 401
　Surgery 406

Ankle and Hindfoot 407
　Ligament, Tendon, and Bursa Pathology 407
　Bone and Joint 415

Forefoot, Midfoot, and Toes 422
　Common Medial Forefoot and Toe
　　Pathologies 422
　Toe Deformity and Fracture 426
　Common Skin Lesion 429
　Common Midfoot Pathologies 429

Neuropathy 431
　Tarsal Tunnel Syndrome (Tibial Nerve Entrapment
　　Neuropathy at Ankle) 431
　Baxter's Neuropathy (Inferior Calcaneal
　　Neuropathy, 1st Branch of Lateral Plantar
　　Neuropathy) 432
　Jogger's Foot (Medial Plantar
　　Neuropathy) 432
　Morton's Interdigital Neuralgia 433
　Anterior Tarsal Tunnel Syndrome (Deep Peroneal
　　Nerve Entrapment Neuropathy) 433
　Superficial Peroneal Nerve Entrapment
　　Syndrome 434
　Saphenous Mononeuropathy 434

Sural Mononeuropathy　*435*
　　Medial Hallucal Neuropathy　*435*
　References　*435*

11. OTHER PAIN SYNDROMES　*441*

Epidemiology　*441*
　Epidemiology of Widespread Pain　*441*
　Epidemiology of Cancer Pain　*441*
　Epidemiology of Common Neuropathic Pain Conditions　*441*

Differential Diagnosis　*441*
　Generalized Musculoskeletal Pain　*442*
　Differential Diagnosis of Diffuse Neuropathic Pain　*442*

Physical Examination　*443*
　Examination for Neuropathic Pain　*443*

Diagnostic Studies　*444*
　Serologic Tests　*444*
　Electrodiagnosis　*444*
　Other Diagnostic Tests　*444*
　Imaging Tests　*444*

Generalized Musculoskeletal Pain　*445*
　Fibromyalgia　*445*
　Polymyalgia Rheumatica (PMR)　*446*
　Chronic Fatigue Syndrome　*448*

Pain Related to Cancer　*449*
　Bony Pain Related to Tumor　*449*
　Muscle and Soft Tissue Pain　*449*
　Joint Disorders/Synovitis (Neoplastic or Paraneoplastic)　*450*
　Neuropathic Pain Related to Tumor　*450*
　Paraneoplastic Peripheral Neuropathy　*451*
　Radiation Plexopathy　*451*
　Leptomeningeal Metastasis　*451*
　Polyradiculopathy　*451*
　Chronic Radiation Myelopathy　*451*

Neuropathic Pain　*452*
　Central Poststroke Pain Syndrome (Thalamic Pain)　*452*
　Spinal Cord Injury–Related Pain Syndrome　*452*
　Complex Regional Pain Syndrome　*453*
　Small Fiber Neuropathy　*454*
　Erythromelalgia　*455*

References　*455*

Index　*457*

Abbreviations

A	Artery	LCL	Lateral collateral ligament
AAP	Acetaminophen	lig	Ligament
Abx	Antibiotic	M	Male
ACL	Anterior cruciate ligament	m	Muscle
AFO	Ankle foot orthosis	MC	Most common
Ant	Anterior	MCL	Medial collateral ligament
ASA	Abnormal spontaneous activity	MNCS	Motor nerve conduction study
ASIS	Anterior superior iliac spine	MSK	Musculoskeletal
BMD	Bone densitometry	MT	Metatarsal
br	Branch	N	Nerve; neuropathy
Ca	Cancer	OPLL	Ossification of posterior longitudinal ligament
CIx	Contraindication		
CMAP	Compound motor action potential	PCL	Posterior cruciate ligament
CV	Cardiovascular	RA	Rheumatoid arthritis
D	Day	SCM	Sternocleidomastoid
Ddx	Differential diagnosis	sec	Seconds
DISI	Dorsal intercalated segmental instability	Sen	Sensitivity
DJD	Degenerative joint disease	SI	Signal intensity
DM	Diabetes	SNCS	Sensory nerve conduction study
DTR	Deep tendon reflex	SNRI	Serotonin-norepinephrine reuptake inhibitors
Dx	Diagnosis	Spe	Specificity
Dz	Disease	Sx	Symptom
E	Exercise	Syn	Syndrome
EMG	Electrodiagnosis; electromyography	Tx	Treatment
esp	Especially	US	Ultrasound; ultrasonography
F	Female	VISI	Ventral intercalated segmental instability
FOOSH	Fall onto outstretched hand	w	With
Fx	Fracture	wk	Week
GRF	Ground reaction force	wo	Without
Ix	Indications	YO	Year old
Jt	Joint		

Preface

This volume is intended for physiatrists, sports physicians, orthopedists, rheumatologists, and primary care physicians. Although there are comprehensive textbooks and abundant literature reviews devoted to musculoskeletal (MSK) medicine, gaps still exist regarding optimal outpatient management for many MSK disorders due to the relative paucity of information on the clinical decision-making process and differential diagnosis and treatment in the practice setting. This book tries to address these gaps by using a uniform approach (based on the symptoms, particularly the location of the pain) to the diagnosis of MSK disorders in different anatomic locations and emphasizing the nonoperative management options applicable to the outpatient clinic.

Each chapter provides a patho-anatomic approach based on the location of pain. This approach can be efficient and intuitive with sound knowledge of MSK anatomy, particularly in the peripheral MSK systems such as the hand and the foot. The author acknowledges the limitations of this approach in some MSK disorders (eg, chronic painful conditions or concomitant multiple pain generators) or in patients with difficulty identifying either surface anatomy or the location of the pain. Epidemiology, mechanism of injury, risk factors, and abnormal biomechanics are often useful information to obtain a relevant differential diagnosis, and each site-specific chapter contains the latest information on all of these topics. In addition, modification of risk factors and education about correct biomechanics are important in the successful management of MSK disorders. Each chapter describes concise physical examinations for each anatomic region and the reader is encouraged to cultivate essential physical examination skills using other available resources and visual demonstration.

Ultrasonography (US) has been increasingly available in the outpatient MSK clinic and has proven to be an important tool both in diagnosis and treatment. This book incorporates point-of-care ultrasound, defined as US performed and interpreted by the clinician at the bedside in the clinical decision-making process. Comprehensive information on the many applications of MSK US, including dynamic images of individual pathology and interventional techniques, is beyond the scope of this book.

Musculoskeletal Injuries and Conditions is not a comprehensive desk reference for all aspects of MSK care; it is rather a clinical guide to the diagnosis and management of MSK complaints routinely encountered in the outpatient clinic. My goal in writing the book is to help in framing a context for developing an initial management plan using flowcharts and providing quality nonoperative care. Indications for surgical referral are included. My intent is to foster an approach to common MSK complaints that can be applied and adapted to the specifics of individual cases. It is up to each clinician to determine the most appropriate treatment for the patient.

Se Won Lee, MD

Acknowledgments

I would like to thank the following colleagues, whose reviews and edits helped make this book possible:

Eun Kwang Byun, MD Private Practice, Orange, California

Richard Chang, MD Assistant Professor, Department of Physical Medicine and Rehabilitation and Orthopedic, SUNY Downstate Medical School

Mohammed Emam, MD Fellow, Sports Medicine, Department of Physical Medicine and Rehabilitation, Montefiore Medical Center/Albert Einstein College of Medicine

Dennis D. J. Kim, MD Associate Professor, Department of Physical Medicine and Rehabilitation, Montefiore Medical Center/Albert Einstein College of Medicine

Jung H. Kim, MD Assistant Professor, Department of Anesthesiology, Mount Sinai St Luke's Hospital/Mount Sinai College of Medicine

Soo Yeon Kim, MD Assistant Professor, Department of Physical Medicine and Rehabilitation and Anesthesiology, Montefiore Medical Center/Albert Einstein College of Medicine

Bittu Kuruvilla, MD Fellow, Sports Medicine, Department of Physical Medicine and Rehabilitation, Montefiore Medical Center/Albert Einstein College of Medicine

Jenna Le, MD Fellow, Musculoskeletal Radiology, Department of Radiology, Montefiore Medical Center/Albert Einstein College of Medicine

Phuong Le, DO Fellow, Pain Medicine, UCLA/VA Greater Los Angeles Healthcare System

Karen Morice, MD Assistant Professor, Department of Physical Medicine and Rehabilitation, Montefiore Medical Center/Albert Einstein College of Medicine

Mooyeon Oh-Park, MD Associate Professor, Kessler Institute of Rehabilitation, Rutgers University Medical School

Rakhi Sutaria, MD Fellow, Sports Medicine, Department of Physical Medicine and Rehabilitation, Montefiore Medical Center/Albert Einstein College of Medicine

Beverly Thornhill, MD Associate Professor, MSK Radiology, Department of Radiology, Montefiore Medical Center/Albert Einstein College of Medicine

Timothy Tiu, MD Attending Physician, Sports Medicine, Department of Physical Medicine and Rehabilitation, Montefiore Medical Center/Albert Einstein College of Medicine

CHAPTER 1

Approach to the Patient With a Musculoskeletal Problem

HISTORY AND PHYSICAL EXAMINATION

CHIEF COMPLAINT

Common chief complaints in outpatient musculoskeletal (MSK) clinic

Pain
- Nociceptive (somatic, MSK) and neuropathic pain
- Combined: common (eg, chronic MSK pain with neuropathic components involved)
- Nonorganic cause of pain: underrecognized

Loss of function
- Disability: restriction or lack of ability to perform an activity (1)
- Neurologic causes or secondary to pain (with MSK causes)

Characteristics of Pain
- Important clues for differential diagnosis and approach to the plan
- Many different ways available to characterize the pain
- Systematic approach recommended to decrease missing information

    Description of pain, "PQRST," by the International Association for the Study of Pain (2)

P—provoke and palliate
- Specify the etiology or contributing factors
- Identify provoking (aggravating) or alleviating (palliating) factors
  - Therapeutic implication by modifying abnormal biomechanics (provoking factors) especially in overuse injury

Q—quality (characteristics)
- Nociceptive (MSK), neuropathic pain or mixed pattern
- Nociceptive, neuropathic (non-nociceptive), mixed, and psychogenic

	NOCICEPTIVE PAIN	NEUROPATHIC PAIN
Characteristics	Aching, dull, and tearing	Electric shock, paroxysmal Pins, needle, burning, tingling, and numbness
Temporal pattern	Worse during the day or at the end of day (activity related) • Inflammatory: at night (second part of the night) ○ Often wake up and move to relieve symptoms	Worse at night and/or when waking up
Contributing factor (provoking)	Mechanical: worse with movement and weight bearing activity • Becomes constant as it progresses • Inflammatory arthropathy: improves with movement ± significant morning stiffness >1 hour, for example, rheumatoid arthritis	Compression or stretching of the peripheral nerve • Helps identify etiology/underlying biomechanics and therapeutic implication by addressing aggravating factors ○ For example, cycling (handle bar) or driving with leaning the elbow on the side: ulnar neuropathy on the wrist and the elbow. Inversion ankle sprain: stretch/injure superficial peroneal N

N, nerve.

1. Approach to the Patient With a Musculoskeletal Problem

- Mixed pattern: chronic nociceptive (MSK) pain has neuropathic pain components
- Psychosomatic pain: no typical presentation or distribution of involvement
  - Complaints are more impressive than the clinical evaluation; do not be judgmental, often responsive to the treatment

R—regional (local) versus diffuse versus referred pain
- Indentify typical pain patterns: the dermatomal pattern (root), peripheral nerve distribution, or sclerotome (frequently overlooked; Figure 1.1)
- Regional/local pain
  - Explains acute/subacute lesions of local MSK structures better
  - Knowledge of the regional/surface anatomy: especially superficial structure (hand and foot) leading to localization of pathology
  - Joint structures as pain generator; different structures have different pain thresholds (contribution)

	PAIN PERCEPTION DURING DIRECT PROBING DURING ARTHROSCOPY (4)	PAIN CORRELATION WITH MRI FINDING IN KNEE OA (5)
Highly painful structure (nociceptive)	Periosteum, subchondral bone, capsule, and fat pad	
Intermediate	Synovium	Cartilage volume/thickness to presence of pain (weak relation)
More controversial as pain generator	Articular cartilage	Meniscal tear in patient with knee osteoarthritis

OA, osteoarthritis.

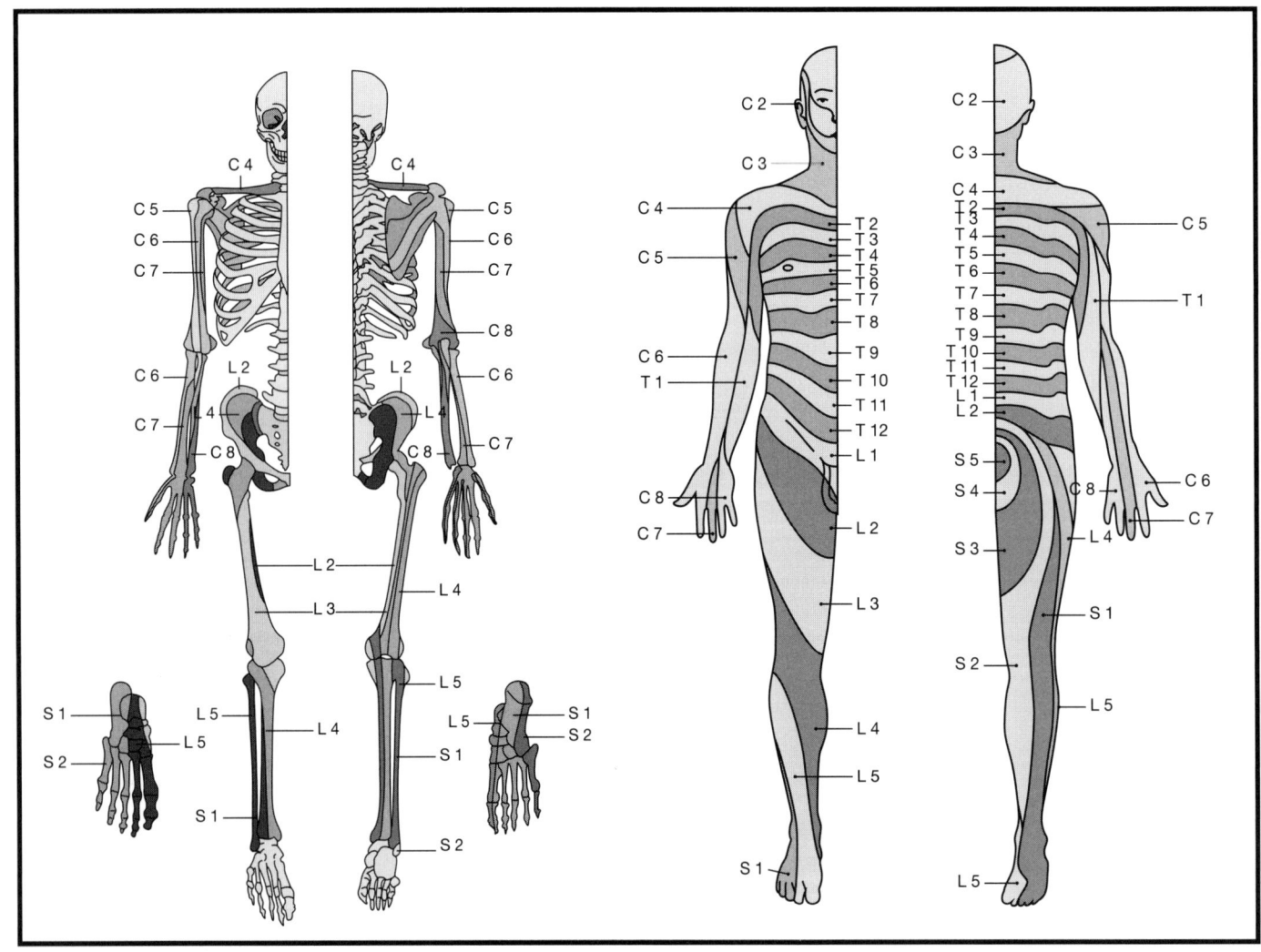

FIGURE 1.1

Typical pain distribution from sclerotome, dermatome, and peripheral nerves.

Source: Adapted from Ref. (3). Werner C, Boos N. History and physical examination spinal disorders. In: Boos N, Aebi M, ed. Springer, Berlin and Heidelberg; 2008:201–225.

(continued)

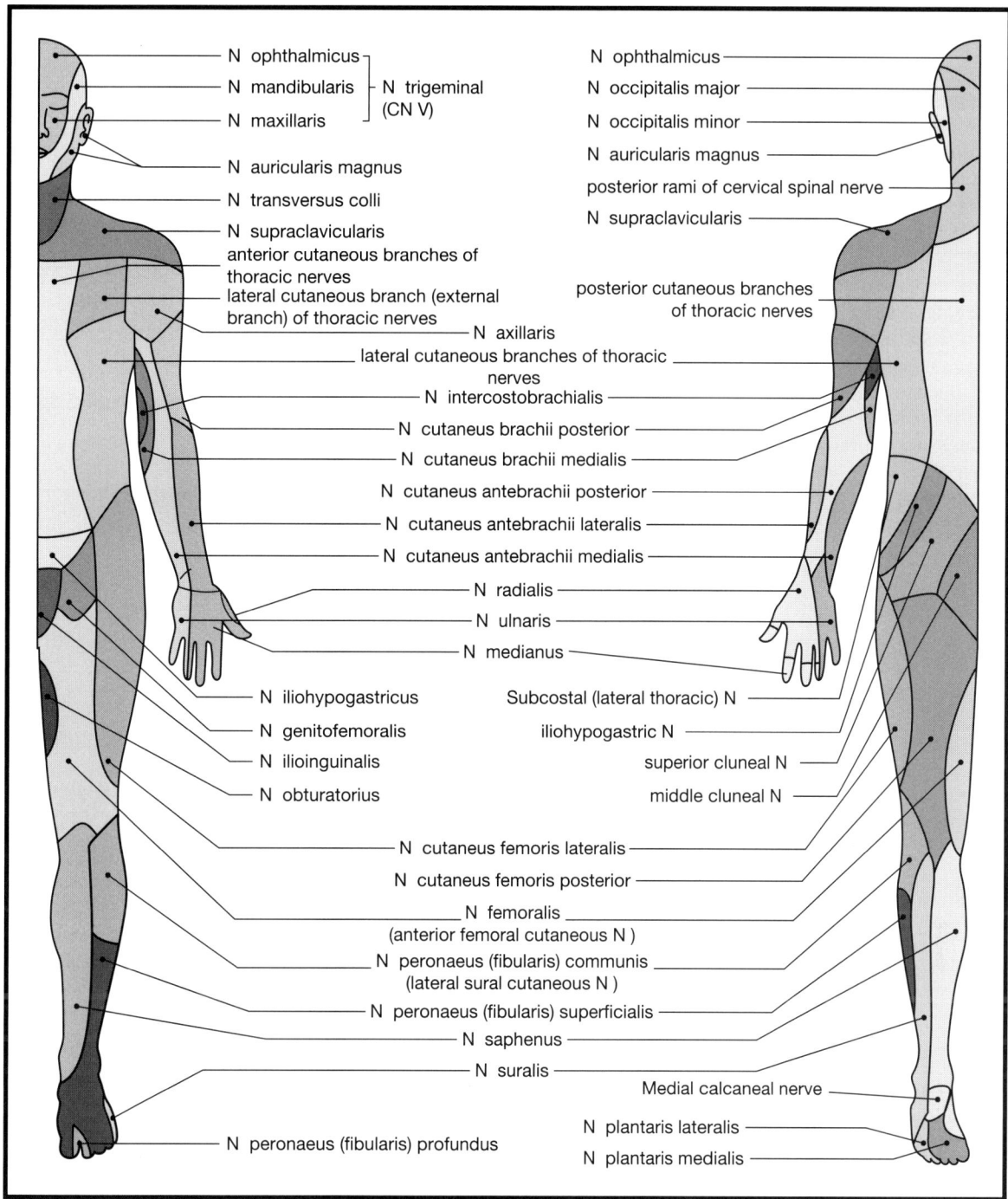

FIGURE 1.1 *(continued)*

N, nerve/nervous.

- Periarticular soft tissue structures as pain generator: often presents with distinct localization
  - Ligament (sprain, tear), bursa (bursitis), muscle/tendon (contusion, strain/tear, rarely myopathy/myositis), subcutaneous tissue (cutaneous nerve, lipoma, etc) and skin (cellulitis)
  - Intra-articular structures (eg, cruciate ligament); not as distinct localization as periarticular structure
- Referred pain
  - Peripheral nerve pathologies
    - Radiculopathy: radiating pain typically in dermatomal distribution (±neuropathic pain)
    - Entrapment neuropathy: in peripheral nerve distribution typically
  - MSK pathologies: less common (sclerotome)
    - Joint pathologies (facet arthropathy, sacroiliac joint complex pathology) and muscle fascia (6) (with trigger point) can present with referred pain (7)
- Diffuse pain
  - MSK pathologies: fibromyalgia most common (MC), polymyalgia rheumatica, metabolic muscle disorders, systematic inflammatory disease (polyarthralgia), and so on
  - Chronic neuropathic pathologies: central nervous system (CNS); central (thalamic) pain, neuropathic pain from spinal cord lesion, complex regional pain syndrome, and so on
- More details are provided in Chapter 11.

S—severity
- Often not as objective as desired
- Useful in the follow-up (FU) of the response to treatment and deciding for initial treatment plan, many different scales available
- Visual analogue scale (most validated, 10 cm), numeric rating scale (0–10, MC used)
  - Numeric rating scale often categorized as mild (1–3), moderate (4–6), or severe (7–10) (8)
  - Minimal meaningful change: 2 to 3 in numeric scale (varies depending on the condition)
- Other scales available: patient's global impression of change, verbal description scale, African palliative outcome scale (APCA), or pain assessment in advanced dementia scale (9) and so on
  - Global impression of change: 1 (very much improved) to 7 (very much worse) (10)
  - Scales for subjective improvement: 0% to 100% improvement (easier for patients to report) on FU or after intervention (procedure)
    - Placebo effect varies depending on the disease and method of placebo; upto 30% (11)

T—temporal, acute, or chronic

	ACUTE PAIN	CHRONIC PAIN
Inciting factor/associated pathology	Clearer inciting factor (trauma, injury, overuse etc)/inflammatory process	Often not identifiable factor/not expected to improve with resolution of inciting factor. Neuropathic pain mechanism added
Healing response	Pain improves as the injury heals. Inflammatory response	Neither pain nor function expected to improve. Pain may limit activities that could improve condition
Recovery	Expected	Either unpredictable or not expected
Psychosocial effects	Limited (acute stress reaction)	Negative effects a prominent feature of disease[a]

[a]Important to recognize stressful life events, depression, and other psychiatric problems, and take history in nonjudgmental fashion.
Source: From Ref. (12). Marx JA, Hockberger RS, Walls RM, Adams J, Rosen P. *Rosen's Emergency Medicine: Concepts and Clinical Practice*. 7th ed. Philadelphia, PA: Mosby/Elsevier; 2010.

Differential Diagnosis Based on Symptoms (13)
Different approaches
- Based on location of pain, mechanism of injury, etiologies, and so on.

Common versus uncommon etiologies (diagnosis)
- Initially focus on the common conditions, then less common etiology if not responsive to treatment for the common diagnosis

Serious versus nonthreatening etiologies
- Serous etiologies: tumor, infection, progressive neurologic, systematic inflammatory arthropathy, or vascular
  - Should not be missed in the differential diagnoses although it is not common or likely considering the related significance of morbidity or mortality
  - Check red flags: unexplained constitutional symptoms (fever, chills, night sweats, unintentional weight loss), rapidly progressive progress, unclear mechanisms, and so on

Valid versus less valid etiologies
- First, focus on the valid (well-accepted) causes of pain, then investigate unusual causes of the pain if you rule out the valid diagnosis explaining the presentation/pain

NEUROLOGICAL IMPAIRMENT

Weakness

Secondary to neurologic versus MSK disorder

	NEUROLOGIC DISORDER	MUSCULOSKELETAL DISORDER
History	Often sensory symptoms coexist (numbness, unsteadiness, tingling, or neuropathic pain). The pain is not usually prominent. Significant weakness (focal, multifocal depending on the pathology). Neuromuscular dysfunction or mild lesion cause fatigue (diurnal variation) rather than frank weakness	Weakness due to pain: pain is significant compared to weakness (usually mild unless severe structural injury presents). Weakness due to instability: often subtle, deterioration in sports performance (in athletes)

- Neurological disorders
  - Categorized into upper (brain, spinal cord) and lower motor neuron disease
  - Upper motor neuron disease: more prominent dysfunction than weakness with coordination (cortical/subcortical/extrapyramidal)

	UPPER MOTOR NEURON DISEASE	LOWER MOTOR NEURON DISEASE
Atrophy/ weakness	Less common Generalized (more than focal/ multifocal): limb (or limbs) involved	More common and significant Focal or regional: more common than generalized (except polyradiculopathy, diffuse peripheral neuropathy, neuromuscular Dz, myopathy)
Other movement disorder pattern	Coordination problems and more functional complaints than neurologic deficit	Less common

Dz, disease.

- Increased tone/spasticity/rigidity in upper motor neuron disease; can be confused with joint contracture or stiffness (can coexist)
  - Often difficult to distinguish from spasticity (high grade): diagnostic motor block can be helpful

Psychogenic (functional) weakness (14)
- Underrecognized.
  - Functional weakness or functional movement disorder: ~5% of neurology patients in Scotland (15)
- Common features
  - Multiple symptoms, including pain and fatigue (very common)
  - A history of other poorly explained chronic symptoms or syndromes: common
    - Irritable bowel syndrome, chronic fatigue syndrome, menorrhagia, or fibromyalgia
  - Mood dysfunction (depressed or anxious): common but not exclusive
  - Only 20% of patients believe that stress is relevant (lower than patients with disease)
  - Common panic symptoms before acute functional weakness (not exclusive)

Sensory Dysfunction
Symptoms
- Can be divided into positive sensory symptoms (paresthesia, dysesthesia, allodynia) and negative symptoms (hypo/anesthesia)
- Positive symptoms
  - Frequently reported by patients with MSK pathologies
    - Often difficult to differentiate from MSK pain (eg, chronic heel pain; Baxter's entrapment neuropathy versus plantar fasciitis or concomitant)
  - Respond better to the intervention than negative sensory symptoms (in entrapment neuropathy)
- Negative symptoms
  - Prominent in hereditary conditions (eg, hereditary sensorimotor neuropathy [Charcot Marie tooth disease]) or severe nerve injuries (complete anesthesia)
  - Patient may not complain about it so much but more functional impact
    - Related to impaired activities of daily living (ADL)/safety (burn), deformity (Charcot neuroarthropathy), and mobility disability (ataxic gait)
  - Difficult to manage

Impaired Function
Disability
- Umbrella term covering loss of function (self-care, ADL)/I (instrumental) ADL, work/occupation, leisure activity (hobby/sports, etc), and restriction of participation (definition from World Health Organization)
- Traditional model: pathology → impairment → functional limitation → physical disability (16)
- Disability often not correlating with impairment

Differential diagnosis
- Onset of impaired function, preceding event, progression, accompanying symptoms (significant pain or no pain), and comorbidities (diabetes, vascular risk factors, family history of neuromuscular disease, etc): important for differential diagnosis
  - Onset: acute (vascular or traumatic > acute inflammatory) versus chronic (slowly progressive or overuse)
  - Progression: monophasic versus stepwise or slowly progressive
  - Comorbidities: elderly patients with multiple vascular risk factors (hypertension, diabetes, increased cholesterol, smoking) → high risk for vascular events (eg, unrecognized stroke)
  - Neurological lesions: related to self-care and mobility disability
    - Subtle neurological dysfunction and nonorganic causes often underrecognized
    - Fine/gross motor dysfunction, coordination, sensation, ataxia: common cause of disability
- Common presentations
  - Difficulty with dressing, showering, feeding, grooming, and instrumental ADL
    - Upper extremity dysfunction (shoulder, elbow, especially hand with impaired dexterity): pain, decreased range, and weakness
    - Differential diagnosis: rotator cuff tear, cervical (C5–6) radiculopathy, brachial plexopathy, muscle disease (myositis [poly or dermatomyositis] or polymyalgia rheumatica), and so on
  - Difficulty with toileting, bathing, and tub transfer: lower extremity dysfunction (hip, knee, and ankle), upper extremity dysfunction and neurological diseases
  - Difficulty negotiating stairs and standing from sitting
    - Proximal (hip/gluteal/thigh) muscle weakness and pain: hip and knee joint pathologies, tendon/bursal pathologies (painful range/blocking with disuse atrophy)
    - Differential diagnosis: lumbar plexopathy/radiculopathy, or muscle disorder (myopathy, polymyalgia rheumatica, etc)
  - Gait dysfunction: check biomechanics section
  - Fall
    - Joint instability: ligament/tendon/muscle pathologies (massive tear/avulsion → pain inhibited, instability,

weakness), joint pathologies (synovitis/effusion, etc → pain, stiffness, contracture/adhesion)
  - Knee buckling or "giving out": lumbar radiculopathy, plexopathy, myopathy, and so on, in addition to knee pain and instability
  - Foot drop/slap: L4–5 radiculopathy, peroneal/sciatic neuropathy, myopathy, tendon rupture, stroke (spasticity, with vascular risk factors) and other neuromuscular disorders, and so on
  - Ataxia: especially recurrent falls; more common; central (especially in recurrent) or peripheral
  - Others: syncope, cardiac, and CNS lesions
  ○ Sphincter control (bladder and bowel) dysfunction
    - Peripheral nerve (autonomic dysfunction), lumbosacral (LS) radiculopathy (cauda equina syndrome), spinal cord lesion (including conus medullaris), or medication induced and other neurological dysfunction
- Evaluation and FU regarding the progression of impaired function: important for treatment/rehabilitation plan
  ○ Scales available: Disability of the Arm, Shoulder, and Hand (DASH), Oswestry low back disability scale, Western Ontario and McMaster Universities Osteoarthritis Scales (WOMAC) for knee and hip osteoarthritis (OA), American Orthopaedic (AO) foot and ankle surgery scale, and so on, based on the anatomical region
  ○ Can integrate the functional activities into the therapy program and for FU of response to treatment

OTHER HISTORY

Flowchart 1.1
- Obtain historical information that can help in differential diagnosis

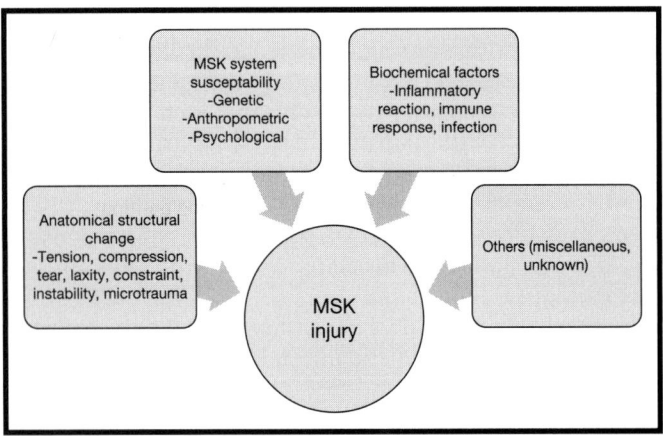

FLOWCHART 1.1
Etiology of musculoskeletal disorder.
MSK, musculoskeletal.
Source: From Ref. (1). Harper JD. Determining foot and ankle impairments by the AMA fifth edition guides. *Foot Ankle Clin*. 2002;7(2):291–303.

Relevant histories for MSK disorders (17,18)

RISK FACTOR	FREQUENTLY ASSOCIATED MSK DISORDERS
Age	Osteoarthritis, and osteoporosis
Gender	Female: rheumatoid arthritis, fibromyalgia, hand and knee osteoarthritis, osteoporosis, and chronic wide spread pain versus male: gout
Family history	Rheumatoid arthritis, osteoarthritis, and osteoporosis
Weight	Obesity: osteoarthritis, back pain, and gout
	Underweight: osteoporosis
Diet/nutrition	Osteoporosis, stress fracture, osteomalacia, and gout
Alcohol abuse	Osteoporosis, gout, increased risk of road traffic injuries
Smoking	Rheumatoid arthritis (17,18) and osteoporosis (19,20)
	Be suspicious of extrinsic causes of pain (cardiovascular, lung, cancer, peripheral arterial disease, etc)
Lack of exercise	Osteoarthritis, osteoporosis, and back pain
Sports injury	Upper and lower limb pain syndromes, back pain, premature osteoarthritis
Work injury	Upper and lower limb injuries, back pain
Medications	Osteoporosis associated with corticosteroids

MSK, musculoskeletal.

Common MSK Disorders Related to Specific Sport/Recreational Activity (21)

ACTIVITY	COMMON DISORDERS	RISK FACTORS
Running	Common injuries in runners • Patellofemoral syndrome (PFS) ~30% (MC) > tibial stress syndrome > Achilles tendinopathy, stress fracture, plantar fasciitis Differences in injury pattern between sprinters, middle-distance runners, and long-distance runners • Hamstring tendon Dx: more common in sprinters • Backache and hip problems in middle distance runners • Foot problems in long distance	Training mile per week (20, 40 miles per week), previous running injury (within 1 year), inexperienced runner (<3 years), training intensity (recent transition)

(continued)

ACTIVITY	COMMON DISORDERS	RISK FACTORS
Football	Lower extremity injury: more common • Medial collateral ligament (MC injury) • Anterior cruciate ligament (most devastating injury) • Quadriceps contusion, turf toe, hip pointer Upper extremity • Shoulder instability (anterior dislocation), Jersey finger, stinger/burner (MC nerve injury, C5–6/upper trunk brachial plexus), cervical cord neurapraxia (involves bilateral extremities) Spondylosis	Offensive lineman for shoulder instability Spinal canal ratio (compared to vertebral body: Torg's ratio) Stinger/burner: defensive player Defensive backs: headache
Basketball	Lower extremity (F > M), ankle (MC, inversion injury), knee (up to 20%), sprain, anterior shin pain, and stress fracture	Landing on another's foot Poor biomechanics/neuromuscular pattern (knee injury)
Baseball	Shoulder (MC): rotator cuff syndrome (impingement, tear), instability, labral tear, glenoid lesion (Bennett) Elbow: osteochondritis dissecans, ulnar collateral ligament injury Little league elbow	Pitcher Training error; overuse Underlying abnormal biomechanics (eg, glenohumeral internal rotation deficit)
Tennis	Elbow; lateral and medial epicondylitis (MC, overuse) Shoulder: rotator cuff Syn. Lower extremity; ankle sprains, medial gastrocnemius tear, medial tibial stress syndrome. Achilles tendinopathy (22)	Backhand stroke (lat. epicondylitis), Forehand stroke (med. epicondylitis) Service (rotator cuff and medial epicondylitis)
Bicycle	Traumatic; distal upper extremities (Fx of scaphoid, distal radius) > AC sprain Overuse: knee pain (patellofemoral syndrome, iliotibial band [ITB] syndrome, hamstring tendinopathy), neck/shoulder (myofascial pain syndrome, hyperextension)	Training error, equipment (eg, positioning of seat; too high or too posterior; ITB syndrome)

(continued)

ACTIVITY	COMMON DISORDERS	RISK FACTORS
Golf	Amateur: lumbar spine injury (MC), follow through, reversed C position Professional: hand/wrist region > lumbar spine Injury • Tendinopathy: MC, Fx of hook of the hamate Shoulder; nondominant; overuse injury, AC joint pathologies	Training error in swing, overuse

AC, acromioclavicular; Dx, diagnosis; F, female; Fx, fracture; M, male; MC, most common.

Relationship between OA and sports/recreational activity
• Intensity and duration of exposure: a risk factor for hip and knee OA in high level athletes
• The risk of OA associated with sport: lesser than that associated with a history of trauma and overweight
• Joint trauma is a greater risk factor than the practice of sport
• No firm conclusion about the possible protective role of sports, such as cycling, swimming, or golf

Common Sports-Related Peripheral Nerve Lesions (23)

SPORTS	COMMONLY AFFECTED NERVE	MECHANISM AND LOCATION
Baseball	Suprascapular nerve	Repetitive stress from the throwing motion
	Axillary nerve	Direct trauma or quadrilateral space syndrome
	Ulnar nerve	Compression at cubital tunnel due to valgus forces
Cycling	Ulnar nerve (cyclist's palsy)	Compression at Guyon canal due to repetitive trauma
	Median nerve (carpal tunnel syndrome)	Compression at wrist due to hand position
	Pudendal nerve	Stretch or compression due to seat position
Running	Interdigital nerves (Morton neuritis/neuroma)	Stretch during push-off movement (forefoot)
	Tibial nerve (Tarsal tunnel syndrome)	Compression at ankle due to repetitive trauma and malalignment
	Medial plantar nerve (jogger's foot)	Local entrapment or external compression (medial plantar midfoot)

(continued)

SPORTS	COMMONLY AFFECTED NERVE	MECHANISM AND LOCATION
Football	Brachial plexus (stinger or burner)	Forceful neck movement during blocking and tackling
Tennis	Radial nerve (supinator syndrome) Suprascapular nerve	Compression due to serving motion
Weight-lifting	Medial pectoral nerve	Extrinsic compression from muscular hypertrophy
Skiing	Femoral nerve/ saphenous nerve	Compression due to hip flexion or ill-fitting footwear (Ski boot compression syndrome)
	Ulnar nerve	Compression at wrist due to poling maneuver

Occupational Risk for MSK Pain (24)

Job title: higher incidence in strenuous and manually intensive work tasks

Physical load (ergonomic stressor): forceful activity, higher repetition, and awkward posture
- The precise nature of biomechanical stresses leading to OA remains unclear
- High loads on the joint, unnatural body position, heavy lifting, climbing, and jumping may contribute to knee and hip OA

Psychosocial factors: low social support at work, and low job control. Less job satisfaction and depressive symptoms. Patients receiving worker's compensation with chronic low back pain have longer length of time to return to work (25).

PAST MEDICAL HISTORY (LIMITED TO MSK PROBLEMS)

Systemic Conditions
- Local pain/presentation can be presentation of systematic conditions, referred pain (from neighboring body part), or regional MSK conditions
- Systematic conditions (rheumatologic, tumor, infection, vascular, inflammatory, etc): review involvement of other joint and other system (neurologic, hematologic, dermatologic, and others)
  ○ For example, rheumatoid disease or inflammatory disease: frequent involvement of multiple joints
- Diabetes mellitus (DM): adhesive capsulitis, peripheral neuropathy (length-dependent, dying-back phenomenon: MC pattern) and diabetic amyotrophy (radiculoplexus neuropathy), entrapment neuropathy (more common), Charcot neuroarthropathy (in foot)
- Cardiovascular history/stroke: shoulder–hand syndrome (complex regional pain syndrome) and immobility-related conditions (tight iliopsoas, tight hamstring, tight gastrocnemius, etc)

History of cancer
- Metastatic lesion to bone (spine, femur, and others) and paraneoplastic syndrome (sensory neuropathy, neuronopathy, neuromuscular dysfunction, etc), chemotherapy-related problem, or radiation plexopathy
- Timely (urgent) work up if red flags exist or systematic treatment required

History of pediatric MSK issues
- OA: for example, hip OA with past medical history of (H/O) hip dysplasia and slipped femoral epiphysis for early onset hip OA
- Tendinopathy with H/O enthesopathy (eg, patellar tendinopathy with H/O Osgood–Schlatter disease, Achilles tendinopathy with h/o Sever's disease)
- Tardy ulnar nerve palsy with H/O elbow fracture/dislocation during childhood

History of trauma or injury
- Late sequels related to fracture/dislocation: posttraumatic arthritis (especially in arthritis resilient joints, such as ulnar-trochlear (elbow) or ankle joint), local nerve irritation (radial neuropathy in humeral shaft fracture or tardy ulnar nerve palsy after elbow fracture), or underrecognized compartment syndrome
- Secondary MSK condition related to iatrogenic nerve injury
  ○ For example, accessory nerve injury with scapular depressed and protracted scapula with myofascial pain syndrome, shoulder impingement syndrome

REVIEW OF SYSTEMS

Constitutional
- Weight loss, night sweat, fever: red flags for cancer, infection, and other systematic disease

CNS
- Headache (cervicogenic; chronic neck pain or Chiari malformation in the context of spinal malformation)

Head, ears, eyes, nose, and throat (HEENT)
- Vision (uveitis; inflammatory arthropathy—rheumatoid arthritis, ankylosing spondylosis, psoriasis, etc.; or visual disturbance—optic neuritis in multiple sclerosis)
- Dry mouth (Sjögren, small fiber neuropathy), and others

Respiratory and cardiovascular
- Chest discomfort/tightness, cough, shortness of breath: shoulder/scapular girdle pain from cardiac/pleural pathologies or myofascial pain syndrome (after cardiac/pleural pathologies ruled out)
- Claudication in the leg and nonspecific abdominal pain: aortic or arterial disease especially with smoking or family history

Gastrointestinal (GI) and renal
- Diarrhea (inflammatory bowel disease: often related to inflammatory arthropathy), medication (Metronidazole: sensory neuropathy)
- Gastritis/ulcer: in nonsteroidal anti inflammatory drug (NSAID) users (or contraindication for NSAID)

- Abdominal pain (upper): rarely referred pain from thoracic (or thoracolumbar) spine pathologies
- Dysuria, frequency (urinary tract infection), can mimic the lower back pain, an etiology of vertebral osteomyelitis
- Renal insufficiency: contraindication for NSAIDs or adjust the dose of the medication

Bowel/bladder dysfunction/saddle anesthesia
- Cauda equina (especially in patients with chronic low back pain) or conus medullaris syndrome
- Pain medication (opioid): more common cause of incontinence (from constipation/fecal impaction)
- Unless specifically asked, can be missed
- Must be evaluated in chronic low back pain, severe back pain (large disc herniation), or any red flags

Skin
- Psoriasis or dry skin (Sjögren's disease) related to arthropathy or small fiber neuropathy

OTHER MSK SYMPTOMS

Joint and Limb Swelling
- Acute-subacute onset
  - Joint effusion (immediate onset → hemarthrosis: associated with intra-articular injury, synovitis, OA flare up) versus periarthrial swelling: focal, bursal effusion or tenosynovitis (26)
- Chronic: often confused with bone osteophyte or deformity and rarely bony tumor

Unilateral limb swelling (27)
- Acute: deep vein thrombosis, ruptured Baker cyst, compartment syndrome, cellulites
- Chronic:
  - Venous insufficiency (MC cause): common with varicosities, hyperpigmentation from hemosiderin deposits
  - Reflex sympathetic dystrophy: rarely bilateral (BL)
  - Pelvic tumor, lymphoma (external pressure on veins), abdominal tumor or radiation; subacute, can be BL
  - Secondary lymphedema (tumor, surgery, infection), congenital venous malformations
  - May–Thurner syndrome (iliac vein compression syndrome)
  - Arterial entrapment syndrome

BL limb swelling
- Subcutaneous/skin
  - Pitting or nonpitting edema
    - Lymphedema: typically painless (secondary: tumor, radiation, infection, filariasis), nonpitting
    - Chronic venous insufficiency: pitting ± low-grade pain
  - Classification based on etiology
    - Idiopathic (adolescent, female <50 years, no signs of systemic or venous insufficiency): cyclic edema (premenstrual), pregnancy related (preeclampsia)
    - Medication (common secondary cause): calcium channel blocker/others anti hypertension medications (HTN meds), prednisone/hormone, NSAID, gabapentin, Lyrica, and others
    - Systematic: heart (heart failure, restrictive cardiomyopathy, pericarditis), pulmonary hypertension (sleep apnea: underrecognized, >45 years), liver/GI (protein losing enteropathy) and kidney (nephrotic syndrome, glomerulonephritis), beri beri (vitamin B1 deficiency), and so on
- Muscle edema
  - Myopathy (28), diabetic muscle infarct (29,30), and myxedema (hypothyroidism)
  - Mimicker
    - Muscle tear with retraction; tendon rupture in the wrist (31), and medial gastrocnemius rupture in the calf
    - Tenosynovitis (eg, extensor tendon in the wrist): inflammatory arthropathy

Joint Stiffness and Contracture (32)

EXTRA-ARTICULAR CAUSES	INTRA-ARTICULAR CAUSES
Heterotopic ossification (ligament, capsule, or muscle) Extra-articular malunion after fracture or arthropathy Soft-tissue contractures following burns	Capsular contractures/adhesion: prolonged immobilization or disuse or others (idiopathic, inflammatory, etc) Articular mal- and nonunions or joint destruction Loss of articular cartilage, intra-articular loose bodies and osteophytes

Snapping (33)
- Differential diagnosis
- Calcification on the muscle and bursa: calcific tendinopathy or bursitis over bony prominence
  - Subcoracoid bursopathy under the coracoid process
  - Rectus femoris calcific tendinopathy (near the origin at anterior inferior iliac spine or reflected head to acetabulum)
- Periarticular soft tissue over the joint: labral tears, intra-articular loose bodies, indirect head of the rectus femoris rubbing with hip joint capsule
- Tendon over benign bony tumor: chondral or osteochondral lesion; osteochondroma

Mechanical Locking of Joint
- Common causes: ectopic materials interposed between the articular surfaces
- Loose body
- Chondral or osteochondral fragments
- Torn meniscus, ligament or rarely tendon swelling (the long head of biceps) or torn tendon

PHYSICAL EXAMINATION

Inspection

Gait and posture
- Quickly evaluate as the patient walks in
- Visually examine the location of interest

Standing posture
- Frontal plane (from the front or back): pelvic obliquity, asymmetric skin fold (in frontal plane, observation from the back) for scoliosis, knee (genu varum/valgum/recurvatum),

hindfoot (calcaneus) eversion/inversion, and forefoot abduction/adduction
- Sagittal plane (observation from the side): lumbar/cervical lordosis and thoracic kyphosis. Knee (genu recurvatum) and patellar location from tibial tuberosity (patellar alta or baja)

Sitting posture
- Head posture (anterior tilted head or dropped head), cervical spine (kyphosis or straight in sagittal plane), and scapular posture (protracted, symmetric), and so on
- Coronal balance in scoliosis (difference from standing posture) can be evaluated

Inspection of individual part (head to toe)
- See individual chapters
- Quick limb and joint inspection for atrophy, masses, edema/fullness, scars/wounds, involuntary movement (tremor, myokymia, or fasciculation, etc), erythema, and so on
- Periarticular swelling
  - Focal (part of joint, often superficial structure like bursal effusion) versus general (joint effusion)
  - Often difficult to recognize in obese person

Palpation

Area of Maximal Pain/Tenderness
- Ask the patient to indicate; if unable, try to palpate locations for common pathologies or specific pathologies suggested by history followed by systemic palpation
- Be aware of bony landmark (surface anatomy in individual chapter) then palpate and describe based on the bony landmark (more consistent)
- Try to be consistent in the pressure of palpation
  - May provide rough idea of severity (or nonorganic: less or no pain on the same amount of palpation on the same location after distraction; may indicate psychological component involvement)
- Soft tissue: tenderness, spasm, guarding, trigger point (with referred pain) or tone
- Joint: swelling/edema, warmth, masses, crepitus, snapping, or mechanical locking

Vascular
- Pulse examination; often misleading; a low reliability
- If suspicious of vascular compromise, consider objective tests

Palpation of cutaneous nerve
- Particularly useful on the dorsum of the hand and foot in the lean person
- In suspected focal nerve entrapment syndrome, palpation can reproduce pain with radiation proximally or distally (Valleix's phenomenon, Tinel sign) ± sensory symptoms
- For example, superficial radial nerve, dorsal ulnar cutaneous and superficial peroneal, or saphenous nerves palpable: useful for nerve conduction study (NCS)

Range of Motion

Difference exists between the normal and functional range of motion (ROM) (less than normal ROM)

- Impaired range required for ADLs can cause increased energy expenditure or compensation from other joints in the proximity

Clinical evaluation
- Goniometer using consistent surface landmark and test positions (increased reliability). Check the joint in the plane of movement. Compare it with the opposite side
- 0° defined as anatomic position
- Normal range of movement: check individual chapter

Variations
- Based on age, gender, conditioning, obesity, and genetics; generally more flexible in younger than in older population and occurs more in females than in males

Limited range in the neighboring joint
- Can be underlying culprit/contributing factor for the pathology (especially overuse syndrome)
- Limitation of wrist joint can be contributing factor for elbow overuse syndrome

Spasticity versus contracture
- Range the joint passively at very low speed → additional ROM is achieved in spasticity versus no difference in contracture
  - Frequently both components exist
- Nerve block can give a further diagnostic value for high-grade spasticity from joint contracture

Common muscle tightness in patients with MSK problems
- Scapular protractor tightness (round shoulder) in shoulder pain: pectoralis major, minor, and subscapularis muscles
  - Distance between midline to medial scapular border: rough idea of progress in FU or dynamic evaluation to ask patient retract, evaluate the distance from resting to contracted position
- Scapular girdle muscle tightness: trapezius (lateral neck flexion), levator scapular (flex the neck toward axilla), and latissimus dorsi/teres major muscles (internal rotator, adductor and extensor), and so on
- Glenohumeral internal rotator tightness: evaluation by sidearm external rotation (with the elbow on the trunk)
- Hip flexor (iliopsoas, and rectus femoris) affecting anterior tilting of the pelvis (therefore increase lumbar lordosis): Ely test
- Hip extensor (hamstring muscle) tightness: loss of lordosis; flat back affecting sagittal balance (stooped posture): popliteal angle for hamstring tightness
- Hip external rotator tightness (tight piriformis, gluteus medius) affecting buttock pain, hip external rotation (promoting pronation response on standing/walking): check side-to-side difference
- Hip abductor (Ober test) and adductor tightness
  - Hip adductor tightness: causing pain in the medial knee (adductor tubercle) as well as groin pain with hip abduction (FABER position)
- Ankle plantar flexor: gastrocnemius (two joint muscle) tighter than soleus
  - Due to subtalar, midtarsal joint compensation, the deficit underrecognized commonly

○ To check ankle tightness, subtalar/midtarsal joint movement should be minimal. Subtalar neutral or slight hindfoot inversion (lock subtalar and midtarsal joint) while dorsiflexing the ankle joint
○ Silfverskiold test for gastrocnemius tightness (34)

Check the details of the examination in individual chapters.

Generalized ligament laxity
- Beighton score (Figure 1.2)

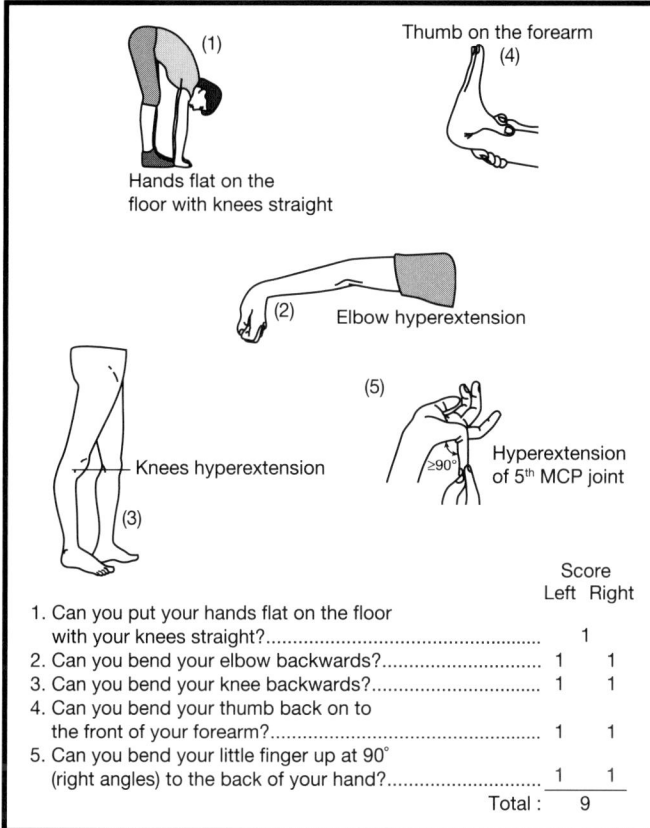

FIGURE 1.2
The Beighton score for generalized ligament laxity.
MCP, metacarpophalangeal.

○ Fifth finger dorsiflexion, thumb to the forearm, elbow hyperextension, knee hyperextension (one for each limb), palm rest on the floor (1)
○ Positive if greater than or equal to 4/9
○ The Brighton criteria (major) for joint hypermobility syndrome
  ▪ Joint pain >3 months in ≥4 joints and Beighton score ≥4/9

PROVOCATIVE TEST

- Special test may not be specific for one pathology
- Often positive for multiple different pathologies (low specificity); therefore, needs some precautions for interpretation

General principles
- Helpful to understand underlying mechanisms
  ○ Shoulder impingement test: for example, Hawkins Kennedy tests: bursa or rotator cuff tendon impingement between greater tuberosity and coracoid-acromial arch by abduction and internal rotation of humerus (by engaging greater tuberosity under the coracoacromial arch)
  ○ Ankle impingement: impingement of the soft tissue between the tibia and talus or calcaneus
    ▪ Aggravation of pain of anterior impingement by dorsiflexion and posterior impingement by plantarflexion
    ▪ Therapeutic implication
      – Avoid dorsiflexion in anterior impingement (heel lift), plantarflexion in posterior impingement (avoid provoking activity: toe walking, eg, Ballet dancer and wearing high heels)
- Be proficient in three to four special tests in common pathologies for time efficiency

Sensitivity and specificity
- Predictive value varies from study to study
- Be aware of different study population, slightly different techniques (with modification) and definition of the test and different gold standards
- Typically, multiple positive tests may provide higher predictive value and specificity

Specific tests: See in the individual chapter

Focused Neurological Examination
Sensory examination
- To find the pattern of abnormality
  ○ Peripheral nerve (individual or multiple) distribution
  ○ Root/plexus distribution: different peripheral nerve of same root or plexus
    ▪ Plexus lesion: often patch involvement
    ▪ Root: dermatomal distribution
  ○ Spinal cord (distal to the level of injury with variation of involvement depending on the location and sensory modality) or brain (contralateral side typically)
- Test different sensory modalities for the nerve fiber of the different size
  ○ Smaller fiber: pins/needle/temperature, lateral spinothalamic tract in the spinal cord
  ○ Larger fiber: proprioception and vibration, posterior column in spinal cord
  ○ Clinical implications
    ▪ Entrapment neuropathy: large fiber usually first involved
      – Two-point discrimination often used before and after the peripheral nerve procedure. Different threshold for normal; palm: 10 mm, foot: 20 mm)
    ▪ Smaller fiber neuropathy can spare larger fiber (usually assessed by NCS and needle electrodiagnosis [EMG]; therefore normal in isolated small fiber neuropathy)
- Occasionally, patient's interpretation is different from the objective examination: hyperesthesia in ipsilateral side may indicate decreased sensation in the opposite side
  ○ Often challenging to interpret

Motor examination
- First, differentiate pain inhibited (usually mild in the area of MSK pathologies) versus true muscle weakness
- True muscle weakness: follows patterns of neuromuscular abnormality similar to sensory examination
  - Upper motor neuron syndrome (hemi, di, quadriparesis/plegia), peripheral nerve (root, peripheral nerve), neuromuscular junction (diurnal variation, fatigue), or muscle (commonly proximal and symmetric but can be distal)
- Evaluate key myotomes
  - Most muscles innervated by multiple roots; therefore, single-level radiculopathy often causes mild/subtle weakness
- Localize the peripheral nerve lesion: root versus peripheral nerve (root lesion; multiple peripheral nerve of same root and not length dependent)
  - Example: mild weakness in ankle dorsiflexion (often presenting as foot slapping)
    - Differential diagnoses: distal peripheral neuropathy (eg, diabetic peripheral neuropathy), peroneal neuropathy, compartment syndrome, lumbar plexopathy or L5 radiculopathy, motor neuron disease, upper motor neuron disease (stroke)
      - If hip abductor (gluteus muscle, tensor fascia lata) is also weak, then differential diagnosis narrowed down to proximal lesion (plexopathy, L5 radiculopathy, and motor neuron disease, etc)
- Pain-inhibited weakness typically shows less severe weakness than neuromuscular dysfunction
  - Quicker response to the treatment: pain relief can improve weakness dramatically but takes longer to improve subtle weakness (or disuse atrophy)

PHYSICAL EXAMINATION	NEUROLOGIC ETIOLOGY	MSK ETIOLOGY
Atrophy	Common in peripheral nerve lesion	Not striking (mild from disuse typically)
Sensory examination	Often abnormal	Normal sensory examination usually
DTR	Decreased in peripheral N lesion and increased in upper motor neuron Dz	Normal examination usually
Passive ROM	Normal passive ROM (unless contracture developed) with impaired active ROM	More pain on passive ROM (worse at the end range)

DTR, deep tendon reflex; Dz, disease; N, nerve; ROM, range of motion.

Functional weakness (35)
- Hoover's sign
  - With the patient seated, weakness of hip extension returns to normal with contralateral hip flexion against resistance
- Dragging gait: patients with acute functional weakness may drag their whole leg behind them with the hip externally or internally rotated (unlike patients with hemiparesis who tend to swing or circumduct their legs)

Deep tendon reflex
- Grading
  - 0: absent, 1: trace or only with facilitation/reinforcement; 2: normal; 3: brisk; 4: sustained clonus (other scales available)
- Facilitation/reinforcement
  - Jendrassik maneuver for knee or ankle jerk: The patient's fingers of each hand are hooked together so each arm can forcefully pull against the other. Pull for a second before tapping
  - Priming: slight ankle plantarflexion (touch the examiner's hand on neutral ankle dorsiflexion) before tapping
- Asymmetric pattern (decreased DTR) often helpful in localizing the specific root lesion. However, MSK injury to the muscle/tendon can also compromise the reflex.
- Difficult to obtain in some patients (in obese or big persons)
  - Needs good hammer (with some weight and soft rubber)
  - Palpation of muscle/tendon contraction also useful for grading

Upper motor neuron signs
- Hoffman reflex: may be more sensitive than Babinski sign for cervical myelopathy (36)
- Can be used in peripheral nerve disorder
  - Presence of Babinski in patient with difficulty dorsiflexing ankle indicates intact peroneal nerve, extensor hallucis longus muscle (in addition to presence of upper motor neuron disease)

CLINICALLY ORIENTED ANATOMY

TENDON AND LIGAMENT

Introduction (31,37)
- Microscopic anatomy: major components of tendon and ligament
  - Collagen
    - Type 1 (MC): principal element, a major contributor for load and tensile strength
    - Type 3: found in immature tendon
      - Smaller, less organized fibrils, may cause reduced mechanical strength
      - Found in insertion sites of highly stressed tendons and in aging
      - Type 3 to type 1 collagen fiber remodeling during recovery
  - Elastin and ground substance
    - Elastin: scarce in tendon, and more common in ligament
    - Water more common than proteoglycans and glycoproteins
    - Decreases with aging → tendon becomes stiffer and tighter
- Gross (macroscopic) anatomic characteristics of tendon (38,39)
  - Synovial sheath

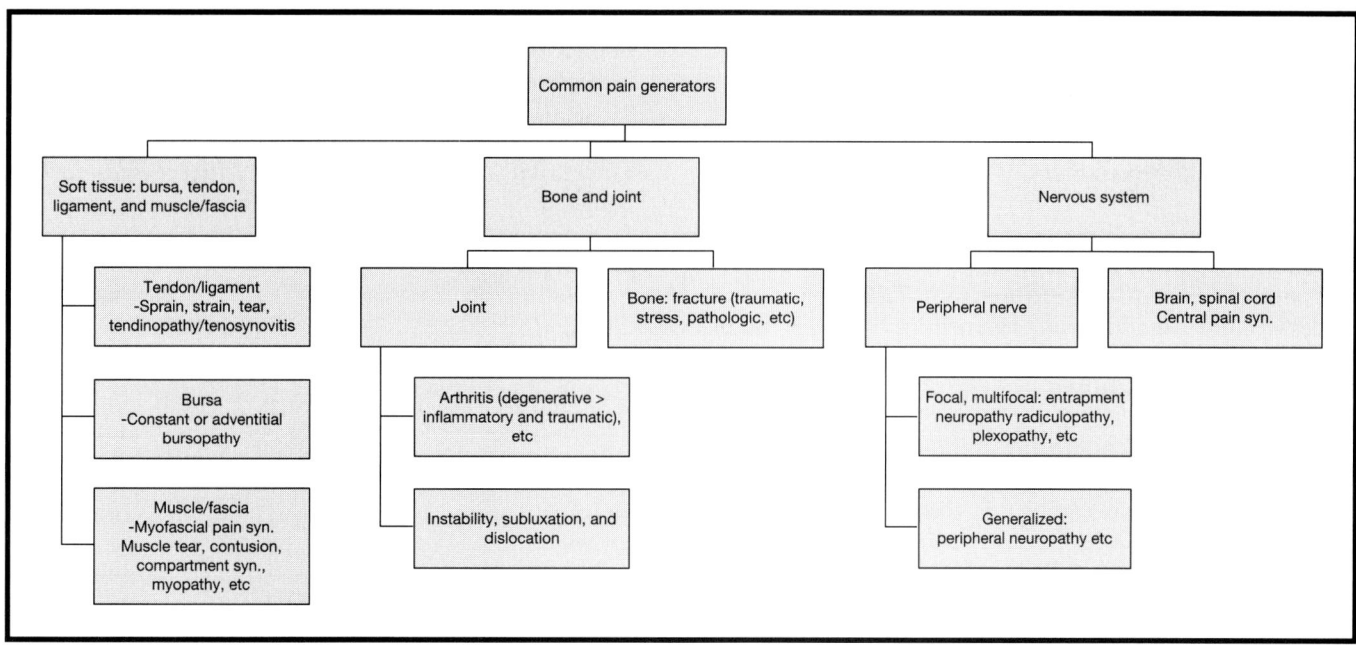

FLOWCHART 1.2
Common pain generator encountered in a musculoskeletal clinic.
syn., syndrome.

- The synovial fluid produced within the tenosynovial sheath
- Inflammation (tenosynovitis) cause tenosynovial effusion. However, presence of effusion doesn't indicate inflammation necessarily
  – Common locations: tibialis posterior, peroneus, and extensor/flexor tendon of the wrist and the hand
- Achilles tendon: no synovial sheath, instead it has paratenon, a thin vascular membrane (no fluid)
  – Site for inflammation (paratendinitis) and important structure for prognosis (intact paratenon: better prognosis in Achilles tendon tear)
- Extracapsular versus intracapsular (rarely, eg, long head of biceps in shoulder and popliteus in knee)
  ◦ Dynamic joint stabilizer
  ◦ Injury can cause intracapsular effusion
  ◦ Tendon as the site for muscle attachment
    - Lumbricals on the flexor digitorum profundus (FDP)
      – Muscle belly rarely located in the carpal tunnel (attached on the flexor digitorum superficialis [FDS]); cause of secondary carpal tunnel syndrome (CTS)
    - Oblique fibers of vastus medialis on adductor magnus and oblique fiber of vastus lateralis on ITB, and so on
      – Adductor magnus and ITB stretching may be required for vastus medialis oblique and vastus lateralis oblique muscle strengthening or optimal functioning
  ◦ Sesamoid bone: provide mechanical advantage and reduce friction on the tendon (decrease excessive wear)
  ◦ Sesamoid pathology: fracture, arthritis or bony lesion (40)
      – Differential diagnosis for tendinopathy
    - Adductor pollicis and flexor pollicis brevis on the base of the proximal phalanges (hand)
      – Differential diagnosis for stenosing tenosynovitis (trigger finger)

- Pisiform in the flexor carpi ulnaris (FCU): FCU tendinopathy and pisiform-hamate arthropathy
- Patellar: patellar tendinopathy and bipartite patellar
- Fabella in the lateral head of gastrocnemius: fabella syndrome
- Tibialis posterior and peroneus longus (PL): accessory navicular and accessory cuboid syndrome
- Sesamoids in the flexor hallucis brevis; sesamoiditis on the plantar medial forefoot pain
- Innervation
  ◦ Increased innervation near the musculotendinous junction
  ◦ Four types of receptors
    - Type 1: Ruffini corpuscles, pressor receptor, sensitive to stretch and adapt slowly
    - Type 2: Vater-Pacini corpuscles, activated by any movement
    - Type 3: Golgi tendon organ, mechanoreceptor
    - Type 4: Free nerve ending mediating pain sensation

Tendon

Characteristics and clinical implications
- Wavy and crimp configuration: shock absorber
  ◦ Length: can elongate up to 70%, break (tear/rupture) at 150%, Figure 1.3
- Spiral configuration
  ◦ Achilles tendon: spiral up to 90° laterally: medial head of gastrocnemius → posterior part of Achilles tendon. Lateral head of gastroc → anterior part of Achilles tendon, soleus (anterior) → medial part of the tendon
    - This arrangement may attribute to a higher rate of med gastrocnemius tear and location of the tendinopathy: concentrated pressure at this point, 2 to 5 cm above the insertion

- The blood supply: longitudinal vessels in the paratenon, intraosseous vessels at the tendon insertion, and vincula circulation
  - Hypovascular zone in tibialis posterior, Achilles and supraspinatus tendons: common sites for pathologies, suggested as one of the mechanisms for degeneration/tear
- Aging tendon
  - An increase in cross-linking promotes stiffness and shortening of these collagen tissues, which results in tight/shortened muscle/tendon and decreased joint ROM
  - Weakening of tendon (and ligament) attachment point to the bone, which makes these areas of attachment much more susceptible to injury

Suggested mechanism of pain after tendon dysfunction
- Overstretch, tear, rupture of tendon and ligament → inflammation of tendon and tendon sheath, and nerve ending irritation
- Neuronal response to tendon injury: nerve ingrowth during initial inflammatory phase, subsequent proliferative and remodeling phase: partially regulated by sensory nerves and glutaminergic system
  - Increased glutamate in patients with painful chronic Achilles tendinosis (41) and painful rotator cuff tear
  - Involvement of nociceptive marker in tendon pain; NK-1, α-2a adrenergic receptor, PGP 9.5, Nav 1.7, and TRPA1 and so on (42)
  - Suggested mechanism of pain improvement from anti-inflammatory medication
- Secondary effect with contracture, fatigue, and weakness (indirect)
  - Neighboring structure injury/overuse by compensation mechanism or abnormal biomechanics and increased risk of injury or impaired function

  - Characteristics of tendinosis
    - High concentration of glycosaminoglycans and increased glutamate concentration
    - Irregular fiber structure arrangement
    - No inflammatory cell infiltrates
    - Increased type 3 collagen and decreased type 1 collagen
    - Chronic tendinopathy often mixed with subtle fibrillar tear, areas of mucoid degeneration with the reparative process

Common site for tendon–muscle injury

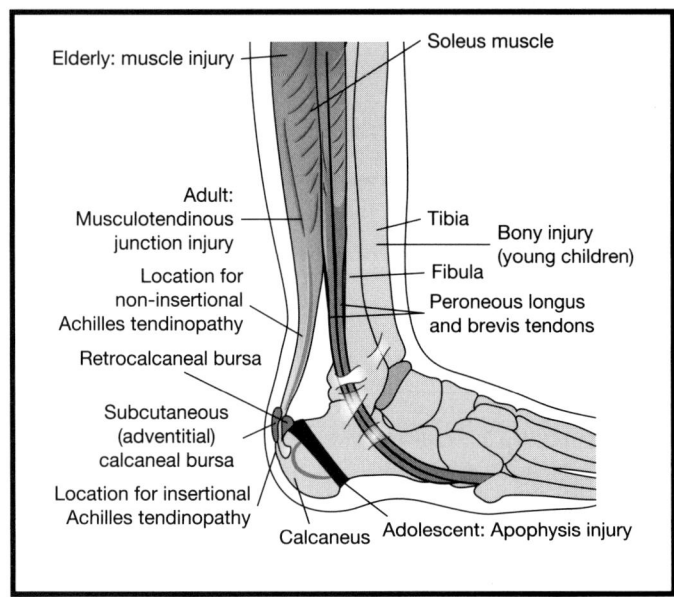

FIGURE 1.4
Different locations of common musculoskeletal injuries based on age.

- Location: varies depending on age group as the area of weakness in the tendon–bone chain changes (Figure 1.4)
- Musculotendinous junction
  - Under greater mechanical stress during the transmission of muscular contractile force to the tendon: slight different location depending on the type of muscle
    - Unipennate muscle (eg, medial gastrocnemius): at the musculotendinous junction (or distal)
    - Circumpennate (eg, tibialis anterior) or bipennate (eg, rectus femoris): proximal to the distal musculotendinous junction or muscle belly
- Osseotendinous junction
  - Tendon strain to load: 3 times greater at the insertion sites than at midsubstance
  - Collagen fiber stiffness is less at insertion sites
  - Four zones; pure fibrous tissue, unmineralized fibrocartilage, mineralized fibrocartilage and bone
    - Lack of transition in surgically reattached tendon: high risk of re-tear
  - Periosteum with osteogenic potential

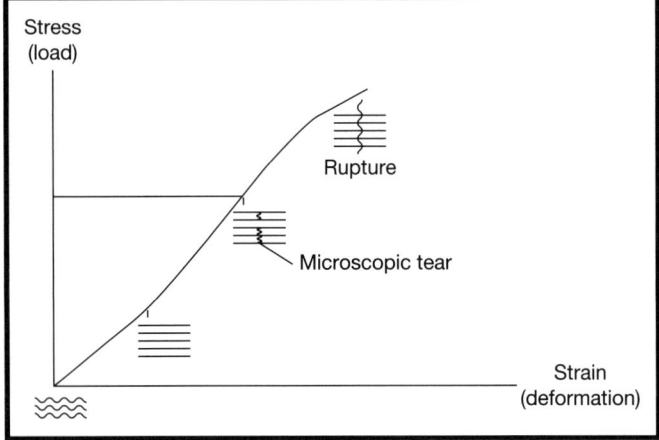

FIGURE 1.3
Tendon and ligament stress–strain relationship curve.

Tendon Pathologies

Classification (38,43)
- Tendon strain, tear, rupture, paratendinopathy (tenosynovitis), and stenosing tenosynovitis
- Tendonitis in acute/inflammatory and tendinosis in chronic/degenerative stages

Predisposing conditions for tendinopathy, tear, or rupture
- Past medical history: DM, chronic kidney disease (CKD), gout, lupus, rheumatoid arthritis (RA), steroid injection, fluoroquinolone antibiotic (Abx), hyperparathyroidism, calcium pyrophosphate deposition disease (CPPD), isotretinoin treatment (Tx), etc
- Genetic susceptibility (44)
  - Implicated in Achilles tendinopathy, rotator cuff, and anterior cruciate ligament injury
    - For example, some genetic polymorphisms in Achilles tendinopathy (the COL5A1; type 5 collagen and TNC genes: regulate tissues' response to mechanical load)
- Biomechanical factors

Intrinsic	Malalignments: excessive ankle pronation, genu valgum/varum, femoral neck anteversion, etc Limb length discrepancy Muscular imbalance and weakness Hypermobility of joints Lack of elasticity (inflexibility)
Extrinsic	Training errors: distance, intensity, hill work, technique, and fatigue Environmental conditions (ground surface, temperature, etc) Footwear and equipment

- High-risk occupation for tendinopathy: meat packers, cashiers, data-entry clerks, musicians, construction workers, electricians, cake decorators, postal workers, assembly workers, punch press operators, and automobile workers (45).

Epidemiology of sports-related tendon injury (46)

ANATOMIC LOCATION	COMMON PATHOLOGIES	SPORTS WITH HIGH INCIDENCE
Shoulder	Rotator cuff tendinopathy, tear/rupture	Throwers and racquet sports (tennis serve, the volleyball hit, and javelin and ball throwing), 35 (40) to 60 years Rupture: M > F, > 50 YO
Elbow	Lateral epicondylitis Medial epicondylitis	30% to 40% of tennis players, golfers, throwers, and pitchers
Posterior thigh	Hamstring tendinopathy, tear, or rupture	Sprinting, hurdling, jumping sports (prevalence upto 50%), and soccer (prevalence: ~20%)
Lateral thigh	Proximal ITB syndrome, distal friction syndrome, enthesopathy	Runners, joggers, skiers, soccer players, circuit trainers, weightlifters, cyclists, and athletes who participate in jumping sports
Anterior knee	Overuse injury Osgood–Schlatter	Soccer (Prevalence: ~20%), long-distance running, volleyball (~10%), orienteering, and ice hockey (7%–8%) Physically active adolescents

(continued)

ANATOMIC LOCATION	COMMON PATHOLOGIES	SPORTS WITH HIGH INCIDENCE
Heel (Achilles)	Overuse tendinosis (MC type: 60%) Insertional tendinopathy (20%) Rupture	Running, orienteering, track and field, tennis, and other ball games Training errors, varus (with rigid subtalar Jt.) or hyperpronated foot (depending on study) Calcaneal apophysitis in younger population Bimodal (4th > 3rd decades), M > F, ball games, different from country to country (soccer, badminton, handball, gymnastic, skiing, etc)

F, female; ITB, iliotibial band; Jt., joint; M, male; MC, most common; YO, year old.

Tendon healing (47)
- Inflammatory (2–4 days), fibroblastic (5 days–4 weeks), and remodeling phase (4 weeks to ~3.5 months)
  - Inflammatory phase for (2–4) days: essential for repair
    - Bleeding and hemostasis
    - Inflammation symptoms and signs: edema, pain, warmth, and redness
    - In chronic tendinopathy: lack of inflammatory cells (inflammatory healing process)
  - Fibroblastic phase
    - Fibroplasia: 4 to 8 weeks, abundant type 3 collagen (immature), granulation tissue, and neovascularization
  - Maturation: remodeling, months to years
    - Type III to I collagen, realigning and remodeling fibers (force magnitude and direction), reduced cellularity, and vascularity
    - Scar tissue: never become normal (with increased risk for reinjury)
- Extrinsic and intrinsic mechanisms
  - The extrinsic mechanism by the activity of peripheral fibroblasts
    - The dominant mechanism contributing to the formation of scar and adhesions
  - Intrinsic healing by proliferation of epitenon and endotenon tenocytes and the activity of the fibroblasts derived from the tendon: a normal gliding mechanism especially if tendon sheath is preserved
  - Tendon injury with injury to the synovial sheath combined with immobilization leads to extensive adhesions
  - Different healing pattern in particular location of injury: for example, extrinsic healing mechanism has a bigger role than intrinsic healing mechanism in the rotator cuff tendinopathy

Ligament

Characteristics and clinical implications (48,49)
- Hypertrophied components of the fibrous joint capsule, more interweaving of collagen fibers
  - Less homogeneous histological and sonographic appearance (compared to the tendon), vary in size
- Provide stability (physical restraint) between bones permitting a limited range of movement
  - Passive stabilizer, aided by the capsule
- The collagen in ligament: more elastic than that in tendon because more flexibility is necessary

- Important in sensorimotor control of joint movement (50)
  - Mechanoreceptor near the insertion of ligament to the bone
    - Large joint: more prevalent Golgi-like endings to detect extreme ROM, for example, cruciate ligament of the knee
    - Ankle: free nerve endings are a dominant mechanoreceptor (than Ruffini endings)
    - Located near the insertion of the ligament to the bone, mediate noxious stimulus as well as proprioception
    - Decrease free nerve ending and Ruffini ending: contribute to the lack of balance and coordination in ligament injury

Ligament Pathologies

Ligament sprain presentation
- Acute (pain, ecchymosis, swelling, etc) versus chronic (pain, instability, decreased performance, etc)
  - Abnormality in motor function (decreased performance) after ligament injury (51)
    - Loss of/altered ascending afferent feedback (disruption of mechanoreceptor → mechanical instability with excessive movement) and pain → CNS reorganization and altered neural activation
    - Reduced muscle strength and altered muscle activation

Common ligament injuries
- Shoulder: acromioclavicular (AC) for example (coracoclavicular [CC]), sternoclavicular ligaments
- Elbow: ulnar collateral ligament
- Wrist (scapholunate ligament), hand (dorsoradial/oblique beak ligament for carpometacarpal [CMC] joint and collateral ligament for 1st metacarpophalangeal [MCP] joint)
- Sacroiliac (SI) joint and sacrococcygeal ligament
- Knee: anterior cruciate ligament/posterior cruciate ligament (ACL/PCL), medial collateral ligament, lateral collateral ligament
- Ankle (anterior talofibular ligament, syndesmosis)
  - Lateral ankle ligament tear/sprain: MC sport-related injury
- MC location of ligament injury: intraligamentous (preserving vascularity and nerve ending at the bony insertion, better in recovery)

Evaluation
- Clinical diagnosis: grading; microscopic, partial, and full thickness tear (check lateral ankle ligament injury section)
  - Tear usually accompanied by bleeding
    - Intra-articular: hematoma (acute or subacute swelling) and extra-articular: swelling with ecchymosis
  - Clinical grading system: often inaccurate and variable interrater/intrarater reliability
- Imaging: often unnecessary except complex injury or chronic injury
  - Ultrasound (US): ideal for superficial ligament, limited in intra-articular, or deeply located ligaments
    - Advantage: able to do dynamic examination, more accessible
  - MRI: gold standard for intra-articular structures (eg, the cruciate lig assessment), evaluate other structures (including cartilage, bone, such as bone edema or fracture etc) for preoperative planning

Healing of ligaments (52)
- Overlapping phases of healing-retraction, inflammation (formation of blood clot, resorption), cellular proliferation (fibroblast produce collagen) and remodeling
- Relatively hypocellular and hypovascular → lower healing potential
- Healed ligament
  - Suboptimal biomechanical properties with scarring: increased strain under constant or repetitive low stress
  - Biological differences: ↑ glycosaminoglycan content, ↓ collagen fibers, abnormal collagen cross-linking different collagen types and predominance of small diameter collagen fibrils

MUSCLE AND FASCIA

Muscle

Characteristics and clinical implications
- Forty- to forty-five percent of body mass, muscle pain: very common, 60%–85% of population experience back pain
- Categorized into striated (skeletal and cardiac) versus nonstriated (smooth) morphologically
  - Classification of skeletal muscle
    - Fusiform muscle (biceps brachii): greater tensile force than pennate (sartorius and rectus abdominis)
    - Pennate: unipennate (eg, gastrocnemius) and bipennate (eg, rectus femoris); muscle fibers oriented obliquely to the epimysium
      - Pennate angle: functional characteristics of muscle, varies depending on muscle contraction intensity and fiber length, and increases with contraction

Pain sensation of the muscle injury (53)
- Poorly localized (compared to cutaneous pain), tearing, cramping, pressing, and referred pain
- Nociceptor
  - A delta (group III): high threshold mechanoreceptor by strong local pressure, rapid, acute, and sharp muscle pain
    - Involved in spontaneous pain and dysesthesia
  - C (group IV): polymodal, range of stimuli, delayed, diffuse, dull, or burning pain
    - Mediators: substance P, calcitonin gene-related peptide and somatostatin
    - Hyperalgesia in response to inflammation

Compartmental anatomy
- Important to understand cross-sectional images in MRI, US, and needle localization in EMG and for injection (54) (Figure 1.5)
- Mid arm level
  - Anterior (biceps, brachialis and coracobrachialis, musculocutaneous nerve) and intermuscular septum (median/ulnar nerve)
  - Posterior (triceps and radial [posterior to lateral])
- The forearm level
  - Volar: superficial (FCR, FCU, FDS, pronator teres [PT]), deep (FDP, flexor pollicis longus [FPL]) and median nerve (between FDS and FDP) ulnar nerve (under FCU)
  - Lateral/mobile wad (brachioradialis [BR], extensor carpi radialis [ECR], radial nerve)
  - Dorsal (extensor carpi ulnaris [ECU], extensor digitorum communis [EDC], extensor digitorum minimi [EDM], supinator, posterior interosseous nerve [PIN])

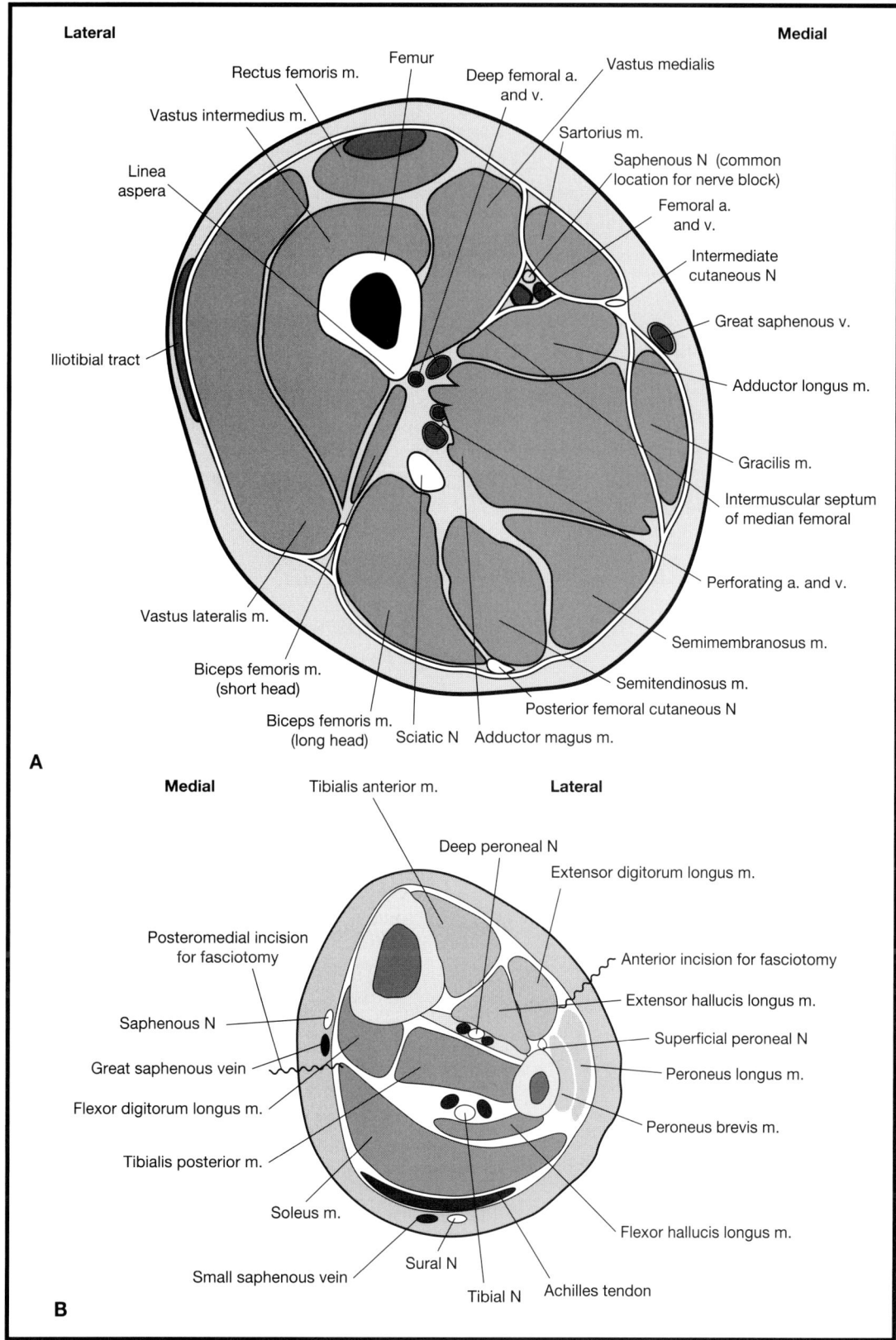

FIGURE 1.5

Compartmental anatomy of upper and lower extremities. (A) Distal thigh; (B) mid-leg; (C) mid-arm; and (D) mid-forearm.

a., artery; m., muscle; N, nerve; syn., syndrome; v., vein.

Source: Adapted from Ref. (54). Patel KM, Major NM. Compartmental anatomy. In: Davies AM, Sundaram M, James SLJ, eds. *Imaging of Bone Tumors and Tumor-Like Lesions*. Springer Berlin Heidelberg; 2009: 665–676.

(continued)

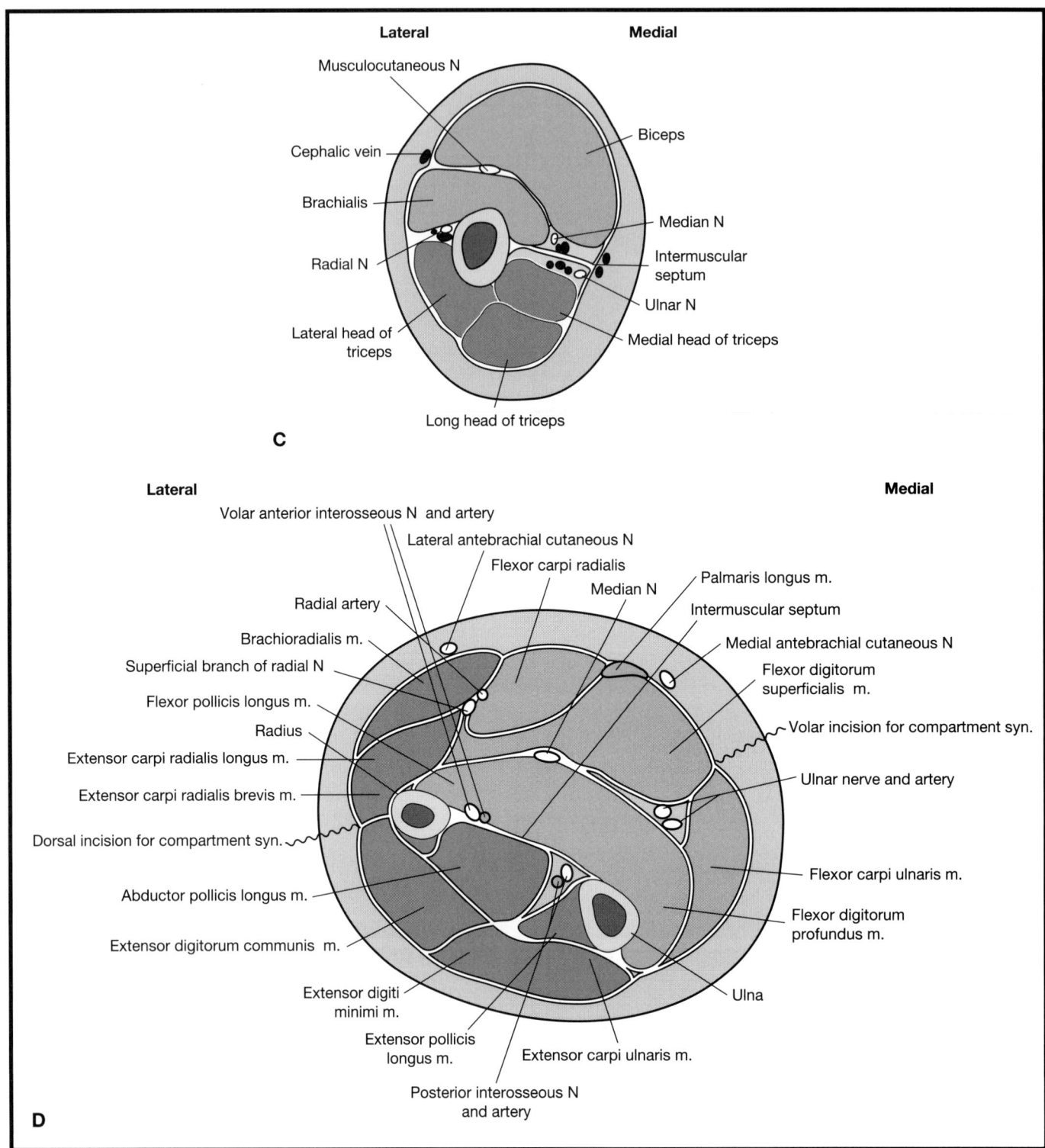

FIGURE 1.5 *(continued)*

- Thigh level
  ○ Anterior (quadriceps and sartorius), posterior (hamstring, sciatic nerve between medial and lateral hamstrings) and medial (adductor and gracilis)
  ○ Saphenous nerve (anterior under the Sartorius muscle then course between anterior and medial compartment)
- Leg level
  ○ Anterior (TA, extensor hallucis longus [EHL], EDL, and peroneus tertius), lateral (PL and peroneus brevis [PB]), superficial posterior (soleus, gastrocnemius, plantaris), and deep posterior (tibialis posterior [TP], flexor hallucis longus [FHL], and popliteus tibial nerve)
    ▪ Superficial peroneal (between lateral and anterior), deep peroneal (anterior) nerves
- Muscle variation and prevalence

UPPER EXTREMITY	PREVALENCE IN %	CLINICAL IMPLICATION
Biceps	8–20	
Pronator teres	8	Pronator teres syndrome
Anconeus epitrochlearis	5–25	Cubital tunnel syndrome
Palmaris longus	11–13	
Flexor digitorum superficialis	14	
Abductor digiti minimi	24	
Lumbrical	20	Carpal tunnel syndrome

LOWER EXTREMITY	PREVALENCE IN %	CLINICAL IMPLICATION
Piriformis	15	Piriformis syndrome
Gastrocnemius	3–5	
Peroneus quartus	10–22	MC variant muscle of ankle (55)
Accessory flexor digitorum longus	2–8	Tarsal tunnel syndrome
Accessory soleus	1–6	Tarsal tunnel syndrome or bulging mass in the medial ankle

MC, most common.

  ○ One of the differential diagnoses of a soft tissue mass

Classification of muscle injury (56)
- Muscle trauma; indirect (strain) and direct (contusion, crush) trauma
  ○ Muscle strain (57)
    ▪ More common in type II fibers, biarticular muscles, and during eccentric contraction
    ▪ Commonly injured muscles: rectus femoris, medial gastrocnemius, biceps brachii, and hamstring muscles
  ○ Healing after muscle strain (58)
    ▪ Destructive phase: hematoma formation → myofibrillar necrosis and inflammatory response (put the limb in the position of muscle stretching, so it may decrease hematoma formation) (59)
    ▪ Repair phase: phagocytosis of necrotic tissue and regeneration of myofibers and formation of fibrous tissue (~1 week)
      – Brief immobilization (depending on the grade of injury), no longer than needed for the scar to bear the pulling force without re-rupture → early mobilization
    ▪ Remodeling: maturation of regenerated muscle tissues and reorganization of scar tissue
- Delayed onset muscular soreness
  ○ Twenty-four to seventy-two hours after exercise, especially after unaccustomed eccentric exercise, for several days to a week
    ▪ Mechanism: muscle damage (eccentric exercise; more structural damage to the muscle banding pattern, including disruption of sarcomere Z line)
    ▪ The release of nociceptive sensitizing substances during repair and prostaglandin-induced swelling
    ▪ Type 1 (oxidative) muscle; more preferentially involved
- Chronic exertional compartment syndrome (60,61)
  ○ Reversible ischemia secondary to a noncompliant osseofascial compartment that is unresponsive to the expansion of muscle volume occurring with exercise
  ○ Diagnosed by compartmental pressure study after exercise (see Chapter 9)
  ○ Complications: acute compartment syndrome, muscle herniation through fascial defect; for example, tibialis anterior irritating superficial peroneal nerve at the distal leg
- Rhabdomyolysis, myonecrosis, inflammatory, or other myopathy
  ○ Inflammatory myopathy
    ▪ Polymyositis, dermatomyositis, inclusion body myositis, and so on
    ▪ Infectious myopathy (viral, pyomyositis, toxoplasmosis, trichinosis, etc)
  ○ Rhabdomyolysis (±underlying myopathy) (62)
    ▪ Common causes: alcohol abuse, muscle overexertion, muscle compression, and medication or illicit drugs
    ▪ In recurrent rhabdomyolysis, workup for the underlying myopathies necessary
      – Myophosphorylase deficiency (McArdle disease), phosphofructokinase deficiency, carnine palmitoyltransferase deficiency, mitochondrial myopathies
      – Fatigue/myalgia with exercise in milder form
    ▪ Malignant hyperthermia syndrome, drug and toxin
  ○ Other myopathies
    ▪ Myotonic dystrophy and fascioscapulohumeral dystrophy: chronic pain is common (>50%)
    ▪ Muscular dystrophy (Becker, limb girdle, 1A, 1C, 2D, 2H)
    ▪ Myopathies with tubular aggregates or tubulin reactive crystalline inclusions
    ▪ Neuromyotonia with internalized capillaries: exertional myalgia, responsive to steroid (17)
    ▪ Myoadenylate deaminase def.: exercise intolerance, cramps and muscle pain
    ▪ Selenium or vitamin D deficiency

Referred muscle pain (18)
- The size of referred pain is related to the intensity and duration of ongoing/evoked pain
  ○ Patients with chronic MSK pains have enlarged referred pain areas to experimental stimuli. Proximal spread of referred pain; common but very rare in healthy individuals

- Possible mechanism: temporal summation and central hyperexcitability
- Modality specific somatosensory changes occur in referred areas emphasizing the importance of using multimodal sensory test modalities for assessment

Fascia

Classification (19)
- Superficial fascia: blood vessels and nerves to and from the skin
  - Immediately below the skin: a layer of areolar connective tissue
- Deep fascia
  - Aponeurotic fascia: composed of two to three layers of parallel collagen bundles separated by thin connective tissue
    - Richly innervated, especially in the superficial sublayer (the capsule of corpuscles and free nerve endings). Examples: thoracodorsal, fascia lata, crural fascia etc
  - Other deep fascia (epimysial fascia and specialized deep fascia): paratendon, periosteum, and neuromuscular sheath
    - Epimysial fascia: the thin collagenous layers that are strictly connected with muscle, same arrangement as aponeurotic fascia with free nerve endings particularly around the vessels, but homogeneously throughout fibrous components
    - Age-related increase in the stiffness in the epimysium; impaired lateral transmission
    - Different portion of fascia is stretched on different angle of range (therapeutic implication for therapy)

Mechanism of fascial pain (20)
- Overloaded muscle fiber → involuntary shortening, loss of oxygen and nutrient supply and an increased metabolic deficiency in local tissue
- Abnormal depolarization of motor end plates and prolonged muscle contractions → localized adenosine triphosphate (ATP) energy crisis that is associated with sensory and autonomic reflex due to central sensitization
- Ingrowth of nociceptive fibers
  - Different fascia has different intensity of free and encapsulated nerve endings (Ruffini and Pacinian corpuscles); abundant in thoracolumbar fascia and less in some area (bicipital aponeurosis and tendinous expansion of pectoralis major)
- An alteration of the viscosity, fibrosis, or adhesions can create nerve stretch inside the epineurium with impaired intrafascial gliding

Diagnostic approach
- Clinical diagnosis: local pain of the muscle fascia ± referred pain
  - Palpation of trigger points (active and latent): problem with inter/intrarater reliability with characteristic referred pain
  - Pain often coming from several concurrent sources deeper to fascia: from joint, muscle, and ligaments (63)
- Diagnostic imaging: not established yet
  - Electrodermal instrumentation, thermography, ultrasonography, and MRI: none satisfactory (64-67)
    - US and MRI: experimental in diagnosis but US is used to guide a needle in deeply located muscle
    - Measure soft tissue stiffness and thickness of fascia
    - Dynamic ultrasonography (speckle tracking) methods to appreciate the gliding between different structures

BURSA

Characteristics and clinical implications (68)
- >140 bursae described in human body
- Composed of fibrous, areolar, adipose tissue, and synovial cells
- Locations of common bursal pathologies in major joint complex
  - Shoulder: subacromial/subdeltoid, subcoracoid/subdeltoid bursa
  - Elbow: olecranon, bicipitoradial bursa
  - Hip: trochanteric, iliopsoas, ischial bursa
  - Knee: suprapatellar, prepatellar, popliteal, and anserine bursa
  - Ankle: retrocalcaneal, superficial calcaneal, intermetatarsal bursa

Classification
- Constant: formed during embryologic development, sack-like structures lined with endothelial cells, or no minimal effusion physiologically
- Adventitial: myxoid degeneration of fibroid tissue usually by friction

Etiologies
- Trauma (hemorrhagic), inflammation (eg, RA and spondyloarthropathy), infection, and crystal deposition

Presentation
- Local pain, aggravated by the position of pressure or impingement ± other structural conditions (tendinopathy, arthritis) ± swelling or warmth (in acute lesion)
- Correlation of pain with bursal inflammation
  - Pain correlates with proinflammatory markers and pain chemicals/cytokines, substance P in bursal tissue (69)
    - Positive inflammatory cells in subacromial bursal tissue: constant shoulder pain and night pain
    - Negative inflammatory cells in subacromial bursal tissue: only with movement (overhead)

Diagnostic approach
- Usually clinical with imaging study to confirm
- US: bursal effusion, increased thickness (often not present, not very sensitive) ± increased vascularity on Doppler
- MRI findings of bursal enhancement or thickening: common, not necessarily correlating with pain (70)

BONE AND JOINT

Bone

Basic anatomy of axial skeleton
- Cortical and cancellous bone
  - Cortical: low porosity, high mineral content, higher stiffness, withstanding greater stress, less strain
  - Trabecular: high porosity, low mineral content, withstanding more strain, shock-absorbing capability
  - Vertebrae: mostly trabecular versus long bone; more cortical bone than vertebrae
- Spine: anterior arch (vertebral body and anterior 1/3 of the pedicle) and posterior arch (posterior 2/3 of pedicle, lamina, and process)

Pain-sensitive structures in spine (71)
- Skin, subcutaneous tissue, and adipose tissue
- Capsules of facet and sacroiliac joints
- Ligaments: longitudinal spinal, interspinous (mainly posterior), flaval (minimal innervation), and sacroiliac
- Periosteum: vertebral bodies and arches
- Dura mater and epidural fibroadipose tissue
- Arterioles for joints and cancellous bone and veins (epidural and paravertebral)
- Paravertebral muscles: perivascular unmyelinated nerve endings in the adventitial sheaths of intramuscular blood vessels

Basic anatomy of appendicular skeleton (72)
- Compact cortical layer and spongy, interior trabecular meshwork (Figure 1.6)
  ○ Cortical bone: diaphysis, resist compression, or shearing force better than tension forces
  ○ Cancellous (trabeculae) bone: metaphysis and epiphysis: measured by bone mineral density
  ○ Ratio of cortical versus trabeculae: 4:1 in adults
  ○ Resist compression > tension > shear (weakest) force
- Periosteum becomes weaker and less osteogenic with age: slower fracture healing and contributes to delayed union and nonunion with aging

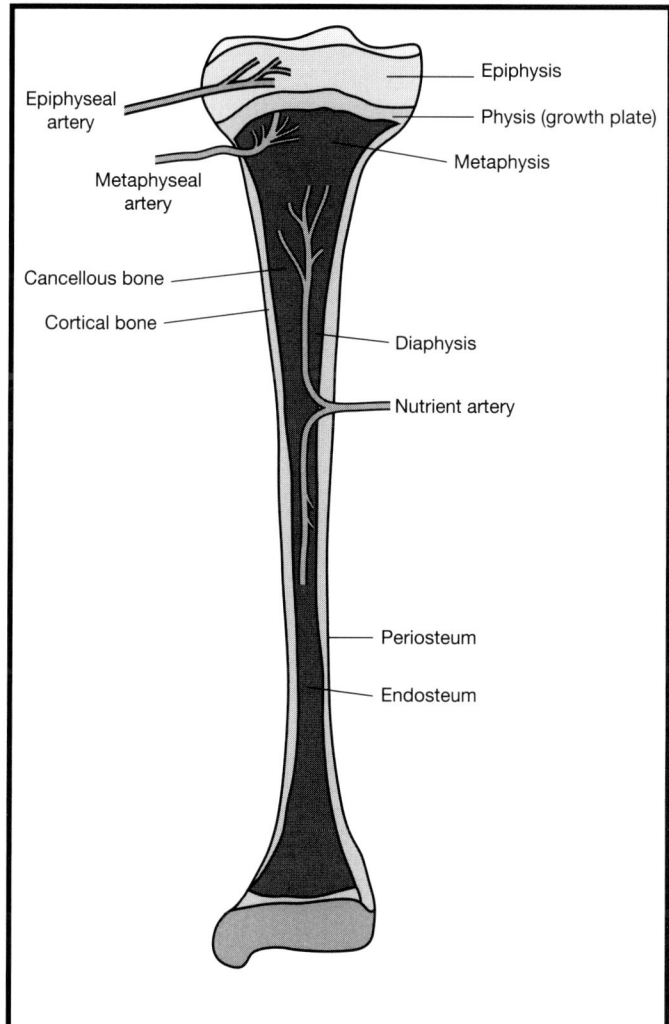

FIGURE 1.6
Anatomy of bone.

- Innervation (73)
  ○ Periosteal nerves: sensory nerves, including pain fibers
  ○ Vasomotor nerves with arteries in the Haversian canals
  ○ Sympathetic fibers
  ○ Neurotransmitters: dopamine and serotonin, cannabinoids related to bone integrity (osteopenia in animal models)

Fracture
Introduction
- Classification: many different systems available
  ○ Complete versus incomplete (periosteum remains intact, eg, Greenstick by angular force, compression fracture), buckling (torus; one cortex compacted and the opposite cortex is intact)
  ○ Transverse (usually by direct blow or purely angular, usually aligned) or spiral (oblique) by twisting force → fracture along the shear line, difficult to align, and unstable
  ○ Comminuted: more than two fracture segments
  ○ Avulsion: by avulsion force through enthesis
- Common (subtle) fracture patterns encountered in the outpatient clinic
  ○ Fatigue fracture: overuse; normal bone density
  ○ Insufficient fracture: low bone density (BMD; osteoporotic) or metabolic disease
  ○ Pathologic fracture; metastasis

Bone healing (21)
- Depends on the extent of the injury; primary site (periosteum; precursor cells into the chondroblasts and osteoblasts) or secondary sites (bone marrow, endosteum, small blood vessels, and fibroblasts)
- Healing of fracture: initially fibrocartilaginous callus then bony callus formation in 3 to 4 weeks and firm union in 2 to 3 months usually
- Types of bone healing
  ○ Primary: slow, no callus in rigid compression fixation, with direct and intimate contact between the fragments
  ○ Secondary: reactive (1–2 weeks), reparative phase (weeks to months, callus formation, lamellar bone deposition) and remodeling phase (months to years; remodeling to original bone contour)
- Weight bearing: weight bearing as tolerated (WBAT) if there is the evidence of callus formation

Complications
- Immediately after the fracture
  ○ Neurologic and vascular injury: neurapraxia by stretching (common mechanism)
  ○ Fat embolus: 4 hours to 4 days after the trauma (rare, but can be fatal)
  ○ Compartment syndrome: mild case often underrecognized
    ▪ Symptoms and signs subtle: 5 Ps (pain, pulselessness, paralysis, paresthesia, and pallor) can be unclear due to pain medications, fracture pain
    ▪ For example, displaced supracondylar fracture of the humerus → Volkmann's contracture (involving anterior compartment, anterior interosseous artery)
  ○ Infection
  ○ Deep vein thrombosis
- Late onset
  ○ Avascular necrosis: especially scaphoid fracture, femoral head, talar head fracture, etc

- Posttraumatic arthritis: for example, common cause of ankle arthritis and elbow arthritis
- Delayed union, malunion, or nonunion
- Complex regional pain syndrome

Stress (Fatigue) Fracture

Introduction
- Stress fractures divided into fatigue fracture and insufficiency fractures
  - Fatigue fracture: prolonged cyclical mechanical stress on normal bone
    - Specific site at particular sports: 10% of all sport related injury, MC in tibia
  - Insufficiency fracture; physiologic stress on abnormal bones
    - Elderly, particularly in patients with tumors
- Risk factors of stress fracture (fatigue)
  - Extrinsic risk factors (74)

LOCATION OF STRESS FRACTURE	ACTIVITY FREQUENTLY INVOLVED
Ulna-coronoid (elbow) joint	Pitching
Humerus-distal diaphysis	Throwing
Ribs	Carrying heavy objects, golf
Lower cervical spine	Clay shoveling
Lumbar spine (spondylolysis)	Lifting, ballet
Obturator ring	Bowling, gymnastics
Femur diaphysis and neck	Ballet, running
Tibia, distal fibula	Running (distance, eg, >40 miles/wk)
Proximal fibula, calcaneus	Jumping
Tarsal navicular	Marching/running
Metatarsal diaphysis	Marching

- Others: training variables in runner, shoes >6 months etc
  - Intrinsic risk factors
    - Smaller calf girth/tibial width and less muscle mass in the lower limb, poor muscle endurance
    - Abnormal biomechanics: leg–leg discrepancy, foot mechanics (pes cavus and planus/hindfoot eversion), genu varum and femoral anteversion, excessive hip adduction
    - Gender, bone density, other comorbidities, and so on

Presentation
- Insidious onset of pain over 2 to 3 weeks: often correlates with a recent change in training habits or equipment
- Check known endocrinopathies (eg, DM), autoimmune and eating disorders, depression, malabsorption syndrome, bariatric surgery, and gastroesophageal reflux disease
- Dietary history should include questions regarding the intake of calcium, vitamin D, protein, and alcoholic and caffeinated beverages

Diagnostic approach
- Clinical diagnosis confirmed by imaging study
- Plain x-ray: usually normal initially. Repeat in 1 to 2 weeks
- MRI or technetium 99m bone scan
  - MRI can give further information; for example, tension versus compression site

Pathologic Fracture

Introduction
- Fracture related to tumor (75)
  - Primary versus metastatic (more common)
  - Common bony metastatic cancers: breast, lung, kidney, prostate, thyroid, and myeloma
    - Common in long bone (femur and humerus): 10% to 30% with bone metastasis
  - Risks for pathologic fracture
    - Painful lesion >2.5 cm in diameter, occupy >50% bony cortical diameter, involve >50% medullary cross-sectional area, first 6 to 8 weeks with radiation therapy
  - Other pathologic fracture: osteoporotic fracture, check lumbar spine section

Diagnostic approach
- High clinical suspicion: prompt imaging study if red flags are present
- Initially x-ray, then consider advanced imaging
  - Typical locations associated with pathologic fractures: subtrochanteric femur, junction of the humeral head and humeral metaphysis, and the spine
    - ≥10% not confidently detected by plain x-ray
  - Sclerotic lesion by prostate, breast, colonic, bladder, and soft tissue sarcoma
  - Osteolytic lesion: myelomas (punched out), renal, hepatocellular cancer, lymphoma, and leukemia
  - Mixed pattern: MC
- Radiologic findings helpful to differentiate pathologic from fatigue fracture (74)

DIAGNOSTIC IMAGING	STRESS (FATIGUE) FRACTURE	PATHOLOGIC FRACTURE
Radiographs and CT	Endosteal thickening Benign periosteal reaction Absence of any aggressive features	Endosteal scalloping (focal resorption of the inner margin of cortical bones) Aggressive periosteal reaction Soft tissue mass Aggressive bone marrow pattern of destruction Mineralized matrix
MRI	Linear or band-like signal abnormality Surrounding bone marrow T2 abnormality (edema) Absence of or ill-defined T1 bone marrow abnormality	Well-defined T1 bone marrow abnormality Massive muscle edema Soft tissue mass

Pediatric Bony Injury

Introduction
- Long bone in children: metaphysis, physis (growth plate, not stable or strong) and epiphysis (less resistant to shear and tensile forces) (76)

- Common pediatric bony injury
  ○ Growth-related problem
    ▪ Coalition: talocalcaneal and calcaneonavicular coalition; pain when ossified
    ▪ Accessory ossicles: separate ossification center extra-chondrally, 8 to 10 years, for example, trigonum and navicular
  ○ Overuse injuries (77)
    ▪ Apophysitis at junction between a tendon/musculotendinous unit and the epiphysis; Osgood–Schlatter, Sinding Larsen Johansson, Sever's disease, and Iselin's disease (5th metatarsal)
    ▪ Osteochondroses and osteonecrosis (at ossification center): little leaguer's elbow (capitellum), Konig disease (femoral condyle, medial > lateral), talus (posteromedial > anterolateral), Kohler's disease (navicular) and Freiberg's disease (2nd metatarsal).
    ▪ Stress fracture: tibia (metaphyseal–diaphyseal junction), fibula and the metatarsal bones

Presentation
- Unique pediatric fracture
  ○ Torus (buckle) fracture: compressive fracture leading to failure of the bone at the junction of the metaphysis and diaphysis, because of the porous nature of the bone, stable and heals well with splinting or casting
  ○ Greenstick fracture: incomplete fracture in the shaft of long bone, disruption of cortex (bending of bone; one side is fractured), immobilization if minimal angulation
  ○ Supracondylar fracture: 3 to 11 years old, fall on outstretched hand or direct trauma, higher risk of complication (especially neurovascular → referral for surgical fixation)
- Salter–Harris epiphyseal fracture
  ○ Physes close at 14.5 years in girls and 17 years in boys: differently at different bones
  ○ Twenty percent of pediatric fracture involves the growth plate

Diagnostic approach
- Clinical suspicion confirmed by radiologic test
- Salter–Harris epiphyseal fracture (Figure 1.7)

TYPE	CHARACTERISTICS
1	Through physis; x-ray is usually negative • Best prognosis; growth arrest rare
2	Through physis and metaphysis: MC (~75%), excellent prognosis, and possible joint instability • May have growth arrest
3	Through physis and epiphysis sparing the metaphysis: greatest risk to joint integrity • Intra-articular fracture; uncommon
4	Through all; poor prognosis (growth arrest and articular cartilage congruity) with loss of blood supply
5	Compression (crush) fx of physis; rare, usually diagnosed retrospectively
6	Injury to the perichondrium: angular deformity may occur

MC, most common.

Joint

Introduction
- Classification based on the anatomy
  ○ Diarthrodial joint
    ▪ Movement (sliding, spinning, and rolling) depending on the shape of joint surfaces
    ▪ Cartilage and synovial fluid (hyaluronate): little wear and tear despite enormous loading and motion
    ▪ Plane (or gliding): flat articular surfaces, limited motion by the articular capsule, gliding, or sliding
    ▪ For example, proximal tibiofibular, intercarpal, intermetacarpal, and AC joints
    ▪ Hinge (ginglymus): movement around the one axis (like door hinge), flexion, and extension
    ▪ For example, elbow (humeroulnar), ankle, knee, interphalangeal joint

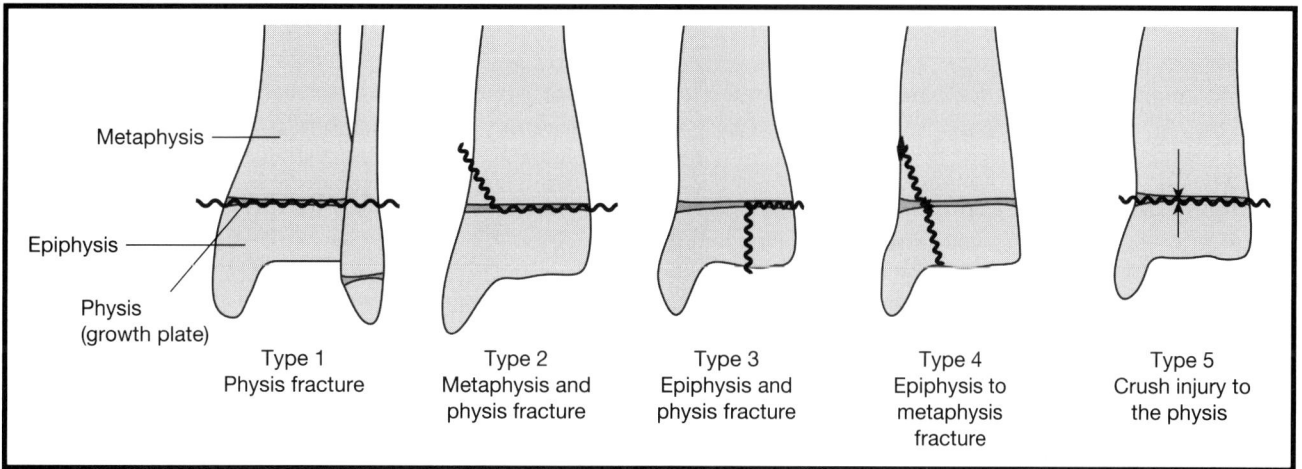

FIGURE 1.7
Salter–Harris epiphyseal fracture classification.

- Pivot (trochoid): central bony pivot turning within a bony ring, movement around one axis, allow rotation only
- For example, radioulnar (proximal and distal) and atlantoaxial joint
- Ellipsoidal (condyloid): reciprocal convex and concave, biaxial at right ankle to each other without axial rotation
- For example, radiocarpal, atlanto-occipital, and MCP joints
- Saddle: trapezio-1st metacarpal, ellipsoidal joint function and circumduction
- Ball and socket: rotation (shoulder) and circumduction (MCP); shoulder, MCP, and hip joints
  - Fibrous: non-movable, syndesmosis, inferior tibiofibular, and tympanostapedial syndesmosis
  - Cartilaginous
    - Synchondroses (immobile): costochondral joint and epiphyseal plate
    - Symphyses: joined by a plate of fibrocartilage and slightly movable. Example: pubic symphysis, and intervertebral disc
- Joint constraint and stability
  - Passive stabilizer (static)
    - Capsuloligamentous structures: change in length, line of action, and material properties of the tissue
    - Joint articulation surface (concavity compression), negative intra-articular/intracapsular pressure
  - Active stabilizer: muscle–tendon unit
- Innervation of joint: Hilton's law
  - Joint innervated by sensory nerve across the joint and any nerve innervating the muscle across the joint
    - All the motor nerves innervating the adjacent muscles that induce motion of the joint contribute to the joint innervation
    - Neuropathy involving both sensory and motor nerve innervating the muscle can cause joint pain (pain from motor nerve involvement; not typical neuropathic).
- Proposed mechanism of pain in degenerative arthritis
  - Cystic degeneration of the subchondral bone: the synovial fluid forces its way into small cracks in the subchondral bone, with creating caverns in the spongiosa (trabecula)
    - Subchondral bone is richly innervated by nerves transmitting pain sensation (in contrast with cartilage); therefore, repetitive high fluid pressure in the subchondral bone could be an explanation for pain perceived by the patients

Effects of aging on bone and joint
- A decrease in cross-linking in bone tissue with age. The inflexibly and shortened tendon can cause more than usual stress on the weakened bone attributing to a fracture
- Changes in cartilage tissue
  - Difficult to determine if this is due to normal aging or to injury
  - Increase in cartilage stiffness with aging, due to increased cross-linkages in the collagen tissue
  - Decrease in strength but no normal thinning of the cartilage with aging

Evaluation of Arthropathy

Common presentation of joint pathology (78)
- Pain, swelling (effusion), tenderness, deformity, and/or warmth

Demographics
- Age
  - OA, pseudogout; more prevalent in older age versus traumatic arthropathy, psoriatic arthritis (PsA), reactive arthropathy, and ankylosing spondylitis (AS) in younger age group
- Premenopausal women more common than men in systemic lupus erythematosus (SLE) by 9 times and RA by 3 to 4 times
- Race and ethnicity
  - Caucasians: polymyalgia rheumatica and Wegener granulomatosis
  - African: higher sarcoidosis and SLE

Classification based on number of joints involved

MONOARTICULAR	OLIGOARTICULAR (2–4 JOINTS)	POLYARTICULAR
OA	OA	OA
Gouty arthritis: acute gout or Pseudogout; can be oligoarticular	Rheumatic fever (can be symmetric polyarticular)	RA
Infectious	Reactive arthritis (ReA), Behçet disease	SLE
• Bacterial arthritis (gonorrheal, nongonococcal, lyme disease, mycobacterial infection); can be asymmetric oligoarthritis	Ankylosing spondylitis	Still disease
	Psoriatic arthritis; can be polyarticular	Behçet disease
	Arthritis associated with inflammatory bowel disease (IBD)	Sarcoid arthritis (SA)
• Viral arthritis: HIV or Parvovirus B19 infection; can be symmetric polyarticular		

OA, osteoarthritis; RA, rheumatoid arthritis; SLE, systemic lupus erythematosus.

Classification based on underlying pathology
- Arthralgia versus inflammatory arthritis
  - Arthralgia: joint pain without signs of inflammation (swelling, warmth, etc), pain for <15 minutes typically
- Infectious versus noninfectious arthritis

	INFECTIOUS	NONINFECTIOUS
Constitutional symptoms	Fever (high grade), chills	Constitutional symptoms with low-grade fever in inflammatory arthropathy ReA if previous urethritis and uveitis
Risk factors	Skin infection, risky sexual behavior, vaginal or urethral discharge, exposure to gonorrhea, recent IA steroid injection Osteomyelitis, age >60 years	Trauma Family history of inflammatory arthritis
Patterns of joint involvement	Single usually Can be migratory; for example, gonorrhea, lyme	Multiple (migratory in rheumatic Dz)
Pain	Acute, significant local pain, constant	Aggravated by motion and weight bearing (especially OA) Morning stiffness (RA)
Comorbid conditions	DM, concurrent RA, immunosuppression, sickle cell disease, chronic renal disease	
Progression	Rapid progression Atypical in fungal infection or tuberculosis (from endemic country)	

DM, diabetes mellitus; Dz, disease; IA, intra-articular; OA,; RA, rheumatoid arthritis; ReA, reactive arthritis.

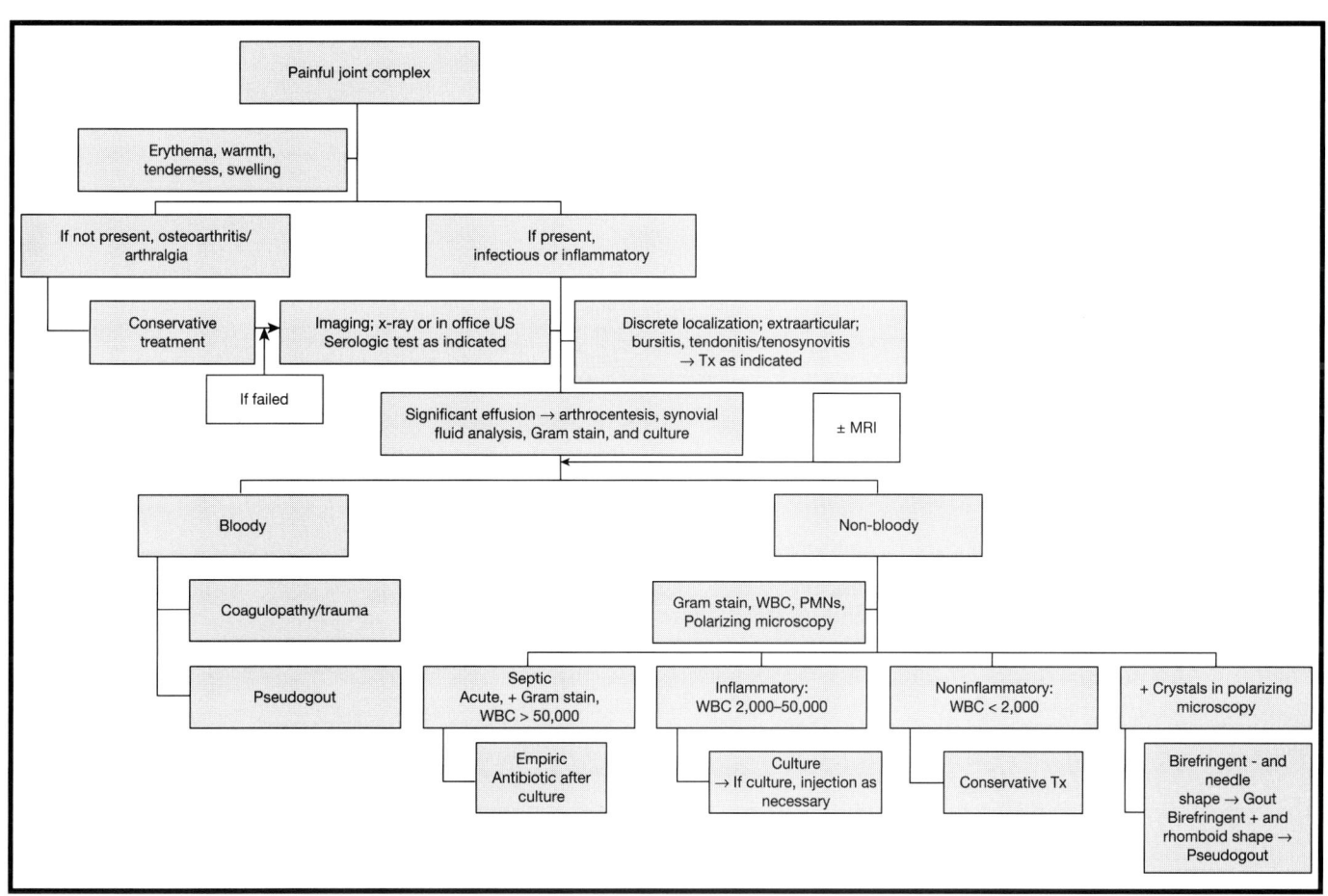

FLOWCHART 1.3
Approach to painful joint.
+, positive, –, negative; Tx, treatment; US, ultrasound; WBC, white blood cells.

NERVOUS SYSTEM

Introduction (79)
- Central (brain and spinal cord) and peripheral nerve system (anterior horn cell in ventral horn in spinal cord and distal including root, plexus, and peripheral nerve)
- Ascending pathway

LOCATION	ANATOMY, PHYSIOLOGY, AND CLINICAL IMPLICATION
Peripheral receptors	Nociceptor • Found in skin, connective tissue, blood vessels, periosteum, and most of the visceral organs • Formed by peripheral endings of sensory neurons • Polymodal nociceptors (to C fibers): mechanical, chemical and thermal stimuli • High threshold mechanical nociceptors (HTM) and myelinated mechano-thermal (MT) nociceptors (to A δ fibers) Transmission • Tissue damage • Mast cell, neutrophil, and macrophages → TNF-α, IL-1β (COX-2 → PGE 2 → PGE receptor), IL-6 (cytokine receptor), nitric oxide, bradykinin, nerve growth factor, protons (Trk A receptor extracellular signal related kinase 1, 2) • Protein kinase A, C, phosphorylation • Action potential → activate or sensitize neurons Acute nociceptive (noxious), inflammatory/joint (inflammation and tissue damage), neuropathic (nerve damage), noninflammatory and non-neuropathic pain Therapeutic implication involving this level: local anesthetics, capsaicin, nitrite patch, anticonvulsants, NSAIDs involved in this level
Peripheral N	Aβ fiber (large thick myelinated)—nonnociceptive pain • Normally response to nonpainful stimuli (mechanical) • Can be recruited to pain processing over time Aδ nociceptive fibers (conduction velocity [CV], 15 m/sec): nociceptive, a sharp, well-localized pain sensation • Heat, cold, high-intensity mechanical stimuli Nociceptive C fibers (CV: 0.5–2 m/sec): a dull, burning, or aching and poorly localized pain • Heat, mechanical, or chemical stimuli • Limited evaluation by conventional nerve conduction velocity (NCV) studies that measure large myelinated fibers Sympathetic and parasympathetic nerves Common pathologies involving this level • Focal: nerve entrapment syndrome, mononeuropathy/neuritis or traumatic nerve injury or neuroma • Diffuse: peripheral neuropathy with DM, HIV, chronic kidney disease, etc • Multifocal/regional: amyotrophy (radiculoplexus neuropathy, brachial, lumbosacral), mononeuritis multiplex etc Therapeutic implication involving this level: local anesthetic, opioid, TENS, nerve block, and sympathetic nerve block
Dorsal root ganglion	The first order neurons; cell bodies of the nerve fibers; located in superficial layers (rexed laminar I, II) and deep (V) of the dorsal root ganglion • Aδ fibers terminate primarily in I and V • C fibers in lamina II Neurotransmitters • Excitatory: glutamate and substance P • Inhibitory: GABA, glycine, endocannabinoids, opioids, monoamines and descending inhibitory (NE[1] and 5-HT[1]) Compression of dorsal root ganglion increases activity in Aδ fiber and C fibers Pathologies involving this level • Ganglionopathy: inflammatory response of ganglion, not length dependent and often severe. Symptoms may begin from upper extremity or with severe sensory deficit (ataxia in addition to numbness, tingling paresthesia) Therapeutic implication involved at this level: opioid, local anesthetics, A two agonist and NSAIDs Sympathetic (paravertebral ganglia including stellate ganglion and others), prevertebral (including celiac etc): site for sympathetic nerve block
Spinal cord	The second-order neurons in the dorsal horn (gray matter) • Respond only to noxious stimuli (nociceptive specific neurons) and others (wide dynamic range [WDR] neurons): respond to both nociceptive and non-nociceptive sensory stimuli • Substantia gelatinosa and nucleus proprius Cross in the anterior white commissure of the spinal cord and ascend as the spinothalamic tract in the opposite anterolateral quadrant This tract is somatotopically organized, with sacral elements situated posterolaterally and cervical elements more anteromedially Therapeutic implication involved at this level: spinal cord stimulator

(continued)

LOCATION	ANATOMY, PHYSIOLOGY, AND CLINICAL IMPLICATION
Brainstem	The ventral posterolateral (VPL) nucleus (3rd order neuron) of the thalamus as the neospinothalamic pathway • Mediate fast and well-localized pain sensation The periaqueductal gray: spinoreticular pathway • Paleospinothalamic tract: fibers from brainstem join with fibers from the spinothalamic tract to project to the central or laminar nuclei of the thalamus and constitute the paleospinothalamic tract • Slow and poorly localized pain and emotional response to pain stimulation Pathologies involving this level: central (thalamic) pain syndrome
Cerebral cortex	A multidimensional integration of sensory-discriminative, cognitive, and affective motivational axes Primary sensory cortex (basic pain processing) and secondary sensory cortex and insula (dorsal posterior for higher function of pain perception) Nociceptive matrix: posterior insula, parietal operculum, mid cingulate, and primary sensory/motor, (S1, M1) posterior parietal cortex • Orienting, withdrawal, and sensory encoding Emotional aspects of pain perception are mediated by the anterior cingulate cortex and the posterior insula and parietal operculum. Chronic pain: brain dysfunction and reorganization • Functional MRI and PET scan in research setting to investigate the brain pathway (80,81) Neuropathic pain pathologies involving this level: central pain syndrome (poststroke pain) Therapeutic implication involving this level: opioids, $\alpha 2$ agonists, NSAIDs, tricyclic antidepressants (TCA), selective serotonin reuptake inhibitors (SSRIs), serotonin norepinephrine reuptake inhibitors (SNRIs)

DM, diabetes mellitus; GABA, gamma-aminobutyric acid; N, nerve; NSAID, nonsteroidal anti-inflammatory drug; TENS, transcutaneous electrical nerve stimulation.
Source: Refs. 82 and 83.

- Descending pathway
  ○ Somatosensory cortex to thalamus and limbic forebrain to brainstem (corticobular fibers/tract)
    ▪ Second- and third-order matrix involved in descending control
    ▪ Second-order matrix: anterior insula, anterior cingulate, dorsolateral prefrontal cortex, posterior parietal cortex (attentional-perceptive)
      – Top-down attentional modulation, access to consciousness, cognitive control, and vegetative reactions
    ▪ Third-order matrix: perigenual cingulate, orbitofrontal, anterolateral prefrontal cortex, ventral striatum (affective-reappraisive)
      – Internal state, emotional modulation, reassessment, and delayed perception.
      – Example: not feeling pain or less pain under stress
  ○ Brain stem to spinal cord (dorsal horn; dorsolateral funiculus) to synapse with incoming primary afferent neuron, second-order pain transmission neuron, or interneurons
    ▪ Periaqueductal gray region of the midbrain (opioid receptor), medullary reticular formation (serotonin) and the locus ceruleus (norepinephrine)
    ▪ Release neurotransmitters serotonin (5HT) and norepinephrine (NE) in the spinal cord
    ▪ Activate interneurons in the spinal dorsal horn to release opioid peptides

Common pathologies for neuropathic pain
- Entrapment neuropathy (84)
  ○ Clinical stages: mostly unpredictable progression and individual variation (85)
    ▪ Initially pain at rest, worse at night (intraneural microvascular perfusion changes disappears with activities), and intermittent paresthesia
    ▪ Progress to constant, numbness, pain during the day, and weakness (segmental demyelination)
    ▪ Advanced to constant pain, sensory loss, and muscle atrophy (nerve fiber degeneration)
      – Asymptomatic (improving pain) with declined inflammatory response, and atrophy of the nerve
      – Possibly cortical or proximal sensitization (86): similar to complex regional pain or chronic neuropathic pain
  ○ Large myelinated fiber involvement earlier than small fibers; role for routine EMG test
  ○ Anatomically, proximal (to the entrapment) swelling/enlargement: accumulation of axoplasm, nerve swelling (edema) or fibrosis following chronic inflammatory changes, increased perineurial and endoneurial fibrosis
    ▪ Basis for imaging diagnosis (US and MRI)
- Radiculopathy
  ○ Common etiologies
    ▪ Mechanical (more common): disc disease and spondylosis
      – Rarely metastatic disease, Pott's disease, primary tumor etc
    ▪ Nonmechanical (rare): DM (MC for non-mechanical etiology), infection, such as lyme, HIV, syphilis, tuberculosis, abscess, sarcoidosis, metastasis, arachnoiditis, and so on
  ○ Common locations
    ▪ Cervical radiculopathy: C7, C6, C8, and C5 in descending order
    ▪ LS radiculopathy: L5 > S1; MC level, 62% to 90% of all radiculopathy
    ▪ Thoracic radiculopathy (87): unusual, T 11–12 (MC level)
- Traumatic nerve injury or Neuroma (88)
  ○ Pathophysiology
    ▪ Traumatic nerve injury → proximal stump degeneration and regeneration → proximal nerve fibers sprout into regenerating units with upregulation of neurotrophin, neural cell adhesion molecules, cytokines, and so on in the microenvironment → adhesion and traction on nerve
    ▪ Abnormal connection between Aβ fiber and nociceptive fibers (A δ and C), overall sensitization and hyperexcitability, ephaptic transmission, and causing centralization
  ○ Presentation of neuroma (89)
    ▪ Gradual onset of neuropathic pain, worse with movement, occasionally pressure or tension
    ▪ Tenderness with referred/radiating pain, confirmed by imaging-guided nerve block

Evaluation (localization based on the symptoms and signs)

- Anatomy-based differential diagnosis and localization (in the axis of root, plexus, and peripheral nerve branch): examples
  - Sensory symptoms in lateral hand and fingers: C7–6 radiculopathy versus CTS versus plexus lesion (less common, lateral cord, upper and middle trunk)
    - If radial or musculocutaneous nerve involved, proximal lesions are favored; plexus or root
  - Sensory symptoms in medial hand/finger: C8–T1 radiculopathy versus brachial plexus lesion (lower trunk, medial cord; thoracic outlet syndrome, or tumor infiltration) versus ulnar neuropathy
    - If medial antebrachial cutaneous nerve (favor proximal lesion) or radial nerve, extensor indicis (EI) or abductor, or extensor pollicis are involved, lower trunk or root lesions are favored
  - "Sciatica": L5–S1 radiculopathy versus sciatic nerve lesion versus peripheral neuropathy versus tarsal tunnel syndrome (or interdigital neuritis)
    - If gluteal muscle is involved, root or plexus lesions are favored
  - Hip and thigh weakness: L3–4 radiculopathy versus lumbar plexus lesion versus femoral neuropathy versus myopathy
    - If hip adductor is involved, root or plexus lesions are favored. If hip abductor is involved as well, myopathy or MSK lesion is favored
- Possible mechanism based on the onset of symptoms
  - Acute/immediate; vasculitis or traumatic, onset over days: inflammatory, over a longer period: entrapment or compressive neuropathy
- Nerve fiber size involvement based on sensory symptoms
  - Large diameter (myelinated); vibration, position sensation, light touch; involved earlier in entrapment/compressive neuropathy
    - Decreased proprioception (ataxia)/vibratory sense, areflexia
    - Pain can occur with axonal degeneration
  - Small fiber (A delta and unmyelinated C fiber) for pain, temperature and autonomic (90)
    - Presents with burning and pins/needle pain, and dull aching
    - Autonomic symptoms (small fiber involvement): vasomotor, sweating (increased or decreased) or skin changes/decolorization, orthostatic dizziness/hypotension, and bowel/bladder dysfunction
    - Not assessed by routine NCS. May require skin biopsy for epidermal fiber density or quantitative sudomotor tests
- Motor symptoms: negative (weakness) and positive (cramps, fasciculation, myokymia, etc)

Diagnostic approach

- Nerve conduction study (NCS) and needle EMG if large diameter fiber or motor segment involvement is suspected
  - Sensory NCS (important to differentiate preganglionic (root, motor neuron lesion) versus postganglionic (plexus or peripheral nerve)
    - Normal in preganglionic lesion (because dorsal ganglion is intact to maintain the integrity of sensory nerve versus motor neuron is located in the ventral horn of the spinal cord) and neuromuscular junction/muscle disease
  - Mild lesion or cutaneous nerve entrapment (branches) is limited by NCS/EMG evaluation
    - Often imaging-guided diagnostic block with ~1 mL of lidocaine can be useful
- Small fiber neuropathy evaluation limited by EMG/NCS (usually negative in isolated lesion) (91)
  - Sympathetic skin response during routine NCS: semi-quantitative, low sensitivity, often not correlating with clinical manifestation
  - Referral to epidermal nerve fibers in skin biopsy or for quantitative sensory testing, quantitative sudomotor axon reflex test, cardiovagal, and adrenergic autonomic testing
  - Workup for potential causes of small fiber neuropathy

PATHOLOGIES	EVALUATION
DM	Fasting glucose, Hb_{A1C}, 2-hour glucose tolerance test
HIV	HIV-1/2 Antigen/antibody immunoassay, HIV 1 nucleic acid test
Alcohol	History
Sjögren's syndrome	ANA, SS-A/Ro, SS-B/La Ab, Schirmer tear test, Rose-bengal corneal staining
Toxin (pharmacologic, environmental)	History and toxicology test
Monoclonal gammonopathy	Serum and urine protein electrophoresis, quantitative immunoglobulin
Hyperlipidemia	Fasting lipid profile
Familial "burning feet" neuropathy	Family history (autosomal dominant) (92)
Systemic amyloidosis	Serum and urine protein electrophoresis, nerve/muscle biopsy, abdominal fat or rectal biopsy
Familial amyloidosis	Transthyretin gene
Tanglier disease	Alpha (high density) lipoproteins
Fabry's disease	Alpha galactosidase assay
Hereditary sensory neuropathies	History and genetic study

Ab, antibody; ANA, antinuclear antibody; DM, diabetes; SS, Sjögren's syndrome.

BIOMECHANICS

INTRODUCTION (49,93)

Biomechanics: the study of continuum mechanics
- Loads, motion, stress, strain of solids, and fluids of biological systems and the mechanical effects on the body's movement, size, shape, and structure

Kinematics: study of motion, the geometric and time-dependent aspects of motion (without analyzing the forces causing the motion)
- Body motion analysis in both 2-D and 3-D space
- Motions: rotatory (angular), translatory (linear)—gliding, curvilinear (rotatory and translatory motion combined)
- Location of motion (plane): transverse (axial), frontal (coronal), and sagittal plane
- Direction of motion based on the different plane: flexion/extension (sagittal), abduction/adduction (axial), inversion/eversion (coronal)
- Quantity of motion: linear distance, arc, speed etc

Kinetics: the study of the forces and moments causing movement

- Kinetic analysis: measure force (eg, ground reaction force), joint moment (eg, turning, twisting or rotational effect of a force), power and torque (special type of a moment)
  - Ground reaction force (GRF): force to resist body's downward movement (by gravity), affected by body posture
    - Overall body posture affecting the GRF location
    - GRF located outside the base of support → unstable
  - Moment arm: distance from fulcrum of movement to the muscle
    - Longer the moment arm: the better mechanical advantage for the same amount of tendon or muscle force, more tendon excursion for the same amount of joint rotation
    - Determine potential force generation
- External (gravity, wind, water etc) and internal force (body source, muscle, bone etc); friction, shear, and contact
- Force vector defines point of application, action line, and magnitude
- Equilibrium: forces acting on an object sum to zero
- Center of pressure (COP): the mean of all of the vectors of the forces acting on the bottom of the foot during the stance phase of gait. Force and vectors measured by force plate
  - Center of mass (COM): weight average of the segment centers of mass.
  - COM within the base of support by limits COP displacement → unperturbed standing balance

CLINICAL APPLICATION (63,94)

Clinical application of Newton's law
- Law of inertia (Newton's 1st law): objects resist initiation of motion or a change in direction of motion
  - Eccentric contraction (requiring more force) to slow down inertia during gait (swing and initial stance phase)
- Law of acceleration (Newton's 2nd law): acceleration of an object is proportional to the unbalanced forces acting on it and inversely proportional to the mass of the object, or a (acceleration) = F (force)/m (mass). Force = acceleration × mass
  - Impact of body weight (mass) on force (motion)
  - Sagittal and coronal balance with gravity to pull down (increased acceleration with longer lever arm to center of mass)
    - Decrease force by decreasing lever arm length
    - For example, cane in the hip pain, correct lifting technique toward the axis (near plum line) and correct head posture in muscle strain or myofascial pain of cervical spine extensor muscles
- Law of reaction (Newton's 3rd law): every action has opposed and equal reaction (reaction force)
  - Ground reaction force (upward force) on walking (downward force)
    - Force plate (gait analysis) measures the ground reaction force

Physiologic diversity of movements
- More than one MSK movement strategy available for a certain task
  - Common strategy exists for a certain task, but not universal
  - Therefore, detailed description for the injury mechanism is important for diagnosis
  - Therapeutic implication to modify motor task to avoid pain
- Compensatory mechanism is essential for coping with the consequences of injuries or diseases to the MSK system: recognition important for the diagnosis

Recognition of abnormal biomechanics
- Important to understand the mechanical aspect of pain generation/aggravation and intervention (to correct false biomechanics and minimize painful compensation mechanism)
- Any injury or lesion of the individual elements of the MSK system will change the mechanical interaction and cause degradation, instability or disability of movement
- Proper modification, manipulation, and control of the mechanical environment can help prevent injury, correct abnormality, and speed healing and rehabilitation

Skeletal muscles
- Factors for the maximum tension generation potential
  - Muscle mass or volume: proportional to its work capacity
  - Cross sectional area of muscle
    - In agonist/antagonists for any joint, muscle with bigger cross sectional (with some variability depending on the types of skeletal muscle) dominates resting position
    - Balancing this asymmetry by stretching and strengthening the smaller cross sectional muscle can improve abnormal posture and biomechanics with reduction of pain (eg, impingement syndrome with shoulder retractor strengthening)
  - Length of muscle fiber: mechanical advantage in 80% to 120% of length (decrease if the length is beyond this range)
- Two joint muscles: more vulnerable for injury
  - Couple the motion of the two joints in that they cross and redistribute muscle torque, joint power, and mechanical energy throughout a limb
    - Muscle activation of two joint muscles: effected by direction of force rather than direction of movement (shortening or lengthening of muscle) (95)
    - Shortening velocity of biarticular muscles is less than that of monoarticular muscles (concentric contraction)

Clinical application of each joint: See individual chapters

GAIT CYCLE

Terminology
- Step length: the distance between the point of initial contact of one foot and the point of initial contact of the opposite foot
- Stride length: the distance between successive points of initial contact of the same foot
- Cadence (walking rate): steps per minute
- Foot angle or toe out: an angle between the line of progression and a line drawn between the midpoints of the calcaneus and the second metatarsal head

Phases and timing of gait cycle (see following table)
- Stance and swing phase: 60% or 40% as speed increases, it reverses (decrease stance phase)
- Double limb support: 20% (lowest center of gravity)
- Single limb support: 40%: important for safety (falls)
- Foot flat to heel off: the longest period in the gait cycle; related to forefoot pain (metatarsophalangeal [MTP] joint extension)
- Velocity
  - Free speed: the individual's comfortable walking speed. High individual variability up to 20%
  - Increase speed: typically from increased cadence and step length

PHASES	POSITION	MUSCLE ENGAGED

Initial contact	Calcaneus: a slightly inverted position
	• Pronatory force on the calcaneus and subtalar joint by vector of ground reaction force behind the axis of the ankle joint
	• Pronation of the subtalar joint
	  ○ Unlock the midtarsal joint (parallel of talonavicular and calcaneocuboid joint alignment) → more flexible and facilitating adaptation to terrain.
	  ○ Accommodate the functionally longer leg (from various pathologies, eg, tight Achilles)
	• Inversion of longitudinal axis of midtarsal joint (medially pulling ankle dorsiflexor)
	• Once the forefoot contacts the ground, friction prevents adduction, and tibial internal rotation is absorbed by subtalar pronation.
	Hip flexed 25°, knee slightly flexed
		Erector spinae, gluteus maximus, hamstring
		Quadriceps prevents buckling
		Ankle dorsiflexor: eccentric (most active in early stance)
		• Tibialis anterior, extensor hallucis longus: eccentric contraction of ankle dorsiflexor: supination of the longitudinal axis of the midtarsal joint

Loading response	Pronation response Hip flexed 25°, knee flexed 10°–20° and ankle PF 15°	Eccentric contraction of pretibial muscles (ankle dorsiflexor, anterior compartment) E Spinae, G Max, hamstring Quadriceps: eccentric contraction
Mid stance—2nd rocker	A period of single support External rotation moment of tibia (from pelvis swing during contralateral limb advance) → coupling movement; supination of the subtalar joint (assisted by tibialis posterior, flexor digitorum longus [FDL], flexor hallucis longus [FHL], gastrocsoleus muscles [GCS]) → two midtarsal joint: out of parallel (intersect) →increased rigidity of midtarsal joint Ankle: from 8° of plantarflexion to 5° of dorsiflexion Hip neutral, knee flexed 15°	Eccentric contraction of soleus and gastrocnemius (soleus then gastrocnemius) Tibialis posterior (TP): prevent the foot from everting past neutral position Peroneus longus (PL): balance the TP: plantarflex 1st ray Gluteus medius-minimus: maximal activity
Terminal stance—3rd rocker	Supination (terminal stance to initial swing) Relatively rigid midfoot and forefoot • Windlass effect (MTP dorsiflexion → tighten plantar fascia) • Midtarsal joint (talonavicular and calcaneocuboid joint) intersects (supination from tibial external rotation) → midtarsal joint become rigid → lever arm for push up • 1st ray stabilized by extrinsic and intrinsic foot muscles Hip extended, knee nearly extended Ankle dorsiflexed to 10°–20°	Eccentric contraction of soleus and gastrocnemius • To minimize passive ankle dorsiflexion: additional 5° DF • Gastrocnemius: maximal resisting knee hyperextension • Foot intrinsic muscles (to support arch) 1st ray stabilizing muscles • Peroneus longus: plantarflex the first ray and stabilize it against the proximal tarsal bones • Peroneus brevis: compresses the cuboid into the calcaneus • FHL, FDL: supinate the oblique axis of midtarsal joint • Abductor hallucis: plantarflex the first ray Adductor/iliopsoas muscles begins to activate
Preswing	Continued tibial advancement combined with GCS contraction Tibia: maximally externally rotated at toe off Hip extended 10°, knee flexed 40° and ankle plantarflexed 10°	GCS contraction → generation of a flexion torque at the knee (by gastrocnemius) Concentric contraction of pretibial muscles for ground clearance during swing phase Adductor/Iliopsoas: max active to resist hip extension Quadriceps
Swing	Subtalar and midtarsal joint: initially pronate due to extensor digitorum longus (EDL), later in swing, with combined activation of tibialis anterior (TA), resupinate in preparation for initial contact	

MTP, metatarsophalangeal.

Clinical implications of spatiotemporal parameters of gait

PARAMETERS	CLINICAL IMPLICATIONS
Gait speed	Correlated with function and degree of some musculoskeletal disorders • Slower speeds often being correlated with foot pain and poorer function Correlated with general outcomes in elderly patients; mortality, dependency, institutionalization, cognitive dysfunction
Stride length	Correlated with antalgic gait (shortened stride lengths), control of gait and steadiness during gait Correlated with general outcome measures in elderly patients (mortality, dependency, and institutionalization)
Cadence Step or stride width Single limb/double limb support Stance time	Correlated with function and functional improvements following intervention for foot and ankle conditions

Inman's six determinants of gait
- Six determinants
  - Pelvic rotation (limit center of gravity [CG] rise) and pelvic tilt (limit CG rise and absorb shock: midstance phase)
  - Early knee flexion (limit CG rise and absorb shock) and late knee flexion: stance phase
  - Weight transfer from heel to flat toe (stance)
  - Lateral displacement of the pelvis toward the stance limb: normal knee valgus helps
    - Two inches vertical/lateral displacement
- Clinical implication
  - Any pathology increasing center of gravity (vertical and lateral) displacement increase energy cost of ambulation
  - Most efficient gait is achieved by minimizing vertical and lateral excursions of the body's center of gravity
    - CG
      – Highest in midstance (single limb support) and lowest in double support (initial contact)
      – Running: highest in flight phase and lowest in midstance of single limb support

GAIT DYSFUNCTION

Antalgic Gait (96,97)
Characteristics
- Slow gait speed, limited ROM, unable to bear full weight, short step length on the uninvolved leg
- Compensation mechanism to avoid pain
  - Compensated Trendelenburg, mild hip external rotation (decreased joint capsule tension) with forefoot abduction, shorted single leg stance with knee flexion (decreased full extension), and lateralization of the foot weight bearing

Common underlying causes
- Lower extremity joint pain: OA, inflammatory arthropathy and others (avascular necrosis [AVN], synovitis, etc)
- Lumbar spinal stenosis: claudication, prefer forward bent posture (stooped posture) to preserve central canal space, "shopping cart sign"

Gait dysfunction with hip pathologies
Trendelenburg gait
- Characteristics
  - Trendelenburg: bend the trunk to painful side (compensated), center of mass closer to the joint → decreased hip abductor activity → decreased joint compressive/reactive force. Normal up to 5°
  - Compensated (trunk tilt toward the weak side) and uncompensated (opposite)
  - Hip pain, hip abductor contracture, motor neuron disease, L5–S1 radiculopathy, LS plexopathy, gluteal neuropathy or myopathies (polymyositis, dermatomyositis)
- Waddling gait
  - Lumbar lordosis, swaying, symmetric, and wide based
  - BL gluteus medius weakness
  - Hip extension weakness: posterior trunk lean/backward thrust lurch

Gait with hip flexion contracture: more prominent in later half of stance, compensated by lumbar extension (hyperlordosis), and crouch gait pattern

Scissoring gait: adductor spasticity from upper motor neuron syndrome

Gait dysfunction with knee pathologies
Gait with knee flexion contracture: functionally short leg, reduction in contralateral step length (more obvious in middle stance phase)

Knee instability: excessive flexion (buckling), hyperextension (recurvatum), varus and valgus
- Knee pain (MC cause), quadriceps weakness (from neurological causes: L3–4 radiculopathy, plexopathy, femoral neuropathy and myopathy, amyotrophy or disuse atrophy)
- Knee recurvatum: can cause anterior knee pain due to Hoffa's fat pad impingement or posterior knee pain

Gait dysfunction with ankle and foot pathologies
Equinus
- Compensated by over-pronated gait and/or knee recurvatum
  - Overpronation can cause pain proximally: buttock (SI joint dysfunction), lateral hip/knee (ITB tightness), and medial knee (pes anserine stretching)
- Mechanical disadvantage with standing from sitting; standing requires ankle dorsiflexion to move the center of mass forward

Calcaneal gait (heel walking) (98,99)
- Characteristics
  - Foot flat on the ground in the later stance phase (instead of heel off)

- Late (delayed) heel rise, excessive ankle dorsiflexion, excessive knee flexion, short step on the contralateral side
- Increased pressure to the plantar heel, pain, callus, or ulceration on the heel, can cause anterior ankle impingement
• Common etiologies: rare
  - Weakness of ankle plantarflexion (gastrocsoleus): chronic Achilles tear/rupture, tethered cord, and spinal lipoma etc

Intoe gait
• Characteristics: unilateral or BL internal rotation of the long axis of the foot to the line of progression (the direction in which the child is moving)
• Common etiologies
  - Femoral anteversion/torsion (MC reason for age 3–10 years)
  - Hallux varus, metatarsus adductus, talipes equinovarus, cavus, tibia torsion, or femoral anteversion

Ankle–foot instability
• Common etiologies: chronic ligament injury or muscle tear/atrophy/insufficiency
• Secondary to other deformity: excessive equinus, varus, equinovarus, valgus, equino/pes planovalgus

Foot drop/slap from ankle dorsiflexion weakness
• Characteristics
  - Steppage pattern: resulting from foot drop, excessive flexion of hips and knees when walking, short strides, tripping
  - Foot slap: inability to control eccentric ankle dorsiflexion at the initial loading response (mild weakness compared to the steppage pattern)
  - Foot dragging: upper motor neuron syndrome from extension synergy/spasticity
• Differential diagnosis: L4–5 radiculopathy, LS plexopathy, sciatic nerve, common/deep peroneal neuropathy, peripheral neuropathy (length dependent; DM and HIV etc) and myopathy (inclusion body myositis), functional weakness

Swing phase problem

Limb clearance problem: equinus foot deformity, foot drop, stiffness, limited hip flexion, hip adduction, and pelvic drop

Limb advancement problem: flexed knee, limited hip flexion, contralateral hip extension, and adducted hip

Excessive Pronation and Supination During Gait
Common pathologies by both conditions
• Foot pathologies: functional hallux rigidus, metatarsalgia, plantar fasciitis, and midtarsal arthropathy
• Proximal limb pathologies: ITB syndrome, SI joint dysfunction and back pain

PRONATION; FUNCTIONAL LEG SHORTENING		SUPINATION	
PES PLANUS	COMMON PROBLEMS	PES CAVUS	COMMON PROBLEMS
Forefoot abduction	Pain from wearing foot orthotics (if inadequately designed), AFO (lateral forefoot irritation, medial midfoot/sole irritation)	Forefoot adduction	Callus formation, MTP overloading/pain
Midfoot DF, navicular dropping	Aggravate tibialis posterior insufficiency Lateral hindfoot (calcaneocuboid arthropathy or impingement syndrome)	1st metatarsal head plantarflexion Midfoot PF	
Calcaneal eversion (normal 5–10 valgus)	Subtalar arthropathy	Calcaneal inversion	Subtalar arthropathy Inversion ankle sprain Peroneus tendinopathy
Tibial/femur internal rotation	Saphenous N irritation Pes anserine tendinopathy Tight hip external rotator (piriformis syndrome)	Tibia/femur external rotation Knee hyperextension	Anterior knee pain (Hoffa's fat pad impingement)

AFO, ankle foot orthosis; DF, dorsiflexion; MTP, metatarsophalangeal; N, nerve; PF, plantar flexion.

Unsteady (Ataxic) Gait (100)
Characteristics: wide based with truncal instability (trunk sway) and irregular lurching steps, which results in lateral veering and if severe, falling. Impaired tandem stance and gait

Common etiologies
• Midline cerebellar disease or loss of proprioception (sensory ataxia; posterior column of spinal cord, sensory neuronopathy, or neuropathy)

Running (101)
• Characteristics versus walking (Figure 1.8)
• Gait cycle change with increased velocity (decreasing stance phase and increasing swing phase)
  - No double stance phase
    ▪ Judging for race walking (if no double stance → not walking)
    ▪ Stance phase: 60% in walking versus 30% in running and 20% in sprinting

- Overlap of swing phase rather than stance phase
  - Float phase (two float phases)
  - Decreased CG with increased speed
  - Decreased base of support
- Requires more ROM of all lower limb joints, pelvis, and lumbar spine (especially sagittal)
  - Increased GRF with more loading on the joint (knee and hip), increased pelvic rotation (adductor works as hip flexor → can cause overuse)
  - Requires greater eccentric muscle contraction
- Forward momentum from swing leg and arms (rather than stance leg in walking)
- Initial contact varies, depending on speed; location of foot pain may vary

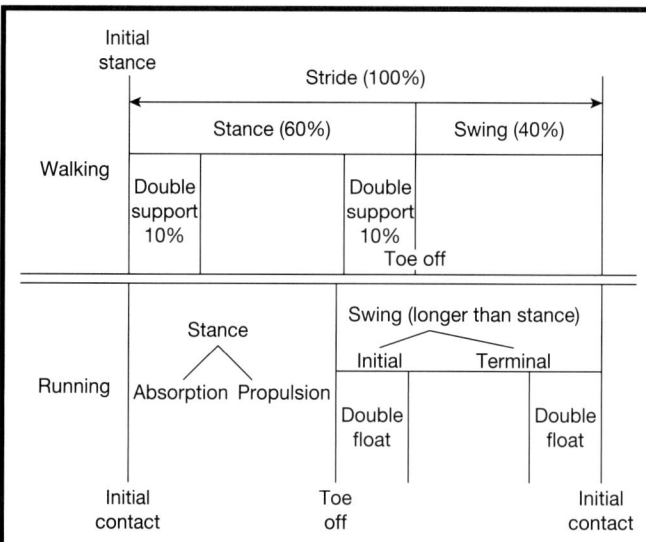

FIGURE 1.8
Gait cycle: walking and running.

Sprinting: no heel contact, >10 mph

Stair Climbing

- 15° or 20° more knee and hip flexion compared with level walking.
- Hip joint load: descending ~2.6 times (×) body weight (BW), ascending ~2.5 × BW, and level walking ~2.4 × BW
- Peak patellofemoral contact force: 8 × level walking

Dominant role of knee during weight acceptance and pull up with supporting roles by the hip and ankle

- Elliptical exercise (EE) compared to level walking (102)
  - Smaller loading at heel strike when compared to level walking and reduced vertical ground reaction force
  - Greater compensatory hip flexor and knee extensor moments (103)

WORKUP

MSK IMAGING (FLOWCHART 1.4)

Indications
- Based on American College of Radiology Appropriateness Criteria, available free online at www.acr.org/Quality-Safety/Appropriateness-Criteria

Acute trauma to shoulder, wrist, hand, hip, knee, ankle, or foot
- Imaging is indicated for high-energy trauma and may be considered in low-energy/minor trauma in specific populations with risk factors (eg, osteoporosis, other metabolic disease, or metastatic disease)
- Specific recommendations/guidelines are available for certain situations
  - For example, Ottawa ankle/knee rule (1): improves sensitivity and decreases overall usage of radiographs

Chronic pain in joints
- May try conservative treatment first if there are no red flags

Suspicion for diseases with significant morbidity ("red flags")
- AVN of the hip
- Ankle fracture
- Stress or insufficiency fracture (including sacrum)
- Osteoporosis
- Primary bone tumors, soft tissue tumors, and metastatic bone disease
- Osteomyelitis versus Charcot neuroarthropathy in patients with DM

Persistent or worsening symptoms after surgery
- Should consult with operating surgeon if available

Neurological symptoms/signs
- Common indications: ataxia, focal neurologic deficits, low back pain with variants, myelopathy, or plexopathy (brachial or LS)
- Start with plain radiographs before getting cross-sectional imaging (MRI)
  - If there are red flags or symptoms progress, immediate workup and timely management are key (eg, suspicion for cauda equina syndrome)
- Suspected spine trauma (cervical or thoracolumbar)
  - Plain radiographs may not suffice → consider CT or MRI

RADIOGRAPHS

Plain Radiographs

- Precautions: test for pregnancy in premenopausal females, and be aware of special radiation reduction protocols for the pediatric population (for more info, see www.imagegently.org)

34   1. Approach to the Patient With a Musculoskeletal Problem

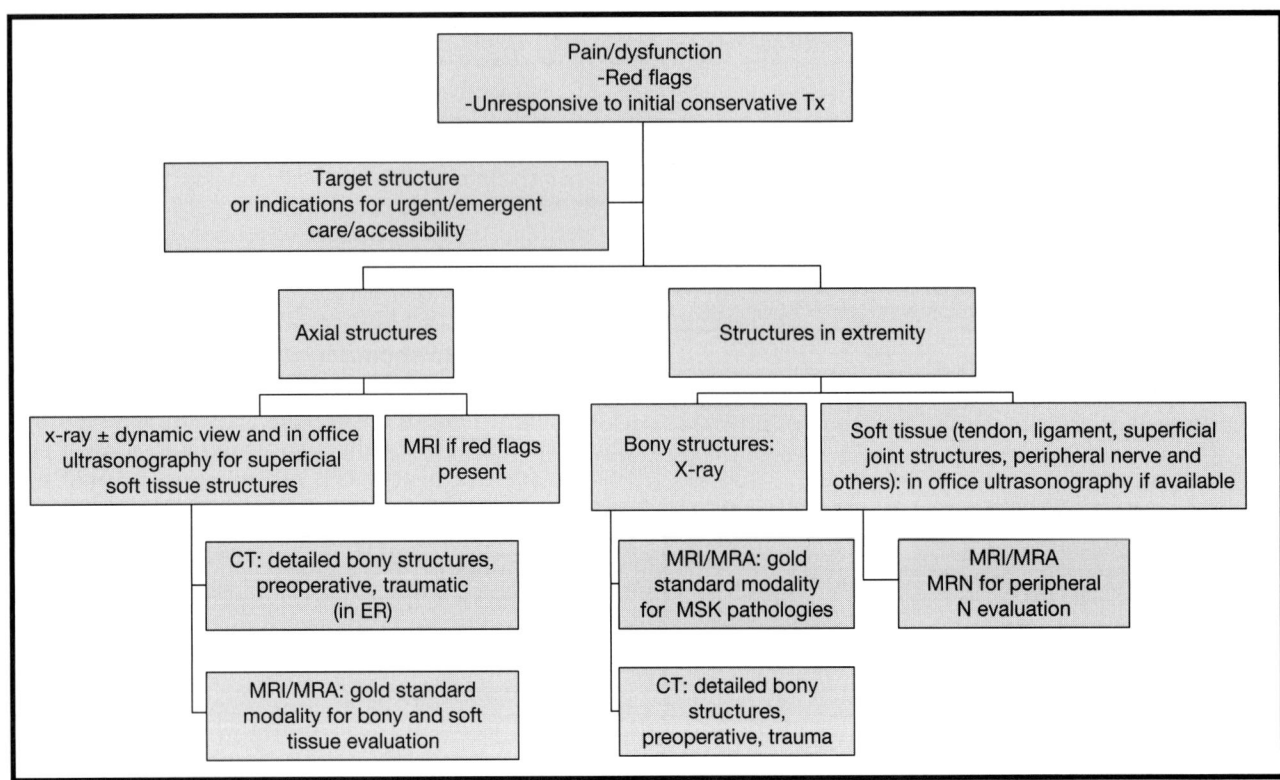

FLOWCHART 1.4
General guidelines for musculoskeletal imaging.

ER, emergency room; MRA, magnetic resonance arthrography; MRN, magnetic resonance neurography; N, nerve; Tx, treatment.

Indications
- Routine plain radiographs (see following table)

REGION	ROUTINE VIEWS	ADDITIONAL VIEWS AND COMMON INDICATIONS
Cervical spine	AP and lateral	Open mouth view: to evaluate C1 and C2 Oblique views: to evaluate facets/uncovertebral joints Flexion/extension views: for suspected instability or ligamentous insufficiency • Indications include Down syndrome, rheumatoid arthritis, etc. • Contraindicated if there is altered MS or a neurologic deficit
Shoulder	Externally rotated, internally rotated, and scapular Y view	Externally rotated view: greater tuberosity is seen in profile Internally rotated view: lesser tuberosity is seen in profile Good for visualizing Hill–Sachs lesions (posterosuperior humeral head impaction Fx) Scapular Y view: to evaluate for subluxation or dislocation (humeral head should project over the "Y" of the glenoid) AP oblique (Grashey) view: to minimize overlap of humeral head and glenoid Supraspinatus outlet view: to evaluate shape of acromion (flat, curved, or hooked)

(continued)

REGION	ROUTINE VIEWS	ADDITIONAL VIEWS AND COMMON INDICATIONS
Elbow	AP and lateral	AP view: look for irregularity along the capitellum, indicating an osteochondritis dissecans Lateral view: look for loose bodies; also look for the "sail sign" (uplifted anterior fat pad), indicating a joint effusion Oblique view: to evaluate olecranon and radial head Gravity stress view: for suspected ligamentous instability
Wrist and hand	PA, lateral, and oblique	Carpal tunnel view: for suspected hook-of-hamate fracture Roberts view (true AP): to evaluate 1st carpometacarpal joint AP view with ulnar deviation: to evaluate for ulnocarpal impaction or scapholunate instability Clenched-fist AP or PA view: to evaluate for scapholunate instability
LS spine	AP and lateral	Oblique views: to evaluate for spondylolysis Flexion/extension views: to evaluate for instability of a spondylolisthesis Coned-down views: may increase sensitivity
SI joints	AP and oblique	Modified Ferguson view: the x-ray beam is angulated cephalad to optimize visualization of the SI joints
Hip	AP (including the pelvis) and frog-leg lateral	Cross-table lateral view: for patients who cannot tolerate frog-leg positioning due to pain or trauma Dunn/modified Dunn view: for suspected cam-type femoroacetabular impingement
Knee	AP (obtained during standing if possible) and lateral	Axilla view (AKA sunrise view): to assess patellofemoral joint Merchant view (AKA modified sunrise view): for suspected patellar tilt or subluxation
Ankle	AP, lateral, and mortise	Mortise view: good for assessing for syndesmosis injury or talar dome abnormality (eg, osteochondritis dissecans); can also see a 5th metatarsal base avulsion Fx
Foot	AP, lateral (standing), and oblique	Harris Beath view: to assess calcaneus and middle facet of subtalar joint (eg, if talocalcaneal coalition is suspected) Broden view: also used to assess subtalar joint Medial oblique view: for lateral structures Lateral oblique view: for medial structures

AKA, also known as; AP, anterior posterior; Fx, fracture; LS, lumbosacral; PA, posterior anterior; SI, sacroiliac.

Stress Radiographs (2)

Indications
- Suspicion for ligamentous laxity or joint instability

Characteristics
- Performed with either manual force or device
- Advantages: quick, convenient, and inexpensive
- Disadvantages: technique (operator)-dependent, limited by individual (patient) variability, and provides only indirect evidence of ligamentous injury, with lack of a gold standard

Common examples
- Cervical and lumbar spine: obtain flexion-extension lateral stress views
- AC joint: obtain views with and without 5-kg weight (normal AC distance: <8 mm)
- Elbow: assess for valgus instability by measuring ulnohumeral distance with and without Telos stress device
- Wrist: obtain clenched-fist AP view to assess interosseous membrane integrity in setting of distal radioulnar joint injury, to assess integrity of first MCP joint ulnar collateral ligament, and to assess for scapholunate instability
- Pelvis: assess for instability with single leg stand; use push–pull (push on one extremity while pulling on the contralateral extremity) to assess for vertical instability
- Hip joint: use stress views to assess for instability in setting of acetabular fracture or impingement
- Knee: assess for patellofemoral instability by applying valgus/external rotation stress with/without quad contracture or by pushing patella medially–laterally; can also use stress views to assess posterior cruciate ligament and medial collateral ligament
- Ankle: widening of medial joint space or syndesmosis with external rotation force may indicate syndesmosis injury
- Foot: weight-bearing views with abduction–adduction of the forefoot to assess for Lisfranc joint instability

X-ray findings in common musculoskeletal disorders (3)

MSK DISORDER	RADIOLOGIC FINDINGS
Osteoarthritis (OA)	Joint space narrowing (best assessed with weightbearing x-rays of the weightbearing joints), osteophytes, subchondral sclerosis and cystic change
Rheumatoid arthritis	Juxtaarticular osteopenia, periarticular soft tissue swelling, marginal erosions, joint space narrowing, and subluxation
Gout	Juxtaarticular erosions with a "punched-out" appearance, sclerotic borders, and overhanging edges
Calcium crystal deposition disease (CPPD)	Calcium crystal deposition in the soft tissues (cartilage, menisci, etc) Joint space narrowing, osteophytes, and subchondral cysts in a distribution that is not typical for osteoarthritis (eg, CPPD frequently affects the MCP joints, whereas OA rarely does)
Psoriatic arthritis	Pencil-in-cup deformity (expansion of the base of the distal phalanx with destruction of the head of the middle phalanx), acroosteolysis, and whole-digit soft tissue swelling ("sausage digit")
Lupus arthropathy	Joint subluxations without erosions, joint space narrowing, or other articular cartilage involvement
Septic arthropathy	Initially: imaging may be normal, or there may be periarticular soft tissue swelling and/or joint space widening with effusion With progression: joint space narrowing, poorly defined erosions, and marginal erosions as uncovered intracapsular bone is destroyed Osteomyelitis: focal osteopenia, periosteal reaction, bone destruction, and sequestrum formation
Neuropathic joint	Initially: imaging may be normal With progression (which can be very rapid): severe cartilage loss, fragmentation of subchondral bone with pathologic fracture → disintegration of joint structure and juxtaarticular cortical bone loss ("4 Ds": destruction, density, debris, and dislocation)

MCP, metacarpophalangeal.

ADVANCED IMAGING

US versus MRI in MSK conditions (3)

	US	MRI
Indications	Evaluate soft tissues (superficial structures particularly) Assess for synovitis in inflamed joints, bursae, and tendon sheaths (look for effusions and synovial thickening on grayscale images, synovial hyperemia on Doppler images) Monitor response of synovitis to treatment	Gold standard MSK imaging modality for inflammatory, infectious, and destructive Dz Assess all structures in arthritic diseases, including intra-articular structures and subchondral cysts/edema (4) Monitor treatment efficacy (not common/practical due to high cost and limited availability)
Advantages	Easy accessibility (in office) Dynamic assessment Better spatial resolution: 0.2–0.4 mm (5–13 Hz) in superficial structures Imaging guidance for diagnostic/therapeutic steroid injections/blocks to joints, bursae, and tendon sheaths	Can assist in formulating a more complete differential diagnosis Can assess disease activity in clinically difficult cases or joints Has potential for prognostication under different therapeutic regimens
Disadvantages	Technical limitations (not all joint areas are accessible to the ultrasound beam) Operator dependence	Potential for allergic reaction to contrast and nephrogenic systemic fibrosis in renal patients Higher cost/lower availability Longer examination times → a few joints per session

Dz, disease; MSK, musculoskeletal; US, ultrasound.

CT versus MRI in MSK conditions (5)

	CT	MRI
Advantages	Rapid acquisition time Less sensitive to motion than MRI Superior osseous images: better detection of calcification and ossification Less artifact from metallic foreign bodies or prostheses than MRI Good patient tolerance	Anatomic and pathologic information (proton density, T1, T2, chemical shift) Better tissue contrast than CT Direct multiplanar imaging No ionizing radiation
Disadvantages	Anatomic information predominantly; less pathologic information than with MRI Ionizing radiation Limited imaging planes (but reconstructions can be made in any plane using reconstruction software)	Longer acquisition time than CT More sensitive to motion than CT Lower resolution for cortical bone or calcification than CT Considerable signal loss from metallic foreign bodies or prostheses Some problems with claustrophobia, although lessened with large-bore or open MRI scanners

Computed Tomography

- Superior to MRI in delineating the frequently encountered anatomical deformities, structural bone damage, sequestra, or bone callus formation
- Preoperative planning with 3D reconstructions

Indications

- Suspected fracture (cervical spine fracture, sternoclavicular fracture/dislocation, pelvic fracture, etc) in acute trauma or ER setting
- Chronic back pain after instrumentation (if MRI is contraindicated); subtle fracture (pars fracture)
- Suspected hematoma in patients on anticoagulation (eg, CT pelvis for evaluation of femoral neuropathy with mild right thigh/hip weakness)

CT myelogram

- When MRI is contraindicated or limited by artifacts
- To evaluate the bony neural foramina and spondylosis (best seen on axial CT images and sagittal reformations)
  - Can evaluate intraforaminal or far lateral disc abnormalities

Common artifacts

- Streak artifact: occurs at interfaces between tissues of very different attenuation: for example, linear streaks around metal prostheses
- Other artifacts: ring, metal, and out of field artifact

Magnetic Resonance Imaging

- Gold standard in MSK imaging despite issues with accessibility and, infrequently, patient's inability to tolerate MRI (6)

Indications (7)

- Characterize and assess the extent of a lesion
- Evaluate a mass (soft tissue mass or bony mass) or intra-articular/intracortical lesion
- Surgical planning

Contraindications and adverse effects

- Some (but not all) metallic objects, pacemakers, hearing aids, and spinal cord stimulators (check with the manufacturer), ferromagnetic foreign bodies in the eyes
  - More MRI-compatible implants are being manufactured over time
- Claustrophobia (open MRI is available, but its downside is lower resolution/image quality)
  - May need anxiolytics (alprazolam or lorazepam)
- Nephrogenic systemic fibrosis with gadolinium contrast (very rare)
  - Risk in patient with renal insufficiency
  - Gadolinium is contraindicated if GFR <30 mL/min/1.73 m^2
  - If GFR is between 30 and 60, then a half dose of gadolinium may be considered, and IV fluid before contrast administration may also be helpful
  - Cardinal features: thickening and hardening of the skin in the trunk and extremities, marked expansion, and fibrosis of the dermis associated with CD34-positive fibrocytes.
    - Systemic fibrosis can involve muscle, fascia, lung, and heart

Basic MRI principles

- Images are produced by energy emitted by tissues and liquids (eg, fat, muscle, spinal cord, edema, cerebrospinal fluid [CSF]) after stimulation of their protons by radiofrequency (RF) waves in the presence of a magnetic field
- Determinants of signal intensity (brightness)
  - Different sequence techniques (T1-weighted, T2-weighted, etc)
  - T1 and T2 characteristics of tissue: intrinsic properties of the proton molecular environment in tissue or fluid
  - The proton density of the tissue
- Spin echo images: produced by repetitive use of a 90° excitation pulse along with a refocusing pulse. Of importance is the amount of time allowed the excited spins to relax (TR) and the length of time between the excitation and refocusing pulse (TE)

	ADVANTAGES	HIGH SIGNAL (BRIGHT)	LOW SIGNAL (DARK)
T1 weighted– short TR and short TE	Good anatomic detail Detection of fat or subacute hemorrhage Gd-DTPA (contrast) enhancement (with fat saturation) Detection of marrow pathology	Adipose tissue (short T1, long T2) Gd-DTPA (contrast) Some stages of hemorrhage (eg, subacute hemorrhage in the brain) Melanin	Air Calcification Some tumors Some stages of hemorrhage (eg, acute or chronic hemorrhage in the brain)
T2 weighted– long TR and long TE	Detection of fluid and many pathologic processes (because many pathologic processes are associated with edema)	Edema (ie, water; long T1 and long T2), as in inflammation or infection Many tumors Subacute blood (methemoglobin)	Air Calcification Fibrous tissue Hemosiderin Flow voids (ie, fast-flowing blood in vessels) Proteinaceous fluid

Gd-DTPA, gadolinium-diethylenetriamine pentaacetic acid; TE, the length of time between the excitation and refocusing pulse; TR, amount of time allowed for the excited spins to relax.

Tissue signal intensity (5,8)

TISSUE	T1-WEIGHTED IMAGE	T2-WEIGHTED IMAGE
Fat	High	Low
Cortical bone/fibrocartilage	Low	Low
Fatty bone marrow	High	Low
Red bone marrow	Intermediate	Intermediate
Muscle	Low to intermediate	Low to intermediate
Tendon/ligament/meniscus	Low	Low
Fluid	Low	High
Rapidly flowing blood within vessels	Low	Low
Subacute hemorrhage (3–7 days)[a]	High	High
Chronic hemorrhage (>14 days)[a]	Low	Low
Intervertebral disc (normal)	Low	High
Desiccated disc	Low	Low

[a]Determining the age of a hemorrhage is an imprecise process, especially in musculoskeletal (MSK) imaging; these guidelines are relatively accurate for determining the age of a brain hemorrhage, but have limited accuracy in determining the age of a hemorrhage in the soft tissues.

Commonly used MRI sequences (8)

MRI SEQUENCES	COMMENT
STIR	A fat suppression technique that is relatively invulnerable to metal artifact when compared with other fat suppression techniques Better evaluation of marrow and soft tissue pathology Denervated skeletal muscle, being high in extracellular water content, looks bright on STIR as on T2-weighted images

Postcontrast	Pinpoints areas with increased vascular permeability (eg, areas with inflammation) or areas with impairment of the blood–brain/nerve barrier
	• Can help distinguish postoperative scar versus residual disc extrusion
	• In the setting of infection, can be used to evaluate for abscesses and sinus tracts and to distinguish viable versus nonviable (necrotic) tissue
	• Mass evaluation
	  ○ Can help distinguish cystic versus solid, viable tumor versus necrosis
	  ○ Pitfall: fibrovascular tissue in organizing hematomas may show enhancement
	  ○ Contrast enhances the signal intensity of well vascularized or edematous tissues on T1-weighted images, enhancing the demarcation between tumor and muscle, or between tumor and edema
	• Multiple sclerosis (in 4–6 weeks) and neurosarcoidosis

MR arthrography	Distention of a joint with a solution containing dilute Gd-DTPA Common applications • Evaluation of labral tears in the shoulder and hip • Evaluation of meniscal tear (contrast extends into the tear) versus healed meniscal scar in patients with a history of prior surgery Exam must include T1W images, with fat saturation so that Gd-DTPA can be distinguished from fat (eg, in the subacromial/subdeltoid bursa in the shoulder) A T2W sequence in at least one plane is also necessary to detect edema, cysts, and other T2-sensitive abnormalities in the soft tissues or marrow
DTI	Underlying principle: water molecules in white matter nerve tracts have *anisotropic* diffusion properties (ie a preferred orientation of movement), as opposed to *isotropic* diffusion (equal preference for movement in all directions) in surrounding tissues Used to evaluate brain or spinal cord intrinsic lesions
MR myelography	Noninvasive method for evaluating intraspinal structures that does not require contrast Advantages: relatively short acquisition time, comparable to CT myelography and conventional myelography in demonstrating damage to intraspinal structures Disadvantages: artifacts; difficulty in determining the exact level of injury, because no bony landmarks are included
MR neurography	Distinguishes nerve fibers from surrounding structures, and the various structures within the perineurium from each other Common applications • Neoplasm (both primary and secondary), radiation fibrosis, vascular abnormalities, and swelling of the nerve trunks in the posterior triangle of the neck following trauma • Traumatic nerve injury (9) • The optimal neuroimaging study for assessing all portions of the BP

BP, blood pressure; DTI, Diffusion tensor imaging; Gd-DTPA, gadolinium-diethylenetriamine pentaacetic acid; STIR, short-time (tau) inversion recovery sequences.

Common artifacts
- Magic angle artifact: hyperintense signal in tightly bound collagen at 54.7° to the main magnetic field (on coronal and oblique T2W sequences), which may be mistaken for tendinopathy or tear
  - Can cause signal change in the rotator cuff tendon, peroneal tendon, etc
- Motion and metal artifact (reduced in T2 fast spin echo technique): distortion of image
- Others: black boundary artifact at muscle-fat interfaces (often called "India ink artifact"), chemical shift artifact, dielectric effect artifact, etc

Common MRI findings

TISSUE	T1-WEIGHTED IMAGES	T2-WEIGHTED IMAGES
Tendinopathy/ligament sprain	Intermediate	Intermediate
Torn tendon/ligament	Intermediate	High
Calcification	Variable	Variable
Edema	Low	High
Fracture	Linear band of low signal	Surrounding area will demonstrate high signal compatible with edema
Bone metastasis Lytic	Low	Intermediate to high
Sclerotic	Low	Low
Cyst; simple – complex	Low, intermediate, or high	High
Abscess	Low	High
Degenerated	Intermediate to low	Low

MSK tumors
Benign versus malignant tumor
- MRI findings are often nonspecific and can be misleading, so clinical correlation is important, and a further confirmatory test (like biopsy) may be required

BENIGN	MALIGNANT
Smooth, well-defined margins, small size, and homogeneous signal intensity, particularly on T2-weighted images	Larger (eg, >5 cm) and more likely to outgrow their vascular supply, with subsequent infarction and necrosis, presenting as heterogeneous signal intensity on T2W images
	Deep (rather than superficial) with centripetal growth and surrounding edema, which manifests as increased T2 intensity in skeletal muscle surrounding the mass
	Bone or neurovascular involvement

MRI findings in tumors
- The majority are nonspecific, but the following characteristics are specific (10):

CLASSIFICATION	COMMON TUMORS	CHARACTERISTICS OF COMMON TUMORS
Vascular lesion	Hemangioma Hemangiomatosis (angiomatosis) AV malformation Lymphatic malformation	AV malformation in the spine • High signal on T1W images (because of fat content) different from nonhemorrhagic metastases: low signal, similar to or lower than hematopoietic marrow • Soft-tissue extension and spinal cord compression
Bone and cartilage forming lesions	Myositis ossificans Panniculitis ossificans	Myositis ossificans • Initially, edema-type change in the muscle. Cortical bone developing around the edges of the lesion is of low-signal intensity on all sequences. • In mature lesions, the center of the area becomes filled with bone trabeculae surrounded by fatty bone marrow
Fibrous lesions	Superficial fibromatosis (plantar fibromatosis/ Dupuytren's contracture) Elastofibroma Musculoaponeurotic fibromatosis (desmoid tumor)	Fibrous tumors • Elongated spindle cells (fibroblasts) with varying amounts of collagen • Relatively hypointense on all MRI sequences • Enhancement can be limited because of the relatively hypovascular nature of the tumor • Proton density image: best demonstrate the lesion • MRI frequently underestimates the full extent
Lipomatous lesions	Lipoma Lipomatosis Hibernoma Intramuscular lipoma Neural fibrolipoma Lipoblastoma Lipoblastomatosis Liposarcoma Parosteal lipoma	Lipoma • When encapsulated, MRI can delineate a surrounding fibrous capsule of low-signal intensity on all sequences • Thickened septa or nodular nonfatty components suggest a well-differentiated liposarcoma • Intermuscular lipomas may have a dumbbell shape; intramuscular and well-differentiated liposarcoma are often spherical masses

(continued)

CLASSIFICATION	COMMON TUMORS	CHARACTERISTICS OF COMMON TUMORS
Peripheral nerve lesions	Neurofibroma and schwannoma MPNST	Malignant nerve sheath tumor • Characteristic features include large size, heterogeneity, perilesional edema, and intratumoral necrosis (which manifests as an irregular/nodular peripheral enhancement pattern)
Synovial lesions	Pigmented villonodular synovitis Giant cell tumor of tendon sheath Synovial chondromatosis Synovial cyst	Pigmented villonodular synovitis • A nodular lesion with areas of hemosiderin (low signal on all sequences) and hemorrhage (low signal with "blooming" on GRE sequences). Joint effusions and bony erosions are well demonstrated. • Contrast enhancement • The differential diagnosis: haemophilia and synovial hemangioma (rare, characterized by phleboliths in soft tissue)
Tumor-like lesions	Aneurysm Abscess Bursitis Calcific myonecrosis Diabetic muscle infarction Ganglion Hematoma Myxoma Pseudoaneurysm	

AV, arteriovenous; GRE, gradient echo sequence; MPNST, malignant peripheral nerve sheath tumor.

Dual-Energy X-Ray Absorptiometry

Indications
- Different guidelines available (eg, National Osteoporosis Foundation guidelines)
- Women ≥65 years and men ≥70 years, regardless of clinical risk factors
- Younger postmenopausal women, women in the menopausal transition, and men aged 50 to 69 years with clinical risk factors for fracture
- Adults with a fracture after the age of 50 years
- Adults with a condition (eg, rheumatoid arthritis) or taking a medication (eg, glucocorticoids in a daily dose ≥5 mg prednisone or equivalent for ≥3 months) associated with low bone mass or bone loss

Measurement of bone density (BMD)
- Lumbar spine: measure BMD from L2 to L4 and compile the scores
- Hip: measure BMD from femoral neck, trochanter, and intertrochanteric region and compile the scores
- The same dual-energy x-ray absorptiometry (DEXA) instrument should be used for serial BMD testing whenever possible

Interpretation

	DEFINITION
T score	BMD relative to normal young matched controls (25 years old)
Z score	BMD relative to similar-aged patients For premenopausal women, men younger than age 50 years, or children
Osteopenia	L2–L4 lumbar density of 1–2.5 standard deviations below the peak bone mass of a 25-year-old individual (T score: −1 to −2.5)
Osteoporosis	L2–L4 lumbar density > 2.5 standard deviations below the peak bone mass of a 25-year-old individual (T score < −2.5)

BMD, bone density.

- Different guidelines using different anatomic regions for osteoporosis
  - The WHO for the femoral neck. Other recommends to use the lowest T score of the lumbar spine (L1–L4), total proximal femur, femoral neck, or one-third radius

Point-of-Care (POC) Ultrasonography

- Ultrasonography performed and interpreted by the clinician at bedside (11)
- Common utility by clinicians
  - Guidance for injection, diagnostic, and screening (eg, thyroid mass)

Indications (12)
- Soft tissue with/without concomitant bone (not the primary modality) injury
- Tendon or ligament (not intra-articular) pathology
- Joint complex: arthritis, synovitis, or crystal deposition disease, intra-articular bodies, or joint effusion
- Nerve entrapment, injury, neuropathy, masses, or subluxation; superficial nerves particularly
- Evaluation of soft tissue masses, swelling, or fluid collections
- Detection of foreign bodies in the superficial soft tissues
- Planning and guiding an injection in deeper structures or obese patients
- Imaging guidance for high-risk procedure
  - Nerve (trunk) block; especially proximal nerve or deeply located nerve
  - Injecting a biologic (viscosupplementation, platelet rich plasma or stem cell)
  - Soft tissue lesion, and evaluate anatomic variations and pathology
- Postoperative or postprocedural evaluation.

Limitations
- Inability to evaluate intra-articular or intracortical structure
- Subtle pathology without gross structural change: no equivalent of tissue edema or contrast enhancement for infection or tumor
- Depth of the tissue (decreased resolution for deeper structures)
- Tattoo or foreign body: no visualization underneath because of postacoustic shadowing

Challenges
- Limited field of view (microscopic or narrow): difficult identifying the structure without the knowledge of area of scanning.
  - Identify the lesion of interest by physical examination then scan the area of interest (unlike x-ray to give the general anatomic view) and scan based on protocol (same order)
- Variability between manufacturers; difference in gray scale and resolution
- Operator dependence with steep learning curve (especially in diagnostic scanning)

Basic procedure/knobology (13)
- Choose transducer (linear transducer for most MSK pathologies versus hockey stick for superficial structures in foot and hand versus curvilinear [not commonly used, for deeper structure])
- Adjust the frequency depending on the depth of the structure: 8 to 13 Hz for most MSK structures
  - Higher frequency → lower penetration (less optimal for the deeper structure) with better axial resolution
- Position patient: make scanning structures taut
  - Can press the soft tissue gently; however, it may affect the measurement of soft tissue or superficial bursitis (with effusion), can be collapsed
- Orient the probe: left and right or proximal/distal (mirror like image preferred: left side of the probe points left side of the screen)
- Adjust the depth/focus zone (hardware specific, some manufacturers have automatic focus function)
  - Focus: narrowest band of the US beam affecting lateral resolution
  - Adjust gain: brightness (most machine has auto gain function)
- Follow protocol for scanning: The American Institute of Ultrasound in Medicine (AIUM) guideline and dynamic maneuver if necessary
- Scan contralateral side for comparison

Basic interpretation: echogenicity (brightness)
- Mechanisms for hyperechogenicity; the extent of US reflection
  - Sound waves reflects at boundary between two media difference of acoustic impedance (AI) of the two tissues at the interface; makes echogenicity (more reflection)
    - AI: the resistance of a tissue to passage of US wave
      - Increased AI mismatch → increased return of US wave to the probe: hyperechoic
    - Example: hyperechoic in border of air–skin (unless using gel to decrease AI mismatch between skin and air) and muscle–bone (hyperechoic with most beams reflected with postacoustic shadowing)

BODY TISSUE	ACOUSTIC IMPEDANCE (106 RAYLS)	SPEED (M/SEC)
Air	0.0004	331
Fat	1.34	1,450
Liver	1.65	1,570
Blood	1.65	1,570
Muscle	1.71	
Bone	7.8	4,080

  - Angle of incidence; angle between the structure and US beam; anisotropy effect (hypoechoic if the angle of incidence is not 90° because the beam does not return to the probe)
  - Tissue interaction
    - Specular reflection: flat, smooth interface, for example, bone, diaphragm, and gallstone: strong specular reflection
    - Diffuse reflection: weaker, for example, scattering
- Hyper (bright), iso, hypo, and anechoic (dark) depending on the brightness

ECHOGENICITY	NOTE
Anechoic	No reflection of US beam, fluid and blood-filled structures (beam passes easily) • Vein: easily collapsed by compression
Hypoechoic	Solid organ, muscle
Hyperechoic	Strong specular reflection, diaphragm, gallstone, bone, pericardium

US, ultrasound.

STRUCTURES	ECHOGENICITY	NOTE
Dermis	Echogenic	
Subcutaneous fat	Hypoechoic Hypoechoic with irregular hyperechoic lines	Lipoma: similar echogenicity to the adjacent fat, hypovascular, homogeneous
Nerve	Hyperechoic/hypoechoic (nerve fascicle)	Honeycomb appearance in short axis Long axis view: continuous hypoechoic elements with hyperechoic perineural connective tissues

(continued)

STRUCTURES	ECHOGENICITY	NOTE
Tendon	Predominantly hyperechoic (can be hypoechoic because of anisotropy)	Short axis: "broomstick" appearance Long axis view: fibrillar echotexture with discontinuous hyperechoic speckles In normal conditions, color and power Doppler does not detect flow signals inside tendons because of the small vessel size and slow flow
Muscle	Hypoechoic outline with short streaks of hyperechoic lines; the outline of a muscle layer (the fascial sheath; hyperechoic) "starry night" in short axis	Hyperechoic lines (in normal muscle) • Epimysium, perimysium (inside the muscle), internal aponeurosis (thicker than perimysium/fibroadipose septa) Atrophy and muscle pathology Increased echogenicity (because of fatty infiltration; can be compared with neighboring muscle of different innervation or contralateral asymptomatic side) and decreased size
Bone	Hyperechoic lines with a hypoechoic shadow	Reverberation effect (with mirror image)

Common artifacts (14)

COMMON ARTIFACTS	CHARACTERISTICS
Posterior acoustic enhancement artifact	Deep to the fluid-filled structure → hyperechoic region (contrast effect) May not detect if fluid is small or spread over a large area For example, ganglion cyst and peripheral nerve sheath tumor
Acoustic shadow artifact	Hypoechoic bone shadow deep to bone outline: gas (high absorption), bone surface (high reflection) or calcification For example, calcific tendinopathy (sometimes no shadowing in soft or small calcification by partial volume artifact) Partial volume artifact: when the ultrasound beam is wider than the scanned structure or the structure itself is just partially sectioned so that it is surrounded by tissues with different acoustic impedance Lateral (edge) shadowing: occurs at the edge of structure (especially round), foreign body, torn Achilles or patellar tendon by combination of refraction/reflection when the ultrasound beam is tangential to tissues with different acoustic impedance
Reverberation artifact	The reflection of the ultrasound beam several times back and forth between two nearby interfaces For example, needle injection or foreign body (woodstick) • Mirror artifact: duplication of the image occurring when the beam meets a highly reflective interface causing reflection and reverberation phenomena • Rain effect artifact: a reverberation artifact because of the gain curve. When soft tissue overlies a fluid collection. Can be mistaken as complex effusion
Anisotropy	Changes in echogenicity depending on the angle of incidence (the US beam) Hyperechoic when perpendicular to the surface of the tendons, and easily hypoechoic if the transducer is slightly tilted, because of the resulting oblique incident angle of the beam Common in short axis scanning of tendon
Refraction artifact	Refraction: a change in the direction of sound transmission after hitting an interface of two tissues with different speeds of sound transmission Incorrect localization of a structure on US image; for example, duplication of aorta or kidney with refraction artifact during scanning through the midline abdomen

US, ultrasound.

Common US findings

COMMON PATHOLOGY	FINDINGS
Tendinosis	Diffuse increase in thickness; useful to compare the contralateral asymptomatic side Heterogenous hypoechogenicity Accompanying findings • Diffuse wall thickening of neighboring bursa or paratendon • Increased vascularity, rounded, and irregular border
Partial tear	A hypoechoic/anechoic area located inside the tendon or at its bursal or articular aspect that is manifested in two perpendicular planes or as a mixed hypo-hyperechoic area Located at the level of the critical area—less sensitive in partial tear
Complete tear	Anechoic/hypoechoic gap with muscle/tendon retraction (more on contraction), and hematoma (mixed echogenicity or hypoechoic later in the periphery, as it resolves) • False negative: synovial tissue and debris mimicking intact tendon in complete tendon tear/rupture

(continued)

COMMON PATHOLOGY	FINDINGS
	○ Check with the longitudinal view (absent fibrillar pattern) and compression (compressible in tear with debris, hematoma, or granulation tissue)
Bursitis	Bursal thickening with/without effusion Septic bursitis: hyperechoic foci of gas with comet tail artifacts within a mixed hypoechoic and isoechogenic
Ganglion	Well-defined anechoic structure with posterior acoustic enhancement
Erosive arthritis	Defect in the echogenic subchondral plate with accompanying synovitis Cautious of pseudoerosion in metacarpal head (notch seen normally) (15)
Osteoarthritis	Periarticular osteophyte/cortical irregularity, narrowed joint space, and effusion (16) Simple effusion: anechoic
Rheumatoid arthritis (104)	Synovitis (effusion with increased vascularity), tenosynovitis (increased tendon thickness with tenosynovial effusion and increased vascularity), bursitis, bony changes (erosion and cartilage thinning)
Entrapment neuropathy	Hypoechogenic enlargement of nerve (entrapped site or immediately proximal) (105)
Neuroma	Oval-shaped hypoechoic enlargement (loss of normal architecture) with reproduction of symptoms in sonopalpation

Joint effusion evaluation

EFFUSION	US FINDINGS AND DIFFERENTIAL DIAGNOSES
Simple	Anechoic

Heterogeneous	Nonhomogeneous echogenicity of fluid and/or echogenic spots
	• Protein-containing materials, cartilage fragments, crystal aggregates, and calcified loose bodies or after injection
	• Recurrent effusion: fine particulate debris floating in the synovial fluid, long-standing or recurrent effusion
	• Infectious or hemorrhage
	Complex effusion: joint recess compressible, redistribution/motion of joint recess, Doppler: not increased.
	Synovitis and synovial proliferation
	• Synovial pannus (inflammatory arthropathy, eg, RA)
	  ○ Hypervascular (active) from hypovascular (inactive) pannus (Doppler)
	  ○ Monitor the response to therapy based on a decreased hyperemia by Doppler although varies in each Dz
	• Noninflammatory synovial proliferative disorders
	  ○ Pigmented villonodular synovitis

(continued)

EFFUSION	US FINDINGS AND DIFFERENTIAL DIAGNOSES
	○ Synovial osteochondromatosis (hyperechoic and possible shadowing similar to intra-articular body) Rice body • Release of subset of loose bodies: difficulty to distinguish from hypertrophied synovium • Characteristic of rheumatoid arthritis

Dz, disease; RA, rheumatoid arthritis.

Soft tissue mass evaluation

- Limited role: distinguish solid versus cystic mass and vascular versus nonvascular
  ○ Often difficult to distinguish soft tissue hematoma versus other mass
- Solid mass
  ○ Differential diagnosis with complex effusion: increased vascularity in Doppler favoring tumor
  ○ Examples
    ▪ Lymphoma: heterogeneous, predominantly hypoechoic, with possible increased through transmission
    ▪ Hemangioma: variable and heterogeneous appearance, ranging from hypoechoic to hyperechoic, infiltrating the involved soft tissue
- Common subcutaneous mass (21)
  ○ Lipoma: elongated isoechoic or echogenic mass commonly in the subcutaneous tissues (±striated echoes inside the mass)
  ○ Ganglion cyst: anechoic amorphous mass with relatively sharp borders and protrusion towards the joint
  ○ Epidermal cyst: round to oval structure along with post acoustic enhancement and lateral shadowing, central hypo/anechoic lesion owing to their contents as well as partial indentation to the dermis
  ○ Tumor
    ▪ Benign tumors; rather echogenic versus metastatic lesion (eg, melanoma); anechoic spherical lesion often with posterior acoustic attenuation with partial or even extensive vascularization
- Lymph node: oval shape with an echogenic (interfaces between the fatty tissue and sinusoids) central hilum and hypoechoic rim
  ○ Anterior cervical node: commonly encountered during anterior neck scanning
    ▪ Enlarged with infection (mononucleosis, URI, etc), malignancy (squamous cell cancer of head and neck, lymphoma and leukemia, etc)
  ○ Epitrochlear lymph node in the medial elbow: lymphoma, sarcoidosis, reactive inflammation from distal infection or inflammation, and cat scratch disease (22)
  ○ Inguinal lymph nodes (horizontal and vertical node groups): up to 1 to 2 cm in diameter in many healthy adults
    ▪ Benign reactive and infection (MC cause for lymphadenopathy) and possibly cancer (lymphomas, penile, vulvar, testicular cancer, etc)
  ○ Malignancy: absence of the echogenic hilum, thickening of the hypoechoic cortex and a peripheral or mixed pattern of vascularity on Doppler
- Foreign body

○ Glass: hyperechoic foreign body fragments with a hypoechoic halo and posterior reverberation
○ Metal: hyperechoic metal with various degree of posterior reverberation artifact and heterogeneous shadowing

Bony evaluation
- X-ray, CT, and MRI are better imaging modality. Cortical bone can be evaluated while evaluating the soft tissue not as a primary imaging modality for bony pathologies
  ○ Order x-ray for gross bony anatomic view
  ○ More sensitive in early stress fracture and detection of small osteophyte and avulsion fracture
- US findings of bony pathologies
  ○ Fracture: step off with hyperechoic callus formation (on healing) and hypoechoic soft tissue swelling
    ▪ Fracture nonunion in instrumentation: if hyperechoic nail/foreign body (with reverberation artifact) seen, indicating no overlying callus formation
  ○ Exostosis (Osgood–Schlatter syndrome in tibial tuberosity, Haglund deformity in posterior calcaneal tuberosity)
    ▪ Irregular hyperechoic bony formation with/without postacoustic shadowing
  ○ Osteomyelitis: cortical irregularity (bone destruction) and hypoechoic abscess and cortical destruction with adjacent hypoechoic soft tissue swelling; MRI if suspicious
  ○ Evaluation of hardware with neighboring structures (irritating tendon ± bursitis irritated by hardware)

Muscle evaluation
- US findings of common muscle injury (23)
  ○ Muscle contusion (extrinsic injury): focal isoechoic muscle swelling (often difficult to identify) with hematoma (both hypo and hyperechoic)
  ○ Strain/tear (intrinsic): disruption of pennate pattern or internal aponeurosis with hematoma, discontinuity of the perimysium at the myotendinous or myofascial junctions
  ○ Myositis: increased echogenicity (also in denervated muscle from other etiologies) with decreased volume with atrophy
  ○ Muscle infarct: rare, thigh (MC location) and DM (MC etiology)
    ▪ Hypoechoic and swollen lesion with hyperechoic fibroadipose septum and epimysium throughout (can distinguish soft tissue abscess with no fibroadipose septum) ± subfascial fluid

Peripheral nerve disorder evaluation (24)
- US of entrapment neuropathy (25)
  ○ Focal nerve enlargement (fusiform) just proximal to the site of entrapment
  ○ Typical findings (MC used criteria): cross sectional area ≥2 standard deviation above the mean reference value or 1.5 to 2 times or greater than unaffected portion of the same nerve in the same site
  ○ Other supporting findings: change in echotexture (hypoechoic), shape (flattening and pinching at the site of entrapment), fascicle size and vascularity, and change (decrease) in mobility
- US of traumatic neuropathy (26)
  ○ Supplementary tool to the neurophysiologic study
    ▪ Assessment of nerve continuity/discontinuity (axonotmesis vs neurotmesis)
    ▪ Especially where the NCS is limited (eg, proximal nerve lesion or in multiple sites of injury)
  ○ Identify etiology (bone fragments, hardware, and others) of nerve injury
- US of nerve sheath tumor (schwannoma, neurofibroma, and malignant peripheral nerve sheath tumors) evaluation
  ○ Indicated in atypical presentation of localized/regional neuropathy or screening tool before MR neurography
  ○ Schwannoma: predominantly hypoechoic with internal homogeneous echoes with increased through transmission
- US versus MRI
  ○ If the lesion is identified by bedside MSK US, then additional diagnostic information or tissue characterization may not be required
  ○ MRI/magnetic resonance neurography (MRN) indicated if the nerve of interest is not visualized or a lesion is not identified, or if additional information (other structures), tissue characterization, or preoperative planning is needed

	ULTRASOUND	MRI/MR NEUROGRAPHY (27)
Advantage	Immediately available	Better evaluation of surrounding structure Tissue signal change, enhancing lesion for infection or tumor infiltration (indicative of disruption of blood nerve barrier) Can evaluate fascicular pattern
Disadvantage	Deeper structure, limited evaluation of surrounding structure (bony, intra-articular), tissue edema, etc	Accessibility, dynamic view Smaller sized nerve (2–3 mm) evaluation
Normal nerve finding	Honeycomb appearance Less anisotropic than tendon	Isointense to skeletal muscle in T1/2 weighted image Fascicular appearance: nonbranching, relatively straight course in most parts, and lack of flow voids (signal loss).
Abnormal nerve	Increased cross-sectional area ± increased vascularity on color-Doppler US Qualitative changes in echogenicity, hyperemia, mobility, and fascicular pattern	Focal or diffuse enlargement • Larger than the adjacent artery Loss of fascicular pattern T2 hyperintensity (becoming similar to adjacent veins) Asymmetric hyperintensity Perineural strand/disruption of fat plane Enhancement in infection or tumors

US, ultrasound

SCANNING PROTOCOL, MODIFIED FROM AIUM PROTOCOL (12)

Shoulder

Two views (long and short axis) for each structure required

SHOULDER		
REGION	**POSITION**	**TARGET STRUCTURES TO SCAN**
Anterior	Forearm supination	Biceps long head, tendon/tenosynovium (Figure 1.9) Subscapularis T, subcoracoid bursa Dynamic maneuver with external/internal rotation for biceps subluxation/dislocation and subcoracoid impingement
Lateral	Crass position (internal rotation, extension/hand on the back)	Supraspinatus T: transverse "tire on a wheel," sagittal/oblique sagittal plane orientation of the probe for longitudinal scan (Figure 1.10) Infraspinatus T: can be evaluated from the posterior aspect Subacromial–subdeltoid bursa Dynamic view by gradual abduction (oblique coronal) for subacromial impingement
Superior		AC joint with cross arm adduction (dynamic maneuver with crossing the arm to the midline) (Figure 1.11) Suprascapular notch
Posterior	Neutral to internal rotation of arm	Infraspinatus, teres minor • Transverse view, infraspinatus: tendinous vs. teres minor: still muscular near the attachment site Posterior glenohumeral joint with labrum Spinoglenoid notch (immediately medial to the GH joint) Humeral head and hyaline cartilage External and internal rotation: pocketing of effusion/fluid at posterior glenohumeral joint capsule

AC, acromioclavicular; AIUM, The American Institute of Ultrasound in Medicine; GH, glenohumeral; POC, point of care; T, tendon; US, ultrasound.

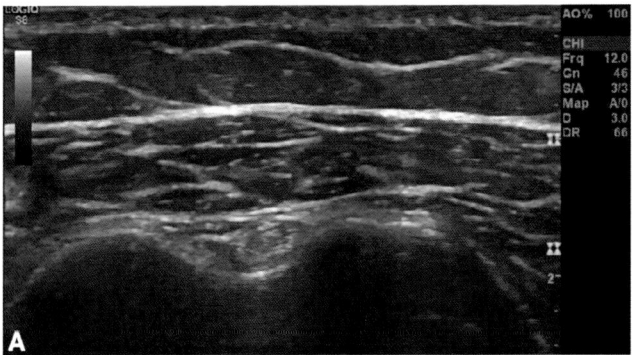 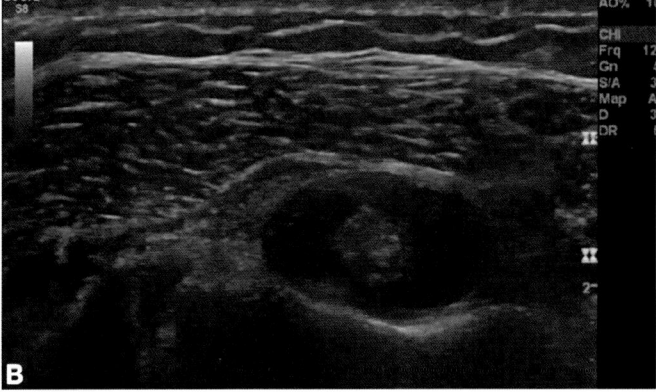

FIGURE 1.9
Normal (A) and common abnormal finding (B) of transverse US view of long head of the bicep tendon in the anterior aspect of the shoulder. Effusion in the bicipital tenosynovium (B) can be observed with glenohumeral joint effusion, adhesive capsulitis (common underlying cause), or bicipital tenosynovitis.
US, ultrasound.

(continued)

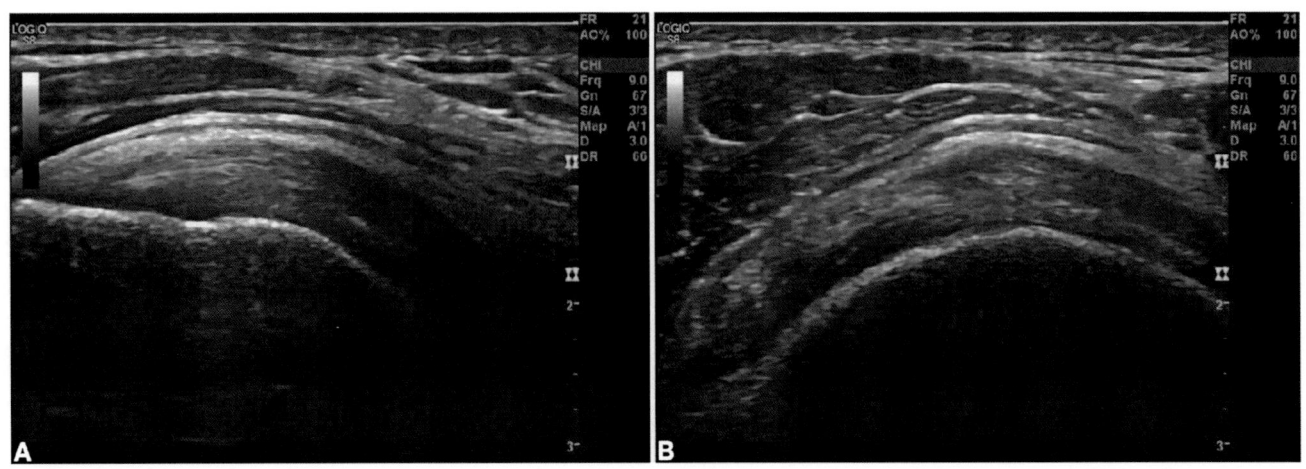

FIGURE 1.10
Normal (A: longitudinal; B: transverse US view) and abnormal finding (C: longitudinal; D: transverse) of supraspinatus tendons in the antero-lateral aspect of the shoulder. Absence of supraspinatus tendon and sagging of superficial deltoid muscle is characteristic of full thickness supraspinatus tear.
US, ultrasound.

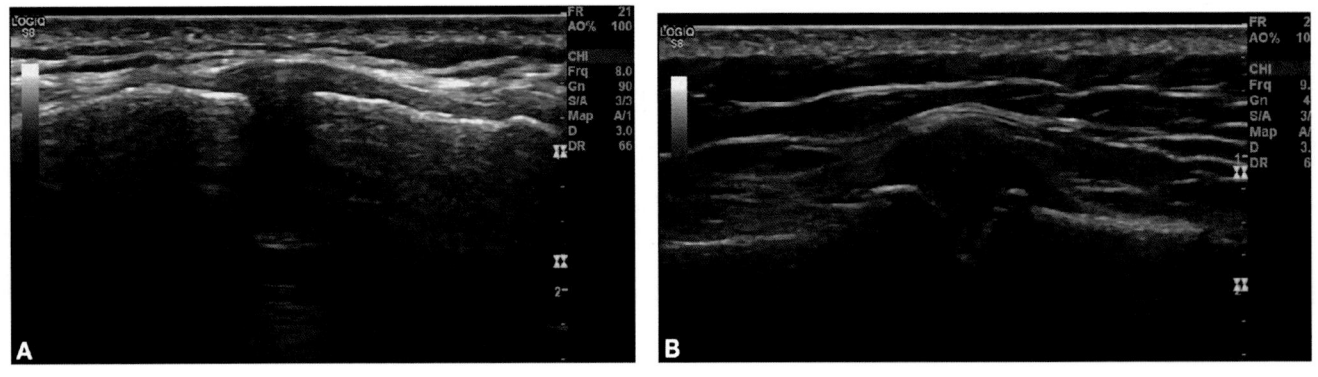

FIGURE 1.11
Normal (A) and abnormal finding (B) of longitudinal US view of acromioclavicular joint. Bulging of the joint capsule and bony irregularity consistent with degenerative acromioclavicular joint disease.

Elbow

ELBOW	
REGION	**STRUCTURES**
Anterior	Position: elbow extended with slightly supinated Brachialis muscle: over the elbow joint (anterior recess) Biceps tendon • Insertion; often difficult to visualize (on radial tuberosity); forearm supinated Median N: between brachialis and pronator; difficult to visualize often, med to brachial A Radial N: between brachialis and brachioradialis, check bifurcation into PIN
Medial	Position: forearm supinated Common flexor T: parallel to the forearm in long-axis view (with elbow flexion) Ulnar collateral ligament: slight oblique angle (distal to medial/anterior) to long axis of the common flexor tendon Ulnar nerve situated on the retrocondylar groove: hypoechoic normally due to wavy course (Figure 1.12)
Lateral	Position: elbow flexion with forearm pronated Common extensor T: parallel to the forearm in long-axis view (Figure 1.13) Radial collateral ligament under the common extensor tendon Radial head, annular recess, capitellum Radial N and posterior interosseous nerve
Posterior	Position: 90° elbow flexion Posterior joint recess: Olecranon fossa and fat pad Triceps muscle and tendon Olecranon bursa: abnormal if effusion presents
Dynamic	Ulnar collateral ligament injury/tear by valgus stress with measuring distance of ulnohumeral joint space Ulnar nerve snapping/dislocation on the medial condylar side of retro-condylar groove to ant (volar) aspect ± medial head of triceps M snapping with elbow flexion

M, muscle; N, nerve; PIN, posterior interosseous nerve; POC, point-of-care; T, tendon.

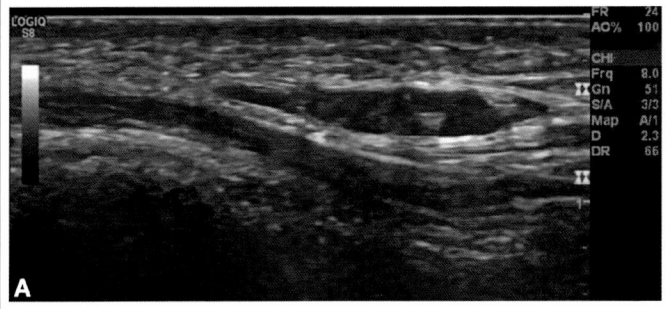 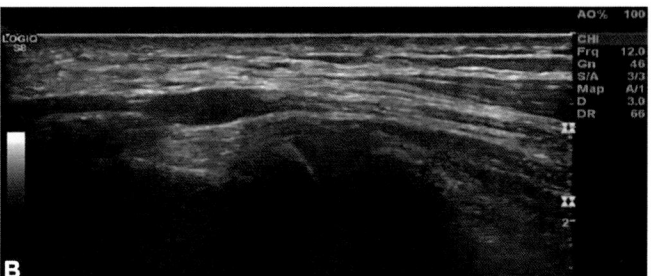

FIGURE 1.12
Normal (A) and abnormal finding (B) of the ulnar nerve in the medial elbow. Focal enlargement of the ulnar nerve at the retrocondylar groove in longitudinal view suggestive of ulnar entrapment neuropathy at elbow.

(continued)

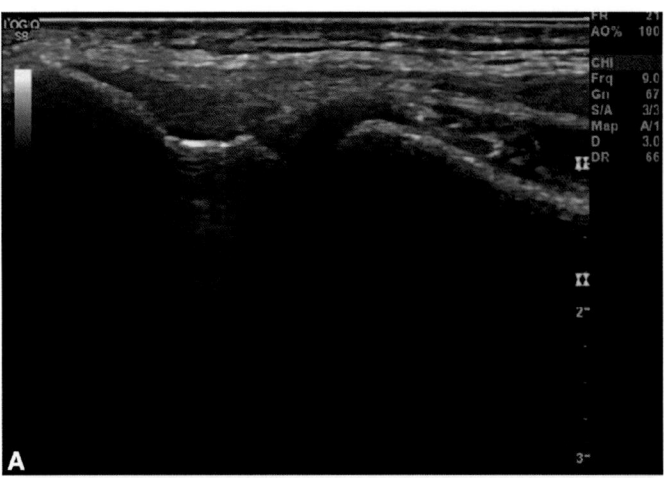

FIGURE 1.13
Normal (A) and common abnormal finding (B) of longitudinal US view of the common extensor tendon in the lateral elbow. Heterogenic echogenicity with increased vascularity suggestive of lateral epicondylitis.
US, ultrasound.

Wrist and Hand
AIUM guideline divides volar, ulnar, and dorsal

WRIST AND HAND		
REGION		**STRUCTURES**
Volar	Middle	Median nerve: ulnar to the flexor carpi radialis, under flexor retinaculum or transcarpal ligament Flexor tendons (inside carpal tunnel: flexor pollicis longus and flexor digitorum superficialis and profundus) Volar joint recess (radio-scaphoid)
	Radial	Scaphoid (bilobar shape), scaphotrapezium, trapezium-1st metacarpal (basal joint, abductor pollicis longus insert on base of 1st MC) Flexor carpi radialis (lies on top of scaphoid at the wrist)
	Ulnar	Ulnar artery and nerve (medial to the ulnar A) under the flexor carpi ulnaris (FCU) tendon Pisiform (FCU insertion) and hamate (1 fingerbreadth radial/distal; landmark for distal carpal tunnel and Guyon's canal)
Dorsum	Radial	Lister's tubercle of the radius (between 2nd and 3rd dorsal compartment) Extensor tendons (1st dorsal compartment; APL, EPB on the radial styloid process) (Figure 1.14) Dorsal joint recess
	Middle	Scapholunate lig.: check the interval distance Extensor tendon (EDC, EI), EDM on radioulnar joint Carpal bone (osteophyte, carpal boss)
	Ulnar	Triangular fibrocartilage complex Extensor carpi ulnaris on the ulnar groove
Dynamic		ECU tendon subluxation with pronation and supination

APL, abductor pollicis longus; ECU, extensor carpi ulnaris; EDC, extensor digitorum communis; EDM, extensor digiti minimi; EI, extensor indicis; EPB, extensor pollicis brevis; MC, metacarpal.

(continued)

Workup 49

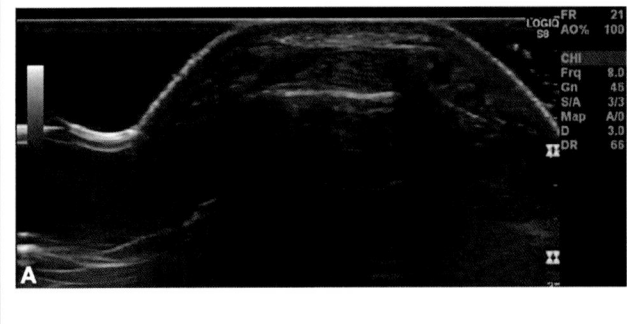
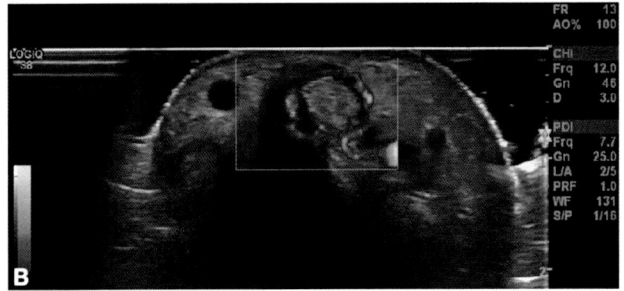

FIGURE 1.14
Normal (A) and abnormal finding (B) in the radial aspect of the wrist. Increased thickness of tendon, tenosynovium, and vascularity noted on the 1st dorsal compartment suggestive of de Quervain tenosynovitis.

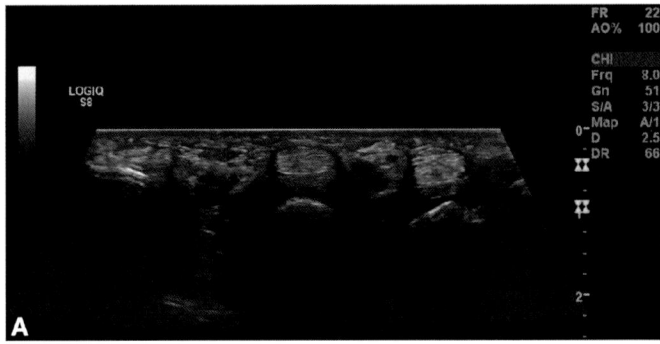
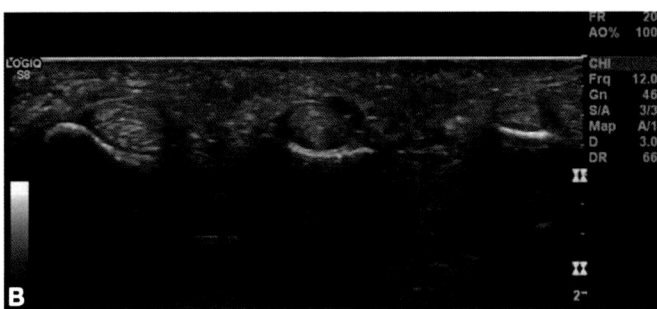

FIGURE 1.15
Normal (A) and abnormal finding (B) of transverse US view of the flexor tendons in the volar aspect of the hand/finger. Focal thickening of A1 pulley suggestive of stenosing tenosynovitis causing triggering.

US, ultrasound.

Finger

FINGER	
LOCATION	STRUCTURES
Volar	Flexor tendons (tenosynovial effusion or retinacular cyst) Pulleys: thickened pulley (A1 on MCP level for trigger finger) (Figure 1.15) Volar plate on the joint and joint recess
Dorsum	Extensor tendons: 1st column (APL, EPB) to 6th column (ECU) (Figure 1.16) Joint recess
Lateral	Collateral ligament (ulnar collateral ligament of the 1st MCP for Skier's thumb) Finger collateral ligament

AIUM, The American Institute of Ultrasound in Medicine; APL, abductor pollicis longus; ECU, extensor carpi ulnaris; EPB, extensor pollicis brevis; MCP, metacarpophalangeal; US, ultrasound.

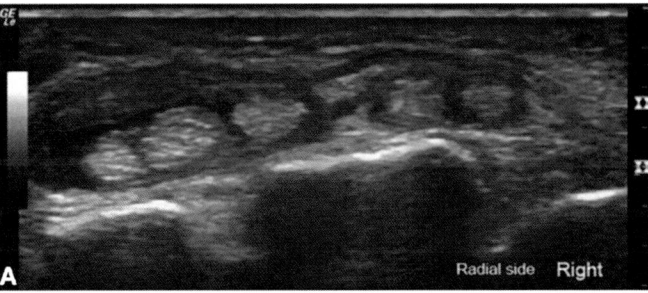
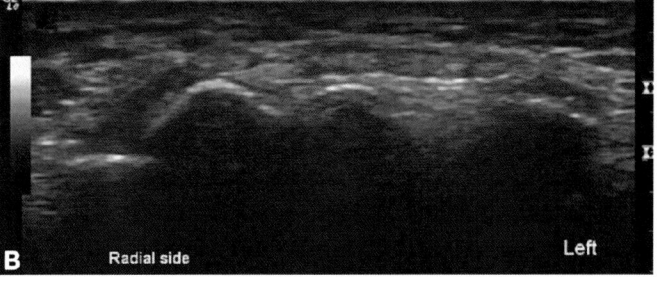

FIGURE 1.16
Normal (B) and abnormal (A) finding of transverse US view of extensor tendons in the dorsal aspect of the hand. Increased size of the tendon and effusion in the tenosynovium suggestive of extensor tenosynovitis.

US, ultrasound.

Hip and Thigh

HIP AND THIGH	
REGION	STRUCTURES
Anterior	Position: supine with slight hip abduction Sagittal oblique plane for long axis view of hip joint Hip joint: acetabulum, anterior part of labrum, capsule, anterior recess on the head–neck junction (Figure 1.17) Iliopsoas, iliopectineal eminence, sartorius, rectus femoris (direct and indirect head), vastus medialis, vastus intermedius, vastus lateralis
Medial	Position: frog leg (hip external rotation with 45° knee flexion) Femoral artery, vein, and nerve Hesselbach's triangle (bordered by rectus abdominis, inguinal lig and inferior epigastric vessels) for direct inguinal hernia Adductor longus, brevis muscle, attachment to pubic tubercle Gracilis Obturator nerve • Anterior branch between adductor long. and brev. • Posterior branch between adductor brev. and magnus Pubic symphysis
Posterior	Position: prone (with hip flexion with pillow underneath) Semimembranosus attachment to ischial tuberosity Conjoint tendon of semitendinosus and long head of biceps femoris to ischial tuberosity (medial/superficial to semimembranosus attachment to ischial tuberosity) Sciatic nerve: lateral to ischial tuberosity then courses between medial and lateral hamstring
Lateral	Position: lateral decubitus Gluteus medius, minimus muscle and tendons Greater trochanter: anterior (gluteus minimus), lateral (medius), and posterior facet (trochanteric bursa on posterior facet under gluteus maximus muscle) (Figure 1.18)
Dynamic	Snapping hip with the movement • Iliopsoas tendon over the iliopectineal eminence • Iliotibial band friction on the greater trochanter • Rectus femoris direct/indirect head on the acetabulum or in-between

US, ultrasound.

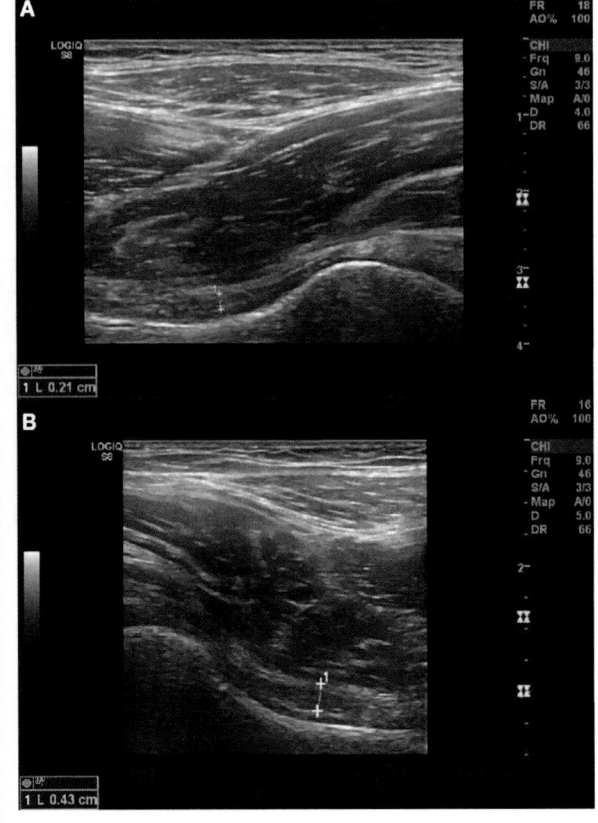

FIGURE 1.17

Normal (A) and abnormal (B) finding of longitudinal US view of proximal femur in the groin. Slightly increased thickness in the anterior capsule suggestive of mild joint effusion.

US, ultrasound.

(continued)

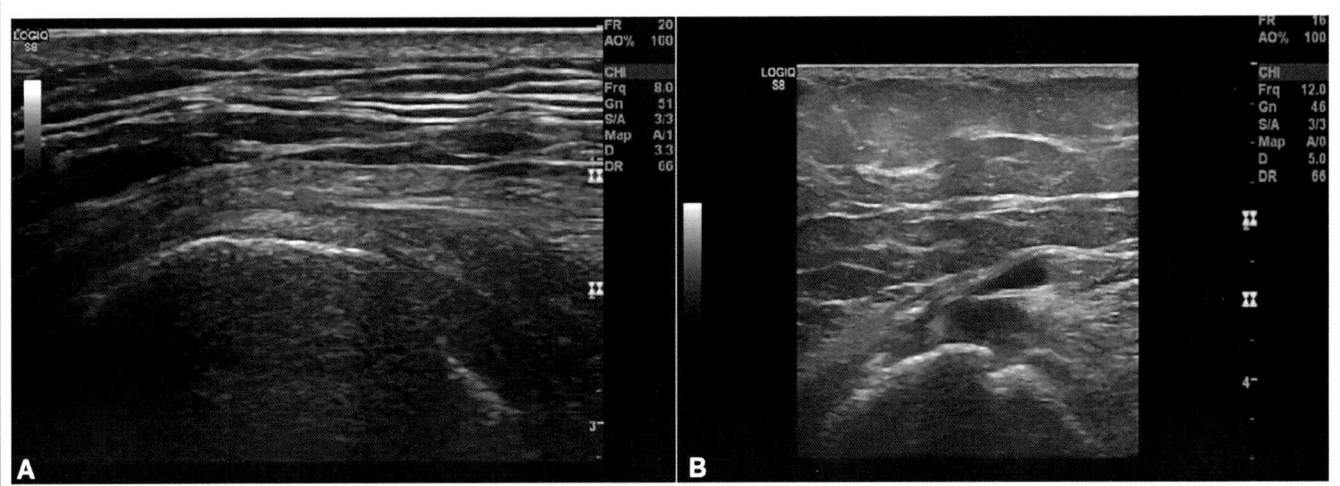

FIGURE 1.18
Normal (A) and abnormal finding (B) of transverse US view of the greater trochanter in the lateral hip. Anechoic effusion suggestive of trochanteric bursitis.
US, ultrasound.

Knee

KNEE	
Anterior	Position: Knee slightly flexed (~30° with the pillow under) Quadriceps muscle and tendon Patellar tendon and deep inferior patellar bursa effusion Patellar retinaculum Suprapatellar recess between suprapatellar fat and prefemoral fat pad (Figure 1.19) Femoral trochlear cartilage and intercondylar groove with knee hyperflexion
Medial	Position: leg externally rotate Medial collateral ligament; deep meniscofemoral/ meniscotibial ligament and superficial ligament Medial femorotibial joint Medial meniscus: body and anterior horn (Figure 1.20) Pes anserinus (superficial to medial collateral ligament) Medial patellofemoral ligament/retinaculum, possible medial plica Saphenous nerve/infrapatellar branch between vastus medialis and sartorius muscle
Lateral	Position: leg internally rotated Iliotibial tract over the lateral femoral condyle inserting on Gerdy's tubercle (Figure 1.21) Popliteus on the popliteal fossa in the lateral femoral condyle Lateral meniscus; body and anterior horn Lateral collateral ligament (posterior to ITB and oblique direction to the fibular head, inverted Z with ITB, lateral collateral ligament and biceps femoris tendon) Biceps femoris insertion to the fibular head Common peroneal nerve: easily visible at slightly superior and posterior to fibular head
Posterior	Baker's cyst between medial gastrocnemius and semimembranosus (Figure 1.22) Meniscus; posterior horns Posterior cruciate ligament (often difficult to visualize) Neurovascular structures: popliteal artery and tibial nerve Fabella in the lateral gastrocnemius tendon
Dynamic	Iliotibial band friction on the lateral femoral condyle Varus and valgus stress test Medial plica on the medial femoral condyle with knee flexion and extension

ITB, Iliotibial band; US, ultrasound.

(continued)

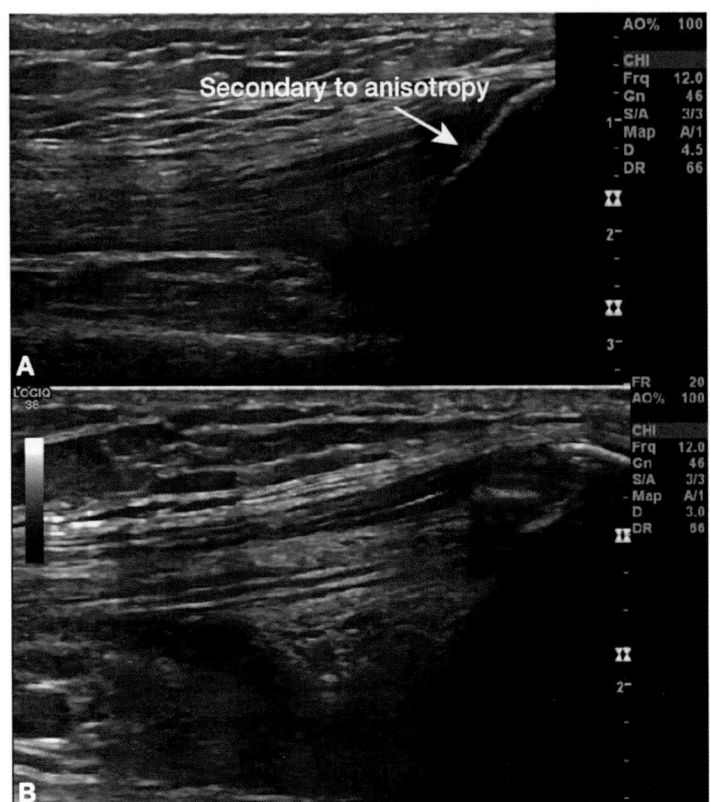

FIGURE 1.19
Normal (A) and abnormal finding (B) of longitudinal US view of the quadriceps tendon in the anterior knee. Calcification in the quadriceps tendon to superior pole of the patellar suggestive of quadriceps tendinopathy with mildly increased effusion in the suprapatellar recess.

US, ultrasound.

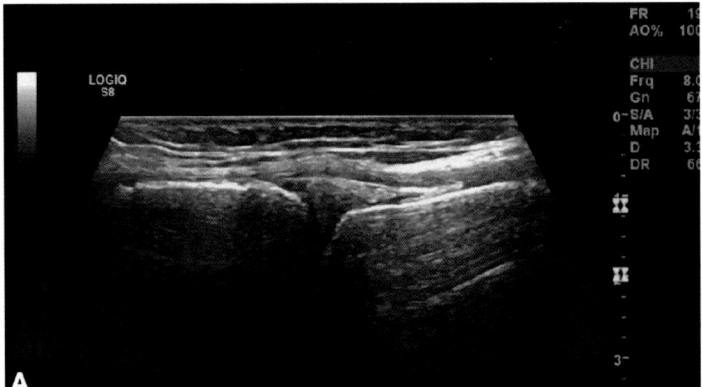

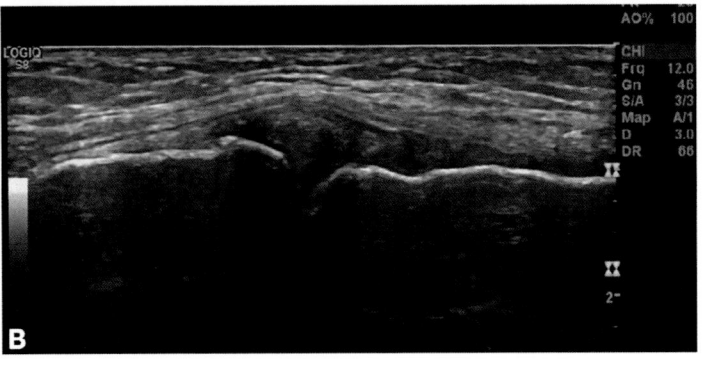

FIGURE 1.20
Normal (A) and abnormal finding (B) of longitudinal US view of the medial knee (femorotibial) joint. Displaced medial meniscus with small osteophyte in the medial knee joint consistent with degenerative joint disease.

US, ultrasound.

(continued)

Foot and Ankle

FOOT AND ANKLE	
Anterior	Position: supine with ankle plantarflexion/knee flexion
	Anterior tibiotalar joint recess with plantarflexion (more sensitive for effusion) (Figure 1.23) talonavicular, naviculocuneiform, cuneiform–metatarsal, metatarsophalangeal joints
	Tibialis anterior, extensor hallucis longus, extensor digitorum longus tendons
	Dorsalis pedis artery and deep peroneal nerve
	Superficial peroneal nerve (between peroneus muscle and extensor digitorum longus muscle distal shin)
Medial	Position: external rotation of the leg with pillows under the lateral ankle
	Tibialis posterior tendon on the medial malleolus (Figure 1.24)
	Flexor digitorum longus tendon
	Tibial nerve branching into medial, lateral plantar N, inferior calcaneal, and medial calcaneal N
	Flexor hallucis longus muscle/tendon (groove between posteromedial and postero-lateral talar processes)
	Flexor retinaculum (on tarsal tunnel)
	Deltoid ligament
Lateral	Peroneus longus and brevis; at the level of retromalleolar groove and the peroneal tubercle (peroneus longus on the plantar to the peroneal tubercle and brevis above it)
	Anterior talofibular ligament; parallel to the sole of the foot
	Calcaneofibular ligament (deeper to the peroneus longus and brevis tendons)
	Anterior tibiofibular ligament of the syndesmosis complex
	Subtalar joint (under calcaneofibular ligament)
Posterior and calf	Achilles tendon (Figure 1.25)
	Retrocalcaneal bursa; immediately anterior (deeper) to the Achilles tendon insertion to the calcaneus
	Os trigonum (posterolateral talar process)
	Soleus
	Medial and lateral heads of gastrocnemius
	Plantaris (medial aspect of Achilles tendon)
	Tibial N in soleal sling
Heel	Position: prone with knee flexion (or on the pillow under the ankle)
	Plantar fascia at medial calcaneal tuberosity (US; Figure 1.26)
	Distal plantar fascia (for fibromatosis)
Forefoot	Scanning from dorsal aspect: dorsal joint recess and interdigital space
	Scanning from plantar aspect
	• Sesamoid
	• 1st and 2nd MTP (volar plate) from plantar aspect
	• Interdigital nerve (for Morton's neuroma (ankle 90° dorsiflexion) with pressure from the dorsum, often difficult to visualize)
Dynamic	Ankle inversion and anterior drawer for ATFL ligament tear and calcaneofibular ligament
	Tibia external rotation for syndesmosis widening (anterior inferior tibiofibular joint)
	Ankle eversion and dorsiflexion for evaluation of peroneal tendon snapping

ATFL, anterior talofibular ligament; MTP, metatarsophalangeal; N, nerve; US, ultrasound.

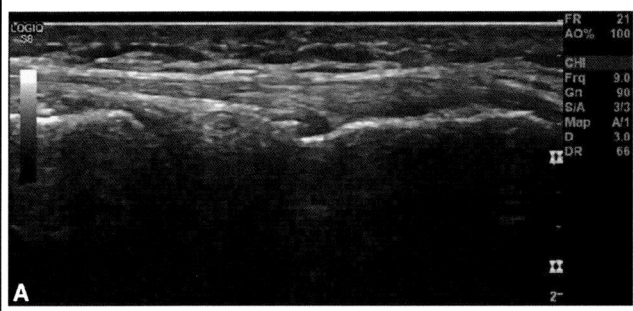
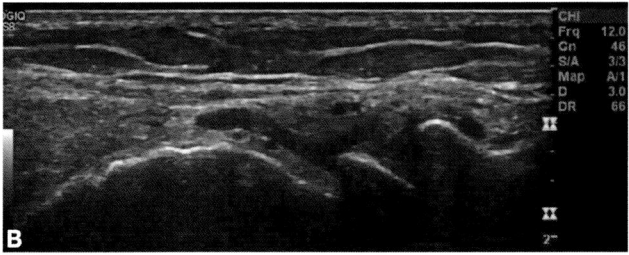

FIGURE 1.21
Normal (A) and abnormal finding (B) of longitudinal US view of lateral knee (femorotibial) joint. Osteophytes in the lateral femoral condyle, tibia, joint effusion, and decreased joint space consistent with degenerative joint disease.
US, ultrasound.

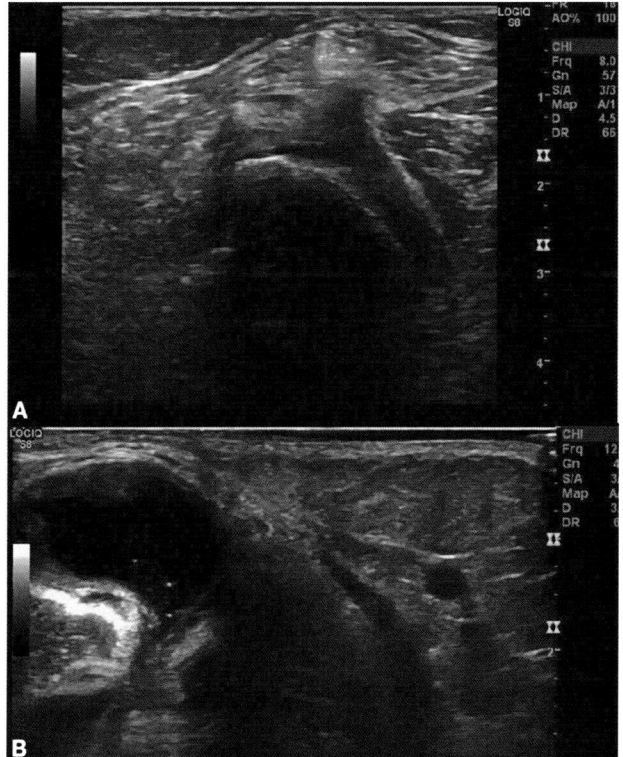

FIGURE 1.22
Normal (A) and abnormal finding (B) in the posterior aspect of the knee. Anechoic cyst between the medial gastrocnemius and semimembranosus tendon (hypoechoic due to anisotropy) with neck and base of the cyst suggests Baker's cyst.

(continued)

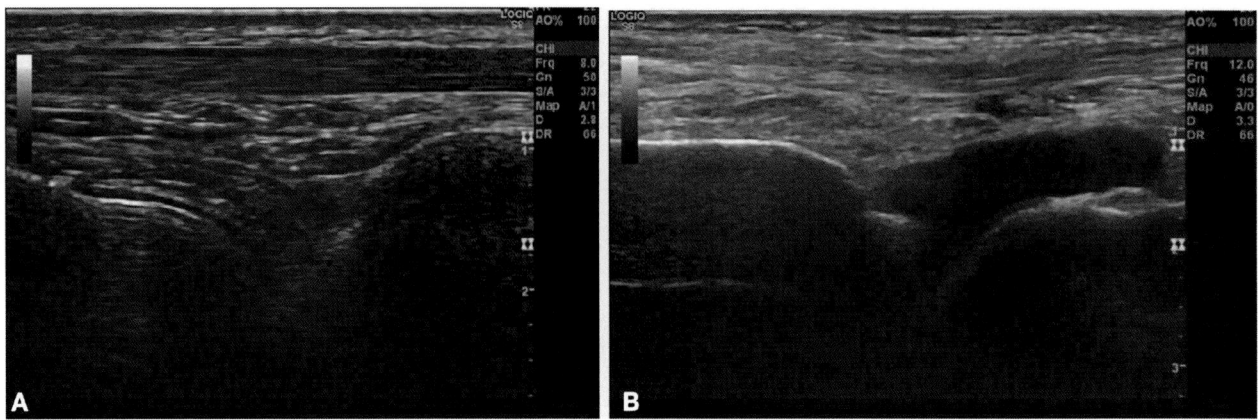

FIGURE 1.23
Normal (A) and abnormal finding (B) of the anterior tibiotalar recess of the ankle joint. Anechoic effusion was noted in the anterior recess.

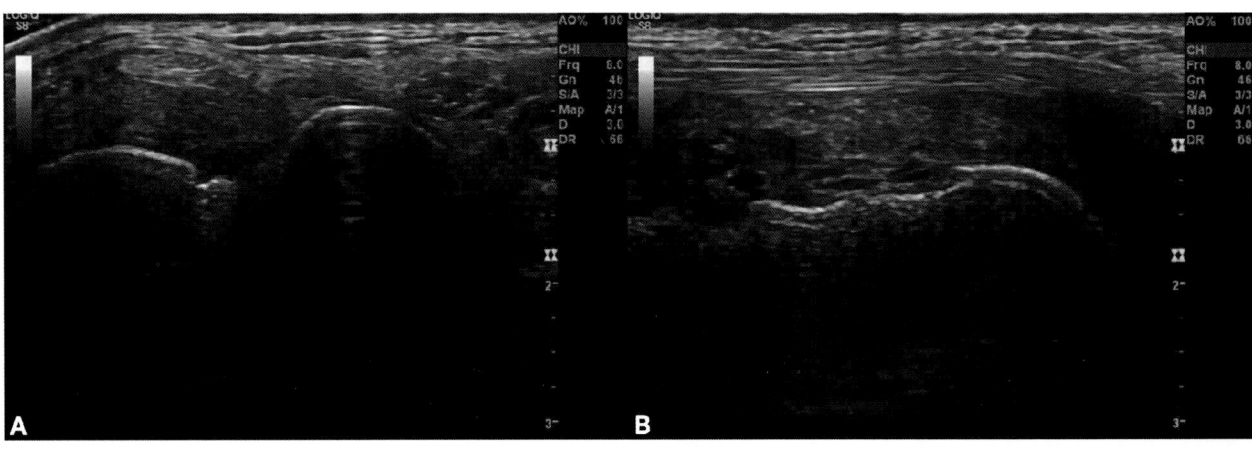

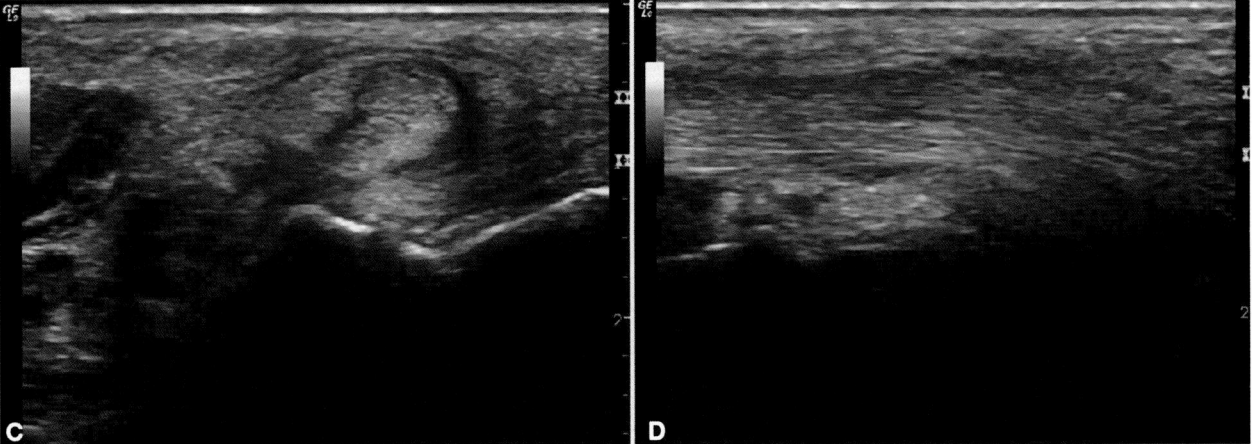

FIGURE 1.24
Normal (A, B in transverse and longitudinal views) and abnormal finding (C, D in transverse and longitudinal views) of tibialis posterior tendon in the medial ankle and hindfoot. Transverse US view of tibialis posterior tendon (C) showing anechoic cleft with increased diameter of the tibialis posterior tendon suggestive of tibialis posterior tendinopathy with split tear.
US, ultrasound.

(continued)

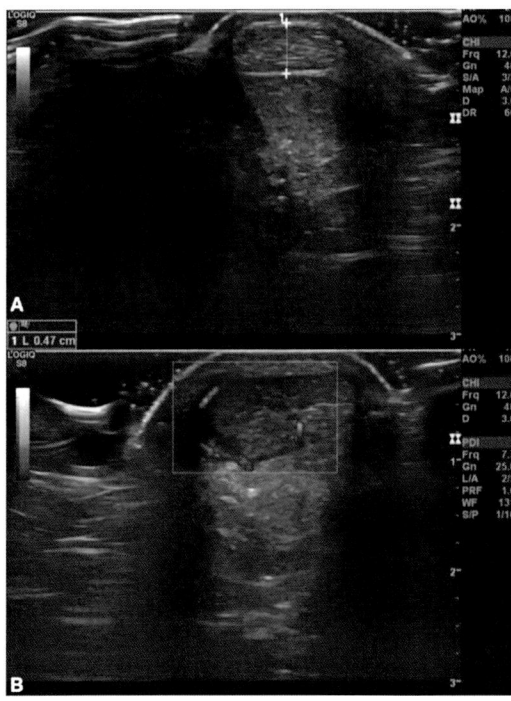

FIGURE 1.25
Normal (A) and abnormal (B) transverse US view of Achilles tendon in the posterior ankle. Increased diameter, heterogenic echogenicity, and increased vascularity suggest Achilles tendinopathy.
US, ultrasound.

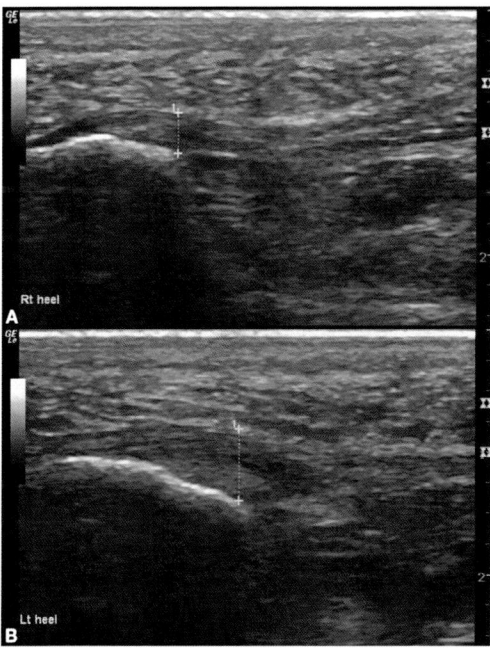

FIGURE 1.26
Normal (A) and abnormal (B) finding of longitudinal US view of plantar fascia in the plantar heel of the same person. Increased thickness with heterogenic echogenicity was noted in the symptomatic side (in the left side) compared with the contralateral asymptomatic side.
US, ultrasound.

US-guided injection (28–30)

PROS	CONS
Improved accuracy	Operator dependence
Improved localization	Time consuming
Avoiding vascular or intraneural puncture	Sterility (extra cost for probe cover)
	Need longer needle, longer trajectory (especially in in-plane view)

Role in diagnostic injection
• If there is no pain relief from injection to the structure with accurate localization → not likely pain generator (without guidance, it's difficult to validate the accuracy even in experienced hands because of normal anatomic variations)

Practical tips for scanning and guidance (32)
• Heel toe maneuver: in structure around the curve to decrease the anisotropy, press down one end compared with the other to make it parallel
  ○ Tilt the probe to make it more parallel to the needle
• Do not advance until the tip of the needle is identified or confirmed
  ○ Find the needle; rotate the stylet, jiggle, give small dose of injectate
  ○ The length of needle and angle of insertion give rough estimate of the needle tip location (depth)
• Avoid transducer sliding, tip of the needle; not necessarily where it is in the monitor, keep the target in the middle
• Walk-down technique in out-of-plane view; initially shallow angle to progressively steeper angle (45°–75°) to the target
• Move one thing at a time (either probe or needle, not together)

Technologies to improve image quality

Matrix (array) probe (33)
• More element (crystals); all channels are dedicated to transmit US pulses, improve contrast resolution, higher sensitivity and penetration, and provide harmonic capabilities

Harmonic (tissue) image
• Images created from returning harmonic waves generated within the tissue with specific transmitted frequency and built up with depth to a point of maximal intensity
• Advantages: higher resolution and decreased near-field artifacts, reverberation artifact, clutter, and off-axis scatterers

Spatial compounding image
• Electronic steering of US beams from an array transducer to image the same tissue multiple times by using parallel beams oriented along different directions. The echoes from these different directions averaged together (compounded) into a single composite image
• Advantages: reduction of image artifacts (eg, speckle [look less grainy], clutter, noise, angle-generated artifacts), sharper delineation of tissue interfaces, and better discrimination of lesions (margin definition) over the background, as well as improvement in detail resolution (lateral resolution) and image contrast

Beam steering
- Steer the beam electronically to perpendicular axis of the scanning structure
- Advantage: to decrease anisotropic artifact in structures, such as tendons or ligaments, which are examined with an incidence angle far from 90° because of their oblique course from surface to depth (distal biceps tendon, Achilles and supraspinatus tendon insertion, etc)

US elastography (34)
- Allows the qualitative visual or quantitative measurements of the mechanical properties of tissue
- With stress applied to tissue, measures changes (tissue displacement) depending on the elastic properties of tissues
- Strain EUS; low-frequency compression of the soft tissue (MC used)
  - A compressive force is applied to tissue causing axial tissue displacement (strain), which is then calculated by comparing the echo sets before and after the compression
  - Most often, red is used for encoding soft tissues, blue for hard tissues, and yellow/green for tissue of intermediate stiffness (depending on setting)
  - Indication: evaluation of mass for malignancy
- Experimental: tendinopathy (increased stiffness), muscle pain (trigger point with increased stiffness), myopathy, and marker for response after Botox injection, soft tissue evaluation (skin involvement in sclerosis, evaluate rheumatoid nodule vs tophi and discrimination of soft tissue mass)

OTHER WORKUP: LABORATORY INVESTIGATION

- Not indicated for arthropathy initially unless red flags present or suspicion for systematic disease
- Complete blood count (CBC), blood chemistry, and urine analysis
  - HIV, Hep B and C, lyme disease, and human leukocyte antigen (HLA) B 27 if indicated by history
  - Uric acid: little diagnostic value with asymptomatic hyperuricemia
- Synovial fluid analysis by arthrocentesis
  - Contraindications for arthrocentesis; bacteremia, joint prosthesis and overlying soft tissue infection
  - Send fluid analysis for white blood cell (WBC) count, cultures, gram staining, synovial fluid analysis, and polarized light microscopy
- Serologic test for polyarthralgia

DIAGNOSIS	TYPICAL CLINICAL SYMPTOMS	DIAGNOSTIC TESTS
Rheumatoid arthritis	Symmetric joint involvement, morning stiffness, anemia, serositis	CBC, ESR, CRP, RF, anti-CCP antibodies
Systemic lupus erythematous	Facial malar rash, photosensitivity, painless oral ulcers, serositis, seizure or psychosis in the absence of other causes	ANA, anti-ds DNA, anti-Sm, complement (C3,C4,CH50)
Ankylosing spondylitis	Progressive stiffness of the spine in a young adult	HLA-B27
Sjögren syndrome	Parotid gland enlargement, lymphadenopathy, dryness of eyes, mouth mucosal ulceration	ANA, anti-Ro (anti-SSA), anti-La (anti-SSB)
Reactive arthritis	Keratoderma blennorrhagicum, circinate balanitis, conjunctivitis	Screening for gonococcus or Chlamydia trachomatis, HLA-B27
Psoriasis	Silvery skin plaques on extensor surfaces, and involvement of DIP joints	Skin biopsy
Lyme	Erythema migrans, bilateral Bell's palsy, arrhythmia (heart block)	IgM and IgG antibodies to Borrelia burgdorferi, ECG
Sarcoidosis	Erythema nodosum, bilateral ankle arthritis, lymphadenopathy, scleritis	Chest radiograph, CBC, serum ACE level, lymph node biopsy
Inflammatory bowel Dz	Abdominal pain with loose stools, perianal disease, weight loss, erythema nodosum, anemia	Colonoscopy
Drug-induced lupus	Discoid rash after recent medications like minocycline, hydralazine	ANA, antihistone antibodies

ACE, angiotensin-converting enzyme; ANA, antinuclear antibody; anti-ds DNA, anti-double stranded DNA; anti-Sm: anti-Smith; CBC, complete blood count; CCP, cyclic citrullinated peptide; CRP, C reactive protein; DIP, distal interphalangeal; Dz, disease; ESR, erythrocyte sedimentation rate; HLA, human leukocyte antigen; IgG, immunoglobulin G; IgM, immunoglobulin M; RF, rheumatoid factor; SS, Sjögren syndrome.

TREATMENT

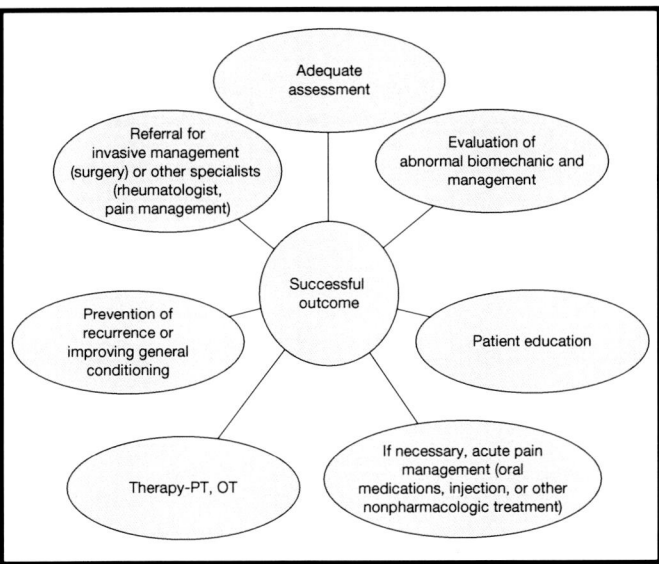

FLOWCHART 1.5
Treatment overview in musculoskeletal disorders.
OT, occupational therapy; PT, physical therapy.

PATIENT EDUCATION (104; FLOWCHART 1.5)

Objectives of education
- To prevent or reduce the impact of MSK disorders and complications
- Exercise education to reduce the morbidity and mortality associated with cardiovascular disease, diabetes, and respiratory diseases in addition to MSK disorders

Lifestyle modification
- Maintains an ideal body weight, balanced diet with adequate calcium and vitamin D, regular exercise, avoidance of smoking and alcohol abuse, and a safe and ergonomically suitable work environment
- Strengthening exercise
  ○ Functional outcome is more related to muscle strength
    ▪ Strength: usually decreased in painful conditions directly or indirectly from disuse
  ○ Different modes available (isometric or water-based initially, then progress to resistive and eccentric strengthening; usually needs education/therapy sessions, can be injurious)
    ▪ Maintain flexibility and ROM as much as possible

Exercise and arthritis (106)
- Patients with OA in general can pursue a high level of physical activity and continue to engage regularly in recreational sports provided the activity is not painful and does not predispose to trauma
- Radiographic or clinical OA: not a contraindication to promoting activity in patients who have a sedentary lifestyle
- Exercise and other structured activities have favorable effect on pain and function in the sedentary patient with knee OA
  ○ Dynamic exercise favored over static mode
  ○ Availability, preference, and tolerance being the criteria for the choice of an exercise
  ○ Frequency: at least 1 to 3 times/week
- No scientific argument to support halting exercise in case of an OA flare-up
- The OA patient who practices a sport at risk for joint trauma should be encouraged to change sport (not high-level evidence-based recommendation)

Recovery after soft tissue injury
- Objective: to improve compliance and education for rough time frame and plan
- Phases of recovery
  ○ Inflammatory (2–3 days), fibroblastic (5 days to 4 weeks), and remodeling phases (4 weeks to ~ 3.5 months)
  ○ Inflammation for (2–4) days: essential for repair
    ▪ Bleeding and hemostasis
    ▪ Inflammation: edema, pain, warmth, redness, and dysfunction
    ▪ In chronic tendinopathy: lack of inflammatory cells (inflammatory healing process)
  ○ Fibroblastic phase
    ▪ Fibroplasia: 4 to 8 weeks, type 3 collagen (immature), granulation tissue, and neovascularization
    ▪ Risk of re-injury/regression: be cautious to prevent re-injury during this period
    ▪ Intervention: graded rehabilitation (stretching, ROM, and strengthening initially) and may initiate gradual return to play
  ○ Maturation: remodeling, months to years
    ▪ Type III to I collagen, realign and remodel fibers (force magnitude and direction), reduced cellularity and vascularity
    ▪ Scar tissue: never become normal → increased risk for re-injury
    ▪ Subtle change in muscle imbalance, neuromuscular deficit, kinetic chain dysfunction/technique alteration
    ▪ Intervention: neuromuscular training, perturbation/agility training, sports-specific training and maintain general endurance/aerobic capacity, return to play

PHARMACOLOGIC MANAGEMENT

General Principles
- Choose pain medications based on adverse effect/side effect profile/comorbidities (renal, liver, and CV risk factors), etiology (inflammatory or not), less to more potent
- Understand pharmacokinetics and prescribe the dose accordingly
- Nonpharmacological management can be applied at the same time depending on the cost and availability

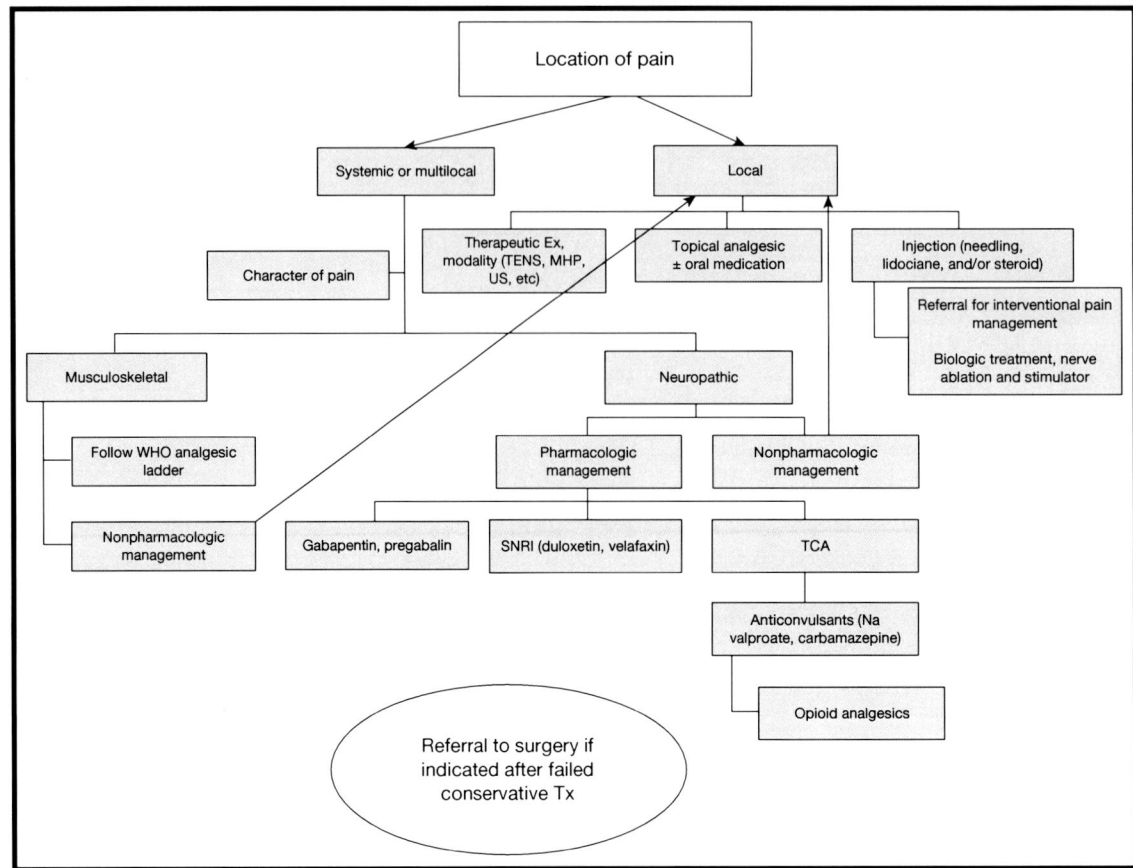

FLOWCHART 1.6
General principle of treatment for common painful conditions in the outpatient clinic.

MHP, moist heating pad; SNRI, serotonin-norepinephrine reuptake inhibitors; TCA, tricyclic antidepressant; TENS, transcutaneous electrical nerve stimulation; Tx, treatment; US, ultrasound.

WHO ANALGESIC LADDER, 2002		
Step 1	Nonopioid medications ± adjuvants • Acetaminophen (64); upto 650 mg × 5/d • NSAID	NSAID (diclofenac 75 mg bid) (65) better than AAP in osteoarthritis of the knee and hip (66,67)
Step 2	Add "weak" opioid for moderate pain ± adjuvants • AAP + codeine: Tylenol #3® • AAP + hydrocodone: Vicodin®	Equianalgesic dose to 30 mg of morphine 200 mg of codeine 30 mg
Step 3	Start "strong" opioid ± Adjuvants • Morphine • Hydromorphone (Dilaudid®) • Methadone • Oxycodone (Percocet®) • Fentanyl patch (Duragesic®)	Equianalgesic dose to 30 mg of morphine 7.5 mg 20 mg 30 mg 12.5 mcg/hr

AAP, acetaminophen; NSAID, nonsteroidal antiinflammatory drug.

Mechanism of actions for commonly prescribed medications

CLASS	TARGETS	MECHANISMS	FUNCTIONAL CONSEQUENCES	SIDE EFFECTS
NSAIDs	Cyclooxygenases (COX-1,2)	↓ Prostaglandin ↓ Thromboxanes	↓ Sensitization of sensory neurons ↓ Inhibition of spinal neurons	Nonselective: gastrointestinal ulcers, perforation, bleeding, renal impairment COX-2: thrombosis, myocardial infarction, and stroke
Opioids	G-protein–coupled μ δ κ-receptors	↓ cAMP ↓ Ca2+, ↑ K+	↓ Excitability of peripheral and central neurons ↓ Release of excitatory neurotransmitters	μ, δ: sedation, nausea, euphoria/reward, respiratory depression, constipation κ: dysphoria/aversion, diuresis, sedation

cAMP, cyclic adenosine monophosphate; NSAID, nonsteroidal antiinflammatory drug.

Commonly Used NSAIDs (107)

CATEGORIES OF NSAID		DOSE
Salicylates	Aspirin	3–4 g/d in divided doses
	Salsalate	Salicylic acid, 1,500 mg bid
	Diflunisal	Dolobid® 500–1,000 mg in two doses
Propionic acids	Ibuprofen	Motrin® 800 mg qid
	Naproxen	Naprosyn® 500 mg bid
	Fenoprofen	Nalfon® 300–600 mg tid-qid
	Ketoprofen	Orudis® 50 mg qid or 75 mg tid
	Flurbiprofen	Ansaid® 200–300 mg in two to four doses
	Oxaprozin	Daypro® 600–1,800 mg/d
Acetic acids	Arylalkanoic acids	Diclofenac (Voltaren®): 75 mg bid
		Indomethacin: 25–50 tid to qid
		Sulindac (Clinoril®): 150–200 mg bid
		Tolmetin (Tolectin®): 600–1,800 mg in three to four doses
	Pyrroles	Ketorolac 10–20 mg initially followed by 10 mg q6 PRN (max: 40 mg/d)
	Pyranocarboxylic acids	Etodolac (Lodine®) 300 (bid or tid)–500 bid
	Naphthylalkanone	Nabumetone (Relafen®) 1,000–2,000 mg/d
Enolic acids	Meloxicam	Mobic® 7.5–15 mg qD
	Piroxicam	Feldene® 20 mg qD
Fenamic acids	Meclofenamate	200–400 mg in three to four doses
	Mefenamic acid	500 mg initial dose, followed by 250 mg q 6 hour (<1 week)
Selective COX-2 inhibitors	Celecoxib	Celebrex® 100–200 mg bid
Sulphonamides	Nimesulide	100–200 mg one to two times a day
Pyrazolidinediones	Phenylbutazone	400 mg initially then 100 mg q 4 hours (<1 week)

COX-2, cyclooxygenase 2

Common side effects
- NSAIDs: GI side effect, cardiovascular (including HTN), renal side effects, swelling or rash
  - NSAIDs can increase the risk of MI and strokes as early as after first week
  - Pregnancy: generally avoid: may be related to cardiac defect (in early pregnancy)
    - Cyclooxygenase-2 (COX-2) inhibitor: category C (adverse effect in animal study, no data from human studies)
- Neuropathic medications: suicidal thoughts, swelling, dizziness, sleepiness, etc
- Check the medication side-effect profiles and also consider interaction in patients with medications that may interact with NSAIDs

Other Medications for MSK Pain

Glucosamine and chondroitin
- Proposed mechanisms
  - Glucosamine: may restore and repair the extracellular matrix by acting as a substrate for the formation of chondroitin sulfate and to stimulate the synovial production of hyaluronic acid
  - Chondroitin sulfate: may initiate synovial fabrication of hyaluronic acid
- Indications
  - Knee OA: glucosamine: no difference from placebo in WOMAC scale (108,109)
    - Glucosamine 1,500 mg/chondroitin 1,200 mg daily may be effective in moderate to severe knee pain (110)
  - Ankle OA: not yet proven
- Precaution/adverse effect; allergy to shellfish, may affect insulin resistance and affect cholesterol

Topical analgesics
- Lidocaine or lidocaine creams/patches (5%) q 12 hours, lidocaine/prilocaine (EMLA cream)
  - Possible CNS side effects related to topical analgesics
- NSAIDs (diclofenac): bioavailability and plasma concentration (5%–15%); indication: cutaneous or muscle pain
  - Less systemic side effect (but exist)
- Capsaicin cream
  - Reversibly depleting sensory nerve endings of sub P by reducing the density of epidermal nerve fibers

- Intense burning sensation at the beginning (especially in moist area, may put EMLA cream together): bouts of sneezing
- Glycerol trinitrate
  - Off label use for chronic tendinopathy, nitric oxide molecules to induce fibroblast proliferation and collagen synthesis (in a rat model)
  - 0.1 mg/hr: can increase to 0.2 mg/hr, cut in ¼ (5 mg/24 hours patch) and place it where it hurts
  - Indications: lateral epicondyle, Achilles tendon, and possible subacromial region
  - Adverse effects: headache and dizziness (cautious in patients with cardiac risk factors)

Medication for Muscle Cramps (111)

MEDICATION	TYPICAL DOSE	SERIOUS SIDE EFFECTS	COMMON SIDE EFFECTS
Quinine sulfate	260 mg q.h.s.	Thrombocytopenia, disseminated intravascular coagulation, hemolytic–uremic syndrome, hepatotoxicity, interstitial nephritis, ototoxicity	Headache, hypoglycemia, nausea/vomiting, dysphagia, rash
Gabapentin	300 mg q.h.s.	Stevens–Johnson syndrome (rare)	Ataxia, dizziness, somnolence, blurred vision, diplopia, nystagmus, fatigue, myalgia, tremor, peripheral edema
Vitamin E	1,000 I.U. q.h.s.		GI distress

GI, gastrointestinal.

Muscle (Skeletal) Relaxant

- Central (spasmolytics) (112)
  - Antispasmodic: metaxalone (Skelaxin® 800 mg, 3–4/d), methocarbamol (Robaxin® 750–1,500 mg, 3–4/d), carisoprodol (Soma® 250–350 mg tid), chlormezanone, mephenesin; meprobamate,
  - Benzodiazepine: diazepam 2 mg to 10 mg 3–4/d
  - GABA: baclofen (Lioresal®, 5 mg tid upto 80 mg/d)
  - Tizanidine: α2 adrenoreceptor agonist
- Peripheral
  - Neuromuscular: depolarizing/nondepolarizing, dual action; primarily used for general anesthesia
  - Directly acting
    - Dantrolene interferes with the release of calcium through the sarcoplasmic reticulum calcium channel

Neuropathic Pain Medications

Approach to neuropathic pain (113–115)

Step 1	Assess pain and establish the diagnosis of NP Establish and treat the cause of NP Identify relevant comorbidities (eg, cardiac, renal, hepatic disease, depression, gait instability) requiring the dose adjustment or additional monitoring Explain the diagnosis and treatment plan Can initiate referral to comprehensive pain management center
Step 2	Initiate symptomatic treatment • Ca^{2+} channel α2-δ ligands: gabapentin (1st choice) or pregabalin • Tricyclic antidepressants (secondary amine TCA; nortriptyline, desipramine or SNRI: duloxetine, venlafaxine) • Localized or peripheral NP: topical lidocaine used alone or in combination with one of the other first line Tx • Carbamazepine: 1st choice for trigeminal neuralgia • Acute NP, cancer pain, episodic exacerbations: opioid or tramadol maybe used alone or combination • Nonpharmacological treatment
Step 3	Reassess pain- and health-related quality of life frequently • If substantial pain relief (average pain reduced to ≤3/10) and tolerable adverse effects, continue Tx • Partial pain relief (average pain ≥4/10) at target dosage after an adequate trial, add one of 1st line Tx • If no or adequate pain relief (eg, <30%) at target dose after an adequate trial, switch to an alternative first line medication
Step 4	If trials of 1st line medications alone and in combination fail, 2nd or 3rd line medication or referral

NP, neuropathic pain; SNRI, serotonin-norepinephrine reuptake inhibitors; TCA, tricyclic antidepressant; Tx, treatment.

Symptomatic approach based on mechanism of NP (116)

SYMPTOMS		MECHANISM	TARGET	MEDICATION
Spontaneous shooting pain (paroxysmal pain)		PN hyperexcitability ectopic impulse generation, oscillation in dorsal root ganglion • Ectopic impulse generation, oscillation in dorsal root ganglion	Na^+ channel	Selective Na^+ channel blocker • Lidocaine, carbamazepine, oxcarbazepine, lamotrigine, tricyclic antidepressant (TCA)
Sympathetic-mediated pain	PN nociceptor sensitization	Noradrenaline, histamine α receptor H1 receptor	α receptor Histamine receptor	Sympathetic N block TCA: H1 receptor antagonist α receptor antagonist (phentolamine)
Allodynia	Heat	PN nociceptor sensitization; reduced threshold to heat, cold, mechanical stimuli	TRPV1 receptor	Capsaicin cream
	Cold		TRPM8 receptor	Possibly menthol
	Static mechanical (nonpainful static pressure)		ASIC receptor	

Spontaneous ongoing pain
• Allodynia (dynamic mechanical)
  ○ Pain by nonpainful light touch such as stroking skin with brush, cotton swab, or gauze
• Punctate mechanical hyperalgesia
  ○ Normally tingling but not painful stimuli cause pain
  ○ Pricking of the skin with sharp stick, safety pin
		Central dorsal horn hyperexcitability
		Central sensitization on spinal level
		Ongoing C input → ↑synaptic transmission
		Amplification of C fiber input
		Gating of A β fiber input (mechanical dynamic hyperalgesia)
		Gating of A δ fiber input (mechanical punctate hyperalgesia)
			Presynaptic μ receptor, Ca^{2+} channel
			Postsynaptic NMDA, NK1 receptors, Na^+ channel intracellular μ
				μ receptor agonists: opioid
				Ca^{2+} channel blocker: gabapentin, pregabalin
				NMDA receptor antagonists: ketamine, dextromethorphan
				Selective Na^+ channel blocker: carbamazepine

		GABAergic	GABA B receptor	Baclofen
		Change in the supraspinal descending modulation (inhibitory control; noradrenaline, 5-HT decrease)	α2 receptor 5-HT receptors	α2 receptor agonist: clonidine NA/5-HT reuptake blocker: TCA, venlafaxine, duloxetine
		PN nociceptor sensitization Inflammation within nerves, cytokine release	Cytokines	Cytokine antagonists, cyclooxygenase blocker, TNF-α antagonist, NSAIDs

5-HT, 5-hydroxytryptamine receptors; ASIC, acid sensing ion channel; GABA, gamma-aminobutyric acid; NMDA, N-methyl-D-aspartic acid or N-methyl-D-aspartate; NSAID, nonsteroidal antiinflammatory drug; PN, peripheral nerve; TCA, tricyclic antidepressant; TNF-α, tumor necrosis factor.

Commonly used NP medications (113)

MEDICATION	MODE OF ONSET	SIDE EFFECTS	PRECAUTIONS	OTHER BENEFITS	EFFICACY	STARTING DOSE/ MAXIMAL	TITRATION	DURATION OF ADEQUATE TRIALS
Tricyclic antidepressants								
Nortriptyline Desipramine	Serotonin and/or Norepinephrine reuptake inhibitor, block of Na channels, anticholinergic	Sedation, anticholinergic effects (eg, dry mouth or urinary retention, weight gain	Cardiac disease (ECG), glaucoma, seizure disorder, use of tramadol	Improvement of depression and sleep disturbance	A: diabetic neuropathy, PHN B: SCI/CPSP, chronic radiculopathy	25 mg at bedtime/150 mg daily	Increase by 25 mg every 3–7 days as tolerated	6–8 weeks (at least 2 weeks maximum tolerated dose)
SSNRI								
Duloxetine	Inhibition of both serotonin and norepinephrine reuptake	Nausea	Hepatic dysfunction, renal insufficiency, alcohol abuse, use of tramadol	Improvement of depression	A: diabetic neuropathy	30 mg once daily/ 60 mg twice daily	Increase by 60 mg once daily after 1 week as tolerated	4 weeks
Venlafaxine			Cardiac disease, tramadol, withdrawal with abrupt discontinuation			37.5 mg 1 or 2× a day/225 mg	Increase by 37.5 or 75 mg	4–6 weeks
Ca²⁺ Channel α2-δ Ligands								
Gabapentin	Decrease release of glutamate, NE, and sub P with ligands on α2-δ subunit of voltage Ca²⁺ channel	Sedation, dizziness, peripheral edema	Renal insufficiency	No clinically significant drug interactions	A: diabetic neuropathy, PHN, Ca associated neuropathic pain	100–300 mg 1 to 3 times a day/3,600 mg, reduce if impaired renal function	Increase by 100–300 mg tid 1–7 days as tolerated	4 weeks

(continued)

MEDICATION	MODE OF ONSET	SIDE EFFECTS	PRECAUTIONS	OTHER BENEFITS	EFFICACY	STARTING DOSE/ MAXIMAL	TITRATION	DURATION OF ADEQUATE TRIALS
Ca^{2+} Channel α2-δ Ligands								
Pregabalin		Sedation, dizziness, peripheral edema	Renal insufficiency	No clinically significant drug interactions, improvement of sleep disturbance and anxiety	A: diabetic neuropathy, PHN, SCI	50 mg tid or 75 mg bid/200 mg tid or 300 mg bid, reduce if impaired by renal function	Increase by 100–300 mg tid 1–7 days as tolerated	4 weeks
Topical lidocaine								
5% lidocaine patch	Block of Na$^+$ channels	Local erythema, rash	None	No systemic side effects	PHN	1–3 patches/3 patches	None	2 weeks
Opioids								
Morphine, oxycodone, methadone, levorphanol	μ receptor agonist, (oxycodone: also causes k receptor antagonism)	Nausea, vomiting, constipation and dizziness	Substance abuse, suicide risk, driving impairment	Rapid onset of analgesic effect	A: diabetic neuropathy, PHN, phantom pain B: chronic radiculopathy	10–15 mg morphine every 4 hours as needed	After 1–2 weeks, convert to long acting opioids/ transdermal applications, use short acting drug as needed	4–6 weeks
Tramadol	μ receptor agonist, inhibition of NE and serotonin reuptake		Substance abuse, suicide risk, driving impairment, concomitant use of SSNRI, TCA (serotonin syndrome)		A: diabetic neuropathy, phantom pain B: SCI, cancer associated neuropathic pain	50 mg 1 or 2/d/400 mg daily	Increased by 50–100 mg every 3–7 days	4 weeks

A, good scientific evidence; B, some scientific evidence; CPSP, central post stroke pain; PHN, postherpetic neuralgia; SCI, spinal cord injury; SSNRI, selective serotonin and norepinephrine reuptake inhibitors; TCA, tricyclic antidepressant.

Commonly used opioid analgesics (12)

NAME	INITIAL ORAL DOSE	DURATION	EQUIPOTENT PO DOSE (TO 50 MG OF MORPHINE)	COMMENTS
Morphine	0.5 mg/kg	3–4 hr		Standard opioid for comparison
Hydromorphone	0.075 mg/kg	2–4 hr	7.5 mg	Inactive metabolites make it superior in patients with renal or hepatic disease
Methadone	0.2 mg/kg	4–8 hr	20 mg	Used for opioid addiction treatment and chronic pain, half-life longer than duration of action
Fentanyl	3 µg/kg	0.5–1.5 hr	NA	Transcutaneous patches (q 72 hrs) commonly used. Transmucosal or nasal form available
Oxycodone	0.15 mg/kg	3–4 hr	15 mg	Excellent bioavailability makes it an effective oral agent
Codeine	2.5 mg/kg	2–4 hr	200 mg	Pronounced peripheral effects (constipation, nausea and vomiting, cough suppression)
Hydrocodone	5–15 mg	3–4 hr	30 mg	Commonly used in preparations with acetaminophen, more potent than codeine
Meperidine	3 mg/kg	2–3 hr	300 mg	Toxic metabolite normeperidine accumulates at normal doses
Oxymorphone	0.1 mg/kg (rectal)	3–4 hr	10 mg (PR)	Rectal dosing more predictable than other agents
Propoxyphene	1 mg/kg	2–4 hr	100 mg	Combination with acetaminophen inferior to acetaminophen alone, no indications for use
Alfentanil	NA	8–12 min	NA	Short duration because of redistribution, duration of action increases with the size of the dose
Sufentanil	NA	1–1.5 hr	NA	Minimal cardiovascular side effect
Nalbuphine	0.1 mg/kg	3–4 hr	NA	Mixed agonist/antagonist, decreased respiratory depression relative to other opioids, limited analgesic effect, used in perinatal period

LOCAL INTERVENTION

Injection

Common indications
- Pain from the following
  - Joint pathologies; inflammatory arthropathy (pseudogout, adjuvant Tx for RA), symptomatic OA flare up, adhesive capsulitis, and so on
  - Bursal pathologies; subacromial, trochanteric, pes anserine, retrocalcaneal bursitis
  - Tendon (tenosynovium, paratendon) pathologies; de Quervain tenosynovitis, stenosing tenosynovitis (trigger finger), and painful ligament sprain
  - Peripheral entrapment neuropathy: CTS, meralgia paresthetica, superficial peroneal neuropathy, and so on
  - Others; ganglion cyst and fascial defect (tear)
  - Epidural/axial joint (facet joint)/selective nerve block injection
  - Muscle and myofascial pain syndrome

Type of injectate
- Steroid
- Local anesthetics: lidocaine, bupivacaine
- Viscosupplementation (117)
- Biologics; hyperosmolar agents (prolotherapy), platelet rich plasma, and stem cells
- Alcohol/phenol for nerve block

Practical injection techniques
- Anatomic knowledge is the key for successful injection and decreases local complications
  - Individual variation of anatomy limits blind (anatomic landmark based) injection sometimes
- Many different approaches available
  - Several approaches for each structures: choose the approach based on individual patient's condition and experience/preference of physician
    - Subacromial or GH joint: posterior versus anterior and lateral approach
    - Elbow joint: lateral versus posterior to the olecranon
    - Knee joint: superolateral versus superomedial, infrapatellar, and so on
  - Shorter needle trajectory (distance) from the skin to the target preferred
    - Imaging guidance (US guidance) may require longer trajectory of needle especially in in-plane approach
  - Try to go away from the important neurovascular structures rather than approaching them

- Negative aspiration (to avoid intravascular injection) and resistance-based injection (to avoid tendon or ligament injection)
  - Withdraw the needle slightly if significant resistance (to push injectate) met
  - Significant resistance can be felt when the needle hits the bone or tendon normally; however, it may not be when using large bore needle or in osteoporotic patient
  - A small-bore needle preferred for patient comfort (and often not able to penetrate the tendon/ligament) but often difficult to advance in deeper structure (too flexible)
    - 25 to 30 G, 1 to 1.5 inch needle for superficial structures (or in lean patient), 22 G, 3.5 to 5 inch needle: deeper structures, 21 G or bigger for aspiration
  - When in doubt or for patients with red flags, do not inject patient (unless work up done or already established patient), especially steroid injection to the joint (especially when septic joint cannot be ruled out)
    - Aspiration for fluid analysis and culture
- Be cautious of neurovascular structures at the injection site (imaging guidance can be helpful)
  - Subdeltoid bursa: deltoid artery (branch of thoracoacromial A)
  - Long head of biceps: anterior circumflex humeral artery
  - Lateral elbow: radial nerve and radial recurrent A
  - de Quervain tenosynovitis/CMC joint: superficial radial nerve/artery
  - Hamstring and piriformis: sciatic nerve and inferior gluteal A for piriformis (medial side)
  - Medial knee injection: infrapatellar branch of saphenous nerve or genicular artery
  - Tibiofibular joint: common peroneal nerve, popliteus tendon/tenosynovium; common peroneal, lateral collateral lig
  - Plantar fascia: medial plantar nerve (medial approach), first branch of lateral plantar nerve, fat pad
  - Retrocalcaneal bursa: sural nerve and Achilles tendon

Skin preparation
- Aseptic or sterile fashion recommended in most cases

	CLEAN	ASEPTIC	STERILE
Procedure space	On ward or at beside	Dedicated area	Dedicated room
Gloves	Clean or none	Sterile	Sterile surgical
Hand hygiene before the procedures	Routine	Aseptic, for example, alcohol	Surgical scrub Iodophors, chlorhexidine
Skin antisepsis	No	Alcohol	Long-acting agent
Sterile field	No	No	Yes
Sterile gown, mask, head covering	No	No	Yes

- Chloroform (2% chlorhexidine gluconate and 70% isopropyl alcohol [ChloraPrep®]): more effective than iodine-based prep (10% povidone–iodine (scrub care skin prep tray) for infection related in surgical incision (118).

Aspiration
- Fluid analysis (49)
  - Check cell count/differential, gram stain, cultures, crystal examination (polarizing microscopy)

JOINT PATHOLOGY	CELLS/MM³	POLYMORPHONUCLEAR CELLS (%)
Septic	>50,000	>75
Inflammatory	2,000–50,000	>70
Noninflammatory	<2,000	<25

- Techniques
  - Use large bore needle (21G or bigger) on the sterile field
  - One extra needle puncture: helps to aspirate (pressure flow) especially in ganglion cyst (thicker viscosity), not in patients suspicious of infection
  - Smaller needle trajectory recommended if possible

Dry needling/fenestration (119)
- Common indications: myofascial pain syndrome (trigger point injection) (120) and tendinopathy (tendon fenestration)
- Mechanisms
  - Cause bleeding and trigger inflammatory healing response
  - Possibly genetic change and mechanical loading (in rat model)
- Pain reduction as well as histological changes

Image-guided injection
- Comparison with anatomic landmark-based injection (121)

REGIONS	IMAGING ACCURACY % (NO. OF STUDIES, NO. OF PARTICIPANTS)	NO IMAGING ACCURACY % IN LARGEST SIZED STUDY (NO. OF STUDIES, NO. OF PARTICIPANTS)
Subacromial	100 (3, 10–60)	29–100 (7, 10–221)
AC joint	100 (3, 44–110)	39–55 (5, 39–55)
Elbow	100 (2, 1)	25–100 (4, 25–90)
Knee	95–100 (3, 19–75)	40–100 (8, 10–585)

AC, acromioclavicular.

Steroid Injection

Commonly used steroid injection (122)

DURATION OF ACTION	TYPE OF STEROID	BRAND NAME	SOLUBILITY	ANTI-INFLAMMATORY POTENCY	SERUM HALF-LIFE (HR)/AVERAGE ACTION OF DURATION. TYPICAL DOSE CRYSTAL STRUCTURE
Intermediate acting	Methylprednisolone	Depo-Medrol®	Slightly soluble	5	18–26 hr/7–84 d, 40–80 mg for large joint Small, pleomorphic tendency to agglutinate, strong birefringence
	Prednisolone tebutate	Hydeltra-TBA®	Relatively soluble	4	18–36 hr, 2–3 hr/10–15 d. 10–25 mg for large joint Small pleomorphic tendency to agglutinate, strong birefringence
	Triamcinolone	Kenalog®; triamcinolone acetonide	Relatively insoluble	5	88 min/14 d, 20–40 mg for large joint Similar to Depo–Medrol with a strongest tendency to agglutinate and slightly stronger birefringence
		Aristospan®, triamcinolone hexacetonide		5	88 min/8–90 d, 20–40 mg for large joint 15–60 µm rod shaped, negative birefringence, difficult to distinguish from Na+ urate
Long acting	Betamethasone	Celestone Soluspan®	Combination	20–30	6.5 hr/ 9 d
	Dexamethasone	Decadron®	Soluble	20–30	36–54 hr/NA

NA, not available information.

Precautions for intra-articular steroid injection (123)
- Repeat no more often than every 3 months, and no more frequently than three times a year in a weight-bearing joint (eg, the hip, knee, and ankle) to minimize glucocorticoid-induced joint damage
- Avoid more than one large joint injection each time: more likely suppress hypothalamic–pituitary–adrenal axis
- Arthrocentesis before injection may be more effective in pain reduction
  ○ Triamcinolone hexacetonide, which, among the injectable glucocorticoids, is the least soluble preparation, may have the longest effect
- Relative rest for 24 hours: may decrease systemic side effect or articular damage

Adverse effects related to steroid injection (124,125)
- Long-term detriment of tendon: especially lateral epicondylitis (126)
- Infection (1/13,900–77,300 or rarer), disturbance in the menstrual pattern, hot flush–like symptoms the day of or the day after injection, and hyperglycemia in patients with DM
- Local complications
  ○ Subcutaneous fat tissue atrophy (especially after improper local injection), local depigmentation of the skin, tendon slip and rupture, and lesions to local nerves (with improper local injection)
- Pregnancy: avoid in early pregnancy, teratogenic effect too low to be detected in humans, but has caused cleft lip and palate in animal study (consult with obstetrician)
- Osteonecrosis: very rare in intra-articular injection (127)
  ○ Steroid (oral route)-induced bone disorder
    ▪ Suggested mechanisms: small vessel occlusion by fatty emboli, impedance of sinusoidal blood flow secondary to rise intraosseous pressure, decrease osteoblastic activity
  ○ More common with PO corticosteroid >25 mg to 40 mg/d

Other Injection Procedures

Viscosupplementation (injection of hyaluronic acid derivatives) (128)
- Hyaluronic acid: an endogenous proteoglycan that can be found in synovial fluid and serves as a backbone for proteoglycans in cartilage matrix
  ○ Short-term effect by elastoviscous fluid in the joint (mechanical)
  ○ Unclear mechanism of pain relief

- Clinical indications: limited evidence (117)
  - Knee (129,130): more effective than placebo in 5 to 13 weeks after injection
  - Hip: significant benefit for 3 month to 1 year (in observational study), no difference between the medications (131)
  - Ankle (132): positive outcome in cohort study
  - Upper extremity joints: elbow; unclear benefit (133), hand (CMC joint; may be longer lasting effect at 6 months in hyaluronan) (134)
  - Contraindications: protein/avian allergies (except Euflexxa®), pregnancy or nursing, pediatric patients, joint infection, bacteremia, and local overlying skin disease

Prolotherapy (135,136)
- The injection of an irritant into a joint space, ligament, or tendon insertion site as a complementary medical treatment, with the main goal being pain relief
  - To stimulate/trigger a natural healing response (inflammatory cascade) at the site of painful soft tissue and joints
  - Proliferation of fibroblasts, deposition of collagen healing
- Injectate
  - Hyperosmolar dextrose: MC used (eg, 12.5% dextrose and 0.5% lidocaine)
    - Hypertonic atmosphere, which leads to cell rupture, upregulates expression of platelet-derived growth factors
  - Morrhuate sodium (14.7%): attract inflammatory mediators, vascular sclerosant
  - Phenol–glycerine–glucose: cellular irritant
- Indication
  - Chronic low back pain (LBP): conflicting evidence regarding the efficacy of prolotherapy injections for patients with chronic nonspecific LBP
    - Positive effect in SI joint and coccygodynia
  - Chronic tendinopathies
    - Lateral epicondylitis, otherwise low level evidence for Achilles tendinopathy, plantar fasciitis, and hip adductor tendinopathies.
  - OA: knee and finger OA
- Contraindications and adverse effects
  - Absolute contraindications: an overlying cellulitis or septic joint
  - Adverse effects include mild pain or bleeding at the injection site or the development of a postinjection flare, similar to corticosteroid injections. These usually are self-limited and often resolve within 1 or 2 days
- Injection: a series of two to five monthly injections of a topical anesthetic and solution of other medicines

Platelet-rich plasma injection
- Mechanism
  - Platelets produce growth factors that assist in repair and regeneration of tissue
    - Elevated platelet concentration stimulate proliferation, extra fibrillar matrix formation of collage and differentiation mesenchymal stem cells at the injury site
  - Autologous blood products of platelets at supraphysiologic level ➔ release of growth factors and other bioactive factors from its alpha granules ➔ unclear mechanism of exact repair and regeneration of tissue (137)
- Indication: lateral epicondylitis (138), patellar tendinopathy (139), rotator cuff tendinopathy, and OA (138,140)
  - Lateral epicondylitis: PRP better than cortisone at 2 years (success rate 77% in PRP vs 43% in cortisone), level 1 study (141)
  - Knee OA: better pain reduction than placebo and viscosupplementation (or similar to viscosupplementation); limited evidence (142,143)
  - Achilles (noninsertional) tendinopathy: no added benefit compared to saline injection (144)
  - Hamstring muscle injury: no significant difference from placebo injection (145)
  - May consider in younger athletes (or who does not want a steroid injection), or failed other modality (such as steroid injection, viscosupplementation)
- Techniques
  - Blood drawing from the vein ➔ centrifuge (to separate the PRP, two steps centrifugation) then inject
  - Usually given with imaging guidance (US)
  - Not recommend to use NSAIDs concomitantly
  - Support weight bearing or decrease activity for 1 to 2 days (for PRP to settle down): especially with tenotomy (no evidence)
- Complications: possibly marked pain response (can last upto 3–4 weeks), otherwise similar to other injection

Stem cells
- Classification
  - Adult stem cells: hematopoietic (for blood products) and mesenchymal stem cells (MSC) from bone marrow derived MSCs or adipose derived stem cells
  - Autologous or allogenic stem cells
- Indications: limited evidence
  - Studies are being done in animals, and limited basis in humans to conclude (146)
  - Done in refractory lateral epicondylitis, refractory patellar tendinopathy and plantar fasciitis
- Techniques (147)
  - Harvest
    - Bone marrow; good chondrogenic and osteogenic potential; preferred
    - Adipose: lower chondrogenic potential (addition of bone morphogenetic protein (BMP) or transforming growth factor (TGF)-beta)
    - Synovial; greater chondrogenic, but less osteogenic potential
  - Stem cells amplification
    - Concentrated: obtained in fewer passages, cons: heterogeneous composition
    - Expanded: pros: higher MSCs number, cons: contamination risk during amplification
  - Process
    - Intra-articular injection: easy application, but no precise onsite delivery
    - Surgical delivery: direct delivery on lesion site. Cons: invasive delivery approach

1. Approach to the Patient With a Musculoskeletal Problem

Diagnostic nerve block with anesthetic

NAME	POTENCY (LIPID SOLUBILITY)	SPEED OF ONSET (MIN)	DURATION OF ACTION (MIN)	MAXIMAL DOSE[a] (MG/KG)
Lidocaine	3	10–20, rapid	60–200	3–5 1.5 times more toxic than procaine (127)
Mepivacaine	2.4	10–20, very rapid	60–180	5, less potent than lidocaine, less toxic
Bupivacaine	8	15–30	180–360	1.5–3, chondrotoxic and tenotoxic
Ropivacaine		15–30	180–360	3, less chondrotoxic and tenotoxic than bupivacaine (148)
Procaine	1	Slow	60–90	Solutions of 0.5%–2%, used in infiltration and blocks

[a]Maximal dose without epinephrine for axillary nerve block. Doses of lidocaine and mepivacaine can be increased to 7 to 8 mg/kg if epinephrine is added. Lower doses may be toxic if infiltrated subcutaneously, as for intercostal nerve blocks, larger doses of lidocaine and mepivacaine may be tolerated if given by epidural injection.

- Complications of nerve block (149)
  - Systemic: rare except using large volume or axial injection (epidural; spill to the artery to the brain)
    - CNS (seizure) and cardiovascular
    - Lidocaine: cardiac contractility depression (cautious when used more than 20 mL of 1%). Bupivacaine: more disruption of cardiac conduction
  - Local (150)
    - Direct nerve injury; use blunt needle and may inject small dose while advancing slowly (to push the nerve away) or imaging guidance
    Be aware that intraneural injection may not be so painful (just brief paresthesia only)
    - Local nerve ischemia; especially when giving rapid injection
    - Local motor nerve block: dose related, more common with higher concentration (2% lidocaine)
    - Chondrotoxicity: with high dose of bupivacaine in intra-articular injection (in animal model) (151)

Nerve-sclerosing therapy (152)
- Ethyl alcohol (alcohol) block
  - Great affinity to the nervous tissue and when injected in proximity to the nerve → induce dehydration, necrosis, and precipitation of the cell protoplasm → Wallerian degeneration (chemical neurolysis)
  - Alcohol inhibits neurotransmitter receptor function
  - A 30% (~100 mM) solution is preferred
    - A nervous signal inhibition occurs at 80 mM to 120 mM (higher than 20%)
    - Mixture of 100% 0.1 mL alcohol diluted in 0.4 mL of 0.25% bupivacaine (then 20%)
  - Adverse effects: dysesthesia

Different type of neurolysis (see following table)

	ALCOHOL	PHENOL	PULSE RADIOFREQUENCY (153,154)
Mechanism	Nerve coagulation and muscle necrosis by denaturing proteins - At low concentration (5%–10%): blocks Na^+ and K^+ channel acts as a local anesthetic - 35% alcohol (in animal): demyelination mostly in small fibers without axonal damage - 50%–100%: neuronal Wallerian degeneration	<2%: work as local anesthetic Immediate anesthetic effect 5%–7%: denature proteins, effect develops over about 2 days Long lasting: 6–18 months	Selective heating of nervous system (low energy, high frequency, 100–500 KHz) → denervation, impeding nociceptive input Active phase of 20 ms followed by 480 ms of silent phase, temperature ≤42°C
Disadvantage	Slower action More irritating (sclerosing effect) for soft tissues More likely to cause painful neuritis	Higher risk of NP	Localized pain (1%, at needle entry more than 2 weeks)

Source: Adapted from Refs. 155 and 156.

US-guided nerve block (157,158)
- Indications
  - Diagnosis and therapeutic injection for pain from the peripheral entrapment neuropathy
    - Occipital nerve (occipital headache, neck pain), suprascapular nerve (shoulder pain), CTS, cheiralgia paresthetica (superficial radial nerve, wrist pain), PIN block (wrist pain), superior cluneal nerve (buttock pain), lateral femoral cutaneous nerve (meralgia paresthetica), saphenous nerve (medial knee pain), superficial peroneal nerve (dorsum of the foot/ankle pain), sural nerve (lateral ankle pain), and inferior plantar nerve (Baxter's, deep plantar heel pain)
  - Nerve block for spasticity
    - Musculocutaneous nerve block for elbow flexor spasticity, anterior interosseous nerve block for forearm flexor spasticity, femoral and obturator nerve block for adductor spasticity, tibial nerve block for equinus or equinovarus deformity
- Characteristics and advantage
  - US-guided nerve block: faster onset, longer duration, and improved block quality with reduced amounts of local anesthetic, compared with stimulator-guided injection
  - Vessels and nerves are easily identified, and the risk of intravascular and intraneural injection of local anesthetic may be diminished
- Technique
  - In plane (long axis) and out of plane (short axis), perpendicular to the US beam, incidence of US beam to the needle (90°), use shortest path
  - Jiggling (rotate the needle with in and out movement) or hydrolocalization (fluid around the target structure with post acoustic enhancement)
  - Can use stimulator (approximately 0.5 mA to achieve motor twitch): close approximation of the needle tip to the nerve

Other Interventional Procedures

Fluoroscopy-guided steroid injection
- Facet joint injection and medial branch block for diagnosis of facet mediated axial back pain (159)
  - If responsive to diagnostic injection ➔ ablation of medial branch
- Epidural steroid injection or selective nerve block (160)
  - Unclear evidence of superiority over the placebo for radiculopathy: may be effective for short-term pain relief
  - No clear evidence for low back pain without radiation
  - Epidural steroid + lidocaine: no significant benefit over lidocaine in symptomatic spinal stenosis (161)
  - Incorrect placement of needle in 25% to 40% without imaging guidance

Spinal cord stimulation (162)
- Indications; recalcitrant neuropathic pain from postlaminectomy (failed back) syndrome, complex regional pain syndrome, recalcitrant pain from radiculopathy, postherpetic neuralgia, intercostal neuralgia, and phantom pain
- Contraindication: psychiatric disorder (psychosis, schizophrenia, substance abuse, depression/anxiety), infection, coagulopathy, cognitive dysfunction, obliteration of spinal cord
- After interdisciplinary evaluation (including psychological evaluation), lead insertion under local anesthesia (under fluoro guidance) ➔ trial stimulation ➔ if effect documented, implant impulse generator under general anesthesia by surgery and programming

Peripheral nerve stimulation (163,164)
- Indications: failed other treatment for neuropathic pain from posttraumatic neuralgia, postsurgical neuropathic pain, occipital neuralgia, postherniorrhaphy inguinal neuralgia (ilioinguinal/iliohypogastric neuralgia), genitofemoral neuralgia, postherpetic neuralgia, coccygodynia, complex regional pain syndrome (CRPS) type 2, and headache
  - Larger area of pain (multiple peripheral nerves) can be an indication for spinal cord stimulation
- Contraindication: similar to spinal cord stimulator
- Local anesthetic block to predict success for peripheral nerve stimulator, transcutaneous electrical nerve stimulation (TENS) does not have a clear predictive value
- Try trial stimulator for 2 to 14 days

Cryoneuroablation (cryoanalgesia) (165)
- Indication: chronic neuropathic pain recalcitrant to other modalities (chronic craniofacial neuralgia, chest wall pain from neuroma, persistent pain after rib fracture, post herpetic neuralgia, neuralgia, etc)
  - After successful diagnostic block (0.2–0.8 mL of lidocaine) for sensory nerve lesion
- Contraindications: similar to other injection, risk of hyper/depigmentation at the cryolesion site, alopecia (at the eyebrow in supraorbital cryolesion)
- Liquid nitrogen in a hollow tube insulated at the tip to freeze a temperature of −190°C
  - Mechanism; conduction block (similar to the local anesthetic), ice crystal vascular damage to the vaso nervorum ➔ severe endoneural edema ➔ wallerian degeneration but the myelin sheath and endoneurium intact

PHYSICAL AND OCCUPATIONAL THERAPY

Indications
- Common indications for physical therapy (PT): mobility/balance training, therapeutic exercises of lower extremity/pelvic/spine/shoulder dysfunction, manual therapies, education for taping and different modality (ultrasound, transcutaneous electric stimulation, and other heating modalities)
- Common indications for occupational therapy (OT): fine motor skills, ADL, instrumental ADL training, ergonomic evaluation, upper extremity therapeutic exercise (shoulder, elbow, and hand), splinting/wheelchair evaluation/driving evaluation (in some institutions), and neuromuscular training
  - Hand therapy, lymphedema management requiring additional training and certification
- Overlap between PT and OT in some area of MSK problems such as neck, shoulder, elbow pain, and others
- Frequency: two to three times weekly for 6 to 12 times (frequency and numbers are often limited by insurance carrier ➔ transition to home exercise program: important)

- Stretching and improving range after modality as strengthening requires more time (although patient feels quick improvement of strength from better recruitment/firing pattern of motor units)
  - Focus on education of therapeutic exercise rather than passive modality (often available for use at home)
- Specify the practical goal and specific protocol (therapeutic exercise, modality, etc): helps to guide therapists although it can be modified based on their assessment
- Important to communicate with the therapist regarding the details of exercise and check the patient for compliance especially when the patient is not making progress

Follow-ups after PT and OT
- Reevaluation after the first-planned sessions (8–12 sessions)
- To reassess and plan the following step after the completion of therapy and education
  - Review the home exercise program, plan for the transitional place/gym in the community to continue the exercise program or aerobic endurance exercise
- Review component of therapeutic exercise, compliance, and problem with exercise
  - Communicate with the therapist
  - Compliance of patient improves with repetition of plan and consistency from physician and therapist

Common problems and limitations (166)
- No home exercise program. The effect of training: lost after 4 to 8 weeks
  - When training is reestablished, the rate at which training effects occur do not appear to be faster
- Overtraining fatigue syndrome
  - Particularly in young athletes or population with sports activity
  - Prolonged decreased sport specific performance, usually lasting >2 weeks
  - Possible underlying mechanism: premature fatigability, emotional and mood changes, lack of motivation, infections and overuse injuries
- Medical clearance for exercise (167,168)
  - Evaluate the individual risk and exercise program
  - Indications for exercise stress test: H/O CAD or MI, high-risk occupation, valvular heart disease, or arrhythmia or pacemaker, two or more CV risk factors, DM older than age 35 years, DM >10 to 15 years, end stage renal disease (ESRD), pulmonary disease (cystic fibrosis, asthma, interstitial lung disease, chronic obstructive pulmonary disease [COPD])
  - Consider referral to cardiac rehab or monitored setting
  - Emphasis for warm up and cool down

Therapeutic Exercise

Flexibility exercise
- Introduction
  - Tight muscle related to MSK problems or pain (examples illustrated in each chapter)
  - Stretched muscle to a greater than normal length → new sarcomere added
    - Muscle in stretched position if possible (especially during immobility)
    - Muscle permanently lengthened from increase in number of sarcomeres
    - Muscle at rest; tendency to be shortened. Muscle in shortened position → sarcomere at the end of muscle fiber disappears
  - Muscle–tendon unit: 95:5 ratio (muscle stretching is effective way for flexibility)
  - Muscle tendon feedback control system
    - Stretch initially → muscle spindle activate → contract
    - Stretch >6 seconds → Golgi tendon organ (inhibit muscle contraction) fires → relaxation
  - Independent factor in physical fitness (with strength, power, endurance, and coordination)
  - Minimal flexibility during age 10 to 12 years because of growth spurt (muscle/tendon unable to catch up)
- Therapeutic implication
  - Inflexibility: prevalent in most MSK problems and aggravating factor
    - Engaging patient education at early stage also improves compliance as most patients understand this concept well
    - Musculotendinous tightness concomitant with contracture/stiffness of the joint
      - Stretching of musculotendinous component increases ROM of the joint (also delineate the tightness component from contracture)
  - Flexibility to prevent injury: controversial
    - Stretching exercise may be detrimental before high velocity, impact exercise
    - Stretching is most effective during the cool down phase (with increased body temperature)
- Exercise prescription
  - Different types of stretching
    - Ballistic: bouncing or jerking maneuver, less efficient, may cause injury
    - Passive: concern for increased risk of injury in recreational or competitive athletes
    - Static: 15 to 60 seconds, three to five repetitions
    - Neuromuscular facilitation; hold relax, or contract relax technique by muscle length-tension thermostat; more efficient
  - ROM exercise
    - Generally start with active assisted ROM → active ROM → passive ROM
    - Emphasis for ROM exercise in the inpatient, deconditioned patient or patient with impaired mobility
      - Important to prevent contracture and stiffness (even a few times a day can be very effective)
    - Proprioceptive neuromuscular facilitation (PNF): after antagonist muscle is activated (→ relaxation of agonist) followed by stretching agonist
    - For examle, 6-second contraction followed by 10 to 30 seconds assisted stretch for PNF, three to five repetition >3/wk
  - Focus on end range; can use muscle energy principle
  - Static, dynamic, and PNF stretching of major muscle groups including the low back and posterior thigh to a mild degree of discomfort

Manual therapy
- Commonly used therapeutic exercise to increase flexibility/mobility and decrease pain, combined technique; indirect then direct techniques (166)

- Direct and indirect technique
  - Direct technique: moves the body part(s) in the direction of the restrictive barrier
    - Thrust (impulse, high velocity, low amplitude: a quick but forceful thrust applied externally for restriction of motion)
      - Precaution in older or frail patients (osteoporosis, any bony disease, tumor, instability, anticoagulation, etc)
    - Articulation (low-velocity, high-amplitude), rhythmic oscillation applied to a joint to restore neutral mechanics to that joint
    - Muscle energy (direct isometric), contract–relax: contract the shortened muscle to relax/stretch
    - Direct myofascial release (load [stretch] tissues, hold and wait for release)
  - Indirect technique: moves the body part away from the restrictive barrier
    - Strain-counterstrain
      - Identify a tender point located in the muscle belly, tendon, or dermatome of the shortened/tight muscle
      - Move the body part(s) in a direction of freer motion (also the direction of the original injury) until tenderness in the tender point is absent or minimal
      - Hold for 90 seconds. Return to the original position slowly
    - Indirect balancing
      - Move the body part(s) away from the restrictive barrier and in a direction of freer motion
      - The proper position is obtained when tension is equal on all sides of the dysfunction. Hold, and wait for release
    - Indirect myofascial release and craniosacral (to release restrictions around the spinal cord and brain) (169)
    - Combined approach
- Sacroiliac mobilization (170,171)
  - Sacroiliac joint dysfunction (or pelvic malalignment) or sacroiliac immobility often related to low back/buttock pain
    - Mobilization of SI joint by contraction of muscle attached to sacrum or ilium
    - With fixed insertion of muscle, contraction mobilizes bone muscle originates: gluteal M contraction on hyperflexed hip; shin to the chest → will mobilize the ilium because the femur is fixed
  - High-velocity, low-amplitude thrust with the patient in the side-lying position

Stabilization exercise
- Scapular stabilization exercise
  - Functionally unstable scapula or scapular dyskinesia: related to suboptimal shoulder function (decreased performance) and predisposes the individual to shoulder injury
  - Indications: shoulder impingement syndrome/rotator cuff syndrome, myofascial pain syndrome, adhesive capsulitis, and glenohumeral internal rotation deficit (172,173)
- Core stabilization exercise (174,175)
  - Address dysfunction from intrinsic neuro-muscular control and extrinsic motor behavior
  - Common indications: low back pain (core system dissipate the loading to the spine), pelvic, gluteal region pain and dysfunction

Education (biomechanics and home exercise program)
- Back school
  - Group classes providing education about back pain including anatomy, biomechanics, advice about proper lifting technique, ergonomic training and advice about exercise and active lifestyle, ~1 hr/wk for two sessions (176)
- Home exercise program: different exercise programs specific to the disease with repetitions in addition to aerobic endurance exercise, especially for patients with sedentary lifestyle
- Energy conservation technique
  - Indicated in chronic disabling conditions from MSK (eg, RA), neurologic and neuromuscular diseases

Proprioception/neuromuscular control exercise
- Clinical implications in MSK pathologies
  - Impaired from injury or disease (underrecognized)
    - Knee and ankle ligament injury → decrease proprioception → increased risk of joint damage, reinjury and falls
    - Repair (even surgical repair) does not repair proprioception
    - Strength does not guarantee good neuromuscular control
  - Overuse of the proximal stabilizer/neighboring body segment (unrelated to the demand of the task) for precise mechanism can aggravate the condition or delay the recovery
- Exercise
  - Promoting position sense without visual input (eye closed) to enhance joint function
  - Unidirectional board initially then multidirectional board, carioca (sideways running), and backward running
  - Elastic bandage (by stimulation of proprioceptors in the skin) or kinesiotaping

Strengthening exercise
- Mechanism (often useful to educate the patient)
  - Immediate improvement after starting strengthening exercise by neural adaptation
    - Within the first few weeks of a training (early strength/tension gain); recruit larger motor units with higher frequency
  - Muscle hypertrophy: time for hypertrophy varies on age and comorbidities
    - After 6 to 7 weeks of resistance training
    - Increase of cross sectional diameter, more common in fast twitch (type 2A) and by increasing myofibril (actin/myosin), rare in increase of muscle fiber
- Different mode and protocol: none superior to the other
  - Isometric at initial phase: no intentional joint motion, may reduce pain, edema, and atrophy
    - Exercise at different angle of joint position (different fiber recruited at specific angle)
  - Isotonic: active ROM, eccentric then concentric: better carry over than the opposite way
  - Isokinetic: same speed, variable loading, safe in high rate (compared to isotonic exercise), needs equipment such as Cybex, etc
  - Resistive strengthening exercise (different mode available): progressive resistance (MC mode)
    - Specific strengthening exercise involve specific type of muscle fibers recruitment
      - Type 2 muscle cells are recruited first in high velocity (eg, plyometric) activities (vs type 1 muscle fiber

recruited first like Henneman size principle in gradual increase in strength)
- Different principles available: no superiority over the other
  – DeLorme: 10 repetition, 50 → 75 → 100% (of 10 repetition maximum) in each set
  10 repetition maximum: heaviest weight for 10 consecutive repetitions
  – Oxford: the opposite of DeLorme: 100% → 75 → 50%
  – Daily adjusted progressive resistance exercise methods
  – Exercise to the point of muscle fatigue
- Eccentric (lengthening contraction) strengthening (177)
  – Recommended for most of tendinopathy: epicondylitis (lateral and medial), noninsertional Achilles tendinopathy and other tendinopathy
  – Informed to exercise through pain so long as it was not "disabling"
  – Resistance can be increased when the training session could be completed pain free
  – Cautious of injury especially with fast eccentric contraction
- Exercise with elastic band: modified, dynamic resistive exercise
  – Thera-band®: elastic bands made of rubber latex. Come in different colors with a specific force of resistance (178)
  – Cautious at the beginning; mismatch of the band can cause pain or injury
- Plyometric training (at the later/advanced stage of therapy)
  – A brief, explosive maneuver consists of an eccentric muscle followed by a concentric contraction, vary in intensity (ground reaction force of four to five times of body weight)
  – For example, 2 feet in place jumps to hopping and bounding for maximum distance, jumps from boxes of varying height
  – Improved muscle strength, performance, and decreased injuries, initially with caution (166)
○ American College of Sports Medicine (ACSM) Guideline for strengthening exercise
- Frequency: ≥2/wk, duration <1 hour
- Dynamic exercise, low to moderate speed, through a full ROM
- Normal breathing (breath holding can increase blood pressure [BP] with heavy resistance exercise)

Exercise Prescription

Introduction
- Indications
  ○ Maintenance exercise program after PT and OT as the MSK pain improves/recovers from injury
  ○ Anyone who does not do exercise routinely or with sedentary lifestyle
- Exercise can prolong life span by modifying risk factors for chronic disease
- Cardiovascular/endurance/strengthening/flexibility exercise for lifetime

Cardiovascular endurance training
- Benefits: control diastolic BP, glucose control and improve aerobic capacity
  ○ No change in systolic BP, lipid profile, and body fat loss
- Prescribe mode, intensity, duration of time, frequency, and progression
  ○ Mode: large muscle group in rhythmic aerobic activity
  ○ Intensity guideline
    - Subjective: rating of perceived exertion (Borg scale; a range of 12–16; somewhat hard [13] to hard [15] to very hard [104])
    - Objective: heart rate (HR) based
      – HR max: 220-age or HR reserve method (Karvonen method)
        → 70% to 85% of HR max; similar to 55% to 75% of VO_2 max
        → Target HR: (HR max − HR rest; HR reserve) × 0.5 to 0.85 (50%–85%) + HR rest.
      – 60% to 70% × HR max, 70% to 80%, 80% to 90%, respectively for unconditioned, intermediate and advanced fitness
    - Vigorous cardiovascular exercise: increase aerobic fitness more effectively than moderate intensity exercise, greater cardioprotective benefits (179)
    - Vigorous: either ≥6 metabolic equivalents (METs) (walking at 4 mph: 4.5–5.5 MET, shoveling snow: 6–7 MET, >6 MET: jogging, running, rope jumping, calisthenics) or ≥60% of aerobic capacity (VO_2 max)
  ○ Duration: 20 to 60 minutes of continuous aerobic activity. For deconditioned, multiple, short duration exercise session <10 minutes
  ○ Frequency: 3 to 5 d/wk, more frequent for deconditioned

Special Groups
Obese patients
- Decrease the risk for cardiovascular disease ± weight reduction, and successful weight management requires a lifelong commitment
- Goal: frequency ≥5/wk, 55% to 85% of maximal HR, ≥30 (upto 90) minutes each time, with progressive resistive exercise, 2–3/wk (180)
- Nonweight bearing activity at the beginning if pain in the lower extremity (eg, pool exercise)

Seniors (181)
- Balanced exercise program of both endurance and resistance, for example, ≥2/wk for frail elderly
- Endurance exercise (walking, cycling, and dancing) to improve aerobic capacity
  ○ Starts with 40% of max HR and short duration (5–10 min) with warm up and cool down
  ○ Risks: cardiac event and worsening MSK pain (knee, hip, and ankle pain in weight-bearing exercise)
- Resistance exercise to increase muscle mass and strength
  ○ Fewer repetitions with moderate gradually to high resistance, increase weight slowly, and load around 40% to 50% of baseline
  ○ Risks: fracture of osteoporotic bone and exacerbation of underlying joint disease

Patients with MSK pathologies
- OA
  ○ Strengthening, low-impact aerobic exercise, and neuromuscular education; strongly recommended

- Specific types of exercise
  - Cardiovascular land exercise: strong recommendation and high-quality research
  - Aquatic exercise: strong recommendation with moderate quality
  - Tai Chi, kinesthesia, and balance exercise: weak recommendation and low quality

Patients with neuromuscular disease (182)
- Moderate intensity aerobic endurance training to improve cardiopulmonary condition
- Low-intensity resistance exercise for individual with strength ≥3 (antigravity strength)/5
- High resistance exercise: should be avoided (no more advantage over a moderate resistance but cause more injury)

Pregnant patients (183)
- Aerobics, resistance training, swimming ± impact activities
  - Weight-bearing to nonweight bearing exercise as pregnancy progresses (cycling and swimming in second half of pregnancy), stretching exercise
  - Avoid collision sports and deep-water diving
  - Hydrate adequately, avoid extreme weather, wear loose-fitting clothes
  - Stop exercise if tired, dizzy, nauseated, overheated, or short of breath
- ≥30 minutes of moderate exercise on most days
- Safe therapeutic exercise
  - Core exercise: abdominal curl, crunches in first trimester, modified squat
  - Stretching: hamstring, tailor/cobbler position and tailor press
  - Pelvic floor, buttock, and abdominal strengthening: Kegel exercise, pelvic tilt, lateral bends
- Contraindications: preeclampsia/eclampsia, premature rupture of the membranes, antepartum hemorrhage, placenta previa, vasa previa, incompetent cervix/cerclage, significant maternal cardiac disease, restrictive lung disease, fetal growth restriction, chronic placental abruption, multiple gestation

Modality (166)

- Main therapeutic implication: provide temporary relief of pain
- Factors to consider in selection: target tissue (depth), heating/cold, intensity, comorbid conditions with history of cancer, age (epiphyses), and pregnancy

Prescription
- Indication, modality of choice, location, intensity, duration, and frequency
- Commonly used modalities (see following table)

MODALITY		CHARACTERISTICS	CONTRAINDICATION
Cold Modality		Immediate cutaneous vasoconstriction and delayed reactive vasodilatation Decreased acute inflammation Neuromuscular • Decreased muscle stretch reflex amplitudes • Increased maximal isometric strength and decreased muscle fatigue • Temporarily reduced spasticity Joint and connective tissue • Increased joint stiffness and decreased tendon extensibility Miscellaneous • Decreased pain • General relaxation	Cold intolerance/hypersensitivity/Raynaud disease or phenomenon Cryotherapy-induced neurapraxia or axonotmesis • Conduction block and axonal degeneration with prolonged cold exposure Impaired sensation, cognitive/communication dysfunction Arterial/hematologic disease
	Ice massage	Localized symptoms for 5–10 minutes per site	
	Spray and stretch	Ix: myofascial pain syndrome Unidirectional application ethyl chloride spray on trigger area and extend to the reference zone with passive stretching, 4 inches/s	
Hydrotherapy	Contrast bath	Hot (42–45°C/~110°F) then cold (8.5–12.5°C, ~50°F) water for 30 minutes and 10 minutes Immersion in hot water, followed by alternating immersions of 1 minute in cold and 4 minutes in hot water and ending the session Cyclic vasoconstriction and vasodilatation produced by the temperature extremes; decrease pain and swelling	
	Contrast bath	Ix: rheumatologic disease, neuropathic pain, or other chronic pain syndromes such as complex regional pain syndrome Contraindication similar to cold and heat modality	

(continued)

MODALITY			CHARACTERISTICS	CONTRAINDICATION
Heat			Musculoskeletal pain, contracture, muscle relaxation and chronic inflammation Hemodynamic • Increased blood flow, bleeding, acute inflammation/edema • Decreased chronic inflammation Neuromuscular • Increased nerve conduction velocity Joint and connective tissue • Increased tendon extensibility/increased collagenase activity • Decreased joint stiffness and pain	General heat precautions • Acute trauma, inflammation, edema • Impaired circulation • Bleeding diatheses • Large scars • Impaired sensation • Malignancy • Cognitive or communication deficits that preclude reporting of pain
Sup. Heat		Hot colloid pack	After several minutes, check the skin 30 minutes → 1°C increase	Focal pressure from lying on a hot pack; increase heating (due to decreased carry away of the heat) or pressure sore
		Radiant heat (infrared)	Intensity determined by distance (multiplied by 4) and angle of delivery (perpendicular; highest). Put the heater at 30–60 cm from the body	Precautions: light sensitivity, skin drying, and dermal photoaging
		Fluidotherapy	Superficial dry convective heating with forced hot air and a bed of finely divided solid particles The massaging action and the freedom to perform ROM exercises. Common indications: hand and wrist pain	General heat precaution Cross contamination (infected wound)
		Paraffin bath	By conduction Dipping, immersion, and brushing Common indications: scleroderma (with friction massage) and RA	Open wound Impaired sensation Similar precaution to TENS
		Transcutaneous electrical nerve stimulation (TENS)	High frequency (50–100 Hz)/low voltage; pain modulation by gait theory Low frequency (1–4 Hz)/high voltage; acupuncture like, increase endorphin release Hypoalgesia; last up to 5 minutes after cessation Common indications: knee pain/osteoarthritis, myofascial pain and low back pain	Near pacemaker Pregnancy Near carotid sinus
Deep		Ultrasound	Deeper structure (eg, hip joint), 0.5–2 W/cm² temperature upto 46°C, Mode: continuous or pulse, around 1 MHz Indications: MSK pain, bony nonunion, and chronic wound healing	Near brain, eyes, reproductive organs Pregnancy or during menstruation Near pacemaker Near laminectomy sites Malignancy Skeletal immaturity Methyl methacrylate or high-density polyethylene (in joint arthroplasty)
Others		Iontophoresis	The migration of charged particles across biologic membranes under an imposed electrical field The ionic solution to be iontophoresis is placed on the electrode of the same polarity A direct current, typically between 10 and 30 mA	Open wound Impaired sensation Similar precaution to TENS
		Phonophoresis	The use of ultrasound for transdermal migration Pulsed mode, 1 MHz transducer frequency, stroking technique, 1–1.5 W/cm², for ~ 5 minutes per site.	Same as US precaution
		Low energy laser	Deliver <90 mW (vs surgical laser: 10 to 100 + W), intense focal light therapy Wide varieties of equipment/design with conflicting results	Pregnancy, epileptic seizure Pacemaker (for device using electrical stimulation too) Not to the thyroid gland Cancer (radiation therapy), diabetes (uncontrolled) Pediatric

Ix, indication; MSK, musculoskeletal; ROM, range of motion; TENS, transcutaneous electrical nerve stimulation; US, ultrasound.

Extracorporeal shock wave (184)
- Classification: focused (orthotripsy or lithotripsy) versus radial (185)
  - For MSK disorders: orthotripsy or radial
  - High (requiring regional or general anesthesia) and low energy (can be applied in clinic)
- Suggested mechanisms through neovascularization (angiogenic growth factor) and cavitation bubble (when it bursts → force to break down pathologic deposits of calcification and positive effect on inflammatory healing response)
- Indications (186)
  - Plantar fasciitis, lateral epicondylitis, patellar tendinitis, medial epicondylitis, and coccygodynia
    - Achilles tendon; high-energy shock wave, low energy (no difference with placebo)
    - Calcific tendinopathy for shoulder; may require high energy
    - FDA approved for lateral epicondylitis and plantar fasciitis
- Contraindication: neurological/vascular disease, ligament/fascia rupture, open growth plate, pregnancy, implanted metal, anticoagulants, bleeding disorder, or implanted cardiac device
- Application
  - 10 to 20 minutes, three to five sessions, separated over 10 to 20 minutes
  - Discourage taking antiinflammatory or ice

Cervical traction
- Manual cervical traction before home traction
- Supine and head supported by therapist, neck flexed 20° to 25° and traction force
- Mechanical: 10 lbs to 35 lbs (10 lbs is minimum weight to counterbalance a head) for 15 to 20 minutes
  - Different mode: intermittent (using motorized) versus sustained (to induce fatigue in paraspinal M)

Lumbar traction
- Needs a great amount of force (between 60 and 200 lbs or half of patient body weight), not as effective as cervical traction

Alternative Therapies
- No strong evidence of superiority over traditional therapeutic exercise, but if PT or OT program is not successful, consider alternative therapies to patients or completed PT or OT

Acupuncture
- Neurostimulatory technique that induces analgesia and other neurophysiologic effects by inserting small needles into acupuncture points along meridians on the surfaces of the body (corresponding to anatomic locations of the motor points)
- Common indications: MSK pain (OA [187] and short-term pain relief and functional improvement for chronic low back pain [188])
- Contraindications: similar to injection in general

Pilates
- Exercise that promotes rhythmic movement through proximally based strength, flexibility, and coordination
- Common indications: back and neck pain

Feldenkrais
- Use of movement to increase kinesthetic awareness, enabling more functional, efficient, less-painful movement
- Common indications: neck and shoulder pain

Alexander technique
- Psychophysical reeducation methods focusing on kinesthetic awareness, particularly of the head and neck, to improve posture during movement
- Common indications: headaches, arthritis, and chronic low back pain

Yoga
- Mind-body therapy, stretching and breathing, MSK conditions such as back pain, arthritis, and CTS

Tai chi
- Improves balance, flexibility, and cardiovascular fitness in geriatric patients, significant increase in ROM

Water exercise therapy
- Unloading that relied on submergence in water, which can accomplish greater levels of unloading than land-based therapy

ORTHOSES
- Externally applied device used to modify the structural and functional characteristics of the neuromuscular and skeletal systems
- Commonly prescribed orthotics for MSK pain: check individual chapter

Common problems in using orthotics
Compliance
- More extensive/bulky orthotics: less likely to be worn ("best brace is no brace")
  - Consider age, activities, and comorbidities (skin/edema, cardiac status) of patients
  - Custom made orthotics should be cast after edema stabilized or controlled
- Aesthetic concern is important in some patients (eg, job requirement)
  - Ideally trial of brace, or show picture or a sample before ordering orthotics
- Some orthotics need frequent modification or adjustment; better to be seen at specialized orthotic clinic; especially University of California Biomechanics Laboratory orthosis (UCBL), supramalleolar orthosis (SMO), and AFO
- Initially uncomfortable (but shouldn't be painful) to wear any orthotic; increase wearing time gradually
- Consider the future modification
  - Easier to trim the orthotic, but more difficult to add or expand the existing orthotic
  - Prepare some adhesive felt material in the office and prepare heat gun (limited modification possible) in orthotic clinic or send the patient to orthotist for modification with specifics
- Does not overcorrect the deformity: poor compliance with pain

- Goal is to maintain or mitigate progression to further deformity
- Material stiffness: polyethylene < co-polymer < polypropylene < laminated (most stiff)
- Thickness of the orthotics affect the stiffness; thinner orthotic, better tolerated (but may required stiffer material for obese or highly active patient)
- Adding the layer; soft interface, foot insert on AFO, Gillet modification (outside the medial hindfoot plate

Finance
- Important aspect to consider

TREATMENT BASED ON DIFFERENT ANATOMICAL PATHOLOGIES

Tendinopathy (43)
- Relative rest (continue activities if symptoms are not worsening), ice, compression, and elevation (RICE) in the acute stage
- Oral medication
  - Short-term use of anti-inflammatory medications (7–14 days maximum)
    - No evidence of benefit with long-term use and caution for cardiovascular, renal, and GI adverse effects, and so on
  - Acetaminophen for pain control as needed
  - Topical glycerol trinitrate on the point of maximal tenderness—for short term
    - When refractory to anti-inflammatories
    - The most common adverse effect is headache, especially interactions with antihypertensives/antianginal could also possibly be present
- Therapy
  - Cyclic tension applied to healing tendons stimulates the intrinsic healing response
  - Eccentric exercise: not only clinical benefits (↓ pain, ↑ performance), but also improve MRI and histologic findings. However, benefit is not universal in different conditions
    - Midportion (noninsertional) Achilles tendinopathy in athletic population
    - Less effective in less athletic population or other tendinopathy
  - Externally paced resistance training using metronome (189)
    - Either isometric (greater immediate analgesia) or isotonic; no significant difference
- Injection
  - Corticosteroid injections to reduce inflammation in peritendinous structures, but no effect on underlying pathology. Short-term relief of symptoms
  - Platelet-rich plasma (PRP)
    - Autologous whole blood—same goal as PRP, but there is less evidence of its efficacy
  - Prolotherapy—injection of high osmotic pressure, which are thought to cause inflammation and promote healing. More evidence is needed for its recommendation
- Extracorporeal shockwave therapy (ESWT)
  - Hypothesized to disrupt growth of new nerves into the diseased tendon. It may also promote tenocyte proliferation
  - Conflicting evidence and reserved for patients recalcitrant to first-line conservative measures
- Operative management
  - Indication: failure of conservative management
    - Failure rates of surgery can be as high as 20% to 30%
  - Common procedures
    - Tenotomy: trigger angiogenesis that can promote healing. Percutaneously using large bore needle, like 18 gauge under ultrasound guidance and local anesthesia in some cases
    - Open (or arthroscopic/minimally invasive) debridement and excision of degenerated portions of tendon along with release of adhesions: MC procedure with side-to-side tendon repair or end-to-end repair if large areas of tendon are excised (>25%)
  - Postoperative care
    - A short period of immobilization followed by postoperative mobilization techniques to diminish the formation of adhesions and enhance the end result

Ligament injury (190,191)
- Conservative treatment: initial treatment for acute injuries
  - Protection: prevention of further injury and avoidance of potentially aggravating factors
  - Rest: sling in upper limb injuries, immobilization should be minimized
    - Early weight bearing and exercises for ROM, followed by proprioceptive exercises and strengthening of muscles around the affected joint as necessary
    - Orthotic for unstable injuries (usually in chronic case)
  - Ice: reduces swelling and may reduce need for analgesics, compression, and elevation
  - NSAID use for 3 to 7 days for pain control or acetaminiophen
  - Gradual return to full activity/sports; check individual chapter
  - Physical therapy similar to the tendon injury: emphasis on the joint proprioceptive exercise as ligament is important sensory organ (192)
- Operative treatment
  - Indications: high-grade injuries, multiple ligaments injuries, competitive athletes, or cases of chronic instability or failed conservative management
  - Direct repair of injured ligaments
  - Ligament substitution with neighboring ligaments, tendon autografts/allografts or wire loops, or other synthetic materials such as Dacron, Mersilene tape, or polydioxanone (193)

Bursitis
- Relative rest for a few days, activity modification, modality (ice, heating) and NSAID ± education to address underlying faulty biomechanics
- Injection (lidocaine and steroid) ± aspiration of effusion (if significant)
  - US-guided injection if there is minimal amount of effusion (difficult to inject correctly blindly in cases without significant effusion)
- Surgery
  - Common procedure: bursectomy with/without bony resection

Neuropathy
- Management of focal entrapment/regional neuropathy

- Modification of aggravating factor: stop and modify activities worsening symptoms
  - Stop lifting up heavy object or throwing → may stretch brachial plexus with inferior shoulder subluxation or glenohumeral instability
  - Cycling (handle bar) or driving with leaning the elbow on the side: ulnar nerve entrapment on the wrist and the elbow
  - Inversion ankle sprain; stretch/injure superficial peroneal nerve: lateral heel wedge
- Orthotics or bracing in mild cases; for example, cock up splint for CTS, elbow strap with relief for ulnar neuropathy, custom-made relief in foot orthotics
- Nerve block ± hydrodissection (imaging-guided injection preferred): diagnostic and therapeutic injection
- Referral to therapy (improve mobilization of peripheral nerve, or neighboring structures [tendon-gliding exercise]) and education to avoid abnormal compensation strategies or improve ergonomics
- Surgical referral for release if conservative management failed
- Systematic/diffuse neuropathy: symptomatic treatment; check neuropathic pain section

Stress fracture (194)
- General principles (Flowchart 1.7)
  - Decide conservative versus surgical referral
  - Location of the fracture → divide into high-risk and low-risk fracture
    - High risk: femoral neck, tibia diaphysis, navicular, and 5th metatarsal diaphysis
    - Low risk: 2nd to 4th metatarsal, calcaneus, posteromedial tibia, and lateral malleolus
  - Femoral neck (based on x-ray and MRI, send the patient to ortho) and tibial shaft
    - Intramedullary nail; early return to sport, but no significant difference in navicular fracture
  - Low-risk stress fracture: conservative management with splinting and/or functional braces
- Conservative management
  - Rest, ice, compression and elevation (RICE)
    - Immobilization with crutches (practical to give BL because of difficulty using one side) and cast boot as indicated initially
    - Relative rest (avoid offending activity at least 12 weeks (196)
  - Nonimpact exercise: swimming, cycling or water running, and nonweight-bearing stretching
  - Evaluation of intrinsic and extrinsic factors and modification
  - Evaluation of nutritional disorder and eating habits, referral to dietitian
  - DEXA scan, calcium (1,500 mg/d), and vitamin D (800 IU/d)

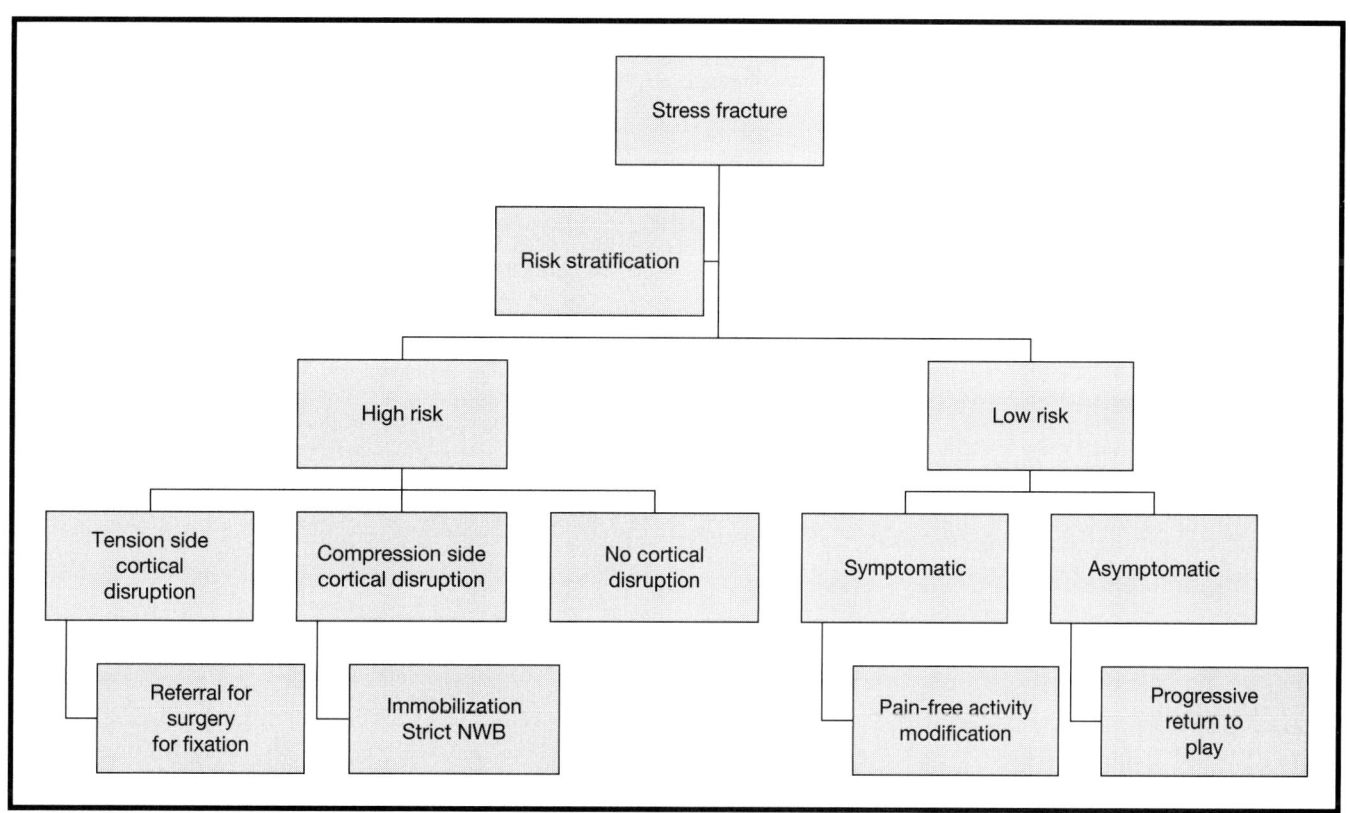

FLOWCHART 1.7
Management of stress fracture.
NWB, non-weight bearing.
Source: Adapted from Ref. (195) McCormick F, Nwachukwu BU, Provencher MT. Stress fractures in runners. *Clin Sports Med*. 2012;31(2):291–306.

- Referral to endocrinology if needed
- Shoe wear change q6 months or 300 to 500 miles for lower extremity injuries related to weight-bearing activity

Other fracture
- General principle of pathologic fracture management (197)
  - Roles and methods of fixation: different from each case, requires immediate mobilization and usually doesn't require fracture healing to achieve stability
  - Bisphosphonate: can decrease the rate of pathologic fractures in general, especially with breast cancer and myeloma
- Metastatic spine disease management
  - Referral to spine surgery, oncology, radiation oncology, and interventional spine management
    - Epidural compression from metastases to the spine and myelopathy, surgical decompression is more effective than radiation
- Rehabilitation for patients with fractures
  - Complications during healing
    - Delayed union, nonunion, malunion, posttraumatic arthritis, growth abnormality (in pediatric fracture), joint stiffness, disuse atrophy, complex regional pain syndrome, etc
  - Pain control, edema control initially: gentle massage and compressive garment
  - General guideline for weight-bearing status
    - Cemented arthroplasty: WBAT versus noncemented; toe touch or NWB in the lower extremities, check with orthopedic surgeon
  - ROM: active assisted exercise, isometric strengthening at least, neuromuscular reeducation, resistive exercises, modality then exercise
  - Mobility, ADL, and IADL training

REFERENCES

1. Harper JD. Determining foot and ankle impairments by the AMA fifth edition guides. *Foot Ankle Clin.* 2002;7(2):291–303.
2. Powell RA, Downing J, Ddungu H, Mwangi-Powell FN. *Pain history and pain assessment.* International Association for the Study of Pain; 2010, Seattle, Washington: IASP, 67–78.
3. Werner C, Boos N. History and physical examination spinal disorders. In: Boos N, Aebi M, ed. Berlin, Heidelberg: Springer, Berlin Heidelberg; 2008:201–225.
4. Hunter DJ, Zhang W, Conaghan PG, et al. Systematic review of the concurrent and predictive validity of MRI biomarkers in OA. *Osteoarthr Cartil.* 2011;19(5):557–588.
5. Hunter DJ, Zhang W, Conaghan PG, et al. Systematic review of the concurrent and predictive validity of MRI biomarkers in OA. *Osteoarthr Cartil.* 2011;19(5):557–588.
6. Benjamin M. The fascia of the limbs and back–a review. *J Anat.* 2009;214(1):1–18.
7. Giamberardino MA, Affaitati G, Fabrizio A, Costantini R. Myofascial pain syndromes and their evaluation. *Best Pract Res Clin Rheumatol.* 2011;25(2):185–198.
8. Krebs EE, Carey TS, Weinberger M. Accuracy of the pain numeric rating scale as a screening test in primary care. *J Gen Intern Med.* 2007;22(10):1453–1458.
9. McLafferty E, Farley A. Assessing pain in patients. *Nurs Stand.* 2008;22(25):42–46.
10. Farrar JT, Young JP Jr, LaMoreaux L, et al. Clinical importance of changes in chronic pain intensity measured on an 11-point numerical pain rating scale. *Pain.* 2001;94(2):149–158.
11. Puhl AA, Reinhart CJ, Rok ER, Injeyan HS. An examination of the observed placebo effect associated with the treatment of low back pain—a systematic review. *Pain Res Manag.* 2011;16(1):45–52.
12. Marx JA, Hockberger RS, Walls RM, Adams J, Rosen P. *Rosen's Emergency Medicine: Concepts and Clinical Practice.* 7th ed. Philadelphia, PA: Mosby/Elsevier; 2010.
13. Bogduk N. The anatomy and pathophysiology of neck pain. *Phys Med Rehabil Clin N Am.* 2011;22(3):367–82, vii.
14. Gelauff J, Stone J, Edwards M, Carson A. The prognosis of functional (psychogenic) motor symptoms: a systematic review. *J Neurol Neurosurg Psychiatr.* 2014;85(2):220–226.
15. Stone J. Functional neurological symptoms. *J R Coll Physicians Edinb.* 2011;41(1):38–41; quiz 42.
16. Escalante A, Haas RW, del Rincon I. A model of impairment and functional limitation in rheumatoid arthritis. *BMC Musculoskelet Disord.* 2005;6:16.
17. Yamout BI, Kyriakides T, Tamim W, Drousiotov A. Myalgia, neuromyopathy and internalized capillaries: a steroid responsive syndrome. *Acta Neurol Scand.* 1995;91(4):294–296.
18. Arendt-Nielsen L, Svensson P. Referred muscle pain: basic and clinical findings. *Clin J Pain.* 2001;17(1):11–19.
19. Stecco A, Gesi M, Stecco C, Stern R. Fascial components of the myofascial pain syndrome. *Curr Pain Headache Rep.* 2013;17(8):352.
20. Malanga GA, Cruz Colon EJ. Myofascial low back pain: a review. *Phys Med Rehabil Clin N Am.* 2010;21(4):711–724.
21. O'Connor F, Sallis R, Wilder R, Pierre P. *Sports medicine: Just the facts.* New York: McGraw Hill Professional; 2004.
22. Abrams GD, Renstrom PA, Safran MR. Epidemiology of musculoskeletal injury in the tennis player. *Br J Sports Med.* 2012;46(7):492–498.
23. Mitchell CH, Brushart TM, Ahlawat S, et al. MRI of sports-related peripheral nerve injuries. *AJR Am J Roentgenol.* 2014;203(5):1075–1084.
24. Shiri R, Viikari-Juntura E. Lateral and medial epicondylitis: role of occupational factors. *Best Pract Res Clin Rheumatol.* 2011;25(1):43–57.
25. Lancourt J, Kettelhut M. Predicting return to work for lower back pain patients receiving worker's compensation. *Spine.* 1992;17(6):629–640.
26. Gupte C, St Mart JP. The acute swollen knee: diagnosis and management. *J R Soc Med.* 2013;106(7):259–268.
27. Ely JW, Osheroff JA, Chambliss ML, Ebell MH. Approach to leg edema of unclear etiology. *J Am Board Fam Med.* 2006;19(2):148–160.
28. McMahon CJ, Wu JS, Eisenberg RL. Muscle edema. *AJR Am J Roentgenol.* 2010;194(4):W284–W292.
29. Parmar MS. Diabetic muscle infarction. *BMJ.* 2009;338:b2271.
30. Aboulafia AJ, Monson DK, Kennon RE. Clinical and radiological aspects of idiopathic diabetic muscle infarction. Rational approach to diagnosis and treatment. *J Bone Joint Surg Br.* 1999;81(2):323–326.
31. Abate M, Silbernagel KG, Siljeholm C, et al. Pathogenesis of tendinopathies: inflammation or degeneration? *Arthritis Res Ther.* 2009;11(3):235.
32. Charalambous CP, Morrey BF. Posttraumatic elbow stiffness. *J Bone Joint Surg Am.* 2012;94(15):1428–1437.
33. Guillin R, Marchand AJ, Roux A, et al. Imaging of snapping phenomena. *Br J Radiol.* 2012;85(1018):1343–1353.
34. DiGiovanni CW, Kuo R, Tejwani N, et al. Isolated gastrocnemius tightness. *J Bone Joint Surg Am.* 2002;84-A(6):962–970.
35. Stone J, Carson A. Functional neurologic symptoms: assessment and management. *Neurol Clin.* 2011;29(1):1–18, vii.
36. Houten JK, Noce LA. Clinical correlations of cervical myelopathy and the Hoffmann sign. *J Neurosurg Spine.* 2008;9(3):237–242.
37. Rees JD, Stride M, Scott A. Tendons–time to revisit inflammation. *Br J Sports Med.* 2014;48(21):1553–1557.
38. Allen GM. *Tendon and ligamentous trauma.* In: Vanhoenacker FM, Maas M, Gielen JL, eds. *Imaging of Orthopedic Sports Injuries.* Berlin Heidelberg: Springer, Berlin Heidelberg; 2007:61–71.
39. Wang JH. Mechanobiology of tendon. *J Biomech.* 2006;39(9):1563–1582.
40. Mellado JM, Ramos A, Salvadó E, et al. Accessory ossicles and sesamoid bones of the ankle and foot: imaging findings, clinical significance and differential diagnosis. *Eur Radiol.* 2003;13 Suppl 6:L164–L177.
41. Ackermann PW, Li J, Lundeberg T, Kreicbergs A. Neuronal plasticity in relation to nociception and healing of rat achilles tendon. *J Orthop Res.* 2003;21(3):432–441.

42. Franklin SL, Dean BJ, Wheway K, et al. Up-regulation of Glutamate in Painful Human Supraspinatus Tendon Tears. *Am J Sports Med.* 2014;42(8):1955–1962.
43. Skjong CC, Meininger AK, Ho SS. Tendinopathy treatment: where is the evidence? *Clin Sports Med.* 2012;31(2):329–350.
44. September AV, Schwellnus MP, Collins M. Tendon and ligament injuries: the genetic component. *Br J Sports Med.* 2007;41(4):241–6; discussion 246.
45. Rozmaryn L. *Tendinopathy in the workplace.* In: Maffulli N, Renström P, Leadbetter W, eds. *Tendon Injuries.* London: Springer; 2005:90–100.
46. Paavola M, Kannus P, Järvinen M. *Epidemiology of tendon problems in sport.* In: Maffulli N, Renström P, Leadbetter W, eds. *Tendon Injuries.* London: Springer; 2005;32–39.
47. Sharma P, Maffulli N. Tendon injury and tendinopathy: healing and repair. *J Bone Joint Surg Am.* 2005;87(1):187–202.
48. Hartright D, et al. *Biomechanical and Clinical Evaluation of Tendons and Ligaments.* In: Walsh WR, ed. *Repair and Regeneration of Ligaments, Tendons, and Joint Capsule.* Totowa, NJ: Humana Press; 2006;185–199.
49. Firestein GS, Budd R, Gabriel SE, O'Dell JR, McInnes IB. *Kelley's Textbook of Rheumatology, 9th ed.* Philadelphia, PA: Elsevier; 2012.
50. Rein S, Hagert E, Hanisch U, et al. Immunohistochemical analysis of sensory nerve endings in ankle ligaments: a cadaver study. *Cells Tissues Organs (Print).* 2013;197(1):64–76.
51. Ward S, Pearce AJ, Pietrosimone B, et al. Neuromuscular deficits after peripheral joint injury: a neurophysiological hypothesis. *Muscle Nerve.* 2015;51(3):327–332.
52. Hsu SL, Liang R, Woo SL. Functional tissue engineering of ligament healing. *Sports Med Arthrosc Rehabil Ther Technol.* 2010;2:12.
53. Mense S. Muscle pain: mechanisms and clinical significance. *Dtsch Arztebl Int.* 2008;105(12):214–219.
54. Patel KM, Major NM. Compartmental anatomy. In: Davies AM, Sundaram M, James SLJ, eds. *Imaging of Bone Tumors and Tumor-Like Lesions.* Springer Berlin Heidelberg; 2009: 665–676.
55. Bilgili MG, Kaynak G, Botanlioglu H, et al. Peroneus quartus: prevalance and clinical importance. *Arch Orthop Trauma Surg.* 2014;134(4):481–487.
56. Bradley WG. *Neurology in Clinical Practice.* 5th ed. Philadelphia, PA: Butterworth-Heinemann/Elsevier; 2008.
57. Draghi F, Zacchino M, Canepari M, et al. Muscle injuries: ultrasound evaluation in the acute phase. *J Ultrasound.* 2013;16(4):209–214.
58. Järvinen TA, Kääriäinen M, Järvinen M, Kalimo H. Muscle strain injuries. *Curr Opin Rheumatol.* 2000;12(2):155–161.
59. Laprade RF, Surowiec RK, Sochanska AN, et al. Epidemiology, identification, treatment and return to play of musculoskeletal-based ice hockey injuries. *Br J Sports Med.* 2014;48(1):4–10.
60. Tzortziou V, Maffulli N, Padhiar N. Diagnosis and management of chronic exertional compartment syndrome (CECS) in the United Kingdom. *Clin J Sport Med.* 2006;16(3):209–213.
61. Wilder RP, Magrum E. Exertional compartment syndrome. *Clin Sports Med.* 2010;29(3):429–435.
62. Sauret JM, Marinides G, Wang GK. Rhabdomyolysis. *Am Fam Physician.* 2002;65(5):907–912.
63. Aptel M, Aublet-Cuvelier A, Cnockaert JC. Work-related musculoskeletal disorders of the upper limb. *Joint Bone Spine.* 2002;69(6):546–555.
64. Voipio-Pulkki LM, Nuutila P, Knuuti MJ, et al. Heart and skeletal muscle glucose disposal in type 2 diabetic patients as determined by positron emission tomography. *J Nucl Med.* 1993;34(12):2064–2067.
65. da Costa BR, Reichenbach S, Keller N, et al. Effectiveness of non-steroidal anti-inflammatory drugs for the treatment of pain in knee and hip osteoarthritis: a network meta-analysis. *Lancet.* 2016;387:2093–2105.
66. Towheed TE, Maxwell L, Judd MG, Catton M, Hochberg MC, Wells G. Acetaminophen for osteoarthritis. *Cochrane Database Syst Rev.* 2006(1):CD004257.
67. Wegman A, van der Windt D, van Tulder M, et al. Nonsteroidal anti-inflammatory drugs or acetaminophen for osteoarthritis of the hip or knee? A systematic review of evidence and guidelines. *J Rheumatol.* 2004;31(2):344–354.
68. Van Mieghem IM, Boets A, Sciot R, Van Breuseghem I. Ischiogluteal bursitis: an uncommon type of bursitis. *Skeletal Radiol.* 2004;33(7):413–416.
69. Santavirta S, Konttinen YT, Antti-Poika I, Nordström D. Inflammation of the subacromial bursa in chronic shoulder pain. *Arch Orthop Trauma Surg.* 1992;111(6):336–340.
70. Hodgson RJ, O'Connor PJ, Hensor EM, et al. Contrast-enhanced MRI of the subdeltoid, subacromial bursa in painful and painless rotator cuff tears. *Br J Radiol.* 2012;85(1019):1482–1487.
71. Devereaux MW. Anatomy and examination of the spine. *Neurol Clin.* 2007;25(2):331–351.
72. Harrast MA, Colonno D. Stress fractures in runners. *Clin Sports Med.* 2010;29(3):399–416.
73. Bunakdarpour A, Reinus WR, Khurana JS. *Diagnostic Imaging of Musculoskeletal Diseases—A Systematic Approach*; New York, NY: Springer Science & Business Media; 2010.
74. Fayad LM, Kamel IR, Kawamoto S, et al. Distinguishing stress fractures from pathologic fractures: a multimodality approach. *Skeletal Radiol.* 2005;34(5):245–259.
75. Cheong HW, Peh WC, Guglielmi G. Imaging of diseases of the axial and peripheral skeleton. *Radiol Clin North Am.* 2008;46(4):703–33, vi.
76. Malanga GA, Ramirez-Del Toro JA. Common injuries of the foot and ankle in the child and adolescent athlete. *Phys Med Rehabil Clin N Am.* 2008;19(2):347–71, ix.
77. Launay F. Sports-related overuse injuries in children. *Orthop Traumatol Surg Res.* 2015;101(1 Suppl):S139–S147.
78. Haile Z, Khatua S. Beyond osteoarthritis: recognizing and treating infectious and other inflammatory arthropathies in your practice. *Prim Care.* 2010;37(4):713–27, vi.
79. Mendell JR, Sahenk Z. Clinical practice. Painful sensory neuropathy. *N Engl J Med.* 2003;348(13):1243–1255.
80. Wager TD, Atlas LY, Lindquist MA, et al. An fMRI-based neurologic signature of physical pain. *N Engl J Med.* 2013;368(15):1388–1397.
81. Peyron R, Laurent B, García-Larrea L. Functional imaging of brain responses to pain. A review and meta-analysis (2000). *Neurophysiol Clin.* 2000;30(5):263–288.
82. Scholz J, Woolf CJ. Can we conquer pain? *Nat Neurosci.* 2002;5 Suppl:1062–1067.
83. Garcia-Larrea L, Peyron R. Pain matrices and neuropathic pain matrices: a review. *Pain.* 2013;154 Suppl 1:S29–S43.
84. Werner RA, Andary M. Carpal tunnel syndrome: pathophysiology and clinical neurophysiology. *Clin Neurophysiol.* 2002;113(9):1373–1381.
85. Lundborg G, Dahlin LB. Anatomy, function, and pathophysiology of peripheral nerves and nerve compression. *Hand Clin.* 1996;12(2):185–193.
86. de-la-Llave-Rincon AI, Puentedura EJ, Fernandez-de-las-Penas C. New advances in the mechanisms and etiology of carpal tunnel syndrome. *Discov Med.* 2012;13(72):343–348.
87. O'Connor RC, Andary MT, Russo RB, DeLano M. Thoracic radiculopathy. *Phys Med Rehabil Clin N Am.* 2002;13(3):623–44, viii.
88. Vernadakis AJ, Koch H, Mackinnon SE. Management of neuromas. *Clin Plast Surg.* 2003;30(2):247–68, vii.
89. Chen PJ, Liang HW, Chang KV, Wang TG. Ultrasound-guided injection of steroid in multiple postamputation neuromas. *J Clin Ultrasound.* 2013;41(2):122–124.
90. Mathias CJ. Autonomic diseases: management. *J Neurol Neurosurg Psychiatr.* 2003;74 Suppl 3:iii42–iii47.
91. Lacomis D. Small-fiber neuropathy. *Muscle Nerve.* 2002;26(2):173–188.
92. Stögbauer F, Young P, Kuhlenbäumer G, et al. Autosomal dominant burning feet syndrome. *J Neurol Neurosurg Psychiatr.* 1999;67(1):78–81.
93. Kontaxis A, Cutti AG, Johnson GR, Veeger HE. A framework for the definition of standardized protocols for measuring upper-extremity kinematics. *Clin Biomech (Bristol, Avon).* 2009;24(3):246–253.
94. Lu TW, Chang CF. Biomechanics of human movement and its clinical applications. *Kaohsiung J Med Sci.* 2012;28(2 Suppl):S13–S25.
95. van Bolhuis BM, Gielen CCAM, van Ingen Schenau GJ. Activation patterns of mono- and bi-articular arm muscles as a function of force and movement direction of the wrist in humans. *J Physiol.* 1998;508(Pt. 1):313–324.

96. Lim MR, Huang RC, Wu A, et al. Evaluation of the elderly patient with an abnormal gait. *J Am Acad Orthop Surg.* 2007;15(2):107–117.
97. Schmid S, Schweizer K, Romkes J, et al. Secondary gait deviations in patients with and without neurological involvement: a systematic review. *Gait Posture.* 2013;37(4):480–493.
98. Sweeting K, Mock M. Gait and posture—assessment in general practice. *Aust Fam Physician.* 2007;36(6):398–401, 404.
99. Salzman B. Gait and balance disorders in older adults. *Am Fam Physician.* 2010;82(1):61–68.
100. Verghese J, Lipton RB, Hall CB, et al. Abnormality of gait as a predictor of non-Alzheimer's dementia. *N Engl J Med.* 2002;347(22):1761–1768.
101. Dugan SA, Bhat KP. Biomechanics and analysis of running gait. *Phys Med Rehabil Clin N Am.* 2005;16(3):603–621.
102. Lu TW, Chien HL, Chen HL. Joint loading in the lower extremities during elliptical exercise. *Med Sci Sports Exerc.* 2007;39(9):1651–1658.
103. Damiano DL, Norman T, Stanley CJ, Park HS. Comparison of elliptical training, stationary cycling, treadmill walking and overground walking. *Gait Posture.* 2011;34(2):260–264.
104. Mody GM, Brooks PM. Improving musculoskeletal health: global issues. *Best Pract Res Clin Rheumatol.* 2012;26(2):237–249.
105. Nguyen BY, Reveille JD. Rheumatic manifestations associated with HIV in the highly active antiretroviral therapy era. *Curr Opin Rheumatol.* 2009;21(4):404–410.
106. Vignon E, Valat JP, Rossignol M, et al. Osteoarthritis of the knee and hip and activity: a systematic international review and synthesis (OASIS). *Joint Bone Spine.* 2006;73(4):442–455.
107. Pangarkar S, Lee PC. Conservative treatment for neck pain: medications, physical therapy, and exercise. *Phys Med Rehabil Clin N Am.* 2011;22(3):503–20, ix.
108. Towheed TE, Maxwell L, Anastassiades TP, Shea B, Houpt J, Robinson V, Hochberg MC, Wells G. Glucosamine therapy for treating osteoarthritis. *Cochrane Database Syst Rev.* 2005(2):CD002946.
109. Sawitzke AD, Shi H, Finco MF, et al. The effect of glucosamine and/or chondroitin sulfate on the progression of knee osteoarthritis: a report from the glucosamine/chondroitin arthritis intervention trial. *Arthritis Rheum.* 2008;58(10):3183–3191.
110. Clegg DO, Reda DJ, Harris CL, et al. Glucosamine, chondroitin sulfate, and the two in combination for painful knee osteoarthritis. *N Engl J Med.* 2006;354(8):795–808.
111. Miller TM, Layzer RB. Muscle cramps. *Muscle Nerve.* 2005;32(4):431–442.
112. Witenko C, Moorman-Li R, Motycka C, et al. Considerations for the appropriate use of skeletal muscle relaxants for the management of acute low back pain. *P T.* 2014;39(6):427–435.
113. Baron R, Binder A, Wasner G. Neuropathic pain: diagnosis, pathophysiological mechanisms, and treatment. *Lancet Neurol.* 2010;9(8):807–819.
114. Dworkin RH, O'Connor AB, Backonja M, et al. Pharmacologic management of neuropathic pain: evidence-based recommendations. *Pain.* 2007;132(3):237–251.
115. Dworkin RH, O'Connor AB, Audette J, et al. Recommendations for the pharmacological management of neuropathic pain: an overview and literature update. *Mayo Clin Proc.* 2010;85(3 Suppl):S3–14.
116. Baron R. Mechanisms of disease: neuropathic pain—a clinical perspective. *Nat Clin Pract Neurol.* 2006;2(2):95–106.
117. Hunter DJ. Viscosupplementation for osteoarthritis of the knee. *N Engl J Med.* 2015;372(11):1040–1047.
118. Darouiche RO, Wall MJ Jr, Itani KM, et al. Chlorhexidine-alcohol versus povidone-iodine for surgical-site antisepsis. *N Engl J Med.* 2010;362(1):18–26.
119. Chiavaras MM, Jacobson JA. Ultrasound-guided tendon fenestration. *Semin Musculoskelet Radiol.* 2013;17(1):85–90.
120. Kietrys DM, Palombaro KM, Mannheimer JS. Dry needling for management of pain in the upper quarter and craniofacial region. *Curr Pain Headache Rep.* 2014;18(8):437.
121. Daley EL, Bajaj S, Bisson LJ, Cole BJ. Improving injection accuracy of the elbow, knee, and shoulder: does injection site and imaging make a difference? A systematic review. *Am J Sports Med.* 2011;39(3):656–662.
122. Hameed F, Ihm J. Injectable medications for osteoarthritis. *PM R.* 2012;4(5 Suppl):S75–S81.
123. Lavelle W, Lavelle ED, Lavelle L. Intra-articular injections. *Med Clin North Am.* 2007;91(2):241–250.
124. Weinstein RS. Clinical practice. Glucocorticoid-induced bone disease. *N Engl J Med.* 2011;365(1):62–70.
125. Seamon J, Keller T, Saleh J, Cui Q. The pathogenesis of nontraumatic osteonecrosis. *Arthritis.* 2012;2012:601763.
126. Coombes BK, Bisset L, Vicenzino B. Efficacy and safety of corticosteroid injections and other injections for management of tendinopathy: a systematic review of randomised controlled trials. *Lancet.* 2010;376(9754):1751–1767.
127. Yamamoto T, Schneider R, Iwamoto Y, Bullough PG. Rapid destruction of the femoral head after a single intraarticular injection of corticosteroid into the hip joint. *J Rheumatol.* 2006;33(8):1701–1704.
128. Strauss EJ, Hart JA, Miller MD, et al. Hyaluronic acid viscosupplementation and osteoarthritis: current uses and future directions. *Am J Sports Med.* 2009;37(8):1636–1644.
129. Cianflocco AJ. Viscosupplementation in patients with osteoarthritis of the knee. *Postgrad Med.* 2013;125(1):97–105.
130. Bellamy N. Campbell J, Robinson V, Gee T, Bourne R, Wells G. Viscosupplementation for the treatment of osteoarthritis of the knee. *Cochrane Database Syst Rev.* 2006(2):CD005321.
131. Rivera F. Can viscosupplementation be used in the hip? An Italian perspective. *Orthopedics.* 2014;37(1):48–55.
132. Lucas Y, Hernandez J, Darcel V, et al. Viscosupplementation of the ankle: A prospective study with an average follow-up of 45.5 months. *Orthop Traumatol Surg Res.* 2013;99(5):593–599.
133. van Brakel RW, Eygendaal D. Intra-articular injection of hyaluronic acid is not effective for the treatment of post-traumatic osteoarthritis of the elbow. *Arthroscopy.* 2006;22(11):1199–1203.
134. Fuchs S, Mönikes R, Wohlmeiner A, Heyse T. Intra-articular hyaluronic acid compared with corticoid injections for the treatment of rhizarthrosis. *Osteoarthr Cartil.* 2006;14(1):82–88.
135. Distel LM, Best TM. Prolotherapy: a clinical review of its role in treating chronic musculoskeletal pain. *PM R.* 2011;3(6 Suppl 1):S78–S81.
136. Rabago D, Slattengren A, Zgierska A. Prolotherapy in primary care practice. *Prim Care.* 2010;37(1):65–80.
137. Middleton KK, Barro V, Muller B, et al. Evaluation of the effects of platelet-rich plasma (PRP) therapy involved in the healing of sports-related soft tissue injuries. *Iowa Orthop J.* 2012;32:150–163.
138. Mishra A, Randelli P, Barr C, et al. Platelet-rich plasma and the upper extremity. *Hand Clin.* 2012;28(4):481–491.
139. Liddle AD, Rodríguez-Merchán EC. Platelet-rich plasma in the treatment of patellar tendinopathy: a systematic review. *Am J Sports Med.* 2015;43(10):2583–2590.
140. Moraes VY, Lenza M, Tamaoki MJ, et al. Platelet-rich therapies for musculoskeletal soft tissue injuries. *Cochrane Database Syst Rev.* 2014;4:CD010071.
141. Daley EL, Bajaj S, Bisson LJ, Cole BJ. Improving injection accuracy of the elbow, knee, and shoulder: does injection site and imaging make a difference? A systematic review. *Am J Sports Med.* 2011;39(3):656–662.
142. Laudy AB, Bakker EW, Rekers M, Moen MH. Efficacy of platelet-rich plasma injections in osteoarthritis of the knee: a systematic review and meta-analysis. *Br J Sports Med.* 2015;49(10):657–672.
143. Lai LP, Stitik TP, Foye PM, Georgy JS, et al. Use of platelet-rich plasma in intra-articular knee injections for osteoarthritis: a systematic review. *PM R.* 2015;7(6):637–648.
144. de Jonge S, de Vos RJ, Weir A, et al. One-year follow-up of platelet-rich plasma treatment in chronic Achilles tendinopathy: a double-blind randomized placebo-controlled trial. *Am J Sports Med.* 2011;39(8):1623–1629.
145. Reurink G, Goudswaard GJ, Moen MH, et al.; Dutch Hamstring Injection Therapy (HIT) Study Investigators. Platelet-rich plasma injections in acute muscle injury. *N Engl J Med.* 2014;370(26):2546–2547.
146. Mautner K, Blazuk J. Where do injectable stem cell treatments apply in treatment of muscle, tendon, and ligament injuries? *PM R.* 2015;7(4 Suppl):S33–S40.
147. Filardo G, Madry H, Jelic M, et al. Mesenchymal stem cells for the treatment of cartilage lesions: from preclinical findings to clinical application in orthopaedics. *Knee Surg Sports Traumatol Arthrosc.* 2013;21(8):1717–1729.

148. Piper SL, Kramer JD, Kim HT, Feeley BT. Effects of local anesthetics on articular cartilage. *Am J Sports Med.* 2011;39(10):2245–2253.
149. Greensmith JE, Murray WB. Complications of regional anesthesia. *Curr Opin Anaesthesiol.* 2006;19(5):531–537.
150. Bowens C Jr, Sripada R. Regional blockade of the shoulder: approaches and outcomes. *Anesthesiol Res Pract.* 2012;2012:971963.
151. Piper SL, Kramer JD, Kim HT, Feeley BT. Effects of local anesthetics on articular cartilage. *Am J Sports Med.* 2011;39(10):2245–2253.
152. Fanucci E, Masala S, Fabiano S, et al. Treatment of intermetatarsal Morton's neuroma with alcohol injection under US guide: 10-month follow-up. *Eur Radiol.* 2004;14(3):514–518.
153. Cahana A, Van Zundert J, Macrea L, et al. Pulsed radiofrequency: current clinical and biological literature available. *Pain Med.* 2006;7(5):411–423.
154. Choi WJ, Hwang SJ, Song JG, et al. Radiofrequency treatment relieves chronic knee osteoarthritis pain: a double-blind randomized controlled trial. *Pain.* 2011;152(3):481–487; 1933–1934; author reply 1934–1936.
155. Kong KH, Chua KS. Neurolysis of the musculocutaneous nerve with alcohol to treat poststroke elbow flexor spasticity. *Arch Phys Med Rehabil.* 1999;80(10):1234–1236.
156. Kocabas H, Salli A, Demir AH, Ozerbil OM. Comparison of phenol and alcohol neurolysis of tibial nerve motor branches to the gastrocnemius muscle for treatment of spastic foot after stroke: a randomized controlled pilot study. *Eur J Phys Rehabil Med.* 2010;46(1):5–10.
157. Tagliafico A, Bodner G, Rosenberg I, et al. Peripheral nerves: ultrasound-guided interventional procedures. *Semin Musculoskelet Radiol.* 2010;14(5):559–566.
158. Brull R, Perlas A, Chan VW. Ultrasound-guided peripheral nerve blockade. *Curr Pain Headache Rep.* 2007;11(1):25–32.
159. Binder DS, Nampiaparampil DE. The provocative lumbar facet joint. *Curr Rev Musculoskelet Med.* 2009;2(1):15–24.
160. D'Orazio F, Gregori LM, Gallucci M. Spine epidural and sacroiliac joints injections—when and how to perform. *Eur J Radiol.* 204;84(5):777–782.
161. Friedly JL, Comstock BA, Turner JA, et al. A randomized trial of epidural glucocorticoid injections for spinal stenosis. *N Engl J Med.* 2014;371(1):11–21.
162. Wolter T. Spinal cord stimulation for neuropathic pain: current perspectives. *J Pain Res.* 2014;7:651–663.
163. Hadzic A. Peripheral nerve stimulators: cracking the code–one at a time. *Reg Anesth Pain Med.* 2004;29(3):185–188.
164. Deogaonkar M, Slavin KV. Peripheral nerve/field stimulation for neuropathic pain. *Neurosurg Clin N Am.* 2014;25(1):1–10.
165. Trescot AM. Cryoanalgesia in interventional pain management. *Pain Physician.* 2003;6(3):345–360.
166. Braddom RL, Chan L, Harrast MA. *Physical Medicine and Rehabilitation.* 4th ed. Philadelphia, PA: Saunders/Elsevier; 2011:1506.
167. Darrow MD. Ordering and understanding the exercise stress test. *Am Fam Physician.* 1999;59(2):401–410.
168. Fletcher GF, Mills WC, Taylor WC. Update on exercise stress testing. *Am Fam Physician.* 2006;74(10):1749–1754.
169. Jäkel A, von Hauenschild P. A systematic review to evaluate the clinical benefits of craniosacral therapy. *Complement Ther Med.* 2012;20(6):456–465.
170. Son JH, Park GD, Park HS. The effect of sacroiliac joint mobilization on pelvic deformation and the static balance ability of female university students with si joint dysfunction. *J Phys Ther Sci.* 2014;26(6):845–848.
171. Suter E, McMorland G, Herzog W, Bray R. Decrease in quadriceps inhibition after sacroiliac joint manipulation in patients with anterior knee pain. *J Manipulative Physiol Ther.* 1999;22(3):149–153.
172. Salamh PA, Kolber MJ, Hanney WJ. Effect of scapular stabilization during horizontal adduction stretching on passive internal rotation and posterior shoulder tightness in young women volleyball athletes: a randomized controlled trial. *Arch Phys Med Rehabil.* 2015;96(2):349–356.
173. Moezy A, Sepehrifar S, Solaymani Dodaran M. The effects of scapular stabilization based exercise therapy on pain, posture, flexibility and shoulder mobility in patients with shoulder impingement syndrome: a controlled randomized clinical trial. *Med J Islam Repub Iran.* 2014;28:87.
174. Key J. "The core": understanding it, and retraining its dysfunction. *J Bodyw Mov Ther.* 2013;17(4):541–559.
175. Standaert CJ, Herring SA. Expert opinion and controversies in musculoskeletal and sports medicine: core stabilization as a treatment for low back pain. *Arch Phys Med Rehabil.* 2007;88(12):1734–1736.
176. Heymans MW, van Tulder MW, Esmail R, et al. Back schools for non-specific low-back pain. *Cochrane Database Syst Rev.* 2004;18(4):CD000261.
177. Isner-Horobeti ME, Dufour SP, Vautravers P, et al. Eccentric exercise training: modalities, applications and perspectives. *Sports Med.* 2013;43(6):483–512.
178. Babu AS, Balthillaya GM, Navada R, Kurien A. Theraband exercises with music for persons with haemophilia. *Haemophilia.* 2013;19(6):e359–e360.
179. Swain DP, Franklin BA. Comparison of cardioprotective benefits of vigorous versus moderate intensity aerobic exercise. *Am J Cardiol.* 2006;97(1):141–147.
180. Matus CD, Klaege K. Exercise and weight management. *Prim Care.* 2007;34(1):109–116.
181. Montero-Fernández N, Serra-Rexach JA. Role of exercise on sarcopenia in the elderly. *Eur J Phys Rehabil Med.* 2013;49(1):131–143.
182. Abresch RT, Carter GT, Han JJ, McDonald CM. Exercise in neuromuscular diseases. *Phys Med Rehabil Clin N Am.* 2012;23(3):653–673.
183. DeMaio M, Magann EF. Exercise and pregnancy. *J Am Acad Orthop Surg.* 2009;17(8):504–514.
184. Romeo P, Lavanga V, Pagani D, Sansone V. Extracorporeal shock wave therapy in musculoskeletal disorders: a review. *Med Princ Pract.* 2014;23(1):7–13.
185. Wang CJ. Extracorporeal shockwave therapy in musculoskeletal disorders. *J Orthop Surg Res.* 2012;7:11.
186. van der Worp H, van den Akker-Scheek I, van Schie H, Zwerver J. ESWT for tendinopathy: technology and clinical implications. *Knee Surg Sports Traumatol Arthrosc.* 2013;21(6):1451–1458.
187. Manyanga T, Froese M, Zarychanski R, et al. Pain management with acupuncture in osteoarthritis: a systematic review and meta-analysis. *BMC Complement Altern Med.* 2014;14:312.
188. Liu L, Skinner M, McDonough S, et al. Acupuncture for low back pain: an overview of systematic reviews. *Evid Based Complement Alternat Med.* 2015;2015:328196.
189. Rio E, Kidgell D, Moseley GL, et al. Tendon neuroplastic training: changing the way we think about tendon rehabilitation: a narrative review. *Br J Sports Med.* 2016;50(4):209–215.
190. Fraser-Moodie JA, Shortt NL, Robinson CM. Injuries to the acromioclavicular joint. *J Bone Joint Surg Br.* 2008;90(6):697–707.
191. Morelli V, Bright C, Fields A. Ligamentous injuries of the knee: anterior cruciate, medial collateral, posterior cruciate, and posterolateral corner injuries. *Prim Care.* 2013;40(2):335–356.
192. Polzer H, Kanz KG, Prall WC, et al. Diagnosis and treatment of acute ankle injuries: development of an evidence-based algorithm. *Orthop Rev (Pavia).* 2012;4(1):e5.
193. Dourte LM, Kuntz AF, Soslowsky LJ. Twenty-five years of tendon and ligament research. *J Orthop Res.* 2008;26(10):1297–1305.
194. Dugan SA, Weber KM. Stress fractures and rehabilitation. *Phys Med Rehabil Clin N Am.* 2007;18(3):401–16, viii.
195. McCormick F, Nwachukwu BU, Provencher MT. Stress fractures in runners. *Clin Sports Med.* 2012;31(2):291–306.
196. Ivkovic A, Bojanic I, Pecina M. Stress fractures of the femoral shaft in athletes: a new treatment algorithm. *Br J Sports Med.* 2006;40(6):518–520; discussion 520.
197. Browner, B. D. (2009). *Skeletal Trauma: Basic Science, Management, and Reconstruction.* Philadelphia, PA: Elsevier Health Sciences.

CHAPTER 2

Neck

EPIDEMIOLOGY OF NECK PAIN

NECK PAIN IN THE GENERAL POPULATION

Prevalence
- ~15% (12%–70% depending on studies) in the general population (1)
- ~5 % have activity limitations (2) and 1.7% are limited in their abilities to work
- Chronic neck pain (>6 months): female > male, increase with age (controversial)
  ○ Chronic neck pain: 15% to 40% of patients with acute neck pain after motor vehicle accident (MVA) and 5% to 7%; disability
- New disability claims per year from neck pain (3,4): 600 per 100,000 (5)

NECK PAIN IN ATHLETES (6)

Prevalence and common causes
- Cervical strain/sprain: (most common [MC] cause of neck pain in athletes):
  ○ Whiplash disorder with acceleration–deceleration-type injury
- Stinger/burner syndrome: MC cause of transient neuropathic pain
  ○ Occurs in 65% of college football players, high recurrence rate up to 87%
- Myofascial pain in the neck–shoulder girdle
  ○ Common in cyclists (~60%), caused by hyperextension of the neck in horizontal riding position
- Discogenic neck pain: uncommon

Spinal cord injury (SCI)
- Cervical cord neurapraxia (CCN): 7 per 10,000 football participants (7)
- SCI: rare, mainly caused by spear tackling (axial loading)
  ○ ~80% drop after spear tackling prohibited in 1976

NECK PAIN AT WORK (1)

Prevalence
- Highly prevalent and continues to increase

Risk factors for chronic pain (>6 months)
- Female > male, age, high quantitative job demands, low-coworker support, repetitive work, nonfixed salary, prolonged sitting, poor ergonomics, previous musculoskeletal (MSK) comorbidities, depressive symptoms
- Crane operators (upto 70%), nurses, and office workers

Cervical disc injury
- Higher in drivers than other occupations
- May be related to vibrations and road shocks, twisting and acceleration/deceleration, or whiplash accident rather than heavy lifting (8)

Workplace modifications: No clear evidence that interventions aimed at modifying work stations and worker posture are effective in reducing incidence of neck pain in workers

DIFFERENTIAL DIAGNOSIS

Differential diagnosis based on the location and radiation of neck pain (Flowchart 2.1)

Working definition of neck region: superior nuchal line to T1 spinous process, laterally by medial scapular border

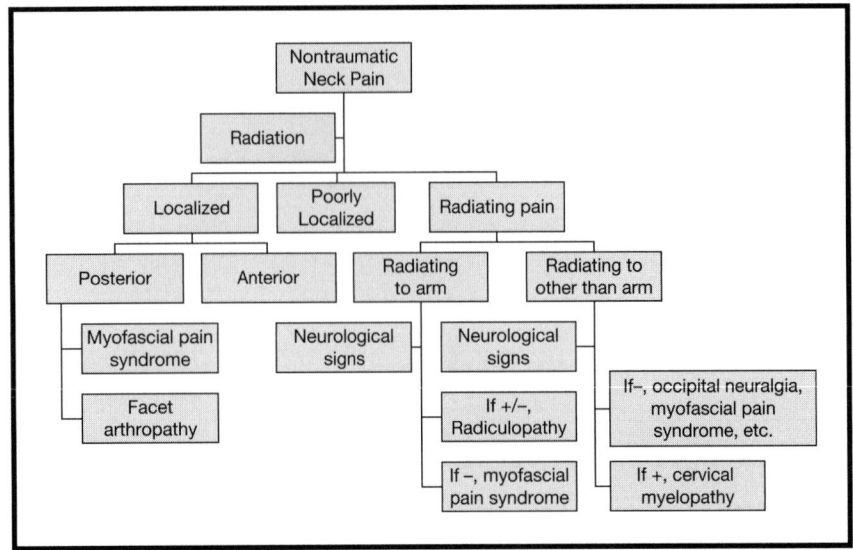

FLOWCHART 2.1
Differential diagnosis of nontraumatic neck pain.

RADIATING NECK PAIN		LOCALIZED NECK PAIN	
Neck pain radiating to arm or upper extremity	Radiating/referred pain to/from other than arm	Localized; posterior Posterior triangle (occipital triangle and supraclavicular triangle)	Anterior neck pain (less common) (8)

• Cervical radiculopathy: dermatomal distribution
  ○ Compressive: disc herniation, spondylosis
  ○ Noncompressive: tumor, sarcoidosis, others
• Myofascial pain with specific referred pain pattern
  ○ Upper trapezius, paraspinal, scalene, scapular girdle muscle
• Thoracic outlet syndrome: symptomatic >> true neurogenic (very rare)
• Brachial plexitis
	• Occipital neuralgia: to posterior head
	• Myofascial pain
	• Cervical plexus lesion: to supraclavicular triangle, lateral neck, and jaw
	• Others: avulsion injury, Schwannoma
		• Muscle strain/myofascial pain without referred pain
		• Cervical facet arthropathy (± referred pain to posterior neck/shoulder/scapular region)
		  ○ Traumatic (whiplash)
		• Degenerative disc disease
		• Rare but morbid conditions[a] (± radiating/referred)
		  ○ Tumor; metastatic
		  ○ Infection (eg, epidural abscess)
		  ○ Vascular: vertebral dissection or carotid artery rupture
		  ○ Rheumatoid arthritis
			• Tendinopathy/tendonitis/strain (scalene muscle and other muscles)
			• Sternoclavicular joint dysfunction
			• Clavicular or 1st rib fracture
			• Supraclavicular neuritis (9)
			• Unusual causes
			  ○ Eagle syndrome (stylohyoid ligament ossification or elongated styloid process)
			  ○ Superior laryngeal neuralgia
			  ○ Carotid artery dissection, infection, tumor
			  ○ Thyroid/cricoid cartilage syndrome

[a]Tumor or infection (<0.4%), vascular disorder (6% of carotid dissection: neck pain as a sole presentation, headache: MC, vertebral artery dissection or aortic aneurysm).
Source: From Ref. (10). Bogduk, N. The anatomy and pathophysiology of neck pain. *Phys Med Rehabil Clin N Am.* 2011;22(3):367–382, vii.

UNUSUAL CAUSES OF NECK PAIN

- Considered if symptoms are not explained by other well-established causes
- Cervical spine: diffuse idiopathic skeletal hyperostosis (DISH), Paget disease, and spondylosis, subluxation of the lateral atlantoaxial joint, joint of Luschka lesion, synovial cyst, subluxation of the facet joints
- Muscle/tendon: torticollis, longus colli tendonitis (retropharyngeal tendinitis), temporalis muscle, hyoid bone or muscle (sternohyoid and omohyoid) syndrome for anterior neck pain
- Soft tissue: infection of the oral cavity, oropharynx, and glands (lymphadenitis, sialadenitis, and thyroiditis); polymyalgia rheumatica
- Referred pain (Figure 2.1)
  ○ Referred pain from temporomandibular joint (TMJ) dysfunction and trigeminal neuralgia
  ○ Migraine headache, basal ganglia disease
- Carotidynia (11,12)
  ○ Dull, throbbing pain directly over the carotid artery (either unilateral or bilateral) with followings
    ▪ Exacerbated with light pressure ± ipsilateral headache, self-limiting <2 weeks
    ▪ One of three findings (tenderness, swelling, and increased pulsations) on carotid artery
  ○ Differential diagnosis: carotid aneurysm, carotid body tumor, carotid dissection, acute carotid occlusion, large vessel vasculitis (giant cell arteritis), and fibromuscular dysplasia
  ○ Workup; emergency room (ER) referral, duplex imaging (initial) for extracranial carotid arteries, and CT or MRI

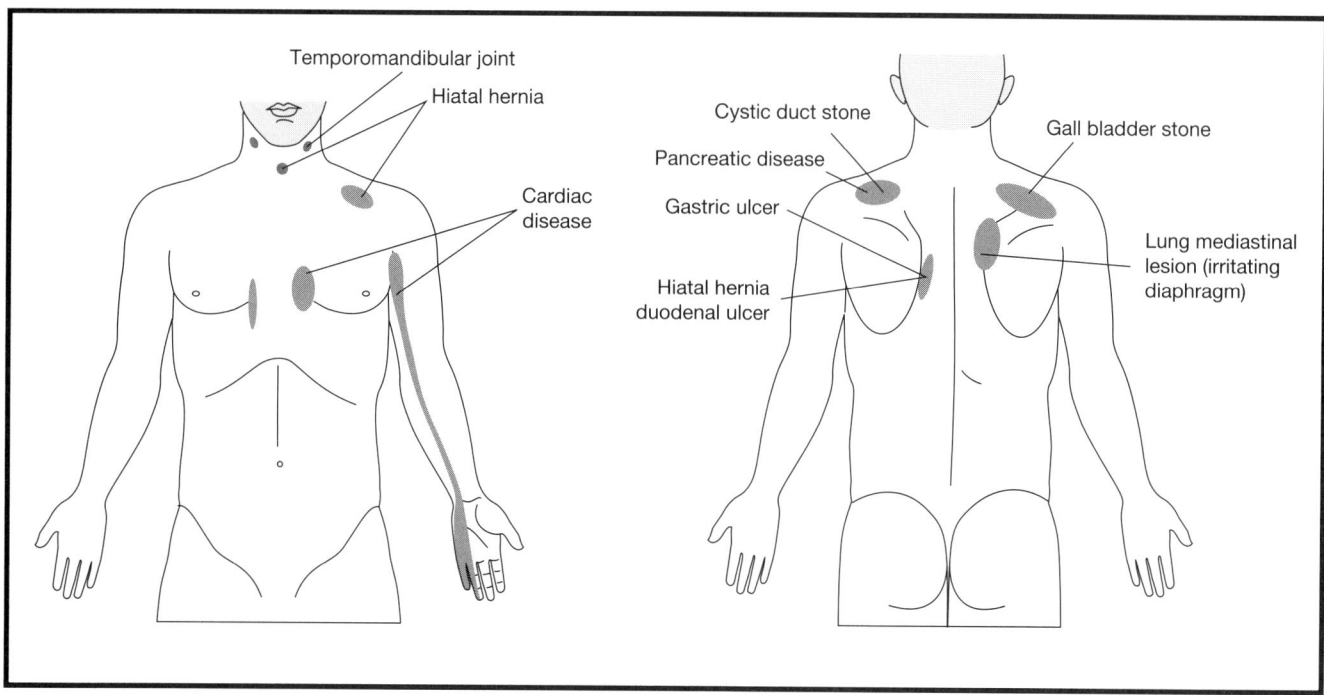

FIGURE 2.1
Extrinsic causes of neck, shoulder, and arm pain.
Source: Adapted from Ref. (13). Firestein GS, *Kelley's textbook of rheumatology.* 9th ed. Philadelphia, PA: Saunders Elsevier; 2012.

NEUROLOGICAL SYMPTOMS ASSOCIATED WITH NECK PAIN

Sensory symptoms
- Differential diagnosis for neck pain with sensory symptoms (numbness, tingling, pins/needles, or burning)
  - Cervical radiculopathy: sensory symptoms present in dermatomal distribution
  - Referred pain from myofascial pain mimicking positive sensory symptoms (Figure 2.2)
  - Concomitant focal entrapment neuropathy (carpal tunnel syndrome [CTS] or ulnar neuropathy) with localized axial neck pain mimicking radiculopathy
  - Other unusual causes
    - Numb chin syndrome (chin and inferior lip): mental/inferior alveolar neuropathy by jaw metastasis or vasculitis (14)
- Differential diagnosis for ataxic gait with/without neck pain
  - Cervical myelopathy: because of alteration of dorsal column; (+) long tract signs (Hoffman's reflex, hyperreflexia, ankle clonus)
  - Chiari I malformation; headache/neck pain is more common than ataxia and scoliosis (next common) (15)

Motor symptoms
- Differential diagnosis for extremity weakness: radiculopathy, myelopathy, radiculomyelopathy, or pain-induced subjective weakness
- Differential diagnosis for regional (neck) involvement: dropped head/neck syndrome, and torticollis/cervical dystonia (stiffness)
  - Differential diagnosis for dropped head/neck syndrome (16)
    - Anterocollis (cervical spine)/anterocaput (head): involuntary, nonfixed anteflexion of the head, frequently associated with pain (17)
    - Motor neuron disease: amyotrophic lateral sclerosis (ALS), postpolio syndrome; 1% of patients with motor neuron disease; presents with dropped head as an early feature
    - Peripheral nerve disease: chronic inflammatory demyelinating polyneuropathy (CIDP)
    - Neuromuscular disease: myasthenia gravis (anti-Ach R Ab+, anti-Musk Ab+), myopathy
    - Myopathy
      – Idiopathic isolated neck extensor myopathy: MC cause of dropped head syndrome
      – Polymyositis, inclusion body myositis
      – Facioscapulohumeral muscular (FSH) dystrophy, myotonic dystrophy, Nemaline myopathy, mitochondrial myopathy, carnitine deficiency, severe hypokalemic myopathy
      – Focal posterior cervical myopathy
    - Others
      – Increased thoracic kyphosis with loss of compensatory cervical lordosis
      – Ankylosing spondylitis
      – Malignancy, Parkinson's disease (18)
- Etiologies of excessive cervical kyphosis
  - Degenerative; normal cervical lordosis decrease with age
  - Neurogenic; dropped head syndrome
  - Traumatic; fracture (burst) and posterior tension band injury (intraspinatus and supraspinatus ligament), jumped facet
  - Congenital
  - Post-laminectomy (less common with instrumentation)
- Etiologies of torticollis (twisting of the head and neck) (17)
  - Nonparoxysmal torticollis (19)

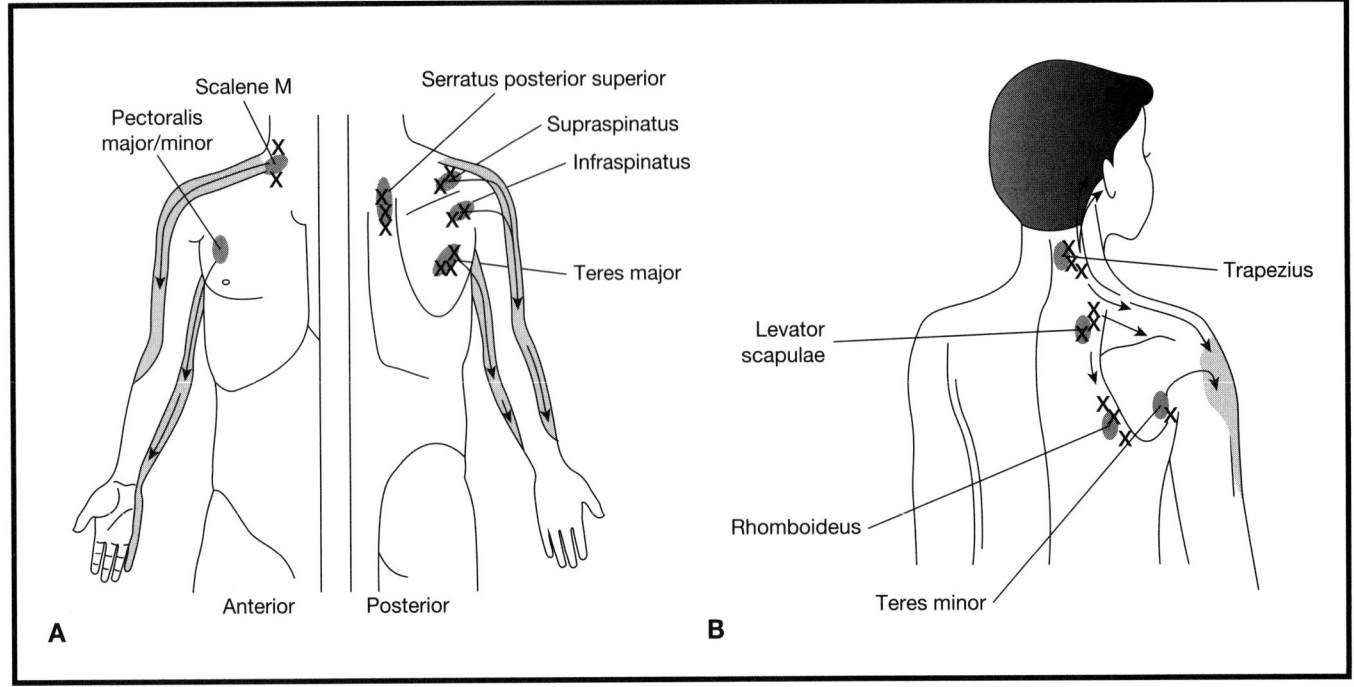

FIGURE 2.2

Typical referred pain patterns from myofascial pain syndrome: (A) trigger points with referred pain below elbow and (B) trigger points with referred pain above elbow.

Source: Adapted from Refs. (20,21).

- Congenital torticollis
  - Breech and difficult delivery; MC cause
  - Incidence: 0.3% to 2% (>80% muscular origin)
  - Other manifestations: congenital hip dysplasia (10%–20%), craniofacial asymmetry (80%), and developmental disorders (eg, attention deficit hyperactivity disorder)
- Osseous torticollis: Klippel–Feil syndrome, cervical vertebral fracture, atlantoaxial rotatory subluxation
- Secondary torticollis: brain lesions in posterior fossa (eg, brain stem, cerebellar tumor) or basal ganglia, hypoxic ischemic encephalopathy, spinal cord lesions (eg, tumor, syrinx), brachial plexus lesion, ocular torticollis (eg, superior oblique palsy, strabismus, spasmus nutans), soft tissue pathology (nonmuscular, infectious: retropharyngeal abscess)
- Paroxysmal torticollis
  - Benign, spasmodic (cervical dystonia), Sandifer syndrome (rare pediatric manifestation of GERD), drug induced (eg, neuroleptics), conversion disorder, increased intracranial pressure (eg, pseudotumor cerebri)
  - Cervical dystonia
    - Incidence ~9 per 100,000, female > male, more common in Whites, onset around 40 years (17)
    - Primary or secondary; Huntington or Wilson disease

Other symptoms

- Differential diagnosis for multiple joint pain (polyarthralgia) with neck pain
  - Systemic inflammatory arthropathy usually accompanied by morning stiffness and other systemic manifestation and associated cutaneous manifestation
    - Rheumatoid arthritis (RA): hand and foot involvement (MC) followed by cervical spine (upper > lower)
    - Ankylosing spondylitis: lumbar spine and chest (limited motion and expansion) involvement (MC) followed by cervical spine
- Cervicogenic headache (22)
  - Location: neck and occipital, unilateral (or bilateral) without side shift, moderate to severe, related to neck movement and posture
  - Involved structures: facet joint (C1–3), uncovertebral joints, disc, cervical/rectus capitis muscle, nerve root, vertebral artery, and ligamentum nuchae
  - Decreased cervical range of motion (ROM), tenderness over C2/3 cervical facet joint
  - Often responsive to occipital N, facet joint, or nerve root blocks
  - Requires work up for brain pathologies
- Pseudoangina pectoris or breast pain: referred pain from C6–7 nerve root irritation (23), unusual cause of chest pain, diagnosis of exclusion
- Altered equilibrium, visual symptoms and hearing: because of irritation of the plexuses surrounding the vertebral and internal carotid arteries
- Differential diagnosis for swallowing difficulty (24)
  - Cervical spine disease: spondylosis, DISH, ankylosing spondylitis

- Mechanical blocking with osteophytes, syndesmophytes
  - Prevertebral abscess
  - Iatrogenic from cervical collar: restrict laryngeal movement
  - Rheumatologic disease
    - Sjögren's syndrome, Behcet's disease, systemic lupus erythematosus (SLE) with xerostomia, ulceration, candidiasis
    - RA involving the TMJ joint (painful mastication)

ANATOMY

REGIONAL ANATOMY (25) (FIGURE 2.3)

Triangles of neck divided by sternocleidomastoid (SCM) muscle
- Anterior triangle of neck bordered by SCM (posterior), mandible (superior), and midline of neck (anterior) (see Figure 2.3)
  - Midline of neck
    - Hyoid cartilage (C3 level), thyroid cartilage (C4–5 level), 1st cricoid ring cartilage (C6 level)
    - Chin with neutral head position (C4 level)
  - Superficial structures
    - Nerves: vagus nerve, hypoglossal (CN 12) nerve, ansa cervicalis
    - Vessels: common carotid artery and internal jugular vein within the carotid sheath
  - Deeper structures
    - Cervical sympathetic chain/ganglion: deep to carotid sheath (not within the sheath) and superficial to longus coli muscle
    - Thyroid gland, superior thyroid artery, superficial laryngeal nerve, inferior thyroid artery, recurrent laryngeal nerve, and thyroid vein
- Posterior triangle of neck bordered by trapezius (posterior border), SCM (anterior), and clavicle (inferior)
  - Superficial structures
    - Nerves: accessory nerve, greater auricular, lesser occipital nerve, supraclavicular nerve, transverse cervical nerve, superficial cervical plexus (exit at the midpoint of posterior border of SCM muscle)
    - Vessels: occipital artery and external jugular vein
  - Deeper structures
    - Nerves: phrenic nerve, transverse cervical artery, brachial plexus (exits between the anterior and middle scalene muscles near the point where external jugular vein crosses the SCM muscle)
    - Vessels: subclavian artery and vein, suprascapular artery

1st rib: palpable at ~3 cm lateral to the insertion of the SCM clavicular head

SPINE COMPLEX (BONE AND JOINT)

C1 (atlas) and C2 (axis) (13)
- C1: no vertebral body, no spinous process, consists of anterior and posterior arch
- C2 has odontoid process (dens), which articulates with the posterior aspect of the anterior arch of the atlas.
- Atlantoaxial joint: true synovial joint, susceptible to inflammatory arthritis (RA)
  - Atlantoaxial joint stabilizer: transverse ligament (principal), alar and apical ligaments (secondary)
  - There is no intervertebral disc between the atlantoaxial and atlanto-occipital joint. Because of the lack of conferred stability from intervertebral discs, destructive inflammatory arthritis involving synovial joints may result in instability

Subaxial cervical spine: C3 to C7 (Figure 2.4)
- Spinous process
  - The C7 spinous process is the largest and the most prominent (easily palpable)
  - The spinous processes of C3 through C6 are bifid, whereas the C7 spinous process usually is not
  - Five articulations between vertebrae: intervertebral disc, two uncovertebral joints (unique in C spine), and two facet (zygapophyseal) joints
- Uncovertebral joint (joint of Luschka)
  - Well visualized in oblique x-ray anterior to the intervertebral foramen (26)
  - Osteophytes from the uncovertebral joint often project into the intervertebral foramen encroaching the cervical nerve root (common in C4–6) and radicular artery
- Transverse process
  - Has anterior and posterior tubercles
  - The discrepancy between the prominent anterior tubercle of the C6 vertebra and the rudimentary anterior tubercle of the C7 vertebra: landmark for ultrasound (US) examination
- Vertebral artery: between longus colli and scalene anterior caudally enter to the transverse foramen between C6 and C7 levels (MC)
- Facet joint (27; Figure 2.5)
  - Diarthrodial, synovial joints with hyaline cartilage, intervening menisci, and joint capsule → susceptible to degenerative changes and inflammatory arthritis
  - The cartilage and the synovial lining are aneural, whereas the joint capsule is highly innervated by the dorsal ramus
  - Joint innervation: dorsal rami of two vertebrae above and below
    - Exception
      - C2–3 innervated by two different branches of C3 dorsal ramus and lesser occipital nerve (branch of C2 ventral ramus)
      - Atlanto-occipital and Atlantoaxial levels by ventral rami of C1 and C2
    - More mechanoreceptors in cervical facet than lumbar facet
    - A delta and C fibers clustered in the dorsolateral aspect of the capsule
  - Facet orientation
    - Cervical: A, B (oblique axial, 45° from the transverse plane, anterior superior to posterior inferior), thoracic: C, D (coronal), lumbar: E, F (oblique sagittal)
    - See Figure 2.5. The orientation of these facet joints influences the ROM of the joint

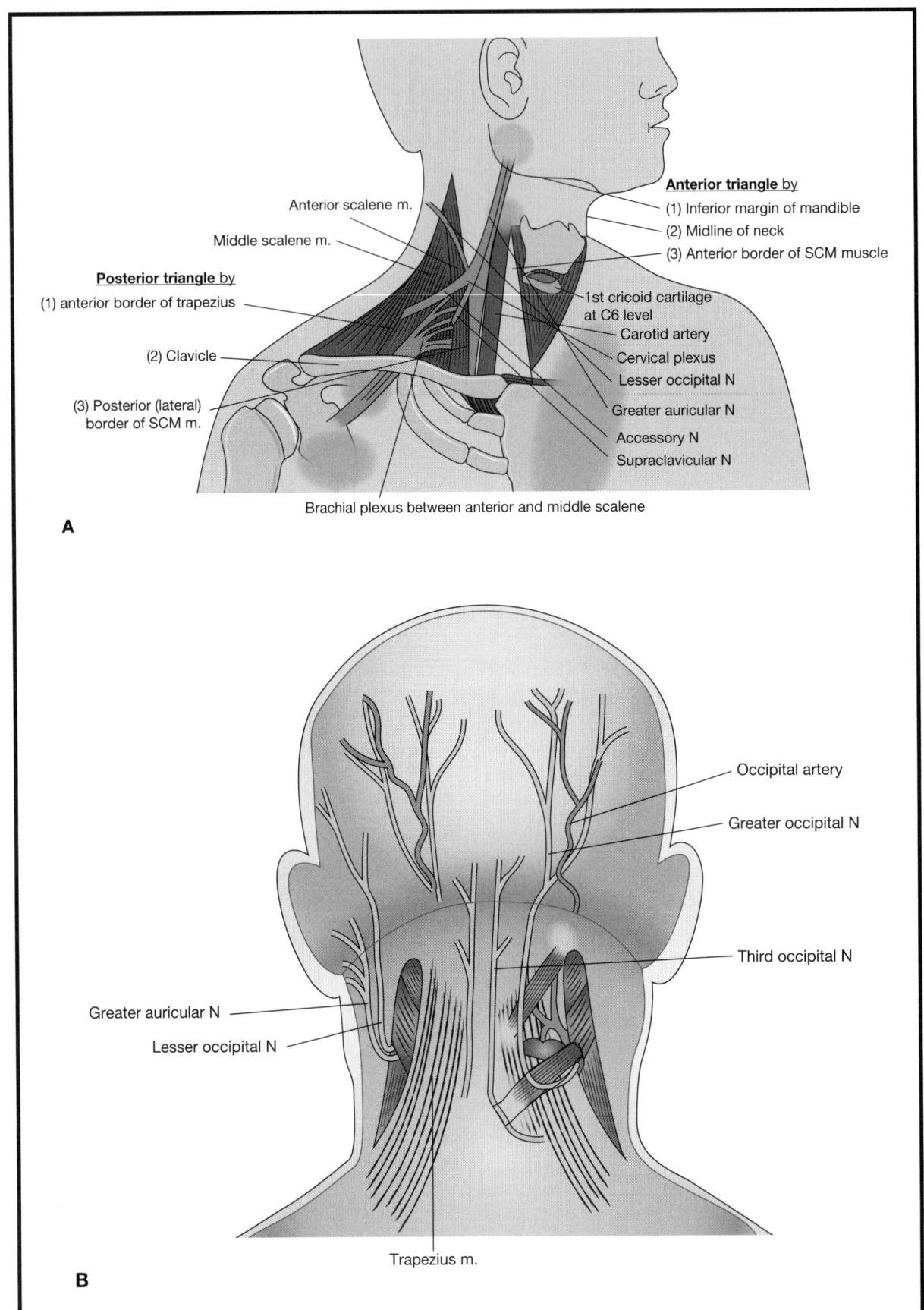

FIGURE 2.3
Surface anatomy of the (A) anterior neck and (B) posterior neck.
Source: Adapted from Ref. (28). Mays MA, Tepper SJ. Occipital nerve blocks. In: Narouze SN, ed. *Interventional Management of Head and Face Pain: Nerve Blocks and Beyond*. New York, NY: Springer; 2014:29–34.

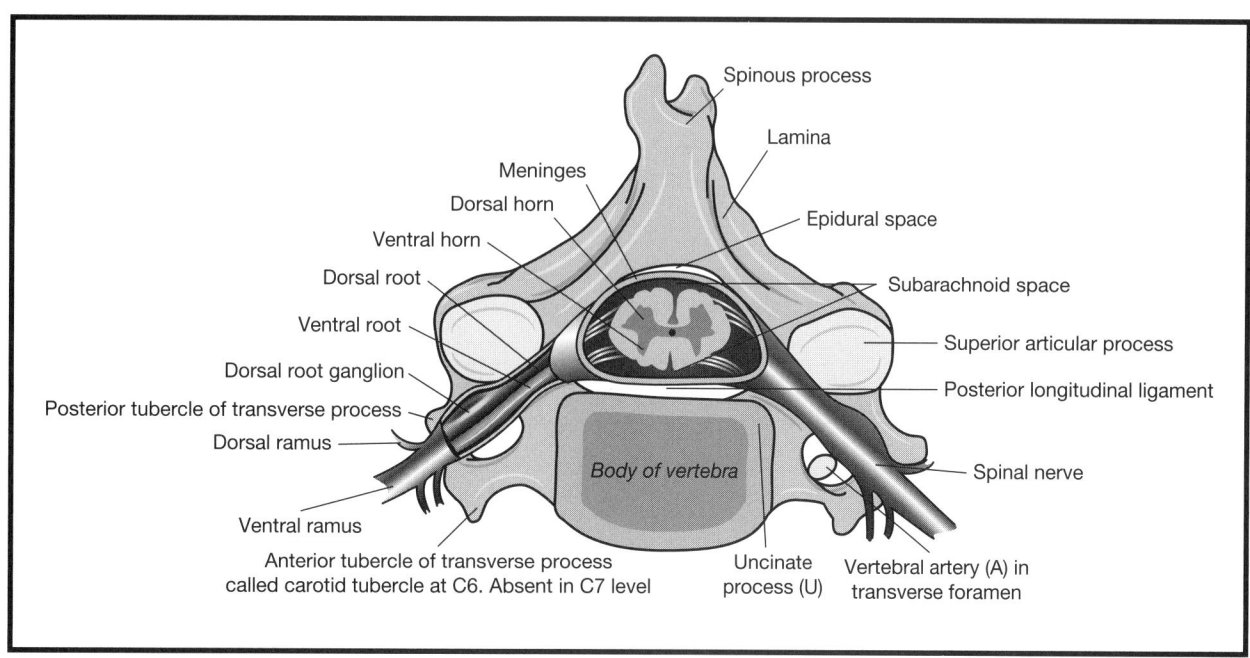

FIGURE 2.4
Cross-sectional view of cervical spine. Uncinate process (U) with uncovertebral joint forms ventral wall of foramen. Spinal nerve exits dorsal to vertebral artery (A).

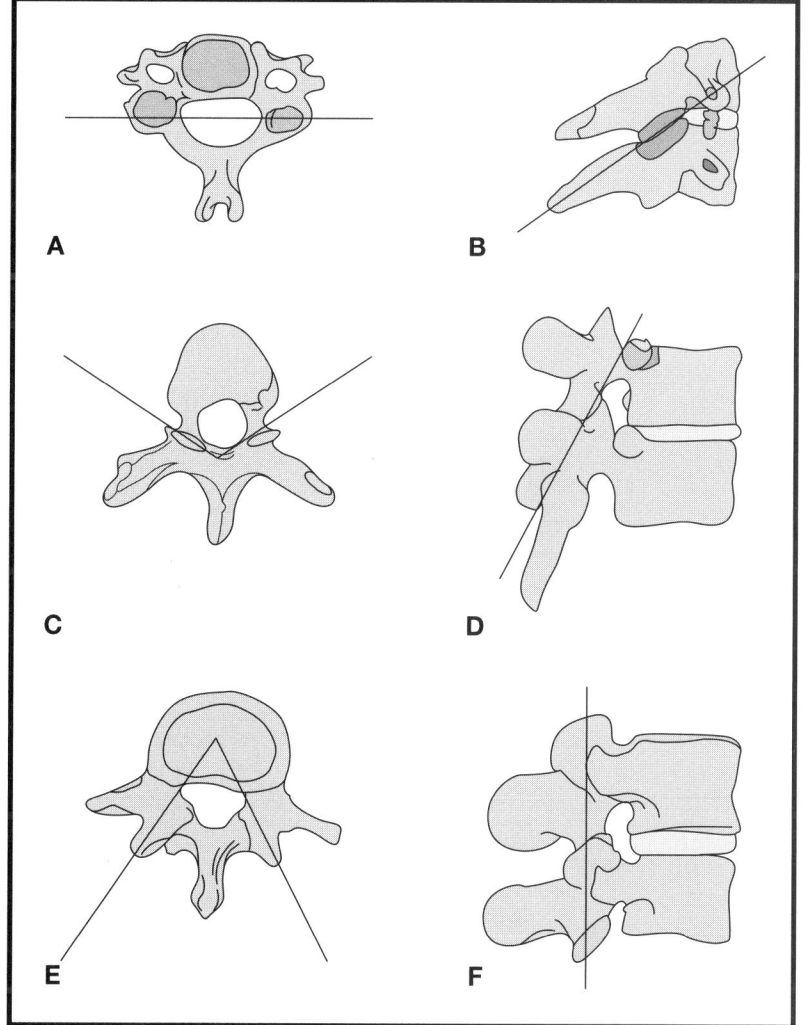

FIGURE 2.5
Facet joint orientation in cervical (A, B), thoracic (C, D), and lumbar spines (E, F).
Source: Adapted from Refs. (29,30).

- Aging changes (31)
  - Start after 2nd decade, cartilage loss, subchondral bone thickening, osteophytes and loss of meniscus, more in the middle and lower segments
- Intervertebral disc (32)
  - Disc consists of the outer annulus fibrosus and the inner nucleus pulposus
    - The annulus fibrosus consists of type I collagen, provides tensile strength
      - Innervated by the sinuvertebral nerve, formed by branches of the ventral nerve root and the sympathetic plexus (33)
    - The nucleus pulposus consists of type II collagen and proteoglycans, which interact with water to resist compressive stress
  - Pressure within the disc is greater with forward flexion and sitting, which can cause discomfort in setting of disc herniation
  - Blood supply: become avascular by 2nd decades, then nutrient supplied by diffusion

Cervical spinal canal and spinal cord
- Lower cervical spine has smaller space for spinal cord than upper cervical spine
  - Spinal cord occupies up to 75% of canal (vs <50% in the atlas level)
  - Biggest diameter of posterior epidural space: C6–7 > C7–T1
- Mid-sagittal diameter is decreased by 2 to 3 mm with neck extension
  - Hyperextension injuries: usually with congenital spinal stenosis, especially in individuals with additional narrowing because of cervical spondylosis → acute cervical myelopathy

LIGAMENT

Atlanto-occipital membrane (dense anterior and thin posterior): limits excessive flexion and extension of atlanto-occipital articulation (about 30°)

Transverse ligament: permit the atlas to rotate around the odontoid process
- A tear in this ligament has the same effect as a fractured odontoid process
- The stability of the atlantoaxial joint depends almost entirely on ligaments
- Frequently dysfunctional in RA and Down syndrome

Posterior longitudinal ligament (PLL): resist hyperflexion, ossification (ossification of posterior longitudinal ligament [OPLL]) can cause cervical myelopathy

Anterior longitudinal ligament (ALL): resist hyperextension

Ligament flavum: thickening can cause spinal stenosis

Supraspinous ligament: C7 to sacrum, above C7: ligament nuchae

NERVE: ROOT AND PLEXUS

Nerve innervation of the spine structure (33)
- Sinuvertebral nerve: innervates anterior vertebral body, external annulus, ALL, PLL, dura mater, and blood vessels
  - Arise from somatic (from ventral ramus) and autonomic root (from vertebral nerve in C1–3 levels or the gray rami communicants from sympathetic trunk and stellate ganglion in the lower cervical level)
  - Innervates more than one level by interconnection with nerves from other levels
- Medial branch of the dorsal ramus: innervates facet (the same level and the level below), interspinous ligament, and deep paraspinals (segmental multifidi and rotators) muscle

Spinal nerve
- C1–7 spinal nerves exit above their corresponding vertebrae, C8 exits between C7 and T1, T1–L5 exit below their corresponding vertebrae
- Dorsal and ventral root → spinal nerve → dorsal and ventral ramus
  - Ventral (anterior) rami form cervical and brachial plexus
  - Dorsal (posterior) rami innervate paraspinal muscles and facet joints, and branch to greater occipital and 3rd occipital nerves
  - Cervical root: tethered in the intervertebral foramen (possible contributor for root avulsion) versus lumbar root: not tethered in the intervertebral foramen
- Cervical plexus (32; Figure 2.6)
  - Ventral primary rami of C1–4
  - Located deep to the internal jugular vein, the deep fascia and SCM and anterior to scalenus medius and levator scapulae (replace with picture)
  - Superficial cervical plexus: outside the prevertebral fascia, posterior margin of middle of SCM muscle
  - Each ventral ramus, except the first, divides into ascending and descending parts that unite in communicating loops
- Dorsal rami from cervical spinal nerves (34) (see Figure 2.3B)
  - Greater occipital nerve: from medial branch of C2 (sometimes C3) dorsal ramus
    - Run over the obliquus capitis inferior/rectus capitis posterior major muscle, pierce through the semispinalis muscle and trapezius aponeurosis
    - Innervates semispinalis capitis exclusively
    - Becomes subcutaneous slightly inferior to the superior nuchal line by passing above an aponeurotic sling composed from the trapezius and SCM muscles. At this point, the greater occipital nerve is immediately medial to the occipital artery
  - Third occipital nerve: from C3 dorsal ramus, ascend the medial to the greater occipital nerve, innervates rostral end of the skin of the neck
  - C3–5 dorsal rami: innervate splenius capitis and facet joints, can cause occiput and posterior neck pain

CERVICAL PLEXUS VENTRAL RAMI OF C1–4	NERVE	ROOT	INNERVATION	NOTE
Superficial (sensory) Ascending Descending (supraclavicular)	Lesser occipital	C2 (3)	Behind the ear Post border of the mastoid process	Emerge from posterior border of SCM muscle (middle)
	Greater auricular	C 2, C3	Skin over parotid gland, inferior to ear	
	Transverse cervical cutaneous	C 2, C3	Anterior neck	
	Supraclavicular (medial, intermediate, and lateral)	C 3, C4	Lower neck and shoulder	
Deep (muscular) Medial Lateral	Spinal accessory	C2, C3, C4	SCM (leaves the posterior aspect of SCM [near the midline, nerve stimulation site]) and trapezius	Course upto foramen magnum (merge with cranial part), down to jugular foramen, course beneath the posterior belly of the digastric muscle
	Phrenic	C 3–5 (4)	Diaphragm	Course anterior to anterior scalene muscle. Deep to carotid sheath
	Ansa cervicalis (loop)	C 1–3	Thyrohyoid (C1), genio-hyoid, sternothyroid, sternohyoid, and inferior belly of omohyoid	Lies superficial to internal jugular vein in the carotid sheath

SCM, sternocleidomastoid.

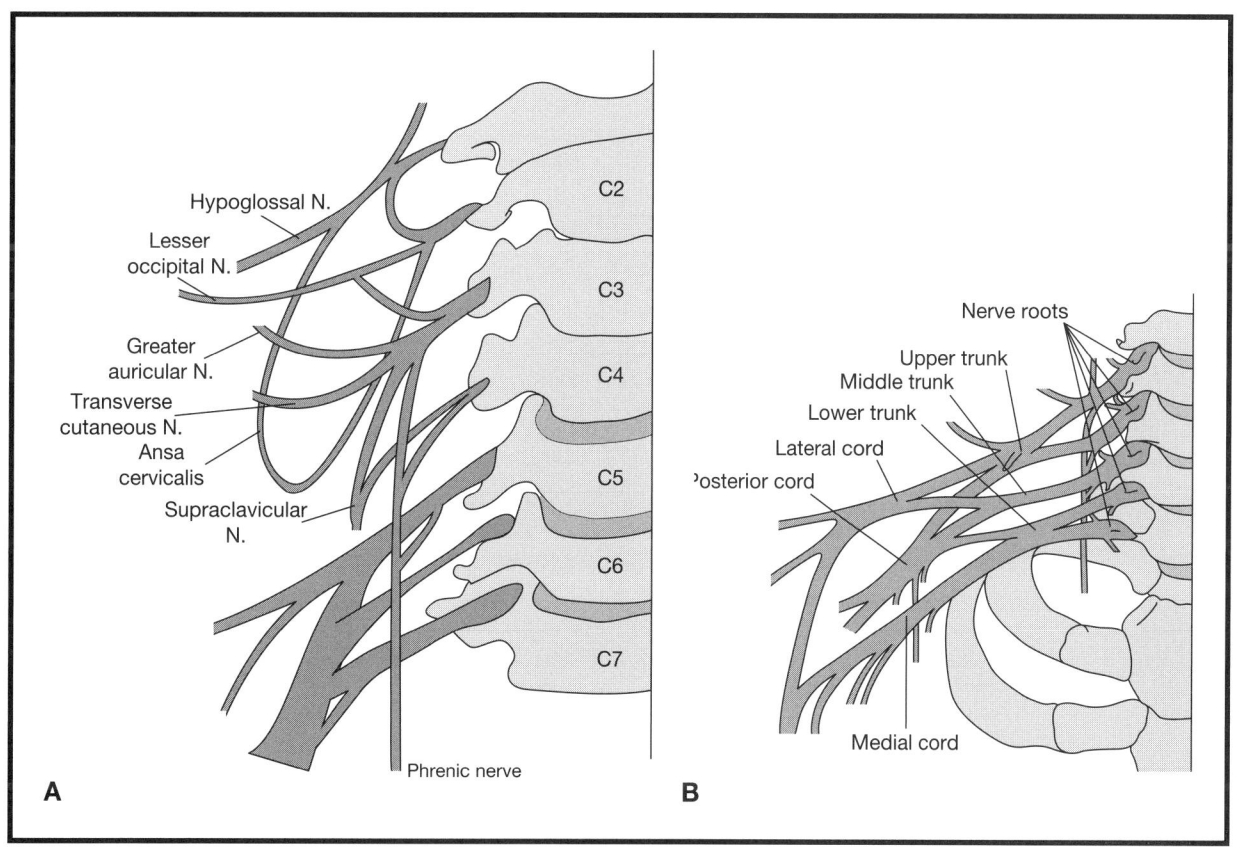

FIGURE 2.6
(A) Cervical plexus and (B) brachial plexus.
Source: Adapted from Ref. (32). Mancall EL, Brock DG, Gray H. *Gray's clinical neuroanatomy: the anatomic basis for clinical neuroscience.* Philadelphia, PA: Elsevier, xiii, 433 pages.

- Brachial plexus
  - Origin: C5 to T1 ventral rami, variations: prefixed (C4 included), postfixed (T1 included)
  - Course: emerges between the anterior and middle scalene muscles, courses behind the clavicle, lies on the serratus anterior and subscapularis muscle and runs with axillary artery
  - Divided by clavicle: trunks above clavicle, cords below clavicle
- Nerve root itself is not pain sensitive, but dural sheath is

MUSCLE

Anterior and anterolateral cervical muscles
- Superficial: platysma, SCM (neck flexion with bilateral contraction, contralateral rotation/ipsilateral flexion with unilateral contraction)
- Anterior deep: longus capitis, colli, rectus capitis anterior, lateralis
- Lateral deep: anterior, medius, and posterior scalene (ipsilateral flexion with SCM)
- Hyoid muscles: muscles for swallowing and synergist for head flexion
  - Suprahyoid muscles (mylohyoid, stylohyoid): pull the hyoid bone upward and forward, widen the pharynx, and close airway
  - Infrahyoid muscles (omohyoid, thyrohyoid, sternohyoid, and sternothyroid): strap muscles of the larynx, return the hyoid bone and larynx back to the original position

Posterior cervical muscles
- Superficial: trapezius muscle
- Intermediate: splenius capitis and splenius cervicis
  - Splenius: acts as a group to extend or hyperextend the head, unilateral contraction rotates and bends head laterally toward the same side
- Deep: erector spinae
  - Iliocostalis cervicis, longissimus capitis/cervicis, and spinalis cervicis (lateral to medial)
  - Primary extensor and controls forward flexion via eccentric contraction
    - Spinalis cervicis: unilateral contraction flex the neck ipsilaterally, bilateral contraction extends the neck
    - Longissimus: capitis extends head and turns face toward the same side; cervicis and thoracis act together to extend vertebral column
    - Iliocostalis: unilateral contraction flex the neck ipsilaterally, bilateral contraction extends the neck
- Transversospinales (from transverse processes to spinous processes of higher level)
  - Semispinalis cervicis/capitis, multifidus, rotator and interspinalis, intertransversarii
  - Flex to the same side and rotate to the opposite side with unilateral contraction. Extension of the vertebral column with bilateral contraction
    - Semispinalis cervicis: acts synergistically with SCM muscles of opposite side
- Suboccipital muscles (rectus capitis posterior minor, major, oblique capitis superior/inferior); innervated by the suboccipital nerve (dorsal primary rami of C1)

Head and neck movement in summary
- Lateral head movement: SCM and scalene muscle
- Head extension: splenius, trapezius, semispinalis, and longissimus muscle
- Head flexion: SCM, synergistic movement with supra and infrahyoid muscle
- Neck flexor: longus capitis and longus coli muscle

MUSCLE	ORIGIN	INSERTION	INNERVATION	ACTION/FUNCTION	COMMENT
Anterior Neck					
Platysma	Deep fascial and skin upon the lower neck and upper chest	Inferior border of the mandible, skin of the face inferior to the mouth	Cervical branch of CN 7	Wrinkle lower face and mouth, draw the corner of mouth inferiorly, depress the mandible	
SCM	Lateral surface of mastoid process of temporal bone and lateral half of superior nuchal line	Anterior surface of manubrium of sternum Superior surface of medial third of clavicle	Spinal root of accessory nerve (motor) and branches from C2 to C4 (pain and proprioception)	Tilt head and flex neck to ipsilateral side, rotate head to contralateral side	Landmark for neck triangle Involved in torticollis

(*continued*)

MUSCLE	ORIGIN	INSERTION	INNERVATION	ACTION/FUNCTION	COMMENT
Scalene anterior	Anterior tubercles of C2–6 transverse processes	Scalene tubercle on the first rib	Direct motor branches from C4 to C6 (ventral rami)	Inspiration with rib mobile (elevate the rib, 1st by scalene anterior/medius and 2nd by scalene posterior)	Brachial plexus emerges between scalene anterior and medius. Can cause thoracic outlet syndrome
Scalene medius	Transverse processes of atlas and axis, post tubercles of transverse processes of C2–7	First rib (posterior to the groove for the subclavian artery)	Direct motor branches from C3 to C8	With rib fixed, bends the cervical spine to the same side and rotate cervical spine to opposite side	Penetrated by the dorsal scapular nerve and long thoracic nerve
Scalene posterior	Posterior tubercles of transverse processes of C4–6	Outer surface of 2nd rib	Direct motor branches from C7 to C8		
Longus capitis	Anterior tubercles of the transverse processes of C3–6	Anterior and basilar surface of the occipital bone	Direct motor branches from C1 to C3	Flex the head and neck with bilateral contraction. Rotate the head ipsilaterally with unilateral contraction.	
Longus colli	Anterior vertebral bodies of T1–T3. Anterior tubercles of the transverse processes of C3–7	Anterior tubercle of the atlas. Anterior vertebral bodies of C2–4	Direct motor branches from C2 to C6	Flex the neck with bilateral contraction	Sympathetic ganglia is located superficial to longus colli muscle within the prevertebral fascia
Posterior Neck					
Trapezius	Medial third of superior nuchal line, external occipital protuberance, lig nuchae, spinous processes of C7–T12	Lateral third of clavicle, acromion and spine of scapula	Spinal root of accessory nerve and branches from C3 to C4	Elevation of scapula (glenoid faces up); upper and lower trapezius. Upper: Shrug shoulder (elevation), rotation of head to opposite side, cervical/head extension. Middle: scapular retraction	Myofascial pain syndrome. Winging of scapula
Levator scapulae	Posterior tubercles of the transverse processes of C1–4	Superior angle and adjacent medial border of the scapula	Dorsal scapular nerve, C4–5 nerves	Elevate, adduct, rotate (glenoid faces down) the scapula, lateral flexion of cervical spine (ipsilaterally) and assist cervical extension	Frequently involved in myofascial pain syndrome

(continued)

MUSCLE	ORIGIN	INSERTION	INNERVATION	ACTION/FUNCTION	COMMENT
Splenius capitis	Ligamentum nuchae and spinous processes of C7–T6	Mastoid process and lateral end of the superior nuchal line	Dorsal rami of C2–6 (mostly C2–3)	Extend head Laterally bend the neck and head, rotate head to the same side with unilateral contraction	
Splenius cervicis	Ligamentum nuchae and spinous processes of C7–T6	Posterior tubercles of the transverse processes of C1–3	Dorsal rami of C2–6	Extend cervical spine Laterally flex head and neck, rotate head to the same side with unilateral contraction	
Spinalis capitis	Transverse processes of C4–T6	Occipital bone (between anterior and inferior nuchal line)	Dorsal rami of cervical spinal nerve	Extend and lateral flexion of the head with unilateral contraction	
Spinalis cervicis	Transverse processes of T1–6	Spinous processes of C2–5	Dorsal rami of cervical spinal nerve	Extend the neck with bilateral contraction	
Semispinalis capitis/cervicis	Transverse processes of C7–T12	Capitis: back of skull between nuchal lines; Cervicis/thoracis: spinous processes of 4–6 vertebrae level above the origin	Capitis: dorsal ramus of C2 Cervicis/thoracis: dorsal rami of spinal nerves C1–T12	Extend the trunk and laterally bend the trunk, rotate the trunk to the opposite side with unilateral contraction	Three parts are named based on their insertions: capitis, cervicis, and thoracis
Suboccipital Muscles					
Rectus capitis major	Spinous process of axis	Inferior nuchal line	Suboccipital nerve (C1)	Extend and rotate head	Rectus capitis minor is deeper and inserts more medial than rectus capitis major
Rectus capitis minor	Posterior tubercle of atlas	Inferior nuchal line medially			
Obliquus capitis inferior	Spinous process of axis	Transverse process of atlas	Suboccipital nerve (C1)	Rotate the head to the same side	Greater occipital nerve (dorsal ramus of C2) ascend superiorly after emerging from the inferior margin of obliquus capitis inferior
Obliquus capitis superior	Transverse process of atlas	Occipital bone above inferior nuchal line	Suboccipital nerve (C1)	Extend the head, rotate the head to the same side	The suboccipital triangle is formed by obliquus capitis superior and inferior and rectus capitis posterior major
Rotatores	Transverse processes	Long rotatores: spinous process of two vertebral level above the origin Short rotatores: spinous process of one vertebral level above the origin	Dorsal rami of C1–L5	Rotate the vertebral column to the opposite side	

SCM, sternocleidomastoid.

FASCIA (35)

Deep cervical fascia
- Encircle the neck completely
- Composed of superficial, middle, and deep layers
- *Superficial layer*: envelops the trapezius and SCM, also called an investing layer
  ○ The superficial layer extends to the trapezius muscle, continues anteriorly over the posterior triangle, and divides to encircle the SCM muscle
  ○ Clinical implication
    ▪ Anatomic basis of the subcutaneous cervical plexus block in the posterior to middle of SCM muscle: no difference in efficacy between the injection under the investing fascia as the anterior triangle may not have deep investing fascia (36)
- *Middle layer*: also called the pretracheal layer
  ○ Encloses the omohyoid and strap muscles and continues laterally to the scapula
  ○ The thyroid gland, larynx, trachea, pharynx, and esophagus are enclosed by the visceral fascia of the middle layer
- *Deepest layer*: prevertebral layer and carotid sheath, barrier for infection
  ○ Prevertebral layer: encloses the scalenus muscles, brachial plexus, sympathetic chain, longus colli muscle, and ALL other structures surrounding vertebral column
    ▪ Anatomic basis for sympathetic nerve block under the prevertebral layer
  ○ Carotid sheath: contains carotid artery, internal jugular vein, and vagus nerve (Figure 2.7)

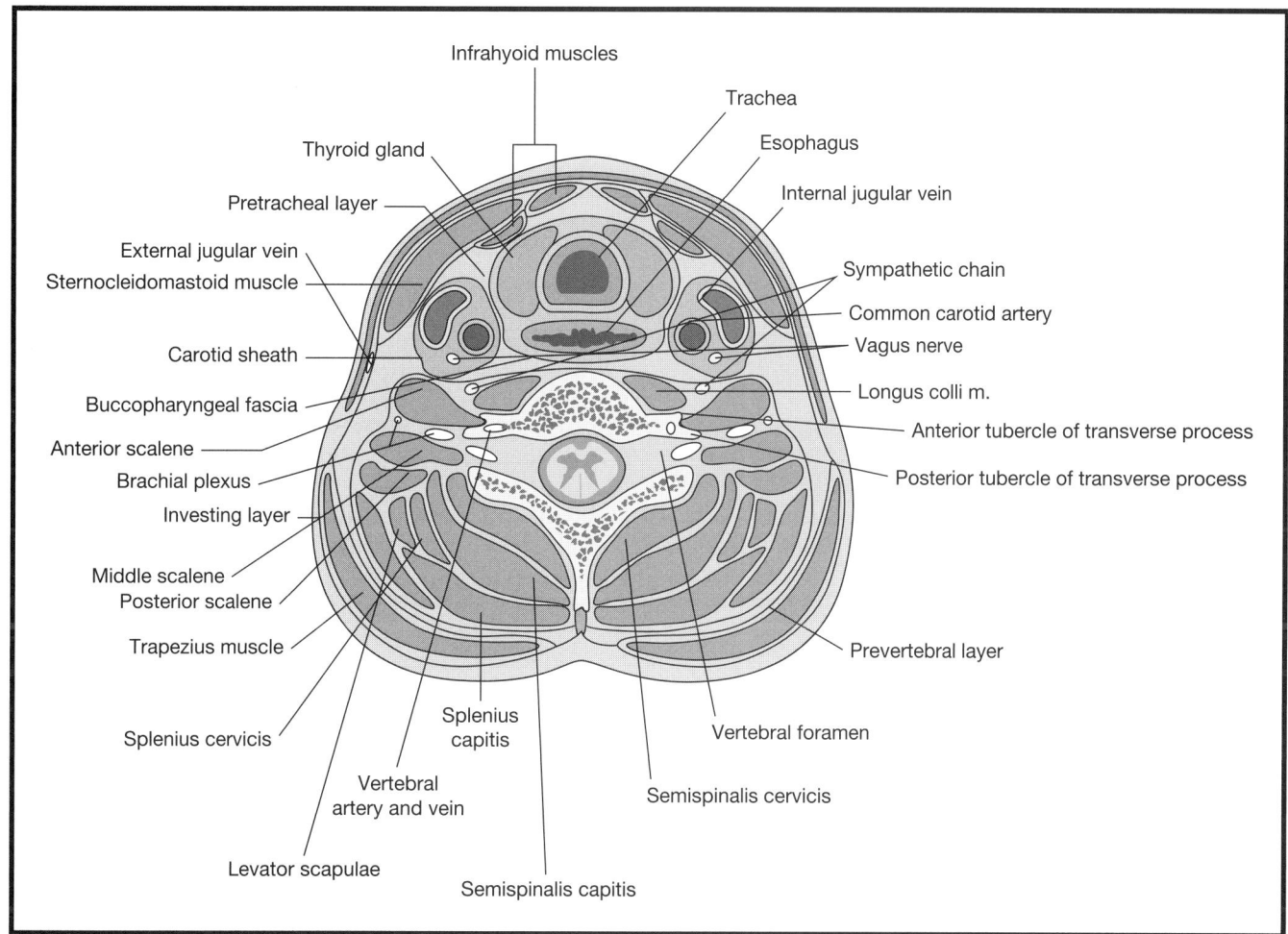

FIGURE 2.7
Cross-sectional view of neck.

BLOOD SUPPLY

Vertebral artery
- Arises from the subclavian artery, courses through the C6 transverse foramen cephalad, passing anterior to the emerging cervical nerve root at each level → lies behind the lateral mass of C1 → enters the foramen magnum and rejoin to form the basilar artery
- Variable presence, more common on the left at C3 and C6 and on the right at C5 and T1
- Anterior spinal artery
  ○ At the level of foramen magnum, branches anterior spinal artery which descends anterior to the spinal cord, takes several radicular arteries, supplies anterior two-thirds of spinal cord
  ○ Radicular arteries (medullary feeder arteries) arise from the vertebral artery at the lower level and ascending cervical artery, enter through neural foramen and join the anterior spinal artery

- Posterior spinal artery: two posterior spinal arteries originate from the posterior inferior cerebellar artery or the vertebral arteries
- Clinical implication in neck pain
  ○ Vertebral artery dissection
    ▪ Severe neck pain with posterior circulation signs such as nystagmus, vertigo, drop attacks, dysarthria, and visual impairment
    ▪ Transient symptoms: associated with head position and a critical reduction in blood flow, can result in a cerebellar infarction (37)
    ▪ Cautious in occipital nerve block near C1–2 level, transforaminal epidural block and stellate ganglion block

Carotid artery (38)
- The right common carotid artery (CCA) arises from the brachiocephalic artery, while the left CCA usually originates directly from the aortic arch
- The common carotid arteries ascend through the mediastinum and lie posterior and medial to the internal jugular veins in the neck. Diameters of the CCA are ~6 to 8 mm
- The CCA bifurcates into the external carotid artery (ECA) and internal carotid artery (ICA) typically at the upper edge of the thyroid cartilage (between C3 and C5)
- The ICA arises posterolateral to the ECA in approximately 90% of individuals; a medial origin is present in the remaining 10%
- Clinical implication
  ○ Carotid dissection; headache (earliest and most common) with/without neck pain

CAROTID DISSECTION	GIANT CELL ARTERITIS
<40 years Neurologic signs suggestive of carotid dissection (such as Horner syndrome or monocular visual loss) CTA may be the test of choice	Older Shoulder pain, neck pain, and pelvic pain (from concomitant polymyalgia rheumatica) Elevations of ESR or CRP MRI to evaluate superficial cranial vessels

CRP, C-reactive protein; CTA, CT angiography; ESR, erythrocyte sedimentation rate.

BIOMECHANICS (39,40)

Cervical spine ROM (41)
- Upper cervical spine: occiput–C2
  ○ Supports the weight of the head and protects spinal cord
  ○ Atlanto-occipital joint: spheroid articulation
    ▪ Approximately 50% of total flexion and extension in the neck
    ▪ Some lateral bending and axial rotation: controversial
  ○ Atlantoaxial (C1–2) joint
    ▪ Restrained by ligaments (cruciate and alar ligament; main motion limiting structures) and tectorial membrane
    ▪ Provides ~50% (50°) of rotatory motion of the cervical spine and 10° flexion–extension
- Other cervical spine
  ○ Has uncovertebral joint: helps for axial loading and stabilize during lateral bending
  ○ Motion stabilized by ALL, PLL, and ligamentum flavum: restrict flexion–extension
  ○ Flexion–extension motion occurs more at lower cervical C5–7 level than upper C2–4 level
- Line of gravity
  ○ Passes auricle of ear, odontoid process of C2, body of C7, anterior to thoracic spine, posterior to L3, mid-femoral head, slightly anterior to knee and ankle joint (thorough calcaneocuboid joint)
  ○ Head forward posture (upper crossed syndrome): straighten cervical lordosis, increase kyphosis of cervicothoracic junction, protracted shoulder
- Coupling motion at cervical facet: lateral bending usually coupled with axial rotation to the same side because of orientation of facet joints
- Vertebral artery can be occluded on full extension and 90° rotation to the opposite site
  ○ Posterior circulation distribution strokes can occur as a result of a variety of athletic injuries and therapeutic chiropractic manipulation
- Pain on rotation may indicate atlanto-occipital joint or rotatory muscle origin versus pain on flexion/extension may indicate subaxial spine or flexor/extensor muscle origin

Role of spinal musculature (42)
- Control the movement of the spine and to contribute essential stabilization to the vertebral column
- Provide proprioceptive feedback regarding the position of the spine in space
- Paraspinal muscle mass decreases with aging → allowing poorly controlled segmental motion → facilitate arthritic changes

Degenerative cascade
- Definition of spondylosis; age-related degenerative changes within the spinal column
- Age-related degeneration: MC cause of cervical spondylosis (43)
- Disc degeneration and cervical spondylosis with aging
  ○ Fibrous nucleus pulposus: loss of water content, protein, mucopolysaccharides, increased keratin sulfate and chondroitin sulfate → loss of elasticity and decreased size
  ○ Loss of annular fiber integrity: loss of load bearing integrity → disc bulging, lax ligaments, and loss of disc height
  ○ Loss of disc height → loss of cervical lordosis with ventral (anterior) compression, and angular change of spinal segment → Progressive kyphosis with vascular and neural compression (44,45)
- Loss of fiber attachment to bone with overload of uncovertebral and facet joints with osteophytes formation
  ○ Up to 70% of axial loading goes to the facet joint in cases of severe disc space narrowing
- Degenerative changes in asymptomatic population
  ○ Imaging findings of degeneration (MRI): 25% in <40 years, ~85% in >60 years (46)
  ○ Some role in occupations or sports activities: for example, rugby, soccer, horseback riding, and so on
  ○ Gender difference: odd ratio for disc degeneration or osteoarthritis (OA): 1.7 and 1.8 for men (47)

- Reason for posterolateral herniation of the disc: lateral to PLL and medial to uncovertebral joints, annulus fibrosus is at its weakest
- C5–6 and C6–7: MC involved level

Whiplash injury (48)
- Mechanism of injury: rear-ended motor vehicle crash (MC)
  - Head motion lags behind the body as a result of the inertia of the head
  - The initial forward acceleration of the torso deforms the cervical spine into a nonphysiologic S-shaped curve; extension at the lower segments and flexion at the uppermost segments
  - The base of the skull is accelerated forward by the neck, causing the head to rotate backward and the upper cervical spine to move into extension
  - As a result of head restraint contact, the head and neck rebound forward into cervical flexion
- The facet joint injury
  - Nonphysiologic pinching motion, with compression posteriorly and distraction anteriorly, usually coupled with shear
  - Facet injuries include capsular strain and tears; bony impingement; synovial fold pinching; and direct-impact injury resulting in contusion, intra-articular hemorrhage, and damage to subchondral bone
- Intervertebral disc injury
  - The anulus fibrosus of the disc and longitudinal ligaments can be disrupted
  - Disc injuries: better correlated with the acceleration of the struck vehicle than with the change in velocity of the vehicle

PHYSICAL EXAMINATION

INSPECTION

Position of head (center of gravity of head at mastoid process/auricle of the ear) in relation to the line of gravity (plumb line): plumb line through C7 vertebral body in normal posture
- Sagittal plane (inspection from the side): forward head position or dropped head
- Coronal plane (inspection from the front/back): scoliosis, torticollis, lateral tilt
- Axial plane (inspection from the top): rotation of the head
  - Torticollis: head toward the shortened muscle while rotating the chin in the opposite direction

Swelling, mass, deformity, scar from previous surgery

Atrophy of muscles: trapezius (accessory nerve injury), winging of scapula (serratus anterior, rhomboid or trapezius muscle dysfunction), deltoid, biceps (C5–6), forearm or hand intrinsic muscles (C8–T1 radiculopathy, cervical myelopathy, motor neuron disease)

PALPATION

Bony structure
- Anterior: hyoid bone, thyroid cartilage (C4–5 level), first cricoid ring (C6), carotid tubercle (anterior tubercle of C6 transverse process, one inch lateral from the cricoid ring); to check palpable mass, tenderness
- Midpoint of the clavicle: brachial plexus beneath it
- Posterior: occiput, inion (superior aspect of superior nuchal line), superior nuchal line, mastoid process, spinous process (C2: highest palpable, C7: most prominent), facet joint (C5–6, MC site for OA; difficult to palpate), superior angle of medial scapular (T2 level)

Muscle and other soft tissue
- Anterior: SCM, scalene (under SCM), and Erb's point (upper trunk of brachial plexus located posterolateral to the SCM; nerve stimulation point)
- Posterior: trapezius, underlying paraspinal, levator scapulae with characteristic referred pain (common sites for trigger point), occiput (tenderness over the occipital nerve with referred pain to frontotemporal region)
- Lymph node palpation (49)
  - Anterior cervical triangle: submandibular and anterior cervical nodes
  - Posterior cervical triangle: posterior cervical and supraclavicular nodes
  - If tender and enlarged (0.5–1 cm depending on location); mostly benign, may needs workup for infections, autoimmune, malignancy and others etiologies

RANGE OF MOTION	
MOTION	ANGLE
Extension	45°
Flexion	45°
Lateral bending	45°
Rotation	80° (to each side)

- Intact passive ROM with decreased active ROM: neuromuscular disease with weakness
- MSK pathologies: usually both active and passive ROM affected
- Head rotation: mostly occurs at the occiput–C3 level

NEUROLOGIC EXAMINATION AND SPECIAL EXAMINATION

Motor and sensory examination of upper extremity
- Motor examination
  - Myotome
    - C5: shoulder abduction and elbow flexion, C6: wrist extension (elbow flexion), C7: elbow extension or wrist flexion, C8: finger flexion (hand grip), T1: finger abduction
- Sensory examination
  - Dermatome
    - C5: lateral arm, C6: lateral forearm, thumb, index finger, C7: posterior forearm, middle finger, C8: medial forearm, ring and little fingers, T1: medial arm

Deep tendon reflexes (DTR)
- C5: biceps, C6: brachioradialis, C7: triceps reflex
- Occasionally scapular and deltoid reflex can be tested; easy to obtain in upper motor neuron disease

PROVOCATIVE TEST		
NAME	DESCRIPTION	SENSITIVITY (SEN) AND SPECIFICITY (SPE) IN %
Cervical Radiculopathy		
Spurling test	Extend and rotate the neck and then apply downward pressure on the head Positive for C6–8 radiculopathy if pain radiates into the distal upper extremity in the same side	Sen: 30–60; Spe: 92–100 (50,51)
Shoulder abduction test	Active or passive abduction of the ipsilateral shoulder with the hand resting on top of the head. Positive if the radicular pain is relieved	Sen: 43–50; Spe: 80–100 (52)
Neck distraction test	The examiner places one hand under the patient's chin and the other hand around the occiput, and then slowly lifts the patient's head Positive if the radicular pain is relieved	Sen: 40–43; Spe: 100
Thoracic Outlet Syndrome (53)		
Adson test	With neck hyperextended and head rotated to the symptomatic side, the radial pulse is palpated during deep inhalation Positive if the pulse disappears and paresthesia develops in the hand of the symptomatic extremity	Sen: 94; Spe: 18–87 (53,54)
Wright's hyperabduction	Radial pulse is palpated at the wrist when the ipsilateral arm is elevated to 90° (or 180°) for 60 s Positive if the pulse disappears	Positive rate: 69 (55)
Roos test	Open and close the fist with the shoulder abduction and elbows at 90° flexion (surrender position) Positive if the patient's usual upper-limb symptoms reproduce within 3 min	Positive rate: 68 (55)
Cervical Myelopathy		
Hoffman's test	Flick the fingernail of the long finger, from dorsal to volar while the hand was supported by the examiner's hand Positive if any flexion of the ipsilateral thumb and/or index finger	Sen: 33 (56); Spe: 59 (57)
Trömner sign	Tap the volar aspect of the distal phalanx of the middle finger Positive if flexion of the thumb and index finger Higher sensitivity than Hoffman (maybe because of the fact that there are no nerve endings in the nail itself) (58)	Sen: 94% and negative predictive value (85%)
Lhermitte's sign	Passive cervical flexion to end range with the patient seated Positive if the presence of an electric like sensation down the spine or in the extremities	Sen: 27; Spe: 28–90

DIAGNOSTIC STUDIES (FLOWCHART 2.2)

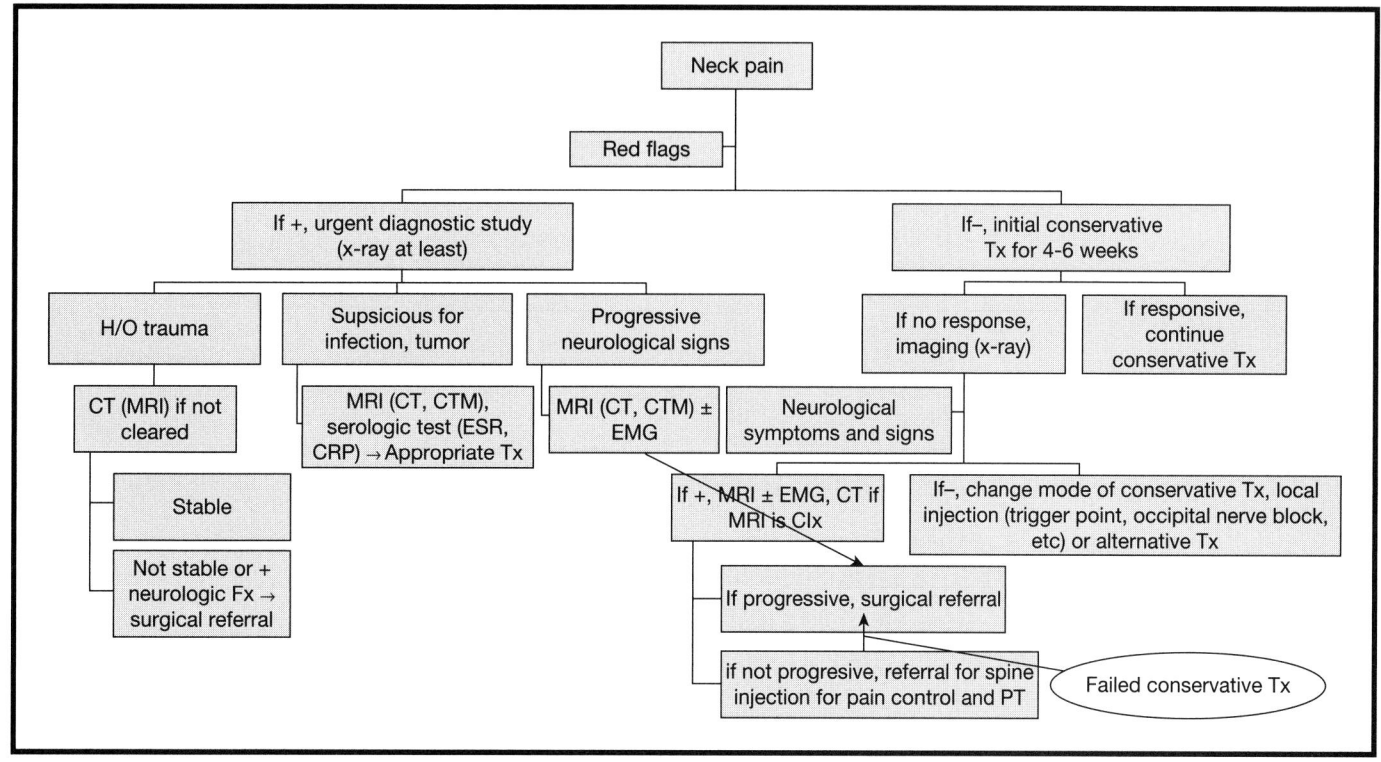

FLOWCHART 2.2
Diagnostic approach and management for neck pain in an outpatient clinic.
CT, CT scan; CRP, C-reactive protein; CTM, CT myelography; Tx, treatment.

PLAIN RADIOGRAPHS (59)

Routine: anteroposterior (AP), lateral, and oblique (for joint of Luschka and intervertebral foramen)
• Lateral view: evaluate for continuity of the anterior vertebral body line, the posterior vertebral body line, the spinolaminar line, and the spinous process line
  ○ C1–2 instability (Figure 2.8)
    ▪ Unstable if anterior atlantodental (dens to anterior arch of atlas) interval >3.5 to 5 mm and posterior (dens to posterior arch of the atlas) atlantodental index <14 mm
    ▪ Commonly seen in Down syndrome, RA, Os odontoideum fracture, and transverse ligament injury
  ○ Torg and Pavlov ratio: sagittal diameter of the spinal canal/the midbody diameter of the vertebral body at the same level. If <0.8: may be predictive of spinal stenosis
    ▪ May not be accurate in large athletes (false positive for spinal stenosis)
  ○ Flexion/extension (instability)
    ▪ Flexion–extension: >3.5 mm of translational displacement or 20° of angular motion: suggesting instability
    ▪ Dynamic view considered in prior surgical fusion, RA or Down syndrome, or other cervical disease

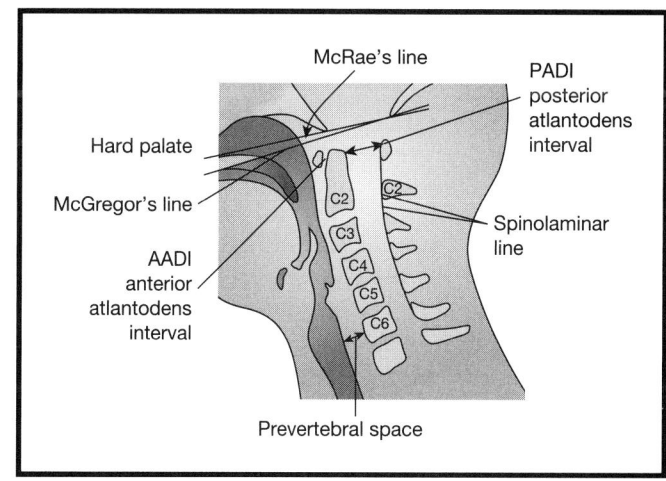

FIGURE 2.8
Radiologic findings utilized in the evaluation of cervical instability.

AADI, anterior atlantodens interval; PADI, posterior atlantodens interval.

- X-ray with history of trauma
  ○ AP, lateral, and open mouth (axis, dens of atlas evaluation)
  ○ Lateral view: evaluate for continuity of the anterior vertebral body line, the posterior vertebral body line, the spinolaminar line, and the spinous process line
    ▪ Signs suggestive of fracture: predendate space <3 mm, the prevertebral soft tissue at C3; usually 3 mm, anterior wedging of >3 mm
  ○ Swimmer's view to evaluate C7–T1
  ○ If suspicion, obtain CT of neck (especially in blunt trauma)

Indications
- Nonspecific neck pain: unhelpful in the diagnosis in most cases
  ○ Consider if (+) red flag signs: age of onset less than 20 years or greater than than 55 years, constitutional symptoms, history of cancer, immunosuppressant, and drug abuse
  ○ Common indications for immediate imaging studies (except trauma)
    ▪ Suspicious of neoplasm: Pain worse at night; unexplained weight loss; history of neoplasm; age >50 years, and so on
    ▪ Infection: fever, chills, night sweats; unexplained weight loss; history of recent systemic infection; recent invasive procedure; immunosuppressed; or intravenous drug use
    ▪ Neurological symptoms and abnormal neurological signs: progressive neurologic deficits; upper and lower extremity symptoms; ataxia, sensory or motor symptoms/signs, bowel or bladder dysfunction; needs MRI (CT if MRI is contraindicated)
  ○ Negative x-ray does not preclude the further workup
- Trauma
  ○ Can be cleared based on history and physical examination if low risk of Nexus criteria and Canadian C-spine rules (all items are met)
  ○ National Emergency X-Radiography Utilization Study (NEXUS) criteria for low risk: the absence of all of the following conditions: midline cervical tenderness, altered level of consciousness or intoxication, abnormal neurologic findings, or painful distracting injuries
  ○ Canadian C spine rules: simple rear-end motor vehicle crash, able to sit in the emergency department, able to ambulate, delayed-onset neck pain, absence of midline tenderness, and ability to rotate neck 45° to the right and left
  ○ Order imaging in clinically relevant trauma; minor trauma in elderly patient or susceptible (eg, ankylosing spondylitis), high risk in Canadian C-spine rules: age >65 years, dangerous mechanism, paresthesias

MRI (34)

Indications
- Evaluation of bony detail, marrow signal, malalignment, stenosis, and radiculopathy
- Evaluation of disc, root, spinal cord (tumor, infarct, inflammation), meninges, infarct, and/or fluid collection

DISC PATHOLOGY	MRI FINDINGS
Bulge	Symmetric extension of annulus beyond the confines of adjacent end plates, displacement of disc comprising >50% of the circumference of the disc
Herniation	Displacement of disc comprising <50% of the circumference of the disc • >25% of spinal canal diameter: more clinically significant (35,36)
Protrusion	Focal area of disc material that extends beyond vertebral margin but remains contained within the outer annular fibers
Extrusion	Herniation of nucleus pulposus beyond the confines of the annulus with disc attached to the remainder of nucleus pulposus by a narrow pedicle
Sequestration	Portion of disc fragment entirely separated from the parent disc

Common findings of disc pathologies (see Figure 6.8)
- Clinical implication of disc pathologies
  ○ Extrusions and sequestration (usually contained gelatinous material of nucleus), may cause chemical radiculitis
  ○ Extruded disc: may improve more significantly because of resorption of proinflammatory materials (37)
  ○ Sequestration (96%) and extrusion (70%): better chance of spontaneous regression (38) than protrusion (41%) and bulge (15%)

Diffusion tensor image (DTI): more sensitive for intrinsic spinal cord abnormalities by spinal stenosis; to evaluate syringomyelia and pre-syrinx

Schmorl's node: herniation of disc into the vertebral end plate; often incidental finding (39)

POINT-OF-CARE ULTRASONAGRAPHY

Indications: to evaluate soft tissue and for guidance for needle
- Diagnostic US: limited in evaluation of the cervical spine bony pathologies and deeper soft tissues
  ○ Limited role in evaluation of facet arthropathy (osteophytes can be visualized)
  ○ Soft tissue: muscle tear if significant, lipoma or other soft tissue mass can be evaluated
  ○ Experimental usage in imaging diagnosis of myofascial trigger point (elastogram to measure stiffness) and anterior and lateral neck: able to measure size of root or plexus (compare the contralateral side)
- US guided injections
  ○ Greater occipital nerve block, facet injection, medial branch block, and RF ablation (fluoroscopy guidance is standard of care)
  ○ Trigger point (indicated for rhomboids, levator scapulae muscle) injection or adventitial bursa injection
- The main disadvantage over the fluoroscopy for cervical epidural: inability to reliably assess for cervical radicular arteries, which have been implicated as the cause of multiple catastrophic outcomes with epidural steroid injections

CT SCAN

Indications
- When MRI is contraindicated
- Detailed bony structures and for surgical planning
- Trauma patient (obtunded patient and in blunt trauma)
- CT myelogram with intrathecal contrast, when MRI is contraindicated or when accurate bony details required for surgery

ELECTROMYOGRAPHY (EMG)

Indications
- Subclinical/clinical motor abnormality (weakness, fatigue, etc), arm pain, or sensory symptoms (paresthesia, numbness) associated with neck pain
- Differential diagnoses of sensory symptoms include: peripheral neuropathy and focal entrapment neuropathy (such as CTS and ulnar neuropathy) in addition to brachial plexopathy
- Value in nonmechanical radiculopathy or brachial plexopathy (amyotrophy): if symptoms and signs of radiculopathy without clear mechanical etiology (such as disc disruption or spinal stenosis)
- Isolated neck pain: EMG is unlikely useful

Nerve conduction studies and needle EMG
- Sensory nerve conduction study (SNCS): lateral antebrachial cutaneous (C5–6) at lateral forearm, median (C6 at 1st and 2nd digits and C7 at 3rd digit), ulnar (C8 at 5th digit), medial antebrachial cutaneous (T1, medial forearm)
  - Normal SNCS findings in radiculopathy (preganglionic lesion) or focal proximal lesion (brachial plexopathy without axonal involvement)
  - Abnormal findings favor peripheral neuropathy (or mononeuropathy), brachial plexopathy, or a concomitant lesion
- Motor nerve conduction study
  - Median at abductor pollicis brevis (C8–T1), ulnar at abductor digiti minimi (C8–T1) and occasionally biceps, deltoid or supraspinatus (C5–6) with Erb's point stimulation
  - Usually normal unless severely affected, F wave (utility is controversial), H reflex (C 7, flexor carpi radialis [FCR], median nerve, often difficult to obtain)
- Needle EMG examination
  - Key findings: abnormal spontaneous activities (ASA), fibrillations in limb muscles of two different peripheral nerves of the same root and paraspinal muscles with decreased motor unit recruitment
    - Examine muscles innervated by one level above and below root (to localize the lesion)
  - Unclear clinical implication of isolated paraspinal muscle ASA findings
  - Pure sensory radiculopathy or mild radiculopathy (focal demyelinating lesion) → negative nerve conduction study and needle EMG study; therefore, EMG test is not to rule out radiculopathy

TREATMENT

NONOPERATIVE MANAGEMENT

Education for nonspecific neck pain (60,61)
- Early mobilization is recommended in general
  - Especially after whiplash injury or minor trauma
  - Brief rest (<4 days)

Oral medication for nonspecific neck pain
- Tylenol, a nonsteroidal anti-inflammatory drug (NSAID) (first choice) then weak opioid (tramadol, Tylenol # 3)
- Topical analgesics: menthol/methyl salicylates, capsaicin, local anesthetics
- Medrol dose pack: may consider for acute radicular pain
- Neuropathic pain medication (tricyclic antidepressants [TCAs], gabapentin, etc) for positive sensory symptoms (ie, pins, needle sensation, tingling, or burning)
- Short-term use of muscle relaxant (up to 3 weeks, especially antispasmodic agents such as cyclobenzaprine, methocarbamol, etc): long-term standing dose is less effective
  - Cyclobenzaprine, tizanidine, orphenadrine: more evidence
  - Carisoprodol (Soma): not used any more because of high addiction rate

Physical therapy (PT)
- Unclear on long-term benefit; after short-term (1–2 months) therapy, continue with home exercise program
- Strengthening and stretching exercises; mainstay of the treatment
  - Diminished deep cervical flexor strength and increased fatigability, delayed cervical muscle contraction with associated movement of upper limb, increased superficial flexor muscle activities in patient with neck pain (62)
  - Cervical stabilization exercise (63)
    - Postural reeducation for balanced position, stretching then cervical isometric to resistive strengthening exercise (supine advanced to sitting and standing) with scapular stabilization exercise and upper extremity strengthening exercise
    - May not be more beneficial over other therapeutic exercise
- Postural education
  - Avoid forward head posture: try to put tragus of the ear posterior to the tip of the acromion
  - Avoid extreme extension (especially in patient with spinal stenosis) and rotation
  - Evaluation of environment at work or daily activities: height of chair, desk monitor, etc
- Home exercise program
- Aerobic endurance exercise
- Myofascial release and manual therapy. Manipulation may be better than mobilization (no clear benefit of one over each other, both transient effect)
- Manipulation and mobilization (manual therapy)
- Modality
  - Transcutaneous electrical nerve stimulation (TENS) unit; high-frequency (60–200 Hz) stimulation gives shorter pain relief. However, low-frequency (<10 Hz) stimulation is more uncomfortable
- Cervical traction; mixed result
  - Absolute contraindications: osteoporosis, cervical infections or malignancies, vascular insufficiency, ligament instability (RA), cervical myelopathy
  - Use ~25 lb with 25° neck flexion
  - Different modes available (continuous, sustained, or intermittent): no clear benefit of one mode over the other

Common office-based procedures
- Trigger point injection: effective, possible iatrogenic pneumothorax in thorax region (eg, rhomboid, levator scapulae)

- Greater occipital nerve block with/without imaging guidance for posterior neck and occipital headache
- US-guided injection (64) for facet joint injection and medial branch block
  - Shown high accuracy and shorter procedure time in some reports, no radiation exposure
  - Highly operator dependent
  - Fluoroscopic guidance is still the standard of care
- Stellate ganglion (inferior cervical or cervicothoracic ganglion) block under US guidance
  - For sympathetic mediated complex regional pain syndrome
  - Needle through anterior scalene muscle target to the longus coli fascial layer at C7 level with precaution to avoid injection to vertebral artery and brachial plexus
  - Successful sympathetic block with ipsilateral Horner's syndrome (ptosis, anhydrosis, miosis, enophthalmos, and loss of ciliospinal reflex on the affected side of the face) and temperature increase in the ipsilateral upper extremity
- Cervical plexus block with/without US guidance
  - Can be used for cutaneous neuralgia
  - Injection point; posterior border/midline of the SCM muscles

Alternative therapy
- Acupuncture; some evidence (not high level) for neck pain, safe and less invasive, and can be used as a useful adjunct therapy
- Exercise with postural treatment (Pilates, yoga, Alexander technique, Feldenkrais pattern) for nonspecific neck pain

Common cervical orthoses

CERVICAL ORTHOSIS	CHARACTERISTICS
Soft collar	Minimal/no restriction of movement Increased sensory feedback, comfort (retain body heat) Not proven to be effective for neck pain
Hard collar Philadelphia collar	For stable cervical injury Rotation and lateral bending is not well controlled compared with flexion/extension Aspen, Miami, and Malibu collars are alternative
Halo vest, SOMI, thermoplastic Minerva body jacket	High cervical fracture, indicated for unstable injury Halo vest (Occipito-C2 stability) for 12 weeks, SOMI (for bedridden patient), Minerva jacket for below C2-level injury

SOMI, sternooccipital mandibular immobilizer.

Interventional procedure with fluoroscopic guidance (rarely use CT guidance)
- Cervical epidural steroid injection; for cervical radicular pain (65)
  - For short-term pain relief
  - Recommend fluoroscopically guided cervical interventions using digital subtraction angiography to avoid unwanted vascular injection
  - Interlaminar approach is preferred for cervical radiculopathy and central canal stenosis
    - Cervical transforaminal ESI: higher risk of arterial puncture and injection (65)
  - Spinal stenosis secondary to disc herniation shows better outcome than osseous etiology
- Facet joint injection, cervical medial branch neurotomy; for facet joint–mediated pain; chronic whiplash injury
- Selective nerve root block (66)
  - Target perineural space surrounding the selected nerve root
  - More diagnostic than therapeutic
    - Diagnostic information obtained by blocking the pain associated with a symptomatic nerve root
    - May be useful for surgical planning

SURGERY

Surgical management
- Decompression
  - Indications: progressive neurologic deficit, spinal instability, persistent pain refractory to conservative treatments
  - Anterior cervical discectomy and fusion (ACDF) (67)
    - More rapid relief (within 3–4 months) for radicular neck pain with maintenance of gains over the course of 12 months compared with PT
    - Short hospital stay (1–3 days) with rapid recovery
    - Usually performed for one- to two-segment disease
    - Potential for accelerated degenerative changes at adjacent levels
  - Posterior spinal fusion (PSF)
    - For more extensive disease involving more than two to three segments
    - More limited ROM postoperatively
    - Potential risk of cervical kyphosis/dropped head syndrome because of loss of neck extensors
  - Others: laminotomy and laminoplasty
- Artificial disc replacement
  - Common indication: single-level disease with minimal facet arthrosis
  - Unclear effect on adjacent-level disease
- Complication of cervical surgery: rare when performed by an experienced surgeon
  - SCI (iatrogenic vs reperfusion injury), C5 nerve root palsy
  - Recurrent laryngeal nerve injury with anterior approach: right more vulnerable than left
  - Horner's syndrome
    - Caused by cervical sympathetic chain injury
  - Bone graft side morbidity (iliac crest with superior cluneal nerve neuropathy)

Return to Play (6)

- Full cervical ROM without pain, >90% strength recovery, and no neurological deficits
- Previous CCN with cervical spinal stenosis (suggested by a Torg ratio <0.5): 75% risk of another CCN if return to contract sport
- Return to contact sport for athletes with known spinal stenosis: debates in regards to increased risk of transient quadriparesis and permanent neurologic injury
- Absolute contraindication for contact sports: neurological symptoms >36 hours, evidence of spinal cord edema, cervical bony abnormalities, spinal fusion surgery above C3-level surgery involving more than three spinal levels (one level below C3 is not contraindication)

- Special populations
  - Down syndrome
    - Upto 30% has atlantoaxial instability and 12% to 16% of these develop neurologic symptoms and signs
    - Check lateral x-ray with flexion/extension view to rule out instability
    - Follow guideline from the organization of each sport
  - RA
    - High prevalence of atlantoaxial instability
    - Can develop cervical cord injury from minor trauma in geriatric population with RA

NERVE AND SPINAL CORD PATHOLOGY

CERVICAL RADICULOPATHY

Introduction (68)
- Incidence: ~80 per 100,000 (population-based study in Minnesota), male > female, common in 6th decade
- MC location: C7 nerve root (70%) > C6 > C8
- MC cause: cervical disc herniation followed by cervical spondylosis
  - Rare causes: intraspinal or extraspinal tumor, nerve root avulsion after trauma, synovial cyst, meningeal cyst, dural arteriovenous fistula, or tortuous vertebral artery

POSSIBLE CAUSES OF CERVICAL RADICULOPATHY, LISTED BY STRUCTURE (10)	
STRUCTURE	PATHOLOGY
Intervertebral disc	Herniation (protrusion, extrusion), sequestration, bulge, osteophyte–disc complex
Facet joint	Osteophyte, ganglion, tumor, RA, gout, ankylosing spondylitis, fracture
Vertebral body	Tumor, Paget's disease, fracture, osteomyelitis, hydatid disease (parasite), hyperparathyroidism
Meninges	Cyst, meningioma, dermoid cyst, epidermoid cyst, epidural abscess, epidural hematoma
Blood vessels	Angioma, arteritis
Nerve sheath	Neurofibroma, schwannoma
Nerve	Neuroblastoma, ganglioneuroma

RA, rheumatoid arthritis.

History and physical examination (69)
- Arm pain more than neck pain ± weakness
  - Arm pain in 99%, sensory deficits in 85%, neck pain in 80%, motor deficits in 68%, scapular pain in 53%
  - Arm pain is usually not dermatomal, but sensory deficit is
  - Less common: anterior chest pain in 18%, headaches in 10%, anterior chest and arm pain in 6%
- Neurologic examination
  - Motor examination
    - Weakness may not be striking because of multiple-root innervation of each muscle
    - (+) Obvious motor weakness: workup for peripheral nerve involvement such as brachial plexopathy
- Sensory examination
  - Distinguish dermatomal versus peripheral nerve distribution
  - Thumb (median/radial nerve vs C6), 3rd digit (median nerve vs C7), 4th digit splitting of deficit in median/ulnar nerve versus C8 (no splitting)
  - DTR; C5 biceps, C6 brachioradialis, and C7 triceps reflex
  - Hoffman test (to rule out concomitant cervical myelopathy or myeloradiculopathy) and plantar scratch test
- Provocative maneuver: low sensitivity and high specificity (70)
  - The Spurling test (for C6–8) and neck distraction test
  - Shoulder abduction sign: relief of arm pain with shoulder abduction (lower cervical root involvement) (52)

Diagnosis
- Clinical diagnosis confirmed by imaging study and EMG test
- Differential diagnosis
  - MSK and other peripheral neuropathy mimicking cervical radiculopathy

LEVEL	MIMICKERS	NOTES
C5	Shoulder pathologies (C5–6)	Impingement syndrome, adhesive capsulitis/GH osteoarthritis, GH instability, biceps tendon disorder
	Suprascapular nerve entrapment	Intact C5 innervated muscles except infraspinatus and supraspinatus. Paralabral cyst: MC cause
C6 or C7	Carpal tunnel syndrome	Intact C6–7 innervated muscles except median nerve innervated muscles distal to carpal tunnel (flexor carpi radialis, pronator teres, extensor digitorum communis/triceps muscles). Abnormal median nerve conduction study
	Lateral epicondylitis/wrist-finger extensor tendinopathy	Reproducible pain/symptom on palpation on lateral epicondyle, positive provocative test (eg, Cozen test)
	Posterior interosseous neuropathy	No cutaneous sensory dysfunction (but complaint of deep wrist pain), elbow extension spared
	Triceps tendinopathy	Worsening pain on resisted elbow extension

(continued)

LEVEL	MIMICKERS	NOTES
C8	Anterior interosseous neuropathy	No cutaneous sensory dysfunction, normal radial or ulnar innervated muscle of C8 myotome (extensor indicis, flexor digitorum profundus to digit 2 and 3)
	Ulnar nerve entrapment	Intact radial/median nerve innervated muscles of C8 (extensor indicis, abduction of thumb)
	Medial epicondylitis/ wrist-finger flexor tendinopathy	Pain/symptom reproduction on palpation on medial epicondyle and positive provocative test

GH, glenohumeral, MC, most common.

- Other neurological causes
  - Brachial plexopathy: thoracic outlet syndrome, Pancoast tumor (lower trunk/medial cord), idiopathic brachial plexopathy (neuralgic amyotrophy)
  - Herpes zoster
  - Peripheral mononeuropathy; long thoracic, accessory, musculocutaneous neuropathy
  - Upper motor neuron involvement; Multiple sclerosis (MS), syringomyelia, elevated intracranial pressure and intracranial tumor
- Vascular pathologies
  - Thoracic outlet syndrome (vascular)
  - Effort-induced thrombosis of the subclavian-axillary vein (71)
  - Aortic arch syndrome
  - Vertebral artery dissection
- Others
  - Referred pain from dental pain
  - Neck tongue syndrome (C2 nerve root compression) (72)
- Imaging study
  - C-spine x-ray
    - Cervical spondylosis (>90% of population has positive imaging finding by 7th decade)
    - Low sensitivity and specificity to diagnose cervical radiculopathy
    - Evaluate C-spine alignment, instability, degenerative disc disease, and arthropathy
  - MRI
    - Imaging modality of choice for cervical radiculopathy
    - Evaluate disc herniation with or without mass effect on the spinal cord or spinal nerve root, spondylotic osteophytes, and intrinsic spinal cord lesions
    - Clinical correlation is critical to avoid false-positive results
  - CT myelogram
    - When MRI is contraindicated
    - Visualize cerebrospinal fluid (CSF) blockage and better distinguish soft tissue from bony pathologies
    - Invasive compared with other modalities
- Electrodiagnosis (73)
  - Indication: clinical evidence of weakness, suspicion of subclinical motor deficit, used to differentiate other lower motor neuron disease or noncompressive radiculopathy (eg, diabetic radiculoplexus neuropathy [amyotrophy], zoster, etc), or concomitant lesions (eg, CTS, ulnar neuropathy or brachial plexus lesion, etc)
  - Typical findings of cervical radiculopathy
    - Normal SNCS (unless concomitant lesion present)
    - Normal motor nerve conductions study in mild to moderate cases because of multiroot innervations of a muscle, abnormal in severe cases or with multiple roots involvement
    - Needle EMG: ASA in two muscles innervated by the different peripheral nerves of the same root with, reduced motor unit recruitment, and paraspinal muscle involvement
  - Negative findings cannot rule out radiculopathy: focal demyelinating lesion, isolated sensory radiculopathy, and chronic lesion (after reinnervation)

Treatment (74,75)
- Conservative management
  - 70% to 80% patients have good to excellent outcomes with conservative treatments within several weeks
  - Maintain normal activities of daily living (ADL) with light stretches combined with modalities (ice/heating pack to the neck). Soft cervical collar is not recommended
  - Medications
    - NSAIDs, short course of tapering oral corticosteroids (Medrol Dose Pak: methyl prednisone)
    - Neuropathic medications: gabapentin, pregabalin, TCAs
    - May consider a short course of narcotic analgesics if not responsive to other medications
  - PT; few sessions will help for concomitant MSK pathologies and education for home exercise program (61)
    - Indication: persistent disability after resolution of acute radicular pain
    - Strengthening exercises of the cervical paraspinal muscles, stretching and strengthening of shoulder girdle muscles
    - Modalities (TENS, heating, etc) as needed
    - Cervical traction: 25° flexion for 15- to 20-minute interval
  - Workstation evaluation and evaluation of ergonomic equipment: telephone headset, slanted writing board, document holder, book stand
- Interventional management (65)
  - Epidural steroid injection if no relief of pain within 4 to 6 weeks
  - The efficacy of cervical epidural steroid injections
    - Uncontrolled studies: good to excellent results in 60% to 76% of patients
    - Unclear in the literature in terms of maximum number of injections or frequency
- Surgery
  - Indication: progressive weakness, concomitant myelopathy with progressive symptoms, intractable pain despite nonoperative managements
- Both anterior (anterior discectomy with or without fusion) and posterior (laminectomy/laminoplasty) approaches

NONCOMPRESSIVE RADICULOPATHY

See Lumbar Radiculopathy section in Chapter 6

C5 (NERVE ROOT) PALSY

Introduction (76)
- Prevalence: rare in general population

○ Not uncommon in patients after cervical spine surgery (5%–6%)
○ More common in patients with OPLL (8.3%) > cervical spondylotic myelopathy (5.6%) (77)
• Pathophysiology/etiology; controversial
○ Inadvertent injury to the nerve root during surgery
○ Traction of C5 root: tethering phenomenon
  ▪ With posterior decompression, extent of posterior shifting of the cord is the greatest at C5 level (apex of decompression), and gives more traction to C5 root than other roots
  ▪ C5 root/rootlet is shorter than other level and anchored anteriorly by protruded C4–5 facet joint, which makes C5 root more susceptible
  ▪ However, there is no correlation between the incidence of C5 palsy and the extent of posterior shift of the cord
○ Spinal cord ischemia because of decreased blood supply from radicular arteries or reperfusion injury of the cord
○ A form of idiopathic brachial plexopathy (78)
• Prognosis: good
○ Motor strength 3–4/5: full recovery (>90%) in 3 to 6 weeks
○ Severe motor weakness <3/5: recovers to functional level (~70%)

History and physical examination (79)
• Weakness in shoulder abduction and elbow flexion (the deltoid and the biceps brachii muscle after cervical decompression surgery without any deterioration of myelopathy symptoms)
• Intractable pain and sensory deficits in the shoulder region (50%)
• Unilateral commonly (~90%), onset within a week, but varies from 2 to 4 weeks after the surgery, can involve other cervical nerves

Diagnosis
• Clinical diagnosis confirmed by EMG test
• Imaging study (MRI) for differential diagnosis
• EMG; often useful to compare preoperative test findings
○ ASA (fibrillation) in a few days after the surgery indicates pre existing pathologies rather than new development as ASA development takes 2 to 4 weeks

Treatment
• Neuromuscular electrical stimulation on the muscles (deltoid and biceps) and shoulder abduction sling. Cervical traction, muscle strengthening exercise (weak muscle and scapular stabilizer), and ROM of shoulder joint
• Rigid external fixation using a halo vest and bed rest if recommended by the surgeon
• Intraoperative monitoring during the surgery for prevention, and foraminotomy in addition to ACDF

GREATER OCCIPITAL NEURALGIA

Introduction (80)
• Unknown prevalence. Underrecognized cause of posterior upper neck pain with headache
• Etiology
○ Trauma, entrapment between muscles, and degenerative spine disease/disc disease affecting C2 dorsal ramus

ETIOLOGY	PATHOPHYSIOLOGY
Trauma	Whiplash and hyperextension injury
Musculotendinous	Semispinalis, trapezius muscle spasm
Osteogenic	Cervical spondylosis, disc disease C1/C2 arthrosis, atlantodental sclerosis Hypermobile posterior arch of the atlas Cervical osteochondroma Osteolytic lesion of the cranium
Vascular	Irritation of the nerve roots C1/C2 by an aberrant branch of posterior inferior cerebellar artery Dural arteriovenous fistula at the cervical level Bleeding from a bulbocervical cavernoma Cervical intramedullary cavernous hemangioma Giant cell arteritis Fenestrated vertebral artery pressing on C1/C2 nerve roots or aberrant artery
Neurogenic	Schwannoma in the area of the craniocervical junction C2 myelitis Multiple sclerosis

History and physical examination
• Shooting or stabbing pain in the neck radiating over the cranium
○ ± Retro-orbital pain (because of overlap of the C2 dorsal root and the nucleus trigeminus pars caudalis, 33%), dizziness (50%), nausea (50%), and congested nose (17%) in connection to CN 8, 9, 10, and the cervical sympathetic nerves
• Physical examination
○ Hypo- or dysesthesia in the area of the occipital nerve as well as tenderness over the course of the occipital nerve
○ Tenderness and positive Tinel's sign (pain on percussion over the nerve reproducing symptoms, Valleix's sign)

Diagnosis
• Clinical diagnosis confirmed by diagnostic block with small volume (~1 mL) of local anesthetics
○ False positive in migraine and cluster headaches
• Differential diagnosis
○ Upper cervical facet arthropathy
○ Myofascial pain syndrome
○ Tumors, infection, and congenital anomalies (Arnold-Chiari malformation)
○ Giant cell arteritis
• Imaging test
○ Cervical x-ray: AP, lateral, and open-mouth view
○ CT and MRI/A of brain to rule out CNS or soft tissue pathologies

Treatment (81)
• PT: therapeutic muscle exercises (myofascial release, stretching, correct posture) addressing suboccipital and trapezius scapular stabilizer, and modalities (TENS and vapocoolant spray)
• NSAIDs, muscle relaxants, TCA (nortriptyline), and anticonvulsants (gabapentin, pregabalin)

- Diagnostic and therapeutic injection (82)
  - Blind injection: be cautious of neighboring occipital artery, ~2 cm lateral and ~2 cm inferior to the external occipital protuberance with 2 to 3 mL of lidocaine, bupivacaine, or mixed, ± steroid
  - US-guided occipital nerve block; to avoid the occipital artery, can use smaller volume (83)
    - Medial to the occipital artery above superior nuchal line
    - Fascial plane block superficial to the obliquus capitis inferior muscle (from C2 spinous process to laterally to C1 transverse process) with patient prone with slight neck flexion
- Pulse radiofrequency ablation, occipital nerve stimulator
  - Indications: recurrent pain with good temporary relief with block
- Occipital nerve stimulator: gate theory mechanism to reduce nociceptive inputs, modulate the trigeminocervical complex in the brain stem, which reduces meningeal vasodilation

SUPRACLAVICULAR NERVE ENTRAPMENT SYNDROME

Introduction (9)
- Rare, unknown prevalence
- Anatomy
  - C3–4 → three branches at the posterior border of the SCM and pierce the deep fascia above the clavicle, transosseous tunnels in the clavicle in 1%
  - Medial branch: innervating sternoclavicular joint and down to the 2nd rib
  - Intermediate branch: clavicle, and anterolateral upper thorax anterior axillary line
  - Lateral branch: deltoid and posterior shoulder and spine of the scapula
- Etiology: trauma, clavicular fracture/healing, iatrogenic, variation of muscles (wide implantation of the trapezius or SCM muscle on the clavicle)

History and physical examination
- Altered sensation, dysesthesia, and chronic pain in the anterior neck and upper chest wall like complex regional pain syndrome
- Decreased neck extension limited with pain

Diagnosis
- Clinical diagnosis, confirmed by image-guided injection or EMG (often technically difficult, compare with opposite side)
- X-ray if history of trauma (clavicle fracture, callus, or malunion) and CT scan (coronal reconstruction for notch/osseous canal)

Treatment
- Lidocaine gel, stretching of the muscle (trapezius and SCM), TENS, and injection (image guidance)
- Referral for excision and decompression if not responsive to the conservative management

CERVICAL MYELOPATHY

Introduction
- Epidemiology: male > female, earlier presentation in female, increases with age
  - Spondylotic myelopathy is most common
  - Myelopathy is the second MC neurological manifestation of spondylosis after radiculopathy
- Etiology
  - Spondylosis, disc herniation, congenital, posttraumatic, OPLL (common in Asia)
    - Radiologic findings for spondylosis: >95% in age above 70 years
  - Other causes: MS, motor neuron ds, vasculitis, neurosyphilis, subacute combined degeneration, syringomyelia, spinal tumors, and so on

History and physical examination (44)
- History
  - Insidious onset, initial deterioration then stable for years, possible acute exacerbation with hyperextension injury
  - Unsteady gait, impaired hand dexterity (difficulty buttoning and writing), weakness, impaired proprioception and coordination, dizziness (because of proximity of cervical mechanoreceptor projection to the vestibular nucleus in the brainstem)
  - Sensory symptoms
    - Axial neck pain: MC
    - Cervical radiculopathy can coexist in ~60%
    - Paresthesia and dysesthesia in the distal upper limbs (mechanical irritation of dorsal root)
    - Burning pain in hands and face with paresthesia and/or dysesthesia: need evaluation for central cord syndrome
  - Bowel and bladder dysfunction in severe case
- Physical examination
  - Lower extremity weakness (more than proximal upper extremities) and intrinsic hand muscle wasting/weakness
    - C3–6 level: decreased hand dexterity, arm weakness, and sensory symptoms.
    - C6–8 level: spasticity and loss of proprioception in legs
  - Sensory abnormality; loss of proprioception
  - Upper motor neuron signs: hyperreflexia, plantar stretch reflex
    - Scapulohumeral reflex: C2–3 involved, tapping of the spine of the scapula or acromion results in scapular elevation and/or abduction of the humerus (84)
    - Hoffman sign, Tromner sign for upper motor lesions (58)

Diagnosis
- Clinical diagnosis confirmed by imaging study or other tests (for nonmechanical myelopathy)
- Differential diagnosis of cervical spondylotic myelopathy (85)
  - Concomitant pathologies including radiculomyelopathy, motor neuron disease, and old stroke
  - Nonmechanical myelopathy (86)
    - Inflammatory: SLE, Sjögren, Behcet disease, sarcoidosis, RA, and ankylosing spondylitis with upper cervical subluxation
    - Demyelinating: MS, neuromyelitis optica, acute transverse myelitis, acute disseminated encephalomyelitis

- Vascular: spinal cord infarct, arteriovenous (AV) malformation, hematomyelia, decompression sickness
- Infection: viral (HIV, human T-cell lymphotropic virus [HTLV], varicella-zoster virus [VZV], West Nile), syphilis, lyme, epidural or intramedullary abscess, osteomyelitis
- Toxic, metabolic and hereditary; B12, folic acid, vitamin E deficiency, copper deficiency, nitrous oxide toxicity, superficial siderosis, hereditary paraparesis, and adrenomyeloneuropathy
- Other lesions: synovial or arachnoid cyst, DISH, Paget disease, OPLL, syringomyelia, and trauma
- Imaging studies
  - X-ray: AP and lateral view
    - Spondylolisthesis, fusion (congenital), and osteophytes
    - Canal size for spinal stenosis: Pavlov ratio (ratio of canal/vertebral body)
    - Flexion/extension view for instability
  - MRI; imaging modality of choice
    - Confirm the diagnosis, document the extent and severity of degenerative changes, and rule out common mimickers
    - Evaluate the causes of cervical cord compression: spondylosis, disc herniation, and OPLL
    - Findings: lack of CSF surrounding spinal cord in the axial view, cord deformation, intrinsic cord signal abnormalities (myelomalacia: progressive cord compression, signal alteration, and atrophy)
      – Smaller cross-sectional area of the cord at the site of compression: more severe symptoms and suboptimal postoperative outcome
      – Focal T2 hyperintensity: controversial as prognostic indicator
  - CT scan in patients with contraindications for MRI; can provide better bony details
  - CT myelogram is as sensitive as MRI

Treatment
- Nonoperative treatments (87) in patients without gait disturbance or pathologic reflexes; improvement in 33% to 50%
  - Avoid hyperextension, heavy lifting, and contact sports (unclear evidence in asymptomatic patient)
  - Epidural steroid injection: controversial (may be helpful for concomitant radiculopathy)
- Surgery
  - Neither MRI signal intensity change nor area of spinal cord involvement can predict surgical outcome
    - More likely related to transverse area of the spinal cord at the site of compression and duration of myelopathy
  - Indication: severe or progressive symptoms, failed conservative managements
  - Anterior versus post approach—determined by the number of stenotic levels, the contour of the cervical spine
- Three or fewer: ACDF (improvement in 85%–99%)
- Three or more, and preserved lordosis: posterior laminoplasty (fewer complications than laminectomy)
- Three or more, loss of lordosis: laminectomy and post-fusion

CERVICAL CORD NEURAPRAXIA

Introduction (88)
- Acute, transient neurologic injury
- Prevalence: 7 per 10,000 football players (7)
- Etiology and risk factor
  - Axial force to the top of the head with neck in slight flexion (cervical spine straight in 30° flexion)
  - Hyperflexion or extension: pincer type cervical spinal cord compression injury
  - Risk factor: cervical stenosis (controversial)

History and physical examination
- Transient neurologic injury, typically resolves within 10 to 15 minutes (can last up to 48 hrs)
- Sensory changes, possible weakness or paralysis in two or more extremities

Diagnosis
- Clinical diagnosis
- Differential diagnosis: burner or stinger (usually not bilateral)
- Imaging study
  - Plain x-ray (screening); Pavlov Torg ratio (canal diameter/AP width of vertebral body <0.8: (consider larger vertebral body in athletes: high false-positive)
  - MRI (89)
    - Frank cervical cord compression in 34% or effacement of the thecal sac (25%)
    - Cervical disc herniation (MC finding, >80%), spinal stenosis: 33% in group with frank cord compression

Treatment
- Reassurance and education for sports participation
- Return to play: 50% overall risk of a recurrent episode with return to football
- Exclusion from return to play to contact sports; ligament instability, neurologic symptoms >36 hours, recurrent episodes or MRI evidence of cord defect, cord edema, or minimal functional reserve

OSSIFICATION OF POSTERIOR LONGITUDINAL LIGAMENT (OPLL)

Introduction (90)
- Prevalence: 0.16 % (non-Asian) to 2.4% (Asian), 2.5% in patients with cervical myelopathy (White). Average onset: fifth to sixth decades, male > female
  - Cervical myelopathy is present in 25% to 45% patients with OPLL
- MC location: cervical (MC: C4–6) > thoracic and lumbar spine
- Type of involvement: continuous > mixed > segmental and others (in Japan)
- Risk factors
  - Associated with DISH, ankylosing spondylitis, and other spondyloarthropathy
  - Progression in ~25% (length) and 13% (thickness); not necessarily exacerbating symptoms (91)

- Symptomatic (myelopathic) if spinal canal is compromised by OPLL >60%: but if less, dynamic factor (ROM) and stability may be important for symptom development
- If no myelopathic signs at presentation, likely remain stable without progression

History and physical examination
- Gradual onset of myelopathic/myeloradiculopathic symptoms with sudden deterioration after trauma
  - Bowel/bladder symptoms in severe cases

Diagnosis
- High index of suspicion confirmed by imaging study
- X-ray: lateral x-ray (lower inter-/intraobserver reliability), maximal spinal canal stenosis (thickest point of stenosis; not associated with the degree of neurologic dysfunction)
- CT: three dimensional construction to show ossified area and location, bone window CT scans; most useful imaging
- MRI: decreased signal intensity in all sequences typically. Often inadequate evaluation for focal ossified lesion. Evaluate the spinal cord: hyperintensity in T2 weighted image (WI) correlating with neurological deficit

Treatment
- Conservative management: immobilization with cervical brace with mandibular support, cervical traction, modification of ADL, avoid contact sports, or strengthening exercise, and avoid extreme neck extension (56)
- Surgical referral for progressive myelopathy, especially in younger population (progression is so slow)
  - Laminectomy ± fusion, laminoplasty, or anterior approach

SYRINGOMYELIA

Introduction (92)
- Definition: fluid-filled cavity in the spinal cord parenchyma or central canal
  - Centromedullary spinal cord syndrome with predominantly sensory symptoms
- Prevalence: 8.4 per 100,000 (Western countries). Commonly at C2–T9 level (thoracic spine: MC)
- Etiology: congenital versus acquired
  - MC congenital causes; myelomeningocele, tethered cord syndrome, Chiari malformation type 1
  - Acquired: spinal canal stenosis, spinal cord tumor, trauma, postsurgical, infectious adhesive arachnoiditis

History and physical examination
- Pain (nonspecific), paresthesia, temperature insensitivity, numbness, and unnoticed hand injuries
  - Often asymptomatic (incidental imaging finding)
- Other symptoms; scoliosis, cutaneous marker, or developmental anomalies
- Spastic weakness of the lower extremities, paresthesia or dysesthesia, and segmental sensory loss in noncommunicating syringomyelia. Long tract sign

Diagnosis
- Clinical suspicion confirmed by imaging study
- MRI
  - Pain or symptoms often does not correlate with size and location of syringomyelia
  - MRI of head; R/O hydrocephalus and Chiari malformation and MRI of lumbar spine to evaluate tethered cord
  - MRI with contrast: for underlying etiologies especially tumor
- Differential diagnosis
  - Hydromyelia: residual fetal configuration of central canal of the spinal cord, syringomyelia can develop in the setting of trauma
  - Other causes of cervical myelopathy

Treatment (93)
- Nonoperative management; observation and symptomatic management of pain and paresthesia
- Referral for surgery: symptomatic patients with progression on serial examinations
  - Address structural abnormalities; decompression of posterior fossa and foramen magnum, laminectomy, lysis of adhesion, syrinx fenestration and shunting
- Shunting strategies: last resorts because of a variety of complications

CHIARI MALFORMATION

Introduction (94)
- The presence of the cerebellar tonsils below the level of the foramen magnum often associated with syringomyelia
- Classification
  - Type 1 (MC): 1 per 1,000 births, downward hindbrain (cerebellar tonsil at least) herniation through the foramen magnum without meningomyelocele
    - Syringohydromyelia and scoliosis; 10% to 20%
  - Type 2: 0.6 per 1,000 births; cerebellomedullary malformation with meningomyelocele
  - More severe, less common, usually diagnosed during infancy and early childhood

History and physical examination
- Headache ± cervical pain (28%–63%): severe and paroxysmal
- Weakness and sensory changes (numbness) with syrinx
- Strider/dyspnea/apnea, dysphagia/sleep disturbance, dysarthria, tongue atrophy, facial numbness (from brain stem involvement), and ataxia and nystagmus (from cerebellar involvement)
- In Chiari II after neonatal presentation: usually with cervical myelopathy, slowly progressive dysphagia. Ataxia and occipital headache/neck pain; common

Diagnosis
- Clinical suspicion confirmed by imaging study
- MRI of brain to rule out hydrocephalus (frequent in type 2, <10% in type 1) or mass in the brain (59)
- MRI of entire spine: syrinx, scoliosis, or other less common abnormality such as tethered cord syndrome

Treatment
- Referral to neurosurgery: surgical treatment if symptomatic
  - To restore normal CSF flow

DROP HEAD SYNDROME

Introduction (95)
- Severe neck extensor muscle weakness/injury, resulting in dropping head in the standing or sitting position, which is correctable by passive neck extension
- Unknown prevalence, but underrecognized. Higher incidence in elderly
- Etiology
  ○ Injury, fatigue/weakness of semispinalis cervicis (main contributor of dropped head), capitis with secondary kyphotic postural changes, and age-dependent loss of tissue elasticity
  ○ Isolated neck extensor myopathy (MC cause), benign course without generalized neuromuscular disorder after exclusion of neuromuscular disease, a diagnosis of exclusion
  ○ Motor neuron disease, peripheral neuropathy (eg, CIDP), myasthenia gravis, myopathy (polymyositis, inclusion body myositis, nemaline myopathy, fascioscapulohumeral dystrophy, Cushing syndrome, myotonic dystrophy, hypothyroid myopathy, etc), malignancy, and Parkinson's disease.

History and physical examination (96)
- Visible deformity (chin on chest), often with thoracic kyphosis ± posterior neck discomfort
- Weakness of the extensor muscles of the neck, with or without involvement of the neck flexors ± other neuromuscular dysfunction
- No sensory abnormalities

Diagnosis
- Clinical diagnosis with workup for underlying etiologies
- Diagnostic workup; imaging study of cervical and thoracic spine, and EMG for underlying neuromuscular dysfunction
- Differential diagnosis; neurologic versus orthopedic conditions (check differential diagnosis section)
  ○ Fixed cervical kyphosis: ankylosing spondylitis, postlaminectomy and posttraumatic kyphosis

Treatment (16)
- Soft collar, baseball cap brace (97), reclined seating and exercise (for neck extensor, mild to moderate resistance; supine and pushing the pillow) and assistive device evaluation (cane or walker)
- In rare cases, surgical correction can be considered for failed conservative management with significantly impaired ADLs

BONE AND JOINT PATHOLOGY

CERVICAL FACET PATHOLOGY

Introduction (42)
- Facet joint: a source of chronic axial neck pain related to trauma in 25% to 66%
- MC location for pain: C2–3 and C5–6 levels (study by facet joint blocks)

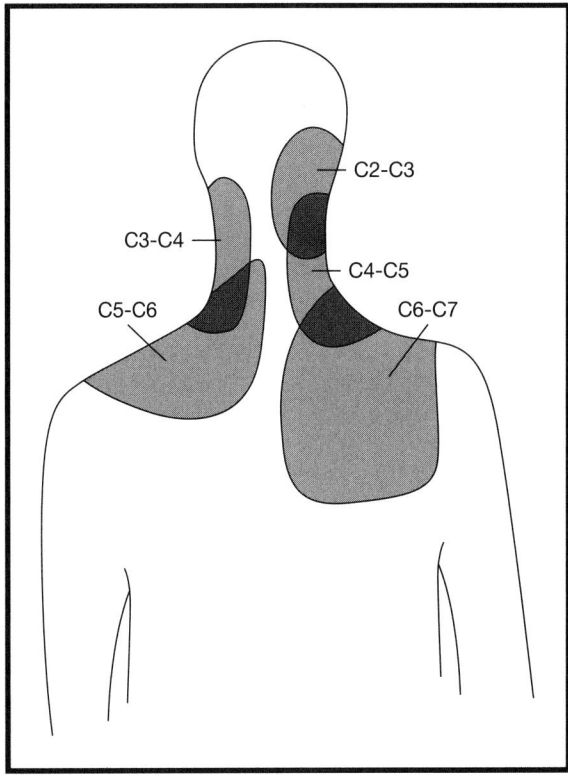

FIGURE 2.9
Pain referral pattern from cervical facet joint injection redirect the lines for clarification.

- Degenerative changes: most commonly at C4–5, followed by C3–4 and C2–3
  ○ Increase with age (widely prevalent in older adults), often asymptomatic

History and physical examination (27)
- Axial neck pain without radiation beyond the shoulders (Figure 2.9)
  ○ Aggravated by rotation and extension movements
- Physical exam (not very specific)
  ○ Tenderness on the cervical facet joint (1.3–2.5 cm lateral to the spinous process, indiscrete bony mass rather than distinct structure)
  ○ Neurological examination and provocative tests for evaluation of differential diagnoses or concomitant pathologies (radiculopathy and myelopathy)
    ▪ Normal in isolated facet pathology

Diagnosis
- Clinical diagnosis confirmed by image-guided injection
- Intra-articular facet joint injection and diagnostic medial branch block
  ○ Pain map from facet joint injection (98): not required for diagnosis
  ○ Medial branch block: single (may have high false positive ratio) versus double block (lidocaine and bupivacaine; different duration of anesthetic, so different duration of response)
- X-ray and MRI (evaluate other differential diagnoses such as radiculopathy, myelopathy, or others): often not correlated with symptomatology

○ Common changes of facet degeneration: narrowing of the facet joint space, subarticular bone erosions, subchondral cysts, osteophyte formation, and hypertrophy of the articular processes

Treatment (99,100)
- NSAIDs for short-term use (cautious of adverse effects, especially in the elderly), opioids (short-term benefit up to 3 months, weak or inconsistent benefit when used chronically)
- Conservative therapy: spine manipulation, acupuncture, massage, PT or cognitive behavioral therapy
- Injection using image guidance; intra-articular injection, medial branch block with local anesthetic ± steroid, radiofrequency ablation of medial branch if responsive to medial branch block

WHIPLASH-ASSOCIATED INJURY

Introduction (27)
- Definition of whiplash: acceleration-deceleration injury results from rear-end or side impact
  ○ MVA (MC cause, 80% of high-speed collision–related injuries). Can be from sports and other injury
  ○ From abnormal motion that occurs within and between individual motion segments
  ○ Not related to the total ROM range of the neck nor the amount of extension or flexion
- Incidence: varies, 1 per 1,000 (insurance claims per year) (101)
- Risk factors: older age, higher mechanical (acceleration-deceleration) forces, seat belt use, poor headrest positioning, poor car seat energy absorption, and improper car design and construction
  ○ Younger age and female associated with filing claims or seeking care
- Pathophysiology (102)
  ○ Facet joint as a pain generator: 50% to 60 % of patients with chronic whiplash-associated injuries
    ▪ Synovial fold impingement, capsular strain, and fracture of facet joints
  ○ Other findings: tear in the ligamentum flavum, disruption of the annulus of the disc and anterior longitudinal ligaments (cadavers study)
- Prognosis
  ○ Most recover, 80% asymptomatic by 12 months, but 15% to 20% symptomatic in 12 months (5% severely affected)
  ○ Outcome predictors (48): variable from study to study
    ▪ Worse outcomes with higher initial intensity of pain, greater pain-related disability, and presentation of cold hyperalgesia
    ▪ Inconclusive: decreased ROM, radicular symptom, degree of property damage in low-speed collisions

History and physical examination
- Neck pain/stiffness/referred pain to the shoulder ± arm pain, paresthesia, jaw (TMJ) pain, headache (referred pain from C2 to C3), dizziness, visual disturbance, and difficulty with memory and concentration
- Nonspecific physical examination: tenderness on the midline cervical spine, restricted ROM as a result of pain and normal neurological examination

Diagnosis
- Clinical diagnosis supplemented by imaging studies and image-guided injections
- Plain x-ray and MRI: usually not specific and often normal
- Cervical facet joint block for diagnosis of facet-mediated pain

Treatment
- Conservative management
  ○ Initial rest for a few days with quick return to ADL recommended (gradually increase activity)
    ▪ Cervical orthosis: no value (cervical collar in mild case → worse outcome)
    ▪ Prevention: active head restraint on rear impact (car design), automobile headrest should be at ear level
  ○ PT: isometric strengthening initially, biomechanic education, modality and home exercise program
    ▪ May reduce pain by 25% to 75% (103)
- Trigger point injection, facet joint injection, and radiofrequency ablation to medial branch if the pain is persistent

DEGENERATIVE DISC DISEASE

Introduction (104)
- Prevalence of symptomatic disc disease: 16% to 50% in chronic neck pain may be explained in part by disc disease (study by discography)
- Anatomy
  ○ Innervation: sensory fibers (outer annulus from dorsal root ganglion) >> autonomic neurons (sympathetic and parasympathetic) (33) → sinuvertebral nerve
- Possible mechanisms of pain: chemical irritation or disc disruption

History and physical examination (29)
- Axial neck pain; deep midline neck pain (similar to facet joint)
- Physical examination: not specific; tenderness on the axial region and pain (nonradiating) on axial loading

Diagnosis
- Diagnosis of exclusion with correlating imaging finding and discography
- Imaging
  ○ MRI: decreased T2 signal intensity, Modic change (not correlating with symptoms).
    ▪ Spondylosis; commonly accompanied (osteophytes, longitudinal ligament calcification, uncovertebral hypertrophy)
- Discography: image-guided injection to nucleus pulposus;
  ○ Limited evidence for diagnostic accuracy, but can be considered after other common generators are eliminated (105)

Treatment
- Conservative management
  ○ Brief rest if significant pain, weight loss, aerobic endurance exercise, and pain medications

○ PT including cervical traction, cervical paraspinal muscle strengthening exercise, and joint proprioception exercise
• Interventional procedure
  ○ Cervical epidural steroid injection: unclear benefit
  ○ Discography: may be considered as a screening tool before cervical fusion
• Surgery: cervical fusion if failed conservative management

RHEUMATOID ARTHRITIS

Introduction (106)
• Prevalence of RA: 0.5% to 1.5% of population, female: male = 2:1
• Cervical spine involvement: 17% to 86% of RA patients depending on diagnostic criteria
  ○ RA involvement; hands and feet > cervical spine
  ○ Atlantoaxial subluxation: 23%, synovitis and pannus formation leading to transverse ligament insufficiency and rupture
    ▪ Erosion of the odontoid process; asymmetric → torticollis
  ○ Atlantoaxial impaction: 26%, follow atlantoaxial subluxation
    ▪ Worse prognosis and much higher risk of myelopathy
  ○ Subaxial subluxation: 19%
    ▪ Weakness of facet capsule and interspinous ligament, late manifestation
    ▪ C2–3 and C3–4: most common level, high risk of myelopathy
• 50% disabled within 10 years

History and physical examination
• Neck pain in 40% to 80% (often asymptomatic), deep aching pain radiating to the occipital, retro-orbital, or temporal area; C2 mediated
• Stiffness, crepitus, and painful ROM
• Sharp Purser test: a clunking sensation during neck extension with spontaneous reduction of atlantoaxial subluxation
• Neurologic examination for deficit in later stages; similar to cervical myelopathy

Diagnosis (107)
• Clinical suspicion confirmed by imaging study
• Imaging: AP, lateral, flexion, and extension view
  ○ Indication for imaging: symptoms >6 months, neurological symptoms and signs, preoperative (precaution for intubation), rapidly progressive carpal or tarsal bone destruction, and rapid function deterioration
  ○ Cranial invagination (atlantoaxial invagination) (108; Figure 2.8)
    ▪ Protrusion of the tip of the odontoid proximal to McRae's line (basion to opisthion) or 4.5 mm above McGregor's line (opisthion to hard plate)
    ▪ Other methods available: Ranawat's method (A) and the Redlund-Johnell method
  ○ Subaxial subluxation (anterior): subaxial instability with anterolisthesis
• Advanced imaging: CT and MRI
  ○ MRI to evaluate soft tissue lesions, neuraxis, epidural tissue, and imaging modality of choice for neural compression
  ○ CT: detailed osseous information

Treatment
• Education: avoid extreme cervical flexion/extension and avoid contact sports
• Referral to rheumatology: disease modifying antirheumatic drug (DMARD); prevent or slow the development of atlantoaxial subluxation (AAS)
• PT
  ○ Strengthening neck muscle (isometric) and postural training
  ○ Soft collar (just for comfort and no limitation of motion or progression)
• Surgery
  ○ Indication for referral
    ▪ Atlantoaxial subluxation; PADI ≤14 mm, >8–10 mm in the anterior atlantodental interval (AADI)
    ▪ Atlantoaxial impaction ≥5 mm above McGregor's line
    ▪ Subaxial subluxation with sagittal diameter ≤14 mm
  ○ Halo vest stabilization often required after surgery

CERVICAL SPINE DISORDER IN DOWN SYNDROME

Introduction (109)
• Incidence of Down syndrome (trisomy 21): 1 per 700 live births, MC genetic abnormalities, increases with maternal age
• Common orthopedic manifestations
  ○ Atlantoaxial instability: 15% to 30 % of Down syndrome, scoliosis and hip abnormalities (5%–8%, dislocation; MC), patellofemoral instability (20%), and foot disorders (pes planus, metatarsus varus)
• Others: intrinsic collagen abnormality or os odontoideum (failure of ossification of the dens to fuse with C2 body)

History and physical examination
• Asymptomatic in most cases
• 12% to 16% of atlantoaxial instability develops symptoms
  ○ Fatigability, neck pain, limited ROM, torticollis, myelopathic symptoms and signs (gait dysfunction, hyperreflexia, and clonus)
• Positive physical examination findings for scoliosis, hip abnormality, patellofemoral instability, and foot disorders (hindfoot valgus, pronation and collapse of the midfoot)

Diagnosis
• Clinical suspicion confirmed by imaging study
• Screening radiographs in all children before anesthesia or procedures that involve significant cervical manipulation
  ○ Screening radiographs: mandatory for high-risk sports
• X-ray: AP, lateral, flexion/extension radiographs, and open-mouth (odontoid) view
  ○ Anterior atlantodental interval (AADI) >4.5 mm is considered abnormal and should warrant further evaluation with MRI
• MRI indicated in patients with neurological deficit

Treatment
• Restriction in sports activity (especially contact sports) (6)
  ○ AADI >4.5 mm disqualifies the athlete for participation

■ Waver option available; check with the specific organization
- Referral for spine surgery in symptomatic patients; usually posterior instrumentation and fusion

KLIPPEL–FEIL ANOMALY

Introduction (110)
- Congenital fusion of several cervical vertebrae often with congenital scoliosis (>50%), rib abnormality, deafness, genitourinary, Sprengel's deformity (upward displacement of scapular), synkinesia, cervical ribs, cardiovascular abnormalities, and torticollis
- Incidence: 1 per 40,000–42,000 births and female > male = 3:2 (111)
- MC location: C2–3 level

History and physical examination
- Mostly asymptomatic (incidental finding during scoliosis evaluation), but increased risk for cervical myelopathy with instability, even with minor trauma
- Pain, limited cervical ROM from fused spine ± neurologic symptoms/signs (radiculopathy and/or myelopathy)
- Classic triad: low posterior hairline, short neck, and limited ROM in 50%
- Examination for other concomitant abnormalities

Diagnosis
- Clinical suspicion confirmed with imaging study
- Type: type 1 (single lesion), type 2 (multiple noncontiguous), and type 3 (multiple contiguous)
- Imaging (59)
  ○ Cervical spine x-ray with flexion and extension view
  ○ Thoracic and lumbar spine x-ray
  ○ MRI (brain and spinal cord) to assess spinal stenosis, syrinx, tethered cord, or diastomyelia
  ○ CT: bony details, cautious (for radiation exposure) in adolescents

Treatment
- Workup for other abnormalities: referral to pediatrician
  ○ Chest x-ray (rib fusion), cardiac US, renal US, and audiology test
- Education: avoid contact sports, or high-risk activity (eg, trampoline, gymnastics) etc
- Spine surgery referral in progressive symptoms and with any trauma
- Controversial for prophylactic procedure even with significant hypermobility

FRACTURE

Introduction
- Epidemiology
  ○ Spinal column injury (fracture or dislocation): ~3% (2%–6%) of blunt trauma (MC cause: car accident)
    ■ May cause SCI in 1%: significantly higher in patients with head trauma and those who are unconscious at presentation
  ○ Bimodal age distribution: young adults between 15 and 29 years of age and in adults >65 years. Male > female. Mortality is significantly higher in elder patients
- Etiology
  ○ Motor vehicle–related accidents (50%): speeding, alcohol intoxication, and failure to use restraints are the major risk factors
    ■ Occupants involved in a rollover accident are at an increased risk of a cervical spine injury
  ○ Other common causes include falls, followed by acts of violence (primarily gunshot wounds), and sporting activities
- Missed or delayed diagnosis of spinal column trauma results in a 7.5-fold increase in the incidence of neurologic injuries
- Injury classification based on mechanism

MECHANISM	FRACTURE

Flexion	Stable
	- Simple wedge (compression) fracture; nuchal ligament intact without posterior disruption
	- Clay-shoveler's fracture
	  ○ Avulsion fracture of the spinous process at the insertion of the supraspinous ligament, usually C7 (C6–T3)
	  ○ Abrupt flexion with heavy upper-body and neck muscles contraction, or direct blow to the spinous process
	Unstable; spine surgery consult
	- Flexion teardrop fracture
	  ○ Flexion with vertical axial compression (eg, diving and MVA) → fracture of anteroinferior aspect of the vertebral body
	  ○ Location: lower cervical level: 70% at C5
	  ○ Significant degree of anterior longitudinal ligament disruption → all 3 columns involved; unstable fracture with high risk of spinal cord injury (MRI or CT required)
	- Bilateral interfacetal dislocation
	  ○ Anterior subluxation (hyperflexion sprain); 20% can cause delayed instability (112)

Other flexion mechanism	Flexion–rotation: unilateral facet dislocation; unilateral jumped facet; bow tie deformity Lateral flexion: uncinate process fracture Isolated transverse process fractures: stable, conservative management

(continued)

MECHANISM	FRACTURE

Vertical compression	- Jefferson burst fracture of atlas (C1)
	  ○ Axial loading with occipital condyle driven into lateral masses of C1
	  ○ 50% involves other C-spine fractures (especially odontoid fracture)
	  ○ Rarely associated with neurologic injury
	  ○ Tx: halo traction and immobilization
	    ▪ If stable: rigid cervical orthosis, less stable: prolonged halo immobilization
	- Vertical laminar fracture
	  ○ Axial loading, with or without rotation, associated with collapse of the vertebral body
	  ○ Isolated lamina fractures: not associated with instability
	  ○ Tx: cervical collar immobilization, followed by dynamic radiographs to rule out instability

Hyperextension	Stable
	- Fracture of posterior arch of atlas
	  ○ Compressed between the occiput and spinous process of C2
	  ○ Transverse ligament and anterior arch of C1; not involved → stable
	Unclear (stability); consult spine surgery
	- Avulsion fracture of anterior arch of atlas
	- Extension teardrop fracture
	- Pillar fracture: hyperextension and rotation (> hyperflexion/rotation). Fracture or separation (pedicolaminar fracture); single lesion often missed in plain radiograph → CT scan (113) and internal fixation/fusion
	- Traumatic spondylolisthesis of C2 ("Hangman's" fracture)
	  ○ Mechanism: extension usually ± traction (like judicial hanging)
	  ○ Fractures of both pedicles of C2 (pars interarticularis) → subluxation of C2 on C3
	  ○ Unstable, but rare neurological deficit as AP diameter of spinal canal is greatest at this level

Injuries by diverse or poorly understood mechanisms	- Occipitoatlantal dissociation and occipital condylar fracture
	- Odontoid (dens) fractures
	  ○ Type
	    1. Type 1: avulsion of the tip of the odontoid process: immobilization, stable; very rare
	    2. Type 2: MC, base of dens with body of C2: unstable, traction, immobilization for 3 months, less likely union
	    3. Type 3: extending to C2 body, treat like type 2
	  ○ Differential with Os odontoideum; separate ossicle with smooth margin separated from foreshortened odontoid peg; asymptomatic presentation to vertebrobasilar ischemia (114)
	    ▪ Referral to surgery if symptomatic

AP, anteroposterior; MC, most common; MVA, motor vehicle accident; Tx, treatment.

History and physical examination
- Neck pain ± neurological symptoms
  ○ Identify underlying risk factors for increased risk of spinal fracture (osteoporosis, ankylosing spondylitis, DISH, etc)
- Physical examination: do not examine the spine first, follow general principal for trauma cases
  ○ Spine precaution in the field
  ○ Neurological examination after stabilizing spine to rule out SCI or other neurological injury (brain injury, intraabdominal or extremity injury)

Diagnosis (115)
- Clinical suspicion confirmed by imaging study
- Imaging indicated unless satisfying Nexus criteria (for low risk) and Canadian C-spine rule for low risk (check diagnostic study section)
- X-ray
  ○ AP, lateral, and open-mouth (odontoid) view
    ▪ Voluntary flexion–extension only: usually not recommended in acute setting. After symptomatic treatment failed (over 2 weeks)
- CT
  ○ Obtunded patient and unclear clinical examination
  ○ 100% negative predictive value for cervical instability (although MRI can detect additional soft tissue lesion)
- MRI
  ○ With neurological deficit, or suspected abnormality on CT
  ○ Can evaluate epidural hematoma, cord edema/compression, root (avulsion)/plexus injury, hematoma, ligamentous, disc lesion, etc

Treatment
- Referral to ER for immediate imaging and ortho/spine surgery consult except stable cases
- Stable
  ○ Minor spinal fracture patterns with no neurologic deficit
    ▪ Symptomatic management for soft tissue injury (strain/sprain) and early mobilization to prevent chronic pain
  ○ If there is any ambiguity regarding spinal stability on plain radiographs, CT scan (and possibly MRI if ligamentous injury is suspected) and spine consult should be obtained
- Unstable: referral to spine surgery

METASTATIC CERVICAL SPINE TUMOR

Introduction (116)
- Primary tumor of the cervical spine: rare
- Metastatic tumor: 20 times more common (117)
  - MC metastatic cancers: breast, prostate, and non-small cell lung cancer
  - MC metastatic areas: thoracic > cervical spine: 8% to 20%
  - Overall: highest in 40 to 65 years of age and male > female

History and physical examination
- Often asymptomatic
- Neck pain without spinal cord involvement
  - Nonmechanical pain: more common than mechanical neck pain
  - Persistent, not relieved by rest, worse at night
  - Pain worse on movement; may indicate instability
  - Often referred pain to interscapular region (118) in 90%
- Neurologic dysfunction in 5% to 10%: root involvement (radiculopathy) more common than cord involvement (myelopathy)
  - May present with weakness, sensory loss, and sphincter dysfunction
- Physical examination: local tenderness on spinous process, neurological examination (to evaluate radiculopathy or other spinal cord syndrome)
  - For example, Brown Sequard's syndrome from intramedullary spinal metastasis (1/3) (> intradural extramedullary metastasis)

Diagnosis
- High clinical suspicion confirmed by imaging study
  - History (new persistent neck pain with h/o cancer → cancer in spine until proven otherwise)
- Imaging; x-ray, MRI with contrast (gold standard), CT (detail of bony anatomy), CT myelogram (for patient with contraindication to MRI), and bone scintigraphy

Treatment (119)
- Multidisciplinary approach; immediate referral to oncology, radiation oncology, and spine surgery
- Nonsurgical intervention; radiation, chemotherapy, hormonal therapy, and high-dose steroid
  - Interventional spine referral for vertebroplasty or kyphoplasty evaluation
- Surgery
  - Indications: neurologic dysfunction, spinal instability, and intractable pain not responsive to medical Tx, radioresistant tumors (renal cell cancer)
  - Palliative surgery with cord decompression and spine stabilization
  - Curative surgery with en bloc tumor radical resection and stabilization
  - Check low back pain section

MUSCLE AND LIGAMENT PATHOLOGY

CERVICAL STRAIN/SPRAIN

Introduction (120)
- One of the most common neck injuries in general population as well as athletes
- Strain: muscle or tendon involvement/injury
  - Eccentric contraction → microscopic or gross tensile failure at myotendinous junction
  - More common in muscle with higher ratio of fast twitch fibers (type 2)
- Sprain (ligament injury): strain usually coexists
  - Children <11 years: more common because of inherent laxity and its shape

History and physical examination
- Pain (localized unless other condition coexists), limited ROM with pain, tenderness on the midline of the posterior neck
- Intact neurological examination

Diagnosis
- Clinical diagnosis
- Imaging: usually not necessary, negative or nonspecific (interspinous widening and loss of cervical lordosis)
  - Possible imaging to evaluate concomitant lesion or differential diagnoses
    - AP, lateral, odontoid (often C7–T1 missing) to evaluate vertebral subluxation, vertebral compression fracture
    - Flexion/extension view (especially in sprain with signs of ligament laxity) (6)
      - Positive (for instability) if >3.5 mm horizontal displacement on flexion/extension view or ≥11° angular rotation, then MRI and consult spine surgery
- Differential diagnosis: facet injury, and cervical disc disease (often concomitant)

Treatment
- Brief rest (for 2–3 days and then early mobilization), ice, pain meds (short-term use of NSAIDs or AAP), or gentle ROM
  - Cervical collar (not more than 10 days); benefit controversial
  - PT
    - Isometric strengthening with gradual increase in resistance. Alternative: early isokinetic strengthening exercise with minimal load (if instrument available)
    - Joint proprioceptive and neuromuscular training
    - Modality: ultrasound (temporary pain relief)
- Acupuncture
- Manipulation; cautious in elderly, focal neurologic deficit, point tenderness over bone, and osteoporosis

MYOFASCIAL PAIN SYNDROME

Introduction (121)
- Working definition: pain, sensory, motor, and autonomic symptoms associated with myofascial trigger points
- Prevalence: lifetime prevalence up to 85% of general population
  - ~20% of the patients in general orthopedic clinic, higher in specialty clinic: 70% to 80% of MSK pains (neurology and pain clinics) (122)

History and physical examination
- Regional muscle pain ± referred pain and paresthesia
  - ± Muscle fatigue, cramps, or subjective weakness (without atrophy)
- Palpation of trigger points: discrete hypersensitive hard palpable nodules located within taut bands of skeletal muscle → local twitch response; a quick, localized contraction of muscle fibers produced by strumming or snapping the taut band in a direction perpendicular to the muscle fibers
  - Active: spontaneous pain ± motor dysfunction (stiffness and restricted ROM)
  - Latent: no spontaneous pain with subclinical motor dysfunction (with taut band, local twitch response ± referred pain on palpation)

Diagnosis
- Clinical diagnosis; reproduction of symptoms by palpation of trigger points ± referred pain
  - Essential features of trigger point (122)
    - Tender point within a taut band of skeletal muscle, characteristic pattern of referred pain, patient's recognition of pain on sustained compression over the tender point, a local twitch response (muscle contraction) within the band of muscle on plucking palpation across the fibers
- Supplementary diagnostic tools (experimental); EMG, ultrasonography (elastogram), pain threshold measurement, and thermographic scanning (123)
- Differential diagnosis or concomitant conditions: facet arthropathy, cervical radiculopathy, occipital neuralgia, and rarely cervical disc disease

Treatment
- Pharmacologic: acetaminophen, NSAIDs, TCA, muscle relaxant, and narcotic (little evidence)
- Trigger point injection
  - Dry needling; highly effective with lasting effect (mechanical stimulation), twitch response, decrease in Sub P and calcitonin gene–related peptide
  - Botox and steroid/lidocaine; no clear benefit over dry needling
  - Complications: rare, hematoma, nerve injury exacerbated pain, pneumothorax; especially in the deeper muscle (rhomboids and levator scapular), and so on
    - US guidance may be useful in the deeper muscle
- Nonpharmacological: manual therapy, massage, spray and stretch, and acupuncture
  - PT: spray and stretching, taping, strengthening (scapular stabilization), correct posture, biomechanics education, and aerobic endurance exercise
  - Modalities (temporary relief of pain)
    - TENS (burst type for 10 min, US, and lower level laser therapy (124)
    - Phonophoresis with hydrocortisone
  - Manual therapy: joint manipulation, strain/counterstrain, ischemic compression and pressure, massage therapy, myofascial release therapy, muscle energy techniques, point pressure release, and transverse friction massage
    - Joint manipulation
      - Atlanto-occipital thrust manipulation technique for the masseter and temporalis muscle
      - Cervical spine manipulation applied at the C3–4 segments: the upper trapezius muscle
    - Strain/counterstrain (SCS)
      - Positional release technique based on the specific positioning of a patient and the affected muscles
    - Ischemic compression
      - Equalizing the length of sarcomeres and reactivating hyperemia in the trigger point region. A spinal reflex mechanism relieves muscle spasms
      - Amount of pressure (until clinician feels the release of) and duration: 60 to 90 seconds
    - Transverse friction massage
      - A deep tissue technique at the site of the trigger point (can mobilize the taut band)
    - Post-isometric relaxation
      - Muscle stretched to the point in which an increase in resistance is observed. Then, the subject performs an isometric contraction of the stretched muscle for 5 to 10 seconds. At the end of each contraction, stretching is passively increased by the therapist

REFERENCES

1. Manchikanti L, Singh V, Datta S, Cohen SP, Hirsch JA; American Society of Interventional Pain Physicians. Comprehensive review of epidemiology, scope, and impact of spinal pain. *Pain Physician*. 2009;12(4):E35–E70.
2. Cote P, Cassidy JD, Carroll L. The Saskatchewan Health and Back Pain Survey. The prevalence of neck pain and related disability in Saskatchewan adults. *Spine (Phila Pa 1976)*. 1998;23(15):1689–1698.
3. Côté P, Cassidy JD, Carroll LJ, Kristman V. The annual incidence and course of neck pain in the general population: a population-based cohort study. *Pain*. 2004;112(3):267–273.
4. Croft PR, Lewis M, Papageorgiou AC, et al. Risk factors for neck pain: a longitudinal study in the general population. *Pain*. 2001;93(3):317–325.
5. Cassidy JD. Saskatchewan health and back pain survey. *Spine*. 1998;23(17):1923.
6. Dorshimer GW, Kelly M. Cervical pain in the athlete: common conditions and treatment. *Prim Care*. 2005;32(1):231–243.
7. Boden BP, Jarvis CG. Spinal injuries in sports. *Phys Med Rehabil Clin N Am*. 2009;20(1):55–68, vii.
8. Aydil U, Kizil Y, Köybasioglu A. Less known non-infectious and neuromusculoskeletal system-originated anterolateral neck and craniofacial pain disorders. *Eur Arch Otorhinolaryngol*. 2012;269(1):9–16.
9. O'Neill K, Stutz C, Duvernay M, Schoenecker J. Supraclavicular nerve entrapment and clavicular fracture. *J Orthop Trauma*. 2012;26(6):e63–e65.
10. Bogduk N. The anatomy and pathophysiology of neck pain. *Phys Med Rehabil Clin N Am*. 2011;22(3):367–82, vii.

11. Stanbro M, Gray BH, Kellicut DC. Carotidynia: revisiting an unfamiliar entity. *Ann Vasc Surg.* 2011;25(8):1144–1153.
12. Barker R, Massouh H. Carotidynia—a valid cause of unilateral neck pain. *Eur J Radiol Extra.* 2009;71(3):e97–e99.
13. Firestein GS, Budd R, Gabriel SE, O'Dell JR, McInnes IB. *Kelley's textbook of rheumatology.* 9th ed. Philadelphia, PA: Saunders Elsevier; 2013.
14. Alentorn A, Montero J, Vidaller A, Casasnovas C. Numb chin syndrome as an early symptom of primary and secondary vasculitis. *Joint Bone Spine.* 2011;78(4):427–428.
15. Carlson MD, Muraszko KM. Chiari I malformation with syrinx. *Pediatr Neurol.* 2003;29(2):167–169.
16. Sharan AD, Kaye D, Charles Malveaux WM, Riew KD. Dropped head syndrome: etiology and management. *J Am Acad Orthop Surg.* 2012;20(12):766–774.
17. Finsterer J, Revuelta GJ. Anterocollis and anterocaput. *Clin Neurol Neurosurg.* 2014;127:44–53.
18. Hogan KA, Manning EL, Glaser JA. Progressive cervical kyphosis associated with botulinum toxin injection. *South Med J.* 2006;99(8):888–891.
19. Tomczak KK, Rosman NP. Torticollis. *J Child Neurol.* 2013;28(3):365–378.
20. Wall PD, Melzack R, Bonica JJ. *Textbook of pain.* 3rd ed. Edinburgh; New York: Churchill Livingstone; 1994: xvi, 1524.
21. Simons DG, et al. *Travell & Simons' myofascial pain and dysfunction: the trigger point manual.* 2nd ed. Baltimore, MA: Williams & Wilkins; 1999: v. 1.
22. Haldeman S, Dagenais S. Cervicogenic headaches: a critical review. *Spine J.* 2001;1(1):31–46.
23. LaBan MM, Meerschaert JR, Taylor RS. Breast pain: a symptom of cervical radiculopathy. *Arch Phys Med Rehabil.* 1979;60(7):315–317.
24. Sheehan NJ. Dysphagia and other manifestations of oesophageal involvement in the musculoskeletal diseases. *Rheumatology (Oxford).* 2008;47(6):746–752.
25. Ihnatsenka B, Boezaart AP. Applied sonoanatomy of the posterior triangle of the neck. *Int J Shoulder Surg.* 2010;4(3):63–74.
26. Hartman J. Anatomy and clinical significance of the uncinate process and uncovertebral joint: A comprehensive review. *Clin Anat.* 2014;27(3):431–440.
27. Gellhorn AC. Cervical facet-mediated pain. *Phys Med Rehabil Clin N Am.* 2011;22(3):447–58, viii.
28. Mays MA, Tepper SJ. Occipital nerve blocks. In: Narouze SN, ed. *Interventional Management of Head and Face Pain: Nerve Blocks and Beyond.* New York, NY: Springer; 2014:29–34.
29. Kikuchi S, Macnab I, Moreau P. Localisation of the level of symptomatic cervical disc degeneration. *J Bone Joint Surg Br.* 1981;63-B(2):272–277.
30. Mathis JM, Shaibani A, Wakhloo AK. Spine anatomy. In: Mathis MJ, Golovac S. eds. *Image-Guided Spine Interventions.* New York, NY: Springer; 2010:1–27.
31. Fletcher G, Haughton VM, Ho KC, Yu SW. Age-related changes in the cervical facet joints: studies with cryomicrotomy, MR, and CT. *AJR Am J Roentgenol.* 1990;154(4):817–820.
32. Mancall EL, Brock DG, Gray H. *Gray's clinical neuroanatomy: the anatomic basis for clinical neuroscience.* xiii, 433 pages; 2011.
33. Bogduk N, Windsor M, Inglis A. The innervation of the cervical intervertebral discs. *Spine (Phila Pa 1976).* 1988;13(1):2–8.
34. Tubbs RS, Salter EG, Wellons JC, Blount JP, Oakes WJ. Landmarks for the identification of the cutaneous nerves of the occiput and nuchal regions. *Clin Anat.* 2007;20(3):235–238.
35. Mills MK, Shah LM. Imaging of the perivertebral space. *Radiol Clin North Am.* 2015;53(1):163–180.
36. Nash L, Nicholson HD, Zhang M. Does the investing layer of the deep cervical fascia exist? *Anesthesiology.* 2005;103(5):962–968.
37. Shah-Nawaz M, Dodwad SNK, Howard S, An, Cervical spine anatomy. In *Textbook of the cervical spine.* Philadelphia, PA: Saunders Elsevier: 2015.
38. Kaufman JA, Lee MJ. *Vascular and interventional radiology.* Philadelphia, PA: Elsevier Health Sciences. 2013.
39. Bogduk N, Yoganandan N. Biomechanics of the cervical spine Part 3: minor injuries. *Clin Biomech (Bristol, Avon).* 2001;16(4):267–275.
40. Yoganandan N, Kumaresan S, Pintar FA. Biomechanics of the cervical spine Part 2. Cervical spine soft tissue responses and biomechanical modeling. *Clin Biomech.* 2001;16(1):1–27.
41. Bogduk N, Mercer S. Biomechanics of the cervical spine. I: Normal kinematics. *Clin Biomech (Bristol, Avon).* 2000;15(9):633–648.
42. Gellhorn AC, Katz JN, Suri P. Osteoarthritis of the spine: the facet joints. *Nat Rev Rheumatol.* 2013;9(4):216–224.
43. Ferrara LA. The biomechanics of cervical spondylosis. *Adv Orthop.* 2012;2012:493605.
44. Harrop JS, Hanna A, Silva MT, Sharan A. Neurological manifestations of cervical spondylosis: an overview of signs, symptoms, and pathophysiology. *Neurosurgery.* 2007;60(1 Supp1 1):S14–S20.
45. Rao RD, Currier BL, Albert TJ, et al. Degenerative cervical spondylosis: clinical syndromes, pathogenesis, and management. *J Bone Joint Surg Am.* 2007;89(6):1360–1378.
46. Triantafillou KM, Lauerman W, Kalantar SB. Degenerative disease of the cervical spine and its relationship to athletes. *Clin Sports Med.* 2012;31(3):509–520.
47. van der Donk J, Schouten JS, Passchier J, van Romunde LK, Valkenburg HA. The associations of neck pain with radiological abnormalities of the cervical spine and personality traits in a general population. *J Rheumatol.* 1991;18(12):1884–1889.
48. Schofferman J, Bogduk N, Slosar P. Chronic whiplash and whiplash-associated disorders: an evidence-based approach. *J Am Acad Orthop Surg.* 2007;15(10):596–606.
49. Bazemore AW, Smucker DR. Lymphadenopathy and malignancy. *Am Fam Physician.* 2002;66(11):2103–2110.
50. Tong HC, Haig AJ, Yamakawa K. The Spurling test and cervical radiculopathy. *Spine (Phila Pa 1976).* 2002;27(2):156–159.
51. Shabat S, Leitner Y, David R, Folman Y. The correlation between Spurling test and imaging studies in detecting cervical radiculopathy. *J Neuroimaging.* 2012;22(4):375–378.
52. Fast A, Parikh S, Marin EL. The shoulder abduction relief sign in cervical radiculopathy. *Arch Phys Med Rehabil.* 1989;70(5):402–403.
53. Ferrante MA. The thoracic outlet syndromes. *Muscle Nerve.* 2012;45(6):780–795.
54. Gillard J, Pérez-Cousin M, Hachulla E, et al. Diagnosing thoracic outlet syndrome: contribution of provocative tests, ultrasonography, electrophysiology, and helical computed tomography in 48 patients. *Joint Bone Spine.* 2001;68(5):416–424.
55. Abe M, Ichinohe K, Nishida J. Diagnosis, treatment, and complications of thoracic outlet syndrome. *J Orthop Sci.* 1999;4(1):66–69.
56. Pham MH, Attenello FJ, Lucas J, et al. Conservative management of ossification of the posterior longitudinal ligament. A review. *Neurosurg Focus.* 2011;30(3):E2.
57. Houten JK, Noce LA. Clinical correlations of cervical myelopathy and the Hoffmann sign. *J Neurosurg Spine.* 2008;9(3):237–242.
58. Chang CW, Chang KY, Lin SM. Quantification of the Trömner signs: a sensitive marker for cervical spondylotic myelopathy. *Eur Spine J.* 2011;20(6):923–927.
59. Laker SR, Concannon LG. Radiologic evaluation of the neck: a review of radiography, ultrasonography, computed tomography, magnetic resonance imaging, and other imaging modalities for neck pain. *Phys Med Rehabil Clin N Am.* 2011;22(3):411–428, vii.
60. Binder A. Neck pain. *Clin Evid.* June 2004(11):1534–1550.
61. Pangarkar S, Lee PC. Conservative treatment for neck pain: medications, physical therapy, and exercise. *Phys Med Rehabil Clin N Am.* 2011;22(3):503–520, ix.
62. Falla D. Unravelling the complexity of muscle impairment in chronic neck pain. *Man Ther.* 2004;9(3):125–133.
63. Dusunceli Y, Ozturk C, Atamaz F, et al. Efficacy of neck stabilization exercises for neck pain: a randomized controlled study. *J Rehabil Med.* 2009;41(8):626–631.
64. Narouze SN, Provenzano DA. Sonographically guided cervical facet nerve and joint injections: why sonography? *J Ultrasound Med.* 2013;32(11):1885–1896.
65. Stout A. Epidural steroid injections for cervical radiculopathy. *Phys Med Rehabil Clin N Am.* 2011;22(1):149–159.
66. Rhee JM, Yoon T, Riew KD. Cervical radiculopathy. *J Am Acad Orthop Surg.* 2007;15(8):486–494.
67. Matz PG, Holly LT, Groff MW, et al.; Joint Section on Disorders of the Spine and Peripheral Nerves of the American Association of Neurological Surgeons and Congress of Neurological Surgeons. Indications for anterior cervical decompression for the treatment of cervical degenerative radiculopathy. *J Neurosurg Spine.* 2009;11(2):174–182.
68. Polston DW. Cervical radiculopathy. *Neurol Clin.* 2007;25(2):373–385.
69. Henderson CM, Hennessy RG, Shuey HM Jr, Shackelford EG. Posterior-lateral foraminotomy as an exclusive operative technique for

69. cervical radiculopathy: a review of 846 consecutively operated cases. *Neurosurgery*. 1983;13(5):504–512.
70. Malanga GA, Landes P, Nadler SF. Provocative tests in cervical spine examination: historical basis and scientific analyses. *Pain Physician*. 2003;6(2):199–205.
71. Hendrickson CD, Godek A, Schmidt P. Paget-Schroetter syndrome in a collegiate football player. *Clin J Sport Med*. 2006;16(1):79–80.
72. Lauder TD. Musculoskeletal disorders that frequently mimic radiculopathy. *Phys Med Rehabil Clin N Am*. 2002;13(3):469–485.
73. Hakimi K, Spanier D. Electrodiagnosis of cervical radiculopathy. *Phys Med Rehabil Clin N Am*. 2013;24(1):1–12.
74. Frontera WR, DeLisa JA. *Physical medicine and rehabilitation: principles and practice*. 5th ed. Philadelphia, PA: Lippincott Williams & Wilkins Health. 2010:v (xxii, 2200, 39).
75. Eubanks JD. Cervical radiculopathy: nonoperative management of neck pain and radicular symptoms. *Am Fam Physician*. 2010;81(1):33–40.
76. Sakaura H, Hosono N, Mukai Y, et al. C5 palsy after decompression surgery for cervical myelopathy: review of the literature. *Spine*. 2003;28(21):2447–2451.
77. Hashimoto M, Mochizuki M, Aiba A, et al. C5 palsy following anterior decompression and spinal fusion for cervical degenerative diseases. *Eur Spine J*. 2010;19(10):1702–1710.
78. Brown JM, Yee A, Ivens RA, et al. Post-cervical decompression parsonage-turner syndrome represents a subset of C5 palsy: six cases and a review of the literature: case report. *Neurosurgery*. 2010;67(6):E1831–43; discussion E1843.
79. Guzman JZ, Baird EO, Fields AC, et al. C5 nerve root palsy following decompression of the cervical spine: a systematic evaluation of the literature. *Bone Joint J*. 2014;96-B(7):950–955.
80. Vanelderen P, Lataster A, Levy R, et al. 8. Occipital neuralgia. *Pain Pract*. 2010;10(2):137–144.
81. Dougherty C. Occipital neuralgia. *Curr Pain Headache Rep*. 2014;18(5):411.
82. Tobin J, Flitman S. Occipital nerve blocks: when and what to inject? *Headache*. 2009;49(10):1521–1533.
83. Cho JC, Haun DW, Kettner NW. Sonographic evaluation of the greater occipital nerve in unilateral occipital neuralgia. *J Ultrasound Med*. 2012;31(1):37–42.
84. Rao RD, Currier BL, Albert TJ, et al. Degenerative cervical spondylosis: clinical syndromes, pathogenesis, and management. *J Bone Joint Surg Am*. 2007;89(6):1360–1378.
85. Toledano M, Bartleson JD. Cervical spondylotic myelopathy. *Neurol Clin*. 2013;31(1):287–305.
86. Rajpal S, Chanbusarakum K, Deshmukh PR. Upper cervical myelopathy due to arachnoiditis and spinal cord tethering from adjacent C-2 osteomyelitis. Case report and review of the literature. *J Neurosurg Spine*. 2007;6(1):64–67.
87. Rhee JM, Shamji MF, Erwin WM, et al. Nonoperative management of cervical myelopathy: a systematic review. *Spine*. 2013;38(22 Suppl 1):S55–S67.
88. Torg JS, Corcoran TA, Thibault LE, et al. Cervical cord neurapraxia: classification, pathomechanics, morbidity, and management guidelines. *J Neurosurg*. 1997;87(6):843–850.
89. Clark AJ, Auguste KI, Sun PP. Cervical spinal stenosis and sports-related cervical cord neurapraxia. *Neurosurg Focus*. 2011;31(5):E7.
90. Saetia K, Cho D, Lee S, et al. Ossification of the posterior longitudinal ligament: a review. *Neurosurg Focus*. 2011;30(3):E1.
91. Matsunaga S, Sakou T. Ossification of the posterior longitudinal ligament of the cervical spine: etiology and natural history. *Spine*. 2012;37(5):E309–E314.
92. Vandertop WP. Syringomyelia. *Neuropediatrics*. 2014;45(1):3–9.
93. Roy AK, Slimack NP, Ganju A. Idiopathic syringomyelia: retrospective case series, comprehensive review, and update on management. *Neurosurg Focus*. 2011;31(6):E15.
94. Hankinson TC, Klimo P Jr, Feldstein NA, et al. Chiari malformations, syringohydromyelia and scoliosis. *Neurosurg Clin N Am*. 2007;18(3):549–568.
95. Petheram TG, Hourigan PG, Emran IM, Weatherley CR. Dropped head syndrome: a case series and literature review. *Spine*. 2008;33(1):47–51.
96. Liao JP, Waclawik AJ, Lotz BP, et al. Myopathic dropped head syndrome: an expanding clinicopathological spectrum. *Am J Phys Med Rehabil*. 2007;86(12):970–976.
97. Fast A, Thomas MA. The "baseball cap orthosis": a simple solution for dropped head syndrome. *Am J Phys Med Rehabil*. 2008;87(1):71–73.
98. Cooper G, Bailey B, Bogduk N. Cervical zygapophysial joint pain maps. *Pain Med*. 2007;8(4):344–353.
99. van Eerd M, Patijn J, Lataster A, et al. 5. Cervical facet pain. *Pain Pract*. 2010;10(2):113–123.
100. Cohen SP, Huang JH, Brummett C. Facet joint pain—advances in patient selection and treatment. *Nat Rev Rheumatol*. 2013;9(2):101–116.
101. Bogduk N, Teasell R. Whiplash: the evidence for an organic etiology. *Arch Neurol*. 2000;57(4):590–591.
102. Bogduk N. On cervical zygapophysial joint pain after whiplash. *Spine*. 2011;36(25 Suppl):S194–S199.
103. Dolman B, Verrall G, Reid I. Physical principles demonstrate that the biceps femoris muscle relative to the other hamstring muscles exerts the most force: implications for hamstring muscle strain injuries. *Muscles Ligaments Tendons J*. 2014;4(3):371–377.
104. Narayan P, Haid RW. Treatment of degenerative cervical disc disease. *Neurol Clin*. 2001;19(1):217–229.
105. Onyewu O, Manchikanti L, Falco FJ, et al. An update of the appraisal of the accuracy and utility of cervical discography in chronic neck pain. *Pain Physician*. 2012;15(6):E777–E806.
106. Kim DH, Hilibrand AS. Rheumatoid arthritis in the cervical spine. *J Am Acad Orthop Surg*. 2005;13(7):463–474.
107. Wasserman BR, Moskovich R, Razi AE. Rheumatoid arthritis of the cervical spine–clinical considerations. *Bull NYU Hosp Jt Dis*. 2011;69(2):136–148.
108. Hohl JB, Grabowski G, Donaldson III WF. Cervical deformity in rheumatoid arthritis. *Semin Spine Surg*. 2011;23:181–187.
109. Amirfeyz R, Aspros D, Gargan M. Down syndrome. *Current Orthopaedics*. 2006;20(3):212–215.
110. Tracy MR, Dormans JP, Kusumi K. Klippel-Feil syndrome: clinical features and current understanding of etiology. *Clin Orthop Relat Res*. 2004;(424):183–190.
111. Samartzis DD, Herman J, Lubicky JP, Shen FH. Classification of congenitally fused cervical patterns in Klippel-Feil patients: epidemiology and role in the development of cervical spine-related symptoms. *Spine*. 2006;31(21):E798–E804.
112. Green JD, Harle TS, Harris JH Jr. Anterior subluxation of the cervical spine: hyperflexion sprain. *Am J Neuroradiol*. 1981;2(3):243–250.
113. Shanmuganathan K, Mirvis SE, Dowe M, Levine AM. Traumatic isolation of the cervical articular pillar: imaging observations in 21 patients. *Am J Roentgenol*. 1996;166(4):897–902.
114. Arvin B, Fournier-Gosselin MP, Fehlings MG. Os odontoideum: etiology and surgical management. *Neurosurgery*. 2010;66(3 Suppl):22–31.
115. Daffner RH, Hackney DB. ACR Appropriateness Criteria on suspected spine trauma. *J Am Coll Radiol*. 2007;4(11):762–775.
116. Molina CA, Gokaslan ZL, Sciubba DM. Diagnosis and management of metastatic cervical spine tumors. *Orthop Clin North Am*. 2012;43(1):75–87, viii.
117. Perrin RG, Laxton AW. Metastatic spine disease: epidemiology, pathophysiology, and evaluation of patients. *Neurosurg Clin N Am*. 2004;15(4):365–373.
118. Sørensen S, Børgesen SE, Rohde K, et al. Metastatic epidural spinal cord compression. Results of treatment and survival. *Cancer*. 1990;65(7):1502–1508.
119. Mazel C, Balabaud L, Bennis S, Hansen S. Cervical and thoracic spine tumor management: surgical indications, techniques, and outcomes. *Orthop Clin North Am*. 2009;40(1):75–92, vi.
120. Zmurko MG, Tannoury TY, Tannoury CA, Anderson DG. Cervical sprains, disc herniations, minor fractures, and other cervical injuries in the athlete. *Clin Sports Med*. 2003;22(3):513–521.
121. Celik D, Mutlu EK. Clinical implication of latent myofascial trigger point. *Curr Pain Headache Rep*. 2013;17(8):353.
122. Cummings M, Baldry P. Regional myofascial pain: diagnosis and management. *Best Pract Res Clin Rheumatol*. 2007;21(2):367–387.
123. Giamberardino MA, Affaitati G, Fabrizio A, Costantini R. Myofascial pain syndromes and their evaluation. *Best Pract Res Clin Rheumatol*. 2011;25(2):185–198.
124. Hakgüder A, Birtane M, Gürcan S, et al. Efficacy of low level laser therapy in myofascial pain syndrome: an algometric and thermographic evaluation. *Lasers Surg Med*. 2003;33(5):339–343.

CHAPTER 3

Shoulder

EPIDEMIOLOGY OF SHOULDER PAIN

SHOULDER PAIN IN THE GENERAL POPULATION

Prevalence
- 20% (1%–67% depending on studies) in the general population
- 1% of adults have disabling shoulder pain (in the United Kingdom; it may vary depending on the definition) (1)
- More common in women, middle-aged and elderly, smokers, those with previous trauma, and wheelchair users
- Common in 50- to 56-year-olds (may be due to normal aging process of the rotator cuff) and in 12- to 18-year-olds (possibly due to computer and mouse use)

SHOULDER PAIN IN ATHLETES (2)

Prevalence
- Varies, 3% to 8% in athletes overall and up to 60% in overhead throwing sports, swimming, or volleyball
- Shoulder: most injured body part in swimmers, third most common (MC) injured area in volleyball players
- Increases with the level of activity and competition (3)
- Signs suggestive of impingement syndrome and instability: very common among athletes

Risk factors
- Overuse/trauma, abundant soft tissue, sports requiring precise neuromuscular coordination
- SICK scapula syndrome: scapular malposition, inferior medial border prominence, coracoid pain/malposition and scapular dyskinesia (SICK), more common in overhead athletes (4)
- Tendon overuse, instability, and trauma in younger athletes versus degenerative changes: mainly in older athletes

SHOULDER PAIN AT WORK (5)

Prevalence
- Common in the workplace, but less commonly caused by work (13% of all shoulder problems presenting to primary care providers are work related)

Risk factors
- High risk for shoulder problems: workers using upper limbs. For example, welders, musicians, sign and brick layers, and workers with pneumatic tools
- Increasing shoulder-related disorders in those who work with computers; especially in younger population
- No readily identifiable cause

Workplace modifications
- No effective ergonomic approaches focusing on primary prevention of shoulder pain at work
- Early return to work likely to have best chance of good vocational outcome

DIFFERENTIAL DIAGNOSIS

MUSCULOSKELETAL (MSK) CAUSES OF SHOULDER PAIN BASED ON LOCATION (FLOWCHART 3.1)

Surface anatomy (Figure 3.1)
- Anterior and lateral
  ○ Coracoid process: 1 inch below the clavicle (at the junction of middle and lateral thirds)
  ○ Greater tuberosity of humerus: same coronal plane as the lateral epicondyle of the elbow, lesser tuberosity; anteromedial to greater tuberosity (expose with external rotation)
- Posterior
  ○ Spine of scapular medially (at T3: root of the spine of scapular), superior angle: T2, inferior border of scapular: T7 level, medial border of scapular depending on the protraction and retraction; about 2 to 3 inches in anatomic position (from midline at T3)
- Superiorly: acromioclavicular (AC) joint

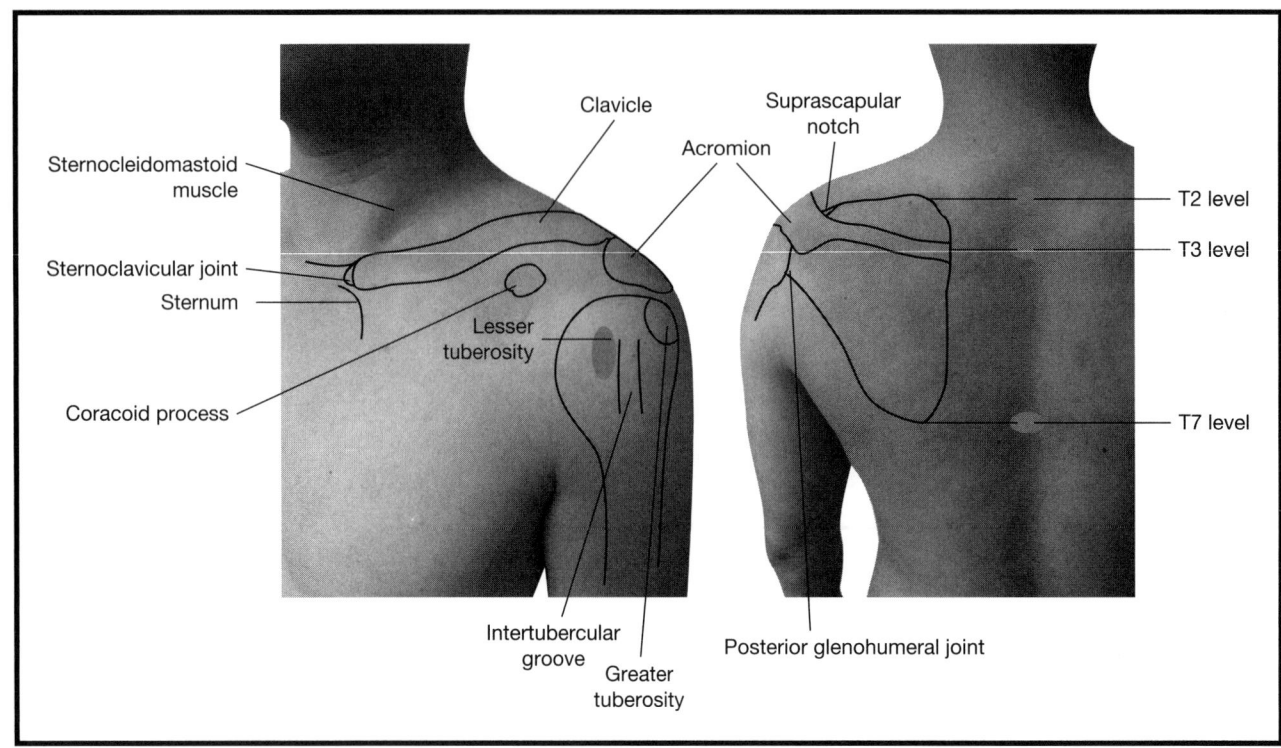

FIGURE 3.1
Surface anatomy of the shoulder (A) anterior and (B) posterior aspect of the shoulder region.

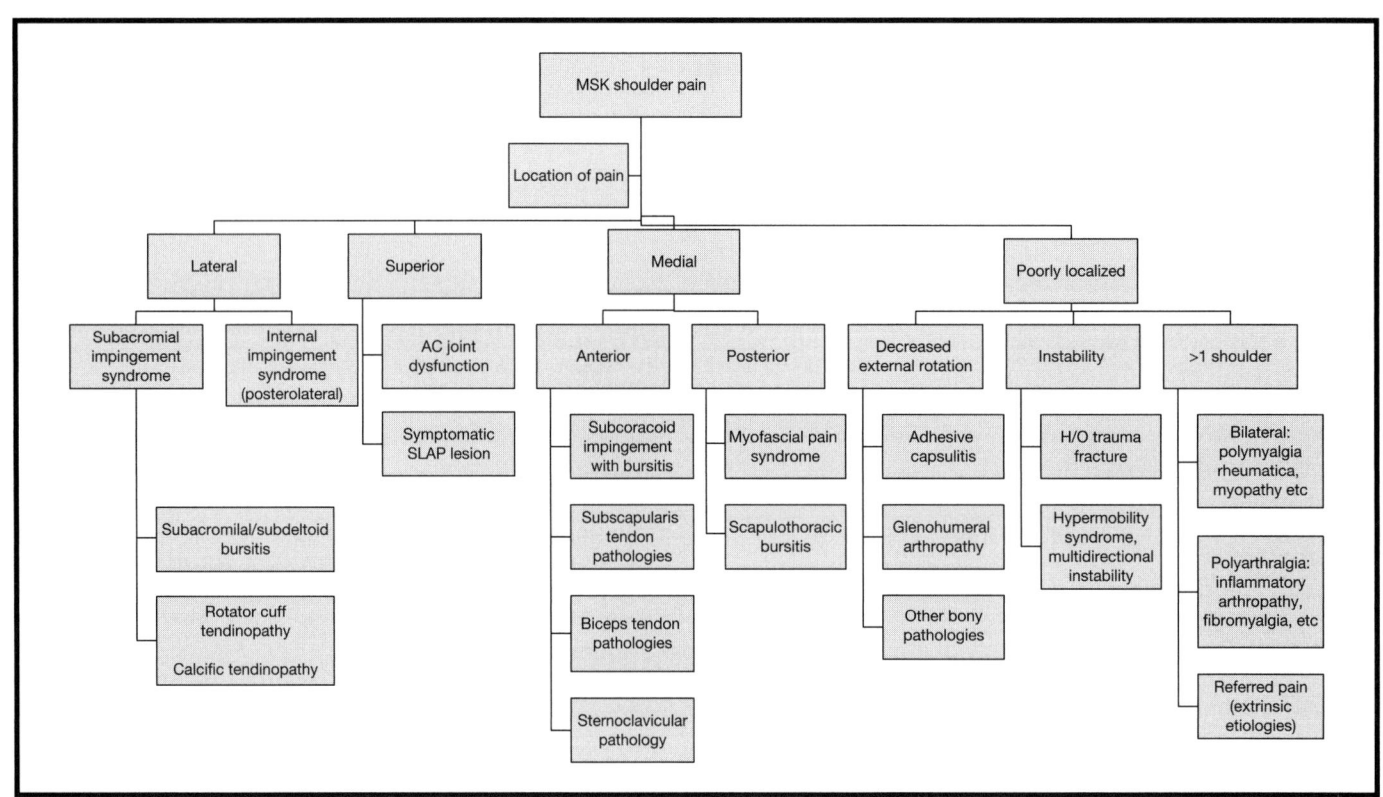

FLOWCHART 3.1
Differential diagnosis of musculoskeletal shoulder pain.

REGION	ANATOMIC STRUCTURE	COMMON MSK DISORDERS
Antero-Lateral	Subacromial space (1 in Figure 3.2)	Subacromial impingement syndrome • Subacromial/subdeltoid bursitis: constant shoulder pain and night pain • Rotator cuff (supra/infraspinatus) tendinopathy/tear: pain with movement (rather than constant). Calcific tendinitis: can be severe, constant temporarily
Superior	Acromioclavicular joint (3 in Figure 3.2) Sup. labrum/supraglenoid tubercle	Degenerative, trauma, distal clavicular osteolysis, and infection Superior labral tear from anterior to posterior (SLAP): often asymptomatic
Antero-medial	Bicipital groove (2 in Figure 3.2)	Bicipital tendinitis and biceps tendon subluxation and tear • Location of tenderness (on bicipital groove) changes with external/internal rotation
	Coracoid process/subcoracoid space	Subcoracoid impingement syndrome Pain/tenderness immediately lateral to coracoid process
	Subscapularis	Tear, tendinosis, subscapularis bursitis • Pain on resisted internal rotation (often not specific)
Medial	Sternoclavicular joint (5 in Figure 3.2)	Degenerative changes (6), trauma, or infection • Pain on the joint with shoulder movement (especially cross-arm adduction)
Posterior	Posterior edge of the acromion (6 in Figure 3.2)	Shoulder impingement; external (subacromial bursitis) Internal impingement between humeral head and glenoid Rotator cuff (infraspinatus) tendinitis/tear, calcific tendinopathy Posterior subluxation of glenohumeral joint; often asymptomatic
	Medial scapular border	Myofascial pain syndrome of rhomboids, trapezius Scapulothoracic bursitis
	Suprascapular notch (7 in Figure 3.2)	Suprascapular N entrapment at suprascapular notch: both supra and infraspinatus muscles involved • Spinoglenoid notch: infraspinatus muscle atrophy (often without pain)
Poorly localized	Glenohumeral joint (4 in Figure 3.2)	Adhesive capsulitis (often diffuse, poorly localized pain), glenohumeral arthritis (OA, inflammatory arthropathy), osteonecrosis, glenoid labral tears, and fracture
	Quadrilateral space (8 in Figure 3.2)	Axillary nerve entrapment (7)

MSK, musculoskeletal; OA, osteoarthritis.

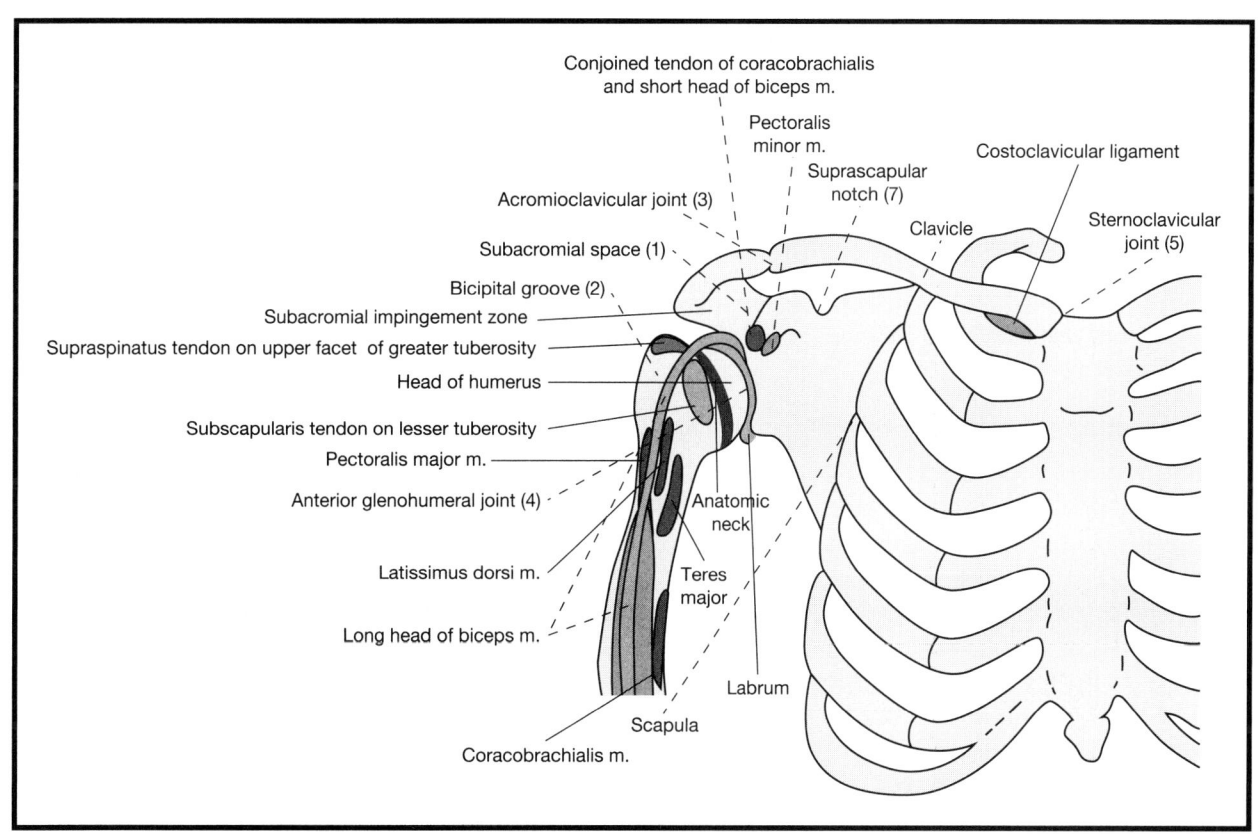

FIGURE 3.2
Bony anatomy of the shoulder.

(continued)

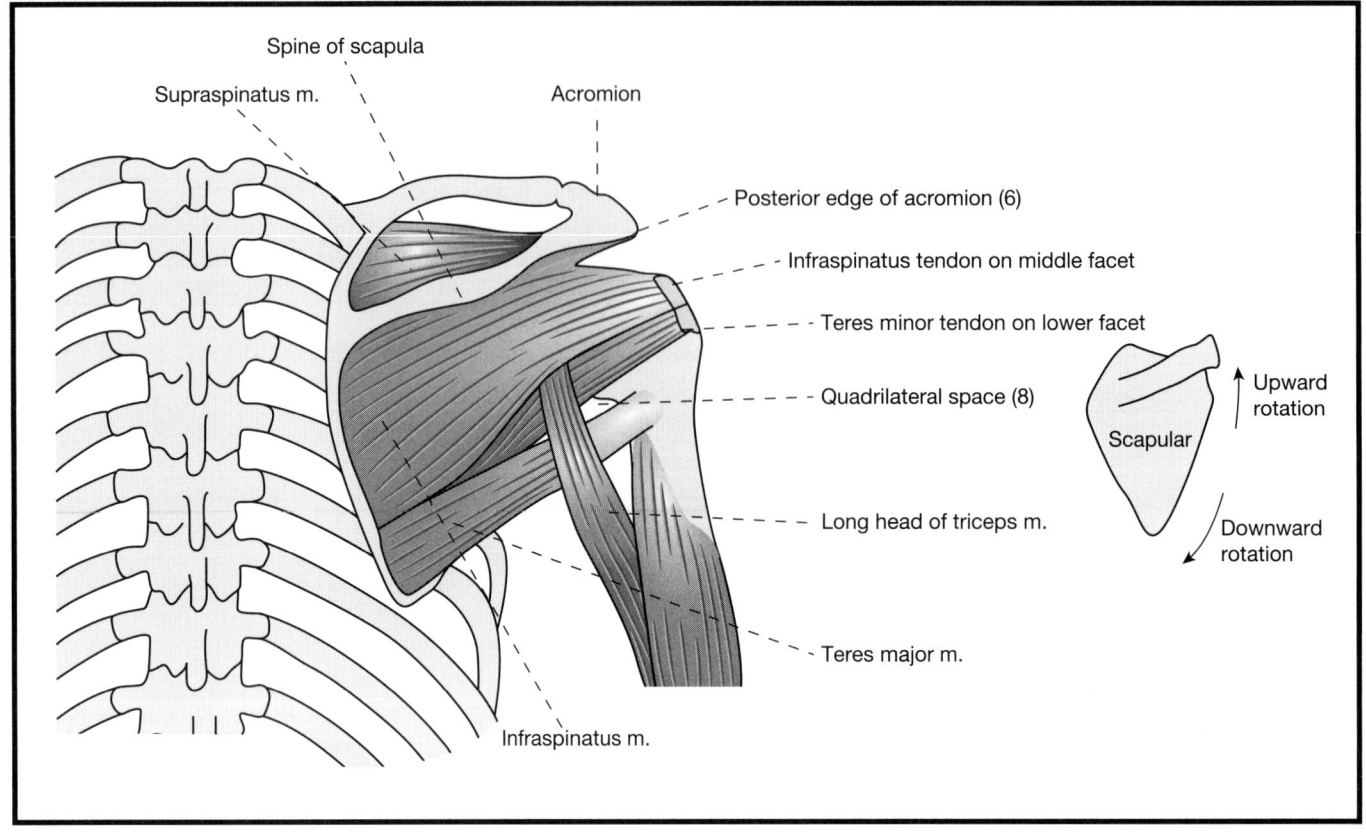

FIGURE 3.2 (continued)

NEUROPATHIC CAUSES OF SHOULDER PAIN

C5, 6 radiculopathy: neck pain more significant than shoulder pain ± sensory (paresthesia, tingling, rarely numbness) and motor symptoms

Brachial amyotrophy: initial severe pain (≥7/10, improved) followed by rapid/significant atrophy and weakness ± persistent sensory symptom

Suprascapular neuropathy: may be isolated atrophy (supra/infraspinatus) ± pain (deep, posterior)

Axillary neuropathy (at quadrilateral space): atrophy (deltoid and teres minor) ± pain (deep)

Mimickers: Myofascial pain syndrome of scapular stabilizer muscle (trapezius, rhomboids, levator scapular etc) with referred pain and cervical facet arthropathy (spondylosis, whiplash, worse with extension/rotation)

EXTRINSIC CAUSES OF SHOULDER PAIN (8)

- Myofascial pain syndrome of neck (paraspinal/suboccipital) muscles (referred pain)
- Hepatobiliary disease
- Diaphragm irritation and pneumonia (atypical pneumonia), and apical lung tumor
  - Risk factors: age, smoking, or constitutional signs/symptoms
- Metastasis; consider if + risk factors, for example, elderly smoker
- Coronary artery disease with known cardiovascular (CV) risk factor

NEUROLOGICAL SYMPTOMS

Sensory symptoms (Flowchart 3.2)
- Cervical spine disease (radiculopathy, facet arthropathy), brachial plexopathy (diabetic amyotrophy; radiculoplexus-neuropathy), suprascapular, axillary neuropathy (positive or negative symptoms), or cerebrovascular accident (CVA; stroke, if + CV risk factors)
- Myofascial pain (with paresthesia, positive sensory, or autonomic symptoms): negative symptoms (numbness) are rare

Motor symptoms
- Weakness and fatigue
- Weakness from MSK disorders: both active and passive range of motion (ROM) involved
  - Tendon tear/rupture with pain
    - Mild weakness unless multiple tendons and muscles are involved. Supraspinatus; minimal contributor to abduction (compared to deltoid muscle)
    - Two heads of biceps brachii; long and short head. One tendon head rupture does not necessarily cause significant weakness
  - Isolated weakness without pain (or minimal pain): decreased ROM presents

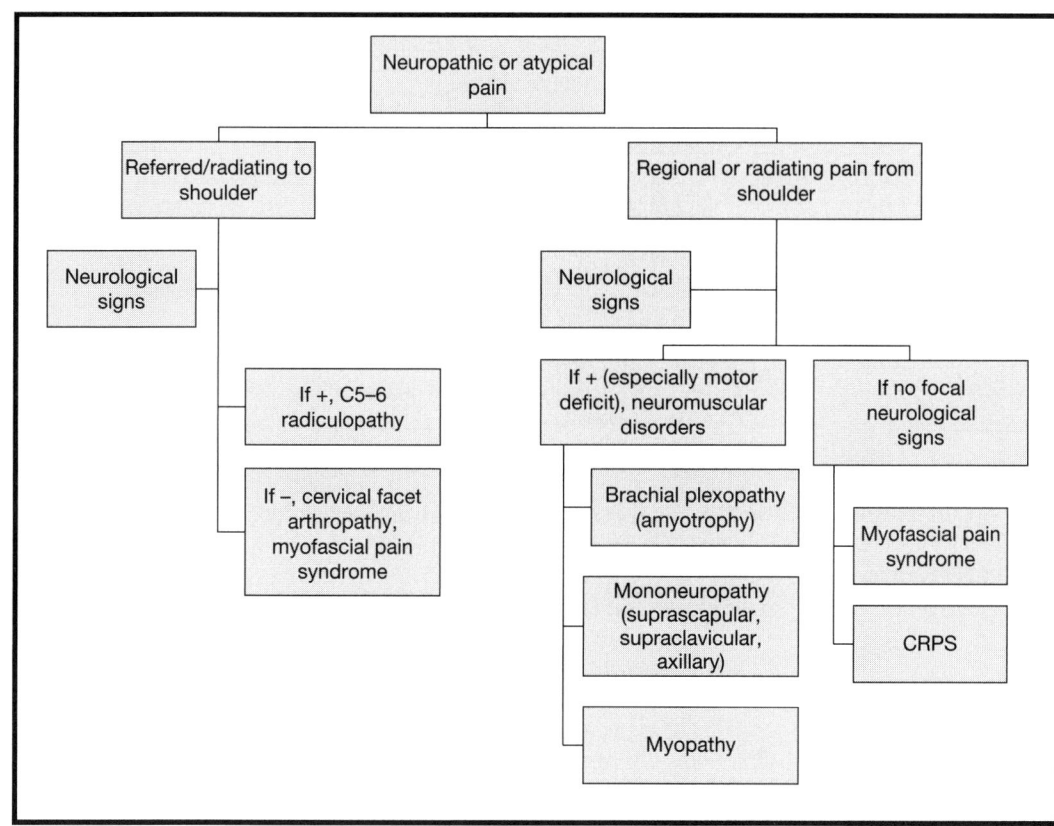

FLOWCHART 3.2 Differential diagnosis of neuropathic shoulder pain.

- Adhesive capsulitis (after initial painful stage, decreased range of motion prominent), massive rotator cuff tear, and joint deformity with contracture
- Osteoarthritis with decreased ROM: global decrease, including external rotation (less severe than adhesive capsulitis)
• Neuromuscular disorders: passive ROM intact unless secondary contracture/stiffness or concomitant MSK lesions exist
  ○ Lower motor neuron disease: cervical (C5–6) radiculopathy, brachial plexopathy, axillary neuropathy, suprascapular neuropathy, rarely motor neuron disease (amyotrophic lateral sclerosis [ALS], spinal muscular atrophy)
    ▪ Significant weakness and atrophy present
  ○ Upper motor neuron disease: stroke, brain lesion (tumor, inflammation, infection, vascular), cervical myelopathy (distal part of extremity than proximal part, inflammatory; multiple sclerosis [MS], tumor, infection, vascular, and idiopathic), ALS
  ○ Muscle disease: minimal sensory symptoms although concomitant lesions or pain (myalgia) can occur with weakness
    ▪ Hereditary (facioscapulohumeral muscular [FSH] dystrophy, myotonic dystrophy) and acquired (polymyositis, dermatomyositis, necrotizing myopathy, etc)
    ▪ Polymyalgia rheumatica: older adults, usually bilateral, with myalgia
• Psychogenic: distraction results in inconsistent findings

SNAPPING SHOULDER

Differential diagnosis based on location (9–11)
• Scapulothoracic articulation (posterior)
  ○ Scapulothoracic dyskinesia with scapulothoracic bursitis, muscle atrophy (from nerve injury or disuse)
  ○ Rotator cuff tendinopathy, tear, and glenohumeral (GH) joint pathology (labral tear, loose body)
  ○ Bony abnormalities
    ▪ Structural spinal deformities (including scoliosis and thoracic kyphosis)
    ▪ Luschka tubercle (6%, a hook-shaped prominence on superomedial angle of scapula)
    ▪ Tumor (including osteochondromas of the rib and scapula; MC benign tumor of the scapulae)
    ▪ Healing fractures of ribs or scapulae with bony angulation or exuberant callus
  ○ Tuberculosis, syphilitic lesions
• Anterior snapping (12)
  ○ GH instability
  ○ Labral tears and intra-articular (IA) loose body (GH joint)
  ○ Chondral or osteochondral lesions
  ○ Bicipital tendon instability and subscapularis tendinopathy
  ○ Bursopathy: subcoracoid bursitis and calcific bursitis

SHOULDER INSTABILITY

Differential diagnosis based on etiology
• Traumatic: soft tissue (capsule, ligament, tendon/muscle) versus bony (Hill–Sachs or bony Bankart lesion)
• Atraumatic: multidirectional instability, neurological (unbalanced muscle pattern: lower motor neuron disease, muscle disease or upper motor neuron disease), generalized laxity

Differential diagnosis based on location
- Anterior instability: MC (≥95%), violent shoulder external rotation/ abduction, fall on outstretched hand
- Posterior: landing on forward flexed and adducted arm above shoulder level
  - Often voluntary, associated with posterior Bankart lesion, and capsular laxity

ANATOMY

BONE, JOINT, AND LIGAMENT

Humerus
- Head and tuberosity
  - Anatomic neck (distinction between the tuberosity and humeral head, 6 mm above greater tuberosity)
    - Lost (flattened) in bony impingement (eg, rotator cuff arthropathy)
  - Neck and shaft inclination: 145° (130–150), angle of inclination
  - Humeral condyle (distal) and head angle; 30°; angle of torsion
    - Increased angle of torsion in retroversion (with decreased external rotation of GH joint in examination) and decreased in anteversion similar to the hip
    - Clinical implication: positive relationship between increased humeral torsion and recurrent anterior dislocation of shoulder
- Bony landmarks (useful for imaging interpretation or MSK ultrasound [US] scanning)
  - Greater tubercle has three facets for rotator cuff tendons (supraspinatus/infraspinatus/teres minor): from anterior/superior to lateral/inferior: upper, middle, and lower facet
  - Lesser tubercle: subscapularis
  - Intertubercular (bicipital) groove: biceps long-head tendon in the groove and distally attachment for tendons from laterally to medially (pectoralis major/latissimus dorsi/ teres major)
  - Deltoid tubercle for deltoid M insertion anteriorly, posteriorly spiral groove for radial N located in the middle of the humerus
- Vascular supply: (13)
  - Anterior circumflex artery; lateral to the biceps long-head tendon; avoid during injection to bicipital groove above surgical neck, main supplier to the humeral head (with posterior circumflex A)
    - Cautious of injury during rotator cuff surgery and open reduction

Scapula
- Suprascapular notch
  - Suprascapular nerve traverses from anteromedial to posterior-inferior-lateral direction
  - Variant; ossified suprascapular ligament → suprascapular foramen; vulnerable to develop suprascapular neuropathy; supra and infraspinatus muscles involved
- Spinoglenoid notch; adjacent to the posterior GH joint; cyst/ganglion in the spinoglenoid notch often originating from labral lesion at the posterior GH joint
  - Isolated infraspinatus muscle involvement
- Scapular tilt: ~30° from coronal plane (lateral side anterior than medial side)

Glenohumeral (GH) Joint
- Glenoid faces posteriorly (~7°) and upward (~5°)
  - If angle decreased → increased risk of recurrent anterior subluxation/dislocation
- Labrum
  - Wedge-shaped fibrocartilage rim attached to glenoid fossa
    - Superior and anterosuperior portion: less vascular; may be more vulnerable to pathology
    - Superior: biceps long head (to the supraglenoid tubercle)
    - Inferior GH ligament: attaches to labrum and glenoid
  - Function: deepens glenoid cavity by 50% (passive stabilizer) and serves as an anchor point (GH ligament and biceps long-head tendon)
- GH ligament
  - Superior GH ligament: superior labrum near biceps to superior part of lesser tuberosity (rotator cuff interval), resists posterior and inferior translation
  - Medial GH ligament: most variable, resists anterior translation
  - Inferior GH ligament: runs mediolaterally from the 3 o'clock to 9 o'clock position and resembles a hammock
    - Primary restraint of anterior-posterior translation in the abducted shoulder (especially 90° ABER [abduction and external rotation])

Acromioclavicular (AC) joint
- A diarthrodial joint with a meniscal homolog (fibrocartilaginous disk: degenerate after 40 years)
- An inherently unstable articulation
- Static stabilizers: AC joint capsule/ligament and the CC ligament (stronger than AC ligament)
  - AC ligament
    - Prevent horizontal plane motion
    - The ligament inserts an average of ~18 mm medial to the AC joint on the clavicular undersurface
      – Aggressive distal clavicle excision (DCE) can destabilize the AC joint and lead to symptomatic posterior impingement against the acromion
  - The coracoclavicular (CC) ligaments
    - Prevent inferior migration of the scapulohumeral complex relative to the clavicle
    - If the AC ligaments are disrupted, the CC ligaments compensate by providing significant restraint to anteroposterior (AP) displacement
    - Composed of the conoid and the trapezoid ligament
      – The conoid ligament: more posterior than trapezoid (important for support against superior displacement)
      – The trapezoid origin on the mid-portion of the inferior surface of the clavicle
- The dynamic stabilizers: the deltoid and trapezius muscles
- AC joint innervated by suprascapular, axillary, and lateral pectoral nerve

Sternoclavicular (SC) joint (14)
- Diarthrodial joint, the articular surfaces of the SC joint covered in hyaline cartilage with an interposed fibrocartilaginous disc and highly incongruent

Anatomy 125

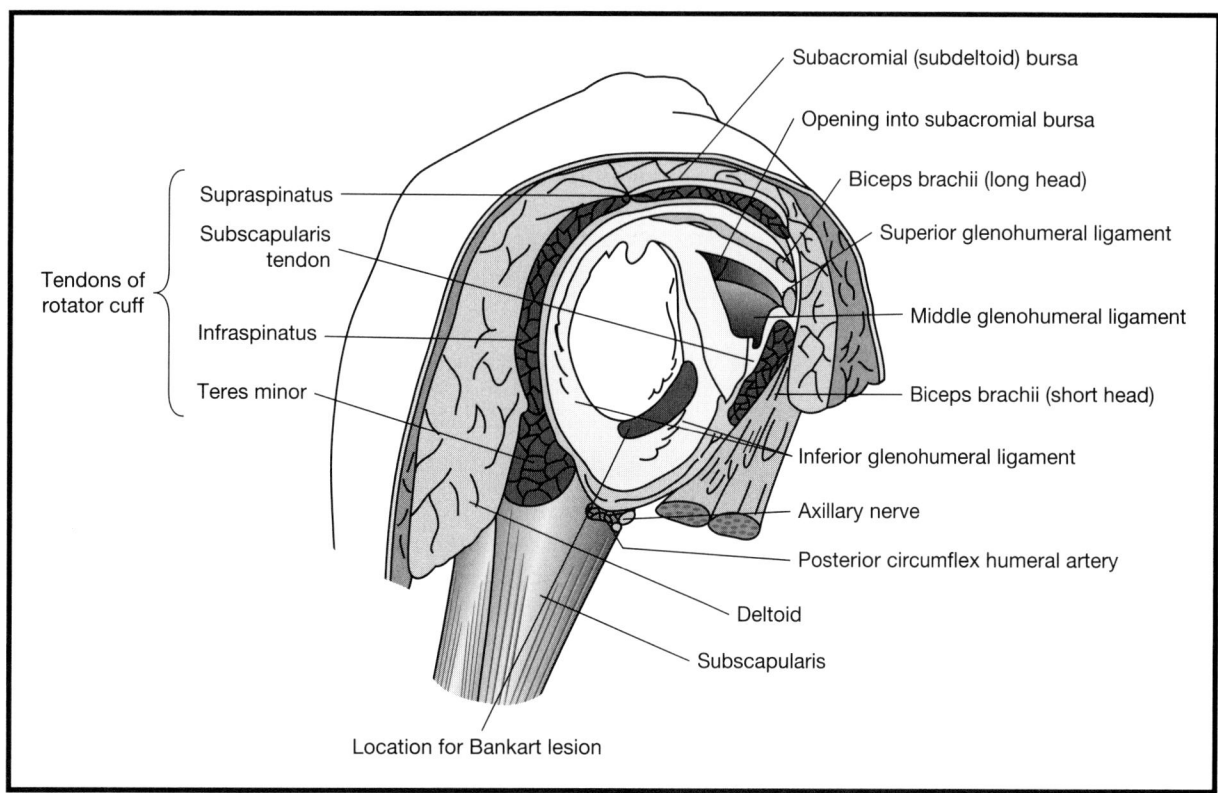

FIGURE 3.3
Glenoid cavity of the scapular and glenohumeral stabilizers (view from the anterolateral aspect).

- A "saddle" (convex in the AP plane, concave in the vertical plane) shape in clavicle and smaller convex shape of the manubrium
  - ROM around the SC joint: nearly freely movable in all planes
    - 35° of elevation, 35° of AP motion, 50° of rotation around its long axis
    - 30° of rotation with shoulder elevation
- Unstable joint: only half of the medial clavicle articulates with the sternum
  - Stability by ligament; the capsular ligament, the IA disc ligament, the interclavicular ligament, and the costoclavicular ligament
    - The capsular ligament is composed of anterior and posterior segments (stronger than anterior resisting superior translation of the medial clavicle)
    - The IA disc ligament resists medial displacement with compression
    - The interclavicular ligament resists superior migration of the medial clavicle
    - The costoclavicular ligament (also known as the rhomboid ligament) is the strongest of the SC ligaments
      - Consists of anterior and posterior fasciculi with an interposed bursa
      - A "twisted" appearance and stability is achieved during rotation and elevation of the distal clavicle

Subacromial/coracoacromial arch space (15)
- Borders of subacromial space
  - The superior border (the roof): the coracoacromial arch—the acromion, the coracoacromial ligament, and the coracoid process
    - The inferior (the floor): the greater tuberosity of the humerus and the superior aspect of the humeral head
  - The space between the acromion and the humeral head: 1.0 to 1.5 cm
    - Containing the rotator cuff tendons, the long head of the biceps tendon, the subacromial/subdeltoid bursa, and the coracoacromial ligament
    - The true height of this space is considerably less than that seen on radiographs (soft tissue is not visualized)
  - The impingement zone: centered on the insertion of the supraspinatus tendon on the greater tuberosity
    - Impingement by the anterior one-third of the acromion, the coracoacromial ligament, and the AC joint rather than by just the lateral aspect of the acromion

Subcoracoid space
- The normal coracohumeral interval, defined as minimal distance between the coracoid process and lesser tuberosity, is in the range of 8.4 to 11 mm
- Involves subscapularis muscle/tendon, subcoracoid bursa and GH joint capsule (16)
- Subcoracoid stenosis: if coracohumeral interval <6 mm. Contribute to subcoracoid impingement syndrome

Rotator cuff interval (17)
- Between inferior edge of the supraspinatus and the superior edge of the subscapularis
  - Medial: superficial; coracohumeral ligament (CHL), deep; superior GH ligament (SGHL) and joint capsule
  - Lateral: four layers

- First layer: superficial CHL fan to subscapularis and supraspinatus tendon
- Secondary layer: subscapularis and supraspinatus
- Third layer: deep CHL
- Fourth layer: SGHL and lateral capsule
• Functions
  ○ Resistance to inferior and posterior translation of the humeral head (especially in flexed, abducted, and external rotated shoulder)
  ○ Prevents excessive flexion, extension, adduction, and external rotation
  ○ Increases stability of long head of biceps tendon
  ○ Limits excessive GH motion
• Clinical implications
  ○ Rotator cuff interval (RI) contracture: thickened and fibrotic RI capsule and CHL
    - Adhesive capsulitis: may be significant inflammation on the bursal side of the RI
  ○ RI laxity: pain and instability (anterior shoulder instability)

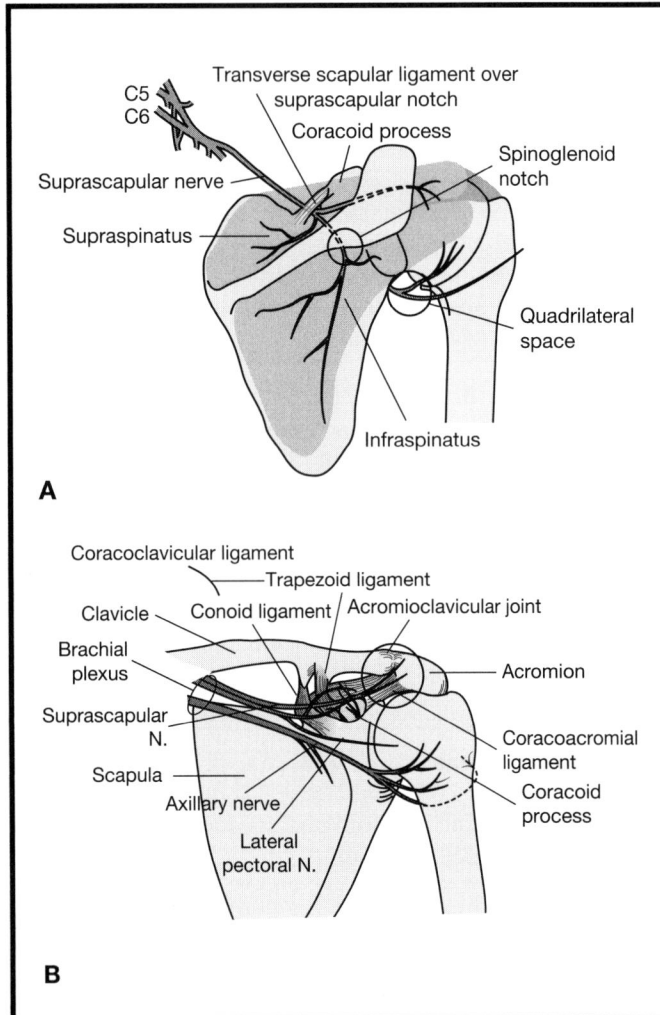

FIGURE 3.4
Nerve innervation around the shoulder joint and common entrapment sites (A) posterior aspect and (B) anterior aspect.

NERVE (18)

Sensory innervation of the human shoulder joint and capsule (19; Figure 3.4)
• Ventral: lateral pectoral, subscapular, axillary, and musculocutaneous N
• Dorsal: suprascapular and axillary N
• Suprascapular N
  ○ Articular (afferent sensory) branch from CHL, AC ligament and joint, GH joint, and subacromial bursa ± cutaneous branch in proximal lateral arm (5/35 in cadaver study)

BURSA

Subacromial subdeltoid bursa (20)
• The largest bursa in the body (21)
• Innervated by suprascapular N. posteriorly and lateral pectoral nerve anteriorly
  ○ Proprioception and nociception (free nerve endings, A δ and C fibers)
• Contains pressure sensitive Pacinian corpuscles and Ruffini endings (mechanical and pressure sensitive)
• Pain correlates with pro-inflammatory markers, cytokines, and substance P in the bursal tissue (6)
  ○ Patients with inflammatory cells: constant shoulder pain and pain at night
  ○ Patients without inflammatory cells: pain only with movement

Subcoracoid bursa (22) (Figure 3.2)
• Located under the coracoid process and the conjoint tendon (of the biceps short head and coracobrachialis), superficial to the subscapularis, and minimizes the friction between the coracoid and the subscapularis tendon
• The subcoracoid bursa occasionally communicates with the subacromial bursa
• It merges with the superior subscapularis recess known as subscapularis bursa (under the subscapularis) in ~30%
  ○ Minimizes the friction of the superficial fibers of the subscapularis against the coracoid

Other bursae around the scapula (23,24)

MAJOR/ANATOMIC BURSAE	
Infra-serratus bursa	Between serratus anterior and the chest wall. Inferior angle of scapula
Supra-serratus bursa	Between subscapularis and serratus anterior
Scapulo-trapezial bursa	Between superomedial scapular and trapezius

MINOR/ADVENTITIAL BURSAE	
Superomedial angle of scapula	Infraserratus and supraserraus bursae
Inferior angle of the scapula	Infraserratus bursae
Spine of scapula; trapezius	Between medial spine of scapula and trapezius

- Scapulothoracic bursa: commonly seen in overhead throwing athletes especially bursa at the inferior angle (pitching), weight training, swimming, gymnastics, football, or local trauma
  - Pain under the scapular, crepitus, grinding, and snapping with/without pain

MUSCLE

GH movement
- Humerus on the glenoid of the scapular; rotator cuff muscle with other extrinsic muscles

MOVEMENT	ABDUCTION	ADDUCTION	FLEXION	EXTENSION	INTERNAL ROTATION	EXTERNAL ROTATION
Muscles	Deltoid Supraspinatus	Deltoid PLT Infraspinatus Coracobrachialis	Deltoid Coracobrachialis Biceps Pectoralis major	Triceps long head Deltoid PLT	Subscapularis Deltoid PLT	SIT Deltoid

PLT, pectoralis major, latissimus dorsi, and teres major: Medially rotate and adduct; SIT, supraspinatus, infraspinatus, and teres minor.

- Pectoralis major and latissimus dorsi: large muscles to adduct and medially rotate the humerus (compared to the small external rotator. Rationale for external rotator strengthening to balance, target for spasticity management)

- Deltoid: all motion of the shoulder
  - Flexion: anterior deltoid, extension: posterior, abduction: middle, adduction: ant + post, internal rotation: anterior, external rotation: posterior

Scapulothoracic movement (scapula on the trunk/ribs)

	PROTRACTION	RETRACTION	ELEVATION	DEPRESSION
Muscles	Serratus anterior	Rhomboids (major, minor)	Upper trapezius Levator scapulae Rhomboids	Lower trapezius Pectoralis minor latissimus dorsi

MUSCLE	ORIGIN	INSERTION	INNERVATION	ACTION	COMMENT
Rotator Cuff Muscles					
Subscapularis	Medial two-thirds of the costal surface of the scapula (subscapular fossa)	Lesser tubercle of the humerus	Upper and lower subscapular nerves (C5,6)	Medially rotates the arm, assists extension of the arm	Involved in subcoracoid impingement syndrome
Supraspinatus	Supraspinatus fossa	Greater tubercle of the humerus (highest facet)	Suprascapular nerve (C5,6) from the upper trunk of the brachial plexus	Abducts the arm (initiates abduction) minimally	MC torn rotator cuff tendon Positions the humeral head on the glenoid

(continued)

MUSCLE	ORIGIN	INSERTION	INNERVATION	ACTION	COMMENT
Infraspinatus	Infraspinatus fossa	Greater tubercle of the humerus (middle facet)	Suprascapular N (C5–6)	Laterally (externally) rotate	Isolated atrophy in suprascapular neuropathy at spinoglenoid notch
Teres minor	Upper two-thirds of the lateral border of the scapula	Greater tubercle of the humerus (lowest facet)	Axillary N (C5–6)	Laterally rotates the arm	Stabilizes the head of the humerus in the glenoid fossa during abduction & flexion of the arm
Scapular Stabilizers					
Serratus anterior	Ribs 1–8 or 9	Medial border of the scapula on its costal (deep) surface	Long thoracic N (C5–7)	Moves the scapula forward; inferior fibers rotate the scapula superiorly	Winging of the scapula Nerve arises directly from ventral root (involvement indicates root level vs plexus)
Latissimus dorsi	T7 to the sacrum, posterior third of the iliac crest, lower 3 or 4 ribs, sometimes from the inferior angle of the scapula	Floor of the intertubercular groove	Thoracodorsal nerve (C7,8) from the posterior cord of the brachial plexus	Extends the arm and rotates the arm medially	Thoracodorsal nerve block for spasticity of upper extremity (for adducted/internally rotated arm)
Trapezius	Medial third of the superior nuchal line, external occipital protuberance, ligamentum nuchae, spinous processes of vertebrae C7-T12	Lateral third of the clavicle, medial side of the acromion and the upper crest of the scapular spine, tubercle of the scapular spine	Spinal accessory (XI), proprioception: C3-C4	Elevates and depresses the scapula (depending on which part of the muscle contracts), rotates the scapula superiorly, retracts scapula	In chronic rotator cuff tear (supraspinatus), trapezius is used for comparison in US or MRI for secondary change of supraspinatus (fatty infiltration) Involved in winging of scapula
Rhomboid major	Spines of vertebrae T2-T5	Medial border of the scapula inferior to the spine of the scapula	Dorsal scapular nerve (C5)	Retracts, elevates, and rotates the scapula inferiorly	
Rhomboid minor	Inferior end of the ligamentum nuchae, spines of vertebrae C7 and T1	Medial border of the scapula at the root of the spine of the scapula	Dorsal scapular nerve (C5)	Retracts, elevates, and rotates the scapula inferiorly	

(continued)

MUSCLE	ORIGIN	INSERTION	INNERVATION	ACTION	COMMENT
Levator scapulae	Transverse processes of C1-C4 vertebrae	Medial border of the scapula from the superior angle to the spine	Dorsal scapular nerve (C5); the upper part of the muscle receives branches of C3 & C4	Elevate scapular	
Pectoralis major	Medial 1/2 of the clavicle, manubrium & body of sternum, costal cartilages of ribs 2–6, sometimes from the rectus sheath of the upper abdominal wall	Crest of the greater tubercle of the humerus	Medial and lateral pectoral nerves (C5-T1)	Flexes and adducts the arm, medially rotates the arm	Clavicular head; lateral pectoral N (C5,6) Sternocostal head; medial pectoral nerve (C7-T1)
Pectoralis minor	Ribs 3–5	Coracoid process of the scapula	Medial pectoral nerve (C8, T1)	Draws the scapula forward, medially, and downward	Tightness implicated in subacromial impingement syndrome (decreasing subacromial space)
Teres major	Dorsal surface of the inferior angle of the scapula	Medial lip of intertubercular groove	Lower subscapular nerve from the posterior cord of the brachial plexus, C5/6	Adducts the arm, medially (internally) rotates the arm, assists in arm extension	Teres major inserts beside the tendon of latissimus dorsi, and assists latissimus in its actions
Others					
Serratus posterior superior	Ligamentum nuchae, spines of C7 and T1-T3	Ribs 1–4, lateral to the angles	Branches of the ventral primary rami of spinal nerves T1-T4	Elevate the upper ribs	A respiratory muscle, embryologically related to the intercostal muscles, not the deep back m.

BIOMECHANICS (7,25)

SHOULDER MOVEMENT (26,27; FIGURE 3.5)

- GH and scapulothoracic joint motion together to achieve the abduction movement
  - Decreased GH joint movement compensated by excessive scapulothoracic movement: often underrecognized and it can cause secondary myofascial pain in the scapular stabilizer
- Normal shoulder abduction requires scapula rotating upwardly and externally, and tilting posteriorly
  - Protracted scapular decreases subacromial space by decreased upward rotation and decreased posterior tilt of scapula → promoting impingement syndrome

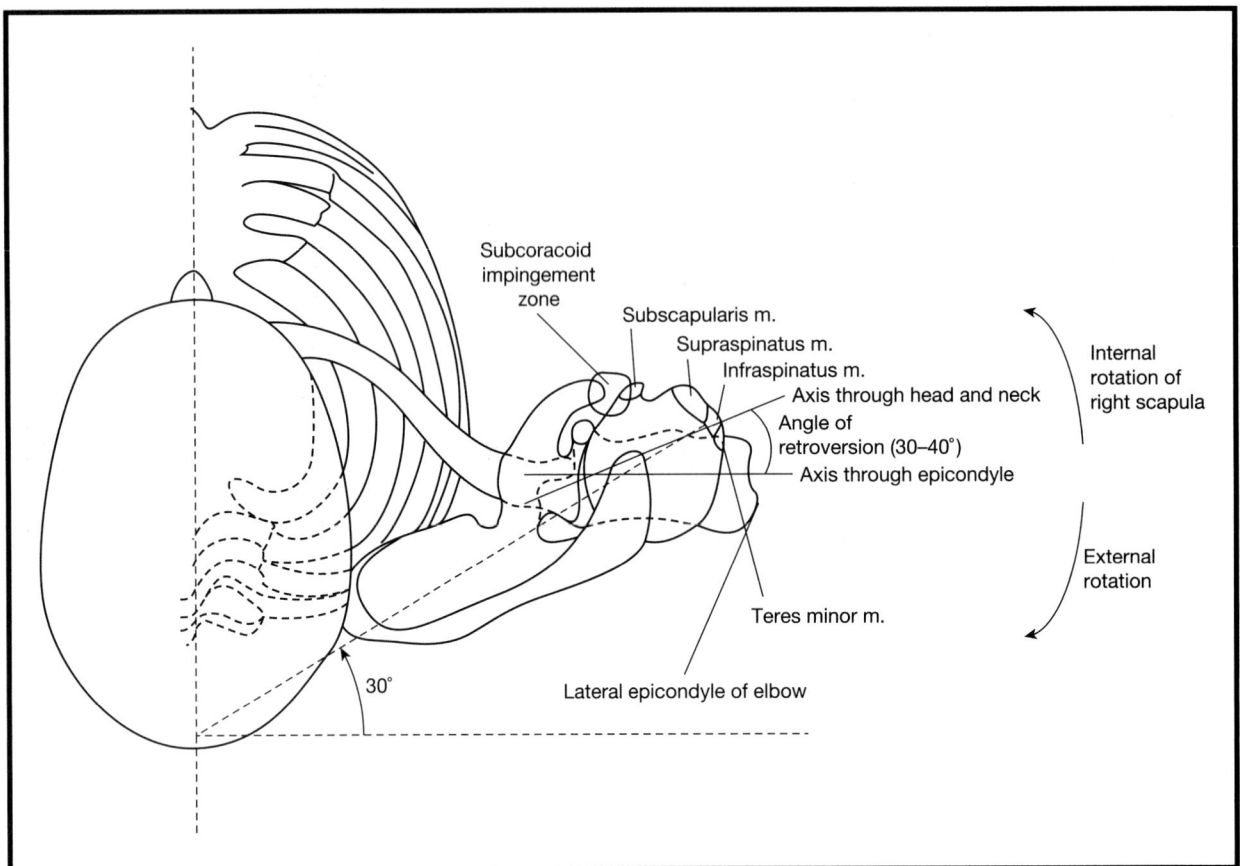

FIGURE 3.5
Scapular plane and angle of torsion.

○ In GH instability: decreased upward rotation and increased internal rotation of scapula
- Abduction requires external rotation to clear the greater tuberosity from impingement
  ○ Decreased external rotation (in GH arthritis and adhesive capsulitis) limit abduction

SUBACROMIAL IMPINGEMENT

Decreased distance between humerus and coracoacromial arch

- Supraspinatus tendon tear: elevates the humeral head to the coracoacromial arch (vicious cycle)
- Scapular stabilizer weakness; scapula protracts and depresses the acromion
- Scapular protraction and anterior tilting of the scapular common in impingement syndrome

Peak forces under acromion: occur between 85 and 135° of elevation (≈painful arc sign)

Main area of increased contact: anteroinferior part of the acromion (hooked or curved shape)
- The subacromial space is decreased when the anterior aspect of the acromion is more prominent

SUBCORACOID IMPINGEMENT: ROLLER WRINGER EFFECT (28)

- The coracoid process impinges on the superficial surface of the subscapularis tendon, applying a tensile load (stretch) to the deep surface or undersurface of the tendon → tensile undersurface fiber failure

SUPRASCAPULAR NERVE TRACTION WITH SCAPULA POSITION

- Sling effect: under the suprascapular ligament
- Scapular protraction and abduction: increased distance between the cervical spine and suprascapular notch (especially if tethering exists)

BIOMECHANICS OF THROWING (29; FIGURE 3.6)

PHASE	ENGAGED MUSCLES	POTENTIAL INJURIES
Windup	Rotator cuff muscles: inactive during this phase	
Cocking	Early cocking: deltoid Late cocking: high torque with supra/infraspinatus/teres minor activation	Anterior subluxation, internal impingement, glenoid labrum lesions Increased risk with glenohumeral internal rotation deficit
Acceleration	Triceps: early activation Late muscle activation • Pectoralis major • Latissimus dorsi • Serratus anterior	Shoulder instability Labral tears Overuse tendinopathy Tendon rupture
Release and deceleration	Eccentric contraction of all muscles is required to slow down arm motion Highest torque phase Most harmful	Labral tear (especially with biceps anchor, type 2 SLAP lesion) Subluxation of the long head of the biceps by tearing of the transverse ligament Lesions of the rotator cuff (teres minor), such as undersurface tears or tensile overload
Follow-through		Labral tear (with biceps anchor, type 2 SLAP lesion) Abnormal glenohumeral kinematics caused by tight posterior glenohumeral joint structures forcing the humeral head anteriorly and superiorly into the acromial arch during this phase

SLAP, superior labral tear from anterior to posterior.

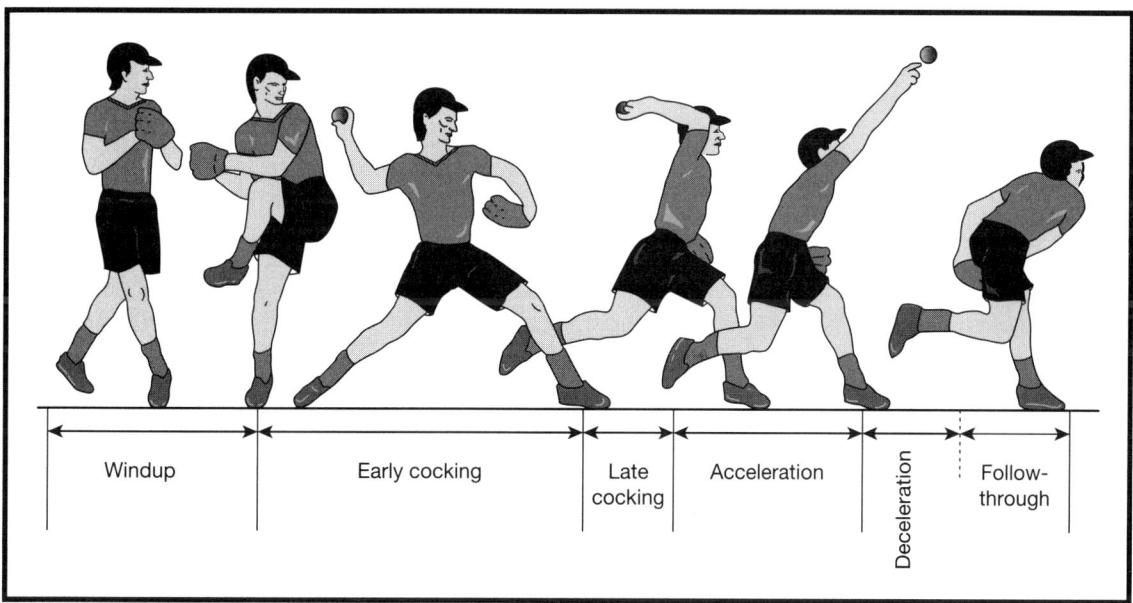

FIGURE 3.6
Six phases of the baseball pitch.

SHOULDER STABILITY (30)

Static stabilizer (see Figure 3.3)
- Position of glenoid: face posteriorly and superiorly (cephalad)
- Joint capsule and negative IA pressure
- Labrum: deepens glenoid by 50%
- GH ligament
  ○ Superior, middle, inferior GH ligament
  ○ Inferior GH ligament: primary restraint of anterior-posterior translation in the abducted shoulder (especially 90° ABER)

Dynamic stabilizer (more important)
- Rotator cuff muscles, biceps, triceps, deltoid, and scapular stabilizer
  ○ Proprioception by joint capsule

PHYSICAL EXAMINATION

INSPECTION

Scapular position
- On seated and standing and inspect scapular positioning after undressing
- Asymmetry of the scapula or prominent medial border and inferior angle: winging of scapula

	LONG THORACIC	SPINAL ACCESSORY	DORSAL SCAPULAR
Rest	Whole medial border prominent Medial translocation	Prominent inferior angle Pure lateral translocation	
Increased by	Forward flexion	Abduction	
Decreased by	Abduction	Forward flexion	Overhead activity

- Less common causes
  - Brachial plexus injury: Erb's palsy (arm internally rotated and adducted, "waiter's tip")
  - Sprengel's deformity: undescended scapular
- Normal variant: throwing athletes have slight depression of the scapular in the dominant side

Other physical findings
- Scar, ecchymosis, erythema, rashes, deformities, shoulder height, etc
- If spine of scapula is visible; consider possible muscle atrophy of either supra/infraspinatus or trapezius M
- Atrophy
  - Significant atrophy with weakness (in relative short time): consider neuromuscular causes (disuse atrophy in chronic rotator cuff tears, not dramatic)
    - With trauma/acute event: traumatic root avulsion, radiculopathy, brachial plexopathy, suprascapular N injury or other mononeuropathy, and chronic tendon rupture
    - Without trauma: brachial amyotrophy or diabetic/non-diabetic radiculoplexus neuropathy
    - Symmetric atrophy or winging: limb girdle muscular dystrophy, fascioscapulohumeral muscular dystrophy, acquired myopathy, and peripheral neuropathy (diabetes [DM] cachexia), etc
    - Asymmetric: DM amyotrophy, cervical radiculopathy, suprascapular neuropathy: infraspinatus atrophy if lesion is at spinoglenoid notch
- Swelling: often difficult to recognize the swelling depending on the body habitus
  - Often indicated by loss of clear bony landmark in lean person
  - Joint effusion; usually subtle vs bursal effusion; more prominent, or symptomatic on either impingement position or direct palpation

PALPATION

Bony landmarks
- On sitting with forearm neutral
- Anterior: bicipital groove (often difficult to palpate), lesser tuberosity (subscapularis, externally rotate to expose, orthogonal to the medial epicondyle), and greater tuberosity (supraspinatus insertion, usually same plane with lateral epicondyle)
  - Internal/external rotation will help to differentiate the tuberosity vs fixed acromion/coracoid
  - Antero-medial: coracoid process (about an inch below the clavicle)
  - Anterolateral: supraspinatus insertion
- Superior: AC joint (palpation with gradual flexion or extension of the arm)
  - Palpate the dislocation and gap of the joint (may be difficult to palpate the gap with effusion and osteophyte; bump)
    - Start palpation from medial one-third of the clavicle
- Posterior: scapular (resting position: medial border; ~3 inches from the midline, superior angle of scapular; second rib and inferior angle; seventh rib), spine of scapula: third thoracic vertebra, GH joint
- Medial: SC joint; clavicle protruded normally

Trigger points
- Look for specific referred pain pattern (see Figure 2.3 in Neck section)

RANGE OF MOTION

Normal and functional ROM (31) (see following table)

	ROM (FUNCTIONAL ROM) °		ROM (FUNCTIONAL ROM) °		ROM (FUNCTIONAL ROM) °
Flexion	180 (120)	Abduction	180 (120–130)	External rotation	60–90 (45)
Extension	45–60 (40–45)	Adduction	45–60 (30)	Internal rotation	80–100 (45–55)

Apley "Scratch test"
- Abduction and external rotation (ABER) to reach opposite scapula: be cautious in patients with anterior subluxation/instability)
- Adduction and internal rotation to reach the inferior angle of the scapula: pain in impingement syndrome

Normal scapulothoracic motion and GH joint articulation
- GH painful arc: 45 to 60° to 120° (when surgical neck strikes the acromion; full abduction is possible when humeral external is rotated), usually at 85°, AC joint painful arc: 170 to 180° abduction
  - If paradoxical, exaggerated scapulothoracic movement → adhesive capsulitis and GH osteoarthritis
- Cautious of trunk rotation when evaluating shoulder ROM (eg, trunk rotation instead of shoulder externally rotation)

GH internal rotation deficit
- Loss of internal rotation >30 to 40° relative to the expected gain in external rotation, compare it to the opposite site, common in overhead throwers
- Tight posterior capsule and anterior capsule stretched
- Associated with internal impingement, GH instability, and increased incidence of SLAP lesion

- Check the AC joint (AC sprain) and SC movement/pain and pain on GH joint movement

STRENGTH OF ROTATOR CUFF MUSCLES

Supraspinatus
- Open (full) can test: resisted abduction with thumb up rather than thumb down
- Jobe's test: resisted abduction to 90° on the scapular plane; with ~30° tilt (anteriorly) from frontal plane and thumb down (internally rotate the arm): often limited with pain from impingement

Infraspinatus
- Resisted arm external rotation

Teres minor
- Resisted arm external rotation with the arm in 90° abduction

Subscapularis
- Arm internal rotation with elbow at side in 90° flexion
- Lift off test: hand brought around back to region of lumbar spine, palm facing outward
  - Test patient's ability to lift hand away from back (internal rotation). Confounded by other muscles. More accurate if the tested hand can reach the contralateral scapula

SPECIAL TESTS (32)

NAME	DESCRIPTION	SENSITIVITY (SEN) AND SPECIFICITY (SPE) IN %
Subacromial Impingement Test (33)		
Neer's test	Stand behind the patient and passively elevate the arm in the scapular plane while stabilizing the scapula. Positive with pain elicited in the arc between 70–120°	Sen: 75–88 Spe: 31–51
Hawkins' test	The patient is examined in sitting position with shoulder forward flexion at 90° and elbow flexed to 90°, supported by the examiner. The examiner then stabilizes scapular holding the spine of scapula while internally rotating the arm. Positive with pain or symptom reproduction. More specific for impingement under the coracoacromial arch	Sen: 83–92 Spe: 38–56
Empty can	To assess the deltoid and supraspinatus M strength as well as impingement. With the arm at 90° of abduction and neutral rotation, the shoulder is then internally rotated on scapular plane with the thumb down. Apply downward force against resistance. Check side to side	Sen: 18–79 Spe: 38–100
Painful arc	Actively elevate the arm in the scapular plane until full elevation is reached then bring the arm down in the same arc. Positive if pain or painful catching occurs between 60° and 120° of elevation (34)	Sen: 60–70 Spe: 40–80
Drop arm test	The examiner abducts the patient's shoulder to 90° and then asks the patient to slowly lower the arm to the side. Positive if the patient is unable to return the arm to the side slowly/smoothly or has severe pain when attempting to do so	Sen: 10–25 Spe: 70–80 PPV: 100

+ **Hawkins', painful arc test, decreased infraspinatus M strength:** very high likelihood for impingement
+ **Drop arm test, painful arc test, decreased infraspinatus M strength:** likelihood ratio of 15 for full-thickness tear

(continued)

NAME	DESCRIPTION	SENSITIVITY (SEN) AND SPECIFICITY (SPE) IN %
Glenohumeral Instability		
The apprehension test	The patient in the supine position and the involved shoulder in 90° of abduction, the arm is externally rotated beyond 90° Positive when the patient is apprehensive or feels as if shoulder will dislocate as the humeral head begins to subluxate anteriorly	Sen: 69 Spe: 50
The relocation test	Patient with shoulder in 90° abduction and external rotation (apprehension position), a posteriorly directed force applied on the humerus. Positive if the sensation of apprehension is relieved (Fowler's sign) (35)	Sen: 30–68 Spe: 44–100
The sulcus sign	Apply axial downward traction with the arm at the side. Positive if a gap is observed between the humeral head and anterior-inferior aspect of the acromion indicating multidirectional instability High false positive in asymptomatic patients	Sen: 90 Spe: 85
Anterior and posterior drawer tests	Patient supine and the arm abducted to 45°, neutral rotation, and elbow flexed. The examiner grasps the proximal arm at the deltoid insertion and stabilizes the limb by grasping the patient's wrist with the opposite hand. Grade 0: mild translation (0%–25%), grade I: 25–50%, grade 2: reducible translation over the rim (50%), and grade III: locking of the humeral head over the rim High false positive (up to 50%) (36)	Sen: 20–50 Spe: 70–80 in traumatic anterior instability (37])
Load and shift test	The patient is seated or standing with the arm to be tested fully relaxed at the side. While stabilizing the scapula with one hand, the examiner grasps the proximal humerus with the other hand and applies force anteriorly and posteriorly. The degree to which the humeral head shifting over the anterior and posterior glenoid rim is measured. Comparison with the contralateral side for side-to-side variation (32).	Sen: 91 Sep: 93
Biceps Tendon		
Speed test	Resisting shoulder flexion with the elbow fully extended and supinated Positive if pain is generated in the bicipital groove Higher sensitivity and specificity for anterior SLAP lesion (38)	Sen: 68–90 Spe: 13–55
Yergason test	With the elbow pronated and flexed at 90°, the examiner resists the patient's attempt to supinate and externally rotate the arm, while palpating the bicipital groove Positive if dislocation of the biceps tendon is felt or pain occurs in the bicipital area without dislocation	Sen: 37 Spe: 86
Ludington test	Place both arms behind the head and isometrically contract the biceps Positive if pain or subluxation is reproduced The "Popeye" sign indicates biceps tendon rupture	
SLAP lesion		
O'Brien test	With the arm forward flexed to 90°, adducted 10–15°, and maximally internally rotated (thumb down), the examiner applies a downward force to the fully extended arm Positive if pain or clicking is "inside" the shoulder and pain is reduced with the arm maximally supinated No relief of pain in maximally supinated → suggests AC joint pathology (39)	Sen: 32–100 Spe: 13–98.5
Anterior slide test	Place the patient's hands on lateral hips with the elbows facing posteriorly The examiner stabilizes the scapula with one hand, and with the other hand placed on the patient's elbow, applies an anteriorly and superiorly directed force to the arm Positive with pain, pop, or click in the anterior shoulder (40)	Sen: 8–78 Spe: 84–91
Crank test	With the patient standing or supine, the arm is elevated to approximately 90° in the scapular plane, and the elbow is flexed. While applying an axial load to the humerus with one hand, the examiner's other hand maximally internally and externally rotates the arm → Positive with pain, pop, or clunk Positive predictive value: 94%, negative predictive value: 90% (41)	Sen: 46–91 Spe: 56–100

(continued)

NAME	DESCRIPTION	SENSITIVITY (SEN) AND SPECIFICITY (SPE) IN %
Clunk test Compression-rotation	The patient is supine with arm fully abducted. The examiner circumducts the humeral head in an attempt to entrap a torn labral fragment. One of the examiner's hand is placed posterior to the humeral head to apply anterior pressure while the other hand is placed at the level of the humeral condyles to provide rotation and axial loading → Positive with clunk or grinding reproducing the patient symptoms	Sen: 80 Spe: 19–49
The Kim test for posteroinferior labral lesion	To evaluate posterior instability (posterior inferior labral lesion) Patients are seated and shoulder is abducted to 90° and then moved to 45° forward diagonal flexion while simultaneously applying a downward and posteriorly directed force to the upper arm and pushing the elbow towards the shoulder joint (42) Positive if a sudden onset of posterior shoulder pain occurs	Sen: 90 Spe: 94
Acromioclavicular Joint		
Cross arm adduction test	Shoulder is positioned in 90° of forward flexion and is forcefully adducted across the body toward the opposite shoulder. Positive with reproduction of patient's pain Sensitive to shoulder impingement syndrome (sensitivity: 82, specificity: 27.7) (43)	Sen: 77 Spe: 79
Paxinos test	Places the thumb over the posterolateral corner of the acromion and the index and long fingers of the ipsilateral or the opposite hand superior to the mid portion of the ipsilateral clavicle Then, the examiner applied pressure to the acromion with the thumb, in an anterosuperior direction, and inferiorly to the midpart of the clavicular shaft with the index and long fingers Positive if pain is felt or increased pain in the AC joint	Sen: 79, Spe: 50(44)
Thoracic Outlet Syndrome		
Roo's test	With the forearms flexed to 90°, the arms laterally abducted to 90° and externally rotated, the patient opens and closes the hands every 2 seconds for 3 minutes. Positive if the symptoms are reproduced, if the patient is unable to maintain the position, or the radial pulse is diminished	
Adson maneuver	The radial pulse is palpated as the patient inspires while maintaining the symptomatic extremity at the side, the neck hyperextended, and the head rotated toward the symptomatic side Positive for vascular thoracic outlet syndrome with alteration or obliteration of the radial pulse or change in blood pressure. Often positive in healthy asymptomatic persons	
Wright maneuver	The radial pulse is palpated while the symptomatic limb is held overhead and abducted (to 180°) with the elbow flexed and the upper extremity externally rotated. This position is maintained for 60 seconds. Positive if the patient's symptoms are reproduced (may be more sensitive in the lesion between the pectoralis minor and rib cage)	

PPV, positive predictive value.

DIAGNOSTIC STUDIES

PLAIN RADIOGRAPHS (38)

Indications
- History of trauma: rule out fracture and dislocation
  - AP and axillary view (if limited, then apical oblique or outlet view)
  - Bankart lesion: west point (axillary lateral) view to evaluate glenoid rim
  - Hill–Sachs lesion: Stryker Notch view (also for coracoid process) on the posterior superior humerus
  - Abnormal if >2 cm acromion-humerus distance
- Persistent pain (despite initial conservative management), ± decreased range to evaluate inflammatory or degenerative joint disease
  - AP tangential view (neutral, internal, external rotation) and outlet view (acromion type)
- If + instability: Bernageau projection (optima visualization of anterior-inferior glenoid rim, Hill–Sachs lesion; apical oblique, and the Stryker/West Point view)

Limitations
- Low capability to assess soft tissues (except tendon calcification), articular cartilage, IA lesion or bursal effusion, glenoid labrum, or marrow

Individual views
- Routine
  - AP: GH joint relation. Grashey (true AP, AP of the shoulder in the plane of scapulae)
  - External rotation: greater tuberosity, calcific tendinopathy, cystic change
  - Internal rotation: light bulb shape of humeral head, impaction fracture (Hill–Sachs lesion; posterolateral indentation fracture) can be seen
  - Axillary view: (orthogonal to AP) perpendicular to the horizontal axis of GH joint: check subluxation and glenoid pathology (glenoid rim fracture)
    - Difficult if the patient cannot fully abduct
- AP with stress (10–20 lbs weight): CC distance <25% site-to-site difference; normal
  - Evaluate AC dislocation or separation or shoulder and clavicle fracture
- Instability
  - West Point axillary lateral: anterior inferior glenoid rim fracture (bony Bankart lesion)
  - Stryker notch view: Hill–Sachs lesion, posterior exostosis and osteophyte; Bennet lesion
- Impingement syndrome
  - Supraspinatus outlet view: subacromial space. Can be limited because of thoracic kyphosis or superimposition of adjacent osseous structures, such as the clavicle, ribs, or scapular body
  - 30° caudal tilt view (Bernageau view): anterior-inferior subacromial spur, CC ligament ossification, acromial spur
- Outlet view (scapular Y view): for both impingement and instability
  - Subluxation/dislocation: humeral head should be at bifurcation of Y normally
  - Acromion type (type 1 to 3, AP, lateral) and outlet of the supraspinatus tendon
- The serendipity view (medial 1/3): SC joint
- Lateral 1/3: Zanca view; clavicular fracture

POINT-OF-CARE ULTRASONOGRAPHY (39)

Indications
- To evaluate soft tissues, effusion, and superficial joint structures

Findings
- Rotator cuff pathology; tendinosis (including calcific tendinopathy) and tear (partial, full thickness, complete, massive) and subdeltoid bursitis (with increased thickness or effusion)
  - Accuracy can be similar to MRI (in experienced examiner)
  - Muscle atrophy and fatty infiltration: in chronic tear/rupture, denervation from C5–6/brachial plexus (upper trunk)/suprascapular N lesion or other neuromuscular disease
    - Compare involved muscle with neighboring muscle innervated by different nerve (eg, supraspinatus with trapezius and infraspinatus with teres minor) in suprascapular N or teres minor vs infraspinatus (in quadrilateral syndrome)
- Biceps long-head tendon pathology; biceps tendinopathy, tenosynovitis, tendon tear/rupture, subluxation, or dislocation
  - Biceps tenosynovial effusion: from GH joint effusion than isolated tenosynovitis (has to confirm no effusion in GH joint)
- Joint and bony pathology
  - AC joint: effusion with capsular bulging and irregularity/osteophyte
  - GH joint: congruence of anatomic neck, torn rotator cuff tendon, irregularity of the greater tuberosity. Calcification of the articular cartilage (chondrocalcinosis)
    - Posterior GH joint effusion (not sensitive because effusion is more common in axillary recess due to gravity in sitting position)
  - Hill–Sachs lesion; defect in the posterior lateral humeral head (impaction fracture; loss of globular shape of humeral head)
- Ganglion on spinoglenoid notch; paralabral cyst with labral tear
  - Differential with vein engorgement
  - External rotation; joint fluid location may make a labral tear more conspicuous
- Dynamic examination of rotator cuff muscles (40) in subacromial (abduction) and subcoracoid impingement syndrome (internal/external rotation)

Limitations
- Limited evaluation of the IA/intracortical pathologies (labrum [limited view]), IA portion of the biceps tendon
- Intracortical/marrow lesion: nondisplaced fracture, tumor, cyst, or avascular necrosis (AVN)
- Operator dependence
- Patient with tattoo or morbidly obese patient

Protocols
- Based on The American Institute of Ultrasound in Medicine (AIUM); see pages 45 and 46 in Chapter 1

MRI/MRA (41)

Indications
- Rotator cuff and IA (labarum)/intracortical (bone marrow) pathologies
- Evaluation of mass, infections, patient with history of cancer (42)

Interpretation and common findings (43)
- Coronal oblique for supraspinatus and axial view for the labrum evaluation
- T1 weighted image (WI) ideal for anatomy. In fat-suppressed T2 WI: increased signal indicates edema or effusion
- Bony: osseous outlet and acromion shape (anterolateral aspect: flat and curved types are associated with high incidence of impingement)
- Labrum; improved imaging with MRA, proton density protocol
  - Low signal intensity in all sequences (fibrocartilage), triangular appearance arising from glenoid
  - T2 weighted coronal images for superior labrum (axial for evaluation of biceps anchor)
  - Labral tear: high signal intensity in T2 or contrast extending into the labrum
  - Often difficult to distinguish from normal variant or subtle tear

- Capsule or ligaments: adhesive capsulitis (thickening of rotator cuff interval), instability (GH ligament avulsion)

Limitation: partial thickness rotator cuff (relatively poor sensitivity); improved by MRA

Artifact: signal change within obliquely oriented structure; less specific due to magic angle effect and partial volume averaging ➔ check in other planes

MRA (43,44)

- Direct contrast injection (by instilling dilute gadolinium (Gd) diethylenetriaminepentaacetic acid (DTPA) into the shoulder joint) or indirectly (by giving Gd DTPA intravenously and obtaining images following exercise of the muscles around the joint)
- Common indications: evaluation of GH instability and suspected labral lesions
  ○ MRA is better than MRI in full and partial thickness rotator cuff tendon tear as well
- T1 weighted images with fat saturation in all planes and abduction external rotation stress imaging to detect nondisplaced anteroinferior labral tears and partial thickness articular surface tears

CT SCAN

- Provides detailed bony anatomy: fracture of the scapula and proximal humerus, prosthesis, or intracortical lesion

Indications
- When MRI is contraindicated
- Evaluate scapular and proximal humeral fracture
- Suspicion of posterior dislocation or medial head of the clavicle with possible vascular compression
- CT arthrogram: evaluate rotator cuff or labrum in a patient who is contraindicated for MRI (Flowchart 3.3)

TREATMENT

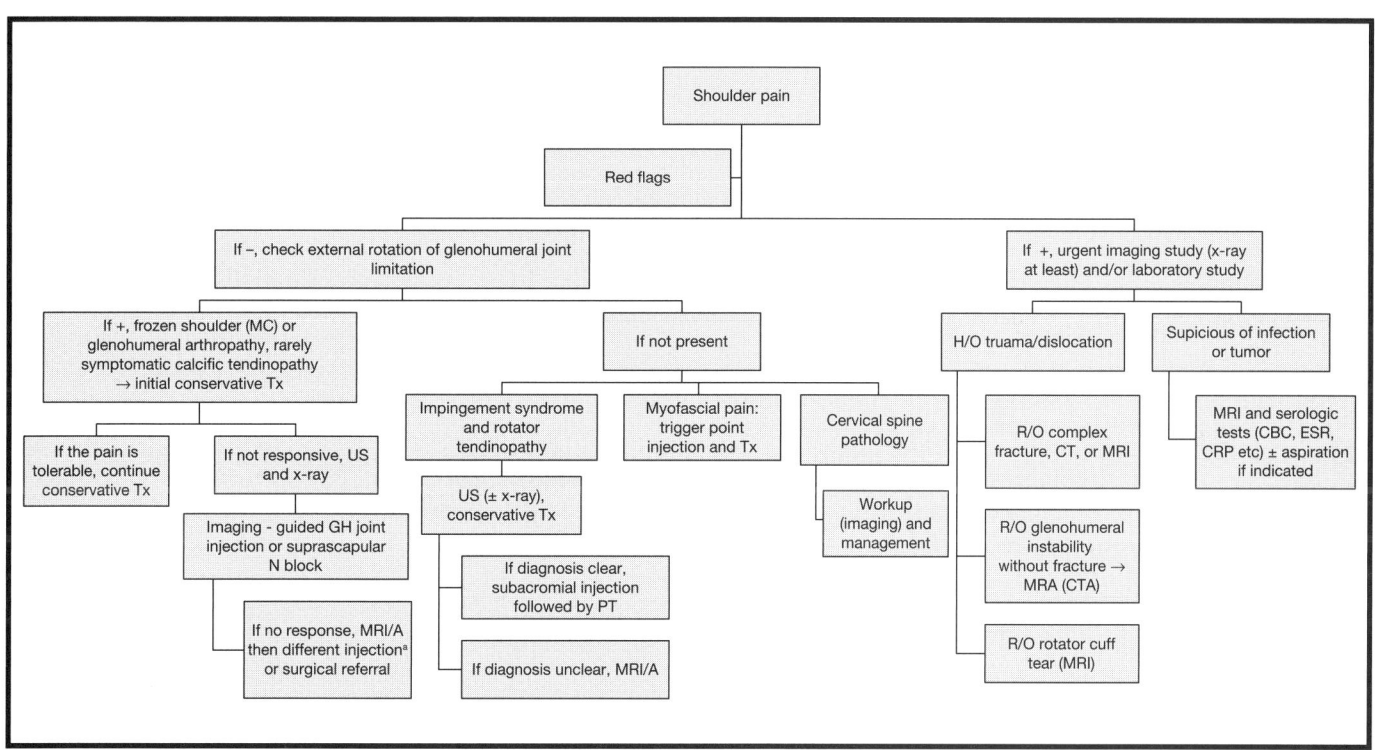

FLOWCHART 3.3
Diagnostic approach and management of shoulder pain in outpatient clinic.
aLarge volume glenohumeral (GH) joint injection, viscosupplementation or plasma-rich plasma if indicated.
CBC, complete blood count; CRP, C-reactive protein; CT, computed tomography; CTA, CT arthrogram; ESR, erythrocyte sedimentation rate; GH, glenohumeral; H/O, history of; MC, most common; MRA, magnetic resonance arthrogram; PT, physical therapy; R/O, rule out; US, ultrasound; Tx, treatment.

NONOPERATIVE MANAGEMENT (FLOWCHART 3.3)

Physical and occupational therapy and education
- Recognize/addresss scapulothoracic dyskinesia/dysfunction: very common, especially in shoulder impingement syndrome (45,46) and myofascial pain syndrome
  ○ Scapular stabilization exercise
    ▪ Stretching of scapular protractor, such as pectoralis major, minor, and subscapularis
    ▪ Strengthening scapular retractor and scapular stabilizer: relatively small muscles, such as rhomboids, and serratus anterior
    ▪ Correct posture education
- Address myofascial components, because of high concomitant myofascial pain syndrome

- Myofascial release using different techniques: spray and stretch, using golf ball, and kinesiotaping
- Stretching of the joint capsule
  - Sleeper's stretch: lying on the ipsilateral side and push the arm to increase internal rotation by rolling the body to prone position: Internal impingement/GH internal rotation deficit
  - Side arm external rotation exercise in adhesive capsulitis (to stretch anterior capsule and rotator cuff interval)
- Postural and biomechanic education can be emphasized especially for young office workers, although ingrained habits are difficult to modify
  - Correct posture education/reminder; chin back, "at attention" posture
  - Aerobic endurance exercise often beneficial
- Modalities for temporary pain relief

Oral medication
- Acetaminophen (AAP), nonsteroidal anti-inflammatory drug (NSAID), methylprednisone (MedrolDosepak), and short duration of muscle relaxant
- Weak opioid medications if the aforementioned medication is not effective or contraindicated
- Neuropathic pain medication as needed

Injection
- Blind injection
  - Subacromial injection: one finger breadth inferior to the edge of acromion toward the root of the subacromial space (inferior border of acromion); laterally, posteriorly, or anterior approach. Move the needle toward the inferior border of the acromion (walk down from the acromion)
    - Anterior (near the location of the pathology) versus posterior (wide space)
  - GH joint injection: one finger breadth inferior to the posterolateral corner of acromion, insert the needle toward the coracoid process until the needle tip touches the intra-articular cartilage (posterior approach)
    - Image guidance recommended in most cases
  - Accuracy varies depending on experience and patient body habitus: 29% of attempted subacromial injections and 42% of GH injections (47)
- US evaluation and possible injection
  - Recognize neurovascular structures; avoid direct injection, can add mechanical adhesiolysis (in chronic lesions, especially in adhesive bursitis and capsulitis)
  - More accurate compared to blind injection (may be more effective) (48)
- Consider imaging study with a specific indication in mind especially in the elderly because of high asymptomatic rotator cuff degeneration/tears or signs of degenerative arthropathy
  - Often difficult to identify primary pain generator
- Trigger point injection to address myofascial pain component
  - Rare but possible complications, for example, pneumothorax (especially with rhomboids, levator, or even trapezius in thin body habitus)

Common shoulder orthoses

ORTHOSIS	CHARACTERISTIC
Shoulder abduction orthosis	Postural reminder To protect against adduction contracture & stretch internal rotator Often difficult to wear it
Mobile arm orthosis	For profound proximal M weakness with spared elbow motion (eg, cervical spinal cord injury) Forearm trough mounted to a swivel mechanism
Arm sling	To relieve pain from overstretching of shoulder musculature and arm downward distraction • Abduction sling: diagonal force to support the shoulders in abducted position allowing the elbow and forearms to be free • Vertical arm sling (humeral cuff with figure of 8 suspension): vertical upward force to support humerus, free elbow, and forearm

SURGERY

Indications
- No improvement/worsening pain (disabling) despite 4 to 6 months of conservative treatment
- Outcome may be better if the pain generator is clearly identified. Often, image-guided injection is used to identify the pain generator

Subacromial decompression and/or bursectomy
- For impingement syndrome with tendinosis and rotator cuff tear

Rotator cuff repair
- Direct repair or tendon transfer (massive tears)
- Latissimus dorsi transfer in intact subscapularis
- High risk of re-tear or non healing repair (especially in >65 years)

Shoulder arthroplasty
- Hemiarthroplasty
  - Common indication: osteonecrosis with a preserved glenoid
    - Similar to reverse arthroplasty: proximal humerus fractures, cuff-tear arthropathy, inflammatory arthropathy (rheumatoid) with massive cuff tear, insufficient glenoid bone stock
- Total shoulder arthroplasty
  - Requires intact/functional rotator cuff tendons
  - Indications: primary osteoarthritis, posttraumatic osteoarthritis, inflammatory arthropathies, and osteonecrosis with an affected glenoid
- Reverse arthroplasty
  - Use of a convex glenoid (hemispheric ball) and concave humerus; allows deltoid muscle to act on a longer fulcrum and greater mechanical advantage

○ Contraindications: deltoid insufficiency (axillary N palsy), acromion deficiency, glenoid osteoporosis, and infection

TENDON AND BURSA PATHOLOGY

Clinical diagnosis (for mechanism)
- Mechanism (and presentation) based on history and physical examination
- Impingement syndrome (typically from overuse and/or spur), traumatic, idiopathic or secondary to abnormal GH or scapulothoracic movement/instability

Structural diagnosis
- Requires imaging to confirm the diagnosis
- Rotator cuff tendinopathy/calcific tendinopathy, tear; partial, full thickness, massive
- Biceps tendinopathy (tendinopathy, tear, dislocation, tenosynovitis)
- Subacromial, subcoracoid subdeltoid bursitis and scapulothoracic bursitis
- Often unclear role as a pain generator especially in the elderly population with high asymptomatic imaging abnormalities

Both ways of description are often used interchangeably by clinicians: for example, impingement syndrome with rotator cuff tendon/bursa involvement (tendinopathy/calcific tendinopathy, tear, subacromial/subdeltoid bursitis, etc)

IMPINGEMENT SYNDROME

Differential diagnosis
- External impingement: very common
  ○ Subacromial impingement from coracoacromial arch: much more common than subcoracoid impingement (under coracoid process)
  ○ Etiology based: primary (aforementioned) vs secondary (abnormal GH or scapulothoracic movement/instability)
- Internal impingement: less common in general population (may be common in specific population)
  ○ Posterosuperior, anterosuperior, anterior impingement, and entrapment of the long head of biceps tendon from rotator cuff and capsular dysfunction

Subacromial Impingement Syndrome

Introduction (49,50)
- MC cause (45%–65%) of shoulder pain (51,52)
- Common structural pathologies underlying subacromial impingement syndrome
  ○ Subacromial/subdeltoid bursitis, rotator cuff (supraspinatus: MC) tendinopathy, partial or full thickness rotator cuff tear
- Etiology
  ○ Impingement from anterior inferior acromion, coracoacromial ligament, and AC joint
  ○ Secondary causes: instability, calcific rotator cuff tendon (supra and infraspinatus), tuberosity fracture nonunion/malunion, a mobile os acromiale, and iatrogenic factors
  ○ Predisposing factors: sports or work-related activities involving overhead motions

History and physical examination
- Pain in the anterolateral aspect of the shoulder
  ○ Insidious onset, gradually over several months typically
  ○ Acute traumatic subacromial/subdeltoid bursitis may develop into an chronic impingement lesion
- Physical examination
  ○ Inspection: scapular dyskinesia or winging (predisposing factor), visible supra/infrascapular fossa (in concomitant chronic tendon tear), rupture of long head of biceps (palpable mass distally or prominent muscle belly compared with the contralateral side, usually secondary or concomitant with impingement syndrome)
  ○ Tenderness on greater tuberosity/supraspinatus insertion ± mild tenderness on AC joint, intertubercular groove: not specific
  ○ ROM (painful arc sign): Neer test and Hawkins' test (sensitive but not specific)
    ▪ If ROM is decreased globally, especially external rotation more than internal rotation, consider adhesive capsulitis or GH arthropathy as primary culprit
  ○ Neurological examination: muscle strength, sensory examination/Spurling test (R/O cervical radiculopathy)
    ▪ Rotator cuff muscle strength deficit; usually subtle in impingement syndrome, usually limited by pain (in painful arc)

Diagnosis
- Clinical diagnosis
  ○ Confirmed by relief of pain from image-guided injection of small volume (1–2 cc) of 1% lidocaine into the subacromial space (bursal); not necessary for diagnosis
    ▪ Repeat impingement sign/test (direct palpation of the joint, internal rotation of the extended arm, and adduction of the arm across the chest)
    ▪ Not specific; however, no relief of pain/painful examination is against clinical diagnosis (especially with image-guided injection)(53)
- Differential diagnosis
  ○ Adhesive capsulitis, rotator cuff arthropathy, and inflammatory arthropathy; global decrease in ROM
  ○ AC arthritis: differential diagnosis with 0.5 to 1 mL 1% lidocaine injection to AC joint capsule
  ○ GH instability (with secondary impingement syndrome): more common in overhead sports athletes, <40 years old
  ○ Coracoid impingement syndrome
  ○ Calcific tendinitis: (often significant stiffness): often underlying cause of impingement syndrome
  ○ Biceps tendinopathy: consider after treatment of impingement syndrome as pain generator (less common as isolated pain generator)
  ○ Cervical radiculopathy (C5,6), brachial plexopathy (idiopathic), and nerve compression (suprascapular neuropathy and rarely axillary neuropathy at quadrilateral space)
  ○ Polymyalgia rheumatica (older patients, bilateral)
- Imaging study to evaluate structural pathologies
  ○ US (54)
    ▪ Primary imaging modality without history of trauma
    ▪ Subdeltoid bursa: bursal thickening/effusion (teardrop sign)

- Rotator cuff tendon: full-thickness/complete rotator cuff tears and calcific tendinopathy
  - Often limited in patients with inability to do extension and internal rotation (crass position), and limited evaluation of tendon under the acromion
  - May be difficult to differentiate partial thickness tear versus tendinosis
- Bicipital tendon tear, tendinopathy, tenosynovitis, and subluxation/dislocation
- Joint: AC joint degenerative change (prevalent in older adults with bulging capsule). GH joint effusion; unusual (55)
- Dynamic examination for impingement: grade 0 to 4:2: soft tissue impingement, 3: upward migration of the humeral head (56)
○ X-ray: AP, axillary, supraspinatus outlet, and 30 caudal tilt view, often negative
- AP view: subchondral cysts or sclerosis of the greater tuberosity (chronic rotator cuff tendinopathy), spur formation on the anterior edge of the acromion, osteoarthritis (OA) of the AC joint, calcific tendinopathy, bony instability of GH joint (an osseous Bankart lesion or a Hill–Sachs lesion), or the GH joint arthropathy
- Axillary view: Os acromiale (unfused acromial epiphysis: 1%–15%)
○ Indication of advanced imaging
- Usually not necessary initially except when red flags are present in history or physical examination
- Persistent pain after a trial of conservative treatment
○ MRI/A
- Indicated early if red flags (fever/chills/systemic manifestation, h/o cancer, erythema etc) present
- To evaluate partial tears and small full-thickness tears (difficult to differentiate small tear from tendinitis), MRA is more reliable for partial thickness tear
  - Unclear clinical implication for differentiation of small tear vs tendinopathy
- Better bony evaluation and evaluation of IA or intracortical lesions
  - AC joint: unfused acromial epiphysis, and anteroinferior acromial morphology, labral, or IA or periarticular bony structure
- Serologic test with red flags: CBC, ESR, CRP, uric acid etc

Treatment
- Nonoperative treatment: mainstay of treatment
  ○ Try minimum of 6 months. The duration of relief varied widely, ranging from 12 to 18 months
  ○ NSAID and modification of activity
  ○ Subacromial injection (landmark-based and US-guided injection if the blind injection did not work or too short duration of relief)
  - US-guided injection with/without hydrodissection (in chronic bursitis with adhesion)
  ○ PT: scapular stabilization, correct posture/biomechanics, and modality as needed
  - Isometric and isotonic muscle-strengthening exercises: 67% with satisfaction, better in patients with a type-I acromion (57)
- Operative treatment: after failed conservative treatment
  ○ Anterior acromioplasty with resection of the coracoacromial ligament: open vs arthroscopic method
  - Poor response in patients with internal impingement, impingement syndrome secondary to GH instability. Subacromial injection may be an indicator for the success
  - No difference in surgical outcome after bursectomy with/without acromioplasty
  - The AC joint resection only if the joint is tender or when inferiorly protruding or osteophytes are contributing to the impingement
  ○ Comparison of open and arthroscopic acromioplasty
  - Similar overall, no differences in ROM, strength, or return to activity at 1-year evaluation
  - Earlier return to normal function after arthroscopy (but can be an inadequate removal necessitating a revision). The open procedure had a longer duration of hospitalization; with an unsatisfactory result receiving Workers' Compensation

Subcoracoid Impingement Syndrome
Introduction (58,59)
- Relatively uncommon, prevalence or incidence not reported; however, under-recognized
- Coracoid impinges on the subcoracoid bursa (causing bursitis), subscapularis tendon (→ tear), and biceps tendon (→ tendinopathy and/or tenosynovitis)
- Etiology
  ○ Idiopathic: congenitally elongated or angled coracoid tip
  ○ Secondary coracoid impingement
  - Rotator cuff weakness (massive tear), scapular dyskinesia, anterior GH instability, space occupying lesion (ganglion) or calcific tendinitis of the subscapularis tendon (60)
  - Trauma: fracture, malunion, displaced fracture of scapular neck
  ○ Iatrogenic: previous anterior shoulder surgery, coracoid transfer and posterior glenoid osteotomy

History and physical examination
- The anterior shoulder pain, dull/aching ± referred pain distally through the biceps muscle belly
- Tenderness near coracoid process, coracohumeral interval ± snapping on GH external/internal rotation ± swelling, scapular dyskinesia, muscle atrophy (rare)
- Reproduction of pain by forward elevation, adduction, and internal rotation (modified Hawkins test)
- Neurological examination; mild weakness for massive rotator cuff, and brachial plexopathy/cervical radiculopathy (motor, sensory, and deep tendon reflex)

Diagnosis
- Clinical diagnosis confirmed with diagnostic injection to subcoracoid region
  ○ Imaging guided, small volume (1–2 mL) may be more specific, blindly to the lateral tip of the coracoid (with arm externally rotated to avoid injection of the subscapularis tendon or biceps tendon)
- Differential diagnosis
  ○ Rotator cuff tendonitis/tear (subscapularis tear/tendinopathy), subacromial impingement, biceps tendinopathy/subluxation/dislocation, anterior shoulder instability, or SLAP lesion

- Often coexisting or contributing as a factor
- Rare: septic arthritis, crystal deposition arthritis, fracture/dislocation, cervical radiculopathy, referred pain from visceral origin: can be poorly localized or vague
- Imaging study
  - Routine x-ray: often unremarkable
  - US (12,22)
    - Subcoracoid bursal thickening, effusion, and/or calcification in the subscapularis tendon
    - Dynamic evaluation: GH external/internal rotation (to see if it reproduces painful impingement and/or snapping)
  - MRI
    - Coracohumeral interval: the coracohumeral distance between the lateral tip of the coracoid and subchondral bone of the humeral head on axial MRI (abnormal if <6 mm)
    - Evaluation of subscapular bursitis/axillary recess, rotator cuff interval structures, labrum, and intracortical lesion (especially with h/o red flag) etc

Treatment
- Nonoperative treatment
  - NSAIDs and patient education: activity modification, avoid repetitive cross-body adduction (pole vaulting, masonry)
  - Physical therapy (PT): scapular stabilization (protractor stretching and retractor strengthening) and rotator cuff strengthening
    - Posture education, stretching of pectoralis minor and thoracic spine mobility
  - Subcoracoid steroid injection (one finger breadth lateral to the coracoid process to the inferior border of the coracoid process with shoulder neutral/external rotation)
    - US-guided injection into subcoracoid bursal space
- Surgical referral: after failed conservative treatment
  - Open or arthroscopic decompression or coracoplasty

Internal Impingement Syndrome

Introduction (61)
- Epidemiology: major cause of shoulder pain in throwing athletes
  - Incidence: not reported, peak in young to middle age, likely under-recognized
- Multifactorial etiology
- Classification (62) and biomechanics

TYPE OF IMPINGEMENT	INVOLVED STRUCTURES	POPULATION AT RISK	UNDERLYING MECHANISM AND RISK FACTORS
Posterosuperior	Articular side posterosuperior rotator cuff (supraspinatus and infraspinatus) between labrum and greater tuberosity, superior labrum anterior and posterior (SLAP), humeral head impaction or subcortical cyst, thickening of posterior capsule	Elite athlete, thrower (tennis, squash, racquet ball, volley ball, etc)	Arm is elevated and ext. rotated related to laxity of anterior capsule (controversial) Glenohumeral internal rotation deficit (GIRD) Suboptimal biomechanics in late cocking, and early acceleration (in throwers) Forklift driver (repetitive rotation of the trunk with the arm rested on the steering wheel)
Anterosuperior	Rotator cuff interval structure (subscapularis, coracohumeral and sup. GH ligament)	Masonry, pole vaulting	Horizontal adduction, externally rotated and forward flexion or repetitive overhead activity
Anterior	Fraying and detachment of SLAP, subscapularis tendon	Non athletic population	Shoulder forward flexion, compressed between sup. humeral head and the glenoid
Biceps long head	Intra-articular portion of long head of biceps tendon between the humeral head and glenoid		Elevation of the arm results in mechanical block

History and physical examination
- Pain in the posterior-superior (diffuse posterior shoulder girdle), anterior-superior or anterior shoulder (anterior coracoid); often difficult to localize the exact location
- Physical examination: shoulder dyskinesia common on inspection
  - Subacromial impingement test (Neer and Hawkins): usually negative (except anterior impingement)
  - Posterosuperior impingement
    - Posterior GH joint line tenderness, laxity (anterior), GH internal rotation deficit/posterior capsule tightness
    - Posterior impingement test: 90° abduction, 10 to 15° extension and maximum external rotation
      - Reproduction of symptom: 75.5% sensitivity, 85% specificity in overhead athletes (63)
      - Jobe relocation test with pushing of humerus posteriorly: reduced posterior shoulder pain in internal impingement (vs relief of pain/apprehension in the

anterior aspect in anterior subluxation/instability) (61)
- Anterior impingement; mimics subacromial impingement; pain with forward arm elevation, no sign of instability
- Biceps long head impingement; pain, locking, and loss of final 10 to 20° of passive elevation

Diagnosis
- Clinical diagnosis confirmed by imaging study
- Differential diagnosis: subacromial/subcoracoid (external) impingement syndrome, SLAP tear and anterior instability (often concomitant)
- X-ray: AP, axillary, scapular Y, West Point, and Stryker notch views
- MRI/MRA

ANATOMICAL REGIONS	FINDINGS
Posterosuperior	Articular-sided partial thickness tear of posterior supraspinatus and infraspinatus, posterosuperior glenoid labral lesion (fraying, tearing, and detachment)
Anterosuperior	Bennet lesion (Type 1–4, biceps subluxation) Type 1: tear of intra-articular fibers of the subscapularis tendon and medial subluxation of the biceps tendon to type 4: tearing of the lateral coracohumeral ligament and anterior extra-articular dislocation of the biceps tendon
Anterior	A partial-thickness subscapularis tendon fraying (20%) and 60% with detachment of the anterosuperior labrum (SLAP)
Biceps long head	Hypertrophic (hour glass) changes of the intra-articular portion of the biceps tendon

SLAP, superior labrum anterior and posterior.

Treatment
- Nonoperative treatment
  - NSAIDs and avoidance of the aggravating position/activity
  - Injection: US-guided injection to extra-capsular (between the rotator cuff tendon and capsule for articular-sided tear) and/or IA (intra-capsular) injection
  - Therapy to enhance dynamic stabilization
    - Posterior capsule stretch ("sleeper stretch") especially internal rotation deficit present
    - Scapular stabilization, dynamic stabilization exercise, and strengthening exercise
- Surgery
  - After failed conservative treatment or early intervention in high-performing/professional athletes
  - Examination under anesthesia, diagnostic arthroscopy, capsular plication, posterior capsular release, debridement (fraying, tearing) versus repair (frank detachment or post instability) of the labral tear

ROTATOR CUFF TENDINOPATHY AND TEAR

Introduction (64)
- Epidemiology (65)
  - Incidence: 1%, prevalence: 39% to 60%, and increases with age (50% at age 80 years)
  - Location and pattern of tear
    - Supraspinatus: MC involved tendon
    - Location of tear: articular-sided tear (cited as MC in clinical study) versus intra-tendinous tear in cadaveric study, likely due to limitation of imaging
      – Bursal tear: more painful
    - Partial tear: MC pattern. Full-thickness tear: 5% to 40%
    - Massive tear if ≥2 tendons detached
  - Concomitant long head of biceps lesion in ~30%
- Correlation with clinical presentation (pain): controversial
  - Asymptomatic tear increases with age (66) and tear itself is not healing usually
    - Not an indication for aggressive intervention
    - Smaller tear: lower risk of progression (<1–1.5 cm full-thickness tear has 25% of progression at 2 years)
    - Fifty percent of asymptomatic full-thickness tears develop symptoms in ~2 to 3 years
      – Larger tear more likely symptomatic over time
  - Forty to fifty percent (in symptomatic full-thickness tear) gets larger
- Etiology and pathophysiology
  - Multifactorial, likely a combination of the following
    - Predisposing factors: smoking, hypercholesterolemia, and family history
    - Chronic dialysis patient; amyloidosis tendinopathy

INTRINSIC (INTRA-TENDINOUS) FACTORS	EXTRINSIC (EXTRA-TENDINOUS) FACTORS

• Aging and shear force
• Muscle weakness and fatigue
  ○ Eccentric (decelerating) internal rotation and adduction overloading the supraspinatus in overhead position
  ○ Swimming, racquet, or throwing sports
• Overuse of the shoulder
  ○ Repetitive microtrauma against the coracoacromial arch
• Degenerative tendinopathy
  ○ Partial tears → proximal migration of the humeral head
	• Glenohumeral instability
	• Degeneration of the AC joint (67) osteophytes (downward)
	• Impingement by the coracoacromial ligament (especially lateral edge)
	• Other causes similar to impingement syndrome
	  ○ Coracoid impingement/stenosis
	  ○ Os acromiale
	  ○ Trauma (tuberosity fracture and malunion), and iatrogenic
	• Calcific tendinopathy

History and physical examination
- Anterolateral shoulder pain (MC, less commonly anterior or posterior) under the acromion if present ± subtle weakness (with performance problems in athletes) unless ruptured
- Inspection
  - Atrophy: unusual except chronic massive tear with disuse atrophy (if significant atrophy over short period present → consider neurological etiologies)

○ Scapular dyskinesia and winging (unusual, as an underlying cause)
- Painful limitation of internal rotation (compared with the other side: posterior capsular tightness, common in overhead thrower) ± snapping shoulder (under the coracoacromial ligament or the undersurface of the acromion)
- Positive shoulder impingement test (Neer, Hawkins, drop arm, painful arc etc)
- Neurological examination: usually unremarkable except mild weakness with pain
  ○ Motor strength: often difficult to isolate rotator cuff muscle strength from extrinsic muscle strength (eg, deltoid)

Diagnosis
- Clinical suspicion confirmed by imaging study
- Differential diagnosis
  ○ Coexisting or underlying causes: shoulder impingement (subacromial/external with bursitis or internal impingement), AC arthritis, GH instability/rotator cuff arthritis
  ○ Brachial plexopathy (diabetic, nondiabetic amyotrophy; radiculoplexus neuropathy) and C5–6 cervical radiculopathy
- Imaging study
  ○ US: ~90% sensitive, and up to 100% positive predictive value by experienced ultrasonographers (68,69)
    ▪ Two orthogonal views (longitudinal and transverse): check size of tear in transverse view, if >2.5 cm in distance mediolaterally suggests full-thickness tear involving infraspinatus)
    ▪ Biceps tenosynovial effusion common (60%)
      – Biceps tenosynovial effusion and subdeltoid bursal effusion: PPV 95% for rotator cuff tear
    ▪ Infraspinatus atrophy: related to poor surgical outcome after repair (70)
    ▪ False positive appearance in musculotendinous junction and false negative by echogenic granulation tissues in full-thickness tear
    ▪ Comparison of US findings between tear and tendinosis

	TEAR	TENDINOSIS
Echogenicity	Anechoic (cautious of echogenic granulation tissue replacing the anechoic gap) with absent fibrillar pattern	Hypoechoic ± disrupted fibrillar pattern
Definition of lesion	Well defined	Ill defined
Thickness	Homogeneous, thin	Heterogeneous, increased thickness
Humeral head/ tuberosity	Bone irregularity	Smooth cortex

  ○ X-ray: sclerosis, cystic change of greater/lesser tuberosity, calcification, narrowed acromiohumeral distance in full-thickness tear; low sensitivity to R/O other bony pathology (with h/o trauma)
  ○ MRI: >90% sensitive and specific; MRA: higher sensitivity and specificity than MRI (particularly useful in small articular-sided tear)

Treatment (65)
- Nonoperative treatment
  ○ Mainstay of the treatment for tendinopathy, partial/small full-thickness tear, all chronic tears in an older age group (older than 65–70 years), and all large irreparable tears with muscle atrophy
    ▪ Tendinosis: ~2/3 improved with nonoperative treatment
  ○ Activity modification
    ▪ Discontinue provoking activity (such as throwing) and avoid overhead activity initially
  ○ Stretching of capsular structure and flexibility exercise as soon as possible
  ○ Gradual strengthening (initially isometric) → eccentric strengthening and plyometric exercise
    ▪ Shoulder girdle strengthening and incorporate core, lower extremity strengthening from the beginning
    ▪ Gradual strengthening of teres minor/infraspinatus muscles
  ○ Sports specific exercise if normal ROM and strength is similar to the opposite side: eg, interval throwing program
- Operative treatment for tear (71)
  ○ Indications: early repair considered if acute tears (<6 weeks) in young active/athletic group (although not limited) and for chronic disabling pain in patients (<65 years old) with tears of substantial size (>1 cm) without significant chronic muscle changes
  ○ Tear size: most important prognostic factor
    ▪ Re-tear; overall 30%, small (<3 cm): 10%, large (>3 cm) or massive; 50% or higher
  ○ Open: subacromial decompression and cuff repair versus arthroscopic technique (preferred)
  ○ In chronic rotator cuff tendinopathy with GH arthropathy; consider reverse shoulder arthroplasty
  ○ Postoperative rehabilitation
    ▪ No strenuous activity for 4 to 6 weeks
    ▪ Passive range of motion (PROM) and pendulum exercise for 6 weeks then active range of motion (AROM) → if full ROM achieved then strengthening exercise (isometric initially)
    ▪ Return to sport participation: 12 M for pitcher, 6 M for other athletes

CALCIFIC TENDINOPATHY

Introduction (72)
- Epidemiology
  ○ Calcification in tendon: common and largely asymptomatic
    ▪ Prevalence: ~10% (2–20%) of asymptomatic population
      – Some may have pain in the past (attributable to calcification)
  ○ Painful calcific tendinopathy: ~7% of patients with shoulder pain
    ▪ More common in 30 to 60 years old (peak in 5th decades), female > male by two times, bilateral in 15% to 25%
- Location: supraspinatus tendon (MC, ~50%), 1.5 to 2 cm from the insertion
- Coexisting with rotator cuff tear in 25% of cases, more painful with smaller calcification

- Pathology
  - Idiopathic (nondegenerative) versus degenerative (fibrosis and necrosis)
  - Mechanism of pain: inflammation around calcium deposits located in or around the rotator cuff tendons, pressure to surrounding structures, impingement like pain by bursal thickening and deposit prominence or stiffening of GH joint (adhesive capsulitis)
- Natural course
  - Pre-calcific stage; asymptomatic fibrocartilaginous transformation within the tendon
  - Calcific stage
    - Formative: ± pain at rest (night) or motion (especially abduction), catching on movement
    - Resting: ± pain
    - Resorptive stage: most incapacitating (extravasation of the calcium crystal into the subacromial bursa)
  - Post-calcific: healing and repair: several months; ± pain

History and physical examination
- Abrupt onset of severe pain, not necessarily activity dependent, stiffness ± swelling (with bursal irritation and with bursal effusion)
- Positive impingement test (Neer and Hawkins) ± decreased ROM (often difficult to distinguish it from adhesive capsulitis)

Diagnosis
- Clinical suspicion confirmed by imaging study
- X-ray: AP, internal/external, scapular Y, and axillary lateral view
  - Degenerative signs in x-ray: rare
- US (69)
  - Hyperechoic lesion in the rotator cuff tendon location with post-acoustic shadowing ± increased vascularity (on Doppler)
  - Evaluation of subdeltoid bursa (effusion), biceps/tenosynovium, and GH joint
- MRI
  - Usually not necessary unless pain is persistent despite the treatment
  - To evaluate differential diagnosis or concomitant lesion: partial rotator cuff tears, intracortical structure, IA structure evaluation
- Serology: normal CBC (WBC) and ESR/CRP (may be mildly elevated)
- Differential diagnosis: adhesive capsulitis, inflammatory (or rotator cuff) arthropathy, septic arthritis, and gout during resorptive phase

Treatment (73)
- NSAIDs, subacromial bursal steroid injection if + impingement sign
- Modalities: US (mixed evidence) and extracorporeal shock-wave therapy
- US-guided needle lavage for resorptive phase (74)
  - Twenty-seven gauge needle with 5 mL 1% lidocaine to skin, subcutaneous tissue, subdeltoid bursa, then 18 G punched into calcification, then inject lidocaine, aspirate, and then change the syringe (filled with lidocaine/saline) → give steroid injection to subacromial bursa (with 2.5 mL of 5% bupivacaine); may be better with warm saline (42°C) (75)
- PT for a few sessions to maintain/improve ROM, scapular stabilization exercise, gradual strengthening exercise of rotator cuff M, pain modality, and home exercise program (HEP)
- Surgery for patient with severe disabling pain who failed conservative management. For formative phase with impingement syndrome

BICEPS LONG-HEAD TENDON PATHOLOGIES

Bicep Long-Head Tendon Disorder
Introduction (76,77)
- Incidence: unknown (78), common in patients with rotator cuff disorders
- Anatomy (79)
  - Posterosuperior labrum and the supraglenoid tubercle → encased within the synovial sheath of the GH joint. Synovial sheath ends in the intertubercular groove
  - Stabilizers: CHL, superior GH ligament (forms reflection pulley for the biceps tendon) and transverse humeral ligament
    - If torn → a slip of supraspinatus tendon is usually torn too
    - Instability common with the subscapularis tear
- Biomechanics and pathophysiology
  - Elbow flexor, supinator, weak shoulder flexor, and decrease torsional rigidity of GH joint
  - Position humeral head on the glenoid (if injured → superior translation of humeral head by 2–6 mm)
    - Similar to supraspinatus tear, humeral head displaced upward from biceps tear/rupture → biceps and supraspinatus further impinged
    - Biceps long-head tear; usually concomitant with rotator cuff tendon tear (supraspinatus tendon > subscapularis tendon) (80)
  - Primary tendinopathy/tear (isolated); less common
    - Etiology: local attrition from periosteitis/bony irregularity, and osteophytes on the intertubercular groove
  - Secondary tendinopathy
    - Similar to rotator cuff impingement syndrome under coracoacromial arch: MC
    - GH joint pathology

History and physical examination
- Anterior shoulder pain on the intertubercular groove ± radiation to the biceps belly
  - Often difficult to distinguish from shoulder impingement syndrome (especially coracoid impingement)
    - More pain with extension (than flexion) and internal rotation
    - ± Painful clicking or snapping especially with overhead position or internal to external rotation
  - Pain often improves with rupture
- Physical examination
  - Focal tenderness on the intertubercular groove, ~7.5 cm distal to acromion with the arm in slight (10°) internal rotation (intertubercular groove faces anteriorly)
    - Tenderness moves with rotation of the arm (as intertubercular groove rotates)
  - Neurological examination: usually normal
  - Provocation test

- Yergason test, Speed test, and Ludington's test; not specific
- Jobe relocation test and O'Brien active compression test for SLAP type 2 lesion
- Subacromial impingement sign: often positive (concomitant)

Diagnosis
- Clinical diagnosis confirmed by imaging study
- Point-of-care US
  - Low sensitivity, unable to evaluate IA portion of tendon, high specificity
  - Tenosynovial effusion (often secondary to GH joint pathology), thickened tendon, tear (partial and complete ± retraction), calcification in the groove, and tuberosity
  - Dynamic view for subluxation with GH rotation (external and internal), dislocation of the tendon deep to the subscapularis (medially)
- X-ray: usually limited except calcification in groove and bony deformity (fracture or osteophytes), cystic change in the lesser tuberosity (subscapularis tendon disorder may be associated with pulley system)
- MRI: similar finding to US and able to evaluate intra-capsular portion, and other peri/IA structures
  - Biceps subluxation and instability classification based on arthroscopic and MRI findings (Bennet): type 1 (IA subscapularis) to type 4 (supraspinatus and lateral CHL lesion)
- IA injection ➔ improvement of pain in the intertubercular groove
  - Less effective with subacromial injection for isolated lesion (but often effective due to high concomitant rotator cuff tendon pathology)

Treatment
- Nonoperative management; improvement in >2/3
  - Brief resting, activity modification and PT
    - PT: posterior capsule stretching and strengthening after ROM exercise
  - Injection: subdeltoid bursa injection (subdeltoid bursa over the biceps tendon under US guidance) as rotator cuff tendinopathy with bursitis is highly prevalent and is often the underlying mechanism for biceps tendon dysfunction
    - If no response ➔ US-guided bicipital tenosynovium injection or intra-capsular (GH joint) injection. Be cautious of lateral humeral circumflex artery in the intertubercular groove

Biceps Long-Head Tear and Rupture

Introduction
- Tear: commonly with tears of supraspinatus or subscapularis, biceps instability (pulley lesion at RI)
- Rupture: rare, usually from progression of chronic partial tear
  - Long-head, IA level more commonly involved. Associated with SLAP lesion
  - Mechanism: fall on outstretched arm (traumatic with SLAP lesion) or repetitive overhead activities (throwing, eccentric force in deceleration phase)

History and physical examination
- Asymptomatic ± pain, audible pop, or ecchymosis at rupture
  - Pain can get better after the rupture in chronic tendinopathy
- Popeye's sign: a soft tissue lump in the middle arm secondary to biceps tendon rupture with retraction
- Strength: elbow flexion (normal to 10% loss) and forearm supination loss (about 20%)

Diagnosis
- Clinical suspicion confirmed by imaging study
- US: empty sac in the intertubercular groove
  - False negative with echogenic debris/granulation tissue, fibrous scarring in the empty groove
    - Supportive finding for tear/rupture: lack of fibrillar pattern in longitudinal scan
  - Retract distally (normally myotendinous junction of long head at the level of pectoralis major tendon insertion, move distally)
- MRA better than MRI (poor concordance rate)
  - SLAP lesion or pulley system; MRA

Treatment (77)
- Nonoperative management: benign neglect with treatment of rotator cuff pathology
  - Isolated rupture: no surgery usually required
- Referral to surgery
  - Indication: high-level athletes or for persistent pain despite conservative management
  - Synovectomy, repair of partial tears or tenodesis (commonly done), resection of the proximal stump (can be entrapped in the joint)
  - Postoperative rehabilitation: sling for 3 weeks (flex/extend arm gently, passive pendulum type ROM immediately), AROM in a month, strengthening of rotator and deltoid in 2 months (M), strengthening of biceps in 3 M, 6 M returning to labor intensive working

Biceps Long-Head Tendon Instability/Subluxation

Introduction (81)
- Stabilizer of biceps long head tendon: "biceps sling": glenohumeral ligament (GHL), CHL, and transverse humeral ligament and shape of the groove
- Etiology
  - Predisposing factor: shallow groove (<3 mm or a flat medial wall)
  - Traumatic causes: a fall on an outstretched arm while the arm is in full internal or external rotation, or falling backward on the hand or elbow
- Medial instability more common than lateral instability
  - Medial dislocation: IA, intra-tendinous, extra-articular
    - Almost always related to a tear of subscapularis except extra-articular dislocation with tendon superficial to subscapularis
  - Lateral instability: in trauma with anterior dislocation and/or fracture of greater tuberosity

History and physical examination
- Pain in the bicipital groove radiating down to the muscle belly
- Clunk of subluxing tendon with abduction (rare in dislocation)
- Limited external rotation because dislocated biceps tendon restraints subscapularis tendon/muscle

Diagnosis
- Clinical suspicion confirmed by imaging study
- US with dynamic evaluation: empty groove with tendon located outside/or on the lesser tuberosity (± tendon thickening and tear of subscapularis tendon)
- MRI: Bennet classification (62)
  - Type 1 (biceps pulley injury involving IA subscapularis tendon) to type 5 (all structures; subscapularis, medial sheath, supraspinatus, lateral CHL involved)
- Arthroscopy: rarely necessary for the diagnosis, dynamic examination with direct visualization

Treatment
- PT focusing on the rotator cuff pathology first, rarely injection for pain control (GH intra-capsular injection with US often helps the anterior shoulder pain or subdeltoid bursa injection)
- Surgery: failed conservative management in concomitant subscapularis tear
  - Internal reconstruction of the rotator cuff interval with superior GHL and CHLs. Tubularization of the tendon and deepening of the bicipital groove
  - Biceps tenodesis (or even tenotomy)

PECTORALIS MUSCLE STRAIN AND TEAR

Introduction (82)
- Pectoralis major tear: rare, peak in 20 to 40 year-old male athletes with weight-lifting exercise
- Etiology: direct blow (crush, motor vehicle, falls) or indirect trauma (rugby, weight lifting: forced abduction with extension or external rotation, rapid eccentric load during flat bench press)
- Location of lesion
  - Muscle belly: common in direct trauma
  - Enthesis: complete tear common in sports injury (anterior shoulder pain; pectoralis minor on the coracoid, pectoralis major to the lateral lib of bicipital groove on proximal humerus)
  - Myotendinous junction: partial tear common in sports injury

History and physical examination
- Tear: sudden pain in the arm and shoulder accompanied by audible pop, followed by swelling and ecchymosis
- Ecchymosis in acute tear/strain, loss of anterior axillary fold and asymmetry, loss of arm adduction (weight lifters), dropped nipple sign (lower than contralateral side in pectoralis major tear)
- Medial shoulder pain (activity dependent) in pectoralis minor enthesopathy and tenderness (83)

Diagnosis
- Clinical diagnosis confirmed by imaging studies and US-guided injection
- US: rapid assessment for tear and US-guided injection for tendinopathy/enthesopathy
- MRI; gold standard, assessment of site and severity and bony structures, surgical patient

Treatment
- Nonoperative treatment: low grade, muscular, musculotendinous tears, older and sedentary patients
- Surgical treatment: complete tendon avulsion at humerus, athletes for early return to sports

JOINT AND BONE PATHOLOGY

AC JOINT SPRAIN AND INJURY (84)

Introduction
- AC injury: 40% to 50% of athletic shoulder injury, concern for later development of OA
- Classification (grading of the degree of injury)

GRADE	CHARACTERISTIC
1	Sprain; no visible deformity
2	Rupture of the AC joint and coracoclavicular (CC) ligament (deltoid and trapezoid) Unstable distal clavicle horizontally with tenderness
3	Rupture of the AC/CC ligament • 100% displacement, severe pain, and tenderness in CC space
4	Clavicle displaced posteriorly • Anterior acromion prominent • Possible sternoclavicular joint and brachial plexus injury
5	Large grade III: coracoclavicular interval: 100%–300% (or >25 mm) vs up to 100% in the III (or ≤25 mm) • Clavicle located subcutaneously
6	The distal clavicle trapped beneath acromion or coracoid process • Rare, caused by high velocity injury

AC, acromioclavicular.

History and physical examination
- Pain in the vicinity of the acromion and clavicle
- Examination on sitting or standing without the support of the arm
  - Inspection; tented skin with dislocation
  - Palpate for tenderness and mobilize (anterior-posterior and adduction-abduction of arm)
- SC joint palpation for concomitant injury
- Neurological examination for brachial plexus injury

Diagnosis
- Clinical diagnosis confirmed by imaging study
- X-ray
  - AP, supraspinatus outlet, axillary, cross-arm adduction AP, and bilateral Zanca view
    - Widen AC joint in type 2, displaced acromion inferiorly (type 3), increased CC distance, posterior translation of lateral clavicle (type 4) on an axillary view
- MRI for the differential diagnosis or for evaluation of ligaments, IA (GH)/intracortical lesion in atypical presentation or persistent pain despite initial management (85,86)

Treatment (87)
- Nonoperative treatment
  - Indications: type 1 and 2, controversial for type 3 (no difference with symptoms in outcome) or chronic conditions
  - Immobilization with sling or immobilizer (up to 10 days for type 1 and 14 days for type 2)
  - ROM exercise if pain resolved, then isometric and gradual strengthening/endurance exercise if ROM is normalized
  - Avoid lifting or contact sports for 2 to 3 months, return to play in ~3 months
  - Steroid injection; may consider after 12 weeks if the pain continues (local anesthetic block before that if needed)
- Surgical treatment
  - Acute type 4 to 6 injury, high-performing athletes with lower grade injury or persistent pain despite conservative treatment
  - No consensus for techniques; goal: restoring and retaining anatomic AC joint reduction
  - Postoperative rehabilitation
    - Limited ROM exercise at 2 weeks restricted beneath the shoulder level, no lifting >5 lbs
    - At 2 to 3 months, screws removed then full ROM with light resistance strengthening 6 to 8 weeks
    - With graft reconstruction; pendulum exercise at 2 weeks, A & PROM exercise at 8 weeks (graft maturation), and light resistance exercise at 3 M

AC OSTEOARTHRITIS (88)

Introduction
- MC pathology of AC joint
- High prevalence of abnormal radiologic finding in asymptomatic population; often difficulty correlating clinically
- Etiology
  - Age-related degeneration of IA disc, posttraumatic arthropathy, distal clavicular osteolysis, joint instability, and impingement

History and Physical Examination
- Pain with P/AROM of the shoulder (especially with overhead, cross-body activities or push-ups) ± mechanical symptoms (popping, catching, or grinding) at AC joint
  - Symptoms can be multifactorial from impingement, biceps pathology, and rotator cuff syndrome
- Physical examination
  - Inspection: swelling, deformity, and prominence of lateral clavicle (instability)
  - Palpation: tenderness and crepitus with ROM
  - Provocation test
    - Cross-body adduction, AC-resisted extension (AC joint pain on resisted extension in 90° forward flexed shoulder) and O'Brien test; if all three are positive, high accuracy and specificity (~90%)
    - Paxinos test
    - Neer, drop arm, and painful arc: often positive (not as sensitive, specific as aforementioned tests)

Diagnosis
- Clinical diagnosis with imaging study
- Differential diagnosis (89)
  - Rotator cuff syndrome/subacromial impingement (often concomitant, caused by AC degenerative joint disease [DJD]), symptomatic os acromiale, and referred pain from cervical spine disease
  - Inflammatory arthropathy and septic arthritis (rare); persistent pain, warmth ± systemic reaction (fever, chills)
  - Superior labrum anterior and posterior lesion

	AC JOINT PROBLEM	SLAP LESION
Pain location	Anterior and posterior aspect of AC joint	Superiorly, deep, or asymptomatic/minimal pain
O'Brien test	Superior shoulder pain in both internal and external rotation of the forearm	Pain in deep shoulder ± click with internal rotation but not external rotation

AC, acromioclavicular; SLAP, superior labral tear from anterior to posterior.

- Imaging
  - X-ray (AP chest, shoulder, Zanca view): joint space narrowing, subchondral cysts/sclerosis, and osteophytes
  - US: similar finding to x-ray with capsular bulging
    - Evaluation of rotator cuff tendons/bursa, biceps tendon/tenosynovium, and joint effusion
    - Dynamic test with shoulder adduction
  - MRI: typically not indicated, consider with atypical presentation or persistent pain despite initial treatment. Evaluate periarticular structures
    - Caudal osteophyte and capsular hypertrophy: may be predictive of response to IA injection

Treatment
- Nonoperative treatment
  - Education and activity modification (avoid/decrease pushing, weight lifting, throwing, or overhead work), brief immobilization (3–7 days in sling with ice as needed) in exacerbation, NSAID, and injection
  - PT for periscapular muscles (scapular stabilizers) and rotator cuff muscle strengthening exercise
  - Injection: volume of 1 mL, may be difficult to inject with smaller gauge needle especially into the bulged capsule
    - US-guided injection: more accurate
- Surgery: disabling pain, loss of function despite full course of nonoperative treatment, and clavicular resection (arthroscopic vs open)
  - Postoperative: P&AROM at 2 weeks, immobilization for ~4 weeks then full ROM, if extensive deltoid detachment,

then active forward flexion and abduction limited for 4 to 6 weeks

DISTAL CLAVICLE OSTEOLYSIS

Introduction (90)
- Common in heavy weight lifting, 28% of elite weight lifters, bilateral in ~80%, average age of presentation: 23 years
- Suggested etiology
  - Repetitive microtrauma during repeated hyperextension of the shoulder (bench press) or chest fly exercises

History and physical examination
- Insidious aching pain aggravated by activity, in particular during flat bench pressing and with dips, flies, and pushups, and pain on adduction
- Point tenderness on AC joint and pain with a cross-body adduction maneuver otherwise not specific, full ROM of GH joint

Diagnosis
- Clinical diagnosis confirmed by imaging study ± diagnostic injection to AC joint
- X-ray (AP views, scapular Y/lateral, Zanca view): rarefaction and subchondral cyst formation along the distal clavicle, acromion; spared (if involved, then consider other disease, such as AC arthritis)
- MRI: often under-recognized with focus on rotator cuff, edema in the distal clavicle and increased T2 signal intensity
- Differential diagnosis: hyperparathyroidism, gout, scleroderma, rheumatoid arthritis (RA), multiple myeloma (MM), infection, and massive essential osteolysis (Gorham's disease)

Treatment
- Avoidance of provocative maneuvers (hyperextension and hyperabduction), modification of weight training, ice massage, and NSAIDs
  - Modification of activities
    - Narrowing the hand space on barbell; <1.5 x biacromial width, do not do near the chest during bench press
    - Power clean; modified to high pull or power pull
- Imaging-guided steroid injection (often effective pain relief up to 6 months)
- Referral for surgery; failure to improve with conservative treatment with correlating imaging, unwillingness to modify the training (91)
  - Distal clavicular resection (open vs arthroscopic)

GLENOHUMERAL JOINT PATHOLOGIES

Adhesive Capsulitis

Introduction
- Prevalence: 2% to 5%, F > M, peak in 40 to 60 years, more common in nondominant side, 20% to 30% develops in the opposite
  - Up to 20% in patients with DM. More common with history of thyroid dysfunction, Dupuytren's contracture, autoimmune disease, treatment of breast cancer, and CVA (spastic phase) and myocardial infarction
  - Rotator cuff lesion; very common ~60% (partial thickness tear of supraspinatus tendon: MC)
- Pathology
  - Hypervascular, hypertrophic synovitis (with rare inflammatory cell) with normal capsular tissue in stage 1 → pedunculated synovitis, perivascular, subsynovial capsular scar in stage 2 → hypercellular collagenous tissue with a thin synovial layer (minimal synovitis) similar to other fibrosing conditions in stage 3 → mature adhesion in stage 4
- Good prognosis usually

History and physical examination (92)
- Painful, gradual loss of both active and passive shoulder motion
- Early loss of external rotation (<15°) with intact rotator cuff examination (although limited due to pain and decreased ROM)

	SYMPTOMS	SIGNS
Stage 1	Pain referred to deltoid insertion, pain at night, duration <3 months	Tenderness on deep palpation Empty end feel at extreme range Full motion under anesthesia
Stage 2	Severe night pain, stiffness (freezing stages)	Motion restricted in forward flexion, abduction, internal and external rotation Some motion loss under anesthesia
Stage 3	Profound stiffness, pain only at the end of range Duration: 9–15 months	Significant loss of motion Tethering at ends of motion No improvement under anesthesia
Stage 4	Profound stiffness with minimal pain	Significant motion loss Gradual improvement in motion

Diagnosis
- Clinical diagnosis with imaging study to evaluate differential diagnoses (such as OA of GH joint)
- Imaging study: usually not necessary
  - US
    - Biceps tenosynovial effusion
    - Reduction of rotator cuff interval ± RI hyperemia
    - The thickness of the CHL: greater in adhesive capsulitis (3 mm) than asymptomatic (1.3 mm) shoulder (93)
  - MRI
    - Thickening of the joint capsule in the axillary recess, enhancement of the RI (with contrast)
    - MRA: increased thickness of the CHL, thickening of the joint capsule in the rotator cuff interval and obliteration of the fat triangle under the coracoid process

- Differential diagnosis: calcific tendinitis, rotator cuff injury, biceps tendinitis, as well as GH or AC arthritis, often concomitant or causes secondary adhesive capsulitis

Treatment (92)
- Education: benign/total neglect of pain (unrestricted activity despite pain), PT, or manipulation
- NSAIDs, or PO steroid for 3 to 6 weeks (or shorter, oral prednisone if patient does not want injection, cautious with cormorbidity eg, high cholesterol and hypertension) (94)
- IA steroid injection under US guidance with steroid, 1% lidocaine and NS total of ~10 mL initially
  - GH joint injection: more efficacious in stage 1 or early stage 2 before developing significant capsular contracture. Unclear long-term benefit
- Suprascapular nerve block, hydrodilation of capsule (about 20 mL without steroid) (95), and adhesiolysis (96) if initial injection is not working
- PT: "neglect" therapy, usually followed by the injection to focus on increasing ROM, capsular stretching, and scapular stabilization exercise
- Surgery referral if persistent disabling symptoms despite the conservative treatment
  - Manipulation under anesthesia
  - Arthroscopic (or open) resection of the capsule (including sup. GH ligament and rotator cuff interval, IA subscapularis tendon)

Rotator Cuff Arthropathy

Introduction (97)
- Rotator cuff insufficiency, diminished acromiohumeral distance with impingement syndrome, and GH arthritis
- ~4% of patients with complete tear of rotator cuff (under-recognized)
- F > M, elderly, dominant side more common
- Proposed pathophysiology
  - Loss of dynamic stability (from rotator cuff insufficiency) → trauma of GH articular cartilage and coracoacromial arch → release of particulate debris into the joint causing crystal-mediated inflammatory cascade (Milwaukee shoulder)

History and physical examination
- Chronic shoulder pain worse at night and with activity and stiffness
- Physical examination
  - Atrophy or swelling (bursal effusion, GH joint effusion communicating with bursa), decreased passive and active ROM (similar to adhesive capsulitis), and weakness (especially external rotation)

Diagnosis (98)
- Clinical diagnosis confirmed by imaging study
- X-ray
  - Superior migration of the humeral head resulting in decreased acromiohumeral distance
  - Osteophytes, joint space narrowing
  - Rounding of the greater tuberosity of the proximal humerus
  - Acetabularization of the undersurface of the acromion
  - Osteopenia of the acromion and proximal humerus
  - GH joint subluxation
- Advanced imaging (US, MRI): usually not necessary, but can confirm massive rotator cuff tear and other IA/intracorticalpathology

Treatment
- Nonoperative management; NSAID, steroid injection to bursa/intra-capsular (often communicating each other) as needed, avoid repeated injection
- Surgery: reverse total shoulder arthroplasty preferred over arthroscopic lavage, arthrodesis, humeral tuberoplasty (71)
  - Indication: persistent disabling pain, impaired ROM despite conservative treatment

SHOULDER OSTEOARTHRITIS

Introduction (99)
- Relatively uncommon compared to the weight-bearing joints (hip and knee)
  - Prevalence: 2% to 16% in older adults (depending on different age groups) (100)
  - One third of patients with shoulder pain >60 years
- Risk factor: age and presence of knee OA

History and physical examination
- Deep aching pain (vague, often nonspecific), often worse at night
- Loss of ROM (usually normal in mild and moderate arthritis)± intermittent locking pain in the mid range
  - Limited in external rotation, bony crepitus, and joint enlargement
  - Compression rotation test: reproduction of pain internally/externally rotate while compressing the humeral head to the glenoid

Diagnosis
- Clinical diagnosis confirmed by imaging study
- X-ray
  - Joint space narrowing, osteophytes, subchondral sclerosis, cyst
  - Grading by Samilson and Prieto
    - Mild arthrosis: <3 mm spur projecting off of the humerus, glenoid, or both
    - Moderate arthrosis: osteophytes measuring between 3 and 7 mm off of the humerus, glenoid, or both, with slight GH joint irregularity
    - Severe arthrosis: osteophytes measuring >8 mm off of the humerus, glenoid, or both, with joint space narrowing and sclerosis
  - US and MRI: intact rotator cuff tendons (vs impaired in rotator cuff arthropathy), crystal deposition in cartilage (in chondrocalcinosis), and MRI for intracortical (AVN) or IA lesion
- Differential diagnosis: RA, crystal deposition disease (pseudogout), rotator cuff arthropathy, septic arthritis, traumatic arthropathy, AVN of humeral head and other causes of shoulder pain (such as adhesive capsulitis, rotator cuff tendinopathy etc; often concomitant)

Treatment
- NSAIDs, PT for ROM, capsular stretching, shoulder girdle strengthening and rotator cuff strengthening
- Steroid injection (imaging guidance preferred); short-term relief of pain and viscosupplementation (with imaging guidance)
- Surgery; >60 years, persistent symptoms despite nonoperative management
  - Total shoulder arthroplasty (if rotator cuff tendon intact) versus reverse shoulder arthroplasty with rotator cuff tear

SHOULDER INSTABILITY

Introduction (101)
- Epidemiology
  - Prevalence ~2 % of general population and bilateral in 16%
    - In older (>40 years), lower rates of primary instability but high rate of rotator cuff disease (with secondary mild instability)
- Risk factors (102)
  - Male, age (bimodal), genetic predisposition, abnormal position of glenoid cavity (posterior instability in excessive glenoid retroversion), hypermobile syndrome, contact sports (as well as butterfly stroke, and gymnastics), etc
    - Risk for recurrence inversely correlating with age: 50% to 75% younger than 25 years
  - Other structural lesions
    - Capsular laxity essential component for multidirectional instability
      - Humeral avulsion of the GH ligament (HAGL); at the attachment of anterior band of inf. GH ligament to the humeral neck
    - Previous injury (dislocation) with decreased bony contact of humerus on glenoid
      - Hill–Sachs lesion (posterolateral humeral indentation fracture); increase risk if >30% of articular surface involved
      - Bankart lesion (anterior inferior capsulolabral avulsion); between glenoid rim and labrum/ligaments; usually after anterior subluxation

History and physical examination
- Sense of instability in specific positions; ABER (in anterior instability) or arm in forward elevation and internal rotation: pushing open door (in posterior instability) ± pain
- "Dead arm" syndrome: brief loss of control in maximally external rotated, abducted, and extension by transient anterior subluxation (103)
  - Pain and paresthesia with carrying heavy objects: traction of brachial plexus in inferior subluxation
- Physical examination
  - Mild tenderness on the GH joint, AC, and SC joint
    - Tenderness on the post aspect of the shoulder (Hill–Sachs lesion)
  - Sulcus sign (with/without inferior traction) and possible atrophy of musculature
  - Loss of passive ER in posterior dislocation
  - Provocative maneuver: anterior apprehension test, Jobe relocation test, anterior and posterior drawer test, load and shift test, and fulcrum test etc
  - Beighton scoring for hypermobility
  - Neurovascular examination: check arm abduction, sensory examination of lateral shoulder (axillary N), and lateral forearm (musculocutaneous N)
    - Anterior dislocation of shoulder: axillary N injury (MC, ~ 15%)
    - Repair of the dislocation: musculocutaneous N damage: MC

Diagnosis
- Clinical diagnosis confirmed by imaging study
- Imaging Studies
  - X-ray with the patient holding 10 to 15 lbs in each arm
    - AP: avulsion fracture in the humeral neck (HAGL)
    - Scapular Y view to check shoulder dislocation/ Axillary view: shoulder dislocation and bony glenoid
    - West Point axillary view (to evaluate Bankart) and Stryker Notch View (Hill–Sachs)
    - Elbow x-ray for loose body (with h/o trauma)
  - US (104)
    - High interobserver variability, varying sensitivity and specificity compared to MRA
    - Anterior (shoulder in ABER with lower frequency probe (5–8 Hz) using axillary approach scanning anterior-labral detachment (Bankart lesion) and effusion
    - Posterior (shoulder in adduction): transverse approach inferior to the spine of scapula: Hill–Sachs lesion and effusion (anterior or posterior translation)
  - MRI/A: gold standard
    - Bony lesion: a glenoid index: ratio of maximal diameter of injured glenoid/uninjured glenoid (<0.75 → may need graft)
    - MRI/A to check ligamentous problem; axillary pouch (normal "U" shape with intact inferior GH ligament to "J" shape in ruptured)
    - MRA with ABER position for labroligamentous complex in unidirectional anterior instability
- Differential diagnosis/concomitant lesion
  - Subacromial impingement, internal impingement, and undersurface rotator cuff tear (often concomitant)
  - SLAP lesions
  - Neurological lesion (can be concomitant); axillary neuropathy

Treatment (105)
- Rehabilitation
  - Precaution in ROM for ~6 weeks; depends on the age, no terminal stretch for 9 to 12 weeks
    - Anterior instability: no Codman (pendulum) exercise for 2 to 3 weeks, avoid external rotation past 45° for at least 3 to 6 weeks, no external rotation and abduction for 8 weeks. Sling: no effect
    - Posterior subluxation: immobilization in neutral rotation for 3 weeks
  - Strengthening of dynamic stabilizer (isometric exercise initially); deltoid, rotator cuff, and scapular girdle M

- Strengthening of infraspinatus, teres minor, and posterior deltoid for ≥6 months
- Scapular band (106); figure of 8 band with anterior strap lower chest wall, improve the effectiveness of scapular stabilization exercise
○ Proprioception exercise to improve muscle coordination and proprioception
○ Return to play: 8 to 10 weeks, no return to contact sport until strength (≥85% of the asymptomatic side, isokinetic measurement ideally) and full pain-free ROM
• Surgery
○ Indication: young or failed rehab treatment (6 months) or if Bankart lesion (>30% of bone loss), Hill–Sachs (>30%–40% of humeral head) or recurrent dislocation in contact sport players
  ▪ First time dislocation: surgery: 14% recurrence versus 80% recurrence without surgery
  ▪ Discouraged in posterior dislocation (25%–50% recurrence with surgery) and multidirectional instability
○ Arthroscopic: capsulolabral complex (with bony deficiency: recurrence risk is 67%)
○ Open: Grade 3, or >1 direction for bony defect or HAGL lesion
○ Thermal shrinkage versus capsular shift (plication)
○ Cautious of musculocutaneous and axillary N injury
• Postoperative rehabilitation
○ Sling protection: 3 weeks, PROM (pendulum); AROM in 6 weeks
○ Terminal stretch and isometric Ex.
○ Return to Sport (107); minimal 14 to 16 weeks, typically 4 to 6 months but up to 9 to 12 months depending on the surgical technique

MULTIDIRECTIONAL INSTABILITY

Introduction
- Incidence: unknown, 7% to 10% of all instability
- Etiology
○ Traumatic (anterior/posterior capsulolabral injury), glenoid dysplasia, retroversion, hyperlaxity of the joint capsule, generalized hypermobility, neuromuscular component, or connective tissue disorder
○ Symptomatic involuntary instability in two or more directions
- Common in second to third decades

History and physical examination
- Vague shoulder pain to symptomatic subluxation and frank dislocation
- Sulcus sign and reduced scapular upward rotation
- Provocative test and increased anterior, posterior GH translation

Diagnosis (108)
- Clinical diagnosis with supplementary imaging findings
- MRI/A: often difficult to interpret findings of capsular widening of the shoulder
○ MRA in ABER position
  ▪ Crescent sign (contrast between the humeral head and the anteroinferior GH ligament (AIGHL)
  ▪ Triangular sign: triangular-shaped accumulation of contrast between humeral head, AIGHL, and glenoid

Treatment (109)
- Nonoperative management: mainstay, 60% to 90% effective; strengthening of the scapular stabilizer and rotator cuff muscles
- Surgical referral when conservative treatment failed: 85% to 90% satisfactory
○ Tightening joint capsule with inferior capsular shift

SLAP (SUPERIOR LABRAL ANTEROPOSTERIOR) LESION (110,111)

Introduction (112)
- Prevalence: 4% to 11 % in shoulder arthroscopy (unknown in general population), associated with rotator cuff pathology in 30% to 40%
○ Common in throwing athletes (pitchers, tennis players, and swimmers)
- Etiology
○ Rotator cuff tear (➔ sup. migration of the humeral head ➔ lifting sup. labrum and biceps tendon)
○ Trauma: fall on outstretched hand or direct blow to the shoulder
○ Overuse injury
  ▪ Overhead throwing (biceps destabilization and posterosuperior impingement)
  ▪ Traction, and torsional peeling (in late cocking phase of pitching) with posterior capsular tightness

History and physical examination
- Nonspecific anterior shoulder pain aggravated by overhead activity, lifting, and pushing
○ ± clicking, popping, stiffness, and instability (giving way with overhead activity)
○ ± "dead arm syndrome" typically with multidirectional instability
- Provocative maneuvers: O'Brien's test, clunk, crank, and anterior slide test

Diagnosis
- Clinical suspicion (high level of suspicion) confirmed by imaging study or arthroscopy
- Imaging study
○ X-ray: AP, axillary, and outlet view for concomitant pathology in AC joint, impingement
  ▪ Usually negative finding in isolated SLAP lesion
○ MRA better than MRI: ~90 % sensitivity, specificity, and accuracy
  ▪ Coronal oblique sequence; contrast in deep cleft between sup. labrum and glenoid or among labral fragments
- Classification by Snyder et al (Figure 3.7)
○ Type 1-IV: I: fraying of the labrum; II: sup. labrum and biceps anchor involved; III: bucket hand tear displaced to the joint; IV: bucket hand tear extend to biceps tendon
○ Type 2: MC, other classification system further divide type 2 (113)

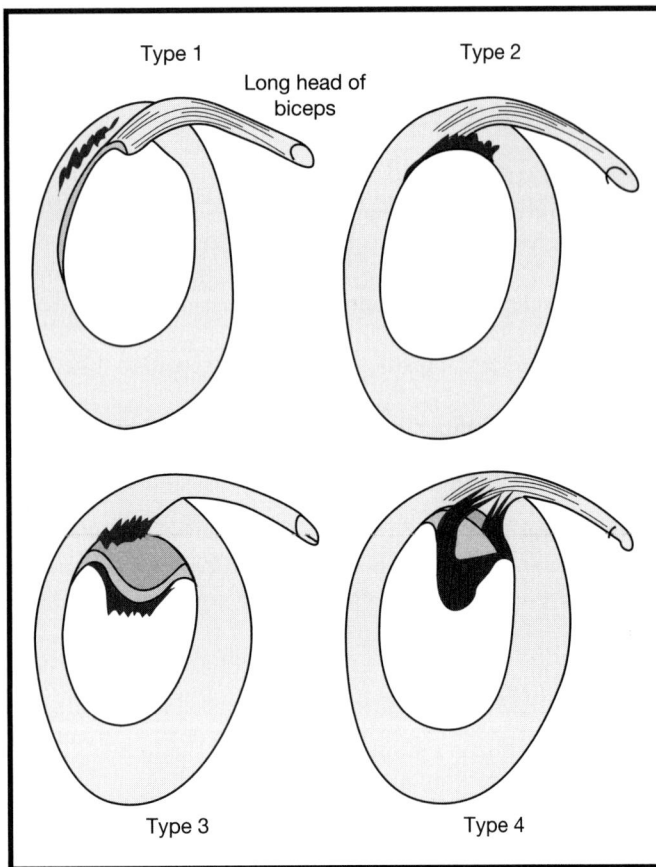

FIGURE 3.7
Classification of SLAP lesions by Snyder.
SLAP, superior labral tear from anterior to posterior.

Treatment (114)
- Nonoperative treatment
  ○ AAP, NSAIDs as needed, avoid activities provoking the symptoms
  ○ PT: Stretching exercise (especially posterior capsule, "sleeper stretch"), address GH internal rotation deficit and strengthening of scapular stabilizer (scapular dyskinesia) and rotator cuff muscle. Neuromuscular facilitation technique
  ○ Avoid shoulder press, bench press
- IA GH injection; diagnose labrum (or IA structure) as pain generator and possible indicator for response to surgery
- Arthroscopic surgery; diagnostic and therapeutic, if the symptom persists despite conservative management
  ○ Debridement, preparation of the superior glenoid for biceps anchor repair and repair of other pathology
  ○ Postoperative rehabilitation: initially passive range (forward flexion) for first four weeks then progressive to AROM, isometric, and then gradual strengthening
  ○ Return to sport around 6 months

BENNETT LESION

Introduction (62)
- Dystrophic/heterotopic extra-articular ossification at the posterior or posteroinferior glenoid rim (near the attachment of triceps M)
- Epidemiology: occurs in young athletes, commonly in baseball players (~20% of professional pitchers)(115), unknown in general population
- Etiology
  ○ Posterior capsular avulsion secondary to traction from the posterior band of the inferior GH ligament
  ○ Overuse: deceleration phase of pitching
- Highly prevalent concomitant rotator cuff tear (undersurface) and posterior labral tear
  ○ Ossification adjacent to torn or degenerated posterior labrum

History and physical examination
- Posterior shoulder pain especially with throwing activities (late cocking, acceleration, or follow through)
- Tenderness at posterior inferior glenoid or GH joint

Diagnosis
- Clinical suspicion confirmed by imaging study
- X-ray (and CT scan; usually not necessary)
  ○ Mineralization of adjacent posterior glenoid and size of ossification; several mms to >1 cm
  ○ Ossification is crescentic +/- fragmentation
  ○ Subchondral sclerosis and cysts
- MRI/A
  ○ Globular to crescent-like ossification within posterior soft tissues, decreased T1 subchondral signal representing sclerosis
  ○ Hypointense T2 signal in the area of ossification at insertion of posterior joint capsule ± adjacent chondromalacia (increased signal intensity in cartilage) and surface irregularity
  ○ Fat suppression: increased signal in surrounding soft tissues representing edema and hemorrhage and torn labrum or markedly heterogeneous
  ○ MRA: associated posterior labral tear with contrast extending into the tear

Treatment
- Nonoperative treatment: PT (similar to SLAP lesion) and NSAIDs, pain may subside with cessation of throwing activity
- Surgical: arthroscopic debridement of soft tissue ossification if failed conservative management (controversial)

RHEUMATOLOGIC DISEASE

Rheumatoid Arthritis (RA) in Shoulder

Introduction (116)
- Epidemiology of RA (117)
  ○ 1% of adults, F:M=2–3:1, peak onset 35 to 60 years
  ○ Genetic: ↑ with class II MHC DRB1, DR4
  ○ Environment: smoking (autoantibody positive disease)
- Shoulder involvement in RA; 65% to 90% reports Symptoms, common in >60 years, underestimated
  ○ Increased with joint destruction in hand/wrist and + rheumatoid factor (RF)
  ○ More than 5 years after onset, 45% has + radiologic involvement of shoulder

History and physical examination
- Pain, swelling, impaired function with morning stiffness (≥1hr)
  ○ Signs of inflammation; often difficult to recognize clinically
  ○ Swelling; subtle unless significant joint effusion or bursal effusion presents
  ○ Joint stiffness/contracture, muscle shortening, bone and deformity; ulnar deviation, swan neck, boutonniere, cock-up deformities (118)
  ○ Erythema and warmth (from superinfected joint)
- Constitutional symptoms: fever, weight loss, and malaise
- Rheumatoid nodule (20%–30%, usually with + RF): subcutaneous nodules on extensor surface along tendon sheath and bursa; also possible in lung, heart, sclera
- Vascular: nail fold infarct, palpable purpura, leukocytoclastic vasculitis
- Extra-articular manifestations
  ○ Ocular: dry eye (keratoconjunctivitis sicca, MC), and redness on sclera (scleritis, episcleritis)
  ○ Pulmonary: cough, shortness of breath (may be suggestive of interstitial lung disease, pleural, bronchiolitis, bronchiectasis)
  ○ Cardiac: asymptomatic (MC), chest pain, pericarditis, myocarditis, valvular/ conduction ds 2/2 nodules

Diagnosis
- Clinical diagnosis supplemented by laboratory/imaging studies
- Lab/radiology
  ○ RF (IgM anti-IgG Ab): 85%, correlate loosely with ds activity, nonspecific (systemic lupus erythematosus [SLE], Sjögren's, subacute bacterial endocarditis, hepatitis, TB, cryoglobulinemia, 5% of healthy population)
  ○ Anti-cyclic citrullinated peptide (CCP) Ab test: more specific
  ○ Hematologic study: anemia of chronic disease, leukemia, lymphoma
    ▪ Felty's syndrome (neutropenia, RF+, splenomegaly) in longstanding seronegative, erosive RA
  ○ ↑ESR, CRP; + antinuclear antibody (ANA) in 15%; ↑ globulin during active disease
  ○ X-ray: periarticular osteopenia, erosion, deformities
    ▪ Different classification based on subchondral geodes, joint space narrowing, osteophytes, effusion, migration of humeral head (upward) or destructive
  ○ US
    ▪ Effusion in posterior recess and bicipital groove. Nonspecific subdeltoid bursitis
    ▪ Evaluate concomitant rotator cuff disease (tendon tear, muscle atrophy) and AC joint degenerative joint disease (DJD)
    ▪ Differential diagnosis with polymyalgia rheumatica: significant effusion in GH joint, bilateral subdeltoid bursal effusion and regional edema
  ○ MRI to evaluate bony and cartilage lesion and rotator cuff evaluation (119)
    ▪ Findings: synovial proliferation, joint effusion, subacromial bursal effusion, muscle atrophy or thinning of the rotator cuff tendon (similar to US) ± edema (increased signal in T2-weighted sequences) in the subchondral bone
  ○ Work up for extra-articular systems: CBC, CXR, referral to ophthalmology and cardiology (echo)

Treatment
- Treatment for RA (check RA of the wrist)
  ○ Initial treatment: NSAIDs (↑CV, gastrointestinal [GI], renal side effect [SE]), COX-2 inhibitor (↑CV SE), low-dose oral steroid, referral to physical/occupational therapy (PT/OT)
  ○ Rheumatology referral for disease modifying anti-rheumatic drugs (DMARD) within 3 months
- IA steroid injection and/or subdeltoid bursal under US guidance; first line without joint space loss in x-ray
- PT/OT with joint protection techniques; scapular stabilization exercise, isometric exercise; cautious of resistive exercise, activities of daily living (ADL) and adaptive equipment evaluation
- Surgery: endoscopic synovectomy (scarce data) and joint arthroplasty (cautious of glenoid loosening)

Crystal-Induced Arthritis (120)

Introduction (121)
- Urate (gout) and calcium pyrophosphate dehydrate (CPPD, pseudogout) crystal deposits causing inflammatory arthropathy
- CPPD is more common in knee > wrists, but shoulder is not uncommon. Urate crystal deposits; uncommon in shoulder joint
- Milwaukee shoulder (122): destructive shoulder arthropathy with large rotator cuff tear
  ○ Some use this term for calcium phosphate crystal-associated destructive arthropathy
    ▪ Common in 60 to 90 years, F > M = 4:1
    ▪ Risk factors: trauma or overuse, CPPD deposition, dialysis, female, and advanced age

History and physical examination
- Rapid onset painful swelling in the dominant side shoulder, but often bilateral involvement
- Warmth on touch without erythema, tenderness, and limited ROM (with pain)

Diagnosis
- Clinical suspicion confirmed by aspiration of joint fluid and crystal demonstration
- X-ray of Milwaukee shoulder
  ○ Joint space narrowing, subchondral sclerosis with cyst formation, destruction of subchondral bone, soft tissue swelling, capsular calcifications, and IA loose bodies
- US: significant effusion, crystal deposition (cartilage-capsule junction and inside the cartilage), marked synovial proliferation, and rotator cuff tear
  ○ US-guided aspiration (for crystal analysis, cell count, and culture): may be hemorrhagic with non inflammatory effusion positive for calcium apatite crystal.
- MRI: US findings + GH joint narrowing, thinning of the cartilage and destruction of subchondral bone
- Differential diagnosis: septic arthritis, neuropathic arthropathy (including syphilis associated), osteonecrosis, or other inflammatory arthropathy

Treatment
- NSAIDs (high-dose aspirin is not recommended because of uricosuric) and IA steroid injection (subdeltoid injection may be OK due to communication) ± imaging guidance
- PT; maintain ROM, scapular stabilization, and rotator cuff strengthening

Amyloid Arthropathy (123)

Introduction (124)
- Rare systemic disorder resembling inflammatory arthritis, from beta2 microglobulin amyloidosis in dialysis and rarely from MM
- Location of common amyloid deposits in bones and joints: hand (carpus), particularly scaphoid, lunate, and capitate
  ○ Shoulder involvement: 68% of amyloid arthropathy, if large subchondral lesions involved; high chance of pathologic fracture
- Risk factors
  ○ Long-term hemodialysis
  ○ MM: 3.5% to 5% develops amyloid arthropathy, other common manifestations of amyloidosis: nephrotic syndrome, cardiomyopathy, and peripheral neuropathy, and carpal tunnel syndrome (125)

History and physical examination
- Symmetric pain with swelling in the shoulders, often lacking acute inflammatory sign
  ○ Multiple joint involvements with symptoms suggestive of carpal tunnel syndrome
- Limited joint motion, shoulder pad sign (periarticular soft tissue amyloid deposition), and subcutaneous nodule in the elbow

Diagnosis
- High clinical suspicion supplemented by imaging study and confirmed by biopsy
- X-ray: often not specific, preservation of joint space or widening (distinguishing from RA)
- MRI: amyloid infiltration within or around the joint: low or intermediate T1 signal and low to intermediate on T2 and joint effusion
- Workup for MM
- Differential diagnosis: RA or other inflammatory arthropathy
- Biopsy of GI (rectal) mucosa and abdominal fat; kappa immunoreactive amyloid deposit (confirmation)

Treatment
- Workup for MM and treat MM if found (oncology referral)
- Low-dose prednisone or IA steroid injection

INFECTIOUS PATHOLOGY

Septic Arthritis

Introduction (126)
- Uncommon: 3% to 5% of all septic arthritis and can be bilateral (more common in weight bearing joint, knee: MC, ~50%)
  ○ Incidence of septic arthritis: 10/100,000, more common in patients with RA and prosthetic joint (up to 70/100,000). Other risk factors: skin infection and HIV
  ○ Higher in young infant or elderly (with chronic medical diseases), mostly hematogenous spread

History and physical examination
- Exquisitely painful shoulder, limited ROM ± local inflammatory signs (swelling, warmth, and erythema)
- Constitutional symptoms and signs: malaise, low-grade fever, less commonly sweats, and rigors
- Physical examination: nonspecific tenderness, decreased ROM ± swelling, deformity, and subluxation of GH joint
  ○ Skin crepitus; subcutaneous emphysema: R/O anaerobic microorganism

Diagnosis
- Clinical suspicion confirmed by laboratory test and synovial fluid culture
- WBC (not always increased), increased ERS and CRP
  ○ X-ray: not specific
- Synovial fluid culture, gram stain (low yield): *S. aureus*. If fluid looks purulent, start treatment empirically

Treatment
- Admit the patient (ER) and ID consult for systemic antibiotic (IV)
  ○ Empiric antibiotic: vancomycin for gram positive cocci, ceftriaxone for gram negative cocci, ceftazidime, cefepime, Zosyn, or carbapenems for gram negative rods. In negative gram stain, vancomycin + either ceftazidime or aminoglycoside (127)
  ○ Immobilize in acute phase of infection
  ○ Aspiration (needle aspiration, arthroscopic or open)
  ○ Referral to surgery (surgical drainage): if not clinically improving, synovial fluid leukocytes not decreasing or when osteomyelitis is suspected)

Lyme Arthritis

Introduction (128)
- Incidence: 7 to 8/100,000, bimodal age distribution (peak in 5–9 and 55–59 years)
- Spirochete (*Borrelia burgdorferi*) transmitted by the tick of the genus *Ixodes* in endemic area (Northeast, Connecticut, check with Center for Disease Control), year round, but mostly during summer (June–August)
- Lyme arthritis; distinguishing feature of late stage (months) lyme disease, 60% of untreated patients
  ○ Shoulder involvement occurs in 30% to 50% of patients with acute Lyme arthritis; knee MC (up to 90%)

History and physical examination
- Expanding rash, erythema chronicum migrans (red macule, 5 to 60 cm size, central clearing occurring 2 to 3 weeks after the tick bite, with arthritis following within a few weeks to 2 years
- Acute pauciarticular and migratory arthritis with large joint involvement, or chronic with inflammatory effusion; progress relatively slowly (not like septic arthritis)

◦ The latter presentation is characterized by pannus formation and articular erosions that are similar to RA

Diagnosis
- Clinical suspicion (high index) with serologic test: ELISA and confirmatory Western blot
- An increased ESR, cryoglobulins containing IgM, and elevated levels of circulating immune complexes are indicators of active disease
- Synovial fluid analysis; often difficult to distinguish from septic arthritis
- Differential diagnosis with bacterial septic arthritis; no fever, normal CRP, no risk factors (such as prosthetic component, RA, HIV), knee involvement (although common in septic arthritis too) favoring Lyme disease

Treatment
- Oral antibiotics: doxycycline 100 mg bid for 28 days or amoxicillin, 500 mg tid for 28 days (ID consult)
- Antibiotic resistant arthritis ➔ may repeat oral Ab again for 4 weeks or intravenous (IV) antibiotic ➔ not responsive then, hydroxychloroquine 200 mg bid and/or consider other pathology
- Referral to surgery (arthroscopic synovectomy) if persistent disabling symptoms for 3 to 6 months

OSTEONECROSIS OF THE HUMERAL HEAD

Introduction (129)
- Second MC site for osteonecrosis after the femoral head, M > F by ~2, common in second to fifth decades (130)
  ◦ Other joint involvement: very common, 90% in steroid use, 75% in sickle cell (femoral head), 29% in Gaucher's disease (autosomal recessive lysosomal storage disease)
- Etiology
  ◦ Corticosteroid use (possibly by ischemia from lipocyte hypertrophy, fat embolism), hemoglobinopathy (embolism), alcohol (fat embolism), Gaucher's disease (ischemia from lipid laden cells, vascular spasm), dysbarism (embolism), connective tissue disease (RA, SLE; steroid, vascular inflammation)
  ◦ Trauma; 3 or 4 part fracture; AVN in 15% to 30% and increased risk of AVN despite open reduction and internal fixation (ORIF)

History and physical examination
- Initially subtle, poorly localized shoulder pain (shoulder girdle, often tolerable until later stage) with difficulty sleeping
  ◦ Can be deep, throbbing, occasional radiation to the elbow
- Physical examination: nonspecific and subtle, ± mechanical symptoms: locking, popping, or painful click (with loose osteochondral fragments)

Diagnosis
- Clinical suspicion confirmed by imaging study
- Imaging study
  ◦ X-ray: AP, scapular, lateral, and axillary view: radiodensity or lucency within the bone, R/O infection, benign or malignant neoplasm, or cysts
    ▪ Can miss stage 1
    ▪ Pelvic radiographs for femoral AVN
  ◦ MRI: a little role if lesion seen in the x-ray. Indicated if negative x-ray or suspicious of other differential diagnoses
- Staging based on imaging studies
  ◦ Stage 1: absent x-ray finding, and increased signal in MRI
  ◦ Stage 2: sclerosis typically in superior portion of the humeral head (subchondral microfracture) without articular collapse
  ◦ Stage 3: crescent sign; external rotation view, some incongruity
  ◦ Stage 4: advanced humeral head collapse with loose bodies or DJD, with spared glenoid
  ◦ Stage 5: degenerative changes in both glenoid and humerus; joint incongruity; humeral head deformity, osteophyte formation, loss of joint space, and cystic changes

Treatment
- Nonoperative management; for stage 1 and 2
  ◦ Risk modification; stop steroid, change to other meds, therapy to encourage maintaining ROM and strengthening shoulder girdle muscles (and rotator cuff muscles)
  ◦ Pain control with NSAID, activity modification (to avoid position to increase joint reactive forces; eg, excessive abduction, extension, and external rotation)
- Referral to surgery: progressive or stage 3
  ◦ Arthroscopy, core decompression (stage 3), hemiarthroplasty (stage 4) and shoulder arthroplasty (stage 5)

LITTLE LEAGUE SHOULDER

Introduction (131)
- Osteochondrosis of proximal humeral epiphysis, epiphysiolysis
- More common in young throwing athletes in 11 to 16 years, M > F
- Etiology
  ◦ Repetitive microtrauma to the proximal humeral epiphysis from large rotational torque during throwing
  ◦ Genetic and environmental factors

History and physical examination
- Progressive pain during throwing motion, usually h/o recent increase in throwing
- Tenderness on the lateral aspect of the proximal humerus
- Common GH internal rotation deficit (side-to-side asymmetry >25° and absolute value <25°)

Diagnosis
- Clinical diagnosis confirmed by radiologic imaging
- X-ray: AP, scapular Y and axillary view
  ◦ Proximal humeral widening: often subtle, check the contralateral side
- MRI
  ◦ Focal widening of the proximal humeral physis in T1, high signal intensity within adjacent metaphysis in T2 weighted image
  ◦ To evaluate other shoulder pathologies

Treatment
- Nonoperative exclusively
- Education for prevention: most important

- Absolute rest for 6 to 12 weeks, NSAIDs initially followed by progressive throwing program/return to play (USA, Baseball Medical & Safety Advisory Committee guideline available) and education on prevention

STERNOCLAVICULAR (SC) SPRAIN/INJURY

Introduction
- Rare injury, 3% of all shoulder girdle injury; high energy trauma; motor vehicle accident (MVA) or contact sports (132)
- Anterior dislocation of clavicle more common than posterior dislocation
  - Posterior dislocation of clavicle: emergency (mediastinal compromise in 30%)
- Anatomy and biomechanics
  - Only joint attaching the upper limb to the trunk
  - Costoclavicular ligament: stabilizing the axis of rotation especially during arm elevation
  - IA (similar to temporomandibular, and facet joints)

History and physical examination
- Pain and deformity (prominence of medial clavicle usually) in high grade injury
  - Pain worse with arm movement or assuming a supine position
  - A bump in the lateral edge of the sternum in posterior dislocation
  - In posteriorly dislocated clavicle; venous congestive symptoms of the neck or arm, dysphasia, cough, hoarseness, or feeling of choking, life-threatening emergency
- Examine entire clavicle and AC joint with frequent dislocation (floating clavicle) and clavicular fracture

Diagnosis
- Clinical diagnosis with imaging study
- AP and serendipity view (oblique view)
- CT scan if patient with suspected mediastinal injuries; occult clavicular fracture, to evaluate degree of dislocation
- Differential diagnosis: Salter Harris type 1 or 2 physeal lesion in young adults
- Classification: type 1 to 3 depending on presence of subluxation (type 2) and complete dislocation (type 3)

Treatment (133)
- Nonoperative treatment: type 1 and 2 and anterior dislocation of type 3
  - Ice for 48 hours, immobilization in a figure of 8 sling less than 1 week for type 1 and 4–6 weeks for type 2, NSAID, then ADL exercise
  - Closed reduction in anterior dislocation: placing the patient in a supine position with conscious sedation, placing a 3- to 4-inch-thick pad between the scapulae, and applying gentle, posterolaterally directed pressure on the medial edge of the clavicle
  - Redislocation: often occurs following reduction in anterior dislocation
  - Avoid contact sports for 3 to 4 months
- Operative treatment
  - Posterior dislocation: general anesthesia with CT surgery consult, risk of vascular injury
    - After reduction, shoulder immobilization for 6 weeks, less likely to re-dislocate
    - Surgery; resection arthroplasty of the medial clavicle with or without reconstruction of the SC ligaments with graft material

SC OSTEOARTHRITIS

Introduction (14)
- Epidemiology
  - DJD of SC joint: common after injury; moderate to severe DJD in 50% of individuals >60 years in postmortem analysis
    - Unclear correlation with clinical symptoms
    - Unknown prevalence of symptomatic SC joint osteoarthritis in general population

History and physical examination
- Anterior upper chest wall pain with arm elevation ± local crepitus and palpable osteophytes
- Symptom generation in SC joint with
  - The push-down test: applying a posteriorly directed force on the medial clavicle
  - Pain with resisted arm abduction

Diagnosis
- Clinical diagnosis confirmed with imaging and imaging-guided injection
- Imaging study: AP and serendipity view (oblique view)
- Imaging-guided injection with small dose <1 mL of injectate volume

Treatment
- Local cryotherapy, activity modification, NSAIDs and, IA corticosteroid injections
- Surgery: resection arthroplasty of the medial clavicle ± reconstruction of the SC ligaments with graft material

FRACTURE

Proximal Humeral Fracture

Introduction (134)
- Four to five percent of all fractures, 75% occurs > age 60 years, and F > M by 3 times
- Shoulder fracture in elderly: third MC after Colles fracture and hip fracture
- Nondisplaced or minimally displaced: MC, 49% to 85%
- Mechanisms: fall onto an outstretched hand (MC)
  - Others: direct blow (onto the shoulder), violent muscle contracture by seizure etc

History and physical examination
- Shoulder pain after trauma. Patient holds the arm (to decrease pain from moving)
- Edema, ecchymosis, and tender to palpation. Concomitant fracture (rib fracture with hemothorax, pneumothorax); not uncommon

- Gross deformity: rare in isolated injury ➜ if present, axillary N or suprascapular N injury; neurological examination (check shoulder abduction and external rotation strength)

Diagnosis
- Classification (by Neer): humeral shaft, head, greater tuberosity, and lesser tuberosity
  ◦ Definition of fragment: >45° angulation or 1 cm displacement
- X-ray: AP, axillary lateral, scapular Y view
- CT if x-ray is not clear or preoperative planning
- MRI in minimally displaced fracture or to evaluate the integrity of rotator cuff in minimally displaced tuberosity fracture (<5 mm)
- Differential diagnosis: rotator cuff injury and AC sprain or dislocation (often concomitant)

Treatment
- Nonoperative treatment
  ◦ Indications: nondisplaced or minimally displaced fracture except fracture of greater tuberosity
    ▪ Sling (and swath) for 2 weeks, elbow, wrist, and hand ROM: immediately, repeat x-ray in a month
    ▪ Mobilization in 5 to 7 days (pendulum exercise) or gentle ROM in 2 weeks then active ROM in 6 weeks
    ▪ Return to work or sports: 6 to 10 weeks (callus formation, near normal range and strength)
- Orthopedic referral
  ◦ Open fracture, with neurovascular compromise, fracture involving anatomic neck (high risk of AVN)
  ◦ Displaced fracture, angulation >20° (in athletes or very active patients)

Scapular Fracture

Introduction (135)
- Common location: body of scapular 50% to 80% and neck 10% to 15%
  ◦ Other area: glenoid, acromion, coracoid process etc
- MC mechanism of injury: direct trauma from a blow or fall
- Frequently associated with other trauma; pneumothorax, rib fracture, pulmonary contusion, clavicle fracture, and brachial plexus injury

History and physical examination
- Pain, hold arm in adduction due to pain ± swelling

Diagnosis
- Clinical suspicion confirmed by imaging study
- X-ray of AP, axillary, and true scapular lateral
- CT scan if glenoid fracture is suspected
- Differential diagnosis with Os acromiale (usually bilaterally)

Treatment
- Nonoperative management; most fractures, ice initially, sling for comfort, and follow up (FU) in 1 to 2 weeks
  ◦ Isolated displaced glenoid neck fracture: reduction not necessary
- Indication for surgical referral
  ◦ Association with displaced clavicle fracture or CC ligament tears
  ◦ Glenoid involved >25%, or humeral head displacement >5 mm
  ◦ Significantly displaced coracoid and body fracture >1 cm
- Return to work/play: at least 8 to 10 weeks after injury

Clavicle Fracture

Introduction (136)
- Five to ten percent of all fractures, commonly in men <25 years, or men >55 years or female >75 years
  ◦ MC pediatric fracture
- MC location: midshaft (thinnest)
- Mechanism of injury/etiology
  ◦ Fall directly onto the shoulder (MC, indirect mechanism), contact sport (direct), MVA (medial one-third)
  ◦ Stress fracture in rowers, gymnasts, and others
- Deforming force: SCM muscle (medial clavicle moves upward) and arm weight and pectoralis (pulling lateral clavicle downward)
- Healing time: up to 6 weeks in children and 12 weeks in adults
- Associated injuries: pneumothorax, hemothorax, and neurovascular injury

History and physical examination
- Pain aggravated by activity, in particular during flat bench pressing and with dips, flies, and push-ups
- Point tenderness, crepitus, or palpable motion of the fractured fragment, ecchymosis initially ± deformity

Diagnosis
- Clinical suspicion confirmed by imaging study
- X-ray (AP with 45° cephalic tilt): minimize the overlap of the ribs and scapula
- CT scan: if x-ray finding is not clear, strong suspicion with normal x-ray, or in medial one-third fracture
- Differential diagnosis (often concomitant)
  ◦ AC separation versus lateral one-third of clavicle fracture
  ◦ SC injury especially with medial one-third of clavicle fracture

Treatment
- Nonoperative treatment: preferred in acute, nondisplaced midshaft clavicle fractures and distal clavicular fractures
  ◦ Arm sling preferred over a figure of 8 bandage: better tolerated with similar outcome
  ◦ Can repeat x-ray in 6 weeks
  ◦ Return to preinjury activity usually in 8 weeks, strenuous or overhead activity: 10 to 12 weeks
  ◦ No contact sports for 8 to 10 weeks
- Referral for surgery
  ◦ Indications: midshaft clavicular fracture (increased risk of nonunion), clavicle shortening >15 to 20 mm, female gender, fracture comminution, complete displacement, greater extent of initial trauma, or older age
    ▪ Young athlete or concerned of visible lump at the site
    ▪ Symptomatic nonunion or malunion increases after 12 weeks
  ◦ Emergent referral to ER when neurovascular injury, open fracture, or tenting of the skin

First Rib Fracture (137)

Introduction (138)
- Rare, <0.1% routine chest x-ray (CXR) has fracture or anomaly of first rib
- Etiology: acute trauma (direct trauma: rare), indirect trauma (MVA and lifting), stress fracture (more common than other rib), congenital (defect between two ossification center)
  - Indirectly by contraction of the anterior scalene
- MC location: at the shallow depression for the subclavian artery (lateral to anterior scalene insertion)
- Complications or concomitant injuries: brachial plexus injury, Horner syndrome, pneumothorax, emphysema, pleurisy, ruptured subclavian A, aortic arch aneurysm, tracheoesophageal fistula or abscess

History and physical examination
- Insidious onset (or acute onset with pop) of shoulder (under the scapula, behind the clavicle) or anterior neck pain radiating to the sternum or pectoral region
- In acute onset, sharp pain with radiation to the ulnar aspect
- Tenderness on the medial to the superior angle of the scapular, root of the neck, supraclavicular triangle or axilla
- Decreased shoulder movement with pain

Diagnosis
- Clinical suspicion confirmed by x-ray or incidental finding
- X-ray (initially can be negative), bone scan, CT, or MRI

Treatment
- Asymptomatic fibrous nonunion: no treatment
  - Pain usually resolves in 2 to 8 weeks
- Immobilization of the shoulder girdle with sling and possible soft neck collar to decrease the pull of the scalene muscle
- Return to sport in 4 to 8 weeks
- Delayed union: 4 to 5 months to heal, up to 9 months
- Surgical referral (excision of the ends of the ribs at the fracture site) for symptomatic nonunion, callus formation for cosmetic concern or rarely compression of neurovascular bundle

NEUROPATHY AND VASCULAR DYSFUNCTION

BRACHIAL AMYOTROPHY (PARSONAGE TURNER SYNDROME)

Introduction (139)
- Idiopathic more common than hereditary (autosomal dominant) by 10 times
  - Incidence: rare disease, 1 to $4/10^5$ per year, but under-recognized. Recurrent up to 25%
  - M > F by 3:2, peak in second to third decades

History and physical examination
- Severe pain (usually numeric pain scale >7/10) at onset lasting days or weeks followed by rapid multifocal weakness, atrophy, and sensory loss
  - Frequently after antecedent event (flu like illness and medical or surgical procedure)
  - Duration of pain and weakness can last for years in 1/2 up to 2/3
- Physical examination
  - Scapular wining or droop, disrupted (often jerky) scapular motion (in abduction and downward movement), paradoxical breathing (with phrenic N involvement, ~7% in idiopathic)
  - Patchy sensory loss (often pinprick sensation than proprioception)
  - Commonly involved muscles (often patchy distribution): shoulder/scapular girdle muscle and anterior interosseous nerve (AIN) innervated muscles (OK sign: flexor pollicis longus (FPL) and flexor digitorum profundus and pronator quadratus, with possibly dull wrist pain)
  - Vasomotor instability in the forearm and hands (upto 15%)

Diagnosis
- Clinical diagnosis confirmed by electromyography (EMG) study
- Nerve conduction study and needle EMG in 3 to 4 weeks after the onset of symptoms
  - Motor and sensory symptoms: sensory symptoms are less severe than sensory nerve conduction study (SNCS) abnormality
  - Abnormal SNCS: study as many nerves as possible
    - Lateral antebrachial cutaneous N in 80%
  - Motor nerve conduction study (MNCS) and needle EMG
    - Normal routine median/ulnar NCS (especially in upper/middle trunk lesion)
    - Brachial plexus study (proximal muscle MNCS): biceps, deltoid, and infraspinatus muscle recording with Erb's point stimulation, check site-to-site amplitude (decreased in axonal lesion). Phrenic nerve study (especially in hereditary involved in 14% vs idiopathic 7%)
    - AIN study recording at FPL or pronator quadratus
    - Needle EMG (if axonal segment involved)
      – Upper plexus: periscapular/peri-humeral muscles (71%) and long thoracic N (50%)
      – Lower plexus: more commonly involved in women (23%) than men (11%)
  - Hereditary form: common involvement outside brachial plexus (56%), related to SEPT9 gene
  - One-third: bilateral, but asymmetrical in severity; check contralateral side
- Differential diagnosis
  - Neurogenic
    - Cervical radiculopathy: sensory and motor in same root level, normal SNCS
    - Mononeuritis: asymmetric involvement, subacute, progressive, often difficult to distinguish
    - Multifocal motor neuropathy: no sensory symptoms, distal predominant, progressive, + anti GM1 Ab
    - Brachial amyotrophic diplegia (no sensory symptoms, painless, and progressive)
    - Hereditary neuropathy with liability to pressure palsies: Often painless, can resolve rapidly, concomitant entrapment neuropathy, polyneuropathy in elderly patients. A/D, PMP gene deletion in chromosome 17
  - Secondary brachial plexopathy

ETIOLOGY	CHARACTERISTICS
Trauma	Temporal relation with trauma (immediate onset > gradual), force direction predicts damage localization
Post radiation	Usually 2–10 years after radiation, slowly progressive, prominent paresthesia, myokymia in needle EMG (not pathognomonic finding)
Post sternotomy or thoracotomy	Immediately after surgery, lower trunk, usually resolves in weeks to months
Neurogenic TOS	Painless wasting of thenar > hypothenar muscles, slowly progressive hyperesthesia in the medial forearm (medial antebrachial cutaneous N) as T1 > C8
Peripheral N tumor	Gradual onset, usually slowly progressive
Pancoast tumor	Insidious onset, progressive pain, lower plexus initially to middle and upper, and Horner syndrome

  ○ MSK disease: rotator cuff syndrome, adhesive capsulitis, and complex regional pain syndrome

Treatment
- Pain management: long-acting NSAID (diclofenac) and opioid analgesic (eg, morphine SR 10–30 mg bid) for acute pain and second phase pain/neuropathic pain: gabapentin, carbamazepine, or amitriptyline
- Therapeutic exercise: scapular stabilization exercise and gradual strengthening (cautious/strengthening weak muscles)
- Education (tucking arm and hand in a coat pocket), sling (hemi-sling), and scapular brace (usually poor compliance)
- Injection: subacromial/subdeltoid or GH joint for adjuvant pain control

CERVICAL RADICULOPATHY

Check spine section
Especially C5–6 radiculopathy

STINGER SYNDROME (BURNER)

Introduction (140,141)
- Common in sports (50%–65% of college football players throughout 4 years), MVA, or other trauma
  ○ Mostly self limited
- Mechanisms
  ○ Extension-induced compression of C5–6 root in neural foramen (similar to Spurling test)
  ○ Mild stretch injury to upper trunk: head forced away from the symptomatic side with ipsilateral shoulder depression
  ○ Compression of the plexus (Erb's point) between the shoulder pad and superomedial scapula in football player

History and physical examination
- Unilateral shoulder pain with paresthesia radiating into the arm (shakes up) ± weakness
  ○ Symptoms resolve within a few minutes most of the time (5%–10% lasting hours)
- Physical examination; usually normal
  ○ Cervical ROM (usually normal), Spurling maneuver (for cervical radiculopathy), and Adson's maneuver (thoracic outlet syndrome; not specific)
  ○ Motor (shoulder external rotator, deltoid, biceps)/sensory/DTR: usually normal

Diagnosis
- Clinical diagnosis
- Diagnostic test: EMG
  ○ Consider if symptoms >2 to 3 weeks
  ○ Usually neurapraxia, focal demyelination (normal NCS, needle EMG usually normal with possibly decreased recruitment), or mixed lesion
  ○ SNCS of lateral antebrachial cutaneous N, radial N to the thumb, median N to the index finger: abnormal if axonal lesion (normal in neurapraxic lesion)
  ○ MNCS of axillary, musculocutaneous, suprascapular, and long thoracic N: usually normal
  ○ Needle EMG: C5–6 root (if paraspinal M involved) versus upper trunk
- Differential diagnosis: spinal cord injury (cervical cord neurapraxia), cervical radiculopathy, idiopathic brachial plexopathy, peripheral nerve injuries, or MSK injuries

Treatment
- Symptomatic treatment (AAP, NSAIDs) and rest from sports activity
- Return to play
  ○ Resolution of symptom (especially radiating arm pain), normal neuro-examination (normal strength), and full pain-free cervical ROM
- Prevention
  ○ Strengthening exercise of neck and shoulder
  ○ Proper sports equipment: high profile shoulder pads (limiting the extent of lateral flexion and extension) ± neck rolls, lifter, and cowboy collar

THORACIC OUTLET SYNDROME (TOS)

Introduction (142)
- Epidemiology
  ○ Prevalence of true neurogenic TOS: 1/million (very rare)
  ○ Nonspecific or vascular thoracic outlet syndrome; more common, young to middle age women
- Classification
  ○ Neurogenic (true vs nonspecific), vascular (arterial or venous), neurovascular and MSK (nonspecific; MC)
  ○ True neurogenic: prominent motor involvement, axonal lesion, involves T1 more than C8 innervated muscles
- Location of compression (in the figure)
  ○ Between the anterior and middle scalene, between clavicle and 1st rib, and between pectoralis minor and rib cages (Figure 3.8)
  ○ Cervical rib: 0.5% to 2% of population

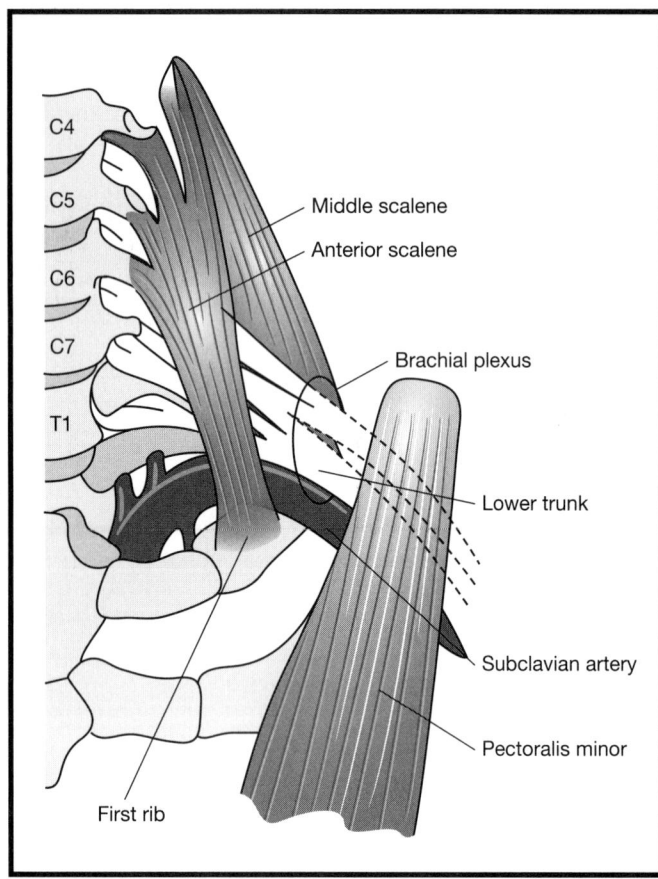

FIGURE 3.8
Location of compression in thoracic outlet syndrome: between anterior and middle scalene, between clavicle (removed in this picture) and first rib, and under the pectoralis minor muscle.
Source: Adapted from Refs. (7) and (143).

History and physical examination
- Pain and paresthesia along the medial aspect of forearm and hand with reduced dexterity
  - Shoulder pain: typically not significant
- Physical examination
  - Provocation test; Adson's, Roo's, and Wright maneuver
  - Abnormal sensory and motor examination in true neurogenic thoracic outlet syndrome
    - Weakness and atrophy in thenar eminence more than intrinsic hand muscle (and hypothenar muscles)
    - Decreased sensation in the medial forearm (medial antebrachial cutaneous N) and in ulnar N distribution

Diagnosis
- Clinical diagnosis confirmed by EMG (for true neurogenic TOS) and vascular study (vascular TOS)
- Nerve conduction study and needle EMG for true neurogenic TOS: axonal lesion in the medial cord and lower trunk brachial plexus
  - SNCS
    - Decreased or absent amplitude in the medial antebrachial cutaneous N and ulnar N (C8/ T1, lower trunk, medial cord) and normal median SNCS (C6/7, upper/ middle trunk, lateral cord)
  - Motor NCS: decreased amplitude in median > ulnar innervated muscles (T1 more involved than C8)
  - Needle EMG: abnormal spontaneous activity (ASA; fibrillation potential)/reduced recruitment in lower trunk innervated muscles (first dorsal interosseous [FDI], abductor pollicis brevis [APB], flexor carpi ulnaris [FCU], extensor indicis [EI]), with normal paraspinal M
  - Differential diagnosis: motor neuron disease, C8-T1 radiculopathy, brachial plexopathy (lower trunk, medial cord), and mononeuropathy (median neuropathy and/or ulnar neuropathy).
- Vascular study, US (144), and MRA (145): low yield usually
- X-ray of chest: fibrous band extending from either an anomalous cervical rib or an abnormally elongated C7 transverse process (cervical rib, 0.5%–2% prevalence, left more common than right)

Treatment
- PT for nonspecific TOS: posture education, myofascial release of scalene muscle, and modality
  - Trigger point injection to scalene muscle (US guidance to avoid brachial plexus injury located between scalene anterior and medius)
- Referral to surgery for true neurological TOS for surgical sectioning of the fibrous band, first rib resection, and scalenectomy

EFFORT THROMBOSIS (PAGET–SCHROETTER SYNDROME)

Introduction (146)
- Spontaneous venous thrombosis of the subclavian–axillary vein associated with repetitive upper extremity activities
- Epidemiology: rare, 2 (1–4)% of all venous thrombosis
  - In young, healthy, and athletic individuals (eg, swimmers, weight lifters, or tennis players)
- Etiology
  - Compression by abnormal cervical ribs, the anterior scalene muscle, clavicle, costoclavicular ligament, subclavius muscle, and first rib
  - Positional occlusion with hyperabduction (late cocking of throwing, ABER)

History and physical examination
- The gradual onset of swelling of the extremity over 1 to 7 days, dull or aching
- Venous engorgement of the arm, discoloration, and mottling of skin, palpable axillary cord, paresthesias, and heaviness or tiredness of the arm
- Normal neurological examination
- Provocative test for thoracic outlet syndrome; may be positive

Diagnosis
- Clinical suspicion confirmed by venous study
- Venography: axillary or subclavian venous thromboses with possible collateralization and recanalization
- Hypercoagulability study with hematology consult

Treatment (146)
- Admit the patient: brief bed rest, elevation of the extremity, and anticoagulation therapy with anticoagulants (heparin or warfarin)
  - Transluminal thrombolytic therapy, followed by 3 months of anticoagulation therapy with warfarin
- Referral to vascular surgery or orthopedic surgery
  - Subsequent trans-axillary first rib resection and thoracic outlet decompression
- Return to activity usually by 1 year following the injury

AXILLARY ARTERY OCCLUSION

Introduction (147)
- Anatomy: the axillary artery is the continuation of the subclavian artery at the outer border of the first rib. Anatomically divided into three segments by pectoralis minor muscle
- Etiology: occlusion under pectoralis minor by compression or trauma
  - Overhead throwing: compression in the late cocking phase of throwing

History and physical examination
- Pain, tenderness over the pectoralis minor, claudication, fatigue, diminished distal pulses, cyanosis, and night pain
  - Feeling cold in the affected extremity
- Late sequel can include embolization to the digits
- Provocative tests, as described for TOS

Diagnosis
- Clinical suspicion confirmed by vascular study
- Cervical spine x-ray to rule out a cervical rib (elongated transverse process of C7)
- Vascular study: Doppler US and photoplethysmography
- An arteriogram in the provocative position (confirmatory test): thrombosis with complete occlusion of the axillary artery or an aneurysmal dilation of the artery

Treatment
- Nonoperative management if there is no occlusion, aneurysm, or embolization
  - Scapular stabilization exercise to maintain the patency of the costoclavicular triangle (anteriorly by middle third of clavicle, posteromedially by first rib, and posterolaterally by upper border of scapula)
- Referral for surgical intervention: thrombectomy, sympathectomy, segmental excision, a bypass procedure with a vascular graft (vein graft), and angioplasty

SUPRASCAPULAR NEUROPATHY

Introduction (148)
- Epidemiology: largely unknown in general population
  - Common in high-level overhead athletes; 13% to 33% in professional volleyball players
- Anatomy of suprascapular nerve
  - Has sensory afferent from CHL, AC ligament and joint, GH joint, and subacromial bursa ± cutaneous branch in proximal lateral arm (5/35 cadaver study)
- Etiology and risk factor
  - Sling effect: can be secondary to depression, retraction, and hyperabduction of the scapular
  - Repetitive overuse, trauma, iatrogenic cause, or microemboli
  - Traction neurapraxia and axonotmesis

History and physical examination
- Pain (often dull) in the posterior aspect of the shoulder ± subtle weakness
- Atrophy (easily visible spine of scapular), weakness (external rotation), tenderness and pain (reproduction of symptoms) on cross-arm adduction test
- Examination for cervical spine pathology: other C5–6 innervated muscles (deltoid, biceps) examination and sensation
- Shoulder impingement test: often positive (concomitant lesion)

Diagnosis
- Clinical suspicion confirmed with EMG
- EMG
  - Normal nerve conduction study (NCS) except MNCS recording at supra/infraspinatus with Erb's stimulation; check site-to-site comparison (not sensitive)
  - Needle EMG: ASA in the supraspinatus and infraspinatus but not deltoid (axillary N, posterior cord, C5/6) or biceps (musculocutaneous N, lateral cord, C5/6)
  - If only involving infraspinatus; the lesion is at spinoglenoid notch (after branching to supraspinatus M) versus suprascapular notch (involving both supra and infraspinatus)
- Imaging Study: US and MRI
  - US to evaluate the ganglion (paralabral) cyst, and fatty infiltration with atrophy of supra and infraspinatus muscles
    - Contrast between trapezius (normal) and supraspinatus muscle (abnormal) or between infraspinatus versus teres minor (unaffected because of axillary N innervation. Normal infraspinatus muscle approximately twice the size of the teres minor)
    - Spinoglenoid ganglion cyst vs vein dilatation: check the Doppler in vein and compressibility (ganglion usually not compressible, often difficult to check blood flow)
  - MRI/A: evaluation of labral lesion (underlying etiology of paralabral cyst), evaluation of rotator cuff tendon and intracortical structures.

Treatment
- Activity modification, scapular stabilization (in PT), and NSAID as needed
- Suprascapular nerve block for pain control at suprascapular notch or spinoglenoid notch (still medication migrates proximally)
  - Coronal plane with slight anterior tilt (parallel to scapular plane), needle away from the notch: decrease the risk of pneumothorax and brachial plexus block
  - US guidance: the concave shape of the floor: can be misinterpreted as suprascapular notch and fascia of the supraspinatus muscle can be misinterpreted by the suprascapular ligament
    - Block at the spinoglenoid fossa: may be effective as the injectate migrates proximally to suprascapular notch

- Aspiration and injection of ganglion cyst
  ○ Aspiration often technically difficult (even using large bore needle)
- Referral to surgery: release of suprascapular ligament, ganglion excision, endoscopic or open surgery

QUADRILATERAL SPACE SYNDROME (147)

Introduction (149)
- Compression of the axillary nerve and posterior circumflex artery within the quadrilateral space
- Unknown prevalence: very rare
  ○ Peak incidence in 20 to 40 years, active athletic population, and more in the dominant shoulder
- Anatomy: quadrilateral space bordered by teres minor, major, triceps (medial head), and lateral head/humerus (neck of humerus)
- Etiology
  ○ Abnormal fibrous bands and muscular hypertrophy, more common in abducted and externally rotated position such as in late cocking (during throwing)
  ○ Space occupying lesion (eg, paralabral cyst)

History and physical examination
- Vague shoulder pain and weakness in forward elevation and abduction
  ○ Often night pain, and decreased performance in throwing athletes
- Neurological examination
  ○ Deltoid weakness/atrophy and subtle weakness in shoulder external rotation (teres minor)
  ○ Normal elbow flexion, lateral forearm sensation, normal DTR
- Provocative test: forward flexion, ABER of the shoulder for 1 to 2 minutes
  ○ Negative Spurling test or test for thoracic outlet syndrome

Diagnosis
- Diagnosis of exclusion confirmed by EMG test and imaging study
- EMG
  ○ NCS usually normal (except deltoid MNCS stimulation at Erb's point, site-to-site comparison)
  ○ Needle EMG: ASA in the deltoid and teres minor muscle
- US
  ○ Evaluation of space-occupying lesion
  ○ Evaluation of deltoid and teres minor muscles for hyperechoic (fatty infiltration) and atrophy (compared to the normal infraspinatus M)
  ○ MRA and subclavian angiography (Seldinger technique): occlusion of posterior circumflex humeral artery in arm ABER position: high false positive
- Differential diagnosis
  ○ C 5–6 radiculopathy and brachial plexopathy: infraspinatus (suprascapular N, C5–6, upper trunk), biceps (musculocutaneous N, C5–6, lateral cord) affected in both conditions (clinically or needle EMG), cervical paraspinal needle EMG to differentiate in-between
  ○ Axillary neuropathy from shoulder dislocation or surgical neck fracture or figure of 8 harness
    ▪ Backpack paralysis: increased risk if ≥30 to 40 kg, compressed by pack or pad

Treatment
- Nonoperative treatment: activity modification, NSAIDs, and steroid injection
  ○ PT: stretching (horizontal adduction), soft tissue massage, and rotator cuff/deltoid muscle strengthening
- Surgery for decompression after failing a 3 to 6-month course of nonoperative treatment or referral if space-occupying lesion is found

REFERENCES

1. Pope DP, Croft PR, Pritchard CM, Silman AJ. Prevalence of shoulder pain in the community: the influence of case definition. *Ann Rheum Dis.* 1997;56(5):308–312.
2. Kjaer M, Krogsgaard M, Magnusson P, eds. *Textbook of Sports Medicine.* Oxford, UK: Wiley-Blackwell Publishing; 2002.
3. Pribicevic, M. The Epidemiology of Shoulder Pain: A Narrative Review of the Literature. In: Ghosh S, ed. *Pain in Perspective*; Rijeka, Croatia: Intech; 2012.
4. Page P. Shoulder muscle imbalance and subacromial impingement syndrome in overhead athletes. *Int J Sports Phys Ther.* 2011;6(1):51–58.
5. Shanahan EM, Sladek R. Shoulder pain at the workplace. *Best Pract Res Clin Rheumatol.* 2011;25(1):59–68.
6. Santavirta S, Konttinen YT, Antti-Poika I, Nordström D. Inflammation of the subacromial bursa in chronic shoulder pain. *Arch Orthop Trauma Surg.* 1992;111(6):336–340.
7. Goldstein B. Shoulder anatomy and biomechanics. *Phys Med Rehabil Clin N Am.* 2004;15(2):313–349.
8. House J, Mooradian A. Evaluation and management of shoulder pain in primary care clinics. *South Med J.* 2010;103(11):1129–35; quiz 1136.
9. Lazar MA, Kwon YW, Rokito AS. Snapping scapula syndrome. *J Bone Joint Surg Am.* 2009;91(9):2251–2262.
10. Chang WH, Im SH, Ryu JA, et al. The effects of scapulothoracic bursa injections in patients with scapular pain: a pilot study. *Arch Phys Med Rehabil.* 2009;90(2):279–284.
11. Gaskill T, Millett PJ. Snapping scapula syndrome: diagnosis and management. *J Am Acad Orthop Surg.* 2013;21(4):214–224.
12. Finnoff JT, Thompson JM, Collins M, Dahm D. Subcoracoid bursitis as an unusual cause of painful anterior shoulder snapping in a weight lifter. *Am J Sports Med.* 2010;38(8):1687–1692.
13. Laing PG. The arterial supply of the adult humerus. *J Bone Joint Surg Am.* 1956;38-A(5):1105–1116.
14. Martetschläger F, Warth RJ, Millett PJ. Instability and degenerative arthritis of the sternoclavicular joint: a current concepts review. *Am J Sports Med.* 2014;42(4):999–1007.
15. Prescher A. Anatomical basics, variations, and degenerative changes of the shoulder joint and shoulder girdle. *Eur J Radiol.* 2000;35(2):88–102.
16. Drakes S, Thomas S, Kim S, et al. Ultrasonography of subcoracoid bursal impingement syndrome. *PM R.* 2015;7(3):329–333.
17. Hunt SA, Kwon YW, Zuckerman JD. The rotator interval: anatomy, pathology, and strategies for treatment. *J Am Acad Orthop Surg.* 2007;15(4):218–227.
18. Lephart, SM, Halata Z, Baumann KL, Costantini A, Giacomo G, Ellenbecker TS. Neuromuscular Control and Proprioception of the Shoulder. In: Giacomo G, Pouliart N, Costantini A, Vita A, eds. *Atlas of Functional Shoulder Anatomy.* Milano, Italy: Springer Milan; 2008: 205–231.
19. Blum A, Lecocq S, Louis M, et al. The nerves around the shoulder. *Eur J Radiol.* 2013;82(1):2–16.
20. Machida A, Sugamoto K, Miyamoto T, et al. Adhesion of the subacromial bursa may cause subacromial impingement in patients with rotator cuff tears: pressure measurements in 18 patients. *Acta Orthop Scand.* 2004;75(1):109–113.
21. Lewis JS. Rotator cuff tendinopathy. *Br J Sports Med.* 2009;43(4):236–241.
22. Drakes S, Thomas S, Kim S, et al. Ultrasonography of subcoracoid bursal impingement syndrome. *PM R.* 2015;7(3):329–333.

23. Manske RC, Reiman MP, Stovak ML. Nonoperative and operative management of snapping scapula. *Am J Sports Med*. 2004;32(6):1554–1565.
24. Kuhn JE, Hawkins RJ. Evaluation and treatment of scapular disorders. In: Warner JJ, Iannotti JP, Gerber C. *Complex and Revision Problems in Shoulder Surgery*. Philadelphia: Lippincott-Raven, 1997: 357–376.
25. Halder AM, Itoi E, An KN. Anatomy and biomechanics of the shoulder. *Orthop Clin North Am*. 2000;31(2):159–176.
26. Struyf F, Nijs J, Baeyens JP, et al. Scapular positioning and movement in unimpaired shoulders, shoulder impingement syndrome, and glenohumeral instability. *Scand J Med Sci Sports*. 2011;21(3):352–358.
27. Kibler WB. Scapular involvement in impingement: signs and symptoms. *Instr Course Lect*. 2006;55:35–43.
28. Lo IK, Burkhart SS. The etiology and assessment of subscapularis tendon tears: a case for subcoracoid impingement, the roller-wringer effect, and TUFF lesions of the subscapularis. *Arthroscopy*. 2003;19(10):1142–1150.
29. Wilk KE, Macrina LC, Arrigo C. 12 - Shoulder Rehabilitation. In: Wilk JRALHE , ed. *Physical Rehabilitation of the Injured Athlete*. 4th ed. Philadelphia, PA: W.B. Saunders; 2012:190–231.
30. Firestein GS, Budd RC, Gabriel SE, et al. *Kelley's Textbook of Rheumatology*. 9th ed. Philadelphia, PA: Elsevier; 2012.
31. Namdari S, Yagnik G, Ebaugh DD, et al. Defining functional shoulder range of motion for activities of daily living. *J Shoulder Elbow Surg*. 2012;21(9):1177–1183.
32. Schultz JS. Clinical evaluation of the shoulder. *Phys Med Rehabil Clin N Am*. 2004;15(2):351–371.
33. Park HB, Yokota A, Gill HS, et al. Diagnostic accuracy of clinical tests for the different degrees of subacromial impingement syndrome. *J Bone Joint Surg Am*. 2005;87(7):1446–1455.
34. Kessel L, Watson M. The painful arc syndrome. Clinical classification as a guide to management. *J Bone Joint Surg Br*. 1977;59(2):166–172.
35. Speer KP, Hannafin JA, Altchek DW, Warren RF. An evaluation of the shoulder relocation test. *Am J Sports Med*. 1994;22(2):177–183.
36. McFarland EG, Campbell G, McDowell J. Posterior shoulder laxity in asymptomatic athletes. *Am J Sports Med*. 1996;24(4):468–471.
37. Farber AJ, Castillo R, Clough M, et al. Clinical assessment of three common tests for traumatic anterior shoulder instability. *J Bone Joint Surg Am*. 2006;88(7):1467–1474.
38. Burkhart SS, Morgan CD, Kibler WB. Shoulder injuries in overhead athletes. The "dead arm" revisited. *Clin Sports Med*. 2000;19(1):125–158.
39. O'Brien SJ, Pagnani MJ, Fealy S, et al. The active compression test: a new and effective test for diagnosing labral tears and acromioclavicular joint abnormality. *Am J Sports Med*. 1998;26(5):610–613.
40. Kibler WB. Specificity and sensitivity of the anterior slide test in throwing athletes with superior glenoid labral tears. *Arthroscopy*. 1995;11(3):296–300.
41. Liu SH, Henry MH, Nuccion S, et al. Diagnosis of glenoid labral tears. A comparison between magnetic resonance imaging and clinical examinations. *Am J Sports Med*. 1996;24(2):149–154.
42. Kim SH, Park JS, Jeong WK, Shin SK. The Kim test: a novel test for posteroinferior labral lesion of the shoulder–a comparison to the jerk test. *Am J Sports Med*. 2005;33(8):1188–1192.
43. Calis M, Akgün K, Birtane M, et al. Diagnostic values of clinical diagnostic tests in subacromial impingement syndrome. *Ann Rheum Dis*. 2000;59(1):44–47.
44. Walton J, Mahajan S, Paxinos A, et al. Diagnostic values of tests for acromioclavicular joint pain. *J Bone Joint Surg Am*. 2004;86-A(4):807–812.
45. Hébert LJ, Moffet H, McFadyen BJ, Dionne CE. Scapular behavior in shoulder impingement syndrome. *Arch Phys Med Rehabil*. 2002;83(1):60–69.
46. Kibler WB, Sciascia A. Current concepts: scapular dyskinesis. *Br J Sports Med*. 2010;44(5):300–305.
47. Eustace JA, Brophy DP, Gibney RP, et al. Comparison of the accuracy of steroid placement with clinical outcome in patients with shoulder symptoms. *Ann Rheum Dis*. 1997;56(1):59–63.
48. Daley EL, Bajaj S, Bisson LJ, Cole BJ. Improving injection accuracy of the elbow, knee, and shoulder: does injection site and imaging make a difference? A systematic review. *Am J Sports Med*. 2011;39(3):656–662.
49. Harrison AK, Flatow EL. Subacromial impingement syndrome. *J Am Acad Orthop Surg*. 2011;19(11):701–708.
50. Chang WK. Shoulder impingement syndrome. *Phys Med Rehabil Clin N Am*. 2004;15(2):493–510.
51. Umer M, Qadir I, Azam M. Subacromial impingement syndrome. *Orthop Rev (Pavia)*. 2012;4(2):e18.
52. van der Windt DA, Koes BW, de Jong BA, Bouter LM. Shoulder disorders in general practice: incidence, patient characteristics, and management. *Ann Rheum Dis*. 1995;54(12):959–964.
53. Gasparre G, Fusaro I, Galletti S, et al. Effectiveness of ultrasound-guided injections combined with shoulder exercises in the treatment of subacromial adhesive bursitis. *Musculoskelet Surg*. 2012;96 Suppl 1:S57–S61.
54. Saeed A, Khan M, Morrissey S, et al. Impact of outpatient clinic ultrasound imaging in the diagnosis and treatment for shoulder impingement: a randomized prospective study. *Rheumatol Int*. 2014;34(4):503–509.
55. Daghir AA, Sookur PA, Shah S, Watson M. Dynamic ultrasound of the subacromial-subdeltoid bursa in patients with shoulder impingement: a comparison with normal volunteers. *Skeletal Radiol*. 2012;41(9):1047–1053.
56. Bureau NJ, Beauchamp M, Cardinal E, Brassard P. Dynamic sonography evaluation of shoulder impingement syndrome. *AJR Am J Roentgenol*. 2006;187(1):216–220.
57. Morrison DS, Greenbaum BS, Einhorn A. Shoulder impingement. *Orthop Clin North Am*. 2000;31(2):285–293.
58. Freehill MQ. Coracoid impingement: diagnosis and treatment. *J Am Acad Orthop Surg*. 2011;19(4):191–197.
59. Paulson MM, Watnik NF, Dines DM. Coracoid impingement syndrome, rotator interval reconstruction, and biceps tenodesis in the overhead athlete. *Orthop Clin North Am*. 2001;32(3): 485–93, ix.
60. Arrigoni, P, Brady PC, Burkhart SS. Calcific tendonitis of the subscapularis tendon causing subcoracoid stenosis and coracoid impingement. *Arthroscopy*. 2006;22(10):1139 e1–1139 e3.
61. Heyworth BE, Williams RJ 3rd. Internal impingement of the shoulder. *Am J Sports Med*. 2009;37(5):1024–1037.
62. Beltran LS, Nikac V, Beltran J. Internal impingement syndromes. *Magn Reson Imaging Clin N Am*. 2012;20(2):201–11, ix.
63. Meister K, Buckley B, Batts J. The posterior impingement sign: diagnosis of rotator cuff and posterior labral tears secondary to internal impingement in overhand athletes. *Am J Orthop*. 2004;33(8):412–415.
64. Matava MJ, Purcell DB, Rudzki JR. Partial-thickness rotator cuff tears. *Am J Sports Med*. 2005;33(9):1405–1417.
65. Tashjian RZ. Epidemiology, natural history, and indications for treatment of rotator cuff tears. *Clin Sports Med*. 2012;31(4):589–604.
66. Kuhn JE. Current concepts: rotator cuff pathology in athletes–a source of pain or adaptive pathology? *Curr Sports Med Rep*. 2013;12(5):311–315.
67. Rineer CA, Ruch DS. Elbow tendinopathy and tendon ruptures: epicondylitis, biceps and triceps ruptures. *J Hand Surg Am*. 2009;34(3):566–576.
68. Sipola P, Niemitukia L, Kröger H, et al. Detection and quantification of rotator cuff tears with ultrasonography and magnetic resonance imaging - a prospective study in 77 consecutive patients with a surgical reference. *Ultrasound Med Biol*. 2010;36(12):1981–1989.
69. Chiou HJ, Chou YH, Wu JJ, et al. Evaluation of calcific tendonitis of the rotator cuff: role of color Doppler ultrasonography. *J Ultrasound Med*. 2002;21(3):289–95; quiz 296.
70. Strobel K, Hodler J, Meyer DC, et al. Fatty atrophy of supraspinatus and infraspinatus muscles: accuracy of US. *Radiology*. 2005;237(2):584–589.
71. Gerber C, Wirth SH, Farshad M. Treatment options for massive rotator cuff tears. *J Shoulder Elbow Surg*. 2011;20(2 Suppl):S20–S29.
72. Hurt G, Baker CL Jr. Calcific tendinitis of the shoulder. *Orthop Clin North Am*. 2003;34(4):567–575.
73. Speed CA, Hazleman BL. Calcific tendinitis of the shoulder. *N Engl J Med*. 1999;340(20):1582–1584.
74. Lerais, J-M, Sarliève P, Hadjidekov G, Riboud C, Kastler B. Aspiration and Lavage of Calcific Shoulder Tendinitis. In: Kastler, B, Barral F-G, Fergane B, Pereira P, eds. *Interventional Radiology in Pain Treatment*, Berlin Heidelberg : Springer; 2007: 145–154.

75. Bureau NJ. Calcific tendinopathy of the shoulder. *Semin Musculoskelet Radiol*. 2013;17(1):80–84.
76. Sethi N, Wright R, Yamaguchi K. Disorders of the long head of the biceps tendon. *J Shoulder Elbow Surg*. 1999;8(6):644–654.
77. Paynter KS. Disorders of the long head of the biceps tendon. *Phys Med Rehabil Clin N Am*. 2004;15(2):511–528.
78. Murthi AM, Vosburgh CL, Neviaser TJ. The incidence of pathologic changes of the long head of the biceps tendon. *J Shoulder Elbow Surg*. 2000;9(5):382–385.
79. Stevens K, Kwak A, Poplawski S. The biceps muscle from shoulder to elbow. *Semin Musculoskelet Radiol*. 2012;16(4):296–315.
80. Beall DP, Williamson EE, Ly JQ, et al. Association of biceps tendon tears with rotator cuff abnormalities: degree of correlation with tears of the anterior and superior portions of the rotator cuff. *AJR Am J Roentgenol*. 2003;180(3):633–639.
81. Ahrens PM, Boileau P. The long head of biceps and associated tendinopathy. *J Bone Joint Surg Br*. 2007;89(8):1001–1009.
82. Haley CA, Zacchilli MA. Pectoralis major injuries: evaluation and treatment. *Clin Sports Med*. 2014;33(4):739–756.
83. Bhatia DN, de Beer JF, van Rooyen KS, et al. The "bench-presser's shoulder": an overuse insertional tendinopathy of the pectoralis minor muscle. *Br J Sports Med*. 2007;41(8):e11.
84. Simovitch R, Sanders B, Ozbaydar M, et al. Acromioclavicular joint injuries: diagnosis and management. *J Am Acad Orthop Surg*. 2009;17(4):207–219.
85. Ernberg LA, Potter HG. Radiographic evaluation of the acromioclavicular and sternoclavicular joints. *Clin Sports Med*. 2003;22(2):255–275.
86. Kim AC, Matcuk G, Patel D, et al. Acromioclavicular joint injuries and reconstructions: a review of expected imaging findings and potential complications. *Emerg Radiol*. 2012;19(5):399–413.
87. Rios CG, Mazzocca AD. Acromioclavicular joint problems in athletes and new methods of management. *Clin Sports Med*. 2008;27(4):763–788.
88. Mall NA, Foley E, Chalmers PN, et al. Degenerative joint disease of the acromioclavicular joint: a review. *Am J Sports Med*. 2013;41(11):2684–2692.
89. Menge TJ, Boykin RE, Bushnell BD, Byram IR. Acromioclavicular osteoarthritis: a common cause of shoulder pain. *South Med J*. 2014;107(5):324–329.
90. Schwarzkopf R, Ishak C, Elman M, et al. Distal clavicular osteolysis: a review of the literature. *Bull NYU Hosp Jt Dis*. 2008;66(2):94–101.
91. Scavenius M, Iversen BF, Stürup J. Resection of the lateral end of the clavicle following osteolysis, with emphasis on non-traumatic osteolysis of the acromial end of the clavicle in athletes. *Injury*. 1987;18(4):261–263.
92. Neviaser AS, Hannafin JA. Adhesive capsulitis: a review of current treatment. *Am J Sports Med*. 2010;38(11):2346–2356.
93. Homsi C, Bordalo-Rodrigues M, da Silva JJ, Stump XM. Ultrasound in adhesive capsulitis of the shoulder: is assessment of the coracohumeral ligament a valuable diagnostic tool? *Skeletal Radiol*. 2006;35(9):673–678.
94. Buchbinder, R, Green S, Youd JM, et al., Oral steroids for adhesive capsulitis. *Cochrane Database Syst Rev*, 2006(4): CD006189.
95. Koh ES, Chung SG, Kim TU, Kim HC. Changes in biomechanical properties of glenohumeral joint capsules with adhesive capsulitis by repeated capsule-preserving hydraulic distensions with saline solution and corticosteroid. *PM R*. 2012;4(12):976–984.
96. Ahn K, Lee YJ, Kim EH, et al. Interventional microadhesiolysis: a new nonsurgical release technique for adhesive capsulitis of the shoulder. *BMC Musculoskelet Disord*. 2008;9:12.
97. Ecklund KJ, Lee TQ, Tibone J, Gupta R. Rotator cuff tear arthropathy. *J Am Acad Orthop Surg*. 2007;15(6):340–349.
98. Macaulay AA, Greiwe RM, Bigliani LU. Rotator cuff deficient arthritis of the glenohumeral joint. *Clin Orthop Surg*. 2010;2(4):196–202.
99. Reineck JR, Krishnan SG, Burkhead WZ. Early glenohumeral arthritis in the competing athlete. *Clin Sports Med*. 2008;27(4):803–819.
100. Oh JH, Chung SW, Oh CH, et al. The prevalence of shoulder osteoarthritis in the elderly Korean population: association with risk factors and function. *J Shoulder Elbow Surg*. 2011;20(5):756–763.
101. Flatow EL, Warner JI. Instability of the shoulder: complex problems and failed repairs: Part I. Relevant biomechanics, multidirectional instability, and severe glenoid loss. *Instr Course Lect*. 1998;47:97–112.
102. Thangarajah T, Lambert S. Management of the unstable shoulder. *BMJ*. 2015;350:h2537.
103. Rowe CR, Zarins B. Recurrent transient subluxation of the shoulder. *J Bone Joint Surg Am*. 1981;63(6):863–872.
104. Simão MN, Nogueira-Barbosa MH, Muglia VF, Barbieri CH. Anterior shoulder instability: correlation between magnetic resonance arthrography, ultrasound arthrography and intraoperative findings. *Ultrasound Med Biol*. 2012;38(4):551–560.
105. Patel RM, Amin NH, Lynch TS, Miniaci A. Management of bone loss in glenohumeral instability. *Orthop Clin North Am*. 2014;45(4):523–539.
106. Tonino PM, Gerber C, Itoi E, et al. Complex shoulder disorders: evaluation and treatment. *J Am Acad Orthop Surg*. 2009;17(3):125–136.
107. McCarty EC, Ritchie P, Gill HS, McFarland EG. Shoulder instability: return to play. *Clin Sports Med*. 2004;23(3):335–51, vii.
108. Schaeffeler C, Waldt S, Bauer JS, et al. MR arthrography including abduction and external rotation images in the assessment of atraumatic multidirectional instability of the shoulder. *Eur Radiol*. 2014;24(6):1376–1385.
109. Warby SA, Pizzari T, Ford JJ, et al. The effect of exercise-based management for multidirectional instability of the glenohumeral joint: a systematic review. *J Shoulder Elbow Surg*. 2014;23(1):128–142.
110. Modarresi S, Motamedi D, Jude CM. Superior labral anteroposterior lesions of the shoulder: part 1, anatomy and anatomic variants. *AJR Am J Roentgenol*. 2011;197(3):596–603.
111. Harwood MI, Smith CT. Superior labrum, anterior-posterior lesions and biceps injuries: diagnostic and treatment considerations. *Prim Care*. 2004;31(4):831–855.
112. Bedi A, Allen AA. Superior labral lesions anterior to posterior-evaluation and arthroscopic management. *Clin Sports Med*. 2008;27(4):607–630.
113. Abrams GD, Safran MR. Diagnosis and management of superior labrum anterior posterior lesions in overhead athletes. *Br J Sports Med*. 2010;44(5):311–318.
114. Keener JD, Brophy RH. Superior labral tears of the shoulder: pathogenesis, evaluation, and treatment. *J Am Acad Orthop Surg*. 2009;17(10):627–637.
115. Wright RW, Paletta GA Jr. Prevalence of the Bennett lesion of the shoulder in major league pitchers. *Am J Sports Med*. 2004;32(1):121–124.
116. Chen AL, Joseph TN, Zuckerman JD. Rheumatoid arthritis of the shoulder. *J Am Acad Orthop Surg*. 2003;11(1):12–24.
117. Scott DL, Wolfe F, Huizinga TW. Rheumatoid arthritis. *Lancet*. 2010;376(9746):1094–1108.
118. Klein-Wieringa IR, Kloppenburg M, Bastiaansen-Jenniskens YM, et al. The infrapatellar fat pad of patients with osteoarthritis has an inflammatory phenotype. *Ann Rheum Dis*. 2011;70(5):851–857.
119. Sommer OJ, Kladosek A, Weiler V, et al. Rheumatoid arthritis: a practical guide to state-of-the-art imaging, image interpretation, and clinical implications. *Radiographics*. 2005;25(2):381–398.
120. Curran JF, Ellman MH, Brown NL. Rheumatologic aspects of painful conditions affecting the shoulder. *Clin Orthop Relat Res*. 1983;(173):27–37.
121. Halverson PB. Crystal deposition disease of the shoulder (including calcific tendonitis and milwaukee shoulder syndrome). *Curr Rheumatol Rep*. 2003;5(3):244–247.
122. Nadarajah CV, Weichert I. Milwaukee shoulder syndrome. *Case Rep Rheumatol*. 2014;2014:458708.
123. Alpay N, Artim-Esen B, Kamali S, et al. Amyloid arthropathy mimicking seronegative rheumatoid arthritis in multiple myeloma: case reports and review of the literature. *Amyloid*. 2009;16(4):226–231.
124. Katoh N, Tazawa K, Ishii W, et al. Systemic AL amyloidosis mimicking rheumatoid arthritis. *Intern Med*. 2008;47(12):1133–1138.
125. Hickling P, Wilkins M, Newman GR, et al. A study of amyloid arthropathy in multiple myeloma. *Q J Med*. 1981;50(200):417–433.
126. Lossos IS, Yossepowitch O, Kandel L, et al. Septic arthritis of the glenohumeral joint. A report of 11 cases and review of the literature. *Medicine (Baltimore)*. 1998;77(3):177–187.
127. Horowitz DL, Katzap E, Horowitz S, Barilla-LaBarca ML. Approach to septic arthritis. *Am Fam Physician*. 2011;84(6):653–660.
128. Smith BG, Cruz AI Jr, Milewski MD, Shapiro ED. Lyme disease and the orthopaedic implications of lyme arthritis. *J Am Acad Orthop Surg*. 2011;19(2):91–100.

129. Gruson KI, Kwon YW. Atraumatic osteonecrosis of the humeral head. *Bull NYU Hosp Jt Dis*. 2009;67(1):6–14.
130. Harreld KL, Marker DR, Wiesler ER, et al. Osteonecrosis of the humeral head. *J Am Acad Orthop Surg*. 2009;17(6):345–355.
131. Osbahr, DC, Kim HJ, Dugas J.R. Little league shoulder. *Curr Opin Pediatr*. 2010;22(1): 35–40.
132. Sewell MD, Al-Hadithy N, Le Leu A, Lambert SM. Instability of the sternoclavicular joint: current concepts in classification, treatment and outcomes. *Bone Joint J*. 2013;95-B(6):721–731.
133. Groh GI, Wirth MA. Management of traumatic sternoclavicular joint injuries. *J Am Acad Orthop Surg*. 2011;19(1):1–7.
134. Melvin JS, Boselli K, Huffman GR. Fractures of the Shoulder and Elbow.In: Pignolo JR, Keenan MA, Hebela NM, eds. *Fractures in the Elderly*. Totowa, NJ: Humana Press; 2011: 187–223.
135. Lapner PC, Uhthoff HK, Papp S. Scapula fractures. *Orthop Clin North Am*. 2008;39(4):459–74, vi.
136. Pecci M, Kreher JB. Clavicle fractures. *Am Fam Physician*. 2008;77(1):65–70.
137. Gregory PL, Biswas AC, Batt ME. Musculoskeletal problems of the chest wall in athletes. *Sports Med*. 2002;32(4):235–250.
138. Sakellaridis T, Stamatelopoulos A, Andrianopoulos E, Kormas P. Isolated first rib fracture in athletes. *Br J Sports Med*. 2004; 38(3):e5.
139. van Alfen N. The neuralgic amyotrophy consultation. *J Neurol*. 2007;254(6):695–704.
140. Shannon B, Klimkiewicz JJ. Cervical burners in the athlete. *Clin Sports Med*. 2002;21(1):29–35, vi.
141. Aval SM, Durand P Jr, Shankwiler JA. Neurovascular injuries to the athlete's shoulder: Part I. *J Am Acad Orthop Surg*. 2007;15(4):249–256.
142. Ferrante MA. The thoracic outlet syndromes. *Muscle Nerve*. 2012;45(6):780–795.
143. Lasanianos NG, Panteli M. SLAP Lesions. In: Lasanianos GN, Kanakaris KN, Giannoudis, VP, eds. *Trauma and Orthopaedic Classifications: A Comprehensive Overview*. London, UK: Springer London; 2015:33–36.
144. Gillard J, Pérez-Cousin M, Hachulla E, et al. Diagnosing thoracic outlet syndrome: contribution of provocative tests, ultrasonography, electrophysiology, and helical computed tomography in 48 patients. *Joint Bone Spine*. 2001;68(5):416–424.
145. Sanders RJ, Hammond SL, Rao NM. Diagnosis of thoracic outlet syndrome. *J Vasc Surg*. 2007;46(3):601–604.
146. Hendrickson CD, Godek A, Schmidt P. Paget-Schroetter syndrome in a collegiate football player. *Clin J Sport Med*. 2006;16(1):79–80.
147. Aval SM, Durand P Jr, Shankwiler JA. Neurovascular injuries to the athlete's shoulder: part II. *J Am Acad Orthop Surg*. 2007;15(5):281–289.
148. Cummins CA, Messer TM, Nuber GW. Suprascapular nerve entrapment. *J Bone Joint Surg Am*. 2000;82(3):415–424.
149. Hoskins WT, Pollard HP, McDonald AJ. Quadrilateral space syndrome: a case study and review of the literature. *Br J Sports Med*. 2005;39(2):e9.

CHAPTER 4

Elbow

EPIDEMIOLOGY OF ELBOW PAIN

ELBOW PAIN IN THE GENERAL POPULATION

Prevalence and common causes
- 7% in 40 to 50 years of age to 14% in people older than 50 years
- Common underlying causes: overuse or trauma (strain, sprain, fracture, and dislocation)

Lateral elbow
- Most common (MC) location for elbow pain
- Prevalence: 1% to 3% in adults of working age (MC cause: epicondylitis)

ELBOW PAIN IN ATHLETES

Prevalence and common causes
- 25% of all injuries in sports occur in the elbow, forearm, and wrist
- Single-stress injury usually caused by contact sports such as football and wrestling
- Repetitive injury: common in tennis (epicondylitis is seen in up to 50% of players, but not necessarily from sports), bowling, cross-country skiing, rowing, and gymnastics
- Highest rate of pediatric elbow injuries occurs in baseball, tennis, and gymnastics

Medial elbow: MC location of elbow pain in young athletes (especially throwing athletes)

ELBOW PAIN AT WORK (1)

Musculoskeletal (MSK) disorders of the elbow
- Usually related to occupational ergonomic stressors
- Ergonomic stressors: repetitive and stereotyped motions, forceful exertions, non-neutral postures, vibrations, or combinations of these exposures (2)

Epicondylitis
- Higher in at-risk industry (up to 29%) than in general population (prevalence: 5%) (3)
- Prevalence varies: 8.9% in meat cutters, ~15% in fish-processing-industry workers
- Risk factors: repetitive movement of hands or wrists, handling loads >5 kg, activities demanding high hand grip forces and the use of vibrating tools

Ulnar neuropathy at elbow (cubital tunnel syndrome)
- More commonly seen in workers who perform repetitive motions, commonly flexed at elbow and directly leaning on elbow (eg, driver)
- Prevalence: 2.8% in workers with repetitive work to 6.8% in floor cleaners

DIFFERENTIAL DIAGNOSIS

MSK and neuropathic causes of elbow pain based on location are listed as follows (4) (Flowchart 4.1 and Figure 4.1):

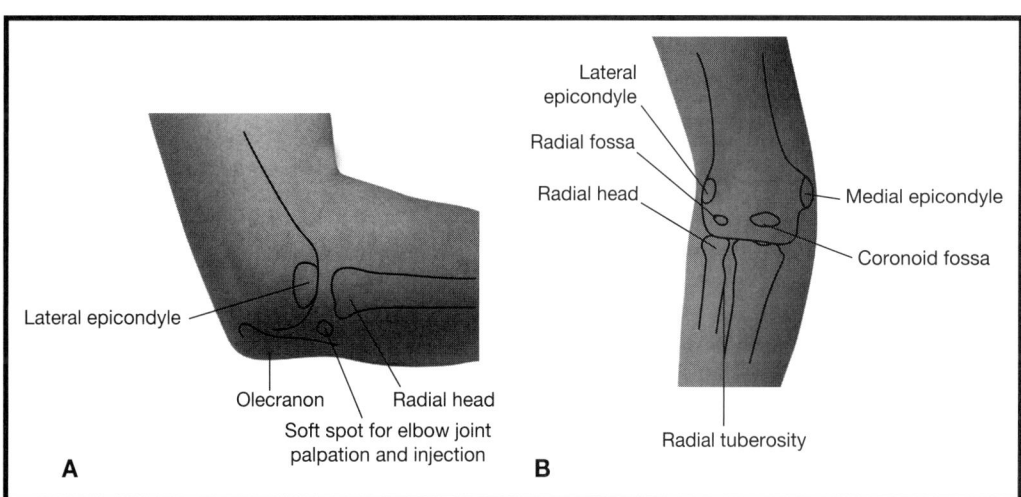

FIGURE 4.1
Surface anatomy of the elbow (A) anterior and (B) posterior views of the elbow.

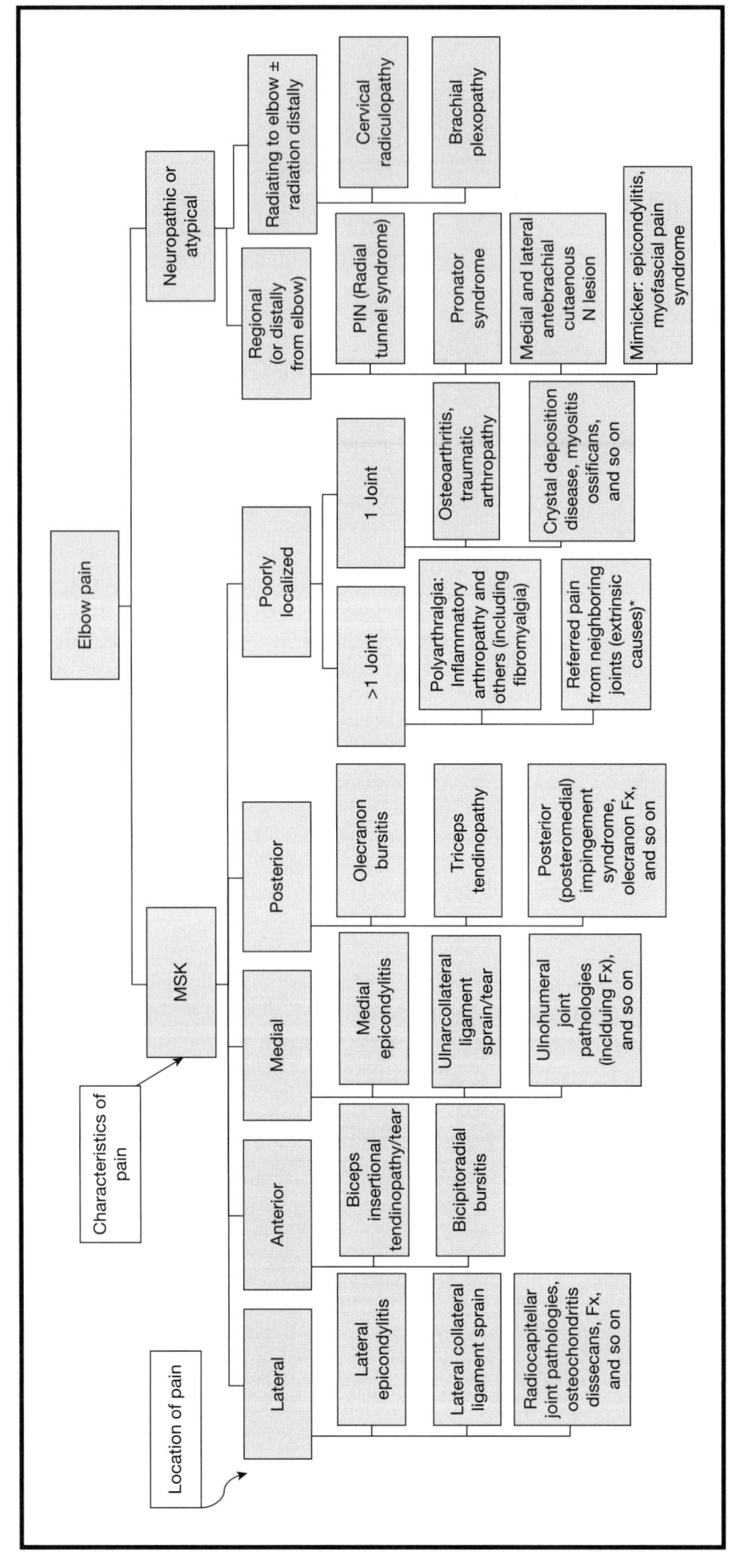

FLOWCHART 4.1
Differential diagnosis of elbow pain.

Fx, fracture; MSK, musculoskeletal; N, nerve; PIN, posterior interosseous nerve.

*Adapted from (5). Simons DG, Travell JG, Simons LS. Travell & Simons' Myofascial Pain and Dysfunction: The Trigger Point Manual. 2nd ed. Baltimore, MD: Williams & Wilkins; 1999:1.

REGION	PATHOLOGIES	CHARACTERISTICS
Lateral	Lateral epicondylitis	Most common pathology
	Lateral collateral ligament pathologies	Consider in recalcitrant lateral elbow pain (failed treatment for lat. epicondylitis)
	Radiocapitellar synovitis, arthritis, and plica	Distal to the lateral epicondyle ± joint effusion
	Osteochondritis dissecans/loose body	History of trauma often present, more common in adolescents
	Crystal deposition disease	Often accompanied with h/o other joint involvement
	Ganglion cyst	Often asymptomatic (incidental finding)
	Radial tunnel syndrome	Radiating pain/paresthesia to the wrist with deep palpation of supinator M and subtle weakness in muscles innervated by the postinterosseous N
	Lateral antebrachial cutaneous neuropathy	Commonly seen as manifestation of brachial plexitis (but can be isolated)
Medial	Medial epicondylitis	Underrecognized, MC cause of medial elbow pain
	Ulnar collateral ligament sprain/tear	Consider if patient not responding to Tx for med. epicondylitis, commonly seen in baseball pitchers and throwers
	Ulnar N subluxation/snapping triceps Syn.	Often asymptomatic
	Valgus extension overload/overuse Syn.	With/without secondary lateral overloading syndrome
Anterior	Biceps tendinopathy	Underrecognized cause of elbow pain (anterolateral) with minimal weakness
	Bicipitoradial bursitis	Swelling, boggy feeling in the cubital fossa (rare)
	Pronator syndrome	Unusual cause of median N neuropathy (motor and sensory symptoms with pain in the hand/fingers)
	Osteoarthritis	Often poorly localized
	Heterotopic ossification in the brachialis M	Recent history of neurologic injury or h/o trauma
Posterior	Olecranon bursitis	Septic bursitis; relatively common
	Triceps tendinopathy	Rare, but underrecognized, in manual or sports activities
	Olecranon stress fracture	Repetitive hyperextension

h/o, history of; M, muscle; MC, most common; med., medial; N, nerve; Syn., syndrome; Tx, treatment.

ELBOW INSTABILITY

Differential diagnosis based on the location
- Lateral elbow instability (6): posterolateral rotatory instability common
  ○ Lateral collateral ligament (LCL) disruption: more stable in pronation
  ○ Dislocation with inadequate ligamentous healing (single trauma): MC
  ○ Valgus instability (usually from chronic overuse), lateral epicondylitis, radial tunnel syndrome, and proximal radioulnar joint instability with radial head dislocation
  ○ Iatrogenic causes: prior lateral epicondylitis release, multiple steroid injections, and radial head excision
  ○ Tardy posterolateral instability: cubitus varus deformity from pediatric supracondylar humerus fracture
- Medial elbow instability (7)
  ○ Medial collateral ligament (MCL) injury/rupture: more stable in supination
  ○ Common flexor-pronator muscle/tendon insufficiency or disruption
  ○ Valgus extension overload in chronic medial insufficiency: posteromedial osteophytes and soft tissue/synovial hypertrophy
  ○ Congenitally shallow ulnohumeral joint

SNAPPING ELBOW (8)

Differential diagnosis based on etiologies

INTRA-ARTICULAR ETIOLOGIES	EXTRAARTICULAR ETIOLOGIES	
	MEDIAL	LATERAL
Radiohumeral menisci interposition (9)	Ulnar nerve snapping	Posterior-lateral rotatory instability
Synovial plica impingement	Snapping of the distal triceps (medial head)	Lateral displacement of the distal triceps M.
Posterolateral elbow rotator instability	The brachialis muscle snapping	Snapping annular ligament over the radial head

STIFFNESS (10,11)

Differential diagnosis based on etiologies
- Traumatic: fracture, dislocation, osteochondritis defect (loose body), crush injuries, and heterotopic ossification

- Atraumatic: rheumatoid arthritis (RA), osteoarthritis (OA), post septic arthritis, hemophilia-associated hemarthrosis, congenital contracture (arthrogryposis), congenital radial dislocationstatus post elective elbow surgery, biceps repair, or elbow arthroscopy

Heterotopic ossification: can occur secondary to burns, head trauma (if combined with elbow trauma: very high), spinal cord injury, trauma, as well as certain surgeries (commonly seen in multiple surgeries 1–2 weeks after trauma)

SITE	AGE AT APPEARANCE	AGE EPIPHYSIS UNITES WITH BODY (YEARS)
Capitellum	18 months	14
Radial head	5 years	16
Medial epicondyle	5 years	15
Trochlear	8 years	14
Olecranon	10 years	14
Lateral epicondyle	12 years	16

ANATOMY

BONE AND JOINT

Bone (12) (Figure 4.2)
- Distal humerus: medial condyle (more prominent, spool-like trochlear) and lateral condyle (spherical capitellum)
  ○ Three fossa: coronoid (trochlear-ulnar side), radial (above capitellar-radial side), anterior, and olecranon (posterior)
- Proximal radius: cylindrical radial head with a concave surface, radial neck angled 15° from shaft
- Secondary ossification centers appear and fuse at predictable ages: need bilateral x-ray to properly evaluate for pathology in pediatric patients (13)

- Tendon attachment site
  ○ Coronoid process of ulnar: insertion of the brachialis tendon
    ▪ Attachment site for anterior bundle of ulnar collateral ligament (UCL): medial facet of the sublime tubercle (~1.8 cm distal to the coronoid tip)
  ○ Tuberosity of the radius: insertion of the biceps tendon

Joints
- Ulnohumeral (coronoid-trochlear) joint: a hinge (also called ginglymus)—allows flexion/extension and dictates carrying angle
- Radiocapitellar and radioulnar joints (also called trochoid joints): allow for axial rotation (pronation/supination) or pivoting at the joint

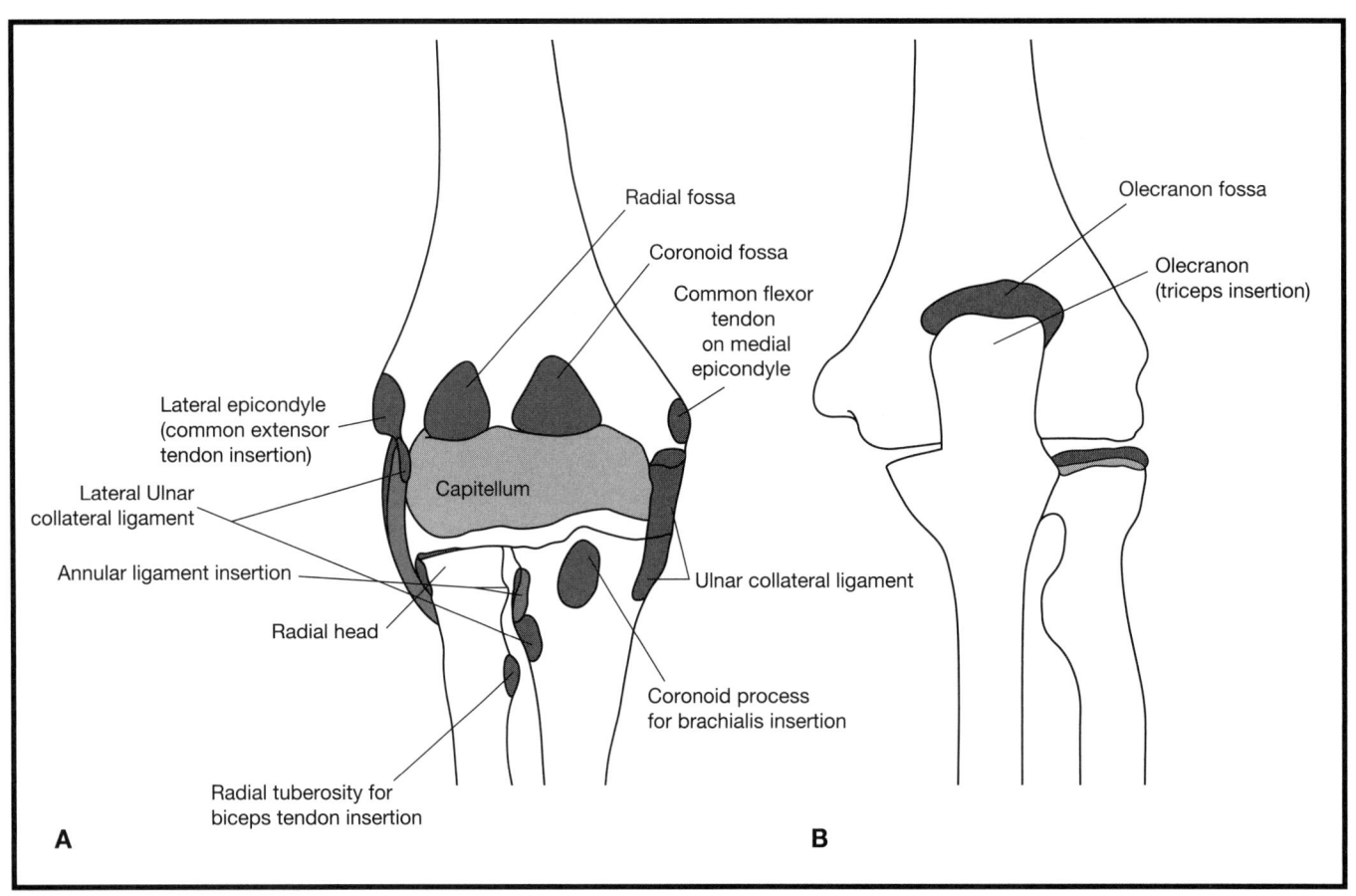

FIGURE 4.2
Bony anatomy of the elbow. (A) Anterior aspect and (B) posterior aspect.
LCL, lateral collateral ligament; LUCL, lateral ulnar collateral ligament; UCL, ulnar collateral ligament.

- Clinical implication
  - Inherent stability at <20° and >120°
  - Carrying angle is formed by the long axis of humerus and ulnar bone
    - Freedom of movement in flexion/extension and pronation/supination

LIGAMENT (FIGURE 4.3)

Medial (ulnar) collateral ligament
- Formed by three bundles—the anterior, posterior, and oblique bands
- Prevents valgus instability, especially the anterior bundle
- Anterior band is attached from the anteroinferior medial epicondyle to the body of the coronoid process
  - Taut in valgus loading in 0° to 85°, during late cocking and early acceleration
  - Common location of tear is midsubstance to proximal
- Posterior band forms the floor of the cubital tunnel
  - Contracture of this band would lead to a significant deficit of flexion
  - Taut in valgus loading in 55° to 145°
  - Experimental sectioning of the posterior band does not increase valgus instability

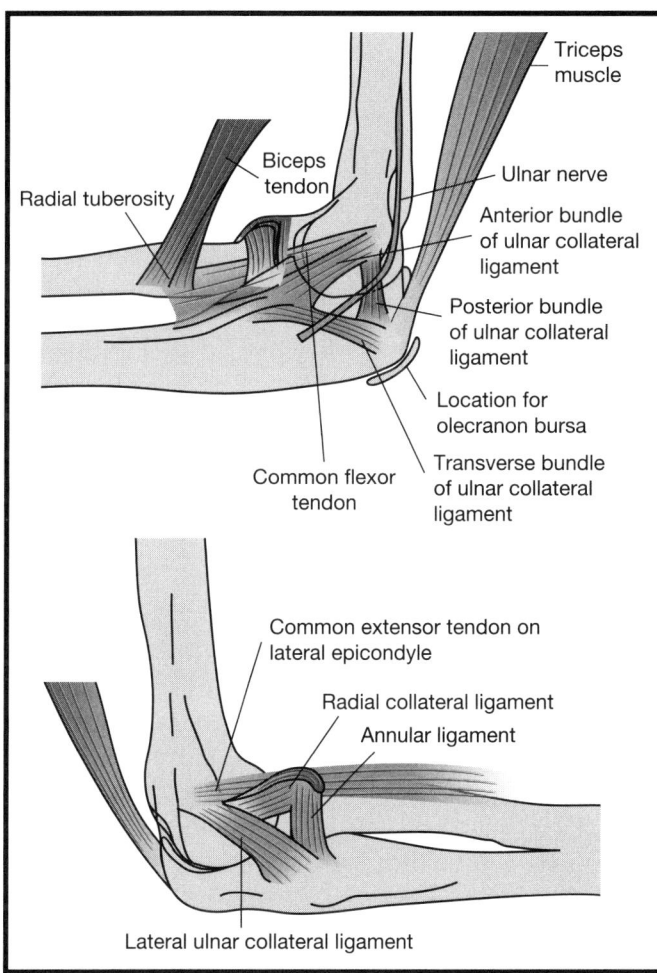

FIGURE 4.3
Lateral and medial elbow ligaments.

Source: Adapted from Ref. (14). Bryce CD, Armstrong AD. Anatomy and biomechanics of the elbow. *Orthop Clin North Am.* 2008;39(2):141–154, v.

Lateral collateral ligament (LCL)
- Lateral UCL
  - From the posteroinferior aspect of the lateral epicondyle, courses along the posterolateral margin of the radial head, and inserts on the supinator crest of the ulna (and partially to the annular ligament)
  - Main function is to prevent posterolateral rotatory instability
  - Common location of injury: avulsion at the humeral origin
- Other LCLs: the annular ligament, radial collateral ligament, and accessory LCL

NERVE

Nerves in the elbow
- The ulnar nerve is located at retrocondylar groove and the cubital tunnel between the two heads of flexor carpi ulnaris (FCU; posteromedial)
- The radial nerve is located at the lateral aspect between the brachioradialis and brachialis
  - Gives off the posterior interosseous nerve, which travels in the radial tunnel between the two heads of supinator to the posterior forearm
- The median nerve lies medial to the biceps tendon and brachial artery
  - Enters the forearm between the two heads of pronator teres (PT)

Joint innervation (15) (Figure 4.4)
- Elbow joint is innervated by multiple nerves: musculocutaneous, median, radial, and ulnar nerve
  - Musculocutaneous nerve/lateral antebrachial cutaneous (LABC) nerve: supplies the anterior radial and ulnar aspect of the joint
  - Median nerve: supplies the ulnar (medial)-anterior aspect of the joint, distal 1/3 of the humerus, and the medial epicondyle
    - Anterior interosseous nerve: supplies the proximal radio-ulnar joint
  - Radial nerve: supplies the anterior-radial aspect and lateral epicondyle
  - Ulnar nerve: supplies the posterior-medial elbow joint, 2 to 3 cm proximal to humeral condyle to the level of the ulnar head of FCU
  - Other contributor is the medial antebrachial cutaneous (MABC) nerve: courses near the ulnar nerve
- Overlapping of innervation
  - Medial (ulnar)/posterior forearm: ulnar and MABC nerve
  - Medial (ulnar)/anterior forearm: median and LABC nerve
  - Radial-anterior forearm: radial and musculocutaneous nerve
- Nerves connected with each other by articular branches plexus

Epicondyle
- Lateral epicondyle: innervated predominantly by radial nerve branches
  - Branches from a radial nerve include a collateral branch, branch to the anconeus branch to the supinator, and the posterior cutaneous nerve
  - Resection of radial nerve branches is performed for recalcitrant lateral epicondylitis
- Medial epicondyle: innervated by the articular branch of ulnar nerve at the ulnar groove

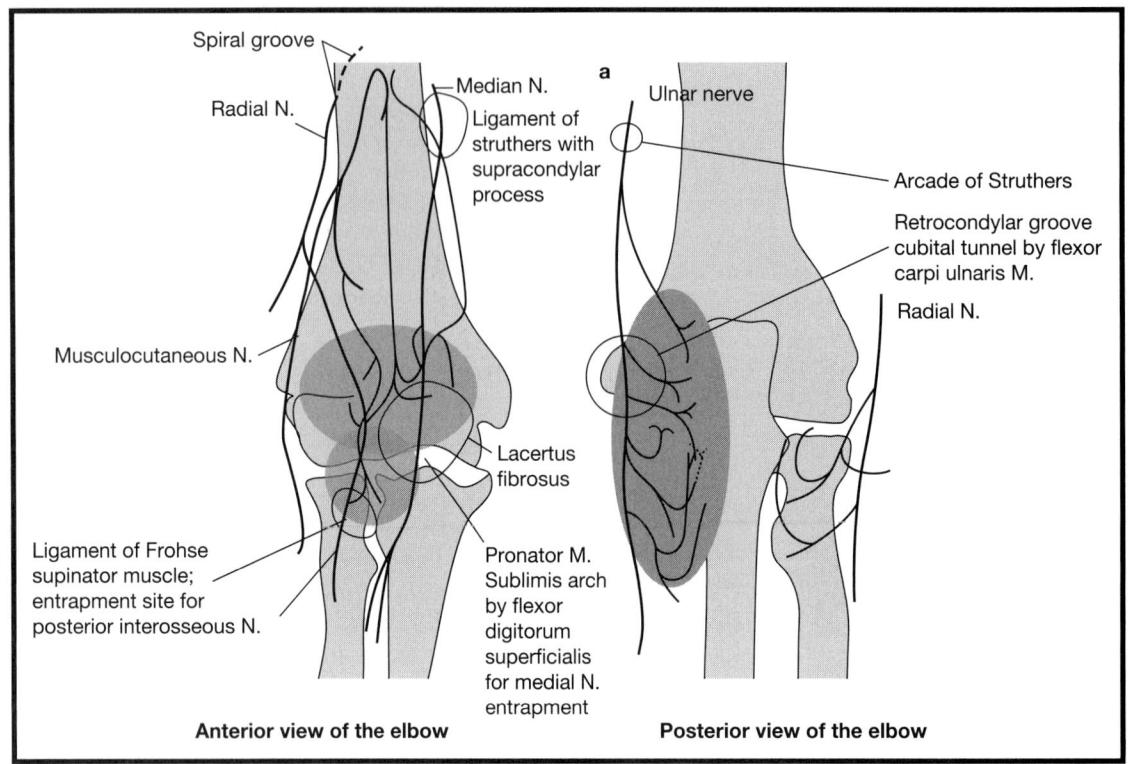

FIGURE 4.4
Nerve innervation of the elbow and site for nerve entrapment.
Source: Adapted from Ref. (16). De Kesel R, Van Glabbeek F, Mugenzi D, et al. Innervation of the elbow joint: is total denervation possible? A cadaveric anatomic study. *Clin Anat.* 2012;25(6):746–754.

MUSCLE

MUSCLE	ORIGIN	INSERTION	INNERVATION	ACTION	COMMENT
Elbow Flexors					
Brachialis	Distal ant. humerus	Coronoid process of the proximal ulnar	Med: musculocutaneous (MSC) N Lat. radial N (C5–6)	Flex elbow	Muscle bulk at the level of elbow joint level (antecubital fossa)
Biceps brachii	Long head: supraglenoid tubercle Short head: coracoid process	Radial tuberosity (proximal radius)	MSC N (C5–6)	Supinate and flex forearm	Short head: part of conjoined tendon to coracoid
Brachioradialis	Lateral condyle	Lateral distal radius	Radial N (C5–6)	Flex elbow	Deforming force in radial Fx
Pronator teres	Humeral head: medial epicondyle Ulnar head: proximal ulna	Lateral radius mid 1/3	Median N (C6,7)	Pronate and flex forearm	Pronator syndrome (proximal median N entrapment)
Elbow Extensors					
Triceps brachii	Long head: infraglenoid tubercle Lateral head: post-humerus (proximal) Medial head: post-humerus (distal)	Olecranon	Radial N (C6–8)	Extends elbow	Medial head M bulk; can cause snapping of ulnar nerve
Anconeus	Posterolateral epicondyle	Posterior proximal ulna	Radial N (C5–6)	Extends elbow	

(continued)

MUSCLE	ORIGIN	INSERTION	INNERVATION	ACTION	COMMENT
Forearm Supinators					
Supinator	Posteromedial ulna	Proximal lateral radius	Posterior interosseous N (PIN), C5–6	Supinates forearm	Supinator syndrome: compression of PIN
Biceps brachii	LH: supraglenoid tubercle SH: coracoid process	Radial tuberosity	MSC N (C5–6)	Supinate and flex forearm	
Forearm Pronators					
Pronator teres	Humeral head: medial epicondyle Ulnar head: proximal ulna	Lateral radius mid 1/3	Median N (C7, 6)	Pronate and flex forearm	Pronator syndrome: median N compression between the two heads
Pronator quadratus	Medial distal ulna	Anterior distal radius	AIN (C7–T1)	Pronate forearm	Primary pronator

AIN, anterior interosseous nerve; ant., anterior; Fx, fracture; Lat., lateral; LH, long head; M, muscle; N, nerve; SH, short head.

Flexor and pronator muscles
- Origin at the medial elbow
- Dynamic support to valgus stress across the medial elbow
- FCU and flexor digitorum superficialis (FDS) over the anterior bundle of UCL: strengthening exercises implicated in medial elbow instability
- The maximal valgus force (290 N) on the medial elbow in the late cocking and acceleration phase in pitching but UCL can hold up to 260 N
- Secondary flexor muscles: PT, extensor carpi radialis longus (ECRL), and flexor carpi radialis (FCR)

Extensor and supinator muscles
- Inserted to the lateral elbow
- Supinator: biceps (major) and supinator. Finger and wrist extensors: weaker supinator
- Secondary extensor muscles: extensor carpi ulnaris (ECU) and FCU

Correlation with ultrasound (US) and MRI (cross-sectional images; Figure 4.5)
- Posterior: triceps tendon; anconeus. Medial: accessory muscle in retro-condylar groove
- Lateral: brachioradialis; ECRL; common extensor tendon; extensor digitorum; extensor carpi radialis brevis; ECU; supinator (superficial head; deep head)
- Anterior: biceps tendon; brachialis; brachial artery and vein; PT (humeral head; ulnar head); common flexor tendon; flexor digitorum profundus; FCU (ulnar head; humeral head); flexor digitorum superficialis; palmaris longus; FCR

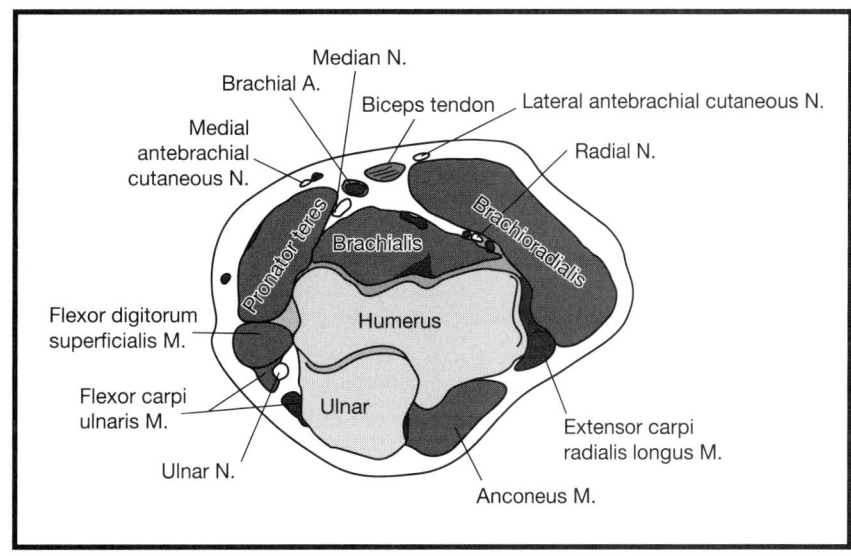

FIGURE 4.5
Cross-sectional image of the elbow showing the relationship of the major nerves around the elbow.

BIOMECHANICS

KINETIC AND KINEMATICS

Loads across the elbow (14,17)
- Loading through radiocapitellar joint (57%) and the ulnohumeral joints (43%)
- Force transmission at the radiocapitellar joint: greatest between flexion and pronation, more than supination
  ○ As elbow flexes from full extension, the contact moves from medial part of trochlear notch to lateral trochlear notch (at 90° flexion) then to the radial head and capitulum (in full flexion)
- Joint force
  ○ Even with falling onto an outstretched hand only from 6-cm height, the axial joint compression is at 50% of body weight
  ○ During a push up, the joint force is 45% of body weight across the elbow
- Elbow in sports activity
  ○ Transfer of energy between the shoulder and elbow during throwing (17)
    ▪ Baseball pitching (rapid extension ~2,400°/s and valgus torque; highest at ball release to prevent elbow distraction)
  ○ Tennis: larger demand on the elbow during serving motion than ground strokes

Kinematics
- Two-degree freedom: flexion/extension by hinge-like motion at ulnohumeral joint and rotational axis at the trochlea and capitellum
  ○ Normal flexion–extension range of motion (ROM): 0° to 150°
  ○ Supination–pronation: axis through distal ulna and the center of the radial head ROM: 75° pronation and 85° supination
- ROM: crucial for activities of daily living (ADL)

ELBOW STABILITY

Stabilizer
- Bony architecture (only at the extremes of flexion and extension) and the stabilizing ligaments/muscles

Bone
- The elbow is a highly congruent, complex hinge joint (ulnohumeral joint)
- Olecranon: 75% to 85% of valgus stress resisted by proximal half of olecranon
- Coronoid (distal half of sigmoid notch): resists 60% to 67% of varus stress

Ligamentous and muscular stabilizer
- The MCL (anterior band) is the main constraint to valgus instability
  ○ Large valgus force is transmitted during throwing (late cocking and acceleration phase)
  ○ MCL; stronger and less elastic than LCL
- The lateral UCL is the main constraint to posterolateral rotational instability (18)
- Posterolateral instability (19)
  ○ MC type of symptomatic chronic instability of the elbow
  ○ When the elbow is extended with the forearm in supination (with arm by the side), the forearm pivots around the medial soft tissue restraints, causing posterolateral subluxation of the radial head with respect to the capitellum
    ▪ The annular ligament remains intact so the radioulnar joint does not dislocate
- Forearm flexor (FCU, lies over MCL): primary dynamic stabilizer against valgus stress
- Posteromedial rotational instability: caused by varus, axial loading internal rotation and coronoid overloading or coronoid fracture and LCL disruption

Elbow stability with forearm rotation
- Elbow: more stable in supination (especially in the setting of coronoid fracture)
- Forearm pronation and supination with decreased valgus laxity compared to the neutral forearm
  ○ Radius moves proximally with pronation of the forearm and distally with supination
  ○ Passive tension in the flexor-pronator muscle with forearm supination
  ○ With passive flexion, the MCL-deficient elbow is more stable in supination, whereas the LCL-deficient elbow is more stable in pronation

ELBOW FUNCTION IN ADL

- Most ADL require 100° of forearm rotation (50° of pronation and supination [slightly more than pronation]) and ~110° (30°–145°) elbow flexion and extension (20)
- Reach the head: 140° of flexion

Loss of forearm pronation: Can be compensated to a certain extent by shoulder abduction; however, there is no effective mechanism to replace supination

Elbow in Sports: Overhead Throwing

- Common cause of overuse injuries in the elbow

Maximal valgus torque
- Occurs during the cocking and acceleration phases of throwing, in which torque peaks immediately before ball release
- Pitching: wind-up, stride, arm cocking, arm acceleration, arm deceleration, and follow-through
- During acceleration the elbow extends from about 110° to 20° at a rate of up to 3,000°/s
- Significant compressive force (500 N) at the radio-capitellar joint: need static stabilizer (ulnar collateral lig.) and dynamic stabilizer (flexor-pronator muscle)

Repetitive stress of valgus extension overload (21)
- Medial tension: MCL sprain, tear, rupture, flexor/pronator tendonitis/rupture, and possible ulnar neuropathy
- Posterior loading: posteromedial osteophyte and olecranon stress fracture

- Lateral compression of radiocapitellar joint: arthrosis, fragmentation (osteochondritis dissecans) [OCD] and loose body

Fall on Outstretched Hand (22)

- Varus extension injury without frank dislocation

Soft tissue injury pattern after a fall: circular from lateral to medial in three stages
- Stage 1: disruption of the lateral ulnar collateral ligament (LUCL)
  ○ Rotatory subluxation of the ulnohumeral joint due to an incompetent LUCL, resulting in posterolateral instability
- Stage 2: disruption of the LCL complex and the anterior and posterior capsule
- Stage 3: partial or complete disruption of the MCL (grossly unstable)

PHYSICAL EXAMINATION

INSPECTION (23)

Carrying angle
- Normally ~5° in male, ~15° in female by long axis of humerus and ulnar
- Cubitus varus (gunstock deformity): history of supracondylar fracture childhood)
- Cubitus valgus in the lateral epicondylar fracture can cause tardy ulnar nerve palsy

Swelling
- Joint effusion
  ○ Flexed elbow on rest: accommodate more fluid with flexion (25–30 mL at 80° flexion) usually at ~ 45° flexion with limitation of extension
  ○ Bulging of soft spot (triangle made up of radial head, lateral epicondyle, and olecranon)
    ▪ Normally subtle concave; compared with the other side
- Bursal effusion: olecranon bursa (posterior and superficial; common) and bicipitoradial bursa (anterior and deep)

Ecchymosis
- Anterior ecchymosis: rule out (R/O) distal biceps rupture (not always present because of lacertus fibrosis)
- Medial ecchymosis: MCL rupture (blood vessels with posterior MCL)

PALPATION

- Palpate for tenderness (systematic way): lateral, medial, posterior, and anterior
- Lateral: epicondyle, radio-capitellar joint, radial head (rotation of the forearm helps to distinguish epicondyle (not rotating) and radial head (rotating))
- Medial: epicondyle and MCL
  ○ Tenderness on MCL: highly sensitive but low specificity for tear
  ○ Retro-condylar groove for ulnar nerve palpation
    ▪ Tinel sign of ulnar nerve on the retro-condylar groove (compare with the other side)
  ○ Snapping or subluxation/dislocation of ulnar nerve and/or medial head of triceps muscle (medially over the medial epicondyle) as elbow flexes gradually
- Posterior
  ○ Triangle of olecranon, medial, and lateral epicondyle on flexion. On extension, malalignment of triangle seen in dislocation (eg, supracondylar fracture)
  ○ Olecranon fossa on flexion of the elbow (site for elbow joint injection)
  ○ Focal swelling ± warmth and/or erythema seen in olecranon bursitis
- Muscle/tendon palpation
  ○ Hook test: distal biceps tendon rupture
    ▪ With the patient's shoulder abducted and the elbow flexed at 90°, the examiner hooks a finger around the lateral side of the distal biceps tendon while the patient actively supinates the forearm. By having the patient supinate the forearm without actively flexing the elbow, an intact biceps tendon becomes more prominent, while the brachialis muscle remains relaxed and is less likely to be mistaken for the biceps tendon
  ○ Lateral to medial at anterior elbow: PT, FCR, PL, and FCU (unable to distinguish by palpation)
  ○ Triceps rupture can be easily overlooked because of continuity of the lateral fascia and anconeus muscle (elbow extensor): often minimal weakness compared to the normal side
- Lymph node palpation: enlarged medial supracondylar lymph node (24)
  ○ Differential diagnosis: skin infection, rarely lymphoma, and skin malignancies

RANGE OF MOTION

Normal and functional ROM

MOVEMENT	ROM (FUNCTIONAL)°
Extension	0–5 (–30)
Flexion	140–160 (130)
Supination	80–90 (50)
Pronation	70–90 (50)

Stiffness frequently defined as loss of extension of >30° and flexion <120°

SPECIAL TESTS

NAME	DESCRIPTION	SENSITIVITY (Sen) AND SPECIFICITY (Spe) IN %
Lateral Epicondylitis (25)		
Cozen test	Resisted radial deviation and extension of the wrist while the examiner resists this motion (performed with fully extended elbow with forearm pronated and fist). Positive with pain at the lateral epicondyle	Sen: 84
Mill's test	Palpating lateral epicondyle with pronated forearm, wrist fully flexed and elbow moved to extension. Positive with pain at the lateral epicondyle	Sen: 53, Spe: 100
Maudsley test	Resisted supination with long finger extension (and for radial tunnel syndrome). Positive with pain at the lateral epicondyle	Sen: 85
Lateral Collateral Ligament (26)		
Posterolateral rotatory-instability test (pivot shift)	Patient supine with the arm over the head. The examiner grasps the patient's forearm and, beginning in full extension and supination, slowly flexes the elbow applying valgus and supination forces and axial compression. Positive with apprehension or dislocation of the radiocapitellar joint	Sen: 38
Chair apprehension signs	Sitting push-up. The patient is seated with elbows flexed to 90°, forearms supinated, and arms abducted greater than shoulder width. A positive test is demonstrated by the reluctance to extend the elbow fully while using arms to rise up from the chair	
Varus stress	The arm is placed in 20° of flexion with slight supination. The examiner gently stresses the lateral side of the elbow joint. Positive if there is excessive gapping on the lateral aspect of the elbow joint	
Medial Epicondylitis		
Resisted wrist flexion and pronation	With the elbow flexed to 90° and forearm supinated, patient makes a fist and flexes the wrist resisted by the examiner. Positive if symptoms reproduced by resisted wrist flexion and pronation. Less pain if performed with elbow in extension	
Medial Collateral Ligament		
Valgus stress test	Valgus stress to elbow at 20°–30° flexion (to unlock the ulnohumeral joint and olecranon) while palpating the medial joint line. Compare with the other side. Positive if pain with laxity is noted compared to the contralateral side. Particularly for anterior band of medial collateral ligament	Sen: 50–66, Spe: 60
Moving valgus stress test	The elbow is brought through range of motion while the examiner applies a valgus force. A positive if the patient experiences pain at midrange of motion (70°–120°)	Sen: 100, Spe: 75
Milking maneuver	Performed by having the patient reach with the contralateral hand under the affected elbow and grasp the ipsilateral thumb. Positive if medial elbow pain reproduced with this maneuver. May be more specific for posterior band of MCL	
Distal Biceps Rupture		
Hook test	With the patient's shoulder abducted and the elbow flexed at 90°, the examiner hooks a finger around the lateral side of the distal biceps tendon while the patient actively supinates the forearm. Positive if unable to hook finger about biceps tendon	Sen and Spe: 100 (27)
Biceps squeeze test	The examiner firmly squeezes the biceps with two hands (one on the myotendinous region of the biceps and the other on the belly of the muscle). Lack of supination of the forearm indicates a positive test (similar to Thompson squeeze test) (28)	Sen: 96
Biceps crease interval test	With slight pronation of the forearm and the elbow flexed at 60° to 80° (to allow for spatial separation), external compression is placed on the biceps muscle and the forearm is supinated if the biceps tendon is intact. Positive if there is no supination of the forearm (28)	Sen: 96, Spe: 80

MCL, medial collateral ligament.

DIAGNOSTIC STUDIES

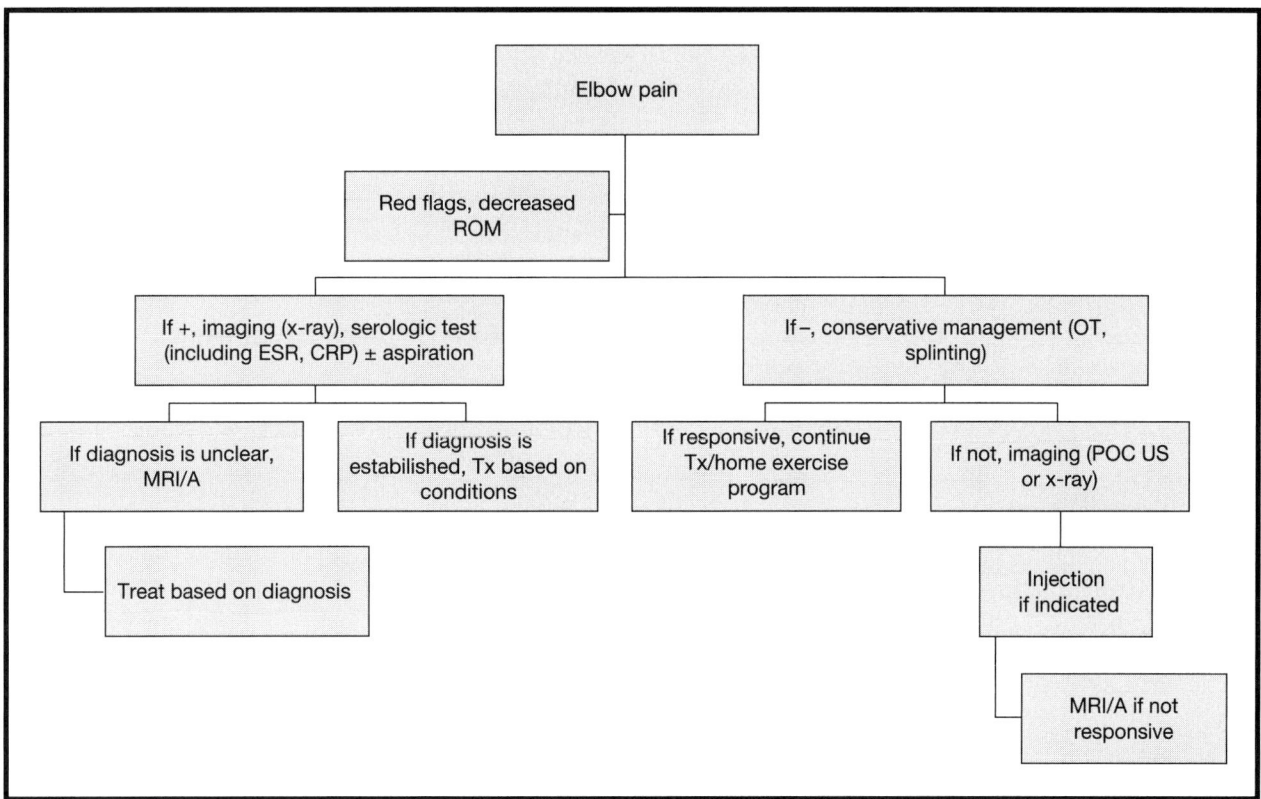

FLOWCHART 4.2
Diagnostic workup and management of elbow pain.
CRP, C-reactive protein; ESR, erythrocyte sedimentation rate; POC, point-of-care; ROM, range of motion; Tx, treatment; US, ultrasound.

PLAIN RADIOGRAPHS (29)

Indications
- Persistent pain (despite initial conservative management) ± decreased ROM to evaluate inflammatory or degenerative joint disease
- Early imaging indicated if trauma, decreased ROM of the joint, and systematic disease (inflammatory, such as RA etc.)
- Useful (not necessarily sensitive) for detecting fractures, arthritis, calcified loose bodies, heterotopic ossification, and destructive processes, such as osteomyelitis and tumors

Limitations: low capability to assess soft tissues (except tendon calcification), articular cartilage, intra-articular lesion, or bursal effusion. Limited in evaluating complex fracture (CT with 3-D reconstruction)

Individual views
- Routine: Anteroposterior (AP) and lateral view
  - True lateral: elbow flexed at 90°
  - Fat pad sign: lucency on the lateral view indicating effusion (especially posterior fat pad sign, anteriorly [sail sign]); indicating ≥5 to 10 mL fluid
  - Anterior humeral line: line drawn along anterior surface of humerus; transects the middle 1/3 of the capitellum on true lateral view. Anteriorly displaced in supracondylar fracture
  - Radiocapitellar line: line drawn along the radial neck; intersect the capitellum. If not, radial head dislocation or subluxation should be considered.
- Oblique view
  - Oblique view with internal rotation to evaluate humeroulnar joint (trochlear notch/coronoid process of ulna) and tip of olecranon process
  - Oblique view with external rotation to evaluate radiocapitellar and proximal radioulnar joints
- Valgus stress radiography
  - Compare with the asymptomatic elbow
  - May be useful in asymmetric medial joint space opening in patients with insufficiency of the MCL
- Bilateral views in pediatric patients
  - Ossification centers: "CRITOE" mnemonic for capitellum, radius, medial (internal) epicondyle, trochlear, olecranon, lateral (external) epicondyle, ossified at 1, 3, 5, 7, 9, and 11 years, respectively, although it can be highly variable

POINT-OF-CARE ULTRASONOGRAPHY (30)

Common indications and findings: soft tissue pain, effusion, and superficial joint structural pain (31)
- Lateral/medial epicondylitis (common extensor/flexor tendinosis [insertional tendinosis]/tear)
- Tendon: partial/full thickness tear of biceps and triceps
- Ulnar and radial collateral ligament tears

- Cubital, bicipitoradial, or olecranon bursitis (bursal effusion)
- Ulnar entrapment neuropathy, posterior interosseous nerve entrapment (radial tunnel syndrome), median neuropathy (ligament of Struthers, PT)
- Soft tissue mass evaluation; ganglion cyst, lipoma, and enlarged lymph node
- Joint evaluation
  - Joint effusion (able to detect 1–3 mL)
    - US elbow flexed at 90°, palm facing the table, posteriorly on the olecranon fossa; more sensitive than x-ray finding of fat pad elevation
  - Synovial hypertrophy and increased vascularity in synovitis
  - Intra-articular loose body; often not sensitive

MRI/MRA (32)

Common indications
- Evaluation of intra-articular or periarticular (eg, ligaments) structure
- Recalcitrant pain (despite conservative treatment) and planning for surgery (providing clearer relationship between the structures) or further evaluation of mass lesion (33)

Evaluation of common abnormal findings
- Muscle, tendon, and ligament pathologies
  - Posterior: pathology for triceps and medial side, for example, accessory muscle in retro-condylar groove (posteromedial)
  - Lateral: common extensor tendon, LCL, supinator (radial tunnel)
  - Anterior: biceps/brachialis insertion, pronator (medially), brachioradialis (laterally), medial and radial nerve
    - Tear/rupture of distal biceps attachment to radial tuberosity and brachialis attachment to coronoid process
  - Medial: common flexor tendon, UCL
- Location of common entrapment neuropathies
  - The ulnar nerve at the retro-condylar groove and cubital tunnel (by the two heads of FCU)
  - The posterior interosseous nerve at the radial tunnel (between the two heads of supinator)
  - The median nerve between the two heads of PT, under lacertus fibrosus, and flexor digitorum superficialis
  - Common abnormal findings: focal enlargement/signal change, increased T2 SI, nonuniform fascicles, subluxation/dislocation, abnormal muscle pathologies (increased T2 SI, atrophy, and fatty infiltration) and underlying structural pathology for entrapment syndrome (aberrant muscle, ganglion cyst, and osteophytes, etc)
- Subtle bony lesion can be seen in Little Leaguer's Elbow: fragmentation or distraction of the medial epicondyle or apophysis

MRA
- OCD, loose body, and plica pain
- UCL and LCL (axial and coronal images)
  - Helpful in patients without joint effusion for subtle ligament tears

CT SCAN
- Performed when evaluating bony structures, when MRI is contraindicated and quicker modality is preferred
  - Osteoid osteoma or myositis ossificans, calcified loose bodies, and fragmented osteochondral lesions
- 3-D construction: for surgical planning, CT arthrogram when MRI is contraindicated

TREATMENT

NONOPERATIVE MANAGEMENT

Education
- ROM/stretching at the end range a few times a day at least, if not contraindicated
  - Prevent elbow flexion contracture (maintain elbow extension)
- Avoid leaning on the elbow (in ulnar neuropathy at retrocondylar groove)
- Gradual increase in resistive strengthening exercise

Physical or occupational therapy
- A, AA ROM exercise ± dynamic splinting or static progressive splinting (less discomfort and better compliance)
- Eccentric strengthening exercise of wrist extensor and flexor usually after stretching with full pain free ROM
- Evaluate ergonomics and abnormal biomechanics (neighboring joint dysfunction, evaluation of sports or work equipment)
- Taping: different methods available, parallel to the common extensor, diamond tape (center on the lateral epicondyle) for lateral epicondylitis or others (34)
- Modality for temporary pain relief

Medication
- Patch/gel (nonsteroidal antiinflammatory drug [NSAID]; diclofenac, lidocaine, capsaicin, and nitroglycerin), acetaminophen, or NSAIDs

Orthotics
- Elbow strap (medial and lateral epicondylitis), elbow hinged orthosis (with/without dynamic control), or wrist splint (often useful for resting wrist flexor/extensor muscles in epicondylitis)

Common elbow orthoses

ORTHOSIS	INDICATION AND PRINCIPLE
Elbow strap (counterforce)	Epicondylitis (lateral and medial) Move functional muscle origin to distally where the strap is located
Articulating elbow orthosis (dynamic elbow splint)	Biceps and triceps tendinopathy Stretching with therapy and after invasive intervention Cautious in spasticity (any joint movement can trigger spasticity)
Elbow pad	Focal pressure relief of ulnar nerve entrapment at elbow

Injection
- Landmark-based injection
  - Elbow joint injection to the soft spot (by triangle of olecranon, lateral epicondyle, and radial head, see Figure 4.1)
  - Olecranon bursal effusion (to bulging mass)
  - Lateral and medial epicondylitis (needling to the bone)
- US-guided injection
  - Common indications: tenotomy (needling or Tenex®, joint injections, small ganglion cyst removal, and injection around the nerve, or when using biologics)

SURGERY

Indications
- Failed conservative treatment for disabling pain
- Contracture: flexion >30° and extension <130°
- Loose body, OCD with pain, and decreased range
- Recalcitrant OA and RA
- Recalcitrant lateral or medial epicondylitis
- Repair of collateral ligament tear (in high-performing athletes or failed conservative management)
- Severe ulnar neuropathy or symptomatic mass (ganglion or soft tissue mass)

Total elbow arthroplasty
- Indications: >65 years old, severe pain throughout ROM/limited motion/functional deficits despite nonoperative interventions, or painful RA (MC)
- Contraindications: aseptic loosening (~5%, clinically), infection, inadequate soft tissue envelope, instability, ulnar neuropathy, triceps insufficiency
- Humeral and ulnar implant ± resection of the head of radius
- Precaution after procedure: avoid lifting >10 lb, repetitive lifting >2 lb after the procedure

TENDON, LIGAMENT, AND BURSA PATHOLOGY

LATERAL EPICONDYLITIS

Introduction
- Epidemiology: 1% to 3% of the population, peak between 35 to 50 years old and male = female
- Pathology: angiofibroblastic tendinosis, degenerative rather than an inflammatory process
  - MC involved tendon: extensor carpi radialis brevis (lateral epicondyle to third metacarpal)
  - Two hypovascular zones: at the lateral epicondyle and 2 to 3 cm distal to the extensor insertion
- Etiology and risk factors
  - Direct trauma, overuse (backhand tennis stroke, more common in novice player), fluoroquinolone antibiotics, and anatomic predisposition
  - Neighboring joint pathologies (rotator cuff pathology, de Quervain tenosynovitis, and carpal tunnel syndrome)
    - Underrecognized shoulder pathology with decreased internal rotation of the shoulder
      - Requires increased wrist flexion with increased eccentric contraction of the wrist extensor muscle (increased risk of lateral epicondylitis) (35)
  - Others: oral steroid treatment, previous history of smoking, and so on (36)

History and physical examination
- Pain and tenderness on lateral elbow (epicondyle) ± referred pain to the wrist
  - Location of tenderness not changing with forearm rotation (supination/pronation) versus rotating tenderness in radial head/neck lesion (radial tunnel syndrome)
- Neurologic test: usually normal
  - Symptomatic posterior interosseous nerve irritation: ~5% of patients with lateral epicondylitis
- Provocative test: Cozen's test, Mill's test, and Maudsley's test

Diagnosis
- Clinical diagnosis supported by imaging study
- Imaging modality to rule out unusual pathologies in recalcitrant case or unresponsive to the typical treatment: do not order initially
  - X-ray: cortical irregularity, spur, and calcification
  - US
    - Common findings: focal hypoechoic swelling with loss of fibrillar pattern in the common extensor tendon origin, calcification of the common extensor tendon, and complete or partial discrete cleavage tears
    - Specific (67%–100%), but not as sensitive (64%–82%) as MRI (sensitivity: 90%–100% and specificity: 67%–100%) (37)
  - MRI: to evaluate intra-articular pathology, radial collateral ligament, or extent of the tear
    - Usually not necessary unless the presentation is atypical or unresponsive to the treatment
    - Common findings: diffuse heterogeneity, increased T2 signal within the extensor tendon, tendon thickening in symptomatic elbows and edema of the common extensor origin (38)
    - Abnormal finding common in asymptomatic population (up to 35%)
- Differential diagnosis (39)
  - Radial tunnel (supinator) syndrome (40)
    - Rare (compared to lateral epicondylitis), radiating pain distally (more common than epicondylitis), tenderness 3 to 4 cm distal to the lateral epicondyle (near the radial neck)
  - Radiocapitellar arthrosis and plica (often concurrent)
    - A painful clicking at terminal extension and forearm supination as well as maximal tenderness over the posterior radiocapitellar joint
  - Osteochondral defect of the capitellum
  - Lateral UCL injury/posterolateral rotatory instability
  - Partial tear of the distal biceps tendon

Treatment
- Benign neglect: initial brief rest (with gradual increase of activity) and observation

- Education on use of sports equipment: for proper tennis racket grip
  - Nirschl technique: circumference of the racket handle should be equivalent to the distance between the proximal palm crease to the tip of the ring finger
- Therapy
  - Isometric and eccentric exercises are better than a contract relax stretching program
    - Initially pain-free resistive strengthening (three sets of 15, bid of wrist curl, elbow flexion/extension, forearm pronation and supination), as well as scapular stabilization
  - Eccentric strengthening exercises using device (Thera-Band FlexBar® or rubber band) and grip strength (2–3 minutes, bid)
  - Deep friction massage (2–3 minutes, bid), ice massage (5 minutes, bid), and stretching (quick varus force to the forearm that is supinated and extended, 30 for 5 reps, tid)
  - Iontophoresis and phonophoresis
- Medications: NSAIDs, diclofenac patch, or topical nitric oxide patch (1/4 of glyceryl trinitrate, 1.25 mg/d patch, cautious of headache or dizziness initially)
- Orthotics: counterforce band and cock-up splint (no significant long-term benefit)
- Injections
  - Steroid injection: for short-term pain relief (not for the long term)
  - Platelet-rich plasma (PRP) injection: for younger athletes and may have longer duration of effect (41)
  - Tenotomy (needling, use large gauge needle) under US guidance
  - Tenex®; ultrasonic percutaneous tenotomy in recalcitrant lateral epicondylitis (42)
- Extracorporeal shock wave
- One year follow-up evaluation success rates for treatments: 69% for injection, 91% for physiotherapy, and 83% for observation (43)

LATERAL COLLATERAL LIGAMENT SPRAIN

Introduction (26)
- Uncommon cause of pain in the lateral elbow ± posterolateral instability
  - Underrecognized often coexisting with lateral epicondylitis
- Anatomy and biomechanics (6)
  - Lateral ulnar collateral ligament (most important lateral stabilizer), radial collateral ligament, and annular ligament work together to stabilize the ulnohumeral and radiocapitellar joints
  - Dynamic posterolateral stabilizers: extensor muscles (ECU) and supinator
    - Radial nerve injury (affecting dynamic stabilizers) can cause instability
- Etiology
  - Trauma (fall on outstretched hand with forearm supinated; MC), elbow dislocation, iatrogenic injury (lateral epicondyle injection and/or radial head fracture with cubitus varus)
  - Delayed onset: cubitus varus (eg, history of pediatric supracondylar humerus fracture), crutch walking, or connective tissue disorder

History and physical examination
- Pain on lateral elbow ± locking, clicking, and snapping
  - Aggravated by activities resulting in supination, extension, and valgus forces, such as carrying a grocery bag with possible elbow giving out
- Provocative test to assess for concomitant posterolateral instability
  - The posterolateral rotatory instability test (pivot shift)
  - Floor push-up test
  - Chair apprehension signs: a sitting push-up

Diagnosis
- Clinical suspicion confirmed by imaging study
- X-ray (stress radiograph during pivot shifting test): slight malalignment of the ulnohumeral joint, overlap of the radial head and capitellum
- US: calcification in LCL located deep to the common extensor tendon, often fibrocartilaginous meniscus homolog (which is attached to the LCL). Loss of continuity and fibrillar pattern, often challenging (44)
- MRI and magnetic resonance arthrography (MRA)
  - Coronal MR is best view for tear of the LCL on humeral attachment. Sagittal MR is best view to see posterolateral subluxation of the radial head with respect to the capitellum (45)

Treatment
- Hinged elbow brace with forearm in full pronation for 4 to 6 weeks in acute sprain/injury
- Strengthening dynamic stabilizers (extensor and supinator muscles) in patient with instability
- Surgery referral if failure to respond to conservative treatment for chronic recurrent lateral instability with impaired ADLs/affecting profession (athletes)

MEDIAL EPICONDYLITIS

Introduction (46)
- Epidemiology
  - Prevalence: 0.3% to 0.6% in men and 0.3% to 1.1% in women, common in 40 to 60 years
    - Twenty percent of all epicondylitis (or more), underrecognized
  - Seventy-five percent in the dominant arms
  - Ulnar nerve and UCL injury often coexist (upto 23%–50%) (47)
- MC involved tendons: PT and FCR muscles
- Etiology and risk factor
  - Activities involving respective forearm pronation and wrist flexion
    - Athletes: pitchers (valgus force at late cocking and acceleration) and also seen in golf (improper swing), tennis, bowling, racquetball, football, archery, weightlifting, and javelin throwing
    - Occupations: carpentry, plumbing, and meat cutting

History and physical examination
- Pain of insidious onset along the medial elbow, worsened by activities (forearm pronation and wrist flexion)
  - ± Tingling, numbness in the medial hand/fingers (due to concomitant ulnar nerve injury)

- Tenderness 5 to 10 mm distal and anterior to the midpoint of the medial epicondyle (overlapping with UCL)
- Symptom reproduction by resisted wrist flexion and pronation

Diagnosis
- Clinical diagnosis supplemented by imaging study
  - X-ray: soft tissue calcification in proximity to the epicondyle (20%–30%) and cortical irregularity
  - US to evaluate the UCL as well as ulnar nerve (focal swelling and subluxation) in addition to common flexor tendon (calcification and hypo/heterogenic echogenicity)
    - Evaluate traumatic tears to the flexor/pronator origin at the epicondyle
  - MRI: if unresponsive to initial management or to evaluate intra-articular/intracortical pathology
  - Electrodiagnosis (EMG) for ulnar neuropathy at elbow if sensory or motor symptoms from ulnar neuropathy persists
- Differential diagnosis
  - UCL injury (often coexist)
  - Ulnar neuropathy and irritation of medial antebrachial cutaneous nerve
  - Medial elbow intra-articular pathology
  - FCR/pronator avulsion: usually concomitant with UCL rupture

Treatment
- Nonoperative management
  - Temporary cessation of offending activities while maintaining flexibility and ADLs
  - PT: initial flexibility (stretching) exercises and then gradually progress to eccentric strengthening exercises of wrist/finger flexor/forearm pronator strengthening
    - Premature discontinuation (of home exercise program) is common reason for failure
  - Counterforce bracing (rarely cause AIN/posterior interosseous nerve [PIN] irritation), night splinting, or ice massage
  - NSAIDs and steroid injection to subaponeurotic recess deep to the flexor pronator mass (no clear benefit for 3 months and 1 year)
  - Prolotherapy or PRP injection if unresponsive or high-performance athlete (with concomitant treatment of UCL lesion)
  - Extracorporeal shock wave therapy
- Surgery: after at least 3 to 6 months trial of nonoperative treatment or may be considered earlier in elite throwing athletes
  - Excision, firm reattachment, and/or repair of the resultant defect
  - Management of any concurrent ulnar nerve or UCL pathology

LITTLE LEAGUE ELBOW

Introduction (48)
- A group of symptoms in the elbow caused by overuse stress injuries during childhood and adolescents
  - Traction apophysitis, medial epicondyle avulsion fracture, OCD
- Etiology and risk factors
  - Repetitive valgus extension overload and compression of the lateral structure (radial head and capitellum)
  - Pitching with fatigued arm, competitively pitching for >8 months/yr, and >80 pitches per appearance

History and physical examination
- Pain ± popping, giving way when throwing
- Point tenderness over the medial epicondyle and pain with resisted flexion and pronation

Diagnosis
- Clinical diagnosis with imaging study for differential diagnosis
- X-ray: normal, avulsion difficult to diagnose, compare with noninvolved side

Treatment
- Complete rest from throwing for 4 to 6 weeks (minimum) ± posterior elbow splint followed by slow progressive throwing program over 6 to 8 weeks
  - Average return to competitive pitching: 12 weeks
- If OCD present, protect elbow for a few months and early ROM in 1 to 2 weeks
- Ortho referral if apophysis is widely displaced. Early ROM exercise recommended
- Prevention: limiting pitching to <105 pitches per game (recommendations based on age: 50 pitches in 8–10 years to 105 pitches in 17–18 years), breaking pitches (ie, curve balls and sliders) should not be thrown until skeletal maturity, no more than 9 months per year

ULNAR COLLATERAL LIGAMENT (UCL) INJURY

Introduction (7,22)
- Most commonly injured ligament in the elbow (18)
  - Common in overhead sports (baseball, tennis, volleyball, golf, javelin, and football)
- MC location of injury: anterior bundle, at the humeral insertion with avulsion of the medial epicondyle
- Etiology: chronic repetitive stress to the elbow
  - Late cocking and acceleration phase in overhead throwing
- Sequels of chronic medial instability from UCL injury (causing valgus extension overload)
  - OCD of the capitellum, radiocapitellar chondromalacia/arthritis, posterolateral synovial plica thickening, posteromedial osteophyte/stress fracture of the olecranon, ulnar neuritis, flexor/pronator weakness

History and physical examination
- Pain (may be minimal, medial elbow initially), impaired performance (loss of control), and instability ± ulnar nerve irritation (by hematoma in acute tear or valgus force)
- Inspection for carrying angle/muscle mass, ROM (elbow flexion contracture common), and normal neurological examination (±Tinel sign for ulnar nerve at retro-condylar groove; not specific)
- Provocation test
  - Static valgus test at 70° to 90°, moving valgus stress test (more accurate), and milk test

Diagnosis
- Clinical suspicion confirmed by imaging study

- X-ray (AP and lateral): avulsion fragment in acute injury, ossification of the UCL, loose bodies, and radiocapitellar or ulnohumeral osteophytes in chronic cases
  - Valgus stress view (negative in partial tears)
- US: elbow slightly flexed (20°–30°) and forearm supinated Normally cord-like structure with broad attachment to the medial epicondyle
  - Injured UCLs: hypoechoic, disrupted fibers (cautious of normal anisotropic artifact), calcification of the ligament, nonvisualization of the ligament
  - Dynamic maneuver with valgus stress (with side to side difference of ulnohumeral joint gap and symptom reproduction)
- MRA: most sensitive and specific.
  - MRI/A: to evaluate differential diagnosis/concomitant pathologies: radiocapitellar impaction, lateral instability patterns, and nonosseous loose bodies

Treatment
- Nonoperative management
  - Temporary cessation of offending activities, NSAIDs, ice/modality, and elbow splint at 90° at night
  - PT: strengthening exercise (pronator, flexor muscle) gradually then return to sports (in 2–3 months) once strength is normalized. General upper body strengthening is important as well
    - Average return to play for thrower: 6 months after the diagnosis. Recommend use of elbow extension braces for throwing and lifting
  - PRP injection to UCL (49)
- Operative management: UCL reconstruction "Tommy John surgery" for high-performing throwing athletes (25% of major leaguers and 10% of minor leaguers have undergone the surgery) (29)

VALGUS EXTENSION OVERLOAD SYNDROME (POSTEROMEDIAL IMPINGEMENT)

Introduction (30)
- Epidemiology: common in throwing athletes (>50% in professional baseball players), swimmers, volleyball players, gymnasts, racquet sports athletes, and golfers
- Pathophysiology
  - Chronic anterior MCL injury → shear force at the posteromedial olecranon → olecranon osteophytes/chondromalacia → common flexor tendinosis and ulnar neuropathy

History and physical examination
- Posterior (posteromedial) elbow pain near elbow terminal extension (pain at ball release in thrower)
- Mild decrease in range (extension; common in dominant throwing arm) with pain otherwise normal
  - Tenderness on posteromedial aspect of the olecranon
  - Symptom reproduction with valgus stress on elbow in 20° to 30° of flexion while forcing the elbow into terminal extension (vs UCL stress test from valgus stress with 0°–20° flexion)

Diagnosis
- Clinical diagnosis supplemented by imaging study
- X-ray: AP, lateral, and axial (check contralateral elbow): posteromedial olecranon osteophytes or loose body
- MRI: if diagnosis is in question or to evaluate concomitant injury (especially MCL injury suspected) or for differential diagnosis
  - MCL attenuation, redundancy, osteophytes on the posteromedial olecranon, and intra-articular loose body
  - Stress fracture of olecranon (pain during or after throwing)
- Differential diagnosis
  - Distal triceps tendonitis: posteromedial pain with resisted arm extension (not necessarily at end range)

Treatment
- Nonoperative management
  - Active rest: resting from throwing and other activities (no throwing for 10–14 days), rotator cuff strengthening, flexor pronator strengthening, and improvement in mechanics → gradual interval throwing program with plyometric exercise
  - Intra-articular steroid injection to control acute pain
- Surgery: in failed conservative management
  - Resection of osteophytes, removal of loose bodies, and debridement of chondromalacia

DISTAL BICEPS TENDINOPATHY/TEAR

Introduction (22)
- Distal biceps tendon rupture: uncommon compared to the proximal rupture, $1.2/10^5$, ~3% of all biceps tendon injury
  - Male > female, peak incidence in 40 to 60 years of age, from single trauma (a sudden eccentric contraction)
  - Full rupture (more common than partial tear) with intact aponeurosis → only mild proximal retraction of muscle (therefore underrecognized)
- Etiologies and risk factors (31)
  - MC activity: weight training (lifting ≥40 kg usually)
  - Minor trauma (incomplete/partial tear) and overuse
  - Systemic risk factors: tendon degeneration and rupture more commonly seen in ankylosing spondylitis (AS), rheumatoid arthritis (RA), acute rheumatic fever, systemic lupus erythematosus (SLE), end-stage renal disease (ESRD), and hyperparathyroidism
  - Local risk factors; hypovascularity and impingement
    - Common location: 1 to 2 cm from the insertion (radial tuberosity): hypovascular zone
    - Impingement between the radius and ulnar during pronation
      - Distance between radius and ulna: decreased from 8 to 4 mm during pronation
    - Impingement by osteophyte-enthesopathy at the radial tuberosity or by bicipitoradial and interosseous bursa

History and physical examination
- Pain on the antecubital fossa (in acute trauma or a rupture) or poorly defined lateral elbow pain (tendinopathy or partial tear)
  - In rupture: "pop," mass in the arm, ecchymosis, and mild weakness with supination (eg, turning screwdriver)
- Provocation tests
  - Hook test, biceps squeeze test, and biceps crease interval test

Diagnosis (32)
- Clinical diagnosis confirmed by imaging
- Imaging study

- US: often difficult to scan in long axis; oblique sagittal (medial-proximal to lateral-distal), tilting down distally
  - Dynamic images (supination and pronation) and compare with the contralateral side
- MRI: can evaluate neighboring structure (bony hypertrophy, bone marrow edema in high-grade tears)
- Differential diagnosis: bicipitoradial bursitis (can be secondary finding), interosseous bursitis, and cubital bursitis

Treatment (33)
- Activity modification, articulating elbow orthotic, and US-guided injection to bicipitoradial or interosseous bursa for pain control. Strengthening exercises of elbow flexor and supinator
- Surgical indication: in acute rupture in high-performing athletes (even during the season as chronic repair/reconstruction not predictable) or in individuals with persistent pain despite conservative treatment, anatomic repair, and/or reconstruction

BICIPITORADIAL BURSITIS

Introduction (50)
- Rare but underrecognized as well
- Etiologies
  - Overuse by repeated pronation/supination
    - Bicipitoradial bursa decreases friction forces between the biceps tendon and the radial tuberosity during elbow movements
  - RA, synovial chondromatosis, synovitis, synovial cyst, and infection

History and physical examination (51)
- Anterior elbow (cubital fossa) pain or discomfort with elbow movements
- Worsening/reproduction of pain with pronation (jamming between biceps tendon and radial tuberosity) ± signs of median nerve irritation
  - Fullness in severe cases

Diagnosis
- Clinical suspicion confirmed by imaging study
- US (effusion surrounding biceps tendon) (52) or MRI to further evaluate neighboring structures (intra-articular and intracortical lesion)
- Differential diagnosis: interosseous bursitis, lipoma, infection, tenosynovitis, ganglion cysts, pigmented villonodular synovitis, or malignant tumor

Treatment
- Nonoperative management with NSAIDs, maintain flexibility, aspiration of the bursa, and steroid injection to the bursa under US
- Surgery if nerve (median or AIN) compression, biceps tendon degeneration/tear, persistent or recurrent symptoms despite conservative management

TRICEPS TENDINOPATHY AND TEAR (22)

Introduction (53)
- Epidemiology: rare
  - Male with heavy manual labor jobs or sports activity: weight lifter (bench pressing), football player, javelin thrower, baseball player, and gymnast
  - Triceps tendon rupture: very rare (<1% of all tendon injury)
    - Partial tear more common than complete tear
- Etiology and risk factors
  - MC mechanism of tear/rupture: eccentric contraction of the elbow (fall on the outstretched hand or direct blow)
  - Risk factors: anabolic steroid use, diabetes, ESRD, lupus, hyperparathyroidism, olecranon bursitis, or steroid injection
- Triceps tendinopathy: often accompanied by posterior impingement, loose bodies, or tennis elbow

History and physical examination
- Posterior elbow pain (especially on resisted extension), mild weakness (with pain), and tenderness
- Snapping triceps syndrome: medial slip or muscle belly detached from the main tendon, snap over the medial epicondyle, may cause ulnar neuropathy (asymptomatic in most cases)
- Rupture
  - Ecchymosis (in acute), defect (later), inability to extend the elbow actively (in full rupture)
  - Modified Thompson test (often difficult due to long lever arm, small cross-section size of triceps compared to gastrocsoleus muscle)

Diagnosis
- Clinical diagnosis confirmed by imaging study
- AP and lateral x-ray (may see flakes sign: flecks or avulsed fragment from olecranon [pathognomic])
  - X-ray of the wrist for concomitant injury
- US: fluid-filled defect within the distal triceps tendon, avulsion fracture, distinguish partial versus complete tear
  - Partial tear: medial side of tendon insertion area is more commonly involved
  - Complete tear: a large fluid-filled gap between the distal end of the triceps tendon and the olecranon process
- MRI for further soft tissue evaluation and associated osseous injuries: radial head fracture, and distal radius fx (CT if MRI is contraindicated)

Treatment
- Nonoperative: good result, splint immobilization for ~4 weeks at 30° flexion, then gradual stretching and strengthening
  - Indications: partial (<50%) or complete within muscle belly, mild weakness, or fatigue
  - Tendinopathy: usually resolve in 3 to 6 months of conservative management (54)
- Surgical if acute complete tear at the tendinous insertion with significant loss of triceps strength or failed conservative treatment in highly active patients with partial tears
  - Earlier (ideally within 2 weeks) intervention, the better outcome

OLECRANON BURSITIS

Introduction (55,56)
- Epidemiology: incidence unknown, male > female, and common in 30- to 60-year age group
- Anatomy

- Olecranon bursa: synovium-lined sac promoting gliding between the olecranon and the overlying skin
- Etiology and risk factors
  - Traumatic, inflammatory, and infectious (20%)
    - Septic bursitis: *Staphylococcus* and other gram-positive organism: MC
    - Trauma/sports: common in football
  - Predisposing conditions: RA, gout, pseudogout, chondrocalcinosis, and pigmented villonodular synovitis

History and physical examination
- Swelling over the proximal olecranon (usually unilateral) ± pain
- Joint mobility: intact; may result in sympathetic effusion in the bursa and extension to the forearm
- Usually not tender (tenderness in only up to 20%–45%), fever (up to 50% in infectious bursa), and erythema (more often in septic form)
- Increased temperature (>2.2°C difference: 100% sensitivity and 94% specificity)

Diagnosis
- Clinical diagnosis confirmed by imaging study
- Imaging: x-ray R/O olecranon fracture, US to confirm and evaluate soft tissue lesion (triceps tendinopathy/tear or joint effusion), MRI in presence of abscess or to R/O osteomyelitis
- Aspiration (18–20 G, usually from lateral approach) for fluid analysis
  - Gram stain (positive in 50%–60%), culture, WBC count (<1,000/mm^3: aseptic; >10,000/mm^3: septic), and glucose level (<50% of serum level: septic)

Treatment
- Ice, compressive dressing, and avoidance of aggravating activity (eg, leaning on elbow)
- Aspiration to R/O infection; 90% resolves in 6 months
- Intrabursal steroid injection: lack of clear benefit, related to the infection, skin atrophy, and chronic pain

BONE AND JOINT PATHOLOGY

OSTEOARTHRITIS

Introduction (57)
- Epidemiology: rare, prevalence of symptomatic elbow OA: 2%
  - Male > female by four times, high incidence in 50s especially with strenuous manual activity
- Etiologies
  - Posterior-medial cartilage defect of the radial head (rare to involve ulnohumeral articulation)
  - Secondary causes
    - Trauma (eg, missed coronoid fracture), OCD, synovial chondromatosis, and valgus extension overload

History and physical examination
- Pain, especially on ROM (end range initially versus mid-range in advanced case or large osteochondral lesion) ± effusion (bulging in lateral soft spot) and crepitus
- Decreased ROM: loss of terminal extension
  - Flexion with impingement type of pain at the end range at early stage
  - If significantly diminished, R/O loose bodies, osteophytes, and capsular contracture
- Neurological examination: check for concomitant ulnar neuropathy

Diagnosis
- Clinical diagnosis supplemented by imaging study
- X-ray: AP, lateral, and oblique
  - Anterior and medial osteophyte involving the coronoid process, posteromedial osteophytes on the olecranon process, and corresponding osteophytes on the coronoid and olecranon fossae
- Advanced imaging; usually not necessary
  - The relative preservation of articular cartilage and the maintenance of joint space with hypertrophic osteophytes formation and capsular contracture
  - CT and MRI in advanced cases; intra-articular loose body (30% missed in plain radiograph)

Treatment
- Nonoperative treatment
  - Short-term rest and NSAIDs
  - Activity modification (often difficult in manual laborers and athletes), dynamic hinged orthotics, static progressive splinting (to address tightness), and OT (unclear benefit, strengthening of elbow flexor, extensor, wrist flexor/extensor strengthening, joint protection technique, and evaluation of adaptive equipment)
  - Viscosupplementation—pain improved at 3 months, but not at 6 months (58).
- Surgical treatment (59)
  - Debridement, osteophytes excision, and contracture release
  - Indication for resurfacing (interposition arthroplasty or total arthroplasty): pain throughout ROM, loss of joint space, and abnormal joint architecture

OSTEOCHONDRITIS DISSECANS OF THE ELBOW (CAPITELLUM)

Introduction (60,61)
- Epidemiology: common in 12- to 15-year-olds when the capitellar epiphysis is almost completely ossified
- MC location in elbow; capitellum
- Etiologies
  - From impaction, shear force from valgus stress (with MCL insufficiency)
  - Increased risk in upper extremity dominant sports: gymnasts (repetitive weight bearing stress on elbow), baseball pitchers (repetitive compression forces), racket sports athletes, and javelin throwers
- Chronic sequels: long-term pain, premature OA, loss of terminal extension, and chronic instability of the radial head

History and physical examination
- Elbow pain (often diffuse, nonspecific), activity-related pain (inflammatory like symptoms after exercise), crepitus, and occasional locking

- Active radiocapitellar compression test: pain/symptom reproduction with active pronation/supination of the forearm with elbow in full extension

Diagnosis
- Clinical suspicion confirmed by imaging study
- Imaging study (62)
  - X-ray: AP, lateral, oblique, and axillary view; radiolucency, rarefaction of the capitellum, flattening and irregularity, sclerotic bone, loose body
  - US: epicondylar fragmentation, detached bony fragment (stable or loose body) in capitellum
  - MRI/A (imaging modality of choice): can check acuity (by bony edema) and additional information for treatment plan (separation, loss of articular cartilage continuity, tracking of fluid, etc)
    - Irregularity of the chondral surface, disruption of the subchondral bone plate, or the presence of a fracture line
- Differential diagnosis
  - Panner disease: self-limiting process in 4- to 8-years-olds
    - Avascular necrosis (AVN) of the capitellum secondary to traumatic injury
  - Little league elbow, pseudo-defect of the capitellum, and hereditary epiphyseal dysplasia

Treatment
- Nonoperative, if articular cartilage is intact (no separation of the fragment): elimination of stress for least 6 weeks (subchondral bone to stabilize), some recommend 6 months for complete healing
  - Hinged elbow brace without restriction for 3 to 6 weeks, start PT in 3 months
  - Return to full activity in 6 months
- Referral to surgery if locking or loose fragment present, or failed conservative management

POSTERIOR IMPINGEMENT OF THE ELBOW

Introduction (63)
- In overhead throwing athletes, or tennis player, rare in general population
- Etiology
  - Repetitive combined hyperextension, valgus, and supination of the elbow → mechanical abutment of bony or soft tissues in the posterior fossa of the elbow → loose bodies and/or osteophyte formation
  - Predisposing factor: ligamentous instability of the elbow, especially ulnar collateral ligament (UCL) insufficiency
    - UCL insufficiency allows for greater shear force and posterior impingement

History and physical examination
- Posterior elbow pain, joint effusion, locking, crepitus, and a decreased ROM, especially extension deficit

Diagnosis
- Clinical diagnosis supplemented by imaging study
- X-ray: an axial view, to detect osteophytes on the olecranon or on the borders of the posterior fossa and stress radiography to document ligamentous laxity or rupture
- POC US: similar to x-ray and soft tissues impingement in dynamic view
- MRI/A: further evaluation of loose bodies (often missed in x-ray and US). CT scan for bony details (if MRI/A contraindicated)

Treatment
- Nonoperative treatment: NSAIDs in combination with rest, ice, compression, elevation, and therapeutic exercises (ROM, strengthening, etc)
- Surgery: arthroscopic or open debridement ± UCL reconstruction if failed conservative treatment

RHEUMATOID ARTHRITIS

Introduction (64,65)
- Elbow involvement in RA: 20% to 65%, rarely occur in isolation (only ~5%)

History and physical examination
- Pain, swelling, and stiffness (synovitis is an early manifestation)
  - Loss of elbow extension and swelling (especially posterolateral) ± painful clicking or snapping as progresses
  - Referred pain to the wrist or wrist pain by posterior interosseous nerve irritation
- Physical examination: complete examination (from neck to fingers) and neurologic examination
  - Other joint involvement is common
  - Effusion, subluxation, and limited ROM
  - Rheumatoid nodules: more common in seropositive disease (preclude more severe erosive lesion), usually asymptomatic (but can ulcerate and cause infection as the skin is fragile)

Diagnosis
- Clinical diagnosis: check hand/wrist RA (American College of Rheumatology criteria) with supplemented imaging of elbow for grading the severity of the involvement
- X-ray: Larsen grading system or Mayo classification
  - Larsen grading: Grade 0 (no change) to V (grossly mutilating changes)
    - Depending on soft tissue swelling, periarticular osteoporosis/erosions with some joint-space narrowing, joint destruction, and collapse
  - Mayo classification (uses a combination of clinical symptoms as well as radiograph assessment)
    - Mayo grades I and II are marked predominantly by synovitis. Type 2: clinical symptoms that cannot be controlled by medication alone
    - Mayo grades III and IV are marked by increasing degrees of joint destruction
- US
  - Common findings: effusion and synovitis (increased vascularity on Doppler) in early stages
  - Used for guidance for injection
- MRI to evaluate disease progression and when indicated for surgery
- Differential diagnosis: psoriatic arthritis, SLE, pigmented villonodular synovitis, and OA

Treatment
- Referral to rheumatology: check other joints, including C spine and hand/wrist
  - Early and aggressive treatment—disease-modifying antirheumatic drugs (DMARDs), biological therapies
- IA steroid injection in early stages ± US guidance
- Occupational therapy (a few sessions)
  - Joint protection education, activity modification, adaptive device evaluation, joint mobilization: balance between rest (causing stiffness) and aggressive exercise (may be detrimental)
- Surgery: synovectomy (± radial head excision) and total elbow arthroplasty
  - Rheumatology consult for scheduling discontinuation of high dose steroid, DMARD (continue low dose), TNF-α antagonist (stop for 4 weeks before and 2 weeks postoperative), and concern for infection

MYOSITIS OSSIFICANS

Introduction (66)
- Definition: abnormal formation of bone in inflammatory muscle
- Rare but underrecognized, commonly involves thigh (vastus lateralis), arm (brachialis), and generally anterior muscle groups rather than posterior muscle groups of the extremities (67)
- Etiology: direct trauma, fractures, dislocations, burns, or neurologic injuries, such as brain trauma or spinal cord injury
  - Three percent of all patients with elbow dislocations without fractures and in 20% of all dislocations with fractures
  - Traumatic myositis ossificans: increased incidence in second to third decades

History and physical examination
- Pain and an enlarging mass/swelling
- ± Tenderness, edema, warmth, redness, fever, and restricted ROM

Diagnosis (68)
- Clinical suspicion confirmed by imaging study
- X-ray: initially normal (faint calcification in 7–10 days) → soft tissue mass with faint peripheral calcification → well-defined cortex with relatively lucent center in 2 months
  - Location: parallel to the shaft of long bones or the long axis of a muscle
- CT (imaging modality of choice): cross-sectional zonal pattern
- US: heterogeneous hypoechoic area (irregular margin) with focal hyperechoic central area initially → hyperechoic calcification with posterior shadowing as it matures
- Differential diagnosis: DVT, infectious disease (cellulites, abscess, or osteomyelitis), or tumor

Treatment
- Indomethacin 25 mg tid for 3 to 6 months, other NSAIDs, bisphosphonates (etidronate, delay the mineralization of osteoid, but can be reversed after discontinuation)
- Referral to radiation oncology for low doses of radiation treatment below 1,000 cGy
- Surgical excision can be considered when the lesions are completely mature on a three-phase bone scan, and there is a normalized level of alkaline phosphatase or the absence of acute symptoms

FRACTURE

Classification (69) (Flowchart 4.3)

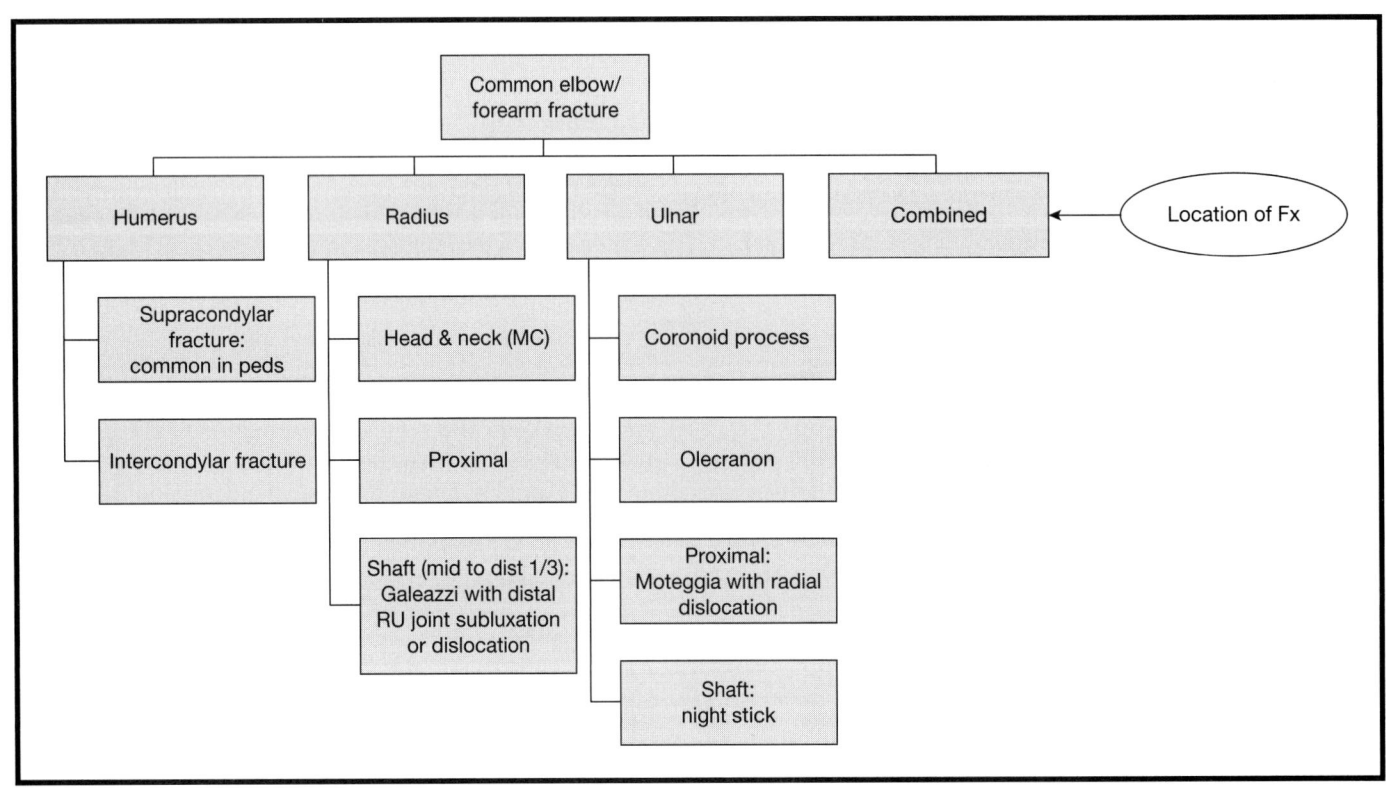

FLOWCHART 4.3
Classification of elbow/forearm fracture.
Fx, fracture; peds, pediatric patients, MC, most common; RU, radioulnar.

Elbow fracture and dislocation
- Elbow fracture: 7% of all fractures (radial head: 20%–30% of all elbow fractures)
- Elbow dislocation: 20% of all dislocations

Radial Head and Neck Fractures
Introduction
- 20% to 30% of all elbow fractures (MC), peak incidence in 30- to 40-year-olds
- Mechanism of injury
  - Fall on outstretched hand (with pronated forearm), axial load across the elbow
- Commonly associated injuries (in ~30%)
  - Elbow: elbow dislocation, ulnar shaft/coronoid fracture, medial (and lateral) collateral ligament injuries
  - Wrist: interosseous membrane injury destabilizing the distal radioulnar joint, distal radial head injury, and carpal fractures
  - Terrible triad: elbow dislocation, radial head fracture, and coronoid fracture

History and physical examination
- Lateral elbow pain, swelling, and limited ROM
- Effusion/hematoma: often requires aspiration and lidocaine block for examination

Diagnosis
- Clinical suspicion confirmed by imaging study
- X-ray: AP, lateral, oblique (radiocapitellar view), will see fat-pad sign (elevation of soft tissue by hemarthrosis)
- CT can be considered for fracture displacement or surgical candidates

Treatment
- Nonoperative: long-arm posterior splint with elbow 90° flexion for minimally displaced <2 mm without mechanical blocks
  - Forearm weakness and loss of extension (10°–15°) is commonly seen (usually functional)
- Referral for surgery: >2 mm displacement, mechanical block to motion, >20% to 30% articular depression, and open fracture

Coronoid Fractures
Introduction
- Coronoid provides up to 50% of elbow stability and prevents posterior subluxation
  - Anterior bundle of UCL and brachialis inserts on the coronoid process
  - Coronoid fractures with dislocation are associated with recurrent instability
- 10% to 15% of elbow injuries
- MC injury mechanism (up to 50%): elbow dislocation with spontaneous relocation and hyperextension
  - Avulsion fracture with brachialis muscle insertion
  - Traumatic shear injury

History and physical examination
- Pain, ecchymosis, swelling over the anterior-medial elbow ± forearm and wrist pain
- Check radial pulse in 90° elbow flexion
- Complications
  - Recurrent elbow instability
  - Elbow stiffness, posttraumatic arthritis, heterotopic ossification

Diagnosis
- Clinical suspicion confirmed by x-ray (AP and lateral) and CT scan if not clear (due to overlapping structures)

Treatment
- <50% involvement of the coronoid can be treated conservatively if the joint is stable
  - Early mobilization to avoid stiffness
- >50% involvement of the coronoid requires surgical intervention

Galeazzi's Fracture
Introduction
- Distal 1/3 of radial shaft fracture with a distal radioulnar joint injury
  - Distal radioulnar joint instability in >50% if the location is <7.5 cm from the joint
- Three times more common than Monteggia fracture
- Reverse Galeazzi: distal ulnar fracture with distal radioulnar joint disruption
- Common mechanisms of injury: direct wrist trauma (dorsoradial aspect) and fall on outstretched hand

History and physical examination
- Pain, swelling, and tenderness with limited elbow ROM (supination and pronation)
- Neurovascular examination (high index of suspicion for compartment syndrome)

Diagnosis
- Clinical suspicion confirmed by imaging study
- X-ray: AP, lateral of elbow, forearm, and wrist
- Findings associated with distal radioulnar joint involvement: fracture of the base of the ulnar styloid, widened distal radioulnar joint, subluxed ulnar on lateral x-ray, and >5 mm radial shortening

Treatment
- Ortho referral
  - Nondisplaced: long-arm cast
  - Displaced: open reduction and internal fixation (ORIF) dynamic compression plate
- Early mobilization if the distal radioulnar joint is stable
  - Unstable radioulnar joint: immobilize the forearm in supination for 4 to 6 weeks in a long-arm splint or cast

- Complications: malunion, a loss of pronation/supination, compartment syndrome, neurovascular injury (iatrogenic), and radioulnar synostosis

Monteggia's Fracture

Introduction
- Proximal 1/3 ulnar fracture and dislocation of the radial head (± fracture)
- Common in children, between 4 and 10 years, rare in adults
- Common mechanisms of injury: fall on outstretched hand with elbow extended and pronated
- Associated injuries: olecranon fracture/dislocation, coronoid fracture, LCL injury, and terrible triad of elbow
- Bado classification (Types 1–4)
  - Type 2 (MC) posterior/posterolateral dislocation of the radial head, with fracture of ulnar diaphysis with posterior angulation by axial loading of the forearm with a flexed elbow

History and physical examination
- Painful swelling at elbow joint, decreased ROM ± radiocapitellar joint dislocation
- Important to check neurovascular status, especially radial nerve/PIN (seen in up to 10% associated with dull wrist pain and weakness of thumb and metacarpophalangeal extension)

Diagnosis
- Early recognition is important as delayed treatment increases complication significantly
- X-ray: AP, lateral, and oblique of elbow, forearm, and wrist
  - Normal: a line drawn through the radial head and shaft, always line up with the capitellum
  - Supinated lateral: lines drawn tangential to the radial head anteriorly and posteriorly should enclose the capitellum
- CT or MRI if x-ray is negative with high degree of suspicion

Treatment
- Close reduction and sugar tongue splint (in supination) and referral to orthopedic, elective ORIF in adults, closed reduction in children usually in OR under general anesthesia
- Postoperative: posterior elbow splint for 5 to 7 days, if radial head unstable then long-arm cast with serial x-rays
- Check PIN/AIN status and radial head instability

Nightstick Fracture

Introduction
- Uncommon isolated fracture of the ulnar shaft (mid-diaphysis), typically a closed fracture
- MC mechanism: direct blow (eg, trying to defend an overhead blow of baton also called "nightstick")

History and physical examination
- Pain and point tenderness over the shaft with swelling

Diagnosis
- Clinical suspicion confirmed by imaging study
- Plain radiographs should include the wrist and elbow

Treatment
- Nonoperative Tx: nondisplaced or minimally displaced (<10° angulation)
  - Posterior splint (to middle upper arm, elbow in 90° flexion) for 7 to 10 days → functional brace 4 to 6 weeks with wrist Ex
- Ortho referral if displacement >50% or with >10° angulation

Olecranon Fracture

Introduction
- Traumatic fracture: bimodal distribution from high-energy injury in the young and falls in the elderly
- Stress fracture from repetitive microtrauma against the olecranon fossa or excessive tensile stress of the triceps tendon

History and physical examination
- Posterior elbow pain during and shortly after sports activity: subtle presentation in stress fracture
- Palpable defect ± inability to extend elbow (may indicate discontinuity of triceps muscle)

Diagnosis
- Clinical suspicion confirmed by imaging study
- X-ray can be normal in stress fracture: additional imaging, such as MRI, CT, or bone scan may be necessary to confirm the diagnosis
- Differential diagnosis: avulsion fractures of the tip of the olecranon and persistent olecranon apophysis

Treatment
- Nonoperative treatment
  - Stress fracture: cessation of sports activity and active rest, bone growth stimulation (unclear benefit)
  - Other fracture: long-arm posterior splint in 45 to 90° for 2 to 4 weeks, start ROM exercises in 3 to 4 weeks, in avulsion fractures avoid prolonged immobilization
- Surgical referral for internal fixation in high demand overhead athletes even in stress fractures
  - Most fractures are intra-articular, so near anatomic alignment required for full ROM
  - Persistent olecranon apophysis may additionally require bone grafting
  - >2 mm displacement in avulsion fractures require ORIF

Supracondylar Fractures in Children

Introduction
- Extra-articular supracondylar fractures: 10% of all pediatric fractures
- MC mechanism: fall on hand or elbow, 98% occur in extension
- Nondominant arm more commonly involved
- Associated injury or complication
  - Compartment syndrome and later Volkmann's contracture
  - Nerve injury
    - Anterior interosseus nerve: MC injured, in up to 50% of completely displaced fractures

- Most recover spontaneously in 3–6 months; neurapraxic lesion MC
    - Radial nerve: injury with posteromedial displacement and lateral spike of proximal fragment
  ◦ Cubitus varus is the MC complication usually due to imperfect reduction. It is usually not associated with a loss of function, but can cause tardy ulnar nerve palsy
  ◦ Arterial injury occurs in 5% of children with supracondylar fractures

History and physical examination
- Severe pain, swelling (minimal with non-displaced fracture) with deformity
- Examination for neurovascular compromise
  ◦ Frequent radial pulse examination: especially with posterolateral displacement and higher grade injuries
  ◦ Intimal brachial artery injury may not present initially
  ◦ Wrist/MCP extension (extensor digitorum communis [EDC]) for radial nerve injury
  ◦ OK sign to test anterior interosseous nerve (flexor pollicis longus, flexor digitorum profundus, and pronator quadratus)
- "Dimple sign": when the fracture ends are caught in the brachialis and subcutaneous soft tissue
- Evaluate for concomitant elbow dislocation
  ◦ With the elbow flexed at a 90°, triangle should be between the two epicondyles and the olecranon
  ◦ The triangle will remain in place with a fracture but be disrupted with a dislocation

Diagnosis
- Clinical suspicion confirmed by imaging study
- X-ray: Gartland classification of fracture
  ◦ Type I: nondisplaced
  ◦ Type II: anterior gapping, rotation malalignment with intact posterior hinge
  ◦ Type III: displaced, no cortical stability, totally unstable

Treatment
- Type I fractures treated with splinting: reduction in 90° elbow flexion to preserve function
- Type II and III require reduction and surgical stabilization
  ◦ After reduction, recheck neurovascular examination and recheck x-ray

Capitellum Fracture

Introduction
- Rare, <1% of all elbow fractures, often associated with radial head fractures
- Little or no soft tissue attachment results in free articular fragment
- MC mechanism of injury: fall on outstretched hand
- Complications: elbow contracture, nonunion, heterotopic ossification, and AVN of capitellum

History and physical examination
- Pain, swelling ± mechanical block (anterior displacement of the articular fragment into fossae [radial or coronoid] blocks flexion)

Diagnosis
- Clinical suspicion confirmed by x-ray: AP and lateral
- Classification
  ◦ Type 1: Hahn–Steinthal fragment, includes a large portion of the capitellum ± trochlear involvement
  ◦ Type 2: Kocher–Lorenz fragment, includes a separation of a small amount of the articular surface of the capitellum
  ◦ Type 3: Comminuted fracture
- CT for further evaluation

Treatment
- Posterior splint immobilization: <3 weeks for non-displaced or <2 mm displaced
- Early motion is key to treatment
- Ortho referral for ORIF, fragment excision, or total elbow arthroplasty

ELBOW DISLOCATION

Introduction (70)
- Second MC dislocation (after shoulder dislocation), 10% to 25% of elbow injury, peak incidence in 10 to 20 years
- Posterolateral dislocation: MC
- Mechanism of injury: axial loading, supination, and valgus force
- Associated injuries: circular disruption of capsuloligamentous cascade (LCL and MCL)

History and physical examination
- Elbow pain, swelling, decreased ROM
- Check skin, neurovascular status, and possible compartment syndrome

Diagnosis
- Clinical diagnosis confirmed by imaging study (x-ray)
- X-ray: AP, lateral, and oblique
- CT scan for complex injury or for evaluation of detailed osseous involvement

Treatment (71)
- Reduction and splinting at 90° for 10 days or hinged brace at 90° for 2–3 weeks for acute simple stable dislocation
- Referral to surgery for ORIF (reconstruction of coronoid, radial head, olecranon) and ligament repair

NEUROPATHY

ULNAR NEUROPATHY

Introduction
- Second MC entrapment neuropathy (after CTS)
  ◦ Incidence: 24.7/100,000 (Italy), male > female (72)
- Location: elbow (MC) followed by wrist (Guyon's canal)
  ◦ Other locations include: above elbow at the Arcade of Struthers (of brachialis and triceps muscle fascia) and the forearm (in patient with arteriovenous shunt; Figure 4.6)
  ◦ Slightly more common in the non dominant hand
- Etiology: no identifiable cause in 30% to 50% (73)

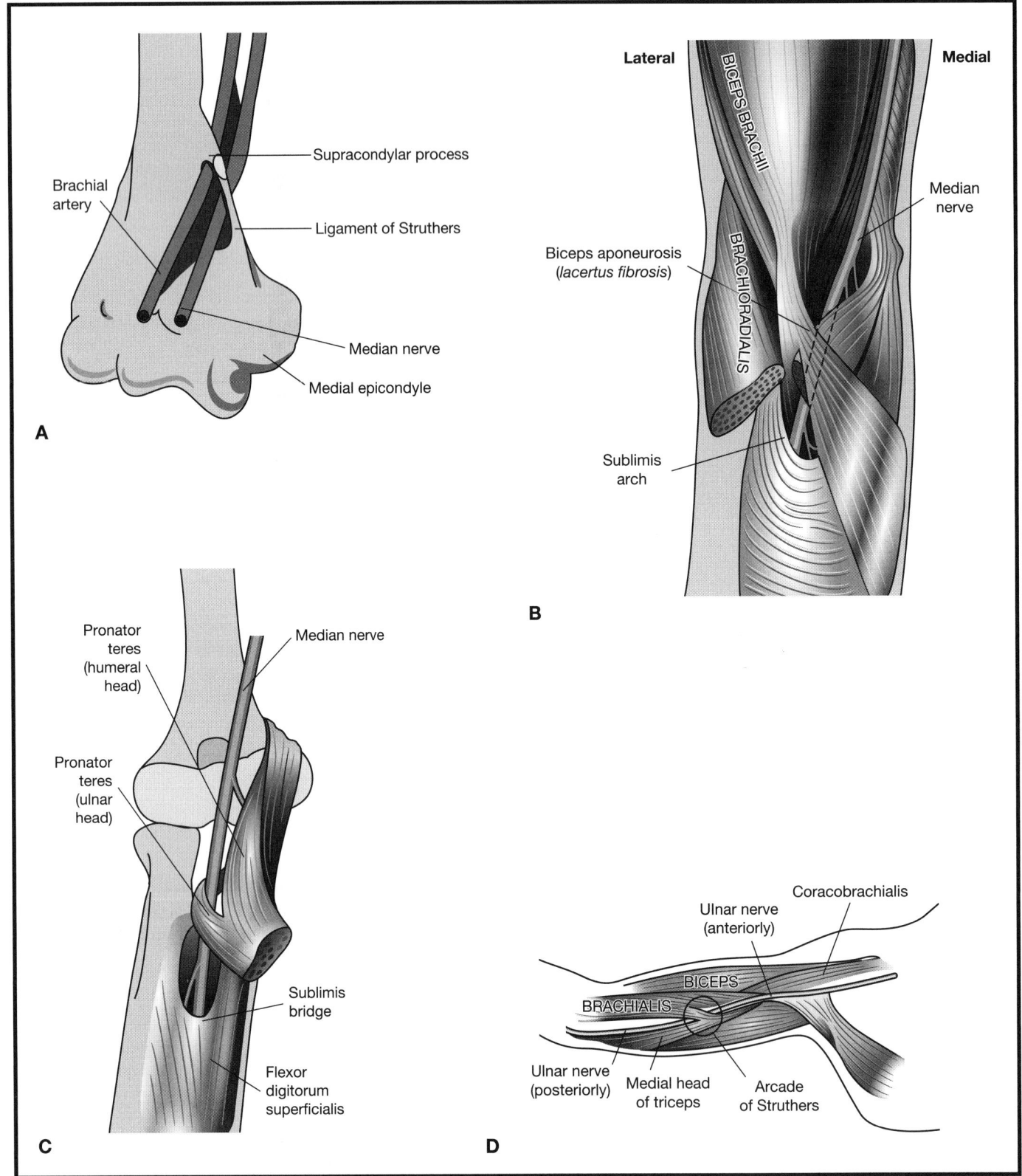

FIGURE 4.6

Locations of common entrapment neuropathies at elbow. (A–C) Median nerve entrapment at ligament of Struthers, lacertous fibrosis, and pronator teres/sublimis bridge of flexor digitorum superficialis respectively. (D–E) Ulnar nerve entrapment by arcade of Struthers and cubital tunnel. (F) Radial nerve entrapment by arcade of Frohse.

(continued)

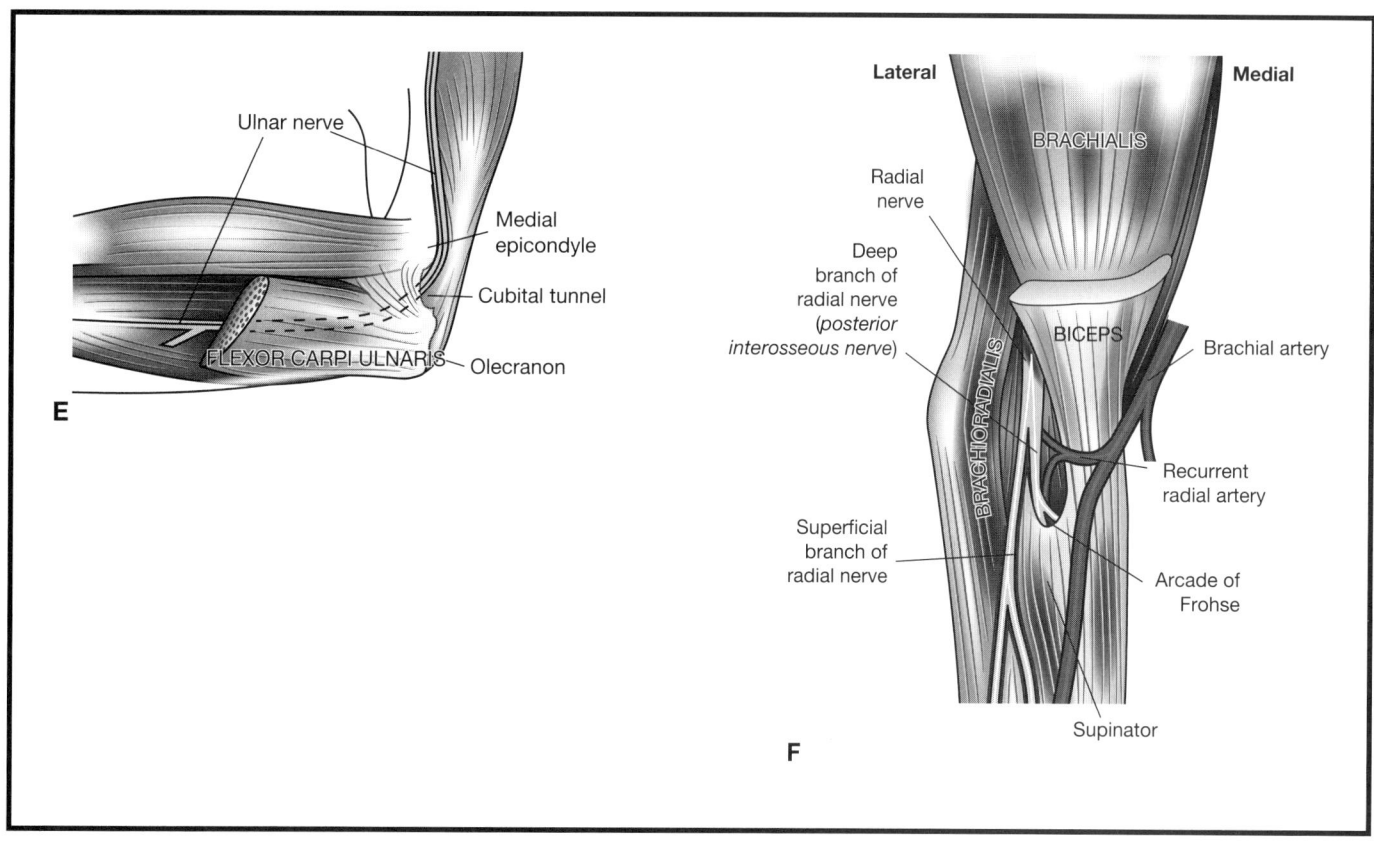

FIGURE 4.6 *(continued)*

○ Retro-condylar groove: MC location in elbow followed by humeroulnar aponeurotic arcade of flexor carpi ulnaris (cubital tunnel): 1 to 2.5 cm distal to medial epicondyle
  ▪ Acute, chronic external pressure, bony or scar impingement, anomalous muscles (anconeus epitrochlearis) or bands, chronic stretch in valgus deformity, and mass
○ Subluxation: unclear role in neuropathy

History and physical examination
- Sensory symptoms (tingling, numbness, neuropathic pain in the medial half of fourth and fifth digits typically, but not always) more common than motor symptoms (weakness) of the hands/fingers
  ○ ± Elbow pain (not typical)
- Sensory examination
  ○ Check dorsum of medial hand sensation (for dorsal ulnar cutaneous innervation): involved in elbow lesion but spared in wrist lesion.
  ○ Medial forearm sensation is spared (medial antebrachial cutaneous nerve coming from the medial cord)
- Motor: intrinsic atrophy (wasting of muscle between the fingers), claw hand deformity (more on the ulnar side, more prominent in wrist lesion compared to elbow lesion)
  ○ Wartenberg sign: slight abduction of fifth finger on resting from unopposed extrinsic muscles with net abduction force

○ Froment's sign: substituting median (AIN) innervated muscle (flexor pollicis longus) when asked to hold a paper with thumb and index finger (instead of using ulnar innervated adductor pollicis muscle)

Diagnosis
- Clinical diagnosis confirmed by EMG study
- Nerve conduction study (NCS): cautious of the temperature (false positive in cold elbow) and elbow position (approximately 90°)
  ○ Sensory NCS
    ▪ Routine sensory: antidromic sensory NCS (fifth digit recording) or orthodromic study
    ▪ Dorsal ulnar cutaneous nerve: if abnormal, suggesting lesion proximal to wrist
    ▪ Medial antebrachial cutaneous nerve: if abnormal, suggesting lesion proximal to ulnar nerve, such as brachial plexus lesion (involving medial cord, lower trunk)
    ▪ Mixed nerve study across the elbow (recording at above elbow with simulation of median and ulnar nerve in the wrist, abnormal if ulnar onset latency is delayed compared to the median latency by >1.4 ms); may be more effective in mild case (only involving sensory)
  ○ Motor NCS
    ▪ Routine motor nerve conduction study (MNCS) recoding at ADM (similar sensitivity to first dorsal interosseous [FDI] recording)

- FDI and ADM latency comparison (abnormal if >2.0 ms) and side-to-side difference of FDI latency >1.3 ms: useful to evaluate isolated lesion involving only deep motor branch in Guyon's canal lesion
- Across the elbow: 10-cm segment with the elbow flexed 70° to 90° (American Association of Neuromuscular & Electrodiagnostic Medicine [AANEM] guideline): positive if
  – CV across the elbow <50 m/s
  – Greater than 10 m/s difference between forearm segment and cross elbow segment
  – Compound motor action potential (CMAP) amplitude drop >20% across the elbow
  – CMAP waveform configuration change
- Inching technique: more sensitive and can localize lesion
- Palmar interosseus and second lumbrical comparison
- Needle EMG
  ○ FDI, abductor digiti quinti (minimi), flexor digitorum profundus fifth digit, and FCU (from distal to the proximal innervation)
  ○ FCU versus FDP; motor branch to FCU is often innervated by ulnar nerve above the elbow
  ○ To rule out more proximal lesion (brachial plexopathy, root, or motor neuron Dz)
    - Medial cord: APB (median, C8–T1), FPL (AIN, C7–8), pectoralis major (medial pectoral nerve, and sternocostal head, C7 to T1)
    - Lower trunk: extensor indicis proprius (EIP) and EDC (radial, PIN, C7–8)
    - C8–T1 Root: paraspinal muscles
- Ultrasonography
  ○ Cross-sectional area
    - Cross-sectional area at the elbow; enlarged if >10–11 mm^2
    - Compare the value with the uninvolved part of the ulnar nerve (usually mid-forearm or arm), focal enlargement if the ratio is >1.5
  ○ Hypoechogenicity: can be normal due to tortuous course around the elbow
  ○ Look for structural findings (for underlying causes): ganglion cyst, lipoma, snapping of ulnar nerve with medial head of triceps, fluid (effusion, hematoma), aneurysm/pseudoaneurysm, or spurs/osteophytes (tardy ulnar nerve palsy) in ulnar-trochlear joint
- Differential diagnosis
  ○ CNS: cerebrovascular accident (CVA), spinal cord lesion involving anterior horn cells (myelopathy, syringomyelia) and multiple sclerosis
  ○ Motor neuron disease (if the sensory involvement is minimal or absent)
  ○ C8–T1 radiculopathy: no splitting of the fourth digit, abnormal spontaneous activity in abductor pollicis brevis (APB), EIP, pectoralis major, and paraspinal muscles with normal sensory nerve conduction study (SNCS)
  ○ Brachial plexopathy
    - Post-median sternotomy, thoracic outlet syndrome and metastasis
    - Medial cord: medial antebrachial cutaneous nerve, APB, pectoralis major involved
    - Lower trunk: medial cord lesion + EIP muscle involved
  ○ Peripheral neuropathy (radial sensory and lower extremity involved)
  ○ Mononeuritis multiplex, hereditary neuropathy liable to pressure palsy, multifocal motor neuropathy, multifocal acquired demyelinating sensory and motor neuropathy (MADSAM), chronic inflammatory demyelinating polyneuropathy CIDP). May need extensive NCS for subclinical lesion
  ○ MSK causes (often coexisting)

Treatment
- Nonoperative treatment for at least 3 to 6 months
  ○ Activity modification: avoid prolonged elbow flexion, triceps extension exercise, and repetitive elbow flexion/extension
  ○ Education: avoid leaning on the elbow
  ○ NSAIDs and steroid injection (no good evidence)
  ○ Bracing: elbow pad during the day and night, splint in elbow extension
  ○ Stretching initially → progressive isometric strengthening and strengthening the dynamic stabilizers of the elbow in 6 weeks
- Surgery if not responsive to conservative treatment or if any structural lesion is identified (74)
  ○ No significant difference between the techniques
  ○ Common reason for surgical failure: failure to release the nerve both proximally and distally properly and failure to address concomitant MSK pathologies
  ○ If subluxation or dislocation, ulnar nerve should be transposed anteriorly

RADIAL TUNNEL SYNDROME

Introduction (22,75)
- Rare, annual incidence: 0.03% (or rarer) (76)
- Location of radial nerve (and/or PIN) compression at the elbow (Figure 4.6)
  ○ Radial tunnel: lateral intermuscular septum between brachialis and brachioradialis muscle
  ○ Arcade of Frohse: fibrous opening in the superficial head of supinator muscle
    - Supinator syndrome: supinator may or may not be involved. Extensor carpi radialis usually spared
    - Up to 5% of patients with concomitant lateral epicondylitis (77)
- Etiology
  ○ Radial head subluxation, Monteggia fracture (proximal 1/3 ulnar fracture and dislocation of the radial head), synovitis, thickening of the anterior capsule of the elbow joints, and compression by the branches of the radial recurrent artery or mass lesion (ganglia)
  ○ Repetitive rotatory movement of the forearm

History and physical examination
- Vague pain in the lateral elbow, discomfort/deep pain in the wrist and weakness of wrist/finger extensors ± numbness in the distribution of the radial nerve (if superficial radial nerve involved)
- Tenderness on the radiocapitellar joint and radial neck, two-finger breadth (~5 cm) below the lateral epicondyle often reproducing the symptoms.

Diagnosis
- Clinical diagnosis confirmed by EMG study (although often negative; so cannot rule out by EMG)
- NCS and EMG (76)
  - SNCS: normal superficial radial, MNCS of extensor indicis (EI)
  - Needle EMG: abnormal spontaneous activity in EI, EDC, and ECU muscles and normal BR (radial), triceps (radial), FDI (ulnar, lower trunk), and paraspinal muscle EMG
- Ultrasonography to evaluate for presence of structural lesion: synovitis (radiocapitellar joint), ganglion, lipoma, or a mass lesion and so on (77)
  - Focal enlargement of PIN compared to the contralateral asymptomatic side
  - Evaluate other concomitant or mimicking MSK lesions
- MRI: allows better evaluation of the pathologies compared to US (especially in structures that are deeply located or between the radius and ulnar)
  - Edema or atrophy within the supinator muscle and extensor muscle innervated by PIN (78)

Treatment
- Wrist splint, activity modification (avoid prolonged elbow extension with pronation and wrist flexion), ergonomic evaluation, modality, and occupational therapy
- US-guided steroid injection (60%–70% improvement in pain) and aspiration of ganglion cyst if present (often technically difficult)
  - Hydrodissection of PIN with normal saline or 5% dextrose at the radial tunnel under US
- Surgery indicated if conservative management fails after 3 to 6 months
  - In wrist drop by severe lesion (very unusual), tendon transfer (PT to ECRL transfer and FCR to EDC transfer) can be considered

POSTERIOR ANTEBRACHIAL CUTANEOUS NEUROPATHY (79)

Introduction
- Isolated: very rare
- Anatomy: branch of radial nerve, arises in the posterior compartment of the arm along with the posterior cutaneous nerve of the arm, often anastomosis with other cutaneous nerve (medial and lateral antebrachial cutaneous nerve)
- Common etiology: iatrogenic after either surgery for lateral epicondylitis or injection

History and physical examination
- Pain, numbness, tingling in the dorsal aspect of the forearm
- Normal motor as well as other sensory examination and DTR

Diagnosis
- Clinical diagnosis confirmed by NCS and/or diagnostic nerve block
- Differential diagnosis: lateral epicondylitis (often coexisting)

Treatment
- Diagnostic nerve block and repeat nerve block if successful (often difficult to identify it even with US)
- TENS or local lidocaine gel, and desensitization

MEDIAN NEUROPATHY AT ELBOW

Introduction (80)
- Rare, incidence/prevalence not established, female > male
  - Diagnosis with skepticism (+ EMG findings are extremely rare; variable frequency)
- Etiology
  - An anomalous ligament of Struthers (proximally, ~1 % of population, ~5 cm above the medial epicondyle, PT muscle involved) (81) (Figure 4.6)
  - Between the two heads of the PT (pronator syndrome)
    - The fibrous band between the superficial and deep heads of the PT M
  - The proximal arch of the FDS
  - The lacertus fibrosus (especially scarred) in the antebrachial fossa or thick bicipital aponeurosis

History and physical examination
- Aching pain on the volar aspect of the forearm, exacerbated by resisted pronation of the forearm (pronator syndrome, forearm pain can be minimal/absent) with paresthesia in the first to third digit and radial aspect of fourth digit, and decreased sensation on the skin overlying the thenar eminence (spared in CTS)
- Physical examination
  - Resisting the patient's hand from pronation with the forearm in a neutral position → pain or paresthesia as the elbow is extended
  - Pronator compression test: pressure over the PT muscle in both upper extremities simultaneously → reproduction of paresthesias in the radial 3.5 digits ≤30 seconds, while the uninvolved limb remains asymptomatic
  - Reproduction of symptoms with resisted elbow flexion at 120° to 130° of flexion with the forearm in maximal supination; if entrapment secondary to lacertus fibrosus
  - Reproduction of symptoms by resisted contraction of the FDS to the middle finger; median N compression at the level of the fibrous arch between the heads of the FDS is suspected

Diagnosis
- Clinical diagnosis confirmed by EMG study (usually normal, positive in <10%) and supplemented by imaging study
- US and MRI for structural lesion or focal nerve swelling
  - Technically difficult to evaluate a focal swelling with US due to the oblique course

Management
- Nonoperative treatment: modification of activities, temporary rest with elbow orthotics, NSAIDs and local steroid injection, ergonomic evaluation, and avoid provoking activities

- Operative treatment if not responsive to conservative treatment or structural lesion/mass is seen: median nerve decompression

OTHER NERVES

Lateral Antebrachial Cutaneous Neuropathy

Introduction (82,83)
- Anatomy: branch of the musculocutaneous nerve, it exits out of the fascia 2 to 5 cm above the elbow crease, between the fascia of the brachialis and biceps tendon, and then divides into anterior and posterior divisions
- Etiology
  - Musculocutaneous N
    - Shoulder dislocation or fracture (MC cause, usually involving other N as well, axillary, suprascapular, or radial N)
    - Entrapment at coracobrachialis in a weight lifter or with other vigorous physical exercises
  - Isolated lateral antebrachial cutaneous nerve entrapment
    - At the elbow: compressed by the biceps aponeurosis and tendon against the brachialis muscle
    - Other causes: hyperextension injury of the elbow (as seen in sports) and antecubital phlebotomy (immediately lateral to the biceps tendon)

History and physical examination
- Pain and burning sensation/dysesthesia in the lateral forearm
- Tenderness of the lateral edge of the biceps tendon reproducing patient symptoms, and decreased ROM of elbow with forearm pronated
- No motor weakness for isolated LABCN lesion (check elbow flexor for proximal nerve [musculocutaneous nerve] lesion or other shoulder and shoulder girdle muscles)

Diagnosis
- Clinical diagnosis confirmed by NCS: check side-to-side difference in latency and amplitude (84)
- Diagnostic block if pain is the prominent symptom (EMG is often negative)
- Differential diagnosis
  - Musculocutaneous neuropathy, brachial plexopathy (upper trunk, lateral cord), C6 radiculopathy
  - Lateral epicondylitis, biceps tendinitis (often concomitant)
  - Pronator syndrome and radial tunnel syndrome

Treatment
- Activity modification and possible diagnostic/therapeutic injection (US guidance, often difficult to find the nerve with US) in the vicinity of compression site
- Referral for surgical decompression in recalcitrant cases

Medial Antebrachial Cutaneous Neuropathy

Introduction (85)
- Isolated: very rare, unknown prevalence
- Etiology
  - Iatrogenic: injection to the medial epicondyle, repetitive elbow flexion/extension, venipuncture (anterior division) in the antecubital region, surgery for ulnar nerve decompression (posterior division), and so on
  - Involvement in brachial plexopathy affecting the lower trunk or medial cord: more common
    - Trauma in which the arm and shoulder are pulled up
    - Invasion of the plexus by a Pancoast tumor at the lung apex
    - Stretch injuries of the lower plexus during chest surgery, such as coronary artery bypass surgery
    - Thoracic outlet syndrome entrapping the lower trunk or medial cord of the plexus

History and physical examination
- Discomfort/pain and numbness/tingling in the medial forearm
- Decreased sensation in the medial forearm
- Motor examination and DTR examination for brachial plexus; usually normal
- Tenderness over the nerve (midline between medial epicondyle or biceps tendon) reproducing the symptoms

Diagnosis
- Clinical diagnosis confirmed by EMG study or image-guided diagnostic block
- NCS and needle EMG R/O brachial plexus lesion or to evaluate cervical radiculopathy (often limited)
- Differential diagnosis: brachial plexopathy, cervical radiculopathy and medial epicondylitis

Treatment
- Good recovery in general, TENS, lidocaine gel, or steroid/lidocaine injection for pain control while recovering
- Workup for other concomitant diagnoses/etiologies

REFERENCES

1. van Rijn RM, Huisstede BM, Koes BW, Burdorf A. Associations between work-related factors and specific disorders at the elbow: a systematic literature review. *Rheumatology (Oxford)*. 2009;48(5):528–536.
2. Punnett L, Wegman DH. Work-related musculoskeletal disorders: the epidemiologic evidence and the debate. *J Electromyogr Kinesiol*. 2004;14(1):13–23.
3. Shiri R, Viikari-Juntura E. Lateral and medial epicondylitis: role of occupational factors. *Best Pract Res Clin Rheumatol*. 2011;25(1):43–57.
4. Wall, PD, Melzack, R, Bonica, JJ. *Textbook of Pain*. 3rd ed. Edinburgh, NY: Churchill Livingstone; 1994:1524.
5. Simons DG, Travell JG, Simons LS. *Travell & Simons' Myofascial Pain and Dysfunction: The Trigger Point Manual*. 2nd ed. Baltimore, MD: Williams & Wilkins; 1999:1.
6. Cheung EV. Chronic lateral elbow instability. *Orthop Clin North Am*. 2008;39(2):221–8, vi.
7. Grace SP, Field LD. Chronic medial elbow instability. *Orthop Clin North Am*. 2008;39(2):213–9, vi.
8. Lasecki M, Olchowy C, Pawlus A, Zaleska-Dorobisz U. The Snapping Elbow Syndrome as a Reason for Chronic Elbow Neuralgia in a Tennis Player—MR, US and Sonoelastography Evaluation. *Pol J Radiol*. 2014;79:467–471.
9. Huang GS, Lee CH, Lee HS, Chen CY. A meniscus causing painful snapping of the elbow joint: MR imaging with arthroscopic and histologic correlation. *Eur Radiol*. 2005;15(12):2411–2414.
10. Nandi S, Maschke S, Evans PJ, Lawton JN. The stiff elbow. *Hand (N Y)*. 2009;4(4):368–379.
11. Kim PD, Grafe MW, Rosenwasser MP. Elbow stiffness: etiology, treatment, and results. *J Am Soc Surg Hand*. 2005;5(4): 209–216.
12. Martin S, Sanchez E. Anatomy and biomechanics of the elbow joint. *Semin Musculoskelet Radiol*. 2013;17(5):429–436.
13. Micheli LJ, Santore R, Stanitski CL. Epiphyseal fractures of the elbow in children. *Am Fam Physician*. 1980;22(5):107–116.
14. Bryce CD, Armstrong AD. Anatomy and biomechanics of the elbow. *Orthop Clin North Am*. 2008;39(2):141–154, v.

15. Wilhelm A. Tennis elbow: treatment of resistant cases by denervation. *J Hand Surg Br*. 1996;21(4):523–533.
16. De Kesel R, Van Glabbeek F, Mugenzi D, et al. Innervation of the elbow joint: is total denervation possible? A cadaveric anatomic study. *Clin Anat*. 2012;25(6):746–754.
17. Loftice J, Fleisig GS, Zheng N, Andrews JR. Biomechanics of the elbow in sports. *Clin Sports Med*. 2004;23(4):519–30, vii.
18. Hariri S, Safran MR. Ulnar collateral ligament injury in the overhead athlete. *Clin Sports Med*. 2010;29(4):619–644.
19. O'driscoll SW, Morrey BF, Korinek S, An KN. Elbow subluxation and dislocation. A spectrum of instability. *Clin Orthop Relat Res*. 1992;280:186–197.
20. Raiss P, Rettig O, Wolf S, et al. [Range of motion of shoulder and elbow in activities of daily life in 3D motion analysis]. *Z Orthop Unfall*. 2007;145(4):493–498.
21. Beltran LS, Bencardino JT, Beltran J. Imaging of sports ligamentous injuries of the elbow. *Semin Musculoskelet Radiol*. 2013;17(5):455–465.
22. Hayter CL, Giuffre BM. Overuse and traumatic injuries of the elbow. *Magn Reson Imaging Clin N Am*. 2009;17(4):617–38, v.
23. Hausman MR, Lang P. Examination of the elbow: current concepts. *J Hand Surg Am*. 2014;39(12):2534–2541.
24. Bazemore AW, Smucker DR. Lymphadenopathy and malignancy. *Am Fam Physician*. 2002;66(11):2103–2110.
25. Saroja G, Antony Leo Aseer P, Venkata Sai, PM. Diagnostic accuracy of provocative tests in lateral epicondylitis. *Int J Physiother Res*. 2014;2(6):815–823.
26. Reichel, LM. Elbow lateral collateral ligament injuries. *J Hand Surg (American ed.)*. 2013;38(1):184–201; quiz 201.
27. O'Driscoll SW, Goncalves LB, Dietz P. The hook test for distal biceps tendon avulsion. *Am J Sports Med*. 2007;35(11):1865–1869.
28. Ruland, RT, Dunbar, RP, Bowen, JD. The biceps squeeze test for diagnosis of distal biceps tendon ruptures. *Clin Orthop Relat Res*, 2005;437:128–131.
29. Conte SA, Fleisig GS, Dines JS, et al. Prevalence of ulnar collateral ligament surgery in professional baseball players. *Am J Sports Med*. 2015;43(7):1764–1769.
30. Dugas JR. Valgus extension overload: diagnosis and treatment. *Clin Sports Med*. 2010;29(4):645–654.
31. Chew ML, Giuffrè BM. Disorders of the distal biceps brachii tendon. *Radiographics*. 2005;25(5):1227–1237.
32. Stevens K, Kwak A, Poplawski S. The biceps muscle from shoulder to elbow. *Semin Musculoskelet Radiol*. 2012;16(4):296–315.
33. Vidal AF, Drakos MC, Allen AA. Biceps tendon and triceps tendon injuries. *Clin Sports Med*. 2004;23(4):707–22, xi.
34. Vicenzino B. Lateral epicondylalgia: a musculoskeletal physiotherapy perspective. *Man Ther*. 2003;8(2):66–79.
35. Laban MM, Iyer R, Tamler MS. Occult periarthrosis of the shoulder: a possible progenitor of tennis elbow. *Am J Phys Med Rehabil*. 2005;84(11):895–898.
36. Titchener AG, Fakis A, Tambe AA, et al. Risk factors in lateral epicondylitis (tennis elbow): a case-control study. *J Hand Surg Eur Vol*. 2013;38(2):159–164.
37. Miller TT, Shapiro MA, Schultz E, Kalish PE. Comparison of sonography and MRI for diagnosing epicondylitis. *J Clin Ultrasound*. 2002;30(4):193–202.
38. Mackay D, Rangan A, Hide G, et al. The objective diagnosis of early tennis elbow by magnetic resonance imaging. *Occup Med (Lond)*. 2003;53(5):309–312.
39. Calfee RP, Patel A, DaSilva MF, Akelman E. Management of lateral epicondylitis: current concepts. *J Am Acad Orthop Surg*. 2008;16(1):19–29.
40. Hariri S, McAdams TR. Nerve injuries about the elbow. *Clin Sports Med*. 2010;29(4):655–675.
41. Judson CH, Wolf JM. Lateral epicondylitis: review of injection therapies. *Orthop Clin North Am*. 2013;44(4):615–623.
42. Seng C, Mohan PC, Koh SB, et al. Ultrasonic percutaneous tenotomy for recalcitrant lateral elbow tendinopathy: sustainability and sonographic progression at 3 years. *Am J Sports Med*. 2016;44(2):504–510.
43. Smidt N, van der Windt DA, Assendelft WJ, et al. Corticosteroid injections, physiotherapy, or a wait-and-see policy for lateral epicondylitis: a randomised controlled trial. *Lancet*. 2002;359(9307):657–662.
44. Stewart B, Harish S, Oomen G, et al. Sonography of the lateral ulnar collateral ligament of the elbow: study of cadavers and healthy volunteers. *AJR Am J Roentgenol*. 2009;193(6):1615–1619.
45. Stevens KJ, McNally EG. Magnetic resonance imaging of the elbow in athletes. *Clin Sports Med*. 2010;29(4):521–553.
46. Ciccotti MC, Schwartz MA, Ciccotti MG. Diagnosis and treatment of medial epicondylitis of the elbow. *Clin Sports Med*. 2004;23(4):693–705, xi.
47. Vangsness CT Jr, Jobe FW. Surgical treatment of medial epicondylitis. Results in 35 elbows. *J Bone Joint Surg Br*. 1991;73(3):409–411.
48. Benjamin HJ, Briner WW Jr. Little league elbow. *Clin J Sport Med*. 2005;15(1):37–40.
49. Podesta L, Crow SA, Volkmer D, et al. Treatment of partial ulnar collateral ligament tears in the elbow with platelet-rich plasma. *Am J Sports Med*. 2013;41(7):1689–1694.
50. Espiga X, Alentorn-Geli E, Lozano C, Cebamanos J. Symptomatic bicipitoradial bursitis: a report of two cases and review of the literature. *J Shoulder Elbow Surg*. 2011;20(2):e5–e9.
51. Kegels L, Van Oyen J, Siemons W, Verdonk R. Bicipitoradial bursitis. A case report. *Acta Orthop Belg*. 2006;72(3):362–365.
52. Le Corroller T, Gaubert JY, Champsaur P, et al. Lipoma arborescens in the bicipitoradial bursa of the elbow: sonographic findings. *J Ultrasound Med*. 2011;30(1):116–118.
53. Yeh PC, Dodds SD, Smart LR, et al. Distal triceps rupture. *J Am Acad Orthop Surg*. 2010;18(1):31–40.
54. Gabel GT. Acute and chronic tendinopathies at the elbow. *Curr Opin Rheumatol*. 1999;11(2):138–143.
55. Aaron DL, Patel A, Kayiaros S, Calfee R. Four common types of bursitis: diagnosis and management. *J Am Acad Orthop Surg*. 2011;19(6):359–367.
56. Del Buono A, Franceschi F, Palumbo A, et al. Diagnosis and management of olecranon bursitis. *Surgeon*. 2012;10(5):297–300.
57. Kokkalis ZT, Schmidt CC, Sotereanos DG. Elbow arthritis: current concepts. *J Hand Surg Am*. 2009;34(4):761–768.
58. van Brakel RW, Eygendaal D. Intra-articular injection of hyaluronic acid is not effective for the treatment of post-traumatic osteoarthritis of the elbow. *Arthroscopy*. 2006;22(11):1199–1203.
59. Gramstad GD, Galatz LM. Management of elbow osteoarthritis. *J Bone Joint Surg Am*. 2006;88(2):421–430.
60. Stubbs MJ, Field LD, Savoie FH, 3rd. Osteochondritis dissecans of the elbow. *Clin Sports Med*. 2001;20(1):1–9.
61. Nissen CW. Osteochondritis dissecans of the elbow. *Clin Sports Med*. 2014;33(2):251–265.
62. Bancroft LW, Pettis C, Wasyliw C, Varich L. Osteochondral lesions of the elbow. *Semin Musculoskelet Radiol*. 2013;17(5):446–454.
63. Eygendaal D, Safran MR. Postero-medial elbow problems in the adult athlete. *Br J Sports Med*. 2006;40(5):430–434; discussion 434.
64. Dyer GS, Blazar PE. Rheumatoid elbow. *Hand Clin*. 2011;27(1):43–48.
65. Studer A, Athwal GS. Rheumatoid arthritis of the elbow. *Hand Clin*. 2011;27(2):139–50, v.
66. Shin SJ, Kang SS. Myositis ossificans of the elbow after a trigger point injection. *Clin Orthop Surg*. 2011;3(1):81–85.
67. Muir B. Myositis ossificans traumatica of the deltoid ligament in a 34 year old recreational ice hockey player with a 15 year post-trauma follow-up: a case report and review of the literature. *J Can Chiropr Assoc*. 2010;54(4):229–242.
68. Tyler P, Saifuddin A. The imaging of myositis ossificans. *Semin Musculoskelet Radiol*. 2010;14(2):201–216.
69. Black WS, Becker JA. Common forearm fractures in adults. *Am Fam Physician*. 2009;80(10):1096–1102.
70. Jennings JD, Hahn A, Rehman S, Haydel C. Management of adult elbow fracture dislocations. *Orthop Clin North Am*. 2016;47(1):97–113.
71. Josefsson PO, Johnell O, Gentz CF. Long-term sequelae of simple dislocation of the elbow. *J Bone Joint Surg Am*. 1984;66(6):927–930.
72. Mondelli M, Giannini F, Ballerini M, et al. Incidence of ulnar neuropathy at the elbow in the province of Siena (Italy). *J Neurol Sci*. 2005;234(1–2):5–10.
73. Landau ME, Campbell WW. Clinical features and electrodiagnosis of ulnar neuropathies. *Phys Med Rehabil Clin N Am*. 2013;24(1):49–66.
74. Palmer BA, Hughes TB. Cubital tunnel syndrome. *J Hand Surg Am*. 2010;35(1):153–163.
75. Rosenbaum R. Disputed radial tunnel syndrome. *Muscle Nerve*. 1999;22(7):960–967.
76. Moradi A, Ebrahimzadeh MH, Jupiter JB. Radial tunnel syndrome, diagnostic and treatment dilemma. *Arch Bone Jt Surg*. 2015;3(3):156–162.

77. Djurdjevic T, Loizides A, Löscher W, et al. High resolution ultrasound in posterior interosseous nerve syndrome. *Muscle Nerve*. 2014;49(1):35–39.
78. Ferdinand BD, Rosenberg ZS, Schweitzer ME, et al. MR imaging features of radial tunnel syndrome: initial experience. *Radiology*. 2006;240(1):161–168.
79. Iyer VG. Iatrogenic injury to posterior antebrachial cutaneous nerve. *Muscle Nerve*. 2014;50(6):1024–1025.
80. Presciutti S, Rodner CM. Pronator syndrome. *J Hand Surg Am*. 2011;36(5):907–909; quiz 909.
81. Lordan J, Rauh P, Spinner RJ. The clinical anatomy of the supracondylar spur and the ligament of Struthers. *Clin Anat*. 2005;18(7): 548–551.
82. Simmons Z. Electrodiagnosis of brachial plexopathies and proximal upper extremity neuropathies. *Phys Med Rehabil Clin N Am*. 2013;24(1):13–32.
83. Davidson JJ, Bassett FH 3rd, Nunley JA 2nd. Musculocutaneous nerve entrapment revisited. *J Shoulder Elbow Surg*. 1998;7(3): 250–255.
84. Spindler HA, Felsenthal G. Sensory conduction in the musculocutaneous nerve. *Arch Phys Med Rehabil*. 1978;59(1):20–23.
85. Jung MJ, Byun HY, Lee CH, Moon SW, Oh MK, Shin H. Medial antebrachial cutaneous nerve injury after brachial plexus block: two case reports. *Ann Rehabil Med*. 2013;37(6): 913–918.

CHAPTER 5

Wrist and Hand

EPIDEMIOLOGY OF WRIST AND HAND PAIN

WRIST AND HAND PAIN IN THE GENERAL POPULATION

Prevalence and common causes
- 3% to 26% (significant hand disability in ~13% elderly population, Rotterdam study) (1)
- Most common (MC) causes of hand pain in elderly: osteoarthritis and rheumatoid arthritis
- Age and Parkinson's disease: significant contributors for hand disability in elderly
- Often coexists with pain in other joints

WRIST AND HAND PAIN IN ATHLETES (2)

Prevalence of wrist and hand injury
- 9% to 25% of all athletic injuries
- 50% involve the fingers (3)
- Sports with higher rates of injuries: football, gymnastics, wrestling, lacrosse, and basketball

Wrist and hand pain in different sports
- Football: 15.8% incidence in national football league (hand sprains: 19%; fracture: 11%; wrist sprain: 10%; and dislocation: 9%)
- Basketball: 10% to 23% for all hand injuries, fractures in two thirds of the total hand injuries (MC-type of hand injury), involvement of scaphoid in 38%, metacarpal in 30%, and phalange in 20%
  - Sprain and dislocation of proximal interphalangeal (PIP) joint: MC
- Golf: wrist involved in 20% of all golf-related injuries
  - Tendinopathy: MC type of injury
  - Hook of hamate: MC site for hand/wrist fracture in golf
- Gymnastics: 46% to 80% prevalence in elite gymnasts
- Boxing: MC musculoskeletal (MSK) injury site (up to 46%) in boxers
- Skiing: Gamekeeper's thumb (ulnar collateral ligament [UCL] tear of 1st metacarpophalangeal [MCP] joint)

Tendinopathy in sport
- Seen in any sport/activity requiring a repetitive motion
  - A tennis serve or volley, a basketball free throw, or "turning the wrists over" as in the completion of a golf or baseball swing: at risk for tendon inflammation, instability, or even rupture
    - Extensor carpi ulnaris (ECU) (4) tendinopathy in elite tennis players
      – Tenosynovitis or tendinitis more common than dislocation of the tendon, subluxation, and ECU rupture
  - Racket sport: de Quervain's tenosynovitis
  - Recreational rock climbing: flexor pulley rupture (A2 and A3 pulley)
  - Rowing and powder skiing: intersection syndrome often seen as it requires repetitive wrist dorsiflexion and radial deviation

WRIST AND HAND PAIN AT WORK (5)

Prevalence
- ~22% complaints of wrist and hand pain over a year: 25% acute injury and 9% chronic pain

Carpal tunnel syndrome (CTS)
- MC reason for worker's compensation claims
- More common in shellfish, fish, other meat-packing industries: 20/1,000 full-time employees
- Risk factors (epidemiologic): repetitive motion, exertion, vibration (presence of multiple risk factors is a strong evidence for increased risk of wrist and hand pain at work)

Other injuries
- Sprain or strains of the wrist and hand: highest reported cases in the upper extremity followed by CTS
  - de Quervain's tenosynovitis and trigger finger: commonly seen
- Risk factors (epidemiologic): repetitive motion, exertion, range of motion (ROM), greater risk if multiple risk factors exist (6)

DIFFERENTIAL DIAGNOSIS

MSK CAUSES OF WRIST AND HAND PAIN BASED ON LOCATION (FLOWCHART 5.1)

Surface anatomy with surface landmark (7) (Figure 5.1)
- Central versus ulnar (medial): midline of 4th digit
- Central versus radial
  - Dorsal landmark: Lister's tubercle
  - Ventral landmark: flexor carpi radialis (FCR) tendon

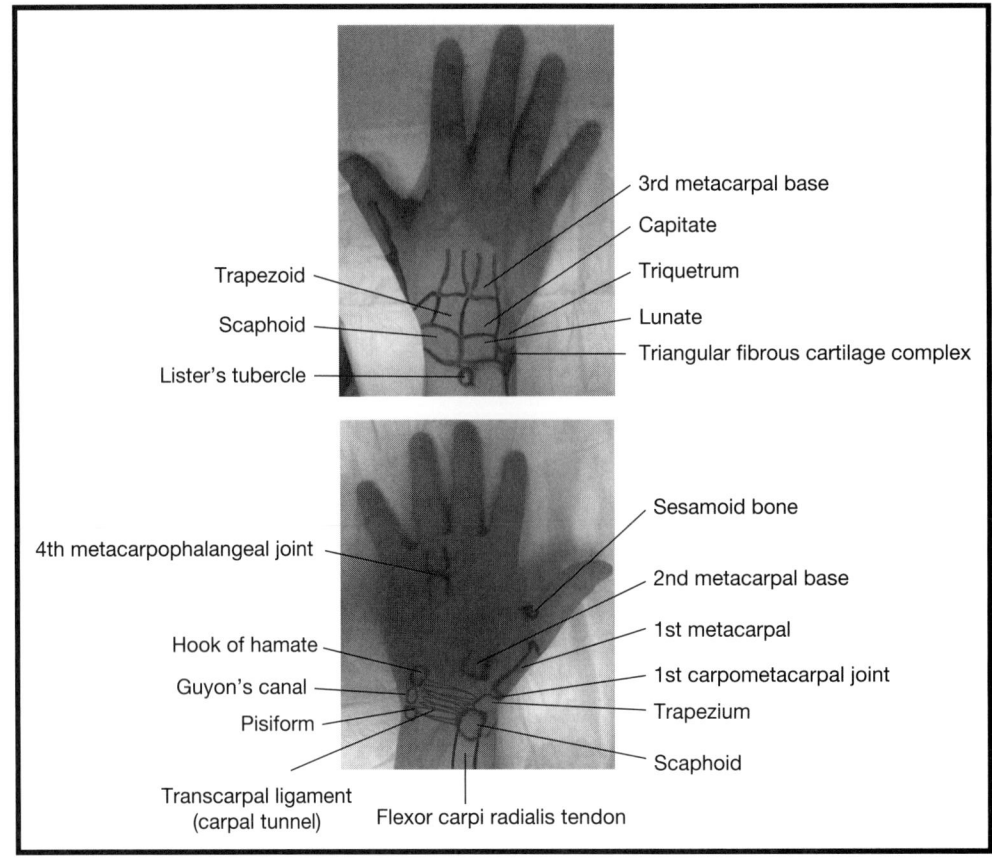

FIGURE 5.1

Surface anatomy of the hand and wrist (palmar aspect and dorsal aspect).

Source: Adapted from Ref. (7). Atzei A, Luchetti R. Clinical approach to the painful wrist arthroscopy. In: Geissler WB, ed. New York: Springer; 2005:185–195.

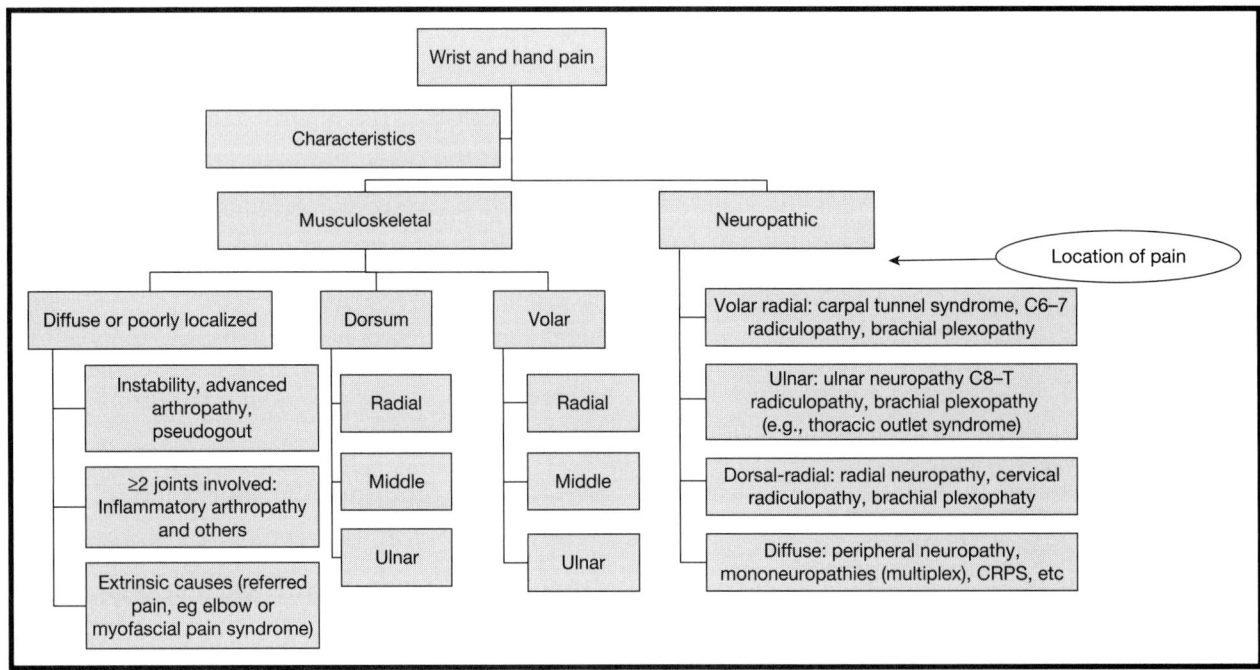

FLOWCHART 5.1

Differential diagnosis of wrist and hand pain.

CRPS, complex regional pain syndrome.
Source: Adapted from Ref. (7). Atzei A, Luchetti R. Clinical approach to the painful wrist arthroscopy. In: Geissler WB, ed. New York: Springer; 2005:185–195.

REGION	STRUCTURE	COMMON PATHOLOGIES (8)
Dorsoradial	Bone	1st carpometacarpal osteoarthritis (OA) (MC site for hand OA) 1st MCP arthritis, wrist arthritis (radial-scaphoid), and scaphoid-trapezium OA Scaphoid fracture, nonunion
	Tendons	1st compartment (abductor pollicis longus [APL], extensor pollicis brevis) and 2nd compartment (Ext. carpi radialis longus and brevis) de Quervain tenosynovitis; MC tendon Dz in wrist Intersection syndrome; 4–8 cm proximal to radial styloid (between 1st and 2nd dorsal compartment) Extensor digitorum brevis manus syndrome (accessory muscle)
	Nerve	Superficial radial neuropathy
Middorsal	Bone	Ganglion; MC from scapholunate Jt. Scapholunate lig. sprain, dissociation/instability Carpal boss
	Tendons	EPL, EIP, EDC tenosynovitis, tear (in rheumatoid Dz) Distal intersection syndrome (EPL and ECRL/B intersection distal to the Lister's tubercle)
Dorsoulnar	Bone	Radioulnar Jt., triquetrum, hamate, 4th and 5th metacarpal bone; carpal metacarpal arthropathy Ulnar triquetral impingement Triangular fibrous cartilage complex tear: between triquetrum and ulnar styloid
	Tendons	5th (Ext. digiti minimi) and 6th dorsal compartment (DC) (Ext. carpi ulnaris; ECU) ECU stenosing tenosynovitis, subluxation/dislocation; from repetitive pronate/supination
	Nerve	Ulnar neuropathy at elbow (spared in Guyon's canal lesion)
Volarradial	Bone	Radius, scaphoid, trapezium, trapezoid, 1st and 2nd metacarpal bones • OA of CMC joint. Wrist and MCP arthropathy • Scaphoid cyst/fracture/AVN
	Tendons	1st dorsal column (APL, EPB); de Quervain tenosynovitis Flexor carpi radialis (FCR) tendinopathy Ganglion cyst originated from flexor tendon Linburg syndrome
Midvolar	Bone	Radius, scaphoid, lunate, capitate, trapezium, 2nd to 4th metacarpal bony pathologies
	Carpal tunnel	Carpal tunnel: FPL, FDS, FDP, median N CTS (often diffuse)
	Tendons	Trigger finger Linburg syndrome
Volarulnar	Bone	Radio-ulnar Jt., pisiform, hamate, 4th and 5th metacarpal bony pathologies Pisotriquetral arthritis Hook of hamate fracture Fracture of metacarpal bone
	Tendons	FCU tendinopathy Trigger finger (stenosing tenosynovitis) at the A1 pulley (at MCP joint)
	Nerve	Ulnar neuropathy (at elbow or Guyon's canal syndrome)

APL, abductor pollicis longus; CMC, carpometacarpal; Dz, disease; ECRL, extensor carpi radialis longus; ECU, extensor carpi ulnaris; EDC, extensor digitorum communis; EIP, extensor indicis proprius; EPB, extensor pollicis brevis; EPL, extensor pollicis longus; Ext., extensor; FCU, flexor carpi ulnaris; FDP, flexor digitorum profundus; FDS, flexor digitorum superficialis; FPL, flexor pollicis longus; Jt., joint; Lig, ligament; MC, most common; MCP, metacarpophalangeal; N, nerve; OA, osteoarthritis; CTS, carpal tunnel syndrome.

NEUROPATHIC CAUSES OF WRIST AND HAND PAIN

- Entrapment neuropathy (local): CTS (MC, volar radial aspect), ulnar neuropathy at elbow (2nd MC, ulnar side), or wrist or superficial radial neuropathy (dorsoradial)
  ○ Cervical radiculopathy (C6: 1st–2nd finger, C7: 3rd finger vs C8: ulnar side, 4th–5th fingers without splitting of sensation in 4th digit)
- Multifocal: mononeuropathy multiplex, hereditarily neuropathy liable to pressure palsy (similar to the common entrapment neuropathy site), and brachial amyotrophy
- Diffuse: diabetic peripheral neuropathy (usually involving distal lower extremities first), sensory neuropathy, or inflammatory polyneuropathy (chronic inflammatory demyelinating polyneuropathy [CIDP] or others)
- Concomitant diffuse neuropathy with entrapment syndrome: amyloidosis, diabetic, and so on

Neurological symptoms

DIFFERENTIAL DIAGNOSIS OF WEAKNESS (±ATROPHY) IN HAND/WRIST MUSCLE	
LOCATION OF INVOLVEMENT	PATHOLOGIES AND CHARACTERISTICS
Central nervous system	Stroke, brain injury, spinal cord lesion/injury • Stiffness and incoordination (clumsiness rather than weakness and atrophy) in brain lesion Cervical myelopathy: related to spondylosis (MC), myelopathic hand
Motor neuron	ALS, primary lateral sclerosis, spinal muscular atrophy (hereditary) • Minimal or no sensory symptoms (exception with concomitant lesion) Syringomyelia (with history of spinal cord injury) affecting anterior horn cells
Root and plexus	Cervical (C8–T1) radiculopathy Brachial plexopathy (thoracic outlet syndrome, metastasis, or median-sternotomy) Klumpke's palsy; C8–T1 involvement; intrinsic hand muscle weakness, numbness, and Horner syndrome (less common than Erb's palsy)
Mononeuropathy	CTS (MC) > ulnar neuropathy > posterior interosseous neuropathy/radial neuropathy
Peripheral neuropathy	Symmetric pattern, length dependent: MC pattern • Dying-back phenomenon: common in diabetic neuropathy, feet usually involved before the hands/fingers Asymmetric pattern: inflammatory neuropathy (CIDP), multifocal motor neuropathy or hereditary neuropathy liable to pressure palsy
Neuromuscular junction and muscle Dx	Typically, more proximal M (including cranial muscle) involved in neuromuscular junction disease Distal muscle involved in some muscle diseases: myotonic dystropy, myofibrillar myopathy, or Welander myopathies, etc • Minimal or no sensory involved

CIDP, chronic inflammatory demyelinating polyneuropathy; CTS, carpal tunnel syndrome; Dx, diagnosis; M, muscle; MC, most common.

DIFFERENTIAL DIAGNOSIS OF FINGER/WRIST DROP

NEUROGENIC	MSK
Presence of tenodesis effect (finger movement by moving wrist → continuity of multijoint muscles) • For example, finger flexion with wrist extension	Absence of tenodesis effect

Upper motor neuron disease
• CVA, spinal cord lesion
Lower motor neuron disease
• Motor neuron disease (focal or early focal)
• C6 radiculopathy/brachial plexus lesion
  ○ Suspect when biceps/deltoid or proximal median N innervated muscles involved (pronator or wrist flexor)
  ○ If there is patch involvement beyond root innervated muscles, favors plexus
• Radial nerve lesion
  ○ Proximal to spiral groove if elbow extensor (triceps) involved
  ○ Posterior interosseous N lesion:
    ▪ Radial deviation (Ext. carpi radialis intact, cutaneous sensory intact on the radial-dorsum of the hand)
• Other neuropathy (multifocal motor neuropathy) or myopathy (distal)
	Tendon rupture
	• Rheumatologic disease; RA
	• Traumatic (immediate or attrition from spur) or iatrogenic (after injection)

CVA, cerebrovascular accident; Dx, diagnosis; MSK, musculoskeletal; N, nerve; RA, rheumatoid arthritis.

SNAPPING (9)

Ulnar side snapping
• ECU subluxation (MC): patient can demonstrate and palpate, reproducible with ulnar deviation and supination
  ○ Sub-sheath tear, common in tennis and baseball players (batting)
• Triangular fibrocartilage complex (TFCC) lesion: often difficult to localize

Dorsal-middle snapping
• Midcarpal instability: radiotriquetral ligament insufficiency → recurrent snapping of the triquetrum
  ○ During ulnar (more than radial) deviation of the wrist, palmar sag of the proximal row with a typical triquetral catch-up clunk generated, confirming the instability
• Boxer's knuckle
  ○ Extensor tendon dislocated ulnarly from disruption of the extensor hood by direct trauma
  ○ Inflammatory joint disease or direct trauma
  ○ Nontraumatic snaps at 5th digit, junctura tendinum (a fascial or tendinous band, linking adjacent extensor tendons) against MCP joint (intact dorsal hood)

ANATOMY

BONE, JOINT, AND LIGAMENT

The proximal carpal row
• Scaphoid, lunate, triquetrum, and pisiform
• Scaphoid

○ A stabilizer of the midcarpal joint, acting as a bridge between the proximal and distal carpal rows (against hand/wrist dorsiflexion)
  ○ Ulnar deviation: scaphoid more longitudinal position (dorsiflexion): lengthen
    ○ Radial deviation: scaphoid palmar flexion
- Intercalated: no tendon insert, movement by mechanical forces from surrounding articulation
- With axial loading, scaphoid: flexion (distal pole; palmar flexion) and lunate/triquetrum (extension)
- Flexion/extension; scaphoid: greatest motion versus lunate: least motion

The distal carpal row
- Trapezium, trapezoid, capitate, and hamate
- Negligible motion in-between, functional single unit bound by stout intercarpal ligaments

Radius: sigmoid notch (articulating with ulna) with variation of morphology

Ulnar: ulnar head covered by articular cartilage, not directly contacting with carpal bones (through TFCC complex)

Joints

Distal radioulnar (RU) joint
- Pivot joint between head of the ulnar and ulnar (sigmoid) notch of the distal radius
- Joint cavity between the fibrous cartilage (disc of TFCC) and the ulnar and radius
- Movement: rotation and translation
- Joint capsule: indefinite, fibrous strand anteriorly, posteriorly fused with the disc below, and form a pouch called recessus sacciformis
- Stabilizer
  ○ Dynamic stabilizer: ECU, flexor carpi ulnaris (FCU), and pronator quadratus
  ○ Static stabilizer: TFCC, interosseous membrane, dorsal/volar RU ligament, UCL, and the joint capsule

Radiocarpal (RC) joint (wrist) (10)
- Ellipsoid joint by the radius, the articular disc (TFCC), proximal row of carpal bones except the pisiform
- Capsule, localized strong bands
  ○ The palmar RC ligament and thinner dorsal RC ligament
  ○ The radial collateral ligament
- Synovial membrane
  ○ Communicate with intercarpal and pisotriquetral joint
  ○ Does not cover the articular disc → communicate with distal radioulnar joint (DRUJ; recessus sacciformis) only when the disc is perforated

Midcarpal (intercarpal) joint
- Ellipsoidal joint between the carpal bones (except pisiform); capitate and hamate by concave socket formed by scaphoid, lunate, and triquetrum
- Plane joint between the trapezium and trapezoid with the scaphoid
- Two degrees of freedom
- FCU extension (pisometacarpal ligament): connect the pisiform to the base of the 5th MC

Trapezio–1st carpometacarpal (CMC) joint
- Biconcave–convex–reciprocal saddle joint
  ○ Unstable joint with loosely arranged capsule
    ▪ 16 ligaments with deep anterior oblique ligament (beak), dorsal radial ligaments as primary stabilizer
  ○ Three planes → 6 degrees of freedom and 90° rotated
    ▪ Flexion/extension (convex of the trapezium), parallel to the palm
    ▪ Abduction/adduction (concave direction), perpendicular to the palm
    ▪ Rotation (oblique)
      – Opposition: flexion and abduction versus reposition: extension and adduction

Other four CMC joints
- Plane (gliding) joint: some gliding motion; more on the 5th (2nd CMC joint: minimal or none)

MCP joint
- Ellipsoidal (condyloid) joint; flexion/extension, adduction/abduction, circumduction
- Fibrous capsule strengthened by the CL, palmar ligament
- Deep transverse metacarpal ligament (connected palmar ligaments of the medial four MCP joints)

IP Joint: hinge (ginglymus) joint

Ligaments of Wrist (11)

Extrinsic ligaments: from the radius or ulnar to carpal bones
- Dorsal ligament
  ○ Dorsal RC ligament: from ulnar and radius, Lister's tubercle to triquetrum and lunate
  ○ Important secondary stabilizer of the scapholunate joint
- Volar ligament: stabilizing the wrist, greater stability than dorsal ligaments
  ○ Radioscaphocapitate (secondary stabilizer for scapholunate joint) and long radiolunate ligament
  ○ The space of Poirier between radiolunate and radioscaphocapitate ligament at the midcarpal joints (interval between the capitate and lunate; poor ligament support → perilunate dislocation/instability)
  ○ Short radiolunate ligament and radioscaphoid ligament

Intrinsic ligaments
- Scapholunate interosseous ligament: rotational stability of the scapholunate joint (dorsal interosseous ligament: thickest, strongest; primary stabilizer), centrally fibrocartilaginous structure (delta shape)
  ○ Injured with excessive wrist extension with ulnar deviation (MC in fall) → tear: more commonly at scaphoid attachment
- Lunotriquetral: thickest and strongest part: volarly, C shape

○ Tear: less common (dorsiflexed wrist in forearm pronated or radial deviation with extreme dorsiflexion); traumatic or degenerative
• Carpal instability: not usually from intrinsic ligament alone; usually from both intrinsic and extrinsic ligament injuries

Triangular fibrocartilage complex (Figure 5.2)
• The central fibrocartilage disc (the meniscal homolog), the dorsal and volar RU ligaments, the ulnolunate and ulnotriquetral ligaments, and the ECU tendon sheath
  ○ TFCC disc: anchored to the articular cartilage of the ulnar side of the distal radius, attached to the ulnar styloid through fibrous bands
  ○ ECU: dorsally, dorsal/ventral RU ligament
• Stabilizer of the DRUJ and a cushion for the ulnar carpus
  ○ Separate the RC from the DRUJ
  ○ Limit pronation/supination/axial migration
  ○ Continuous gliding surface for the RC joint to the ulnocarpal (UC) joint
  ○ Articular surface of the sigmoid notch of radius to the ulnar styloid/UC ligament
• Clinical implications: cause of ulnar-sided wrist pain, instability, and painful decrease in ROM ± snapping

Ligaments of Fingers

Volar plate: thickening of joint capsule volar side of MCP joint and PIP joints (Figure 5.3)
• Thumb: sesamoid bone (two in thumb MP joint, one at thumb interphalangeal [IP] joint, one at 2nd and 5th MP joints)
  ○ Radial sesamoid; more subject to degenerative and arthritic changes
• Tight in MCP extension; prevent hyperextension injury

Collateral ligament
• MCP CL: radial and UCL
  ○ Accessory: fan shape, more volar, tight in extension, valgus, varus stress with extension
  ○ Proper ligament: cord like, more dorsal, tight in 30° flexion, check with 30° flexion
  ○ Injury of UCL in 1st MCP: Gamekeeper's thumb
• Short in flexed IP joint due to oblique direction (keep IP joint straight [in splinting] to prevent contracture), crucial for opposing pinch stability

Retinacular ligament (Figure 5.4)
• Oblique and transverse band
  ○ Retain and position common extensor mechanism (lateral band to the dorsal tip of distal phalanx) during PIP and distal interphalangeal (DIP) joint flexion similar to sagittal band function
• Clinical implication of retinacular ligament dysfunction (Figure 5.5)
  ○ Attenuation of transverse band leads to dorsal translation of lateral bands and a resulting Swan neck deformity (PIP hyperextension and DIP joint flexion)
  ○ Contracture (with attenuation of triangular ligament) of retinacular ligament leads to volar translation of lateral bands, resulting in Boutonnière deformity (DIP joint hyperextension and PIP joint flexion; Figure 5.5)

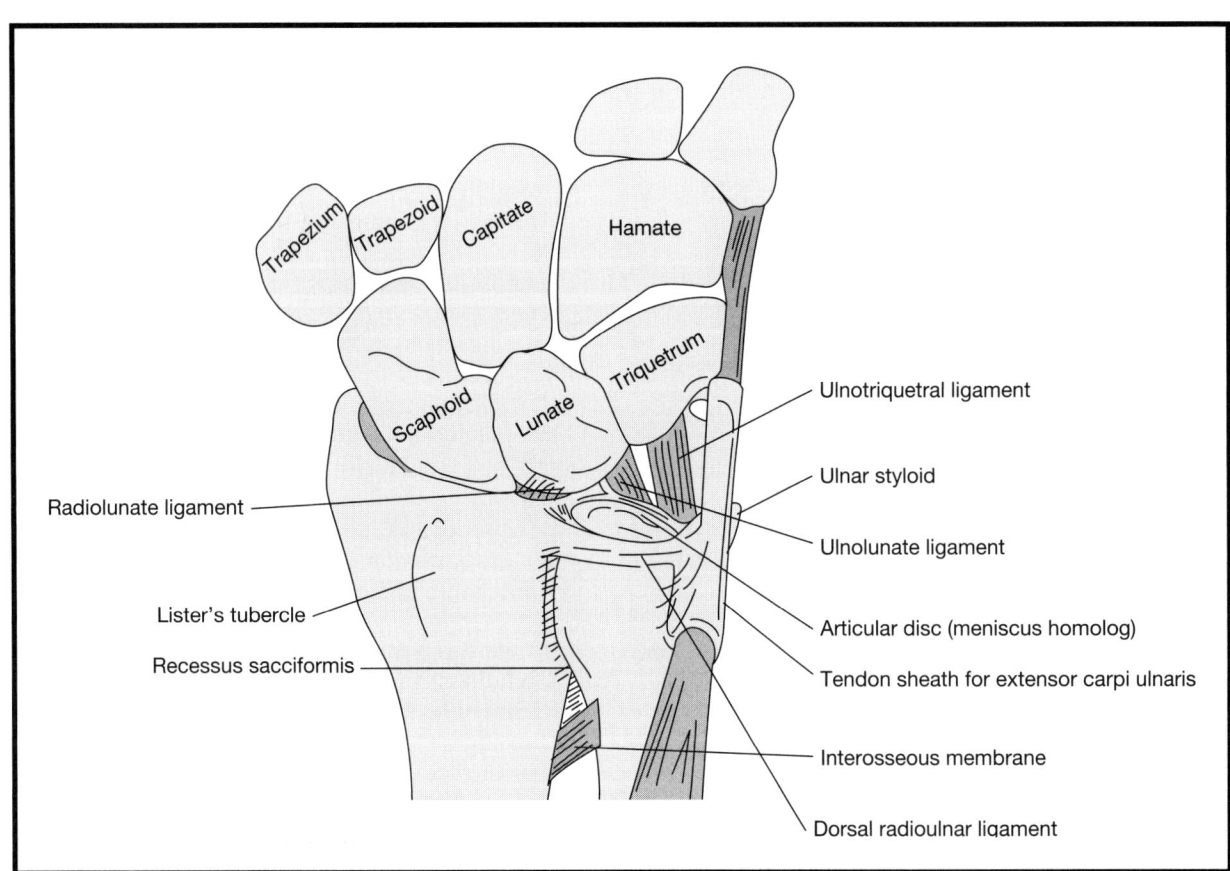

FIGURE 5.2
Triangular fibrous cartilage complex.

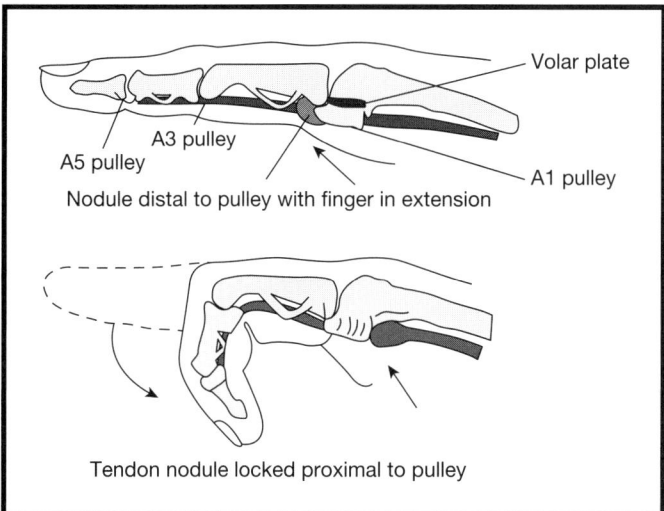

FIGURE 5.3
Pulley system (digital flexor pulley of the finger).

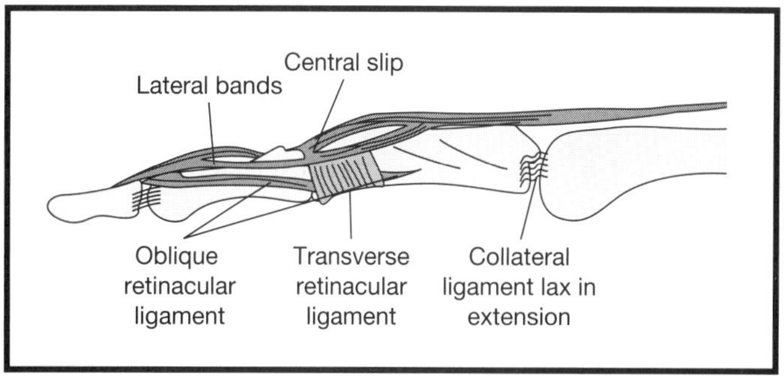

FIGURE 5.4
Collateral ligament and transverse retinacular ligament
Source: Adapted from Ref. (12). Ishizuki M, Sugihara T, Wakabayashi Y, et al. Stener-like lesions of collateral ligament ruptures of the metacarpophalangeal joint of the finger. *J Orthop Sci.* 2009;14(2):150–154.

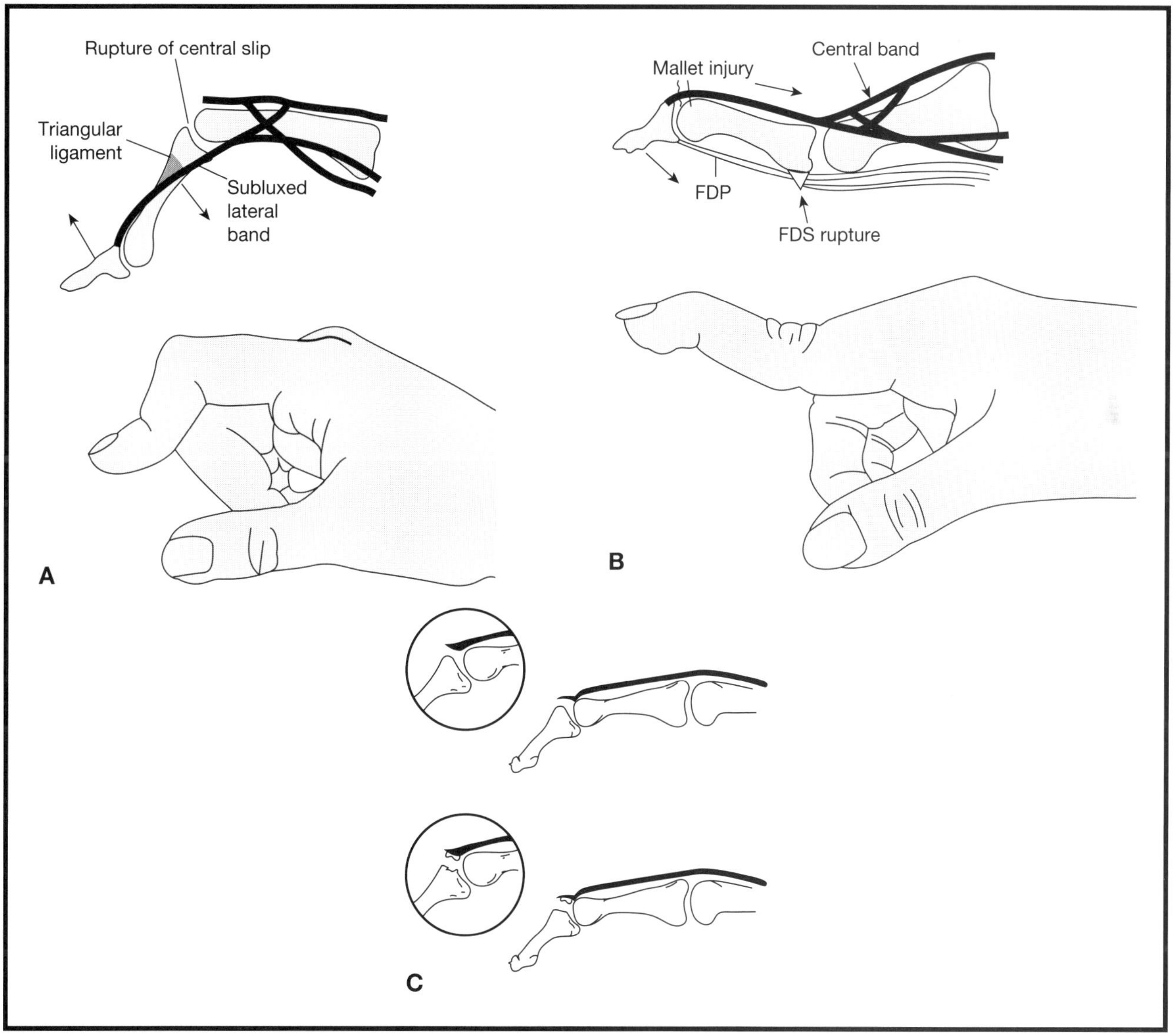

FIGURE 5.5
Common finger deformities. (A) Boutonnière deformity. (B) Swan neck deformity. (C) Mallet finger.
FDP, flexor digitorum profundus; FDS, flexor digitorum superficialis.

Digital cutaneous ligament
- Stabilize the digital neurovascular bundle with finger flexion and extension
- Grayson's ligament: volar to digital nerve; involved in Dupuytren's disease

NERVE

Cutaneous Sensation (13,14)

Median nerve
- Lateral 3.5 fingers (MC pattern, not in everyone) and palmar aspect
- Thenar eminence innervated by palmar cutaneous nerve (branch proximal to carpal tunnel, go over (not inside) the carpal tunnel; spared in typical CTS)

Ulnar nerve
- Medial 1.5 fingers
- Hypothenar eminence and dorsal ulnar aspect (palmar cutaneous of hypothenar and dorsal ulnar cutaneous [DUC] nerve) branching proximal to the wrist spared in ulnar nerve at the wrist (Guyon's canal) lesion
- No splitting of abnormal sensation in 4th digit: can be secondary to variation of ulnar nerve distribution, plexus (lower trunk) or C8 lesion rather than typical ulnar nerve lesion (spared in radial aspect)

Superficial radial nerve
- Adjacent to the radial artery at the mid forearm
- Passes beneath musculotendinous junction of the brachioradialis and the tendon of extensor carpi radialis longus (ECRL; common entrapment site with pronation; Wartenberg syndrome) → emerges 8–9 cm above the radial styloid (possible entrapment by fascial bands) (15)
- Cross (volar to dorsal, superficial to) the 1st dorsal compartment (abductor pollicis longus [APL], extensor pollicis brevis [EPB]) close to the cephalic vein at the wrist (16)

Joint Innervation (Figure 5.6)

Small branch of the superficial radial nerve
- 1st interosseous space dorsally

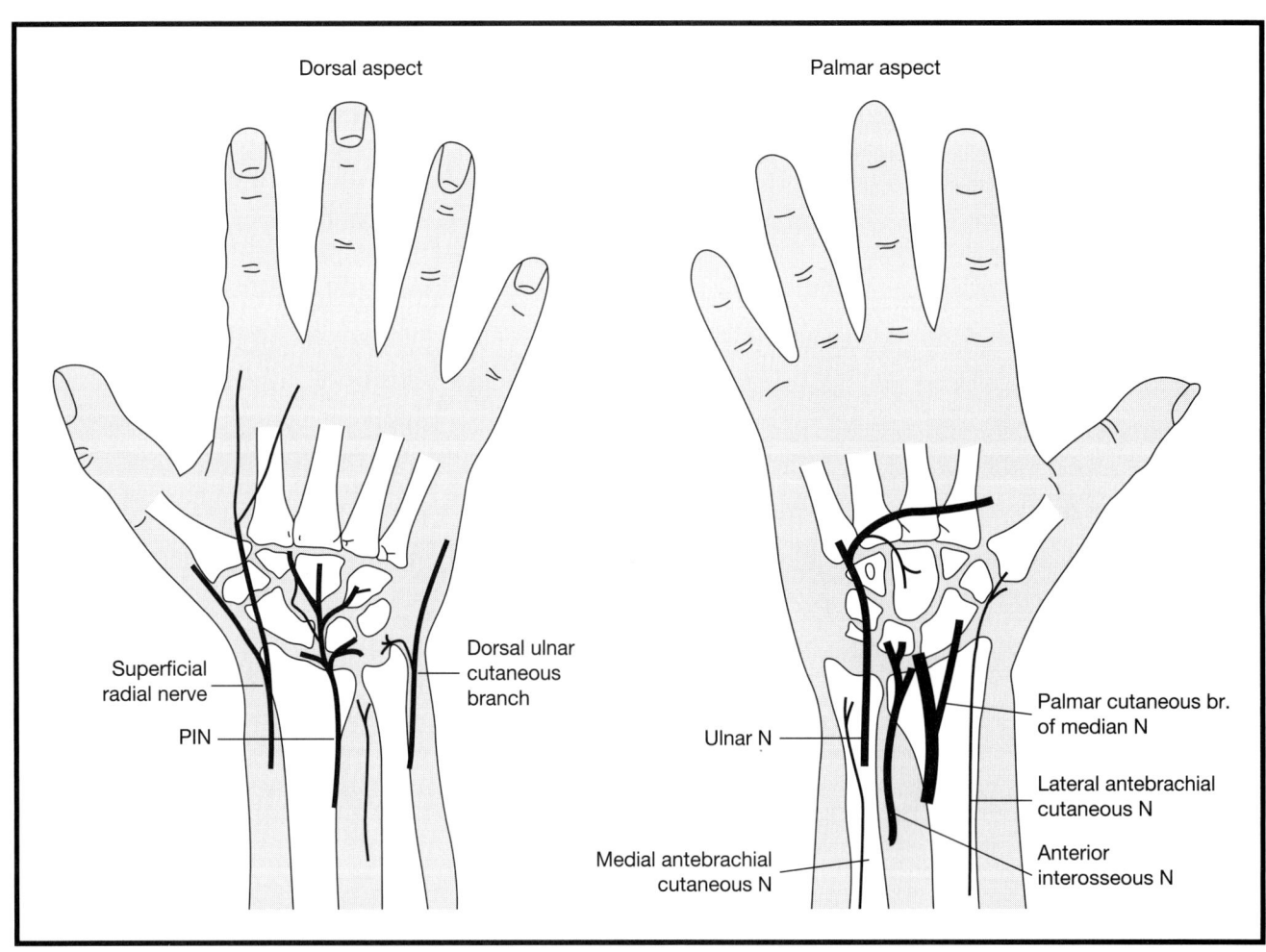

FIGURE 5.6
Nerve innervation of the wrist. The radiocarpal, intercarpal, and carpometacarpal joints are innervated by anterior interosseous nerve (AIN), posterior interosseous nerve (PIN), and ulnar (dorsal and deep branches) nerves.

br., branch; N, nerve; PIN, posterior interosseous nerve.

DORSAL ASPECT INNERVATION	VENTRAL ASPECT INNERVATION
1. *Posterior interosseous nerve*	1. Palmar cutaneous branch of median nerve
2. Superficial branch of radial nerve	2. Anterior interosseous nerve
3. Dorsal branch of ulnar nerve	3. *Lateral antebrachial cutaneous nerve*
4. Perforating branch from the deep ulnar nerve	4. *Deep branch of ulnar nerve*
5. Posterior antebrachial cutaneous nerve	5. Medial antebrachial cutaneous nerve

Italicized terms indicate major contributors.

Posterior interosseous nerve
- Within 1 cm proximal to Lister's tubercle, terminal branch passing deep to the level of the interosseous membrane where it courses before innervating the dorsal wrist capsule
- The terminal branch of the PIN
  ○ The main articular branch to the dorsal aspect of the wrist capsule
  ○ PIN with AIN: innervates three-fourths of the wrist joint capsule
  ○ Location of the nerve block
    ▪ Located in the radial deep aspect of the fourth dorsal compartment (extensor indicis [EI], extensor digitorum communis [EDC])
    ▪ 1.2-cm ulnar to Lister's tubercle and superficial to the periosteum of the radius (17)
  ○ Resection of this terminal branch anywhere along its length provides denervation to the main portion of the dorsal aspect of the wrist capsule

Lateral antebrachial cutaneous nerve
- Innervates radial side of the RC and 1st CMC joint consistently (13)
- Accompanied by radial artery

Ulnar nerve main trunk
- Articular branch to the pisotriquetral joint in ~50%
- Deep branch: 2nd to 4th palmar CMC joints, palmar distal and midcarpal joints

Anterior interosseous nerve
- Provide partial innervation to the palmar RC joint
- In the distal forearm, the AIN runs along the volar surface of the interosseous membrane

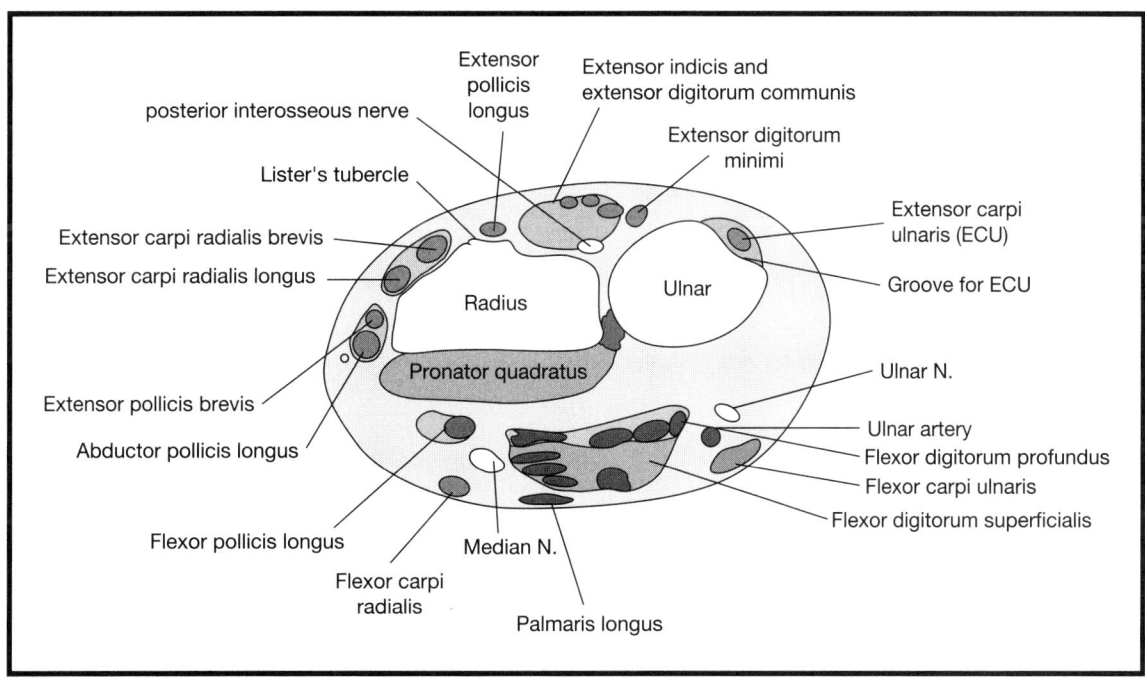

FIGURE 5.7
Wrist compartment (dorsal and ventral compartment).
N, nerve.

MUSCLE

Wrist extensor compartment (Figure 5.7)
- From radial to ulnar; first to sixth dorsal compartments
- PIN except ECRL (radial nerve)
- ECRL/B: C6–7, EDC: C6–8, otherwise: C7–8
- Long extensor (extrinsic); extend MCP, intrinsic (lumbricals, interosseous) extend PIP and DIP
- Extrinsic: finger abduction (as net effect)
- Expansion hood: to extend PIP and DIP joints
  - Central slip: extend PIP, insert to the base of the middle finger
  - Lateral band: extend DIP, insert to distal phalanx, lumbricals, EI, interosseous insert on lateral band

#	MUSCLE	ORIGIN	INSERTION	INNERVATION	ACTION	COMMENT
1	APL	Radius and ulna	Base of 1st MC and trapezium	PIN, C6–8	Abduct/ Ext. thumb CMC Jt	de Quervain tenosynovitis
	EPB	Radius and interosseous membrane	Base of proximal phalanx		Extend thumb MCP Jt	Radial border of snuff box
2	ECRL	Lateral supracondylar ridge of humerus	Base of 2nd metacarpal	Radial, C6, 7 (for ECRL)	Extend (ECRB: prime wrist extensor) and abduct the hand at the wrist	Moment arm for ECRL shorter than ECRB
	ECRB	Lateral epicondyle	Base of 3rd metacarpal	PIN, C6–8 for ECRB		Carpal boss beneath ECRL/B can cause tendonitis
3	EPL	Posterior surface of middle 3rd of ulna	Base of distal phalanx of thumb	PIN, C6–8	Extend thumb IP	Tendon turns 45° on Lister's tubercle
4	EDC	Lateral epicondyle of humerus	Extensor expansions and distal phalanges of fingers	PIN, C6–8	Extend digits	3rd and 4th flexions (EDC maximally stretched) then extend the 2nd digit for isolated EI movement
	EI	Posterior surface of ulnar, interosseous membrane	Extensor hood of 2nd digit			EI; ulnar side to EDC tendon to 2nd digit. Tendon avulsion at central slip: Juncturae tendinae-limiting independent extension of finger (not in EI)
5	EDM	Lateral epicondyle of humerus	Extensor expansion of 5th digit	PIN, C6–8	Extends the 5th digit	
6	ECU	Lateral epicondyle of humerus and posterior border of ulna	Base of 5th metacarpal	PIN, C6–8	Adducts and extends the hand	Subluxation, dislocation (from the groove), tenosynovitis

#, number of dorsal compartment; APL, abductor pollicis longus; ECRB, extensor carpi radialis brevis; ECRL, extensor carpi radialis longus; ECU, extensor carpi ulnaris; EDC, extensor digitorum communis; EDM, extensor digiti minimi; EI, extensor indicis; EPB, extensor pollicis brevis; EPL, extensor pollicis longus; PIN, posterior interosseous nerve.

WRIST FLEXOR						
REGION	MUSCLE	ORIGIN	INSERTION	INNERVATION	ACTION	COMMENT
Radial	Flexor carpi radialis (FCR; Figure 5.7)	Medial epicondyle of humerus	Base of 2nd (80%) and 3rd metacarpals	C6,7, median N	Flex the wrist, and deviate the wrist radially. Weak elbow flex or forearm pronator	Superficial to carpal tunnel. Fibro-osseous canal by crest of the trapezium; site for tendinopathy. Extends finger by tenodesis

(continued)

WRIST FLEXOR

REGION	MUSCLE	ORIGIN	INSERTION	INNERVATION	ACTION	COMMENT
Carpal tunnel	Flexor digitorum profundus (FDP)	Ant. ulnar, interosseous membrane	Distal phalange (ppx) of 2nd to 5th digits	2nd, 3rd: AIN 4th, 5th: ulnar N	Flex DIP, digits, and wrist	Jersey finger (avulsion) Susceptible to Volkmann's contracture
	Flexor digitorum superficialis (FDS)	Medial epicondyle, prox ulna, antero-prox radius	Middle ppx of 2nd–5th digit	C7,8 (T1), median N	Flex PIP, digits, and wrist	
	Flexor pollicis longus (FPL)	Ant. radius, prox ulna	Distal ppx of thumb	C8 (C7, T1), AIN	Flex thumb (interphalangeal joint)	FPL tenosynovitis can cause CTS Susceptible to Volkmann's contracture
Above CTS	Palmaris longus	Medial epicondyle of humerus	Palmar aponeurosis, skin and fascia of palm	C7, 8, median N	Weak flexor of wrist and elbow	Tighten palmar aponeurosis Absent in 15% of people
Ulnar	Flexor carpi ulnaris	2 heads (humeral head on medial epicondyle and ulnar head on olecranon and posterior border of the ulnar	Pisiform, hamate bones and base of 5th metacarpal (anterior)	C8–T1, ulnar N	Flexion of wrist, ulnar deviation of wrist and assist elbow flexion	Roof of the cubital tunnel (Ulnar N at elbow)

Ant., anterior; AIN, anterior interosseous nerve; CTS, carpal tunnel syndrome; DIP, distal interphalangeal; FPL, flexor pollicis longus; N, nerve; ppx, prophylaxis.

Muscle and tendon of hands and fingers

HAND INTRINSIC MUSCLES

MUSCLE	ORIGIN	INSERTION	INNERVATION (C8–T1)	ACTION	COMMENT
Lumbricals	Flexor digitorum profundus (FDP) tendons (radial side of FDP)	Radial lateral band	1,2: Median N 3,4: Ulnar N	Extend PIP, flex MCP Jt.	Inserts on own antagonist M (FDP) 1,2: unipennate 3,4: bipennate
Palmar interossei	Adjacent metacarpal (MC)	Extensor expansion (lat bands)	Ulnar N	Adduct digits	Unipennate M
Dorsal interossei	Adjacent MC	Proximal phalange (ppx) and extensor expansion (lat bands)	Ulnar N	Abduct digits Flex MCP Jt. Weak thumb adduction	Bipennate M
Abductor digiti minimi (ADM)	Pisiform, flexor carpi ulnaris (FCU) tendon	Ulnar side of base of proximal ppx 5th digit	Ulnar N	Abduct 5th finger Flex 5th MCP	Ulnar N and A under it

(continued)

HAND INTRINSIC MUSCLES

MUSCLE	ORIGIN	INSERTION	INNERVATION (C8–T1)	ACTION	COMMENT
Flexor digiti minimi brevis	Hamate, trans carpal ligament	Base of proximal ppx of 5th finger	Ulnar N	Flex MCP of 5th finger	Deep to abductor digiti minimi M
Flexor pollicis brevis (FPB)	1. superficial head: trans carpal lig. 2. deep head: trapezium	Base of thumb proximal phalanx (ppx)	Median N (superficial H) Ulnar N (deep H)	Flex thumb MCP	Dual innervation Superficial head contains radial sesamoid Deep head; often absent
Opponens pollicis	Trapezium	Lateral thumb MC	Median N	Oppose (flex/abduct) thumb	Pronates/stabilizes thumb MC
Adductor pollicis	1. Oblique head: capitate, 2nd/3rd MC 2. Transverse head: 3rd MC	Ulnar base of proximal ppx of thumb	Ulnar N	Adduct thumb, flex thumb MCP	Oblique head converge into a tendon contains sesamoid
Abductor pollicis brevis (APB)	Scaphoid, trapezium	Lat proximal ppx of thumb	Median N	Abduction (perpendicular to the palm)	Primary M in opposition
Opponens digiti minimi (ODQ)	Hamate, trans carpal lig.	Ulnar side 5th MC	Ulnar N	Oppose (flex/abduct) 5th finger	Deep to other M

ADM, abductor digiti minimus; H, head; Jt., joint; Lat, lateral; Lig., ligament; M, muscle; MC, most common; MCP, metacarpophalangeal; N, nerve; PIP, proximal interphalangeal; ppx, prophylaxis.

NO MAN'S LAND

- Zone II: distal palmar crease to the middle crease in the finger (zone I is distal to zone II): A1 pulley to insertion of the flexor digitorum superficialis, unpredictable surgical outcome for tendon repair at this level
- Flexor profundus and sublimis are tightly enclosed within the tenosynovium and inflammatory disease of palm between the distal palmar crease and the crease of the PIP
- Stiffness is common after the surgery

BIOMECHANICS

FOREARM MOVEMENT AND RU JOINT (11, 18)

Ulnar variance: ulnar length (distal end) compared to the radius; varies individually, positive (ulnar longer than radial): pose more loading to UC articulation

In forearm pronation, the distal ulna translates dorsally and distally, whereas in supination, the ulna translates volarly and proximally
- Forearm pronation and ulnar deviation; most pressure to ulnar-carpal/TFCC structures → used in TFCC provocation test

Axial wrist force: through radius (80%–85%) more than ulnar (15%–20%)
- ~50% through scaphoid (scaphotrapezial: 30%, scaphocapitate: 19%), ~30% through the lunocapitate, and ~20% through triquetrohamate joint
- Clinical implication: radial and scaphoid injury more common

ROM OF WRIST AND HAND

- Most activities of daily living (ADL) requires 54° of flexion, 60° of extension, 40° of ulnar deviation, and 17° of radial deviation
- 40° of wrist flexion/extension and radial/ulnar deviation for most of hand placement and ROM
- Flexion ROM contributed by 60% at midcarpal and 40% at RC joints
- Extension ROM contributed by 66% at RC and 33% at midcarpal joints
- Radial deviation: ~90% from midcarpal joint
- Ulnar deviation: 50% to 66% midcarpal and <50% RC joint

Maximal grip strength output at a self-selected optimal wrist position of 35° of extension and 7° of ulnar deviation

Coupled movement: radiodorsal and ulnopalmar motion of the midcarpal joint

Radial deviation: distal carpal row extend and supinate vs flex and pronate with ulnar deviation

PROXIMAL CARPAL MOVEMENTS

Scaphoid: palmar flex (distal flex volarly) vs triquetrum: tend to extend

Lunate: balanced by scapholunate and lunate-triquetral ligament

Lunate-capitate joint: highly mobile and unrestricted (no ligament other than **capsule**)

Dorsal intercalated segmental instability (DISI)
- Lunate dorsally extended position (face dorsally)
- Scapholunate dissociation and scaphoid fracture > scaphotrapezium-trapezoid OA

Volar intercalated segmental instability (VISI) (19)
- Lunotriquetral ligament rupture
- Seen in normal variant or with midcarpal instability

WRIST STABILITY

Lunate
- Proximal row without direct tendon attachment
- Movement affected by link to other carpal bones

Scaphoid
- In the lateral mobile column with trapezium and trapezoid
- Scaphoid position affected by resting forces and radial deviation (link), triquetrum position (opposite to the scaphoid)

BIOMECHANICS OF HAND (20)

- Hand: ~90% of upper limb function
- Thumb: 40% to 50%
- Index digit (lateral, pulp-to-pulp (finger tip) pinch and power grip)
- Middle finger: strongest
- The little finger: power grip

Three biomechanical concepts
- Concepts of link, column, and rows explain motion and role
- Lateral (mobile column: scaphoid-trapezium/trapezoid)—center (flexion/extension: lunate-capitate)—medial column (rotation: triquetrum and distal rows)
- Proximal (lunate) and distal rows: function as a unit, scaphoid connecting both rows
- Three links of chain in radius, lunate, and capitate (center of rotation); intercalated ligament

Hand functions
- Precision grip (21): MCP joints and the radial side and intrinsic muscle
  ○ Flexion at distal interphalangeal joint (DIP) of the index and at interphalangeal joint (IPJ) of the thumb. The ends of the fingernails are brought together as in lifting a paper clip from a tabletop
- Oppositional pinch: dynamometer
  ○ The pulp of the index and thumb brought together with the DIP joints extended. The force to be generated through the thumb opposition, first dorsal interosseous muscle (DI) contraction, and second flexor digitorum profundus (FDP)
- Key pinch
  ○ The thumb adducted to the radial side of the middle phalanx of the index finger
  ○ In ulnar neuropathy → compensate key pinch by thumb and index finger flexion (median nerve innervated muscles)
- Directional grip (chuck grip)
  ○ The thumb, index, and long finger come together to surround a cylindrical object. When using this grip, a combined rotational and axial force is usually applied to the held object (ie, using a screwdriver)
- Power grip
  ○ Hook grip
  ○ Cylindrical grip
  ○ Sperical grip
- Hook grip
  ○ Finger flexion at the IP joints and extension at the MP joints
  ○ The only type of functional grasp that does not require thumb function
- Cylindrical grip: extrinsic muscles, less thumb
  ○ The fingers are fully flexed while the thumb is flexed and opposed over the other digits, as in holding a baseball bat
  ○ Force generated by applying the fingers into the palm
- Span (spherical) grasp
  ○ The DIP and PIP joints flex to ~30° and the thumb is abducted. Force is generated between the thumb and fingers, distinct to cylindrical grasp (only by fingers). Requires the thumb MP and IP stability
- Simpler: thumb finger pinch or digitopalmar grasp
- Forearm position: affects key and fingertip pinches but not the three-jaw chuck pinch
- Measurement: dynamometer, pinch meter
  ○ Normal pinch: 3 to 10 kg and grasp strength: 20 to 40 kg

PHYSICAL EXAMINATION

INSPECTION (22)

Position of the hand
- MCP and IP normally slightly flexed, if one finger extended; rule out flexor tendon injury or tear.
- Normally, all fingers point to scaphoid when flexed PIP joints with DIP extended (cascade sign). If not, check for fracture if history is relevant

Radial side
- Shoulder sign: present if there is radial subluxation of the 1st metacarpal over the trapezium, commonly seen with CMC osteoarthritis
- Osteophytes: scaphotrapezoid osteophyte
- Swelling of 1st dorsal compartment on radial styloid: de Quervain tenosynovitis
- Atrophy of thenar eminence; suspect if the lateral border of the 1st metacarpal is visible

Central
- Carpal boss: prominence in the 2nd or 3rd metacarpal base (seen at dorsum)
- Extensor digitorum brevis (EDB) manus muscle (mild bulging); counterpart of extensor digitorum brevis in foot

Finger
- Palm
  ○ Hill (intermetatarsal space; neurovascular bundle and lumbricals) and valley (flexor tendon)
- Heberden's node in the DIP joint and Bouchard's node in the PIP joint
- Boutonnière deformity and Swan neck deformity (see Figure 5.5)

	BOUTONNIÈRE DEFORMITY	SWAN NECK DEFORMITY
Etiology	RA (weakening of the central extensor attachment [PIP] and volar slip of lateral bands) Damage to central slip (23) and the triangular membrane; injuries to middle phalange (24)	RA (synovitis at PIP) Trauma; ruptured volar plate (dorsal dislocation at PIP) or Mallet finger; ruptured extensor tendon
Characteristics	Unable to flex DIP with straight PIP Ddx with pseudo-Boutonnière deformity (PIP flexion deformity)	Dorsal subluxation of lateral bands Attenuation of the volar plate or transverse retinacular ligament at PIP Rupture of lateral retinaculum of extensor tendon at PIP Contracture of the intrinsic M and deep flexor M and tendon, volar plate, the oblique retinaculum ligament

M, muscle; PIP, proximal interphalangeal; RA, rheumatoid arthritis.

- Intrinsic muscle atrophy and claw-hand deformity
  - Loss of MCP flexion and IP extension (intrinsic hand-muscle dysfunction)
    - Unopposed extrinsic extensor → MCP hyperextension → mechanical advantage to extrinsic flexor (proximal lesion involving FDP; milder deformity) → worsened IP flexion
  - Difficult sweeping the fingers around large objects
  - Wartenberg sign: little finger abduction: unopposed EDM (vs adduction from 3rd palmar interosseous)

PALPATION

Bony landmark; systematically
- Palpate the radial styloid (larger and rounder than ulnar styloid process), and ulnar styloid (distal and deep to the prominent ulnar head)
  - Ulnar variance: palpate the end of radial styloid and ulnar styloid, compare it
- Lister's tubercle; lateral one-third of radial to ulnar styloid (on the dorsum of the radius, at the line drawn between index and middle fingers), lunate (distal and ulnar to Lister's tubercle)—capitate (slightly depressed)—3rd metacarpal in the middorsal (25)
- Radial styloid process, anatomic snuffbox, scaphoid (scaphoid tubercle at distal wrist crease, distal scaphoid tubercle easier to palpate with radial deviation of the wrist), trapezium, and 1st metacarpal bone in the radial aspect
- Ulnar styloid process, pisiform (distal wrist crease), triquetrum (base of pisiform), hook of hamate (one finger breadth distal toward 1st web space from pisiform) in the ulnar aspect

Soft-tissue palpation
- Palmaris longus and FCR (ventrally, prominent with slight wrist flexion)
  - Median nerve located underneath between two tendons at the wrist
- ECU on ulnar groove on the styloid process
- FCU on pisiform
- APL, EPB (1st dorsal compartment) on radial styloid

Range of motion (ROM) (see Figure 5.8)
- Functional ROM for most of ADLs: 50% to 60% of active ROM (26)

Wrist ROM

	ROM° (FUNCTIONAL)		ROM° (FUNCTIONAL)		ROM°
Extension	70 (30–35)	Ulnar deviation	35 (15)	Pronation	75
Flexion	75–80 (10–15)	Radial deviation	20 (10)	Supination	80

Hand ROM

MCP	ROM° (FUNCTIONAL)	PIP	ROM° (FUNCTIONAL)	DIP	ROM° (FUNCTIONAL)
Abduction	20 Thumb: 70	Abduction	20–30	Abduction	20–30
Flexion	90 (60–70)	Flexion	90 (60–90)	Flexion	90 (40–70)

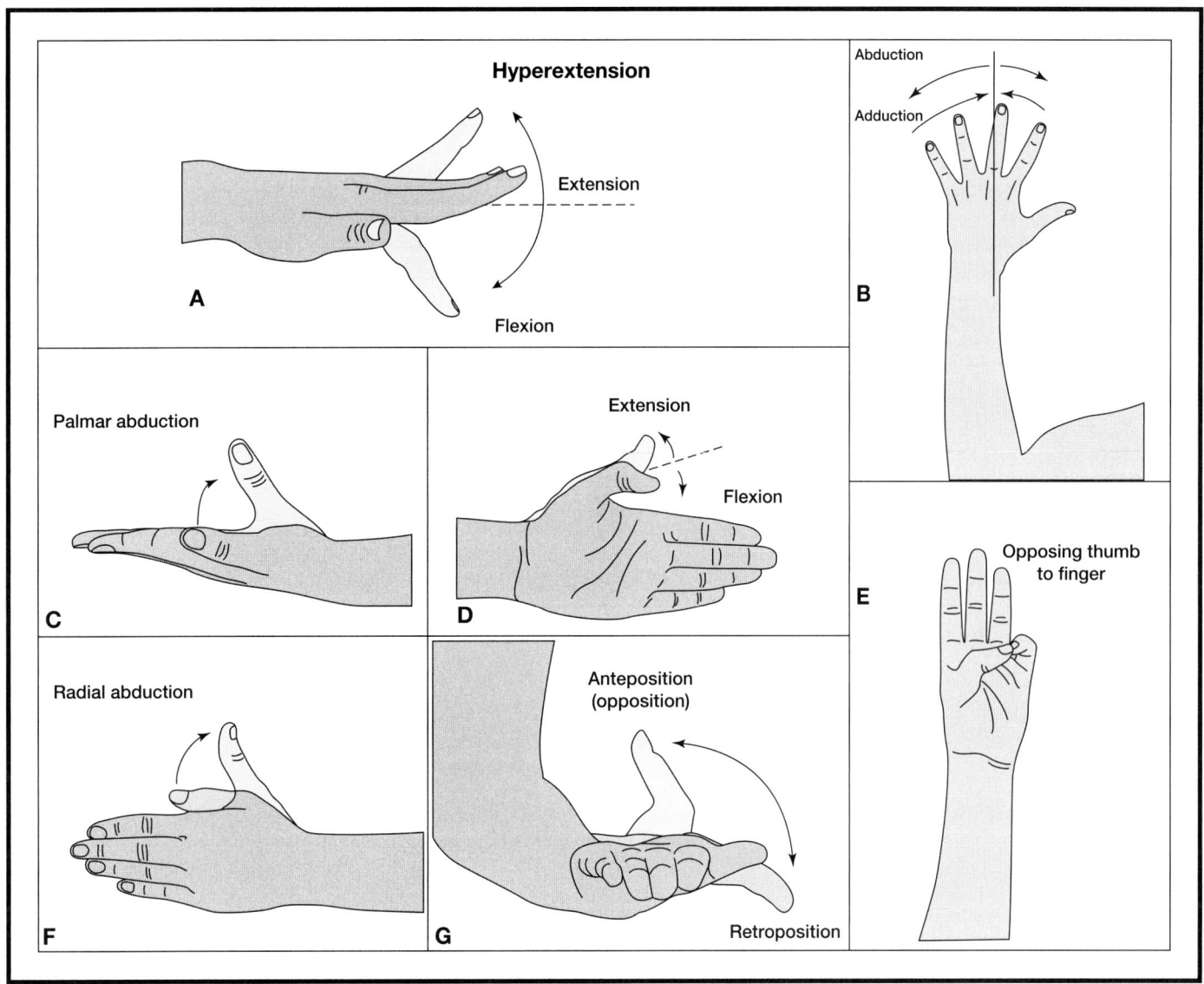

FIGURE 5.8
Different thumb movements.

SPECIAL TESTS OF WRIST AND HAND

	RADIAL	CENTRAL	ULNAR
Dorsal	CMC grind/shear test Tapping of sup radial N	Watson's Litchman's EPL, EIP palpation Radiocarpal subluxation Palpation of carpal boss or aberrant muscle (extensor digitorum brevis manus)	Ballottement (Lunotriquetral) Piano key Ulnocarpal impaction Ulnar styloid impaction ECU palpation, subluxation DUC nerve palpation/Tinel sign
Volar	CMC grind STT joint palpation Finkelstein FCR palpation	Phalen Carpal compression Tinel on median N	Hook of the hamate palpation Pisotriquetral grind

CMC, carpometacarpal; DUC, dorsal ulnar cutaneous; ECU, extensor carpi ulnaris; EIP, extensor indicis proprius; EPL, extensor pollicis longus; FCR, flexor carpi radialis; N, nerve; STT, scaphotrapezium trapezoidal.

NAME	DESCRIPTION	SENSITIVITY (SEN) AND SPECIFICITY (SPE) IN %
Radial		
CMC grind test	Grasp thumb distal to the MCP Jt, and then apply axial compression and rotation to the MCP joint as if "grinding" bones together while examiner's other hand is placed at the CMC joint and shifts the metacarpal base medially and laterally. Positive with pain and crepitus Thumb movement with wrist immobilized: mobilize CMC joint Wrist movement with thumb immobilized: mobilize scaphotrapezium joint (27)	Sen: 40–50, Spe: 80–93
Finkelstein test	Make the fist with thumb inside then deviate the wrist to ulnar side Positive with pain and symptom reproduction Can cause pain on normal hand, so important to compare to the other side	
Central		
Watson's test (scaphoid shift)	Scaphoid stabilized with the thumb over the proximal volar pole with wrist ulnar to radial deviation. Positive with painful subluxation of the proximal scaphoid pole over the dorsal rim of the radius	Sen: ~60, Spe: ~60
Lichtman's test; midcarpal instability	Palmarly directed pressure on distal capitate then wrist axially loaded and passively ulnar deviate Positive with painful catch-up clunk False positive in normal (>50%)	
Ulnar		
Lunate-triquetral Ballottement test (Reagan test)	To evaluate the lunotriquetral interosseous ligament The patient's hand is held in pronation with the fingers toward the examiner. Lunate stabilized by one hand while the other hand shifts the triquetrum in a palmar and dorsal direction Positive with pain or increased translation compared with the contralateral side (28)	Sen: 64, Spe: 44
The Kleinman shear test (or lunotriquetral shuck test)	The patient holds the wrist in a neutral and vertical orientation with the ulnar side facing the examiner. The examiner places a thumb over the dorsum of the lunate and the index finger on the pisiform. Positive if dorsal pressure from the examiner's index finger through the pisiform elicits pain	
Ulnar styloid triquetral impaction test	With the wrist dorsiflexed, the forearm is rotated from a pronated position to supinated position. Positive if the pain or symptom reproduced (22)	
TFCC grind test	To evaluate ulnocarpal impaction or TFCC tear With the forearm in neutral rotation, the wrist is then dorsiflexed maximally and ulnar deviated as the examiner rotates the forearm into pronation. Positive with reproduction of symptoms (pain, click, and crepitus)	
TFCC snap test	With the forearm in neutral rotation and the wrist in ulnar deviation, the wrist is flexed and extended by the examiner with a gentle rolling motion Positive with pain provocation or a painful snap	
Piano keys	To evaluate unstable distal radioulnar joint One hand supports the patient's hand and other hand stabilizes patient's arm. The examiner's index finger then presses down on the ulnar bone Positive if the examiner can press down the ulnar like a piano key	
Pisotriquetral grind test	Translating the pisiform radially and ulnarly while applying dorsally directed pressure. Positive if the patient's symptoms reoccur	

Jt, joint; MCP, metacarpophalangeal; Sen, sensitivity; Spe, specificity; TFCC, triangular fibrocartilage complex.

SPECIAL EXAMINATION OF HAND (FINGER)

MSK examination

NAME	DESCRIPTION
Sweater finger	When the patient makes a fist, the distal phalange does not flex in ruptured flexor digitorum profundus tendon
Elson's test	To evaluate central slip of the extensor hood The patient flexes the PIP 90° on the edge of a table, then extends the PIP while the examiner palpates the middle phalanx → positive if the examiner feels a little pressure (rigid) versus supple if central slip is intact
Boyes test	To evaluate central slip rupture The examiner holds the finger in slight extension at the PIP, and the patient tries to flex their DIP → positive if unable to flex
Bunnell Littler test	To evaluate tight intrinsic muscle or contracture of the joint capsule MCP held in extension by an examiner and then ask the patient to flex the PIP → positive if unable to flex
Lindburg's sign	To evaluate the paratendinitis at the interconnection between FPL and flexor digitorum to index finger The patient flexes the thumb maximally onto the hypothenar and actively extend the index finger → positive if unable to or pain elicited on movement

DIP, distal interphalangeal joint; FPL, flexor pollicis longus; PIP, proximal interphalangeal joint.

Special tests for median and ulnar neuropathy

MEDIAN N		SENSITIVITY (SEN) AND SPECIFICITY (SPE) IN %
Tinel sign	Reproduction of symptoms (tingling or paresthesia) by tapping on the transcarpal ligament (carpal tunnel)	Sen: 74, Spe: 91
Phalen/reverse phalen	Flexion or extend the wrist for 1 minute (flex/extend the wrist at 90° or maximally)	Sen: 50–75, Spe: 33–90
Carpal compression	Direct pressure over the transverse ligament for 30 seconds Sen and Spe can be higher if the wrist is flexed	Sen: 75–90, Spe: ~90
Ulnar N		
Froment's sign	Patient attempts to grasp a piece of paper between the thumb and index finger and the examiner then tries to pull it away; positive if the patient attempts to hold paper with interphalangeal joint flexion	

N, nerve; Sen, sensitivity; Spec, specificity.

- Sensory examination; vibration and/or two-point discrimination
  - Two-point discrimination; more validated for traumatic nerve injury than for CTS
  - Vibration (quantitative vibrometer) had better test for CTS (or stroke of light touch) (29)

Vascular test (30)
- Inspection: splinter hemorrhage (dark spot) in the nail (digital vessel emboli and capillary ischemia)
- Pulsation of radial and ulnar artery pulse; check any mass (aneurysm)
- Allen test to examine the patency of the ulnar and radial arteries
  - The patient opens and closes the fist vigorously several times
  - With the patient's hand tightly closed in a fist, the examiner occludes both arteries simultaneously by compressing the arteries against the underlying bones
  - The patient is instructed to open his or her hand. The examiner then releases pressure from either the ulnar or radial artery and observes blood flow into the pale hand
  - Capillary refill of the palm and digits should be brisk after the pressure had been released. This maneuver is then repeated to assess patency of the other artery. Capillary refill of the digits should also be examined. Normal capillary refill takes fewer than 5 seconds
- Adson maneuver: arm abduction and extension while rotating the patient's head to the ipsilateral elevated arm and extending the neck after a deep inspiration
  - Palpates the radial pulse before and during the maneuver and if it decreases or is completely absent, the maneuver is positive for diagnosis of thoracic outlet obstruction

DIAGNOSTIC STUDIES (FLOWCHART 5.2)

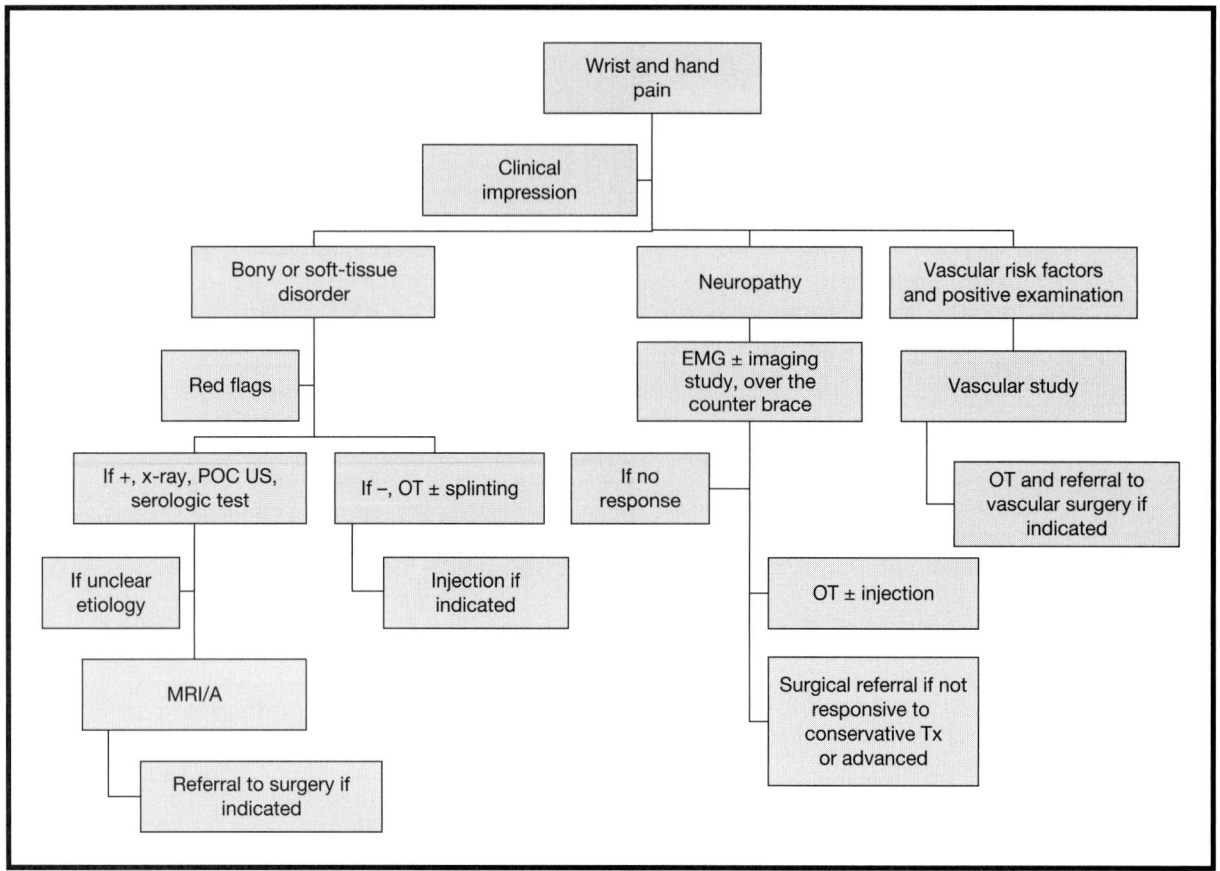

FLOWCHART 5.2
Diagnostic approach and management of wrist and hand pain in outpatient clinic.
EMG, electromyography; OT, occupational therapy; POC, point-of-care; Tx, treatment; US, ultrasound.

PLAIN RADIOGRAPHS (31)

Indications
- History of trauma: R/O fracture and dislocation
- Persistent pain despite the initial conservative treatment to evaluate degenerative joint disease or to evaluate inflammatory joint disease (may not wait for initial conservative treatment trial)

Limitations
- Low capability to assess soft tissues (except tendon calcification), articular cartilage, intraarticular lesion or bursal effusion, and TFCC lesion or marrow

Individual views
- Routine (anteroposterior [AP], lateral, and oblique) (32)
  - AP view of wrist: ulnar variance (by comparing radial and ulnar articular surface), carpal arcs, and joint space for carpal dislocation or dissociation
  - Lateral view of wrist: volar tilt is normally ~10° of the radial surface (suspect radial fracture if not present), scapholunate angle; DISI if >80° (normal 30–60°) or VISI, carpal boss
  - Hand x-ray: PA, lateral, and externally rotated oblique view
    - CMC joint space (if narrowed in especially in 4th and 5th, suspect subluxation/dislocation with relevant history), MCP and IP joint space
    - May also view 1st (base) and 5th metatarsal necks for Bennet fracture/Rolando fracture and Boxer fracture
- Special view
  - Carpal tunnel view to evaluate hook of hamate fracture
  - Roberts view: CMC joint (AP, lateral, oblique)
  - AP with ulnar deviation (ulnar triquetral impaction) or dynamic view for carpal instability
  - Closed fist APs or PAs in both pronation and supination to evaluate scapholunate instability

POINT-OF-CARE ULTRASONOGRAPHY (33)

Indications and findings
- Soft tissues and superficial joint structures
- Soft-tissue pathologies
  - Tendon tear/rupture, tendinopathy, tenosynovitis (34) and ligament tear/rupture
  - Mass: ganglion cyst, lipoma, aneurysm, or foreign body
  - Nerve: focal enlargement in entrapment neuropathy (CTS), generalized enlargement in peripheral neuropathy, rarely nerve tumor, and the like
- Dynamic evaluation of snapping (of ECU over the ulnar groove)
- Role in early detection of bony pathologies (some fracture), effusion and synovitis (in joint), osteophyte, and the like (35)

○ Longitudinal scan (with panoramic view) often easier to visualize the joint structures: hyperechoic subchondral plate, hypoechoic articular cartilage, intraarticular fat pad, joint capsule, effusion, and recess
○ Morphology: highly variable depending on the scanning position (compared to radiography)
• Imaging guidance for injection: carpal tunnel and small joint

Limitations
• The difficulty of accurately imaging some of the intrinsic structures of the wrist including the TFCC as well as its inability to image bone bruises and other subtle bony pathology
• Intracortical structure evaluation also limited

Protocols
• Based on The American Institute of Ultrasound in Medicine (AIUM guideline; see Chapter 1)

MRI/MRA (36)

• Costly, not immediately available, limited dynamic evaluation, but best imaging modality overall

Common indications
• Subtle bony lesion
 ○ Bony cortex and marrow; occult bony injury (occult fracture, bone bruises (contusion), stress (fatigue) fracture, osteonecrosis of the wrist (scaphoid and lunate), bony impaction (abutment) syndrome
• Tendon and ligament injury: TFCC evaluation (magnetic resonance angiography [MRA] preferred) and intercarpal ligamentous injuries
 ○ Great modality for tendon tears and other soft-tissue structures (dorsal hood, pulleys), and other tendon pathologies (tumors). Ultrasound (US) can be used as screening
 ○ Typical findings of ligament disruption
  ▪ Nonvisualization of the ligament, fraying, thinning, and irregularity and fluid signal traversing the ligament on T2-weighted images
 ○ Scapholunate sprain or instability: widening of the space between scaphoid and lunate ± fraying or elongation of the scapholunate ligament
 ○ TFCC (MRA preferred): highly sensitive and specific, difficult to distinguish in aging-induced degenerative thinning and perforation of central portion of TFCC versus pathologic
  ▪ Lower accuracy reported for peripheral (ulnar-sided) TFCC tears
• Mass evaluation: ganglion cysts (trace the base from joint), tumors, or other masses

MRA

• Comparable to conventional angiography in hypothenar hammer syndrome; ulnar artery defect (thrombosis), aneurysm, and the like

CT SCAN

• Useful in supplementing normal or equivocal radiographs in clinically suspected injury

• Accurate for diagnosis of hook of hamate fractures and distal radioulnar joint (DRUJ) subluxation/dislocation
• Helpful in assessment of healing and posttraumatic deformity

ELECTROMYOGRAPHY (EMG)

Indications: clinical/subtle motor abnormality (signs/symptoms), and/or sensory symptoms, neuropathic and radicular pain
• Localize the lesion, assess the severity, and therefore provide prognostic values.

Limitations
• Limited ability to assess the isolated small fiber involvement, sensory radiculopathy, or radiculopathy involving only myelin segments

Nerve conduction studies
• Sensory nerve conduction study (SNCS): 1st digit (C6, median/radial nerve), 3rd digit (C7, median nerve), 5th digit (C8, ulnar nerve), lateral antebrachial cutaneous (C5–6, musculocutaneous nerve), medial antebrachial cutaneous (C8–T1, direct branch from medial cord)
 ○ Typical findings for entrapment neuropathy
  ▪ Demyelinating: focal conduction slowing across the entrapment site ± conduction block (significant decrease in amplitude for a short segment)
  ▪ Axonal: decreased amplitude with distal stimulation (as well as proximal): difficult to localize the lesion
 ○ Normal inpreganglionic lesion (including cervical radiculopathy) or mild proximal lesion (eg, demyelinating lesion in the brachial plexus lesion)
• Motor NCS: median and ulnar nerve (abductor pollicis brevis and abductor digiti minimi, C8–T1)
 ○ Limited evaluation of C6–7 segment (can evaluate the biceps or deltoid but muscles in the hand are C8–T1 innervated)
 ○ Flexor pollicis longus for AIN study
• Needle EMG examination
 ○ Cervical radiculopathy: abnormal spontaneous activities (ASAs); fibrillation in limb muscles of two different peripheral nerves of same root and paraspinal muscles, decreased motor unit recruitment
  ▪ Test 1 spinal (myotomal) level above and below (to localize the lesion)
  ▪ Unclear clinical implication of isolated paraspinal muscle ASA findings
  ▪ Pure sensory radiculopathy or mild radiculopathy (focal demyelination lesion) → negative NCS and needle EMG study; therefore, EMG test is not to rule out radiculopathy
 ○ Focal peripheral entrapment syndrome
  ▪ ASA indicates severe/advanced lesion (axonal involvement).
   – Grading of ASA does not reflect the severity of the axonal lesion. The CMAP amplitude reflects the severity better
  ▪ Reduced motor unit recruitment in neuropathic lesion
   – Valuable in evaluation of severe lesion (presence of motor unit vs absence of motor unit important for prognosis)

TREATMENT

A specific diagnosis is important for the therapeutic plan. There are general recommendations applied in each condition with some exceptions

NONOPERATIVE MANAGEMENT

Education
- Daily ROM: full extension/flexion/radial and ulnar deviation at least 2–3/day, unless contraindicated
  - Maintain wrist extension and ulnar deviation; critical for ADLs
- Stretching of finger flexor or extensor using patient's body weight (gently lean on the palm or the dorsum of the hand on the table)

Rehabilitation
- Therapeutic exercise
  - Tendon-gliding exercise (37)
    - Thumb ROM, three basic fist positions; hook (differential gliding, FDP > FDS), fist (DIP flexion/FDP excursion), and straight fist positions (DIP extension and FDS excursion)
    - FPL gliding by flexion IP and MCP fully
  - Strengthening exercise of wrist/finger flexor, extensor, and hand intrinsic muscles

Edema control (38)
  - Position: hand above the level of heart
  - Wrapping and compressive technique: using Coban (start distally) for finger
  - Compressive/isotoner glove
  - Pneumatic compression sleeves, controlled inflation and deflation
  - Therapeutic massage and lymphatic drainage techniques
  - Scar massage, desensitization exercise, and contrast bath

Oral medications
- Acetaminophen (AAP), nonsteroidal anti-inflammatory drug (NSAID), methyl prednisone (Medrol Dosepak), and short duration of muscle relaxant
- Weak opioid medications if the preceding medication is not effective or contraindicated
- Follow analgesic ladder
- Neuropathic pain medication as needed

Common injections (39)
- Soft-tissue injections (tenosynovium in de Quervain disease, stenosing tenosynovitis, intersection syndrome, FCR tenosynovitis, etc) (40)
- Ganglion cyst aspiration and injection; use 18–21 gauge needle
- Joint injection: CMC joint (cautious of radial A branch and superficial radial nerve), wrist joint injection (radio-scaphoid joint), or IP joint
- Triangular fibrous cartilage complex injection with lidocaine (for diagnosis), steroid or platelet-rich plasma (PRP); US-guided injection under the ECU tendon
- Nerve block
- Carpal tunnel injection; ulnar to (or underneath) FCR (proximal to carpal tunnel; very thin, superficial 2 to 3 mm depth, so be cautious of skin depigmentation)
  - US-guided injection; either radial or ulnar, long or short axis ± hydrodissection of the median nerve
- Superficial radial nerve; cross the 1st dorsal compartment (ventral to dorsal); be cautious when injecting de Quervain tenosynovitis
- Partial wrist denervation: reliable and effective compared to the surgical procedure (41,42)
  - Nerve block of PIN and AIN: 39% to 90% pain relief of wrist pain
  - Kinesthesia is not impaired by the blocking of the nerve

Orthotics (43)
- Functional position; intrinsic plus (for resting wrist hand orthotics; Figure 5.9)
  - Wrist: slight dorsiflexion (20°), ulnar deviation (10°), MCP (45–90°), PIP (0–30°), and DIP (0–10°) flexion
  - Thumb in palmar abduction, 1st web open
  - Lateral ligament in MCP, volar plate, and deep fascial complex: tightened position → less contracture

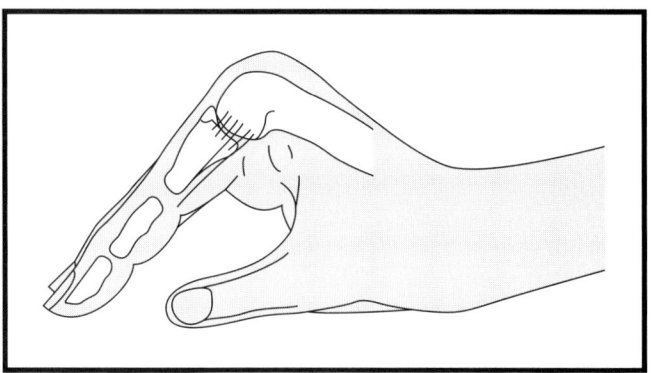

FIGURE 5.9
Functional position of hand and wrist (for immobilization).

- Custom-made orthosis: thumb in opposition position (abduction and flexion toward 5th digit) for 1st CMC OA
  - Different splinting material (for rigidity and surface) available
- Resting-hand splint: paralysis, burn, healing skin graft, Volkmann's ischemia, or painful joints
  - Index through small-finger PIP extension, thumb CMC palmar abduction
  - Different angles of joints for different conditions
- Finger splint
  - Ring orthosis; three-point system to provide dynamic force
  - Aluminum splint (with/without buddy taping) for extensor tendon rupture
  - Stack splint (to prevent DIP flexion) used in mallet finger
  - Boutonnière: PIP extension splint placed for 6 weeks with DIP-free or ring orthosis
  - Swan neck: Bunnell splint (three points, fulcrum in the PIP joint)
- Dynamic wrist hand splint

Commonly used orthosis

PATHOLOGY	MECHANISM AND ORTHOSIS	ADVANTAGES AND DISADVANTAGES
Thumb instability or pain • CMC arthritis • de Quervain tenosynovitis	Immobilize the wrist and CMC joint Thumb adduction stop (to opposition position; allow three jaw chuck) Long opponens thumb spica splint for both Short opponens thumb spica splint for CMC joint pathology	Static, adjustable over time Can grasp with less pain (short thumb spica) Compliance important (especially with long opponens spica)
Mallet finger	DIP extension assist Stax splint	Static Removable; compliance important
Boutonnière deformity	PIP extension assist and DIP extension resist by three-point system Dynamic finger splint (eg, Capener splint)	Removable; compliance important Dynamic splint: using three-point pressure system
Swan neck deformity	PIP extension restriction by three-point system Dynamic finger splint (ring orthosis)	Removable; compliance important
Claw-hand deformity MCP joint extension contracture	Dynamic; passively flex 4th and 5th MCP, prevent shortening of MCP collateral ligament and promote IP flexion Knuckle bender: dynamic Palmar orthosis, static for nighttime	Removable; compliance important Dynamic; may increase or decrease tension on the system by adding rubber bands
Carpal tunnel syndrome	Cock-up splint, wrist neutral position	Best used at night for tolerance, static Allow free thumb movement (can exacerbate basal joint pain)
Rheumatoid deformity	Decrease ulnar deviation and subluxation Static wrist-hand orthotic to wrist extension up to 30°	Modify medial and lateral trims at hand and digits Static, only hold position
Wrist instability	Wrist hand orthosis (with wrist in 20° extension)	

DIP, distal interphalangeal joint; IP, interphalangeal joint; MCP, metacarpophalangeal joint; PIP, proximal interphalangeal joint.

- ○ Provide low-amplitude force over prolonged period
- ○ Force placed by stretched rubber bands commonly, gradual increase in wearing time
- ○ Example: dynamic motion block splint
  - ▪ Kleinert postoperative splint for flexor tendon repair (block extension and resist finger extension by rubber band)
- Static progressive splint (38)
  - ▪ Address joint stiffness by the application of three points of force across the joint
- Buddy taping for CL injury
  - ○ Duration: 3 weeks for partial, 6 weeks for complete tear
  - ○ Tape index to middle, middle to 4th finger (leave index free)
- Compression glove; 10 to 15 mmHg for edema control, 15 to 25 mmHg for scar reduction (44,45)

SURGERY

Indications
- Tenosynovectomy
  - ○ Tenosynovial biopsy: median nerve compression, painful tenosynovial mass, or tendon rupture
  - ○ Indications for flexor tenosynovectomy in the palm: failed conservative management for persistent pain with triggering, tendon rupture, and passive flexion of the fingers that is greater than active flexion
- Wrist arthroscopy for TFCC lesion and repair
- CMC arthritis; resection, arthroplasty
- Resection of ganglion cyst
- Trigger finger release and release of Dupuytren's contracture
- Carpal tunnel or Guyon's canal release

General rehabilitation principles after fracture or surgical procedure (38)
- Therapeutic exercise
  - ○ ROM exercise: A, AA, and passive range of motion (PROM) (with different area of excursion promoted), with greater fracture stability and soft-tissue healing, advanced to strengthening and endurance phase once ROM is normalized
  - ○ Tendon gliding exercises: blocking exercise for isolated joint specific (eg, flex the digit in a proximal to distal manner along the path of least resistance) and differential gliding
  - ○ Strengthening using putty ± neuromuscular electrical stimulation
  - ○ Prevent developing complex regional pain syndrome, desensitization exercise implementing textured dowels, hand immersion, and contrast bath

- Scar massage; direct compression (deep friction as tolerated)
- Splinting; static, dynamic, and static progressive available
- Modality: fluidotherapy, transcutaneous electrical stimulation (to control pain) and neuromuscular electrical stimulation with mixed result (for muscle strengthening and pain control)

Return to play
- No return to play before callus formation after fracture and minimal local symptoms such as edema
- CL injury
  - Stability of joint should not be compromised
  - Acceptable ROM, requirement for grip strength (some exception: nonskilled athletes for early return; for example, using the club cast)
  - Ability to grip and hold on to objects

TENDON AND LIGAMENT PATHOLOGY

WRIST EXTENSOR TENDON DISORDERS

de Quervain's Tenosynovitis/Tendinopathy

Introduction (46)
- Stenosing tenosynovitis of the 1st dorsal compartment (APL/EPB)
- Incidence: female (2.8/1,000 person/year) more common than male (0.6/1,000 person/year), peak in 30 to 60 years (47)
- Anatomic variation in 1st dorsal compartment
  - Septum in the compartment in 34% to 60% of cases with complete compartmentalization of EPB
  - Multiple APL tendon slips: more than one tendinous slip in 58% to 94%
- Risk factor
  - Repetitive grasping/pinching, knitting, and typing, and the like
  - Golf, racquet sports, and fly fishing

History and physical examination
- Pain in the radial wrist (at styloid, anatomical snuff box) ± referred pain to the finger and the forearm (possible irritation of superficial radial nerve)
- Physical examination
  - Tenderness and swelling on the radial styloid process
  - Finkelstein test: can be negative if only EPB is involved
    - Highly sensitive but not specific (positive in normal persons and individuals with arthritis)
  - Pain with resisted thumb extension; less sensitive

Diagnosis
- Clinical diagnosis confirmed by imaging study
- US: thickening of tenosynovium or tendon (heterogenicity) ± increased vascularity
- Differential diagnosis: Intersection syndrome, CMC arthropathy (distally), enthesopathy of APL or superficial radial neuritis (cheiralgia paresthetica)

Treatment (48)
- Steroid injection (±US guidance), 25 or 27 G (for blind injection, total volume 1 mL) with thumb spica splint (49)
  - Skin depigmentation: relatively common (less with US-guided injection and nonparticulate steroid)
- Modification of work and grip as well as adaptive equipment evaluation
- Referral to surgery in recalcitrant cases
  - Persistent pain after surgery → check radial sensory nerve injury or if Finkelstein test + persistently, EPB might not be released or rarely there can be a volar subluxation

Intersection Syndrome

Introduction (50)
- Overuse disorder from friction/entrapment at overlapping of 1st (APL, EPB) and 2nd compartment (ECRL, ECRB) at 4 to 8 cm proximal to radial styloid (or Lister's tubercle)
  - Noninflammatory process of 2nd compartment (tenosynovitis of 2nd compartment at the crossing point) or adventitial bursitis between 1st and 2nd compartments
  - Distal intersection syndrome: adventitial bursitis between 2nd and 3rd compartments (EPL) distal to the Lister's tubercle
- Uncommon in general population (0.2% in patients referred for MRI of wrist), but under-recognized. May be common in sports: prevalence of 11.9% in skiers (from small study, $n = 42$)
- Etiology and risk factor
  - More common in persons involved with hammering, racquet sports, skiing, or in oarsmen (rowing, canoeing)

History and physical examination
- Pain and swelling in the dorsum of the distal forearm (4–8 cm proximal to the radial styloid)
  - ±Crepitus on wrist flexion/extension with tenderness at the intersection
- Weak pinch and diminished grasp
- Finkelstein test: usually positive

Diagnosis
- Clinical diagnosis confirmed by imaging study
- US: scan proximal and distal to see the 1st compartment crossing the 2nd compartment; may show effusion in adventitial bursa. Sono-palpation; discrete tenderness at intersection
  - Distal intersection syndrome: similar finding at intersection of the 1st and 2nd compartments distal to the Lister's tubercle
- MRI; peritendinous edema concentrically surrounding the 2nd and 1st compartments at 4 to 8 cm proximal to Lister tubercle, reactive tenosynovitis, and tissue hyper-edema (51)
- Differential diagnosis: de Quervain tenosynovitis, or extensor tenosynovitis/tendinopathy

Treatment
- Initial rest from aggravating activity, NSAID, activity modification, adaptive equipment evaluation, splint (long-thumb spica splint), and tendon-gliding exercise
- Steroid injection (US guidance) to tenosynovium of 2nd compartment at the tender point

ECU Tendonitis/Tenosynovitis/Subluxation (52)

Introduction (53)
- Anatomy
  - ECU (6th dorsal compartment) traverses the fibroosseous tunnel (separate from extensor retinaculum) at 1.5 to 2 cm of the distal ulna
  - <10% of ECU tendon sheath communicate with DRUJ
- Common in some sports such as tennis (1/18 players/year), golf (8% in professional), and rugby (1/60 players/year) (54)
- Etiology
  - Acute trauma, chronic overuse, and/or inflammatory disease (such as RA) with tethering effect
  - Powerful or repeated pronation from supination
    - Tenosynovitis secondary to unstable retinaculum
  - ECU subluxation
    - Hypersupination (pronation–supination) combined with ulnar deviation and wrist flexion

History and physical examination
- Ulnar-sided wrist pain ± clicking and snapping of the wrist (easily located by patient)
  - In subluxation, pain and clicking reproduced with active forearm supination and wrist extension
- ECU synergy test
  - Pain with ulnar deviation/wrist extension caused by different conditions including TFCC disorders, lunotriquetral arthritis/instability, DRUJ arthritis/instability, and ECU tendon disease
  - Resisted radial adduction of thumb → activate ECU; pain in ECU tendon pathologies but not TFCC or ulnar-sided impingement/abutment (as the space is not narrowed)

Diagnosis
- Clinical diagnosis confirmed by imaging study
- Imaging study
  - US: thickened tendon/hypo/heterogenic echogenicity ± vascularity, thickened tenosynovium, dynamic evaluation for supination/pronation
    - Check position of ECU subluxation in supinated forearm position (subluxation occurs at supination)
  - MRI for differential diagnosis and evaluate TFCC lesion by MRI/MRA and intracortical lesion
- Differential diagnosis
  - TFCC disorders, lunate-triquetral arthritis/instability, or DRUJ arthritis/instability
  - EDM tenosynovitis/tendinopathy, FCU tendinopathy/enthesopathy

Treatment
- ECU tenosynovial injection: proximal to the DRUJ
  - Ulnar (volar aspect) to the ECU tendon, immediately distal to the ulnar styloid (arthroscopic portal 6U), 27 G, 1.5-inch needle with 20 mg of steroid and 0.5 mL of 1% of lidocaine
  - PRP injection (US guidance) between the ECU and TFCC
- Subluxation: long- or short-arm cast/splint and NSAIDs
  - Long-arm casting with forearm pronation and wrist in slight radial deviation and extension for 6 weeks. High-performing athletes or failed conservative treatment → reconstructive surgery

Other Extensor Tenosynovitis or Tendinopathy

Introduction
- The underlying causes: mechanical (overuse or attritional) or nonmechanical (related to inflammatory arthropathy (RA, other rheumatologic) or infectious (with the relevant history)
- Unknown incidence but underrecognized

History and physical examination
- Painful (mild or commonly painless) dorsal wrist mass/puffiness on the dorsum of the hand ± stiffness, and subjective weakness in the handgrip

Diagnosis
- Clinical diagnosis confirmed by imaging study
- Imaging (US) or MRI; tenosynovial effusion ± tendon pathologies (enlargement, tear, rupture)/plain x-ray (for secondary change)
- Serologic test; complete blood count (CBC), erythrocyte sedimentation rate (ESR), C-reactive protein (CRP), rheumatoid factor (RF), anti-cyclic citrullinated peptide antibody (CCP), and the like

Treatment
- Nonoperative management: modification of activity, rest (placement of resting wrist-hand orthosis), anti-inflammatory meds, and US-guided tenosynovial steroid injection if the pain persists
- Referral to rheumatology for further work-up or systemic treatment
- Referral to hand surgery
  - Tenosynovectomy: in failed conservative management, to prevent tendon rupture
  - Tendon rupture: tendon transfer and arthrodesis (55)

Extensor Tendon Tear/Rupture (56)

Introduction
- Classification
  - Inflammatory (tear associated with rheumatoid disease)
    - Relatively common in RA, and disabling condition
    - MC-involved tendons: ECU, EDM, EDC to 4th and 5th digits (31)
    - Pathology: proteolytic effect of pannus, chronic friction over the ulnar head, which is subluxed dorsally
  - Traumatic and overuse
    - EPL: most susceptible (partly due to a course of the tendon from Lister's tubercle with sharp-angle turn)
    - Attritional ruptures of extensor tendons in relation to a spur due to CMC arthritis of the thumb, Kienböck's disease, and osteochondroma of the lunate (32,33)

History and physical examination
- Hand swelling (mild typically), pain ± finger drop
- Absence of extensor tenodesis (vs neurological finger drop; intact tenodesis)

Diagnosis
- Clinical diagnosis confirmed by imaging study and EMG to evaluate differential diagnoses
- Imaging

○ US and MRI: tenosynovial effusion, tendon tear, usually significantly increased vascularity in inflammatory and bony changes. Osteophytes in attritional type, without significantly increased vascularity or tenosynovial effusion.
• NCS and EMG to differentiate peripheral nerve pathologies (C6–7 radiculopathy, posterior plexus lesion, radial nerve and PIN lesion)
  ○ Superficial radial SNCS: differentiate preganglionic lesion (CNS, C6–7 radiculopathy and PIN lesion) versus postganglionic lesion (plexopathy, radial neuropathy)
• Differential diagnosis: neurological conditions; stroke/upper motor neuron (UMN) disease, lower motor neuron disease (brachial plexopathy/plexitis, radial nerve lesion, or posterior interosseous neuropathy)

Treatment
• Referral to surgical evaluation for tenosynovectomy and transfer of tendon
• Splinting (slightly shortened tendon position initially) if surgery is not indicated with ROM (do not perform full extensor stretch at the beginning)

WRIST FLEXOR TENDON DISORDERS

FCR Tendinopathy/Partial Tear/Tenosynovitis

Introduction (34)
• Anatomy
  ○ Located superficial to the scaphoid tubercle (outside carpal tunnel), run through the fibroosseous tunnel of trapezium insert primarily on 2nd and 3rd metacarpal bones
• Unknown prevalence, underrecognized. More common in middle-aged women
• Etiologies
  ○ Overuse, or direct trauma
  ○ OA of CMC, scaphotrapezial joint, scaphoid fracture, or cyst
  ○ Malunited trapezial ridge fracture

History and physical examination
• Pain, swelling, and tenderness along the radiovolar aspect of the wrist
• Pain worsened by resisted flexion and radial deviation, as well as passive wrist extension

Diagnosis (35)
• Clinical diagnosis confirmed by imaging study ± imaging guided diagnostic injection
• Imaging; US and MRI for tenosynovitis, tendonitis, calcification, and tear (US is limited in evaluation at fibroosseous tunnel)
• Differential diagnosis: CMC or trapezium-scaphoid OA, scaphoid cyst, fracture, ganglia, de Quervain tenosynovitis, or Linburg–Comstock syndrome

Treatment (36)
• NSAID, relative rest initially, modify the activity, cock-up/thumb spica splint, and eccentric strengthening exercise
• Injection (US guided to tenosynovium at area of most tenderness or increased thickness/effusion ideally) and sclerosing therapy (polidocanol) (57)
○ Precaution should be taken to avoid the palmar cutaneous branch of median nerve

Flexor Pollicis Longus Tendinopathy/Tenosynovitis

Introduction
• Rare, underrecognized cause of radiovolar wrist/hand pain and secondary cause of CTS
• Etiology: increased in DM and thumb overuse (cell phone texting) (58)

History and physical examination
• Pain (often mimicking CTS) in the volar wrist, radial side of the palm and finger (often more than thumb), swelling, and difficulty moving involved joints with pain
• Tenderness in the volar wrist (at carpal tunnel) and thenar eminence, pain on resisted flexion of the 1st IP joint ± bulging mass and erythema (rare even in infection)
• Positive Tinel and Phalen tests (59)

Diagnosis
• Clinical suspicion confirmed by imaging study
• Differential diagnosis: CTS (secondary CTS), other flexor tendinopathy/tenosynovitis, trigger finger, and wrist arthropathy
• Diagnostic study: imaging study (US or MRI) or EMG (to R/O concomitant or mimicking CTS)
  ○ US: synovial sheath: thin, hypoechoic rim, usually <1 mm normally
    ▪ In tenosynovitis; increased amount of synovial fluid; hypoechoic fluid with irregular tendon margins (60)
  ○ MRI; advantage over US; less operator variability, evaluation of intraarticular and intracortical lesion

Treatment
• Thumb spica splint, OT for activity modification, tendon gliding exercise or modality
• Injection to the carpal tunnel or US-guided injection to the tenosynovium
  ○ Be cautious of infectious tenosynovitis (tuberculosis in endemic region)
• Surgical referral in chronic lesions resistant to conservative management

FCU Tendinopathy

Introduction (61)
• Rare, underreported incidence
  ○ More common in golf and racquet sports
• Anatomy
  ○ Attaches to the pisiform, hamate, and base of the 5th metacarpal bone
  ○ No synovial sheath (therefore, no stenosing tenosynovitis) and tendon follows straight course

History and physical examination
• Ulnar-volar wrist pain, worsened by resisted wrist flexion and ulnar deviation
• Tenderness on FCU (tendinopathy at ~3 cm proximal to the insertion of the pisiform or enthesopathy at the pisiform) ± edema (in acute case) and erythema (rare)

Diagnosis
- Clinical diagnosis confirmed by imaging study
- Imaging
  - X-ray (20° supinated oblique lateral view): calcification, irregularity at pisiform
  - US: calcification in enthesopathy, calcific tendinopathy. Increased thickness (compared to the other side) ± increased vascularity
- Diagnostic injection; imaging guidance with small volume; more specific
- Differential diagnosis: pisotriquetral (PT) arthritis, loose body, ulnar neuropathy at wrist (concomitant or secondary Guyon's syndrome)

Treatment
- Dorsal splint, modify aggravating activities, eccentric strengthening exercises and possible injection for temporary pain control
- Surgical referral in recalcitrant pain despite conservative management

Flexor Tendon Tear

Introduction (55)
- Rupture; rarer although flexor tenosynovitis is common in rheumatologic conditions
  - Flexor pollicis longus; MC tendon to rupture
  - Rupture by bony spur: MC at scaphoid
- Anatomy and biomechanics in flexor tendon in fingers
  - A2 and 4 pulleys: important for finger function; injury → bowstringing of tendon
  - Thumb: A1 and oblique pulley: important, lack vinculum for blood supply
  - From neutral position: 2.5 cm of excursion for extension and 9 cm for flexion
- Prognosis
  - Better prognosis by traumatic or attrition-induced rupture than tenosynovitis
    - Extensive flexor tenosynovitis: adversely affects the outcome
  - Better in the wrist than palm (no man's land)

History and physical examination
- Acute loss of flexion of one or more digits but can be difficult in joint stiffness or instability especially without trauma
- Can be subtle, mild swelling, and mass ± pain

Diagnosis
- Clinical diagnosis confirmed by imaging: US or MRI (check concomitant extensor tendon tear)
- Differential diagnosis or coexisting disease: flexor tenosynovitis in the palm (MC location)

Treatment
- Referral for surgical evaluation
  - Prompt referral to surgery to prevent further tendon damage
  - Reconstruction with a tendon bridge graft, a two-stage flexor graft, a tendon transfer or joint fusion depending on the degree and location of involvement
- If not a surgical candidate, maintain with functional position, or dorsal splint with ROM
- Postoperative rehabilitation (62)
  - Postoperative adhesion: MC complication after surgery
  - Postoperatively, PROM right away, active range of motion (AROM) 14 days postoperation (follow surgeon's protocol)
  - Tendon rupture after primary repair: rare

TRIGGER FINGERS

Introduction (63,64)
- Lifetime risk: 2% to 3%, dominant hand, female > male by six times, and peak in 5th to 6th decades (65)
- MC location: A1 pulley of ring fingers or thumb (at the level of MCP joint, 1–2 cm proximal to the proximal palmar crease)
- Etiology
  - More common with DM (lifetime risk: 10%) and RA
  - Repetitive trauma or space-occupying lesion (retinacular cyst)

History and physical examination
- Triggering/clicking ± pain in the volar aspect, and contracture in advanced case
- PIP contracture and palpate-thickened proximal portion (poststenotic swelling) of the flexor tendon sublimes (superficialis)

Diagnosis
- Clinical diagnosis confirmed by imaging study
- US
  - Increased thickness of flexor tendon (compared with the neighboring tendon or contralateral side)
  - Irregularity or blurring of the tendon margin, loss of fibrillar echotexture, and fluid collection in the tendon sheath
  - Thickening of A1 pulley; hypoechoic lesion (usually difficult to see in asymptomatic person)
- Differential diagnosis: Dupuytren's disease, retinacular cyst, ganglion cyst, tumor of tendon sheath, and RA

Treatment
- Ice, NSAID, and work modification
- PIP extension splint or splinting in 15° flexion of MCP with free PIP and DIP for 3 weeks to 6 weeks
- Steroid injection (0.5–1 mL of betamethasone or triamcinolone + 0.5 to 1 mL of lidocaine) × 1–2 times ± percutaneous tenotomy (66) and ROM (very rare to rupture)
- If not responsive to two injections, additional injections less likely to be effective → referral to surgery

RETINACULAR CYST

Introduction (67)
- Common location: palmar digital sheath in the region of the A1 and A2 pulleys, middle finger
- Isolated or with trigger finger (stenosing tenosynovitis)
- Rare in general, third decade
- Indistinguishable from ganglion cyst histologically

History and physical
- Firm mass in the palm with discomfort or pain during activities requiring forceful grip
- ± Sensory symptoms if irritating the digital nerve

Diagnosis
- Clinical diagnosis confirmed by imaging study
- Imaging: US or MRI
- Differential diagnosis: giant cell tumor of tendon sheath, epidermoid inclusion cyst, granuloma, fibroma, lipoma or neurilemmoma

Treatment
- Aspiration or injection of 1 mL lidocaine and steroid (rupturing the cyst, if not able to rupture, suspect other lesion than ganglion)
- If recurrent, referral to surgery for removal

DUPUYTREN'S DISEASE

Introduction (68)
- Fibroblastic (and myofibroblast) proliferation of the palmar aponeurosis (type 3 collagen)
  - 5% of patients have similar lesion in the medial plantar fascia (Ledderhose disease)
- Prevalence: 0.2% to 56% (northern Europe), male > female: 2–7 times, 40–60s (>50 years), rare in Black and Asian people
  - More common in dominant hand
- Etiology
  - Genetic: A/D with variable penetration
  - Other factors
    - Trauma, diabetes, alcohol-induced liver disease, smoking, HIV, epilepsy, or pulmonary diagnosis
    - Activity (rock climbing and high cumulative exposure to high force or vibration)

History and physical examination
- Tightness of palm/finger (spreading/straightening finger), progressive contracture and impaired ADLs (wash face, shake, clasp, pick up small objects)
  - Functional scale available: a validated Dupuytren-specific subjective assessment scheme
- Isolated or multiple palmar nodules: cord-like induration infiltrating the overlaying skin and extending most often toward the 4th and 5th fingers
- Thickening and contraction PIP 4th or 5th digits of the palmar fascia due to fibrous proliferation
  - MCP and PIP > DIP flexion contracture

Diagnosis
- Clinical diagnosis confirmed by imaging study
- Imaging for differential diagnosis and concomitant pathologies
- Differential diagnosis: Climber's finger: A2 pulley rupture or trigger finger

Treatment
- Modalities including massage, splinting (early stage), steroid injection, and PT
  - Not every nodule progresses (about 50%–69% progress)
- Collagenase clostridium histolyticum (Xiaflex®) injection; risk of tendon rupture

On the following day after injection, work on passive ROM exercises, usually MCP then PIP, not together (can use 1/2 dose for each if planning to inject both)

- Needle aponeurotomy
- Surgery (microneedle aponeurotomy, open fasciotomy, etc)
  - Indication: MCP >30°, PIP joint >25–45° contracture

GAMEKEEPER'S (SKIER'S) THUMB AND STENER'S LESION

Introduction (12)
- Injury of UCL of 1st MCP (thumb)
- Anatomy and biomechanics (Figure 5.10)
  - UCL: proper and accessory CL
  - Dynamic stabilizer: extensor pollicis, flexor pollicis longus/brevis, and adductor pollicis
- MC-injury type at the 1st MCP joint: 86% of all injuries
  - 7% to 32% of all skiing injuries (MC upper extremity injury during skiing) (69)
- Etiology
  - Fall on the abducted thumb (extended, abducted), laxity to radial deviation or fall with holding the pole during skiing
  - Resist excessive valgus opening during forceful grip (holding the game (animal's neck) between the thumb and index fingers, gamekeeper's finger)

History and physical examination
- Pain, swelling, ecchymosis (localized in the ulnar aspect of MCP joint of the thumb), and instability with valgus stress (full extension for accessory CL and 30° flexion for proper ligament)
- Proximal phalanx palmar subluxation with apex ulnar deviation

Diagnosis
- Clinical diagnosis confirmed by imaging study
- X-ray (with stress by patient, R/O avulsion fracture) and MRI R/O Stener's lesion
- US: dynamic (valgus stress, effusion can clarify the ligament injury; hypoechoic lesion can be prominent)
- Classification: three types
  - Type 1: avulsion injury at proximal phalanges
  - Type 2: UCL substance tear
  - Type 3: Stener's lesion: rupturing the ligament leading the proximal ruptured end to displace over the proximal edge of the adductor pollicis aponeurosis
    - → Entrapment of the adductor aponeurosis in the MCP joints → cause sustained laxity → interposition of the aponeurosis prevents healing of the ligament ends

Treatment
- Nonoperative management for type 1 and 2
  - Thumb spica cast or splint (wrist in slight extension and thumb in slight abduction) for 3 to 6 weeks with reevaluation in 2 weeks, then grip-strengthening exercise 8 weeks after injury
- Surgical referral for type 3

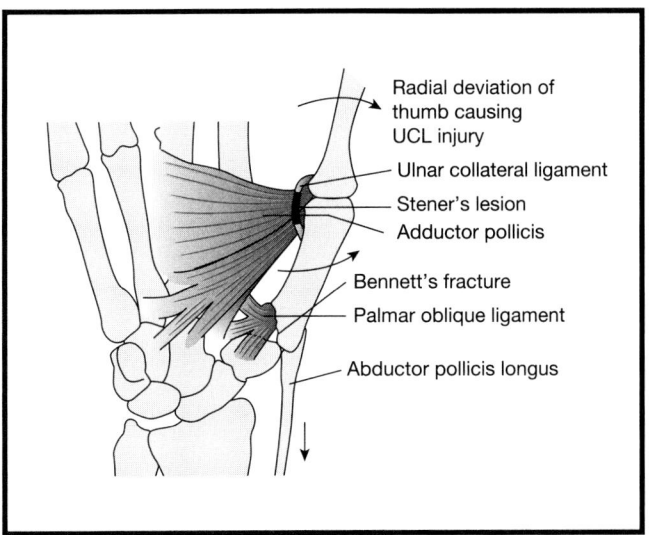

FIGURE 5.10
Common injuries to the thumb (UCL injury and Bennet fracture).

UCL, ulnar collateral ligament.

FINGER SPRAIN AND STRAIN (37)

Jersey Finger

Introduction (70)
- Avulsion of FDP at base of the distal phalanx when grabbing an opposing player's jersey with flexed fingers
- MC location: 4th finger
  - Strength of the FDP insertion of the ring finger is significantly less than that of the adjacent digits
  - During a grip, the distal segment of the ring finger projects further and becomes more prominent secondary to the increased mobility (palmar flexion) at the ring finger CMC joint

History and physical examination
- Pain and tenderness over volar aspect of DIP, slight finger (distal phalange) extension in resting position
- Loss of isolated DIP joint flexion when immobilizing the PIP joint in an extended position
  - Fingertip (DIP) rests at slight extension position compared to the neighboring digit
  - Quadriga effect: active flexion lags in fingers adjacent to a digit with injured or repaired FDP tendon
- ± Palpable flexor sheath for prominence where the tendon end is located and frequently tenderness at the A-1 pulley area if the tendon has retracted into the palm

Diagnosis
- Clinical diagnosis confirmed by imaging study
- X-ray of the hand and finger (PA, lateral, and externally rotated oblique view)
- Ultrasonography and magnetic resonance imaging: usually not necessary

Treatment
- Splint and surgical referral ASAP: direct repair in acute <3 weeks, open reduction internal fixation (ORIF), tendon grafting in chronic injury or DIP arthrosis

Mallet Finger: Baseball Finger

Introduction
- MC-closed tendon injuries among athletes.
- Axial load and forced flexion of the DIP joint → avulsion fracture and extensor tendon rupture (MC mechanism)

History and physical examination
- Finger rest at flexion position and lack of active DIP extension
- Swan neck deformity in chronic stages

Diagnosis
- Clinical diagnosis with x-ray R/O bony injury

Treatment
- Stax splint, splint DIP joint in extension for 6 to 8 weeks
  - Avoid hyperextension, volar splinting less complication than dorsal
  - Progressive flexion exercise at 6 weeks
  - If lesion is >3 months → 8 weeks
- Referral to surgery if chronic injury (>12 weeks): high complication rate or avulsion fracture involving >30% of joint or inability to achieve full extension

Collateral Ligament (CL) Injury Other Than Thumb

Introduction
- Usually at PIP joint ("jammed finger") and MCP
  - Joints other than thumb in 39%
- Forced ulnar or radial deviation at IP joint
- 4th and 5th digits: more likely to have radial CL injuries and 2nd digit more likely to have ulnar CL injury. 3rd digit: equal distribution

Presentation and diagnosis
- Focal pain at the joint, tenderness ± joint instability when grasping objects at CL of MCP joint involved
- Valgus or varus force to interphalangeal joint in 30° of flexion while MCP is in 90° flexion (extended MCP tighten the CL)
  - Compare it with unaffected fingers

Diagnosis
- Clinical diagnosis confirmed by imaging study
- X-ray to R/O avulsion fracture and MRI

Treatment
- Buddy taping (above and below the joint, eg, 4th digit to 5th digit) with AlumaFoam splint for 2 weeks, then PROM
- Surgical referral if the joint is unstable or if injury seen in a child as the growth plate is often involved
  - Radial collateral ligament injury of index finger (needed for pinch stability)

VOLAR PLATE INJURY

Introduction
- MC location: PIP joint
- Without volar plate → the extensor tendons gradually pull the joint into hyperextension (Swan neck deformity in PIP joint involved)
- Etiology: hyperextension of a finger joint

History and physical examination
- Pain and tenderness at volar aspect of PIP and MCP joint
- Check CL
- Joint laxity and swan neck deformity in chronic stages

Diagnosis
- Clinical diagnosis with imaging study (x-ray R/O avulsion fracture)
- US and MRI; sagittal planes of PIP joint: avulsion and proximal migration of the volar plate ± joint effusion, injuries to CL

Treatment
- Progressive extension splint; block splint starting at 30° flexion → in 2 to 4 weeks, then buddy tape
- Referral to surgery if larger fragment (≥40% of articular segment) involved or >30° needed to reduce the fragment

CENTRAL SLIP EXTENSOR INJURY

Introduction
- Central slip: extensor tendon to the PIP joint (continues into two lateral bands to DIP joints)
- Etiology: PIP joint forcibly flexed while actively extended, common in basketball injuries or volar dislocation

History and physical examination
- With PIP in 15° to 30° flexion, unable to extend the joint
- Tenderness on the distal aspect of the middle phalanx
- Boutonnière deformity if not treated
- Elson test and Boyes test (see Physical Examination section)

Diagnosis
- Clinical diagnosis with x-ray R/O bony injury (avulsion fracture) and US/MRI
- Differential diagnosis with mallet finger

Treatment
- PIP joint in full extension for 6 weeks
- Surgical referral if full passive extension is not possible or avulsion fracture involves more than 30% of the joint

NERVE ENTRAPMENT SYNDROME

CARPAL TUNNEL SYNDROME (CTS)

Introduction
- MC entrapment neuropathy, 3% of adults, female > male by ~3 times, peak in the late 50s (71)
  - Commonly coexisting with or mimicking MSK conditions of hand and wrist, and vice versa
- Etiology: unknown but associated conditions including pregnancy, RA, DM, and previous wrist trauma
- Dominant hand more commonly involved than nondominant hand

History and physical examination (72)
- Tingling, numbness at ≥2 of three lateral fingers (1st–3rd) ± 4th or 5th fingers, wrist pain, radiation proximal to the wrist
  - Symptoms correlating with the NCS
- Inspection: atrophy (flattening at thenar eminence or able to see 1st metacarpal bone), thumb abduction strength (other motor strength test: thumb IP flexion: FPL for AIN involvement, indicating proximal nerve lesion)
- Flicker sign, closed fist sign (symptom reproduction with closed fist for 60 seconds); correlate with NCS
- + Tinel sign and − Phalen sign: no correlation with NCS
- Spurling test (cervical radiculopathy), tenderness on the epicondyle (lateral/medial epicondylitis often coexist), CMC grind test (mimicker or coexist), thoracic outlet syndrome

Diagnosis
- Clinical diagnosis confirmed by electrodiagnosis (73)
  - Electrodiagnosis to evaluate other peripheral nerve disorders mimicking CTS (or concomitant) in addition to confirm clinical diagnosis of CTS
    - NCS: sensitivity; 49% to 84%, specificity: 95% to 99% and needle EMG to R/O other differential diagnoses (proximal median neuropathy, brachial plexus lesion, C6–7 radiculopathy)
  - Sensory NCS of median nerve
    - Orthodromic or antidromic at 3rd (C7) and 2nd (C6) digits
      - If wrist to finger segment is abnormal, localize the lesion by midpalm stimulation
      - If normal, may do sensory comparison study (may be more sensitive)
    - Radial-median sensory comparison recording at thumb (with 10-cm proximal stimulation, influenced less from temperature effect, more sensitive). If radial is intact, then generalized neuropathy is less favorable
    - Ulnar NCS (if median NCS is abnormal, it is performed to evaluate for peripheral polyneuropathy)
  - Motor NCS
    - Median nerve recording at abductor pollicis brevis (APB), stimulation at wrist and midpalm to document conduction slowing across the carpal tunnel, often difficult
      - Forearm conduction velocity may be reduced due to a functional large fiber block through the carpal tunnel → measuring smaller (than fastest) fiber conduction velocity
    - Ulnar NCS (if median is involved), median–ulnar comparison study at lumbrical/palmar interosseous.
      - Useful in concomitant CTS in a patient with DM peripheral neuropathy; positive if median latency is delayed than ulnar latency by ≥1 ms)
  - Needle EMG
    - To evaluate C6–7 radiculopathy, especially with SNCS
      - Typical muscles to test: FCR (or PT), EDC/triceps, biceps/deltoid, cervical paraspinal muscles
    - Evaluate motor neuron disease, proximal median nerve lesion (if FCR, FPL involved), brachial plexus pathology (compartment syndrome, thoracic outlet syndrome) or other peripheral neuropathy

- Ultrasonography (74)
  - Cross-sectional area; 11 to 14 mm² at pisiform-scaphoid level, ≥9 mm² (sensitivity 87%, specificity 83%) (75)
  - Ratio: >1.4 to 2.4 (median nerve at wrist compared to median nerve at pronator/mid-forearm where no significant median nerve pathologies present) depending on studies
  - Can evaluate space-occupying lesion (ganglion cyst), amyloidosis, nerve (sheath) tumor, neuroma, and so on (76)
- Other imaging studies: x-ray for square wrist sign (AP wrist diameter/medial–lateral diameter >0.7) or occult bony lesion (especially with history of trauma), MRI R/O other soft tissue, intrabony lesion (for presurgical evaluation) mimicking or co-existing with CTS
- Differential diagnosis (77)
  - MSK causes: CMC OA, FCR/FPL tenosynovitis, scapholunate dissociation, scaphoid/lunate AVN, and the like
  - Neurological causes: proximal median neuropathy (ligament of Struthers, lacertus fibrosis, pronator teres (PT), sublimes of FDS), brachial plexopathy (medial compartment syndrome after catherization), C6–7 radiculopathy, cervical cord lesion (syringomyelia or meningioma affecting the root) or CNS lesions (MS, etc)

Treatment (78)
- Natural course: ~20% improved over 10 to 15 months of follow-up without active intervention (79)
  - 68% of the patients made efforts to reduce occupational and recreational hand stress and 32% changed either hobby or work
- Nonoperative treatment
  - Cock-up splint: ~37% report improvement of symptoms
  - OT: tendon-gliding exercise, education to avoid the provoking symptoms, dexterity exercises
  - Injection (blind vs US-guided): 49% to 81% improvement, varies depending on the study
    - Blind: under the FCR
- Surgery: ≥75% report improvement but leave from the work is days to several weeks (80)
  - Endoscopic versus open; similar
  - Complication and failed carpal tunnel release: 1% to 25% of all carpal tunnel release (81)
    - Permanent complication <1 %, 8% worse
    - Incomplete release of transverse carpal ligament (MC cause)
    - Late complications: complex regional pain syndrome, pillar pain (adjacent to the actual ligament release (82)), neuroma, scar, recurrent or new symptoms
  - US-guided adhesiolysis between the median nerve and scar (by saline ± steroid)

ANTERIOR INTEROSSEOUS NEUROPATHY

Introduction (83)
- Very rare, <1% of neuropathy of upper extremity
- Anatomy: arising at 5 to 8 cm distal to the lateral epicondyle, through or under the PT and then run in the anterior aspect of interosseous membrane
  - Innervates pronator quadrates, FDP (to second and third digits) and flexor pollicis longus
- Etiology: trauma, iatrogenic, or idiopathic (as a form of brachial amyotrophy)
  - Compression: by deep head of PT, FDS tendon to the middle finger or accessory head of FDS, FPL (Gantzer's muscle), tendinous origin of palmaris longus or FCR, ulnar collateral artery thrombosis, aberrant radial artery, and enlarged bicipital bursa

History and physical examination
- Weakness of hand muscles: FPL > PQ and FDP (FDP can be preserved due to cross innervation by ulnar nerve) ± pain, deep wrist and in the forearm (~50% reported in small study)
- Impaired OK sign (flex thumb IP joint [FPL] and index DIP [FDP]), inability to hold a sheet of paper with tip of finger with normal sensory examination and abduction of thumb (median nerve/recurrent motor branch) and finger abduction (ulnar)/extension (radial nerve)

Diagnosis
- Clinical suspicion confirmed by EMG study
- EMG (normal SNCS and routine motor nerve conduction study [MNCS]; median nerve recording at APB and ulnar nerve)
  - AIN study recording at pronator quadratus or FPL study with stimulating at elbow; compare it with the other site
  - Abnormal needle EMG in FDP to 2nd, 3rd digit, FPL, and PQ and normal FDI (C8, T1, medial cord, and ulnar nerve), APB (C8, T1, and median nerve), FCR (C6–7, proximal median nerve), EI or EDC (C7–8, posterior cord, radial nerve)
- Differential diagnosis; flexor tenosynovitis (FPL, FDP), rupture (in RA), and brachial amyotrophy
- Imaging study: US or MRI (to evaluate space-occupying lesion/entrapment site with proximal nerve swelling, muscle denervation, nerve thickness/focal swelling or lesion)

Treatment
- Nonoperative management
  - Usually improves without operative management
  - NSAID as needed and a few sessions of OT (stretching and gradual strengthening exercise)
  - Injection for wrist pain; dorsal to volar approach at 1 cm ulnar and 3 cm proximal to Lister's tubercle (both AIN and PIN) (17)
- Surgical exploration if no improvement or worsening after conservative management for ~2 months (84)

ULNAR NEUROPATHY AT WRIST

Introduction (85)
- Rare, incidence and prevalence: not reported
- Etiology: space-occupying lesions (eg, ganglion cyst), repetitive trauma (occupation: hammering, cyclist), vascular lesions (hypothenar hammer syndrome), aberrancy or deviant hypothenar muscle, calcium deposition disease (CPPD) and calcific tendinopathy (FCU), hook of hamate fracture, and crutch walking (86)
- Classification (Shea and McClain) (87)
  - Type 1: sensory and motor involved, lesion at proximal or Guyon's canal
  - Type 2 (MC): isolated motor involvement, lesion at Guyon's canal: Hook of Hamate at origin of ADM and FDM (IIa: distal to hypothenar muscle)
  - Type 3: isolated sensory involvement, least common
- Association with CTS: disputable

History and physical examination
- Sensory symptoms (ulnar side of 4th and 5th digits in typical cases) and ulnar-sided hand pain
  - Dorsum of the hand and wrist spared due to DUC nerve branches proximal to the Guyon's canal. If involved, suspect ulnar nerve at elbow region
- Motor symptoms: weakness/wasting of 1st DI, intrinsic muscles, hypothenar, and possible thenar (deep head of flexor pollicis brevis muscle)
- Inspection for mass or ganglion cyst
- Sensory examination
  - Intact in the dorsal ulnar aspect of hand (DUC nerve branching above the wrist) and the medial forearm (medial antebrachial cutaneous nerve from medial cord)
  - Sensory examination; the Semmes–Weinstein monofilament test and two-point static discrimination (may be more sensitive)
- Motor strength: side-to-side pinch, Wartenberg sign, and Froment sign (check elbow section)
- Vascular exam (Allen test), and tenderness (hook of hamate)
- Elbow (Tinel sign, subluxation), and cervical spine examination (Spurling test)

Diagnosis
- Clinical suspicion confirmed by EMG
- EMG: American Association of Neuromuscular and Electrodiagnostic Medicine (AANEM) practice guideline. Check the ulnar nerve entrapment at elbow
  - SNCS
    - SNCS recording at digit 5 with wrist stimulation, antidromic or orthodromic
    - Intact DUC nerve (if abnormal, lesion is proximal to DUC branch → ulnar neuropathy at elbow)
  - Motor NCS
    - MNCS recording at abductor digiti minimi (ADM) with stimulation at wrist, below and above elbow (R/O ulnar nerve at elbow)
    - Comparison between ADM and FDI with stimulation at wrist (two-channel recording); if ADM is normal and FDI is prolonged (>2 ms difference compared with ADM), then it suggests lesion at deep recurrent motor branch
  - Needle EMG
    - ADM, FDI involved. Spared FCU or FDP (4th or 5th), APB (median nerve, medial cord, C8–T1), EI (radial nerve, postcord, C8) and lower cervical PS (r/o radiculopathy)
- US
  - To find a mass lesion: aneurysm in the ulnar A, mass (lipoma or ganglion) or, rarely, tumor
  - Check for focal swelling or diameter (between the sites if asymmetrically involved)
- Differential diagnosis
  - UMN lesions: stroke (with vascular risk factors), multiple sclerosis, spinal cord lesion (syringomyelia, cervical myelopathy with myelopathic hand)
  - Ulnar neuropathy: above elbow (arcade of Struthers), at elbow (MC), and forearm (rare)
  - Peripheral neuropathy: motor neuron disease (amyotrophic lateral sclerosis with signs of UMN disease, Hirayama disease), C8–T1 radiculopathy, brachial plexopathy (median sternotomy syndrome, metastatic brachial plexopathy, thoracic outlet syndrome), mononeuritis multiplex, hereditary neuropathy with liability to pressure palsy (typical entrapment site), CIDP (MADSAM; Lewis-Sumner syndrome), multifocal motor neuropathy (unusual location)

Treatment
- Nonoperative management
  - Avoid irritation by modifying the handle bar, the grip of the cane or rolling walker. Wear glove with padding
  - NSAIDs, aspiration, and steroid injection if ganglion cyst presents
- Surgical: if not responsive to conservative treatment
  - Surgical exploration, removal of space-occupying lesion and demonstration of the ulnar tunnel from the standard surgical treatment

SUPERFICIAL RADIAL NEUROPATHY

Introduction (88)
- Cheiralgia paresthetica, Wartenberg syndrome, rare, no prevalence study, female > male
- Common entrapment site: between musculotendinous junction of the brachioradialis and the tendon of ECRL (common entrapment site with pronation; Wartenberg syndrome) → emerge ~8 to 9 cm (distal 1/3 of the forearm) above the radial styloid (possible entrapment by fascial bands) (15)
- Etiologies: de Quervain disease (concomitant in 20%–50%), trauma, tightly worn wrist watch, handcuffs, lipoma, Colles fracture, diabetes, repeated exposure to cold, iatrogenic, tight fascial band, brachioradialis/ECRL, anatomic variation

History and physical examination
- Pain, tingling, pins/needle sensation, and numbness in the dorsum of the hand (dorsal-radial aspect of the wrist, in the lateral three fingers)
- Tinel sign; usually radiate distally (but can radiate proximally). Normal motor examination and deep tendon reflex (DTR)

Diagnosis
- Clinical diagnosis confirmed by sensory NCS (isolated abnormal finding, superficial radial nerve recording at thumb, 2nd metacarpal and 3rd metacarpal bone stimulating at wrist); compare site to site
  - NCS; often negative → imaging guided lidocaine block (0.5–1 mL)
- Differential diagnosis: proximal radial nerve lesion (usually with motor symptoms), C6–7 radiculopathy or brachial plexopathy, de Quervain tenosynovitis (concomitant)

Treatment
- Therapeutic injection (US-guided), lidocaine cream, education for desensitization, and transcutaneous electrical nerve stimulation (TENS)
- Treatment of underlying pathologies (surgical evaluation for persistent pain despite the conservative management)

BONE AND JOINT PATHOLOGY

FIRST CARPOMETACARPAL (CMC) OSTEOARTHRITIS (TRAPEZIOMETACARPAL)

Introduction (89)
- Epidemiology
  - Prevalence: 5% to 7% >70 years old (YO) in United States, more common in 50 to 70 YO, female > male by three to four times
  - Radiologic evidence in 21% to 36% >55 YO female (postmenopausal)
    - Female: greater reciprocal curvature of the trapezium and metacarpal articular surface, lower degree of congruity, smaller surface area → increase contact stress
- Anatomy and biomechanics
  - Major joint stabilizers
    - Anterior oblique ligament (palmar beak ligament), dorsoradial ligament (most important from biomedical study), and APL
    - Abduction combined with slight medial rotation and flexion of the CMC joint at the thumb: increase the stability
- Etiology and risk factor
  - Occupations exposed to repetitive use of hand, family history, maybe obesity and laxity
  - Lateral pinch of thumb and index: causes increased joint compression force by 12 times, palmar side commonly involved

History and physical examination
- History
  - Intermittent aching to severe pain in radial thumb especially with activities requiring opposition
    - Aggravated by writing, opening jars, and carrying heavy objects between thumb and fingers
  - Pain in the thenar eminence, cramping in the 1st web space from joint laxity and synovitis
    - Concomitant CTS (~40% of CMC OA patients: met the criteria of CTS)
- Physical examination (90)
  - Inspection: shoulder sign: step off between 1st metacarpal and trapezium due to dorsoradial subluxation of 1st MC bone
    - Adducted (flexed) CMC joint (metacarpal on the trapezium) with hyperextended thumb MCP joint (as a compensation)
    - Secondary deformity of hyperextension or valgus at MCP and IP joints
  - Palpation: tenderness over CMC joint versus scaphotrapezial joint
  - CMC grind test; axial compression and rotation from MC to trapezium (crank test: axial compression and flexion/extension)
    - Wrist movement affects scaphotrapezial joint more than CMC versus MCP joint movement, which affects CMC more than scaphotrapezial joint
  - Key and tip pinch strength; available objective measurement (dynamometer)

Diagnosis
- Clinical diagnosis supplemented by imaging study
- X-ray; true AP (Robert view, maximal pronation) and true lateral (20° pronation) ± stress view
  - Asymmetric joint narrowing, sclerosis, subluxation, and osteophytes formation
  - Classification based on imaging study
    - Eaton classification based on joint space, subluxation (one third), osteophyte, or loose body size (2 mm) or involvement of periscaphoid joint (stage IV)
- Differential diagnosis (91)
  - Pantrapezial joints (trapezoid-trapezium, scaphoid-trapezium), 1st MCP OA, and radio-scaphoid OA
  - Scaphoid pathology (fracture or avascular necrosis)
  - SL ligament injury, trigger finger, and CTS (can coexist)
  - DeQuervain tenosynovitis, FCR tendonitis, or FPL tendonitis

Treatment (92,93)
- Nonoperative management (94)
  - Occupational (hand) therapy: activity modification (avoid pinching; especially lateral pinching, gripping, lifting and twisting), adaptive equipment evaluation, ergonomic evaluation, and thenar muscle strengthening (dynamic stabilizer, palmar abduction with weight or band)
  - Splinting with long opponens or thumb spica; palmar abduction, slight flexion, and medial rotation
  - Injection
    - Steroid injection followed by 3 weeks of splinting: 40% for subjective relief >12 weeks (stages 1–3)
    - Hyaluronic acid versus corticosteroid (1 mL): faster relief with corticosteroid but hyaluronic acid showed superior pain relief after 6 months
- Surgery
  - Ligament reconstruction with FCR tendon slip and tendon interposition
    - Caution of superficial branch of radial nerve injury and acute CTS
  - Arthroscopy, complete trapezium resection, abduction–extension osteotomy, total joint arthroplasty
  - Postoperative rehab: focusing on achieving abduction

OSTEOARTHRITIS OF THE WRIST

Introduction (95)
- OA: ~5% of patients with wrist x-ray; scaphoid involvement >95%
- Primary idiopathic OA; rarer than secondary OA
  - Trauma-induced OA (96)
    - Ligament injury
      - Scapholunate instability with DISI → dorsal radial subluxation of proximal scaphoid (scapholunate advanced collapse [SLAC])
      - Lunotriquetral dissociation → midcarpal osteoarthritis
    - Fracture-malunion
      - Scaphoid nonunion and advanced collapse after fracture; usually 5 to 10 years after fracture
      - DISI and instability; extension of the proximal pole of the scaphoid → scaphoid-radial styloid joint involvement (stage I), scaphocapitate joint involvement (stage II), and capitolunate joint involvement (stage III)

- RC arthritis (after distal radius fracture, even after the anatomic reduction): usually well tolerated
- Distal radio-ulnar joint OA; axial loading with rotational stress; ulnar-sided wrist pain
  ◦ Others: primary avascular necrosis (Kienböck and Preiser) and deformity (Madelung deformity); rarer

History and physical examination (97)
- Mechanical pain, swelling, ROM limitation, and decreased strength (often subtle)
- Tenderness on scapholunate, scaphoradial joint ± effusion, crepitus

Diagnosis
- Clinical diagnosis supplemented by imaging study
- X-ray: PA, lateral, ± lateral view with 20° to 30° supination (for PT joint)
- MRI for Kienböck disease or if unresponsive to conservative management

Treatment
- Nonoperative management: splint, steroid injection under US guidance, wrist denervation (distal PIN/AIN block; good option for manual laborer with good range or elderly patients)
- Surgical referral in advanced cases and if not responsive to conservative management
  ◦ Scaphoid excision and four-corner arthrodesis, proximal row corpectomies (PRC), total wrist arthrodeses, and total wrist arthroplasty

PISOTRIQUETRAL (PT) ARTHRITIS/INSTABILITY

Introduction (98)
- Anatomy and biomechanics
  ◦ Pisiform: embedded on the FCU tendon, acting as sesamoid
  ◦ PT joint communicate with RC joint in 70% to 80%
  ◦ Wrist extension: PT joint space decrease. Wrist flexion: PT space widens
  ◦ Ulnar deviation of wrist → triquetrum; more ulnar deviation and extension
- Etiology
  ◦ Usually from PT trauma (forceful ulnar deviation and extension of the wrist) with instability
    ▪ Racquet sports (repetitive wrist flexion and direct compression)
  ◦ Primary OA of PT joint: rare

History and physical examination
- Ulnar palmar wrist pain in the vicinity of the pisiform, usually h/o trauma
- Tenderness on pisiform-triquetrum (palpate the pisiform at dorsal/ulnar aspect)
- PT shear test and ulnar impaction test
- Motor and sensory examination for possible concomitant ulnar neuropathy

Diagnosis
- Clinical diagnosis supplemented by imaging study
- X-ray: wrist in 30° supination: early degenerative change at radial distal border of the pisiform joint
- Diagnostic injection (US-guided, small dose, less than 1 mL); maybe low specificity (overflow of injectate and different soft tissues attached to pisiform)
- Differential diagnoses
  ◦ Flexor capri ulnaris pathology (often coexist with PT dysfunction), TFCC lesion, ulnar triquetral arthropathy, or ECU tendon dysfunction

Treatment
- Work modification, glove with padding, corticosteroid injection (with imaging guidance using less than 1 mL, cautious of ulnar nerve in the radial aspect), and splint
- Referral to surgery if the pain continues despite therapy; pisiform excision (risk of ulnar neuropathy)

RHEUMATOID ARTHRITIS OF THE WRIST AND HAND (99)

Introduction (100)
- Epidemiology of RA
  ◦ Prevalence: 1%, female > male by two to three times, peak onset: 35 to 50 (60) YO
  ◦ Multifactorial, ↑ with human leukocyte antigen (HLA) class II major histocompatibility complex (MHC) DRB1, DR4
  ◦ Environment: smoking, silica dust, and the like
- RA involving wrist: very common; >50% of patients with RA have wrist pain within 2 years, 90% wrist involvement by 10 years, >95% bilateral involvement
- Hand and finger involvement: more disabling than wrist
- CTS: common with hyperplastic synovium and thickened transcarpal ligament

History and physical examination
- Pain, swelling, impaired joint function with morning stiffness (≥1 hour)
  ◦ Pain: gradual onset over weeks to months (more common than acute)
  ◦ Swelling (may be secondary to synovitis and tenosynovitis of tendon) ± deformity
    ▪ Joint involvements: MCP joint (especially 2nd and 3rd MCP) and PIP > wrist > knee > shoulders
  ◦ ± Mild weakness; tendon rupture (especially in volar synovitis); underrecognized
- Physical examination
  ◦ Edema/effusion of the wrist/hand (more readily noted in dorsal than palmar/ventral aspect)
  ◦ Deformity; ulnar deviation, swan neck, Boutonnière, cock-up deformities (101)
    ▪ MCP joint; palmar dislocation of the proximal phalanx and ulnar deviation of the finger
    ▪ Zig–zag deformity of wrist-hand: tenosynovitis of ECU and EDC, synovitis of prestyloid recess of the ulna → dorsal displacement of the ulnar (caput ulnar syndrome with stretching of the ulnar carpal ligament) ECU volar subluxation → radial deviation of the wrist → secondary ulnar deviation of the fingers (tenodesis effect) → ulnar translation of the carpals, volar subluxation and supination
  ◦ Neck examination for involvement of cervical spine and examination of other joints for involvement

- Neurological examination: check sensory, motor, provocative test for CTS (common)
  - In motor examination, differentiate with tendon rupture (lack of tenodesis)
- Extraarticular manifestation
  - Rheumatoid nodule (20%–30%, usually RF+): subcutaneous nodules on extensor surface along tendon sheath and bursa; can be found in the lung, heart, and sclera
  - Constitutional symptoms: fever, weight loss, and malaise
  - Ocular: scleritis, episcleritis, and keratoconjunctivitis sicca
  - Pulmonary: interstitial lung disease, pleural, bronchiolitis, and bronchiectasis
  - Cardiac: pericarditis, myocarditis, valvular/ conduction disorder 2/2 nodules
  - Hematologic: anemia of chronic disease, leukemia, and lymphoma
  - Vascular: nailfold infarct, palpable purpura, and leukocytoclastic vasculitis
  - Long-standing seronegative, erosive RA: Felty's syndrome (neutropenia, RF+, splenomegaly)

Diagnosis
- Clinical diagnosis: Revised American College of Rheumatology (ACR) criteria in 2010 (102)
  - Scores ≥6/10 points: "definite RA"

The number and size of involved joints (score 0 to 5, with higher scores for a larger number of small joints affected); 2–10 large joints (1), small joints (2 if 1–3, 3 if 4–10, and 5 if >10 joints involved) Small joint: MCP, PIP, thumb IP, wrist, and 2nd to 5th MTP
Rheumatoid factor or anti-citrullinated protein antibody (2 for +, 3 for a high positive RF (3 × upper normal) or positive anti-CCP
Abnormal sedimentation rate or elevated C-reactive protein (1 point)
Symptom duration ≥6 weeks (1 point)

CCP, cyclic citrullinated peptide; IP, interphalangeal; MCP, metacarpophalangeal; PIP, proximal interphalangeal; RF, rheumatoid factor.

  - Serologic test
    - CBC (mild anemia and leukocytosis)
    - RF (immunoglobulin M [IgM] anti-IgG antibody [Ab], sensitivity: 60% specificity: 80%)
      – False positives are seen with hepatitis C, subacute bacterial endocarditis, sarcoidosis, malignancy, Tb, cryoglobulinemia, Sjögren's, systemic lupus erythematosus (SLE), increasing age, 5% of healthy population
    - Anti-CCP (specific up to 95%–98%): the presence of either RF or anti-CCP ("seropositive RA") is associated with more severe RA
    - ↑ESR, CRP; + antinuclear antibody (ANA) in 15%; ↑ globulin during active disease
- Diagnostic imaging
  - X-ray of wrist and hand
    - Larsen classification: Grade 0 (no change); Grade I (periarticular swelling, osteoporosis, slight narrowing); Grade II (periarticular erosions with some joint-space narrowing); Grade III (moderate joint destruction); Grade IV (severe destruction, collapse, and significant periarticular erosions); and Grade V (grossly mutilating changes)
    - Other: the Wrightington classification specific to wrist
    - Wrist: joint space narrowing at RU and radioscaphoid joint as an early finding, midcarpal involvement seen later
    - Hand: later involves periarticular erosions, especially in MCPs, PIPs, MTPs
  - US and MRI: detecting erosive disease, joint effusion/ synovitis earlier (103)
    - Bare area: where the capsule attaches into the bone; not covered by articular cartilage; bony erosion in early RA
    - US differentiation of pannus (hypoechoic, increased vascularity) versus effusion (anechoic, no vascularity)

Treatment (104)
- Referral to rheumatologist for starting disease modifying antirheumatic drugs (DMARD; methotrexate, hydrochloroquine, sulfasalazine, and leflunomide) or biologic
  - Early diagnosis and Tx→ ↓ ds activity, ↓ radiologic progression, ↑ physical function, ↑ quality of life
  - Initial treatment: NSAIDs (↑ CV ds and other side effect), COX-2 inhibitor (↑ CV ds), glucocorticoid (IA injection, low-dose oral)
  - DMARD within 3 months for all patients
    - Mono treatment with MTX, sulfasalazine, leflunomide, hydroxychloroquin (HCQ) or combination + glucocorticoid or anti-TNF; never use two biologics concurrently
    - Anti-TNF: etanercept, infliximab, adalimumab; screen for tuberculosis
    - Others: azathioprine, penicillamine, gold, minocycline, cyclosporine, and the like
- Nonoperative management
  - Occupational therapy: six to eight sessions
    - Static and dynamic splint: pain relief, no proven benefit to improve function and delaying deformity, splinting in early deformity (ring orthosis, lumbrical bar), Stax splint for mallet finger
    - Joint protection technique, adaptive equipment evaluation (grab bar, universal cuff), ROM exercise (full hand grip, cautious of aggressive stretching exercise) and strengthening exercise (cautious of eccentric or high intensity exercise), hand dexterity exercise, ADL/IADL evaluation/training and education
  - IA steroid injection in addition to DMARDs (imaging guided to the small joint and tenosynovium)
- Referral to surgery: persistent symptoms, synovitis despite 3 to 6 months of conservative treatment or progressive deformity or frank tendon rupture
  - Contraindications: significant comorbidities, poor general health, poor insufficient proximal arm function, previous infection, insufficient bone stock, and long-standing fixed deformity
  - Surgery: synovectomy, tenosynovectomy in early stages, tendon repair/reconstruction, treatment of the arthritic DRUJ, partial and complete arthrodesis of the RC joint, and wrist arthroplasty
  - Joint procedure
    - PIP: prevent hyperextension; flexor sublimis tenodesis or oblique retinacular ligament reconstruction
    - Swan-neck deformity with loss of PIP movement, implant arthroplasty of the PIP joint as well as sufficient

soft-tissue immobilization and release. In late deformities, arthrodesis or arthroplasty
- Boutonnière deformity; early: PIP joint synovectomy. In distal extensor compromise, tenotomy can gain distal IP joint flexion. In late disease, PIP arthrodesis or arthroplasty for fixed PIP flexion contracture

LIGAMENT SPRAIN AND INSTABILITY

Intrinsic ligament (within the carpal bones)
- Scapholunate, lunotriquetral sprain/tears are often under-recognized and can lead to chronic instability (with pain and arthritis)
- Predictable instability pattern: scapholunate → lunotriquetral → midcarpal (SLAC)

Triangular fibrous cartilage complex injury (see page 231)

Extrinsic ligament
- Sprain: usually benign nature
- Dorsal: radiotriquetral and scaphotriquetral (triquetral insertion): common and stable
  ○ Bony avulsion can be seen but underrecognized
- Volar: radiolunotriquetral and scaphocapitate (uncommon but stable)
  ○ Complex: volar + dorsal scaphotriquetral (at scaphoid insertion) ligaments associated with scapholunate instability

Carpal (Wrist) Instability
Classification (105)

	CLASSIFICATION	DESCRIPTION	EXAMPLE
1	Carpal instability dissociative (CDI)	Abnormal kinematics between bones within a carpal row caused by ligament disruption such as a scapholunate or lunotriquetral ligament tear or a fracture (with deformity)	Scapholunate ligament disruption Lunotriquetral ligament disruption Scaphoid (waist) fracture with humpback deformity
2	The nondissociative carpal instabilities (CIND)	Abnormal kinematics between carpal rows caused by extrinsic ligament injuries	Midcarpal instability: palmar, dorsal, or mixed
3	Complex CDI	A combination of CDI and CIND	
4	Adaptive carpal instability (CI)	Carpal malalignment caused by a problem outside the wrist	Distal radial malunion

Scapholunate Sprain and Instability
Introduction (106)
- Scapholunate sprain (MC carpal sprain) can lead to SL instability (MC carpal instability)
- Anatomy: ligamentous scapholunate stabilizer
  ○ Dorsal scapholunate ligament stronger than interosseous and volar components
  ○ Volar radioscapholunate ligament: the strongest ligament
- Etiology
  ○ Fall or direct blow (→ hyperextension of the wrist) or prolonged crutch walking
  ○ Impact load to the base of the hypothenar region with the wrist in extension, ulnar deviation, and supination
  ○ Distal radius fracture or RA, and the like

History and physical examination
- Pain ± swelling over the dorsoradial aspect (or ulnar to the anatomical snuff box), painful click or snapping sensation
- Physical exam
  ○ Tenderness on scapholunate interval (just distal to the Lister's tubercle, prominent in wrist flexion)
  ○ Watson's (scaphoid shift) test: false positive in radioscaphoid arthritis, synovitis, or occult ganglion
  ○ Murphy's sign: for lunate dislocation; if the head of the 3rd metacarpal is leveled with the 2nd or 4th metacarpal bone (sunken 3rd knuckle) during making a fist

Diagnosis
- Clinical diagnosis confirmed by imaging study
- Clinical stages
  ○ Predynamic instability → dynamic instability scapholunate interval (SL) interval widening in ulnar/radial deviation; more common than static → static instability → SLAC: osteoarthritis starting from radial styloid and scaphoid to extend to the midcarpal joint at the advanced stages
- Imaging
  ○ X-ray
    - AP (in full supination) view; gap between scaphoid-lunate >2 to 3 mm, scaphoid (cortical) ring sign; overlap of proximal and distal scaphoid poles
    - Lateral view: DISI (lunate face dorsally), scapholunate angle >70° (normal 30–60°)
    - Clenched fist view: compare with the other side
  ○ US: compare with the contralateral side, SL interval >4 mm; excellent negative predictive value
  ○ MRI arthroscopy: flow to the mid-carpus; sensitivity and specificity 70% and 90%
    - Scapholunate ligament: more commonly injured at scaphoid attachment (wrist extension and ulnar deviation)
    - Lunotriquetral ligament injury: less common

Treatment
- Nonoperative treatment for predynamic, dynamic scapholunate instability
  ○ Cast: "wine waiter's position" wrist in full supination, mild dorsiflexion, and ulnar deviation for 6 to 10 weeks
  ○ Short-arm thumb spica cast/splint, activity modification, pain medication as needed
- Surgical referral for static, complete ligament rupture, or failed conservative treatment

- In acute (<3–4 weeks): closed reduction and percutaneous pinning versus ORIF (K wire and capsulodesis)
- In chronic: no OA; capsulodesis and reconstruction, if OA present, then fusion

Lunotriquetral Sprain and Instability

Introduction (107)
- Less common than scapholunate ligament sprain
- Stabilizer of lunotriquetral joint:
  - Lunotriquetral ligament: volar portion is thicker/more critical than dorsal ligament
  - Dorsal RC ligament
- Etiology: tear or degenerative
  - Ulnar-sided injury leading to perilunate dissociation
    - Lunotriquetral injuries by fall, twisting or sports: isolated lesion rarely leading to instability. With dorsal RC ligament injury can lead to volar intercalated segment instability

History and physical examination
- Ulnar-sided wrist pain elicited by radial or ulnar deviation of the wrist
- Tenderness on the lunotriquetral or scapholunate joint ± clicking (neutral to ulnar deviation with axial compression) or popping
- Lunotriquetral ballottement (Reagan test) and the Kleinman shear test (or lunotriquetral shuck test): check physical examination part

Diagnosis
- Clinical diagnosis supplemented with imaging study
- X-ray: AP and lateral; VISI (volar flexion of the lunate)
- MRI: lunotriquetral ligament injury (sensitivity 82% and specificity 100%)
- US: low sensitivity (25%, because of thinner and deeper location)

Treatment
- Nonoperative treatment: NSAIDs, injection, and splint
- Referral to hand surgery for arthroscopic surgery if failed conservative treatment.

Midcarpal Instability

Introduction (105)
- Uncommon
- Instability between proximal and distal row
- Palmar (ulnar) and dorsal (less clearly defined) midcarpal instability

History and physical examination
- Wrist discomfort/pain with clunking
  - Palmar midcarpal instability; clunking from ulnar deviation and pronation
  - Differential diagnosis with clicking from extrinsic (ECU) subluxation (supination and wrist extension) or distal radio-ulnar joint
- Tenderness over triquetrohamate joint and volar sagging during ulnar deviation and pronation
- Generalized ligament laxity (Beighton score); can be present
- Midcarpal shift test (Lichtman test): high false positive

Diagnosis
- Clinical diagnosis (high index of suspicion)
- X-ray (VISI pattern) or videofluoroscopy, CT, MRI, and US with stress (press down the lunate while push capitate upward)

Treatment
- Nonoperative therapy typically includes splinting and occupational adaptations
- Surgical intervention in failed conservative management: capsular shrinkage, soft-tissue reconstruction, and limited carpal fusion

Triangular Fibrocartilage Complex (TFCC) Lesion

Introduction (108)
- Prevalence of TFCC lesion: common in both symptomatic (27%–49%) and asymptomatic cases (15%–49%) in both affected and unaffected wrists of the same patients (109)
  - Increase with age
  - Difficulty to correlate with symptoms
- Classification

TRAUMATIC	DEGENERATIVE
A. Central perforation	A. TFCC wear
B. Medial avulsion (ulnar attachment) ± distal ulnar fracture	B. TFCC wear and lunate and/or ulnar chondromalacia
C. Distal avulsion (carpal attachment)	C. TFCC perforation + lunate and/or ulnar chondromalacia
D. Lateral avulsion (radial attachment) ± sigmoid notch fracture	D. C and L-T ligament perforation
	E. D and ulnocarpal arthritis

- Etiology
  - Axial load on a pronated wrist: by activities that involve wrist rotation (forceful pronation) and power grip
    - TFCC disc is thinner during forearm pronation
  - Secondary causes: distal radius fracture (radial insertion of TFCC), malunion, distal radius physeal arrest, and proximal radial migration following radial head resection, ulnar styloid fracture
  - Sports: gymnastics, racquet sports, hockey, golf, boxing, water skiing, and pole vaulting

History and physical examination
- Ulnar-sided wrist pain ± clicking, snaps and popping especially with rotation (eg, turning a door or a key)
- Tenderness in the fovea radial to the ulnar styloid (Fovea sign): sensitivity 95%, specificity 86% (110)
- Motor examination: difference in grip strength between hands in pronation and supination
- TFCC (UC) compression test, the piano key sign, and TFCC snap test (see Physical Examination section)

Diagnosis
- Clinical suspicion confirmed by imaging study or arthroscopy (gold standard)

- Differential diagnosis: lunotriquetral ligament sprain, ECU or FCU tendinopathy, and PT joint or midcarpal instability
- X-ray PA; neutral rotation, pronated grip radiograph and lateral view
  - Arthritic changes in the UC joint (distal ulnar, DRUJ, proximal pole of the lunate)
  - Degenerative cysts in the proximal pole of the lunate and the ulnar head
  - VISI: advanced stages
  - Ulnar positive variance (ulnar is longer than radius by >2 mm)
- US: limited evaluation
- MRI/MRA: the diagnosis of TFCC tears with reported sensitivity and specificity of 100% and 93%, respectively
  - Coronal section: low signal biconcave structures normally

Treatment (111)
- Nonoperative management
  - Steroid (or platelet-rich plasma) injection to UC joint, splint immobilization (cast in supination for at least 4 weeks then wrist splint immobilization in another 2 weeks) if DRUJ unstable
- Surgery
  - Indication: unstable and displaced fracture, unstable DRUJ
  - Decompress the UC articulation and remove any degenerative tissue that is causing mechanical symptoms
  - Open diaphyseal-shortening osteotomy
  - Partial ulnar head recession (wafer procedure)

Distal Radioulnar Instability

Introduction (112,113)
- Epidemiology: not studied, rare but underrecognized
- Biomechanics: inherently unstable, allows pronation, supination
- Classification: dorsal, palmar, and multidirectional instability
- Etiology
  - Soft-tissue injury (TFCC, dorsal/palmar RU ligament, interosseous membrane, joint capsule) or fracture (distal part of radius (MC cause) or ulnar)
  - Ulnar impaction (abutment), incongruity, or inflammation

History and physical examination
- Nonspecific pain, swelling, painful clunking sensation worsening with wrist motion ± history of fall (extended and pronated)
  - Pain with pronation and supination; compare side to side
- Tenderness on the fovea (similar to TFCC lesion)
- Subluxation/dislocation: usually dorsal movement of the ulnar particularly in pronation
- Provocation test: piano key test

Diagnosis
- Clinical diagnosis supplemented by imaging study
  - May consider image-guided diagnostic injection to DRUJ to confirm pain generator with small volume of lidocaine
- X-ray (bilaterally); true lateral with forearm neutral; ulnar variance, PA avulsion or nonunion
- Widened radio-ulnar joint, or nonunion
- CT and MRI for congruity of the DRUJ, MRI/A to evaluate TFCC

Treatment
- Acute subluxation and dislocation: reduced with pressure on the ulnar and forceful supination, then casting for 6 weeks
- Functional bracing prefabricated or custom forearm braces (28)
- Surgical referral if no congruity between radio-ulnar joint, locked joint, or failed conservative management

Triquetral Impingement and Ligament-Tear Syndrome (114)

Introduction
- Controversial diagnosis
- Chronic impingement of ulnar sling mechanism on the triquetrum leading to hyperemia and softening of the ulnar slope of the triquetrum
  - Ulnar sling mechanism: ulnar cuff of ligamentous collagen ulnar to the radius including the extensor retinaculum, dorsal extrinsic ligaments, dorsal RU ligament, ECU sheath, volar extrinsic carpal ligament, and ulnolunate and ulnotriquetral ligaments and TFCC

History and physical
- Ulnar-sided wrist pain, more pain with pronation/supination than ulnar deviation ± wrist hyperflexion injury
- Severe tenderness over the triquetrum
- No pain on radio-ulnar compression

Diagnosis
- Clinical diagnosis; diagnosis of exclusion
- Normal radiographs and MRI may show increased T2 signal intensity in the triquetrum

Treatment
- Short period of splint (resting wrist hand) and possible injection
- Referral to surgery if not responsive

GANGLION CYST

Introduction (67,115)
- MC space-occupying lesion in the hand and wrist, more common in 2nd to 4th decades, female > male
- Location of ganglion
  - MC seen around the wrist: 60% to 70% at the dorsum of the wrist and 13% to 20% on the volar aspect of the wrist
  - Dorsal ganglion usually originates from the joint (scaphotrapeziotrapezoidal articulation) with one-way valve system
    - Scapholunate joint: MC
  - Ventral ganglion
    - Location: 2/3 at RC and 1/3 at scaphotrapezoid, between 1st dorsal column and FCR tendon sheath
    - Flexor tendon ganglion: can cause CTS and ulnar neuropathy at the wrist
- Mechanism of pain
  - Irritation of ligament or PIN/superficial branch of radial nerve
  - Larger ganglion usually less painful because it is away from scapholunate interval
- No synovial lining is present within the cyst and cyst may occur from degeneration of periarticular soft tissues

History and physical examination
- Dorsal ganglion: asymptomatic or pain with hyperextension of the wrist
  - 1 to 2 cm cystic mass, aching pain in the wrist (116)
- Ventral ganglion: usually asymptomatic, less mobile in tendon sheath ganglion (associated with tenosynovial disease)
  - Can present as CTS

Diagnosis
- Clinical diagnosis confirmed by imaging study
- US or MRI; for occult ganglion
  - US: posterior acoustic shadow, check septum
    - Doppler (to R/O pseudoaneurysm of superficial radial artery which also has a bruit)
  - MRI: preoperative planning, identifying the origin and concomitant bony lesion

Treatment
- Aspiration (high recurrence of ganglion but can resolve pain) and wrist splint for 1 week
- Referral to surgery for persistent painful ganglion

CARPAL BOSS

Introduction (117)
- Protuberance at the base of 2nd and 3rd metacarpals (at dorsal CMC joint region)
- Uncommon, more likely on the dominant hand, often in early 30s
- MC location: os styloideum on 3rd proximal dorsal metacarpal (>90%), 2nd metacarpal or trapezoid

History and physical examination
- Pain and localized tenderness over the prominence
- Bony, nonmobile prominence on the dorsum of the wrist.

Diagnosis
- Clinical diagnosis confirmed by imaging study
- X-ray: carpal boss view (modified lateral view): the hand and wrist flexed with 30 to 40° of supination and 20 to 30° of ulnar deviation to put the bony prominence in view
- US to differentiate from ganglion and MRI for further evaluation of intracortical lesion
- Differential diagnosis
  - Dorsal ganglion: often mobile, adventitial bursa over the prominence and extensor tendon irritation (often concomitant and source of pain)
  - Benign bony lesions: intraosseous ganglions (the MC bony cystic lesion of the hand and wrist), aneurysmal bone cysts, unicameral bone cysts, enchondromas, osteochondromas, and osteoid osteomas
  - Malignant tumors such as osteosarcomas and metastatic disease or locally invasive tumors such as giant cell tumors

Treatment
- Rest, splint, NSAIDs, and injection with corticosteroid to ganglion or adventitial bursa
- Surgical excision: associated with a prolonged recovery and continued symptoms in a high percentage of patients

TUMOR

Introduction (118)
- 6% of bone tumors occur in the hand
- Most tumors of the hand are benign (95%) except cutaneous malignancies

Common presentation
- Pain, swelling, and mass
- Any unexplained fracture with minor or no trauma; pathologic fracture

Diagnostic imaging
- X-ray
  - Benign tumor: cortical expansion seen within well-defined borders
  - Malignancy: cortical destruction, poorly defined borders, and soft-tissue extension
- CT to further delineate location, size, and bony architecture
- MRI indicated when significant soft-tissue extension is present
- Biopsy: avoid the unaffected site

Treatment
- Individualization based on local tumor control versus hand function, based on tumor size, risk of recurrence, proximity to joint surfaces, and overall predicted function
- Benign tumor: curettage excision, cytotoxic adjuvant agents, and bone graft
- Reconstructive option
- Referral to OT and prosthetic clinic as early as possible

Giant Cell Tumor of Tendon Sheath

Introduction
- Second MC space-occupying lesion of the hand (after ganglion cyst), female > male, peak in 20–50 years of age
- Location: distal radius (MC), the middle phalanx, radial three digits (usually DIP and ventral part but dorsal involvement is not uncommon)
- Known as the localized form of pigmented villonodular synovitis

History and physical examination
- Painless mass in the hand or wrist (volar aspect), slow growing, firmer than ganglion, not visible by transillumination

Diagnosis
- Clinical suspicion confirmed by imaging study and biopsy
- US
  - An extra-articular solid hypoechoic mass with sharp margins, located on the volar aspect of the fingers with lateral and circumferential extension
  - Adjacent to normally appearing flexor tendons
  - Internal echoes and lacks posterior acoustic enhancement (opposite to ganglia). It usually exhibits poor internal vasculature on Doppler
  - Cortical bone erosions of the phalanges secondary to pressure from the overlying lesion in 10% to 50%. ± Eccentric displacement of the digital arteries
- CT scan: more useful for demonstrating cortical destruction and the reactive bony shell

Treatment
- Surgical referral: arthroplasty or arthrodesis for reconstruction of larger defects. Intralesional curettage with the use of adjuvant treatment (eg, cryosurgery, bone cement packing)
- Recurrence rate: <10% (5–50% depending on studies)

Epidermoid Inclusion Cyst
Introduction (67)
- The 3rd MC type of tumor in hand, male > female, commonly seen in laborers
- Etiology: trauma → epithelial cells introduced into the underlying subcutaneous tissues → cyst lined with epithelial cells and filled with keratin

History and physical examination
- Painless mass, slow growing, MC in the fingertip or palm
- Not visible by transillumination, circumscribed, firm, and slightly mobile

Diagnosis
- Clinical suspicion confirmed by imaging and biopsy
- US: hyperechoic mass with posterior acoustic enhancement and a small superficial extension into the dermis

Treatment
- Referral to hand surgery for marginal resection

Glomus Tumor
Introduction (119)
- Arise from the neuromyoarterial glomus, located beneath the nail or over the palmar aspect of the fingertip.
- 1% to 5% of all soft-tissue tumors of the upper extremity, mostly in the nail bed, common in young adults

History and physical examination
- Painful mass in the nail base with excruciating pain exacerbated by local pressure or cold

Diagnosis
- Clinical diagnosis confirmed by imaging and biopsy
- Imaging with US
  - To define the exact location and size of the tumor preoperatively and to detect multiple lesions
  - Small solid homogeneously hypoechoic mass beneath the nail, possibly associated with erosion of the underlying phalangeal bone
  - The high-velocity flow of intratumor shunt vessels makes this lesion a hypervascular mass at color and power Doppler imaging: fairly specific for the diagnosis
- Differential diagnosis: hemangioma and venous malformation

Treatment
- Referral for surgical removal: punching the nail plate and enucleating the tumor, removal of the proximal half of the nail plate or lateral incision in the nail fold. Recurrent tumors are common

Enchondroma
Introduction (120)
- MC primary bone tumor, >90% of bony tumors in the hand
- MC location: proximal phalanges, metacarpals, and the middle phalanx or ulnar digits
- Arise from aberrant cartilaginous foci

History and physical examination
- Pain, localized swelling, and osteoporosis fracture (lytic lesion with thin cortical shell)

Diagnosis
- Clinical suspicion with imaging
- X-ray: a well-defined radiolucent lesion in the diaphysis or metadiaphysis ± a well-defined sclerotic rim. The cortex may have small concavities or may be scalloped in appearance
- Differential diagnosis for malignant transformation to osteosarcoma and chondrosarcoma (30% of enchondromatosis)
  - Ollier disease: nonhereditary condition of multiple enchondromas
  - Maffucci syndrome: multiple enchondroma with hemangiomas

Treatment
- Surgical referral for excision ± grafting

FRACTURE
Phalanges and metacarpals
- MC site for fractures, ~10% of all fractures (121)
- Distal phalanx (MC) > metacarpals
- Phalangeal fracture: more common in children, metacarpal fracture more common in adults

Interphalangeal fracture-dislocations
- Frequent in high-level ball sports (volleyball, football)

General indication for surgery (122)
- Absolute indications: joint dislocation, joint instability, neurovascular injury, or open fractures
- Relative indications: comminution, displacement, and intraarticular involvement

Distal Radial (Colles) Fracture
Introduction (123)
- Epidemiology: MC fracture site in the upper extremity, 1/6 of fractures treated in ER, 10% to 15% in Caucasian women over 65 years
- Mechanism of injury: high-energy fall in youth, in sports and low-energy fall in seniors with osteoporotic bone: fall on outstretched hand (FOOSH)
  - Soccer (increased in artificial turf by five times), skiing/snowboarding, dancing, and rugby, and the like
  - Geriatric populations: risk factors: osteoporosis, recurrent falls, h/o fragility fracture, dementia in >75 years
- Associated injury and complication
  - DRUJ involvement: 5% to 15%, dysfunction of pronation-supination

- TFCC: 45% to 70%; disruption of TFCC and other carpal ligament (scapho-lunate ligament)
- Median neuropathy up to 15% (124)
- Malunion and nonunion; common (rare in minimally or nondisplaced fractures)
- Compartment syndrome
- Arthritis, stiffness
- Underrecognized fracture (especially ulnar styloid)

History and physical examination
- Pain, decreased ROM (check for pronation or supination), swelling, and deformity
- Inspection (silver-fork deformity; Colles fracture), ROM (especially pronation/supination), tenderness for distal RU joint, and dislocation or subluxation

Diagnosis
- Clinical suspicion confirmed by imaging study
- X-ray: true PA and lateral
  - AP: slope of the distal radius (25°), ulnar variance. Lateral; volar tilt of 10°
  - Frykman classification (type 1 to 8) extraarticular (type 1 and 2) intraarticular (type 3 and 4) RC, intraarticular involving distal RU (type 5 and 6), both joints involved (type 7 and 8); a higher number indicates a worse prognosis

Treatment (125)
- Closed reduction with hematoma block (aspiration of blood and 1% lidocaine block under US [126]) with sugar-tong splint (long-arm splint, in neutral or supination to stabilize the DRUJ): limit pronation and supination; FU x-ray q 1 to 2 weeks (to check loss of reduction or shortening)
- Indication for surgical referral: any comminution, any displacement, radial angulation >20°, articular disruption >2 mm (increased DJD)
- Return to play: 3 months after achieving full ROM and strength is near normal
  - Unstable; longer RTP

Pediatric Distal Radial Fracture

Introduction
- Distal metaphysis: MC location, peak incidence: 9 to 14 years, coincide with peak growing spurt (porosity of bone during peak growth)
- Mechanism of injury
  - Fall on extended wrist; simple fall → nondisplaced fracture
  - Fall with forward movement → displaced fracture
  - Fall from a height → concomitant fracture (supracondylar or scaphoid)
- Torus fracture (aka buckle fracture)
  - Simple incomplete buckle fracture of cortex; compression fracture leading to buckle of the cortex (or protuberance) at metaphyseal–diaphyseal junction
- Greenstick fracture
  - Incomplete angulated fracture on cortex caused by severe bending

History and physical examination
- Pain, swelling at the wrist
- Tenderness on the dorsum of the distal radius
- Neurovascular exam: capillary refill, pulse, median, and ulnar nerve

Diagnosis
- Clinical suspicion confirmed by imaging study
- X-ray; AP, lateral and oblique

Treatment
- Torus fracture: immobilization with removable volar splint or casting for 2 to 4 weeks
- Greenstick fracture: sugar-tong splinting for 2 to 3 days followed by short- or long arm cast with close monitoring (orthopedic referral)
- Immediate surgical referral; open fracture, neurovascular injury, compartment syndrome, displaced, Salter-Harris III to V, angulated fracture (15 to 20°, usually need conscious sedation or Bier block for reduction), unstable or complete fracture

Carpal Fracture

Introduction
- Scaphoid fracture: MC
- Other carpal fractures: exceedingly rare, 1.1% of all fractures (127)
- Common mechanism: FOOSH
- Commonly associated injuries: perilunate injuries, axial injury, and avulsion/impaction injuries

Diagnosis
- Standard x-ray frequently insufficient, high index of suspicion
- CT for definite diagnosis

Treatment
- Cast immobilization in nondisplaced fracture, ORIF for displaced or unstable fracture
- Rehab after bony union is confirmed, usually favorable prognosis

Scaphoid Fracture

Introduction (128)
- MC carpal bone fracture. Prevalence: 8 (female) to 32 (male)/100,000, underreported/underrecognized
- MC location in scaphoid: waist (65%). Distal pole: MC in children
- Anatomy: blood supply by retrograde blood flow (80%, distal to proximal) by dorsal carpal branch of the radial artery
- Mechanism of injury: FOOSH (~70%) or forceful dorsiflexion of the wrist
  - Scaphoid; weakest link in the young to middle-aged
    - Longitudinal loading of the scaphoid, producing a flexion moment that is resisted by the constraining intrinsic ligaments and by the radioscaphocapitate ligament crossing the waist
  - Common in skiers, snowboarders, skateboarders, and in participants of contact sports
- Associated injury: scapholunate ligament injury or other ligamentous wrist injury

- Complications: avascular necrosis, scaphoid nonunion, or advanced collapse

History and physical examination
- Painful (often not severe) swelling of the wrist, especially in the area of the anatomic snuffbox
  - Weakness or inability to play sports (baseball) or grip/hold a heavy object associated with pain
- Physical examination
  - Tenderness in the anatomic snuffbox, immediately distal to the radial styloid, over the tuberosity of the scaphoid
  - Pain with ROM, especially extension and radial deviation

Diagnosis
- Clinical suspicion confirmed by imaging study
- Imaging studies
  - X-ray
    - AP, lateral, 45° semipronated, PA in ulnar deviation and clench fist view
    - Repeat in 7 to 10 days with immobilization
  - CT or MRI: waist or proximal pole fracture
  - US: may detect fracture early when the x-ray is negative (129)

Treatment
- If the x-ray is negative; thumb spica splint and reassess q 1 to 2 weeks
- Long thumb spica splint (palmar flexion and radial deviation for 6 weeks then short-arm splint for 3–4 months) for nondisplaced fracture in distal pole or tuberosity fracture; good healing (88%–95%)
- Surgical referral for scaphoid waist and proximal pole fracture or ≥1 mm displacement: ORIF or percutaneous screw fixation
  - Immobilization for 2 to 3 weeks and splint 2 to 3 months
  - Acute lesion: heal uneventfully but chronic lesion; usually not healing well

Triquetral Fracture

Introduction
- 2nd MC carpal fracture, avulsion: MC pattern, common in golf and baseball
- Hyperflexion (dorsal radiotriquetral ligament avulsion) or hyperextension (with ulnar deviation → posteroradial aspect avulsion) of the wrist, direct blow with perilunate dislocation

History and physical examination
- Wrist pain (ulnar aspect) and severe tenderness in ~2 cm distal to the ulnar styloid, swelling, discoloration, and wrist hyperextension

Diagnosis
- X-ray (AP, lateral, and oblique pronated lateral view)
- Differential diagnosis: concomitant pisiform fracture, ligament disruption, or TFCC injury

Treatment
- Volar splint, short-arm cast (immobilization) for 4 to 6 weeks
- May participate in sport if not tender with semirigid cast with padding

- Surgical referral if markedly displaced, persistent pain despite conservative management

Hook of Hamate Fracture

Introduction
- Very rare, 2% of all carpal fractures, underrecognized
- Mechanism of injury
  - Direct hit by baseball bat, golf club, hockey stick
    - Rapid deceleration of the stick, bat, golf club, or racket when tightly held in a clenched fist → impacting the palm, along with the active contraction of the deep flexor tendons
  - Hamate body fractures occur from falls with the wrist in a hyperextended position

History and physical examination
- Pain in the hypothenar aspect of the palm with exacerbation with grip and pressure in the palm, especially when directed over the hamate
- Physical examination (130)
  - Tenderness on the hook of hamate (1 finger breadth diagonal to 2nd digit base from pisiform (prominence at the distal crease)
  - Actively flex the small finger DIP against resistance. Because the FDP of the small finger runs along the radial margin of the hook of the hamate → pain directly over the hamate

Diagnosis
- Clinical suspicion confirmed by imaging study
- Radiographic examination
  - A carpal tunnel view and a semisupinated oblique view
  - CT and MRI are useful diagnostic tests for hook or body fractures of the hamate

Treatment
- Nondisplaced fractures: cast immobilization for 4 to 6 weeks
- Displaced fractures: open reduction and internal fixation or excision

Metacarpal Fracture

Epidemiology (70)
- 2nd MC fracture in hand (up to 1/3) after phalangeal fracture

MC location: 5th metacarpal (50%)
- Neck and shaft: MC site of fracture in the 2nd to 5th metacarpal
- Proximal base in the 1st metacarpal bone

Mechanism of injury
- Direct blow of the hand or indirect force from torsion or bending of the distal finger

Common pattern: dorsal apex angulation
- The more distal the fracture, a greater degree of angulation can be tolerated
- 3rd and 4th metacarpals; more stable than 2nd and 5th because of dual support from the deep transverse intermetacarpal ligaments on the radial and ulnar sides

First Metacarpal Fracture

Introduction
- Classification
  - Type 1, Bennett's fracture: MC, base of metacarpal
    - Intraarticular, proximal part attached to trapezium (by anterior oblique ligament) with subluxation of the distal part by APL (dorsoradially) (Figure 5.10)
  - Type 2, Roland: least common, comminuted fracture involving intraarticular joint
    - Intraarticular, ≥3 fragments, shortened thumb ray due to multiple muscles
  - Type 3 (extraarticular) and Type 4 (proximal epiphysis in children)
- Mechanism of injury
  - Axial load (blow) against partially flexed 1st metacarpal (example, fist fight) or fall with hyperflexed or hyperextended thumb

History and physical examination
- Pain, swelling, painful limited ROM, and subluxation of the metacarpal base

Diagnosis
- X-ray: a true lateral view of the base of the thumb by pronating the hand 30° to the x-ray cassette
- CT scan to delineate the position of the fracture fragment and CMC joint

Treatment
- Ortho referral
  - Short-arm thumb spica splint with wrist 30° extension and free IP joint after anatomic reduction ± traction. Accurate articular reduction for the best functional results
    - Anatomic alignment of the joint surface (important for functional outcome). Percutaneous pinning under fluoroscopic guidance
    - Angulation up to 20 to 30°: well tolerated due to movable nature of thumb
  - Surgical indication: necessary in all intraarticular fractures (Bennett and Roland), in cases when articular alignment is not normal
    - Pinning or screw fixation
    - ORIF or external fixation if fragments are small and comminuted
- Occupational therapy (hand) after cast removed (then on splint), ROM and stretching, strengthening exercise
- Complication: malunion, painful arthritis, and chronic subluxation

Metatarsal Neck Fracture (Boxer's Fracture)

Introduction
- Boxer's fracture: 5th metacarpal neck (and shaft) fracture (street fighter)
  - 2nd metacarpal fracture is more common in Boxer's fracture
- Striking a solid object with a closed fist

History and physical examination
- Painful swelling and deformity (MCP joint depressed by angulation)
  - Distal metacarpal head; displaced volarly (by interosseous muscle) and shaft dorsally
- In chronic untreated case: clawing, cosmetic deformity but good function
- Malrotation; in hook fist position (MCP extension, PIP and DIP flexion), fingernail plane should be toward the scaphoid if there is no rotational deformity

Diagnosis
- Clinical suspicion confirmed by imaging study
- X-ray: AP, oblique, and lateral radiography (measure the angle of displacement)
  - Normal metacarpal angle is 15°; so angulation calculation adjusted for this: if 40° angle observed, angle from fracture is 25°

Treatment
- Reduction and ulnar gutter splint with MCP in 70 to 90° flexion (tightening of CL), wrist extension in 20°, buddy tape (little and ring finger) with PIP joint allowed to move
  - Indications: <10° angulation for 2nd and 3rd MC, <20 to 30° angulation in the 4th and 5th metacarpal bones
- Surgical referral; open fracture, intraarticular, unstable fracture, severely displaced or rotational deformity

OTHER PATHOLOGY

HYPOTHENAR HAMMER SYNDROME

Introduction (131)
- Aneurysm or thrombosis of ulnar artery at the wrist
- Rare in general, male > female by ~9, peak age: 40 to 50's, more common in dominant hand
  - Underrecognized, higher in some occupations (up to 14% of auto mechanics, vibration exposed workers, and auto mechanics)
- Etiology: repetitive/single trauma: hammering, or pushing hard objects, sports (football, baseball, break dancing, golf, basketball, lacrosse, and volleyball)
  - Catching ball → paresthesia in the ulnar digits, pain in the palm
  - Smoking

History and physical examination
- Intermittent, sudden, or gradual onset of ischemic symptoms in the affected fingers
- Hypothenar callus, tenderness (at Guyon's canal), and pulsatile mass in cases of aneurysm formation

Diagnosis
- Clinical diagnosis confirmed by vascular study
- Allen test: occlusion of the radial artery, release of ulnar artery. Positive without flow in ulnar artery (often not sensitive and specific)
- Doppler US, angio (CT, MRA); gold standard

Treatment
- Activity modification, cold avoidance, and smoking cessation
- Rest then padding in the vulnerable sections of the hand with splinting

- Ca^{2+} channel blocker (nifedipine), antiplatelet agent or anticoagulation (check risk benefit ratio), and possibly pentoxifylline
- Referral to vascular surgery depending on acuity and severity of ischemia

REFERENCES

1. Dahaghin S, Bierma-Zeinstra SM, Reijman M, et al. Prevalence and determinants of one month hand pain and hand related disability in the elderly (Rotterdam study). *Ann Rheum Dis*. 2005;64(1):99–104.
2. Rettig AC, Patel DV. Epidemiology of elbow, forearm, and wrist injuries in the athlete. *Clin Sports Med*. 1995;14(2):289–297.
3. Prucz RB, Friedrich JB. Finger joint injuries. *Clin Sports Med*. 2015;34(1):99–116.
4. Filippucci E, Meenagh G, Delle Sedie A, et al. Ultrasound imaging for the rheumatologist XXXVI. Sonographic assessment of the foot in gout patients. *Clin Exp Rheumatol*. 2011;29(6):901–905.
5. Aptel M, Aublet-Cuvelier A, Cnockaert JC. Work-related musculoskeletal disorders of the upper limb. *Joint Bone Spine*. 2002;69(6):546–555.
6. Barr AE, Barbe MF, Clark BD. Work-related musculoskeletal disorders of the hand and wrist: epidemiology, pathophysiology, and sensorimotor changes. *J Orthop Sports Phys Ther*. 2004;34(10):610–627.
7. Atzei A, Luchetti R. Clinical approach to the painful wrist arthroscopy. In: Geissler WB, ed. *Wrist Arthroscopy*. New York NY: Springer; 2005:185–195.
8. Bianchi S, Martinoli C. *Wrist-Ultrasound of the Musculoskeletal System*. Berlin Heidelberg, Germany: Springer; 2007:425–494.
9. Guillin R, Marchand AJ, Roux A, Niederberger E, Duvauferrier R. Imaging of snapping phenomena. *Br J Radiol*. 2012;85(1018):1343–1353.
10. Bookman AAM, von Schroeder HP, Fam AG. 4 - The wrist and hand. In: Lawry GV, Kreder HJ, Hawker G, Jerome D, eds. *In Fam's Musculoskeletal Examination and Joint Injection Techniques*. 2nd ed. Philadelphia, PA: Mosby; 2010:29–43.
11. Kijima Y, Viegas SF. Wrist anatomy and biomechanics. *J Hand Surg Am*. 2009;34(8):1555–1563.
12. Ishizuki M, Sugihara T, Wakabayashi Y, et al. Stener-like lesions of collateral ligament ruptures of the metacarpophalangeal joint of the finger. *J Orthop Sci*. 2009;14(2):150–154.
13. Fukumoto K, Kojima T, Kinoshita Y, Koda M. An anatomic study of the innervation of the wrist joint and Wilhelm's technique for denervation. *J Hand Surg Am*. 1993;18(3):484–489.
14. Skaribas I, Aló K. Ultrasound imaging and occipital nerve stimulation. *Neuromodulation*. 2010;13(2):126–130.
15. Murphy AD, Blair JW. An anatomical variant of the superficial branch of the radial nerve in Wartenberg's syndrome. *J Hand Surg Eur Vol*. 2012;37(4):365–366.
16. Jacobson JA, Fessell DP, Lobo Lda G, Yang LJ. Entrapment neuropathies I: upper limb (carpal tunnel excluded). *Semin Musculoskelet Radiol*. 2010;14(5):473–486.
17. Grutter PW, Desilva GL, Meehan RE, Desilva SP. The accuracy of distal posterior interosseous and anterior interosseous nerve injection. *J Hand Surg Am*. 2004;29(5):865–870.
18. Huang JI, Hanel DP. Anatomy and biomechanics of the distal radioulnar joint. *Hand Clin*. 2012;28(2):157–163.
19. Denti L, Annoni V, Cattadori E, et al. Insulin-like growth factor 1 as a predictor of ischemic stroke outcome in the elderly. *Am J Med*. 2004;117(5):312–317.
20. Duncan SF, Saracevic CE, Kakinoki R. Biomechanics of the hand. *Hand Clin*. 2013;29(4):483–492.
21. Pinchera A, Menzinger G, Greco V, et al. [The metabolism of insulin in human muscle. Study of muscle insulinase activity in the normal subject, the diabetic and in the hyperinsulin subject]. *Folia Endocrinol Mens Incretologia Incretoterapia*. 1962;15:54–65.
22. Young D, Papp S, Giachino A. Physical examination of the wrist. *Orthop Clin North Am*. 2007;38(2):149–65, v.
23. Hopayian K, Song F, Riera R, Sambandan S. The clinical features of the piriformis syndrome: a systematic review. *Eur Spine J*. 2010;19(12):2095–2109.
24. McFarland MB, Langer O, Piper JM, Berkus MD. Perinatal outcome and the type and number of maneuvers in shoulder dystocia. *Int J Gynaecol Obstet*. 1996;55(3):219–224.
25. Hoppenfield S. *Physical Examination of the Spine and Extremities*. Upper Saddle River, NJ: Prentice Hall: 1976: p. 276.
26. Bain GI, Polites N, Higgs BG, et al. The functional range of motion of the finger joints. *J Hand Surg Eur Vol*. 2015;40(4):406–411.
27. Merritt MM, Roddey TS, Costello C, Olson S. Diagnostic value of clinical grind test for carpometacarpal osteoarthritis of the thumb. *J Hand Ther*. 2010;23(3):261–267; quiz 268.
28. Millard GM, Budoff JE, Paravic V, Noble PC. Functional bracing for distal radioulnar joint instability. *J Hand Surg Am*. 2002;27(6):972–977.
29. Hubbard MC, MacDermid JC, Kramer JF, Birmingham TB. Quantitative vibration threshold testing in carpal tunnel syndrome: analysis strategies for optimizing reliability. *J Hand Ther*. 2004;17(1):24–30.
30. Grasu BL, Jones CM, Murphy MS. Use of diagnostic modalities for assessing upper extremity vascular pathology. *Hand Clinics*. 2015;31(1):1–12.
31. Williamson L, Mowat A, Burge P. Screening for extensor tendon rupture in rheumatoid arthritis. *Rheumatology (Oxford)*. 2001;40(4):420–423.
32. Rada EM, Shridharani SM, Lifchez SD. Spontaneous atraumatic extensor pollicis longus rupture in the nonrheumatoid population. *Eplasty*. 2013;13:e11.
33. Singh HP, Srinivasan S, Ullah A. Closed rupture of the extensor indicis and extensor digitorum tendons to the index finger after locking plate fixation of a fracture of the distal radius. *J Hand Surg Eur Vol*. 2013;38(1):86–87.
34. Bishop AT, Gabel G, Carmichael SW. Flexor carpi radialis tendinitis. Part I: Operative anatomy. *J Bone Joint Surg Am*. 1994;76(7):1009–1014.
35. Luong DH, Smith J, Bianchi S. Flexor carpi radialis tendon ultrasound pictorial essay. *Skeletal Radiol*. 2014;43(6):745–760.
36. Gabel G, Bishop AT, Wood MB. Flexor carpi radialis tendinitis. Part II: Results of operative treatment. *J Bone Joint Surg Am*. 1994;76(7):1015–1018.
37. Wehbé MA. Tendon gliding exercises. *Am J Occup Ther*. 1987;41(3):164–167.
38. Hays PL, Rozental TD. Rehabilitative strategies following hand fractures. *Hand Clin*. 2013;29(4):585–600.
39. Gay A, Harbst K, Hansen DK, et al. Effect of partial wrist denervation on wrist kinesthesia: wrist denervation does not impair proprioception. *J Hand Surg Am*. 2011;36(11):1774–1779.
40. Orlandi D, Corazza A, Silvestri E, et al. Ultrasound-guided procedures around the wrist and hand: how to do. *Eur J Radiol*. 2014;83(7):1231–1238.
41. Krimmer H, Wiemer P, Kalb K. Comparative outcome assessment of the wrist joint–mediocarpal partial arthrodesis and total arthrodesis. *Handchir Mikrochir Plast Chir*. 2000;32(6):369–374.
42. Weinstein LP, Berger RA. Analgesic benefit, functional outcome, and patient satisfaction after partial wrist denervation. *J Hand Surg Am*. 2002;27(5):833–839.
43. Singletary S, Geissler WB. Bracing and rehabilitation for wrist and hand injuries in collegiate athletes. *Hand Clin*. 2009;25(3):443–448.
44. Leggit JC, Meko CJ. Acute finger injuries: Part I. Tendons and ligaments. *Am Fam Physician*. 2006;73(5):810–816.
45. Kelly BM, Spires MC, Restrepo JA. Orthotic and prosthetic prescriptions for today and tomorrow. *Phys Med Rehabil Clin N Am*. 2007;18(4):785–858, vii.
46. Ilyas AM, Ilyas A, Ast M, et al. De quervain tenosynovitis of the wrist. *J Am Acad Orthop Surg*. 2007;15(12):757–764.
47. Wolf JM, Sturdivant RX, Owens BD. Incidence of de Quervain's tenosynovitis in a young, active population. *J Hand Surg Am*. 2009;34(1):112–115.
48. McDermott JD, Ilyas AM, Nazarian LN, Leinberry CF. Ultrasound-guided injections for de Quervain's tenosynovitis. *Clin Orthop Relat Res*. 2012;470(7):1925–1931.
49. Jeyapalan K, Choudhary S. Ultrasound-guided injection of triamcinolone and bupivacaine in the management of De Quervain's disease. *Skeletal Radiol*. 2009;38(11):1099–1103.
50. Costa CR, Morrison WB, Carrino JA. MRI features of intersection syndrome of the forearm. *AJR Am J Roentgenol*. 2003;181(5):1245–1249.
51. Browne J, Helms CA. Intersection syndrome of the forearm. *Arthritis Rheum*. 2006;54(6):2038.

52. Ruland RT, Hogan CJ. The ECU synergy test: an aid to diagnose ECU tendonitis. *J Hand Surg Am.* 2008;33(10):1777–1782.
53. Graham TJ. Pathologies of the extensor carpi ulnaris (ECU) tendon and its investments in the athlete. *Hand Clin.* 2012;28(3):345–356, ix.
54. Campbell D, Campbell R, O'Connor P, Hawkes R. Sports-related extensor carpi ulnaris pathology: a review of functional anatomy, sports injury and management. *Br J Sports Med.* 2013;47(17):1105–1111.
55. Ertel AN, Millender LH, Nalebuff E, et al. Flexor tendon ruptures in patients with rheumatoid arthritis. *J Hand Surg Am.* 1988;13(6):860–866.
56. Bianchi S, Martinoli C, Abdelwahab IF. Ultrasound of tendon tears. Part 1: general considerations and upper extremity. *Skeletal Radiol.* 2005;34(9):500–512.
57. Knobloch K, Spies M, Busch KH, Vogt PM. Sclerosing therapy and eccentric training in flexor carpi radialis tendinopathy in a tennis player. *Br J Sports Med.* 2007;41(12):920–921.
58. Akkaya N, Dogu B, Unlu Z, et al. Ultrasonographic evaluation of the flexor pollicis longus tendon in frequent mobile phone texters. *Am J Phys Med Rehabil.* 2015;94(6):444–448.
59. El Miedany Y, Ashour S, Youssef S, et al. Clinical diagnosis of carpal tunnel syndrome: old tests-new concepts. *Joint Bone Spine.* 2008;75(4):451–457.
60. Elhai M, Guerini H, Bazeli R, et al. Ultrasonographic hand features in systemic sclerosis and correlates with clinical, biologic, and radiographic findings. *Arthritis Care Res (Hoboken).* 2012;64(8):1244–1249.
61. Budoff JE, Kraushaar BS, Ayala G. Flexor carpi ulnaris tendinopathy. *J Hand Surg Am.* 2005;30(1):125–129.
62. Skirven TM. Rehabilitation after tendon injuries in the hand. *Hand Surg.* 2002;7(1):47–59.
63. Frontera WR, Silver JK, Rizzo TD. *Essentials of Physical Medicine and Rehabilitation: Musculoskeletal Disorders, Pain, and Rehabilitation.* 2nd ed. Philadelphia, PA: Saunders/Elsevier; 2008:xix, 935.
64. Ryzewicz M, Wolf JM. Trigger digits: principles, management, and complications. *J Hand Surg Am.* 2006;31(1):135–146.
65. Makkouk AH, Oetgen ME, Swigart CR, Dodds SD. Trigger finger: etiology, evaluation, and treatment. *Curr Rev Musculoskelet Med.* 2008;1(2):92–96.
66. Fleisch SB, Spindler KP, Lee DH. Corticosteroid injections in the treatment of trigger finger: a level I and II systematic review. *J Am Acad Orthop Surg.* 2007;15(3):166–171.
67. Nahra ME, Bucchieri JS. Ganglion cysts and other tumor related conditions of the hand and wrist. *Hand Clin.* 2004;20(3):249–260, v.
68. Eaton C. Evidence-based medicine: dupuytren contracture. *Plast Reconstr Surg.* 2014;133(5):1241–1251.
69. Mahajan M, Rhemrev SJ. Rupture of the ulnar collateral ligament of the thumb - a review. *Int J Emerg Med.* 2013;6(1):31.
70. Peterson JJ, Bancroft LW. Injuries of the fingers and thumb in the athlete. *Clin Sports Med.* 2006;25(3):527–542, vii.
71. Bland JD. Carpal tunnel syndrome. *BMJ.* 2007;335(7615):343–346.
72. D'Arcy CA, McGee S. The rational clinical examination. Does this patient have carpal tunnel syndrome? *JAMA.* 2000;283(23):3110–3117.
73. Werner RA, Andary M. Electrodiagnostic evaluation of carpal tunnel syndrome. *Muscle Nerve.* 2011;44(4):597–607.
74. Hunderfund AN, Boon AJ, Mandrekar JN, Sorenson EJ. Sonography in carpal tunnel syndrome. *Muscle Nerve.* 2011;44(4):485–491.
75. Tai TW, Wu CY, Su FC, et al. Ultrasonography for diagnosing carpal tunnel syndrome: a meta-analysis of diagnostic test accuracy. *Ultrasound Med Biol.* 2012;38(7):1121–1128.
76. Chen CH, Wu T, Sun JS, et al. Unusual causes of carpal tunnel syndrome: space occupying lesions. *J Hand Surg Eur Vol.* 2012;37(1):14–19.
77. Amadio PC. Differential diagnosis of carpal tunnel syndrome. In: Luchetti R, Amadio P, eds. *Carpal Tunnel Syndrome.* Berlin Heidelberg, Germany: Springer; 2007:89–94.
78. Bland JD. Treatment of carpal tunnel syndrome. *Muscle Nerve.* 2007;36(2):167–171.
79. Padua L, Padua R, Aprile I, et al; Italian CTS Study Group. Carpal tunnel syndrome. Multiperspective follow-up of untreated carpal tunnel syndrome: a multicenter study. *Neurology.* 2001;56(11):1459–1466.
80. Keith MW, Masear V, Amadio PC, et al. Treatment of carpal tunnel syndrome. *J Am Acad Orthop Surg.* 2009;17(6):397–405.
81. Neuhaus V, Christoforou D, Cheriyan T, Mudgal CS. Evaluation and treatment of failed carpal tunnel release. *Orthop Clin North Am.* 2012;43(4):439–447.
82. Monacelli G, Rizzo MI, Spagnoli AM, et al. The pillar pain in the carpal tunnel's surgery. Neurogenic inflammation? A new therapeutic approach with local anaesthetic. *J Neurosurg Sci.* 2008;52(1):11–15; discussion 15.
83. Ulrich D, Piatkowski A, Pallua N. Anterior interosseous nerve syndrome: retrospective analysis of 14 patients. *Arch Orthop Trauma Surg.* 2011;131(11):1561–1565.
84. Rodner CM, Tinsley BA, O'Malley MP. Pronator syndrome and anterior interosseous nerve syndrome. *J Am Acad Orthop Surg.* 2013;21(5):268–275.
85. Bachoura A, Jacoby SM. Ulnar tunnel syndrome. *Orthop Clin North Am.* 2012;43(4):467–474.
86. Ginanneschi F, Filippou G, Milani P, et al. Ulnar nerve compression neuropathy at Guyon's canal caused by crutch walking: case report with ultrasonographic nerve imaging. *Arch Phys Med Rehabil.* 2009;90(3):522–524.
87. Maroukis BL, Ogawa T, Rehim SA, Chung KC. Guyon canal: the evolution of clinical anatomy. *J Hand Surg Am.* 2015;40(3):560–565.
88. Massey EW. Sensory mononeuropathies. *Semin Neurol.* 1998;18(2):177–183.
89. Yao J, Park MJ. Early treatment of degenerative arthritis of the thumb carpometacarpal joint. *Hand Clin.* 2008;24(3):251–261, v.
90. Tsai P, Beredjiklian PK. Physical diagnosis and radiographic examination of the thumb. *Hand Clin.* 2008;24(3):231–237, v.
91. Van Heest AE, Kallemeier P. Thumb carpal metacarpal arthritis. *J Am Acad Orthop Surg.* 2008;16(3):140–151.
92. Matullo KS, Ilyas A, Thoder JJ. CMC arthroplasty of the thumb: a review. *Hand (NY).* 2007;2(4):232–239.
93. Fuchs S, Mönikes R, Wohlmeiner A, Heyse T. Intra-articular hyaluronic acid compared with corticoid injections for the treatment of rhizarthrosis. *Osteoarthr Cartil.* 2006;14(1):82–88.
94. Towheed TE. Systematic review of therapies for osteoarthritis of the hand. *Osteoarthr Cartil.* 2005;13(6):455–462.
95. Laulan J, Marteau E, Bacle G. Wrist osteoarthritis. *Orthop Traumatol Surg Res.* 2015;101(1 Suppl):S1–S9.
96. Koh J, Dietz J. Osteoarthritis in other joints (hip, elbow, foot, ankle, toes, wrist) after sports injuries. *Clin Sports Med.* 2005;24(1):57–70.
97. Weiss KE, Rodner CM. Osteoarthritis of the wrist. *J Hand Surg Am.* 2007;32(5):725–746.
98. Rayan GM. Pisiform ligament complex syndrome and pisotriquetral arthrosis. *Hand Clin.* 2005;21(4):507–517.
99. Rizzo M, Cooney WP 3rd. Current concepts and treatment for the rheumatoid wrist. *Hand Clin.* 2011;27(1):57–72.
100. Ilan DI, Rettig ME. Rheumatoid arthritis of the wrist. *Bull Hosp Jt Dis.* 2003;61(3–4):179–185.
101. Klein-Wieringa IR, Kloppenburg M, Bastiaansen-Jenniskens YM, et al. The infrapatellar fat pad of patients with osteoarthritis has an inflammatory phenotype. *Ann Rheum Dis.* 2011;70(5):851–857.
102. Aletaha D, Neogi T, Silman AJ, et al. 2010 Rheumatoid arthritis classification criteria: an American College of Rheumatology/European League Against Rheumatism collaborative initiative. *Arthritis Rheum.* 2010;62(9):2569–2581.
103. Filippucci E, Gabba A, Di Geso L, et al. Hand tendon involvement in rheumatoid arthritis: an ultrasound study. *Semin Arthritis Rheum.* 2012;41(6):752–760.
104. Trieb K. Treatment of the wrist in rheumatoid arthritis. *J Hand Surg Am.* 2008;33(1):113–123.
105. Toms AP, Chojnowski A, Cahir JG. Midcarpal instability: a radiological perspective. *Skeletal Radiol.* 2011;40(5):533–541.
106. Manuel J, Moran SL. The diagnosis and treatment of scapholunate instability. *Orthop Clin North Am.* 2007;38(2):261–277, vii.
107. Caggiano N, Matullo KS. Carpal instability of the wrist. *Orthop Clin North Am.* 2014;45(1):129–140.
108. Tomaino MM, Elfar J. Ulnar impaction syndrome. *Hand Clin.* 2005;21(4):567–575.
109. Chan JJ, Teunis T, Ring D. Prevalence of triangular fibrocartilage complex abnormalities regardless of symptoms rise with age: systematic review and pooled analysis. *Clin Orthop Relat Res.* 2014;472(12):3987–3994.
110. Tay SC, Tomita K, Berger RA. The "ulnar fovea sign" for defining ulnar wrist pain: an analysis of sensitivity and specificity. *J Hand Surg Am.* 2007;32(4):438–444.
111. Henry MH. Management of acute triangular fibrocartilage complex injury of the wrist. *J Am Acad Orthop Surg.* 2008;16(6):320–329.

112. Kakar S, Carlsen BT, Moran SL, Berger RA. The management of chronic distal radioulnar instability. *Hand Clin.* 2010;26(4): 517–528.
113. Szabo RM. Distal radioulnar joint instability. *J Bone Joint Surg Am.* 2006;88(4):884–894.
114. Watson HK, Weinzweig J. Triquetral impingement ligament tear (tilt). *J Hand Surg Br.* 1999;24(3):321–324.
115. Gude W, Morelli V. Ganglion cysts of the wrist: pathophysiology, clinical picture, and management. *Curr Rev Musculoskelet Med.* 2008;1(3–4):205–211.
116. Suputtitada A, Yooktanan P, Rarerng-Ying T. Effect of partial body weight support treadmill training in chronic stroke patients. *J Med Assoc Thai.* 2004;87 (Suppl 2):S107–S111.
117. Park MJ, Namdari S, Weiss AP. The carpal boss: review of diagnosis and treatment. *J Hand Surg Am.* 2008;33(3):446–449.
118. Simon MJ, Pogoda P, Hövelborn F, et al. Incidence, histopathologic analysis and distribution of tumours of the hand. *BMC Musculoskelet Disord.* 2014;15:182.
119. Girisha BS, Shenoy MM, Mathias M, Mohan R. Glomus tumor of the nail unit. *Indian J Dermatol.* 2011;56(5):583–584.
120. Henderson M, Neumeister MW, Bueno RA, Jr. Hand tumors: II. Benign and malignant bone tumors of the hand. *Plast Reconstr Surg.* 2014;133(6):814e–821e.
121. Bernstein ML, Chung KC. Hand fractures and their management: an international view. *Injury.* 2006;37(11):1043–1048.
122. Black WS, Becker JA. Common forearm fractures in adults. *Am Fam Physician.* 2009;80(10):1096–1102.
123. Bot AG, Ring DC. Recovery after fracture of the distal radius. *Hand Clin.* 2012;28(2):235–243.
124. Niver GE, Ilyas AM. Carpal tunnel syndrome after distal radius fracture. *Orthop Clin North Am.* 2012;43(4):521–527.
125. Padegimas EM, Ilyas AM. Distal radius fractures: emergency department evaluation and management. *Orthop Clin North Am.* 2015;46(2):259–270.
126. Gottlieb M, Cosby K. Ultrasound-guided hematoma block for distal radial and ulnar fractures. *J Emerg Med.* 2015;48(3):310–312.
127. CoSuh N, Ek ET, Wolfe SW. Carpal fractures. *J Hand Surg.* 2014; 39(4):785–791.
128. Belsky MR. Commentary: scaphoid fracture in an elite or professional baseball player. *Hand Clin.* 2012;28(3):279–280.
129. Hodgkinson DW, Nicholson DA, Stewart G, et al. Scaphoid fracture: a new method of assessment. *Clin Radiol.* 1993;48(6):398–401.
130. DeLee J, Drez D, Miller MD. *DeLee & Drez's Orthopaedic Sports Medicine: Principles and Practice.* 3rd ed. Philadelphia, PA: Saunders/Elsevier; 2010.
131. Ablett CT, Hackett LA. Hypothenar hammer syndrome: case reports and brief review. *Clin Med Res.* 2008;6(1):3–8.

CHAPTER 6

Back

EPIDEMIOLOGY OF BACK PAIN

BACK PAIN IN THE GENERAL POPULATION

Prevalence and common causes
- Up to 80% (14%–85% lifetime prevalence, depending on definition) in the Western world (1)
- Second most common (MC) reason for physician visit (after upper respiratory problems)
  - Male = female, peak incidence between the ages of 30 and 50
- MC cause of work-related disability <45 years and the most expensive cause of work-related disability
- Isolated low back pain (LBP): 85% have nonspecific (no specific pathoanatomical) diagnoses

Risk factors
- Aging (degenerative changes), heavy lifting and twisting, bodily vibration, obesity, and poor conditioning

BACK PAIN IN CHILDREN

- Spondylolysis: 50%
- Mechanical LBP: 25%
- Discogenic: 10%

BACK PAIN IN ATHLETES

Prevalence
- Common cause of pain in young athletes, (2) 1% to 30%, MC cause of missed playing time in professional athletes
- Sprains: MC cause of back pain (3)
- Spondylolysis: peak in ages from 6 to 10 years, prevalence: 4%, repeated hyperextension motions such as gymnastics and diving
- Unclear etiologies: only 15% have precise pathoanatomical diagnosis
- MC: strain/sprain, disc herniation, spinal stenosis, sacroiliac dysfunction, and fracture (compression, sacral stress)

Sports-related rates of LBP
- Higher rates in gymnastics, diving, weightlifting, golf, American football, rowing, and others (ice hockey, rugby, basketball, and racquet sports)
  - Higher in contact sports: football (30% have significant back pain, highest in linemen), ice hockey, basketball, wrestling, and rugby
  - Noncontact sports: 29% professional golfers, 22.5% of spondylolysis in track and field, weightlifters, racquet sports, gymnasts, and divers
- Rare in runners

Risk factors: Hamstring flexibility (spondylolysis), prior back pain (six times higher), improper technique, or poor equipment

Common causes of LBP in mature athletes
- Prevalence of back pain among former elite athletes of all sports is lower than that in nonathletes

BACK PAIN AT WORK (4)

Prevalence
- 14% to 80% in people of working age, depending on the case definition

Risk factors
- Manual work: materials handling, frequent bending or twisting, whole body vibration, carpenter, bus driver, and others
- Physical hard work: different definitions exist, but in general include agricultural, construction, mechanics, fishing, and soldering
- Job dissatisfaction and job control

Work-related factors for lumbar disc disease
- Heavy lifting, frequent bending and twisting

Predictors for disability after LBP at work
- Heavy physical demand, ability to modify work, social support, short job tenure, job satisfaction, and fear of re-injury (5)

SPORTS WITH HIGHER PREVALENCE	COMMON PATHOLOGIES	SUGGESTED MECHANISM
Wrestling, gymnastics Dance and ballet, soccer American football Volleyball, throwing sports Racquet sports	Spondylolysis Spondylolisthesis	Repetitive flexion/extension Hyperextension

(continued)

SPORTS WITH HIGHER PREVALENCE	COMMON PATHOLOGIES	SUGGESTED MECHANISM
Weightlifting American football	Scheuermann's disease	Repetitive loading with flexion
Dancers, gymnasts, and swimmers	Scoliosis	
Weightlifting American football Endplate fracture in skeletally immature athletes	Fracture/ compression fracture	Axial loading
Hockey	Spinous process fracture	Resisted muscle contraction Direct trauma

DIFFERENTIAL DIAGNOSIS

Differential diagnosis based on the location and radiation of pain (Flowchart 6.1) (1,6)

WORKING DEFINITION OF LOW BACK

- Below the 12th rib to the iliac crest (vs buttock: below the iliac crest to the gluteal fold); Figure 6.1
- Patients and clinicians use different definition, description based on anatomic landmark helps to facilitate communication between the patient and clinician

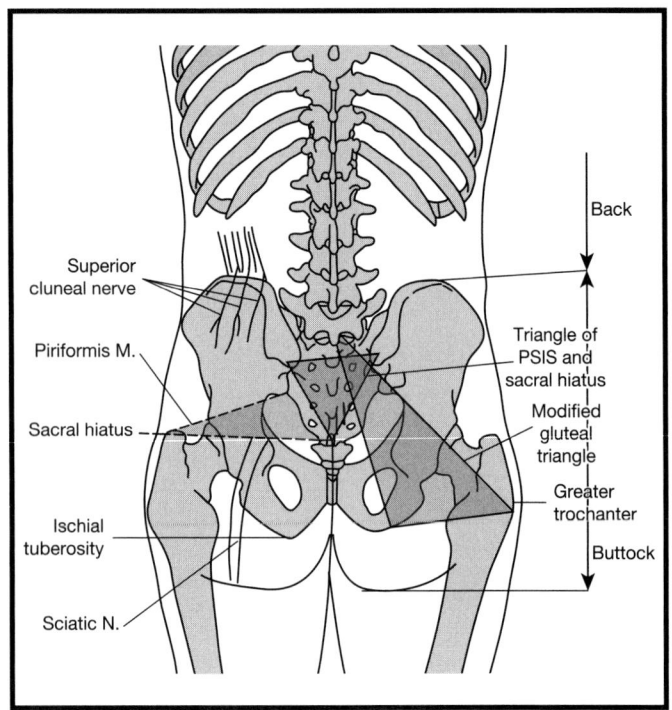

FIGURE 6.1
Surface anatomy of low back.
M, muscle; N, nerve; PSIS, posterior superior iliac spine.
Source: Adapted from Ref. (7). Franklyn-Miller A, Falvey E, McCrory P. The gluteal triangle: a clinical patho-anatomical approach to the diagnosis of gluteal pain in athletes. *Br J Sports Med*. 2009;43(6):460–466.

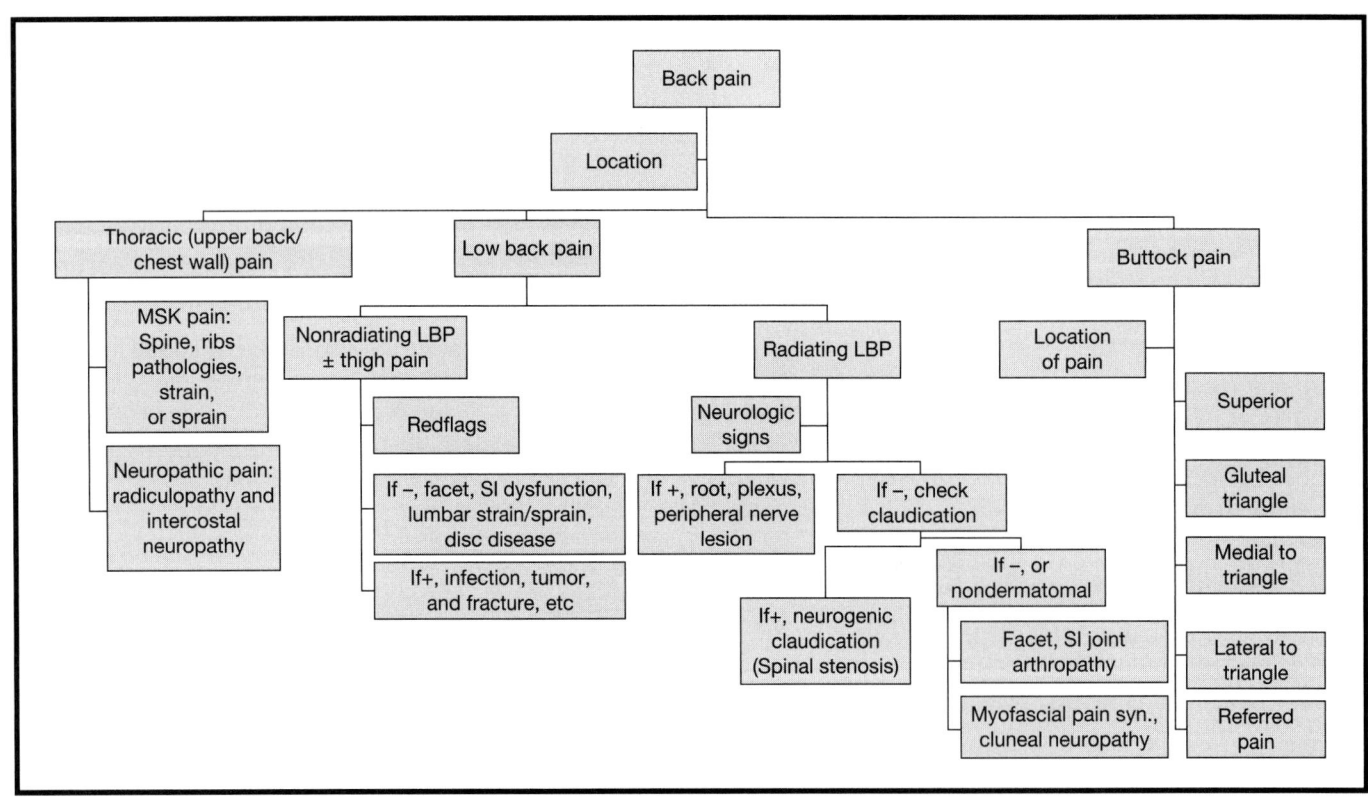

FLOWCHART 6.1
Differential diagnosis of back pain based on the location.
−, negative; +, positive; LBP, low back pain; N, nerve; SI, sacroiliac; syn., syndrome.

RADIATING BACK PAIN BELOW THE KNEE	OTHER LOW BACK PAIN

Radiculopathy (from disc disease, spinal stenosis)
• Sciatica: sensitive and specific for radiculopathy (8)
• Mechanical (MC cause, >90%): discal disruption, spinal stenosis
• Nonmechanical: DM, infectious, tumor etc
Claudication
• Neurogenic: spinal stenosis
• Vascular: peripheral arterial disease
Piriformis syndrome (buttock pain with radiating leg pain)
	Localized (axial pain)
	• Facet joint disease (±referred pain)
	• Degenerative disc disease
	• Vertebral body fracture (±radiculopathy)
	Localized ± referred/radiating pain (proximal to knee)
	• Upper lumbar radiculopathy (to above the knee)
	• Myofascial pain disorder (± referred pain)
	  ○ Quadratus lumborum
	  ○ Gluteus medius (at iliac crest, but more buttock pain); Figure 6.2
	• Sacroiliac joint dysfunction (± referred pain, occasionally distal to the knee)
	• Facet arthropathy
	• Cluneal neuropathy
	• Proximal hamstring tendinopathy (at the ischial tuberosity)

DM, diabetes mellitus; MC, most common.

DIFFERENTIAL DIAGNOSIS BASED ON MODE OF ONSET

- Acute onset: disc disruption or inflammation, vascular process
- Gradual onset: degenerative spondylosis, spinal stenosis
  ○ Preceding events (with trauma or injury vs without clear event)

Unusual causes of LBP

LOCAL CAUSES	REFERRED FROM OUTSIDE THE SPINE (<5%)
Neoplasia • Metastatic cancer • Multiple myeloma • Lymphoma and leukemia • Spinal cord tumor • Retroperitoneal tumor • Primary vertebral tumors Infection • Osteomyelitis, septic discitis, paraspinal abscess, epidural abscess Inflammatory arthropathy • Ankylosing spondylitis • Psoriatic spondylitis • Reiter syndrome • Inflammatory bowel disease Paget's disease	Pelvic organ involvement • Prostatitis • Endometriosis • Chronic (pelvic) inflammatory disease Renal pathologies • Nephrolithiasis • Pyelonephritis • Perinephric abscess GI pathologies • Pancreatitis • Cholecystitis • Penetrating ulcer Abdominal aortic aneurysm/rupture (9) • More abdominal pain and back pain rather than isolated back pain

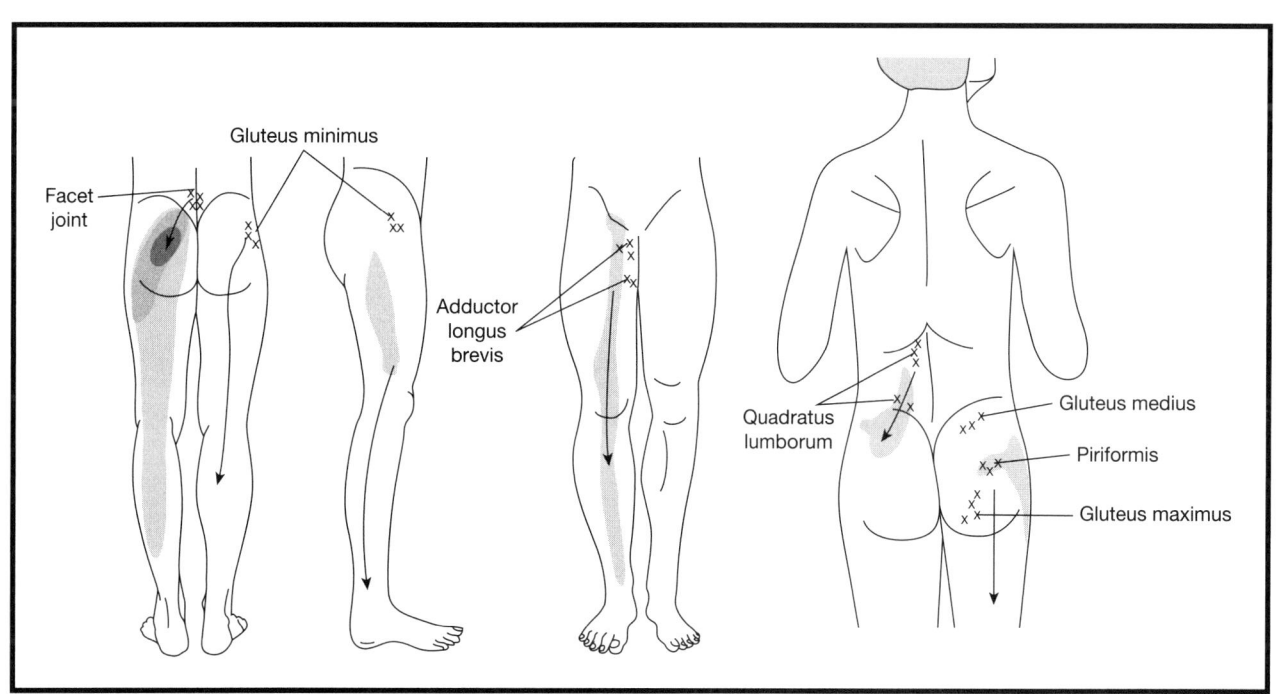

FIGURE 6.2
Pain referral pattern from myofascial trigger point and painful facet joint.

CLASSIFICATION AND DIFFERENTIAL DIAGNOSIS OF SPINE DEFORMITY (10)

Scoliosis: frontal plane deformity ± rotation in axial plane
- Idiopathic: infantile <3 years; juvenile: 3 to 10 years; adolescent (MC): 10 years to maturation
- Degenerative or de novo scoliosis (11)
- Neuromuscular: neuropathic (cerebral palsy, syringomyelia, spinocerebellar degeneration, polio, spinal muscular atrophy, or myelomeningocele) or myopathic (muscular dystrophy, myotonic dystrophy, or arthrogryposis)
- Miscellaneous

Hyperkyphosis: sagittal malalignment; idiopathic, Scheuermann in young adults, and compression fracture in the elderly

Hyperlordosis: spondylolisthesis and back spasm

DIFFERENTIAL DIAGNOSIS OF SEVERE BACK SPASM (12)

- Infectious disease: tetanus
- Toxic disease: strychnine poisoning
- Neoplastic disease: mass-effect causing irritation to spinal nerves or paraspinal muscles
- Vascular disease: spinal arteriovenous malformations and intermittent venous congestion
- Genetic disease: hyperekplexia
- Autoimmune disease: stiff person syndrome, Isaacs's syndrome, spinal multiple sclerosis, paraneoplasia, and myelitis

DIFFERENTIAL DIAGNOSES OF BOWEL AND BLADDER DYSFUNCTION RELATED TO SPINE PATHOLOGIES

Rare but highly morbid conditions such as cauda equina syndrome (CES) (2% of all disc herniation) or conus medullaris should be in differentials (requiring immediate referral to emergency room [ER])

	CONUS MEDULLARIS	CAUDA EQUINA SYNDROME (13)
Pain	Not common. Can be severe, bilateral, and symmetric in perineum or thigh	Severe back and radicular pain (83%–90%)
Onset	Sudden and bilateral	Gradual and unilateral or acute
Bladder/rectal dysfunction	Early and marked involvement	Less marked impairment. Saddle anesthesia and vesicular (urinary retention or incontinence (~55%) >rectal dysfunction (decreased rectal tone) >erectile dysfunction
Sexual function	Erection and ejaculation impaired	Late and less marked
Sensory deficit	Saddle distribution, bilateral, symmetric, dissociation of sensation	Unilateral or asymmetric, sacral N distribution
		Saddle distribution, may be unilateral and asymmetric, no dissociation of sensation
Motor loss	Symmetric, not marked, fasciculation	Asymmetric, more marked, atrophy, no fasciculation
Reflex loss	Only Achilles reflex	Late and less marked

N, nerve.

Other causes
- Iatrogenic from medications; antidepressant (TCA), opioids analgesics (urinary retention), muscle relaxants (retention), and sedatives

DIFFERENTIAL DIAGNOSIS OF CHEST WALL PAIN (FLOWCHART 6.2)

- If there are cardiovascular risk factors or if there is any suspicion, first evaluate cardiac causes and complete the cardiac workup with cardiology consultant
- Incidence of musculoskeletal causes of chest pain
  - 13% to 20% of patients originally thought to be of cardiac origin

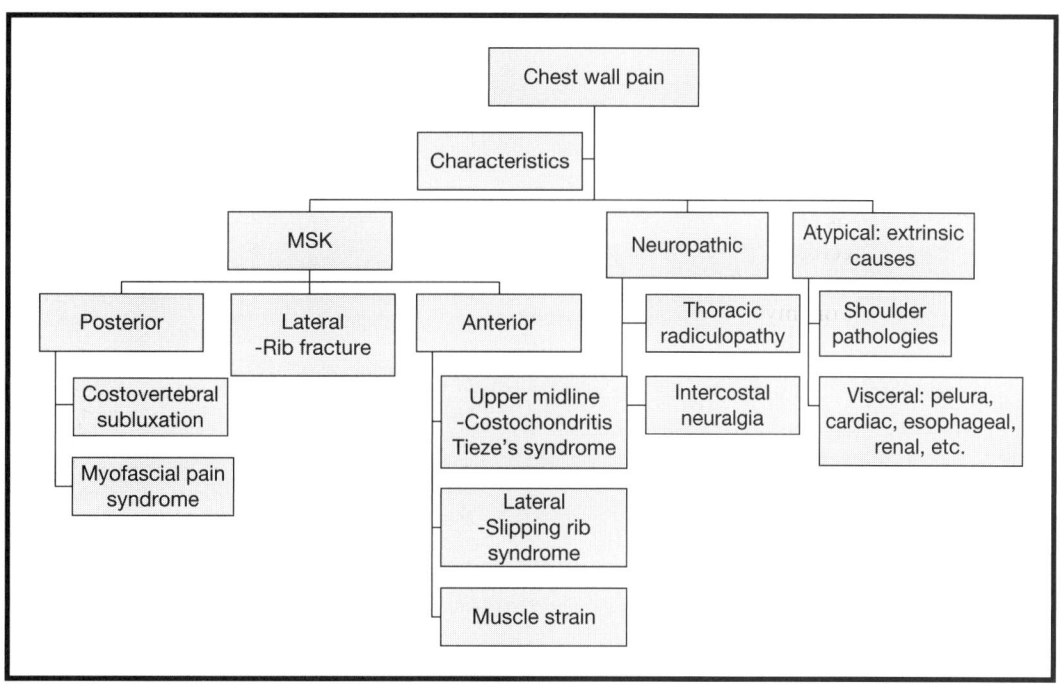

FLOWCHART 6.2
Differential diagnosis of chest wall pain.
MSK, musculoskeletal.

Differential diagnosis based on anatomical structures

ANATOMIC STRUCTURE	PATHOLOGIES	CHARACTERISTICS
Nerve	Intercostal neuralgia (eg, herpes zoster)	Common, thoracic is the MC location, zoster sine herpes (without skin lesion)
	Thoracic spine root lesion (disc, tumor, infection)	Rarer causes: diabetes, sarcoidosis, tuberculosis, and syphilis
	Spinal cord pathology	Myelopathy, dural AVM (lower thoracic), and root sleeves
Rib	Rib stress fracture	Posterolateral angle: MC location
	Slipping rib syndrome	8th to 10th rib; pain under the rib cage and upper abdomen
Sternum	Sternal stress fracture	Anterior chest pain
	Manubrium stress fractures	
	Painful xiphoid syndrome	
Joints	Costochondritis	Upper chest wall
	Tietze's syndrome	2nd and 3rd costochondral junction (upper chest wall)
	Sternoclavicular arthritis	Anterior neck pain
	Manubriosternal arthritis	
	Costovertebral subluxation/arthritis	Posterior upper back pain
	Sternocostal synchondrosis/subluxation	
Muscle	Intercostal muscle strain	MC followed by pectoralis M strain
	Epidemic myalgia	Group B coxsackie virus, intercostal and upper abdominal wall M (severe/ sharp pain)
	Precordial catch syndrome	Diagnosis of exclusion, left parasternal near cardiac apex, increased by deep breathing, no local tenderness
Referred pain (extrinsic causes)	Shoulder pathologies	
	Pleuritis	
	Cardiac conditions	
	Esophageal dysfunction	
	Renal: nephrolithiasis	

AVM, arteriovenous malformation; M, muscle; MC, most common.

DIFFERENTIAL DIAGNOSIS OF BUTTOCK PAIN

Anatomy-based differential diagnosis (see Figure 6.1)

Modified gluteal triangle: Triangle of spinous process of L5, ischial tuberosity, and laterally on the greater trochanter (see Figure 6.1) (7,157)

LOCATION	ANATOMIC STRUCTURE	PATHOLOGIES AND CHARACTERISTICS
Superior	Iliac crest	Thoracodorsal fascia, quadratus lumborum M strain/myofascial pain syn
	Iliolumbar ligament	Iliolumbar lig sprain: mimics or coexists with SIJ pain (158), paraspinal region pain (above the SI dimple)
	Gluteus medius	Myofascial pain syn: often poorly localized, trigger point, dry needling for diagnosis and Tx Gluteus medius strain/tear (muscle belly or near attachment to iliac crest) Pain worse in stance or running and tenderness
	Fat pad	Epi-sacral painful fat pad syndrome (not all fat pads are painful)
	Superficial cluneal N	Iatrogenic superficial cluneal nerve injury from bone graft or muscle injection Superior cluneal nerve entrapment syndrome (at traversing iliac crest) Maigne's syndrome (thoracolumbar transition zone) with irritation of posterior rami T12 to L2
In the triangle	SI joint	SI joint ligament sprain, joint dysfunction, arthritis Pain in the gluteal region (often lower back above iliac crest) ± referred pain (often thigh and rarely the leg)
	Piriformis	Piriformis syndrome (buttock pain ± referred pain or sciatica)
	Obturator internus	Similar to piriformis syndrome; slightly lower than piriformis on the location of local tenderness, difficult to differentiate
	Vessels	Circumflex femoral vein thrombosis Rare, tenderness and pain on resisted flexion without M weakness
Lat to triangle	Femoro-acetabular (hip) joint	Femoroacetabular impingement syn. Degenerative: restriction in daily living, pain on weight bearing +/- clicking or locking
	Femoral neck	Stress fracture Female, change in volume of training, osteopenia/osteoporosis (159)
	Trochanteric bursa Gluteus medius/minimus tendon Tensor fascia lata Iliotibial band (ITB)	Trochanteric tendinobursitis • Pain getting up off bed, tenderness superior and over the GT Gluteus medius (>minimus) tendinopathy/tear TFL/ITB syndrome • Lateral thigh pain worsens with exercise ± snapping hip, sharp burning pain
	Lateral femoral cutaneous N	Meralgia paresthetica • Anterolateral thigh pain/sensory symptoms (tingling, pins/needle sensation)
Med to triangle	SI joint	SI joint/ligament pain Sacroiliitis with/without spondyloarthropathy (AS) • Systemic symptoms (morning stiffness, improvement with mod. activity, diffuse buttock pain, other past medical history such as psoriasis etc.), asymmetric polyarthropathy involving large joints
	Sacrum	Sacral stress fracture • Vague incapacitating gluteal pain, pelvic anteversion, insufficiency versus fatigue fracture, and leg length discrepancy (risk factor)
	Coccyx	Coccygodynia • Dull, achy pain on sitting, sitting to standing
	Pubic ramus	Stress fracture of pubic ramus • Gradual onset, pain standing on one leg and hop, and deep buttock pain

(continued)

LOCATION	ANATOMIC STRUCTURE	PATHOLOGIES AND CHARACTERISTICS
	Sup. (Inf.) gluteal A	Entrapment and endofibrosis • Claudicant gluteal pain on exercise relieved by rest, and smoking Aneurysm of inferior gluteal artery
	Hamstring M/ischial tuberosity	High hamstring syndrome/tear, apophysitis/ischial tuberosity avulsion • Shooting pain following high-energy kick or change of direction Posterior compartment syndrome • Associated with avulsion fracture, sudden tearing pain gradually worsening over 24 hours in acute, more insidious in chronic
	Obturator N	Medial thigh pain on exercise relieved by rest, adductor weakness, superficial dysesthesia, hyperesthesia on med thigh
Referred pain	Disc disease with radiculopathy Lumbar pathology (disc, facet)	LS radiculopathy • LBP radiating down to the leg (below knee) typically • Absence of LBP or leg pain (below knee) doesn't rule out lower lumbar radiculopathy

A, artery; AS, ankylosing spondylitis; ITB, Iliotibial band; LBP, low back pain; lig, ligament; LS, lumbosacral; M, muscle; N, nerve; SIJ, SI joint, sacroiliac joint; syn, syndrome; TFL, tensor facsia lata; Tx, treatment.

ANATOMY

BONE AND JOINT

Spine Complex (14)

Vertebra
- From anterior to posterior: body, pedicle, transverse process (at junction of pedicle and lamina), articular process (facets), lamina (including pars interarticularis), and spinous process (Figure 6.3)
- Characteristics of vertebral anatomy
  - Variation: sacralization of L5 (~17% of population) and lumbarization of S1 (4–6 lumbar vertebrae, less common than sacralization)
  - Vertebral body: taller anteriorly → contribute to lordosis
  - Mamillary process; tubercles on the superior articular processes
  - L5: the largest vertebral body

Intervertebral disc
- Nucleus pulposus and annulus fibrosus (fibrocartilaginous lamina)
- Intervertebral disc accounts for one-fourth the length of the spinal column, partly responsible for physiologic lumbar lordosis
- Nucleus pulposus: gelatinous inner section containing water, proteoglycan, and collagen
- Annulus fibrosus: concentric layers of fibrous tissue and fibrocartilage

Vertebral canal (15)
- Space containing the spinal cord and nerve roots (caudal to L2)
- Spinal canal (central) bordered by
  - Anteriorly: posterior longitudinal ligament
  - Posteriorly: ligamentum flavum, lamina, and facet joints
  - Laterally: pedicles

Lateral canal (16,17)

ZONE	DESCRIPTION	PATHOLOGY CAUSING STENOSIS
Entrance zone	Cephalad (superior) and medial aspects of lateral recess, which begins at lateral aspect of thecal sac and runs obliquely down and laterally toward intervertebral foramen. Same level of nerve root involved, L4 root under L4 superior articular process	Facet hypertrophy, particularly involving superior articular process Developmental problem (short pedicle)
Midzone	Beneath pars interarticularis and just inferior to pedicle Bounded anteriorly by posterior aspect of vertebral body and posteriorly by pars; medial boundary is open to central spinal canal Contains dorsal ganglion and ventral root in extension of dura mater, more sensitive to the stenosis (decreased effective size)	Osteophyte under pars interarticularis Fibrocartilagenous or bursal hypertrophy at spondylolytic defect
Exit zone	Formed by intervertebral foramen Lumbar nerve covered by perineurium	Hypertrophic facet arthritis or subluxation and osteophytic ridge along the superior margin of the disc

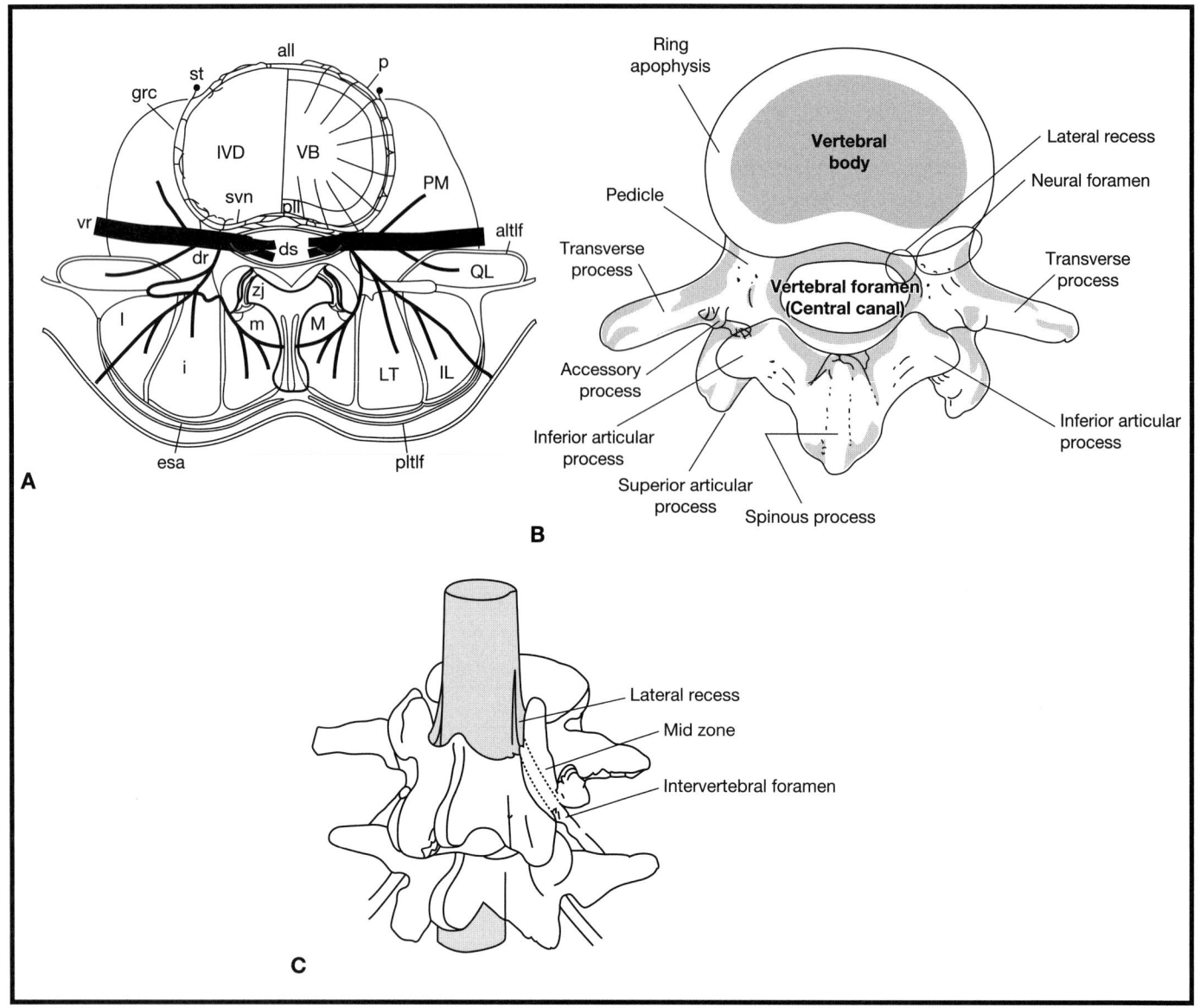

FIGURE 6.3
Bony and soft-tissue anatomy with innervation in the lumbar spine (A and B) and location of lateral stenosis (C).
aCross-sectional view incorporates the level of the vertebral body (VB), and the periosteum (P) on the right and the intervertebral disc (IVD) on the left. all, anterior longitudinal ligaments; altlf, anterior layer of thoracolumbar fascia; dr, dorsal ramus; ds, dural sac; esa, erector spinal aponeurosis; grc, gray ramus communicans; i, intermediate branch; IL, iliocostal lumborum; l, lateral branch; LT, longissimus thoracic; m, medial branch; M, multidus; pll, posterior longitudinal ligament; pltlf, posterior layer of thoracolumbar fascia; QL, quadratus lumborum; st, sympathetic trunk; svn, sinuvertebral nerve; vr, ventral ramus; zj, zygapophyseal joint; PM, psoas muscle.
Source: Adapted from Ref. (18). Suri P, Rainville J, Kalichman L, Katz JN. Does this older adult with lower extremity pain have the clinical syndrome of lumbar spinal stenosis? *JAMA*. 2010;304(23):2628–2636.

Meninges

Dura mater
- The most superficial, becomes epineurium at the dorsal root ganglion
- Ligaments of Hoffman: connect the dura mater and nerve root to the posterior longitudinal ligament

Arachnoid
- Lines dural sac
- Subarachnoid space ends at the dorsal root

Pia mater
- The deepest: forms filum terminale (anchors to the coccyx)

Chest Wall and Thoracic Spine (19)

Thoracic spine
- Upper 10 thoracic vertebrae: costal facet on the anterolateral surface of the transverse process articulating with rib
  - Costal facets: thoracic vertebral body, anterior to the pedicle articulating with ribs
- Smaller clearance between the spinal cord and bony spinal segments (9.2 mm in thoracic spine vs 11.3 mm in the

cervical spine), spinal cord/canal ratio: 0.4 in thoracic spine versus 0.25 in cervical spine
- Primary movements: rotation (8°–9°) and lateral bending (6°)

Ribs (Figure 6.4)
- 1 to 7 ribs: anteriorly with sternum via costochondral cartilage; 8 to 10 ribs: costochondral cartilage with adjacent ribs; 11 to 12 ribs: floating ribs
- 2 to 10 ribs: articulates with vertebral bodies and transverse processes of two vertebrae via the costovertebral and costotransverse (with transverse process) joints

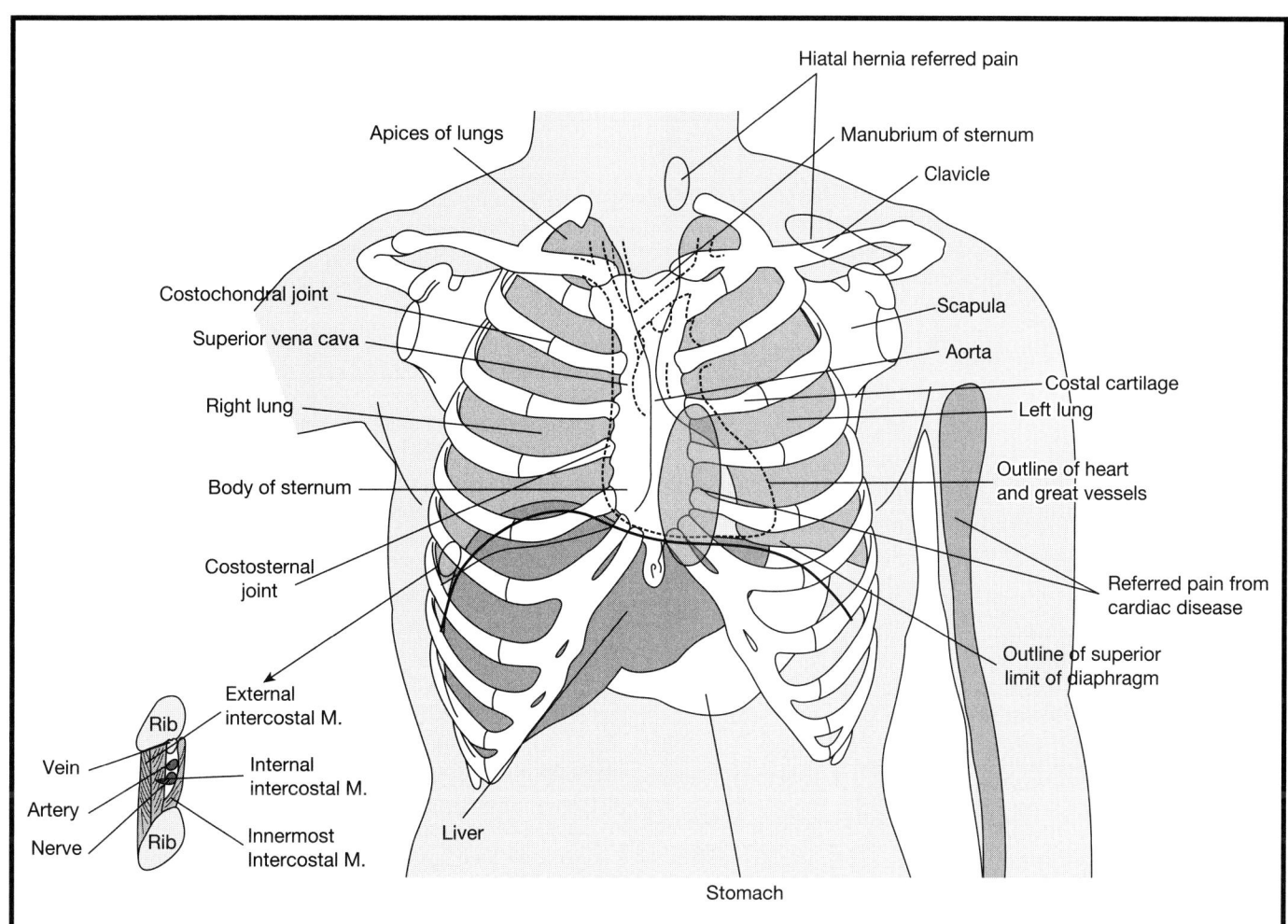

FIGURE 6.4
Anatomy for chest wall pain.
M, muscle.

Thoracic spinal nerves and intercostal nerve
- Ventral rami: no plexus (except T1), continues as intercostal nerves
- T1 (2): supply thorax wall and give branches to brachial plexus
  ○ T1: larger branch to brachial plexus, smaller to the 1st intercostal nerve
  ○ Intercostobrachial cutaneous nerve: axillary sensation (20)
- T3–6: thoracic wall
  ○ Below the intercostal vessels (vein, artery, and nerve), between pleura and posterior intercostal membranes or between internal and innermost intercostal muscle
  ○ Innervates intercostal muscle, subcostal muscle, serratus post, superior, transversus thoracic muscle
  ○ Cutaneous branches: lateral cutaneous and anterior cutaneous branches
  ○ Articular branches to the rib periosteum
  ○ Branches to the parietal pleura
- T7–11: abdomen and peritoneum
  ○ Rectus abdominis and anterior cutaneous branches on the abdominal wall
- T12: subcostal

Sacroiliac Joint (Figure 6.5)

- Five sacral vertebrae and four coccygeal vertebrae
- Large, auricular-shaped, diarthrodial synovial joint

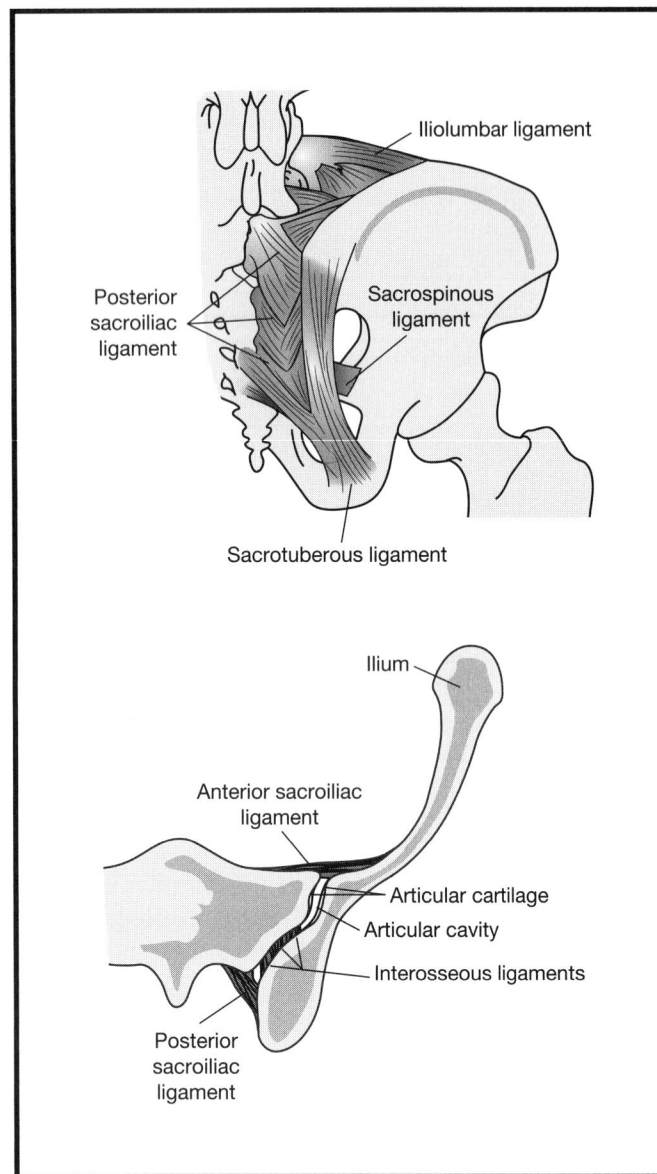

FIGURE 6.5
Sacroiliac joint and ligament.

- The potential for vertical shearing is present in ~30% of sacroiliac (SI) joints, due to the more acute angulation of the short, horizontal articular component
- Part synovial: anterior inferior 1/3, hyaline cartilage on sacrum side, fibroid cartilage on the iliac side
- Part syndesmosis
- Ligament
  - Sacroiliac ligament: primary stabilizer of SI joint
    - Anterior, posterior (sacrum to posterior superior iliac spine [PSIS], short and long) and interosseous
    - More extensive posteriorly, function as a connecting band between the sacrum and iliac because of an absent or rudimentary posterior capsule
    - Main function is to limit motion in all planes of movement
    - In women, the ligaments are weaker, allowing mobility necessary for parturition
  - Sacrotuberous ligament (21)
    - Iliac spine, sacrum to ischial tuberosity
    - Stabilize the sacroiliac joint, provide vertical stability
    - Insertion site for gluteus maximus proximally, distally merge with conjoint hamstring tendon (biceps femoris and semitendinosus)
  - Sacrospinous ligament
    - Ischial spine to sacrum and coccyx
    - Divides sciatic notch into greater and lesser sciatic foramina
- Innervation of SI joint (22)
  - Posterior SI joint: the lateral branches of the L4–S3 (L3–S4) dorsal rami
  - Anterior SI joint: L2 (to L5)–S2 ventral rami depending on the study
    - The anterior SI joint is less innervated
  - Animal study indicates that the SI joints may have lower pain sensitivity than that of the lumbar facet joints

NERVE

Nerve Innervation of the Spine

Somatic nociception
- Sinuvertebral nerve (see Figure 6.3)
  - The posterior longitudinal ligament, posterior annulus, epidural venous plexus, and ventral dura
  - Sinuvertebral nerve → the dorsal root ganglion → the spinal cord and brain
- The dorsal ramus: medial, intermediate, and lateral branches
  - The medial branch of the dorsal ramus
    - The facet joint, lamina, spinous process, and posterior ligaments
    - Supplies the multifidus muscle
    - Mamilloaxillary ligament: can entrap dorsal rami → denervation of paraspinal muscle
  - The intermediate and lateral branches supply lateral muscles and receive supply from the skin (eg, cluneal nerve)

Sympathetic nociception
- The anterior and posterior longitudinal ligaments, annulus, and vertebral body
- Anterior spinal sympathetic ramus (anteriorly)
- The sinuvertebral nerve and white ramus communicans (preganglionic) posteriorly → Paraspinal sympathetic ganglion → grey ramus communicans (postganglionic) → dorsal root ganglion

Possible mechanism of pain from spinal stenosis
- Venous engorgement and arterial insufficiency
- Venous congestion and stagnation → increase epidural and intrathecal pressures → microcirculatory, neuroischemic insults
- Arterial insufficiency: arterial dilatation of the lumbar radicular vessels during lower limb exercise. Loss of reflexic dilatation in spinal stenosis

Lumbar Root and Lumbosacral (LS) Plexus (Figure 6.6)

Ventral root → spinal nerve (with dorsal root) → ventral ramus → lumbosacral (LS) plexus (from spinal cord distally)

Biggest nerve root: L5 with smaller lateral foramen at L5–S1 → one of the reasons for high prevalence of L5 radiculopathy

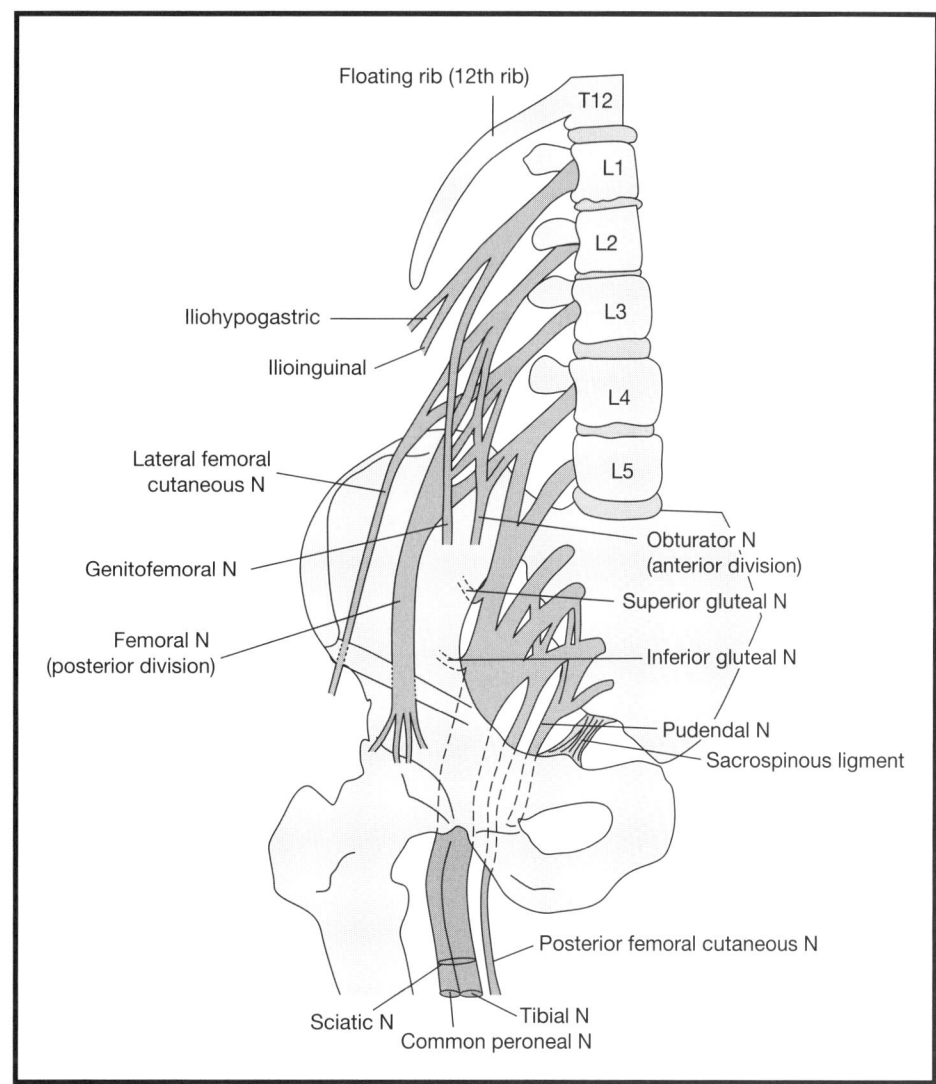

FIGURE 6.6

Lumbosacral plexus.

N, nerve.

Source: Adapted from Ref. (23). Laughlin RS, Dyck PJ. Electrodiagnostic testing in lumbosacral plexopathies. *Phys Med Rehabil Clin N Am*. 2013;24(1):93–105.

	NERVE	NOTES
Lumbar plexus		L1–3, part of L4. Course within the psoas muscle
	Iliohypogastric and ilioinguinal (L1) Genitofemoral (L1–2) Lateral femoral cutaneous (L2–3)	Check groin region (P 302)
	Obturator N (ant. div., L2–4) Femoral (post div., L2–4)	Through obturator foramen Ant. div., post div., innervates hip, knee, and medial thigh sensation Lateral border of psoas major, runs between psoas and iliacus Femoral triangle, lat. to vein and artery Branches: Ant. femoral cutaneous N and saphenous N
Sacral plexus		L4,5 (lumbosacral trunk) and S1–4 In the deeper surface of the piriformis

(*continued*)

NERVE	NOTES
Posterior femoral cutaneous S–3	Inf. cluneal and perineal branches Accompanied by sciatic N
Pudendal S2–4 N to obturator internus L5–S1 N to quadratus femoris L5–S2	Ant div., course below piriformis, lesser sciatic foramen, pudendal canal
Superior gluteal L4–S1 Inferior gluteal L5–S2	Above (cephalad) piriformis, innervates glut. med., min., TFL Below (caudad) piriformis, innervates gluteus maximus Sup and inferior gluteal N: post div.
Sciatic N L4–S3	Tibial (medial/ant. div.) and peroneal (lat./post div.)

Ant., anterior; div., division; glut med, gluteus medius; glut min, gluteus minimus; inf., inferior; lat., lateral; N, nerve; post, posterior; post div., posterior division.

Nerves in the Buttock

Cutaneous nerves (24)
- Superior cluneal nerve: medial (L1), intermediate (L2), and lateral (L3) or T12-L2
  - Course
    - Pass through the psoas major, and paraspinal, posterior to the quadratus lumborum under the thoracodorsal fascia
    - Traverse iliac crest—distance from midline (at the level of PSIS): ~5, 6.5, and 7.3 cm for medial, intermediate, and lateral branches, respectively
      - Injection points (5–8 cm from midline on the posterior iliac crest) for superior cluneal nerve
- Middle cluneal nerve: from posterior sacral foramen, S1–3, S1 most constant and S3 (in 45%)
  - Traverse the paraspinal muscle and tissue overlying the gluteus maximus
  - Less likely entrapped due to shorter length and course through multiple fasciae
- Inferior cluneal nerve (25): from posterior femoral cutaneous nerve from S1–3, comes off with perineal branch (horizontal course medially), reflects cranially between glut. maximus and hamstring muscle

Motor branches (check lumbar spine anatomy)
- Superior gluteal nerve: gluteus medius, minimus and tensor fascia lata
- Inferior gluteal nerve: gluteus maximus
- Nerve to obturator internus (L5–S1)
- Nerve to quadratus femoris (L5–S2)

Pudendal nerve (anterior rami of S2–4): (26)
- Course
  - Pass through greater sciatic foramen (with internal pudendal artery caudal to the piriformis muscle)
  - Posterior to sacrospinous ligament and between sacrospinous and sacrotuberous ligament through lesser sciatic notch and Alcock's canal (the fascia tunnel formed by the duplication of internal obturator muscles, under the plane of the levator ani muscle, on the lateral wall of the ischiorectal fossa)
  - Common mechanism of injury: parturition, bicycle riding, blunt trauma, and penetrating injury
- Three terminal branches
  - The dorsal nerve of the penis, the inferior rectal nerve, and the perineal nerve
  - Sensation around the skin of penis (clitoris), perianal area, and the posterior surface of scrotum or labia majora
  - The external anal sphincter (inferior rectal nerve) and deep muscles of the urogenital triangle (perineal nerve)

ARTERY (27)

Aorta → internal iliac artery → posterior division (superficial gluteal artery) and anterior division (inferior gluteal artery)
- Superior gluteal artery travels through the greater sciatic foramen above (superior to) the piriformis, then divides into superficial and deep division. Supplies the iliacus, piriformis, and obturators
  - Superior gluteal artery in gluteal canal: osseous fibromuscular structure
  - The crest of greater sciatic notch (superiorly), inferior by the arcade of Bouisson (superior border of the piriformis)
- Inferior gluteal artery
  - Inferior gluteal artery: inferior to the piriformis, supplies gluteus maximus and branches to become sciatic artery (runs with sciatic nerve)
  - Aneurysm or pseudoaneurysm can affect the sciatic nerve
- Iliolumbar and lateral sacral artery

Distal aortic occlusion: impotence and buttock claudication

MUSCLE

Paraspinal muscle (Figure 6.3)
- Superficial group: ipsilateral rotation with ipsilateral contraction
  - Erector spinae: iliocostalis, longissimus, and spinalis (lateral to medial)
- Deeper group: deeper to erector spinae, contralateral rotation with ipsilateral contraction
  - Transversospinalis: multifidus (deep to semispinalis) and rotatores
  - Multifidus
    - Local postural muscle, length transducer, or position sensors by way of rich composition of muscle spindles that pass along two or three spinal levels
    - Segmental stabilizer
    - Monosegmental (single root) supplied muscle
- Clinical implications in LBP
  - Pain perception from hypertonic saline injection to paraspinal muscle (28)

- Depth and lateral position may be the most critical descriptors to determine the source of acute lumbar muscular pain
- Overlapping regions of pain may be explained by convergence of receptive fields, innervation of multifidus fascicles at multiple lumbar segments, and convergence of sensory input from different muscles to the same sensory cell bodies (animal study)
- Changes in chronic LBP
  - Have both impaired spinal proprioception and a decrease in paraspinal muscle cross-sectional area (29)
  - Association between decreased paraspinal muscle density and the presence of lumbar spondylosis (30)

Extrinsic muscles

- Quadratus lumborum: flexes vertebral column laterally when acting separately. Together maintains posture. Assists in forced inspiration (31)
  - Cited as a common source of back pain (myofascial pain)
- Latissimus dorsi: adductor and extensor of the shoulder (glenohumeral joint), an extensor and lateral flexor of the back, and is purported to have a bracing effect on the sacroiliac joint, in concert with the gluteus maximus through its action on the posterior layer of thoracolumbar fascia (32)
- Serratus posterior inferior: spinous processes of T11–L2 to inferior borders of 8th–12th ribs, innervated by ventral rami of T9–12 spinal nerves, depresses ribs and counteracts inward pull of diaphragms (assist forced expiration and rotation/extension of the trunk)

Buttock muscles (see the following table)

MUSCLE	ORIGIN	INSERTION	INNERVATION	ACTION	COMMENT
Hip Extensors and External Rotators					
Gluteus maximus	Ilium (medial), dorsal sacrum, coccyx, sacrotuberous ligament and gluteal aponeurosis	ITB, gluteal tuberosity	Inf. gluteal (L5–S2)	Extend, ER thigh (hip)	Gets split in post approach of total hip arthroplasty. On exam: knee flexion isolate the hamstring (during hip extension strength examination)
Obturator externus	Iliopubic rami, obturator memb.	Posterior medial greater trochanter (GT)	Obturator (L3–4)	ER thigh	
Short External Rotators					
Piriformis	Ant. sacrum (2nd–4th, below (caudad) inf. border of SI joint)	Sup. GT (often conjoined with gemelli and obturator internus tendon)	N to piriformis (1st and 2nd sacral nerves)	ER thigh	Landmark for sciatic nerve (under the piriformis >> through, but not superficial to piriformis)
Sup. gemellus	Ischial spine	Medial GT	N to obturator internus, L5–S1	ER thigh	
Obturator internus	Iliopubic rami, obturator foramen, and membrane	Medial GT	N to obturator internus, L5–S1	ER, abduct thigh	Exits through lesser sciatic foramen by curving the post. ischium under the sciatic N
Inf. gemellus	Ischial tuberosity	Med GT	N to quadratus femoris, L5–S1	ER thigh	
Quadratus femoris	Ischial tuberosity	Intertrochanteric crest	N to quadratus femoris, L5–S1	ER thigh	

Ant., anterior; ER, external rotation; GT, greater trochanter; Inf., inferior; ITB, iliotibial band; N, nerve; SI joint, sacroiliac joint; Sup., superior; THA, total hip arthroplasty.

BIOMECHANICS

Kinematic (33)

- Mobility of lumbar spine: varies with age and race
- Range of motion (ROM) of lumbar spine: 50° coronal and 90° sagittal
- Motion: orientation of the facet's joints determines the degree and plane of motion

TRUNK MOTION	MOVEMENT OF INDIVIDUAL COMPONENT
Lumbar extension	Dura lax and fold, PLL bulge, and lig. flavum recoils
Lumbar flexion	Canal widens and lengthens
Lateral flexion	Ipsilaterally: meninges and root lax, intervertebral foramen narrows and contralateral side widens

lig. flavum, ligamentum flavum; PLL, posterior longitudinal ligament.

- Spinal coupling: kinematic phenomenon where movement of the spine in one plane is associated with automatic movement in another plane
- For example: axial rotation with lateral flexion
  ○ Lateral flexion: accompanied by slight ipsilateral rotation
  ○ Axial rotation: lateral flexion in a contralateral direction occurs

LUMBAR SPINE BIOMECHANICS (34)

Sagittal and coronal balance
- If the sagittal and coronal balance is off, energy expenditure is increased
- Line of gravity for sagittal balance reference
  ○ Passing auricle of the ear, odontoid, body of C7, anterior to thoracic spine, posterior to L3, mid femoral head (positive if the line of gravity is forward of the sacrum)
    ▪ Thoracic kyphosis and lumbar lordosis: average 60° (20°–80°), apex at L3
    ▪ With aging, kyphosis increases gradually → increased (+) sagittal balance
- Abnormal sagittal balance
  ○ Severe kyphosis (positive sagittal balance) → hip extension (limiting pelvic tilt by hamstring) compensated by knee flexion
    ▪ Thoracolumbar curve and lumbar curve, worse outcome than thoracic curve (35)
  ○ If pelvis is retrovert (posteriorly tilt) → hamstring shortens → hamstring becomes less mechanically efficient
- If coronal shift >4 cm: poor function and greater pain (implication in surgical correction of adult scoliosis); positive if the center of S1 is right to the C7 plumb line
- Minimizing the center of mass → better for energy efficiency

Disc loads
- Disc loading is increased by
  ○ Rotation adding to flexed posture: disc pressure increases substantially
  ○ Sitting position exerts greater pressure than standing and flexion
- Disc loading with lifting technique
  ○ No significant difference between lifting with knee flexion or knee extension
  ○ Lifting the object close to the body decreases the disc load
- The direction of nucleus pulposus migration changes with the presence of an annular tear (posterior)
  ○ If a tear is present → migrate posteriorly with lumbar extension
  ○ If the annulus fibrosus is intact, it will migrate anteriorly with lumbar extension

Facet joint: transmits ~20% of axial compressive force
- Increase on extension and disc degeneration

Low back in adolescents
- Paraspinal muscle and soft tissue do not grow at the same rate as the bone → fascia and muscle/tendon (eg, hamstring) tightness
- Cartilaginous end plate weaker than nucleus pulposus, excessive compressive forces → end plate to fracture → nucleus herniate into the vertebral body

Degenerative spine cascade
- Anterior intervertebral disc and posterior facet joints are separate but affects each other
  ○ Axial compressive loading → vertebral end plates disruption and degenerative disc disease → posterior facet joint overloading → torsional instability (particularly affected by facet and disc degeneration) (36)
- Intervertebral disc circumferential tear → radial tears (herniation) → internal disruption → loss of disc height (instability) → disc resorption → osteophytes at posterior aspect of vertebral bodies → spinal stenosis

Mechanism for radiculopathy or myelopathy: compression (primary mechanism), often triggered by movement
- Pincer action between hypertrophic encroachment and bony barriers, or space-occupying lesion (tumor) ± edema
- Ischemia: compressive or tensile

Stability of spine
- Working definition of stable spine: no potential for further neurologic loss, progressive deformity, or pain secondary to spinal pathology
- Functional spine unit (vertebral body, disc, and facet joints), ligaments, muscular tendon, abdominal and thoracic pressure, and rib cages
- Denis three-column model of the spine: applicable to trauma cases, not in metastatic cancer

	INVOLVED STRUCTURES	CLINICAL IMPLICATION
Anterior	The anterior longitudinal ligament, the anterior portion of the annulus fibrosus, and the anterior vertebral body	
Middle	The posterior aspects of the vertebral body, the posterior portion of the annulus fibrosus, and the posterior longitudinal ligament	Primary determinant of mechanical stability in the thoracolumbar spine Mid column failure: can cause neurological compromise in 20% (especially with flexion) Indication for immediate surgical referral for stabilization and decompression

(continued)

	INVOLVED STRUCTURES	CLINICAL IMPLICATION
Posterior	The posterior body arch (including the spinous process, the lamina, the facets, and the pedicles) and the posterior ligamentous structures (including the supraspinous ligament, interspinous ligament, ligamentum flavum, and facet joint capsules)	The lack of instability after laminectomy (posterior segment) may indicate the importance of other segment (anterior esp.) However, gross instability develops after fracture–dislocations and severe shear injuries with complete disruption of the posterior ligamentous complex

- Stable versus unstable spine by Denis (37)

SPINE STABILITY	CHARACTERISTICS
Stable	Intact middle column prevents extrusion of bone or disk into the spinal canal and protects against significant subluxation A compression fracture without posterior column involvement prevents abnormal forward flexion
Unstable	Definition: if 2 out of 3 columns are injured Burst fracture with involvement of anterior and middle columns Severe compression fracture with disruption of the anterior and posterior columns A flexion–distraction injury with disruption of the posterior and middle columns • Causes abnormal flexion with a fulcrum at the intact anterior column, which functions as a hinge. Chronic instability and pain may result, however, the injury does not necessarily jeopardize neurologic function.

  ○ Explains chronic instability after spinal injuries (especially resulting in kyphotic deformity); does not explain instability with flexion, extension, rotation, or shear

Biomechanics of Sacroiliac Joint (38)

- Stable joint
- The transmission and dissipation of truncal loads to the lower extremities limits transverse-axis (medio-lateral) rotation, and facilitates parturition
  ○ SI joint is vulnerable to torsion and axial compression (compared to the lumbar spine). Anterior joint capsule: especially weaker point
  ○ SI joint withstands a medially directed force six times greater than the lumbar spine
- SI joint rotates about all three axes, but minimal movements
  ○ Increased movements in all planes with a single leg fixed by 2 to 7.8 times compared to double legs fixed
  ○ Gender difference in movement
    ▪ The main motion: translation in male whereas rotational in female cadavers
    ▪ Higher ROM in female cadavers
- No clear difference in SI motion between symptomatic (pain) and asymptomatic joints
  ○ Unclear relationship of hypermobility and SI joint pain except traumatic instability, multiparity, muscular atrophy, and lower motor neuron disease

PELVIC MOVEMENT	ANTERIOR TILTING OF PELVIS	POST TILTING OF PELVIS
Sacral movement	Sacrum in the counter-nutation position Sacral extension (superior aspect of sacrum tilts posteriorly) relative to the ilium: decreased sacral slope and closed pack position for SI joint	Sacrum in nutation position Sacral flexion (superior aspect of the sacrum tilt anteriorly), anterior rotation of the sacrum in relation to the ilium → increase sacral slope → increase lumbar lordosis
Physiologic	Occurs with trunk extension or hip flexion	Occurs with trunk flexion or hip extension
Pathologic	Tight hip flexor Weak low abdominal muscle Weak gluteal muscle	Tight hamstrings

- Sacroiliac movement and pelvic position
- Age-related changes in the SI joint
  ○ During 3rd and 4th decades, surface irregularities, crevice formation, fibrillation, and the clumping of chondrocytes
  ○ Degenerative changes on the sacral side generally lag 10 to 20 years behind those affecting the iliac surface
  ○ In the 6th decade, motion at the joint may become markedly restricted as the capsule becomes increasingly collagenous and fibrous ankylosis occurs
  ○ By the 8th decade of life, erosions and plaque formation are inevitable and ubiquitous

Lumbopelvic Biomechanics

- Lumbopelvic rhythm
  ○ The kinematic relationship between the lumbar spine and hip joints during sagittal plane movements
    ▪ Bending forward: lumbar flexion (40°) followed by anterior tilting of pelvis and hip joint (70°)
    ▪ Return to erect: posterior tilting at pelvis and at hips followed by extension of lumbar spine
- Clinical application
  ○ Hip movements (hip abduction and adduction) cause angulatory stress on the root (similar fashion to straight leg raise [SLR])

○ In acute sciatica, try to avoid stretching the root-sciatic nerve segment by hip flexion and avoiding ankle dorsiflexion (decreased step length, even tiptoe walking)

PHYSICAL EXAMINATION

INSPECTION

- Curve: coronal plane (scoliosis ± axial rotation) and sagittal plane (hyperlordosis and kyphosis)
  ○ Posterior iliac crest level, and sacroiliac dimple (check secondary scoliosis from pelvic malalignment)
  ○ If suspicious of secondary curve from a leg length discrepancy, check on sitting
  ○ Skin lesion: for example, tuft of hair (meningomyelocele) or cafe au lait spots, etc.
- Step off deformity: suggestive of spondylolisthesis

PALPATION

- Visible dimple (dimples of venus): immediately medial to PSIS (S1–2 level)
- Posterior iliac crest: subcutaneous (highest level with L4 spinous process, L4–5 and L3–4 in female and obese patients)
- Posterior inferior iliac spine: S3 spinous process
- Sacrococcygeal junction (top of the gluteal crease) and coccyx in the gluteal crease
- Ischial tuberosity: at the gluteal fold, on hip flexion (unable to palpate if hip is extended), same line with greater trochanter
- Pubic tubercle: at the level of the greater trochanter on standing
- Sciatic nerve: medial half between the greater trochanter and ischial tuberosity (closer to ischial tuberosity)

Range of Motion

FLEXION	EXTENSION	LATERAL FLEXION	AXIAL ROTATION
40°–60°	20°–35°	15°–30°	30°

NEUROLOGICAL AND OTHER EXAMINATION

- Sensory examination
  ○ Check whether it is peripheral nerve or dermatomal distribution (multiple peripheral N of same root): often difficult and unreliable
    ▪ Dermatome: L1: inguinal region, L2: anterolateral thigh, L3: medial thigh and knee, L4: medial lower leg, L5: lateral lower leg, dorsum of foot, great toe, S1: sole, lateral foot and ankle, S2: medial buttocks, perineal, perianal region
  ○ Central: brain lesion, typically involving unilateral upper, lower extremities and face or spinal cord lesion below the level of spinal cord injury
- Motor examination
  ○ Myotome
    ▪ Hip flexor: L2, knee extensor: L3–4, Ankle dorsiflexor: L5 (L4), greater toe dorsiflexor, hip abductor (L5), ankle plantarflexor: S1
  ○ Hip abduction (to distinguish L5 radiculopathy/plexopathy from peroneal/sciatic neuropathy) versus hip adduction (L2–4/anterior division/obturator) versus hip flexion (L2–4/posterior division/femoral)
    ▪ If all three involved, root lesion is less likely, differential diagnoses include muscle disease or joint problem
  ○ Plantarflexor (S1) weakness: good sensitivity and specificity for LS radiculopathy
  ○ Extensor hallucis longus (EHL) strength can be slightly different from site to site normally
- Deep tendon reflex (DTR): L4: knee jerk, S1: ankle jerk, L5: medial hamstring

Examination for bowel/bladder dysfunction/saddle anesthesia (39)

- Sensation to pinprick in the perianal region (S2–4 dermatomes), perineum, and posterior thigh
  ○ Patients with CES typically have preserved sensation to pressure and light touch, so if discrimination is not made between pinprick and light touch sensation, then the diagnosis may be missed
- A rectal examination to assess the tone and voluntary contracture of the external anal sphincter
  ○ Decreased rectal tone: an early finding in a patient with CES. Check the anal wink
- The bulbocavernosus reflex: a polysynaptic reflex, through pudendal nerve and the sacral spinal cord (S2–4) (40)
  ○ The reflex is performed by applying pressure to the glans penis or clitoris and abnormal if absence of contraction of the anal sphincter
- Palpation of the bladder may reveal a full bladder secondary to urinary retention

Provocative tests (41)

NAME	DESCRIPTION	SENSITIVITY (SEN) AND SPECIFICITY (SPE) IN %
Lumbar Disc Herniation With Radiculopathy		
Straight leg raise test (SLR)	Leg is raised with the knee extended on supine until the patient begins to feel pain, and the type and distribution of the pain evaluated. Positive if the pain is reproduced down the posterior leg below the knee at 30°–70° elevation	Sen: 72–97 Spe: 11–66
Bragard's sign	After a positive SLR, the leg is dropped to a nonpainful range, and the ipsilateral ankle is dorsiflexed, reproducing the leg pain. 94% positive predictive value	Sen: 78–94

(continued)

NAME	DESCRIPTION	SENSITIVITY (SEN) AND SPECIFICITY (SPE) IN %
Cross SLR	Contralateral leg is raised with the knee extended until the patient begins to feel pain in the ipsilateral leg with presenting type and distribution of the pain in the ipsilateral leg evaluated The test is positive if the pain is reproduced between 30° and 70° of elevation	Sen: 23–29 Spe: 11–66
Slump test	The patient is seated with legs together and knees flexed initially. The patient is instructed to slump forward as far as possible. The examiner applies firm pressure to bow the patient's back while keeping the sacrum vertical. The patient is asked to flex the head, and pressure is added to further flex the patient's neck. Lastly, the examiner asks the subject to extend the knee, and dorsiflexion at the ankle is added (42). Positive if presenting type of pain is reproduced	Sen: 84 Spe: 83
Femoral N stretch test	With the patient prone, the knee is passively flexed. Positive if pain is produced in the anterior aspect of the thigh and/or back for upper lumbar root L2–4	Sen: 84–95
Sacroiliac Joint Pathology		
Gillet test	This test is performed with the patient standing, facing away from the examiner, with the feet ~12 inches apart. The examiner places thumbs on each PSIS. The patient is then asked to stand on one leg while flexing the contralateral hip to 90° Positive if the PSIS does not drop (rotate downward); indicates restriction (43)	Sen: 43, Spe: 68
FABER (Patrick)	With the patient supine, the thigh is flexed and the ankle is placed above the patella of the opposite extended leg. As the knee is depressed, with the ankle maintaining its position above the opposite knee, the opposite ASIS is pressed Positive if the patient complains of (back/buttock) pain before the knee reaches the level obtained on normal side (44)	Sen: 82
Gaenslen's test	The patient lies supine, flexes the ipsilateral knee and hip against the chest to decrease lumbar lordosis. The patient is then brought to the side of the table, and the opposite thigh is slowly hyperextended gradually Positive if the hyperextension of the hip reproduces the pain and symptoms (45)	Sen: ~30, Spe: ~70
Fortin finger test	The patient points to the region of pain with one finger Positive if the patient can localize the pain to an area inferomedial to the PSIS within 1 cm, and the patient consistently points to the same area over at least two trials	
Standing flexion test	With the patient standing, facing away from the examiner with his feet ~12 inches apart (approximately equal to the distance between the acetabula). The examiner then places his thumbs on the inferior aspect of each PSIS. The patient is asked to bend forward with both knees extended. The extent of the cephalad movement of each PSIS is monitored. Normally, the PSIS should move equally Positive if one PSIS moves superiorly (cephalad) and anteriorly compared with the other (this is the side of restriction)	
Seated flexion test	Performed with the patient seated with both feet on the floor. The examiner stands or sits behind the patient with the eyes at the level of the iliac crests and places his thumbs on each PSIS; the patient is instructed to flex forward Positive if one PSIS moves unequally cephalad with respect to the other PSIS. The side with the greatest cephalad excursion implies articular restriction and hypomobility. While the patient is seated, the innominates are fixed in place, thus isolating iliac motion	
Piriformis Syndrome		
Freiberg maneuver	Forcefully internally rotate the affected leg while the patient is supine with thigh extended. Positive if pain and symptoms reproduced	
Pace maneuver	Resisted abduction of the hip in the seated position. This activates the piriformis rather than stretching it. Positive if pain and symptoms reproduced	
Beatty	The patient lies with the affected side up with the knee and hip flexed. Resisted abduction of the hip on the affected side Positive if deep buttock pain in those with piriformis, but back and leg pain in those with lumbar disk disease	

(continued)

NAME	DESCRIPTION	SENSITIVITY (SEN) AND SPECIFICITY (SPE) IN %
FADIR (FAIR)	The patient in supine with affected hip in flexion, adduction and internal rotation (FAIR) (46) Positive if exacerbation of pain in the buttock or reproduction of painful symptom	Sen: 88, Spe: 83
Seated piriformis test	The patient is seated over the edge of the table with the hip flexed to 90° and the knee extended. While palpating the sciatic notch, the examiner adducts and internally rotates the limb. Positive if the exacerbation of pain or reproduction of painful symptom	Sen: 52, spe: 90
Ankylosing Spondylitis (47)		
Modified Schober Index	The examiner marks a distance between the midpoint of the PSISs and a point 10cm vertically above when the patient stands erect. Following maximal forward flexion of the spine, the distance between those two points is less than 15cm (normal >15cm) Correlates well with radiologic finding, high specificity (48)	
Finger-to-floor distance	Distance between tip of middle finger and the floor following maximal lumbar forward flexion with knees extended Not specific, no normal range, may be used to track progress over time	
Lumbar lateral flexion	Distance between tip of ipsilateral middle finger and the floor following maximal lumbar lateral flexion, with both feet on the floor, knees extended and without rotation	
Miscellaneous		
Facet loading test	The patient stands up with extension and ipsilateral rotation of the back Positive if axial pain reproduced Limitation: No consistent finding	
Stork test	The patient is asked to stand on one foot and extend their back and repeat on the opposite side Positive if pain in the midline lumbar region • May suggest facet, pars interarticularis or SI joint pathology • Often limited in patients with poor balance, knee, ankle/foot instability, proprioceptive dysfunction	

ASIS, anterior superior iliac spine; FABER, flexion, abduction, and external rotation; FADIR (FAIR), flexion, adduction and internal rotation; N, nerve; PSIS, posterior superior iliac spine; SLR, straight leg raise.

RED FLAGS

- Examination findings
  - Fever, vertebral tenderness, limited spinal ROM (can be secondary to acute pain and muscle spasm), neurologic findings persisting beyond one month (especially progressive), major motor weakness in lower extremities (especially progressive), saddle anesthesia, loss of anal sphincter tone and urinary retention/incontinence
- Historical components suggestive of red flags (49,50)

REVIEW OF SYSTEM	MEDICAL HISTORY
Significant trauma Pain that is increased or unrelieved by rest Unexplained weight loss Fever Bladder or bowel incontinence Urinary retention (with overflow incontinence)	Cancer Immunosuppressive state Prolonged use of steroids Intravenous drug use Urinary tract infection

- Early imaging or serologic study or admit the patient through ER (medical or neurosurgical emergency)

Waddell's sign for psychological (nonorganic) factors in back pain

- Significant if three or more of the following signs (51,52)
  - Tenderness: superficial and diffuse tenderness and/or nonanatomic tenderness
  - Simulation test: production of pain by test that only stimulates a specific movement (LBP with axial loading of head). For example, axial loading on skull causing LBP or LBP with shoulder/pelvis rotation in the same plane (simulated rotation without actual rotation in the lower back)
  - Distraction test: difference (inconsistence of pain) with SLR in supine and sitting
  - Regional disturbances: regional weakness or sensory changes, which deviate from accepted neuroanatomy
  - Overreaction: disproportionate facial or verbal expression
- Clinical implications
  - Do not label patient, consider psychology and psychiatry (interdisciplinary pain management) involvement
  - Psychological evaluation of the spine patient (53) closely linked to transition to chronic pain
    - Depression in 30% to 40% of chronic LBP patients

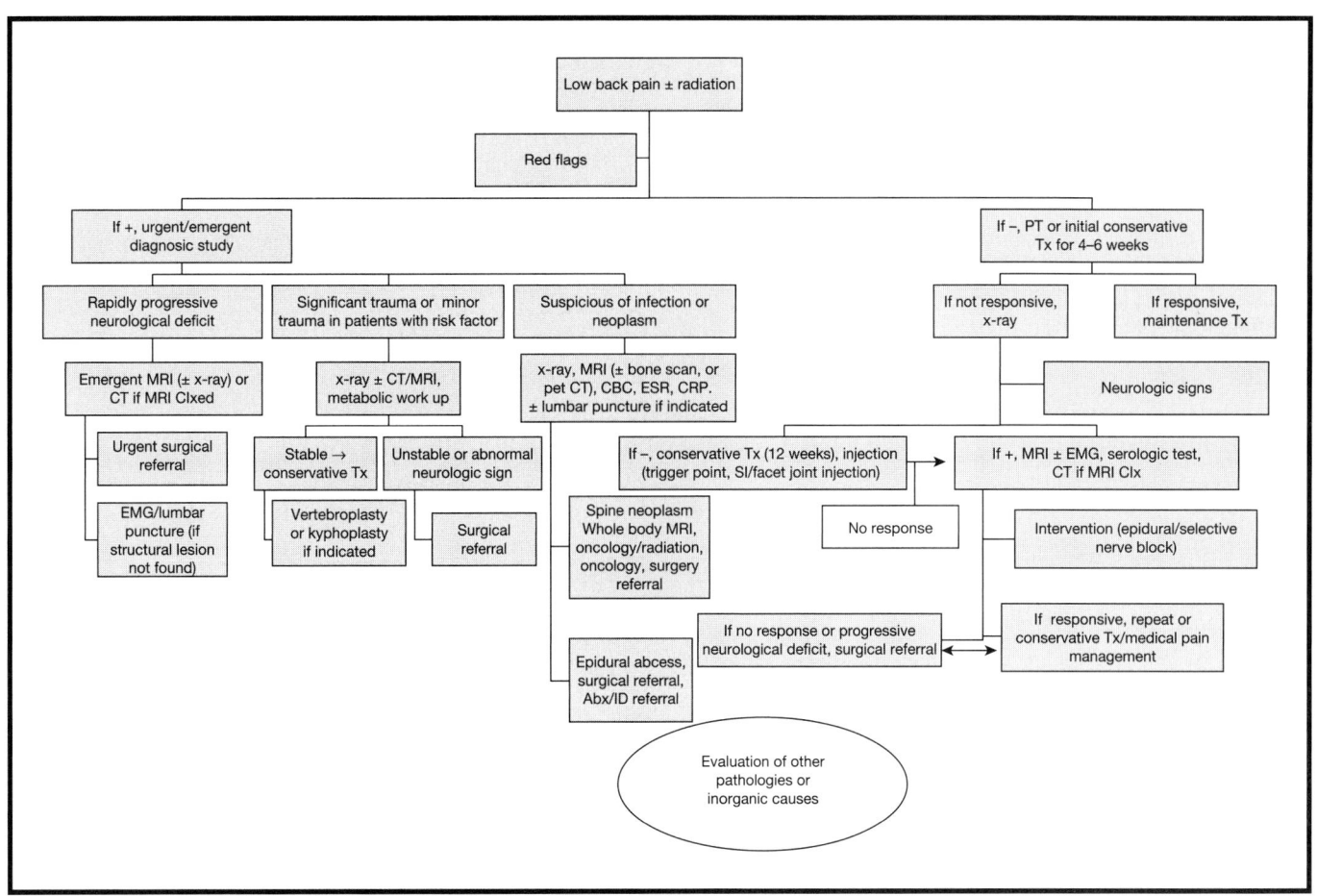

FLOWCHART 6.3
Diagnostic approach and management of low back pain in outpatient clinic.
–, negative; +, positive; CBC, complete blood count; Abx/ID, antibiotic/infection disease; CIx, contraindicated; CRP, C-reactive protein; EMG, electromyography; ESR, erythrocyte sedimentation rate; MRA, magnetic resonance angiography; PT, physical therapy; SI joint, sacroiliac joint; Tx, treatment.
Source: Adapted from Ref. (4). Baker RJ, Patel D. Lower back pain in the athlete: common conditions and treatment. *Prim Care*. 2005;32(1):201–229.

DIAGNOSTIC STUDIES (FLOWCHART 6.3)

PLAIN RADIOGRAPHS (54)

Do not order an imaging study without a proper history and physical examination (55)

Indications
- Persistent pain after 4 to 6 weeks of conservative management in the absence of red flags (56)
  ○ The majority of patients with acute LBP, symptoms, and/or physical exam findings will improve or resolve during a trial of conservative treatment: imaging usually not necessary initially
- LBP with history of trauma or red flags
- Deformity: full-length standing posteroanterior and lateral spine radiographs

Correlation with clinical findings
- Disc degeneration: unclear correlation of findings with patient symptoms
- Metastatic disease: specific but relatively insensitive, 50% of trabecular bone must be lost before a lytic lesion is visible.
- Trauma: not sensitive, wedge fracture to be visualized requires more than 50% loss of height: if suspicious, order CT
  ○ Difficult to distinguish acute versus chronic

Common findings
- Disc degeneration: disc space narrowing, osteophytes, and end-plate sclerosis, indirect sign: facet degeneration (sclerosis and hypertrophy)
- Ossification (ligament)
  ○ Ankylosing spondylitis: syndesmophyte ossification of the outer layer of the annular fibrosis of the disc and the deep layers of the longitudinal ligament
    ▪ Bamboo appearance: syndesmophyte in an ascending symmetric fashion
  ○ Reiter's syndrome and psoriatic arthritis: non-ascending symmetric syndesmophyte formation. Start from the middle of one vertebral body and extend to the same area of adjacent vertebral body
  ○ Diffuse idiopathic skeletal hyperostosis (DISH): hyperostosis affecting the anterior longitudinal ligaments
  ○ Others: ossification of posterior longitudinal ligament and ossification of the ligament flavum
- Fracture

- Compression fracture: loss of anterior, middle, or posterior vertebral body height ≥20%
  - Order x-ray of entire spine for concomitant spine fracture
  - Difficult to differentiate acute from chronic (absence of cortical breaking or impaction of trabeculae in chronic)
  - Often difficult to correlate with symptoms
- The posterior vertebral body angle (PVBA) measured on a lateral plain radiograph (57)
  - The PVBA is the angle formed by either the superior or the inferior end plate and the posterior vertebral body wall, >100° in burst fracture
  - ≥20% of subtle burst fractures can be misdiagnosed on plain radiographs. CT: a better method for evaluating the middle column
- Deformity: sagittal and coronal balance (58,59) (Figure 6.7)
  - To assess regional and global alignment parameters, as well as measurement of pelvic parameters
  - Advanced imaging studies: MRI, CT, CT myelogram, frequently indicated to assess for neurologic compromise and for surgical planning
  - Increased Cobb's angle
    - To measure angulation deformity (in coronal plane, can be used in sagittal for kyphosis)
    - Angle formed by an intersection of two lines parallel to the superior end plate of one vertebra and the other parallel to the inferior endplate of the vertebrae below
  - Rotation
    - 0: no rotation (two pedicles), 1: pedicle toward midline (the other pedicle toward the border), 2: pedicle 2/3 to midline, 3: pedicle in midline (only one visualized), and 4: one pedicle beyond the midline (only one visualized)
  - Sagittal balance indicated by the distance between the C7 plumb line and the posterosuperior corner of S1 in the sagittal plane, and includes both pelvic parameters (pelvic tilt, sacral slope, and pelvic incidence) and the sagittal vertical axis
    - Positive sagittal balance (C7 plumb line anteriorly) → greater pain, lower physical function, poor self-image and poor social function
  - Coronal balance: the distance between the C7 plumb line and the posterior-superior corner of S1 in the coronal plane (+: S1 located right side of the C7 plum line)
    - >4 cm: poor function and greater pain
    - Minimizing the center of mass movement → improve energy efficiency (23)
  - The pelvic incidence: morphological parameter
    - The angle between the line perpendicular to the sacral plate and the line connecting the midpoint of the sacral plate to the bicoxofemoral axis: kyphosis if <35° and hyperlordosis if >85° (check isthmic spondylolisthesis)
  - The pelvic tilt: the angle between the lines connecting the midpoint of the sacral plate to the bicoxofemoral axis and the vertical plane
    - Increased in pelvic retroversion (rotate backward)
    - Reflects hamstring insufficiency → pelvis will be anteriorly rotated in decompensated (insufficient) hamstring (as in compensation mechanism for thoracic kyphosis)
    - As pelvic tilt increases, the center of gravity moves more posteriorly
  - Sacral slope: determine position of lumbar spine
    - If low: more flat back, high: more lordosis

CT SCAN

- Better bony details (for presurgical) and if MRI is not accessible

Indications
- Suspected fracture, follow-up (FU) of a known fracture, skeletal abnormalities such as spondylolysis and spondylolisthesis in operative candidates, congenital vertebral defects, osseous tumor evaluation, and procedures such as lumbar CT myelography (if MRI is contraindicated)
- Limited imaging capacity of soft-tissue structures

MRI

Indications
- LBP with red flags especially malignancy and infection is suspected (with contrast)
- Focal neurological deficit present
- Chronic LBP with unclear etiology

Limitations
- Definitive diagnosis is not achieved in as many as 85% of patients with LBP
- Claustrophobia (open MRI or using sedation as alternatives)

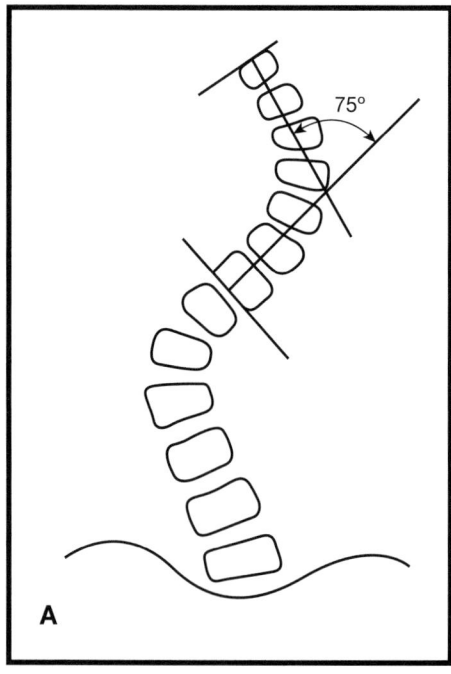

FIGURE 6.7
Plain radiograph of the lower back with angles frequently used in x-ray. (A) Cobb angle formed by the perpendicular lines drawn from the endplates of the most tilted proximal and distal vertebrae to measure the scoliotic curve.

(continued)

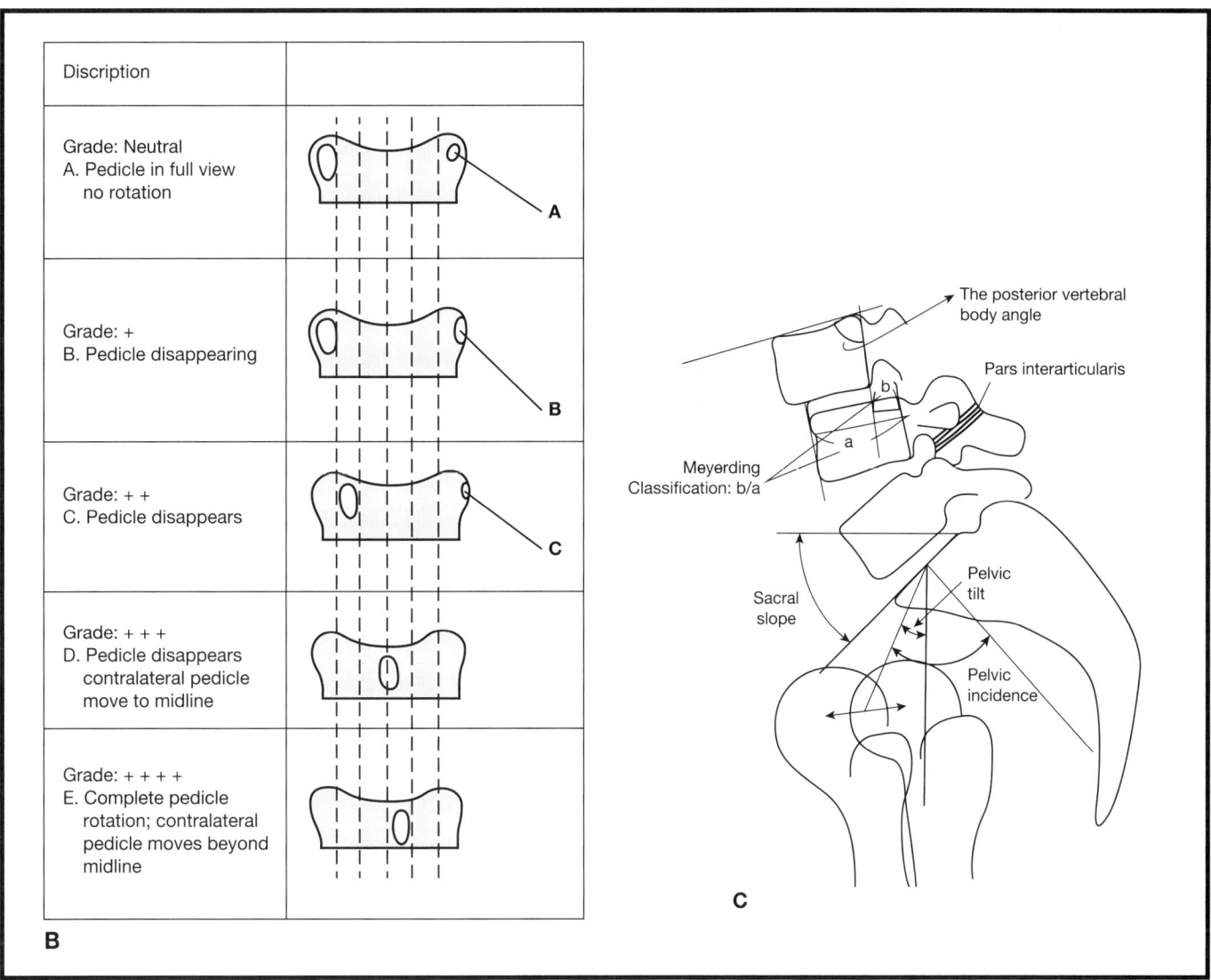

FIGURE 6.7 *(continued)*
(B) Rotation of the spine by pedicle portion. (C) Other measurement.

- Common findings in asymptomatic adults
  ○ Herniated discs (9%–76% depending on ages); bulging discs (20%–81%), degenerative discs (46%–93%), and annular disc tears (14%–56%)
  ○ Spinal stenosis (1%–21%)

Common findings
- Disc pathology

Terminology depending on displaced disc materials

>50% OF CIRCUM-FERENCE OF DISC	<50% OF CIRCUMFERENCE OF DISC → HERNIATION			
Bulge	Protrusion: base > dome		Extrusion: base < dome	
	Broad: 25%–50%	Focal: <25%	Sequestration	Migration

○ Sequestration: portion of extruded disc is displaced beyond the annulus with no connecting disc tissue with the disc of origin
○ Migration: portion of extruded disc is displaced away from tear in the outer annulus
- Location of disc displacement correlating with root impingement (Figure 6.8)
  ○ A far lateral disc herniation (protrusion and sequestration)
    ▪ Isolated to the neural foramen/far lateral region affects the same nerve root/ganglion as it courses beneath the pedicle and beyond (eg, L4 root as it passes beneath the L4 pedicle [black arrow in Figure 6.8])
  ○ Posterolateral (paracentral) disc herniation (protrusion and sequestration)
    ▪ Within the spinal canal (generally medial to the pedicle); traversing the root: that is, L5 as it passes by the L4–5 disc margin [gray arrow in Figure 6.8]
  ○ If the protrusion is both paracentral and foraminal, it can affect the traversing root and the root in the foramen, which gives mixed radicular symptoms

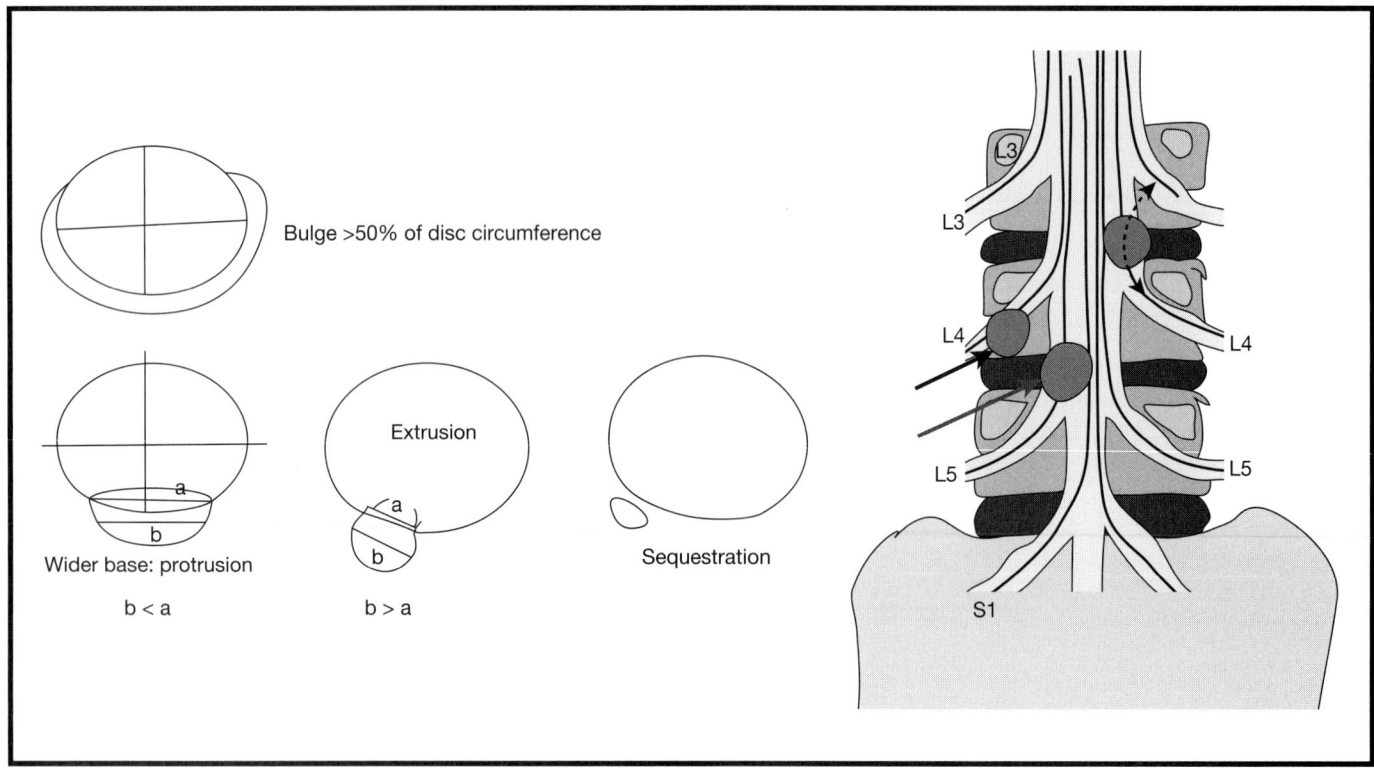

FIGURE 6.8
Classification of disc pathology and its location in relation to corresponding root impingement.

○ A paracentral extrusion that migrates ➔ can affect two roots by projecting inferiorly to the lateral recess or superiorly to the pedicle as demonstrated at L3–4 (curved broken arrows in Figure 6.8) (60)
○ Central: cauda equina syndrome (CES)
• Modic changes (61)
○ Bone marrow and endplate lesion
○ Usually accompanied by degenerative disc disease but not specific

TYPE	T1 WI	T2 WI	CHARACTERISTICS
Type 1	Hypointense	Hyperintense	Vertebral body edema and hypervascularity
Type 2	Hyperintense	Hyperintense	Fatty replacement of the red bone marrow
Type 3	Hypointense	Hypointense	Subchondral bone sclerosis

○ Differential diagnosis
  ▪ Spinal infection: surrounding paravertebral soft-tissue edema and epidural mass effect, erosion of vertebral body and endplates (vs MC: focal and diffuse along the endplates)
  ▪ Tumor
  ▪ Schmorl's node
• Spinal cord findings
  ○ Typical findings suggestive of cord lesion: edema, signal enhancement, and perimedullary dilated vessels
  ○ The spinal cord normally ends at L1–2, seen on thoracic MRI. If the conus medullaris is not seen on thoracic spine imaging, the spinal cord is presumed to be tethered

SEROLOGIC TESTS (62)

Indications
• Identification of visceral and nonmechanical disease suggested by red flags
• Not indicated initially

Laboratory tests
• Complete blood count (CBC), chemistry, erythrocyte sedimentation rate (ESR), C-reactive protein (CRP; infectious/inflammatory disease) for any red flags except trauma or osteoporosis
• ± Rheumatoid factor (RF), antinuclear antibodies (ANA) (rheumatologic disease), urine analysis (UA) (if suspicious of urologic disease), prostate specific antigen (PSA) (prostate cancer), alkaline phosphatase and calcium (metabolic bone disease), vitamin D level

ELECTROMYOGRAPHY (EMG)

Indications
• Subclinical/clinical motor abnormality (weakness, fatigue, etc.), gait dysfunction, leg pain or "sciatica" associated with LBP (with large diameter fiber sensation involved)
• Differential diagnoses of sensory symptoms include: peripheral neuropathy, and focal entrapment neuropathy (although less common in lower extremities)
• Value in nonmechanical radiculopathy or lumbar plexopathy (amyotrophy): if symptoms and signs of radiculopathy without clear mechanical etiology (such as disc disruption or spinal stenosis)

- LBP without leg pain or sciatica: EMG is unlikely to be positive (63)

Nerve conduction studies
- Sensory nerve conduction study (SNCS): sural (S1), superficial peroneal (L5), saphenous (L4), lateral femoral cutaneous N (L2–3)
  - Normal SNCS findings in radiculopathy (preganglionic lesion) or focal proximal lesion (demyelinating)
  - Saphenous and lateral femoral cutaneous nerve conduction study (NCS): technically challenging in some patients
  - Abnormal findings favor peripheral neuropathy (or mononeuropathy), LS plexopathy or rarely a concomitant lesion
- Motor nerve conduction study
  - Tibial at abductor hallucis (S1–2, medial plantar), peroneal (extensor digitorum brevis for L5–S1, tibialis anterior for L4–5), and occasionally femoral (vastus medialis/lateralis or rectus femoris, L2–4)
  - Usually normal unless severely affected, F wave (utility is controversial), H reflex (S1, tibial nerve; once involved, may not recover; would be absent in Achilles tendon injury)
- Needle EMG examination
  - Key findings: abnormal spontaneous activities (ASAs), fibrillations in limb muscles of two different peripheral nerves of the same root and paraspinal muscles with decreased motor unit recruitment
    - Examine muscles innervated by one level above and below root (to localize the lesion)
  - Unclear clinical implication of isolated paraspinal muscle ASA findings
  - Pure sensory radiculopathy or mild radiculopathy (focal demyelinating lesion) → negative NCS and needle EMG study; therefore, EMG test is not to rule out (R/O) radiculopathy

TREATMENT (54)

Outcome measurement scales (55)
- Useful to measure the progress/response to the treatment
- McGill pain questionnaire: instrument designed to measure the three dimensions of pain experience: sensory, affective, and evaluative
- Roland Morris (physical disability), Oswestry Disability Index (functional outcome), etc.

NONOPERATIVE MANAGEMENT

Education
- No bed rest for >2 days for nontraumatic acute LBP without red flags
- Advise patient to remain active
- Back school (56)
  - Education for anatomy, pathologic, ergonomics and correct biomechanics including lifting. For example, do not bend the back, flex the knee, put the lifting object near the center of the body, and the like
  - Practice sessions: correct lifting/functional exercise (increasing the horizontal distance from the trunk → increased risk of developing low back disorders), obstacle course (home and work environment simulation), strengthening and stretching training (33)
  - Can be done in group session or integrated into physical therapy (PT) sessions

Therapeutic exercise (58)
- William exercise (flexion-based): pelvic tilt, knee to chest, partial sit up, hip flexor stretch, and squat exercises especially for patients with spinal stenosis
- McKenzie exercise (extension based): for centralization, lateral based, to restore lumbar lordosis
  - Back conditions divided into three categories: derangement (MC), dysfunction, and postural syndrome
  - Depending on the group, posture correction, performance of end-range repeated movements of the spine, or the use of manual techniques
  - Exercises to centralize the pain, that is, move the pain from the leg or buttock into the lower back. For example, repeated extension in standing and sustained extension in prone position
- Manual therapy (59)
  - Mobilization ± muscle energy technique, manipulation and traction
  - Pelvic mobilization using principle of reversing origin and insertion (fixed insertion then origin) → move axial part rather than peripheral part
- Other typical therapeutic exercises
  - Core stabilization exercise (60)
    - Neuromuscular control, strength, and endurance of muscles in the trunk and pelvis → dynamic stability
  - Lower limb strengthening exercise: shown to decrease incidence of LBP
  - Stretching of iliopsoas/rectus femoris (tight hip flexor causes pelvic anteversion, which promotes lordosis)
  - Modality as needed; superficial heat for acute LBP
- Cognitive behavioral therapy exercise, spinal manipulation (also for acute back pain), and interdisciplinary rehabilitation; moderate efficacy for LBP (of >4 weeks' duration)
- Alternative medicine: acupuncture, massage, yoga (Viniyoga); some benefit for chronic LBP

Oral medication (61)
- Acetaminophen (AAP), nonsteroidal anti-inflammatory drug (NSAID), Medrol Dosepak (methyl prednisone tapering dose), and opioid (do not give opiates in acute LBP before other alternatives have been considered [64])
- Skeletal muscle relaxants: for short-term pain relief
- Neuropathic pain meds: gabapentin, amitriptyline (tricyclic antidepressant [TCA]: for chronic pain), and pregabalin, and the like

Bracing

ORTHOSIS	CHARACTERISTICS AND INDICATION
SI belt	Kinetic feedback, from iliac crests and trochanter SI joint pain or symphysis pubic pain during pregnancy or postpartum
LS belt	Abdominal compression (core stabilization) relieves the pain

(continued)

ORTHOSIS	CHARACTERISTICS AND INDICATION
Lumbosacral corset	Mechanical LBP, extend more than LS belt Pull strap gives mechanical advantage (1 lb of force applied to a pull strap transfers 4 lbs of pressure over the abdomen) With rigid panel (anterior, posterior, or anterior/posterior) • Anterior below xyphoid process and above pubic symphysis • Posterior below scapular to gluteus region, remind to avoid abrupt trunk motion and lift properly • Core reinforce (always needs core stabilization exercise)
Rigid lumbosacral orthotics (LSO)	Sacrum to inferior scapular angle William (extension-lateral control): spondylosis and spondylolisthesis Chairback (flexion-extension-lateral control) and Knight (lateral bar on chairback)
Flexform spinal orthotics (clamshell body jacket)	Lower truncal immobilization for postsurgical thoracolumbar surgery (up to T8) Stable osteoporotic fracture
Other rigid thoracolumbar orthotics (TLSO)	Sacrum to above the inferior angle of scapular Taylor (TLS flexion-extension control); less commonly used than body jacket for kyphosis with stable osteoporotic fracture Jewett (prevent flexion using three-point control at sternum, midback, and pubic symphysis) Others: TLSO with detachable padded shoulder straps

LBP, low back pain; LS, lumbosacral; SI, sacroiliac; TLSO: thoraco–lumbo–sacral–orthosis.

Lumbar epidural steroid injection (fluoroscopic guided)
- Indications: acute or subacute radicular back pain
  - Short-term relief from radicular pain
  - No clear benefit in patients with LBP without radiculopathy
- Controversial value of steroid injection over lidocaine injection (lidocaine vs lidocaine and steroid) (65)
  - In uncontrolled DM patient or patient with problem with steroid → lidocaine alone may be reasonable
- Do not repeat the injection (not shown to improve the outcome) (66)
  - If first injection is not effective, an additional injection within 6 weeks is unlikely to be more effective
  - No impact on the need for surgery
- Interlaminar versus transforaminal approach versus caudal epidural injections
  - Selective nerve block may predict a surgical outcome for pain relief

US-guided lumbar spine procedure (67)
- Not a standard of practice (fluoroscopy-guided is a standard of practice)
- Limitations of US-guided spine procedure: bony artifacts, angle of needle insertion, limited resolution in deep layer, narrow imaging window, and anatomic restriction in degenerative changes and obesity
- Advantages: soft tissue, nerve blood-vessel visualization
- Indications: facet joint injection and caudal epidural in lean person (68)
  - Facet joint injection: oblique parasagittal view, 8–9 Hz, depth 5 cm, in-plane view from lateral to medial
  - Caudal block: identify the sacral hiatus and needle through sacrococcygeal ligament on prone position using in-plane approach using 22 to 25G, 5-cm needle (69)

Facet injection and medial branch block (70–72)
- Only valid method to diagnose pain from the lumbar facet joints; either facet joint injection or medial branch block
  - Medial branch also innervates multifidus muscle and interspinous ligament
- If effective, then consider radiofrequency ablation

SURGERY

Referral to surgery (73,74)
- General indications: failed conservative management or progressive neurological deficits
  - Urgent surgical indication: large midline disc with the following symptoms and signs
    - Bilateral leg weakness (foot drop/slap), especially progressive
      - Often difficult to distinguish pain-inhibited component of weakness
    - New onset bowel/genitourinary dysfunction (CES) with pain
  - Chronic pain with spinal stenosis with/without spondylolisthesis
    - Better symptom relief with surgical management for up to 4 years
    - Isthmic spondylolisthesis: may benefit from surgery
  - Surgical referral for tumor, infection, severe/progressive deformity (scoliosis, kyphosis. See section on specific disease conditions)
- Eventual outcome for radiculopathy is independent of surgery or conservative management in the long term (75,76)
  - Short-term benefit for sciatica in surgery over conservative treatment, unclear for axial LBP

Interventional spine procedure for failed back (postlaminectomy syndrome) surgery (77,78)
- Percutaneous epidural adhesiolysis for epidural fibrosis
- Spinal cord stimulator (SCS)
  - Suggested mechanism: the gate control mechanism and modulation of excitatory and inhibitory neurotransmitter release in the dorsal horn
  - Permanent placement after a successful screening trial
  - More effective for a radicular pain than centralized back pain
  - Current duration of stimulator: 3 to 5 years on average
- Intrathecal analgesic delivery implant systems
  - Typical indication: intractable cancer pain
    - Usually after all other options failed
  - Side effects: urinary retention, constipation, equipment malfunction and catheter tip granuloma, and tolerance

BACK PAIN

NERVE AND SPINAL CORD PATHOLOGY

LS Radiculopathy with Disc Disease

Introduction (79)
- Prevalence: 3% to 5%, male = female, males more likely in 40s, females in 50s to 60s
- MC location: L5 MC than S1

History and physical examination
- Sciatica: back and leg pain, often variable presentation
  - Pain exacerbated by recumbent position → inflammatory, neoplastic, or nonmechanical
- Dermatomal distribution of paresthesia: more specific
- Sensory, motor, and DTR

ROOT LEVEL	LOCATION OF PAIN	SENSORY CHANGES (PARESTHESIA)	MOTOR (INVOLVED MUSCLE)	MUSCLE STRETCH REFLEX
L1	Inguinal region	Inguinal region		
L2	Groin, anterior thigh	Anterolateral thigh	Hip flexor (Iliopsoas)	
L3	Anterior thigh to knee, anterior leg	Medial thigh and knee	Quadriceps, iliopsoas, hip adductors	
L4	Medial leg	Medial lower leg	Quadriceps, TA, hip adductor	Knee joint
L5	Lateral thigh and lower leg, dorsum of foot	Lateral lower leg, dorsum of foot, great toe	Hip abductor, toe extensor (EHL) and flexor, ankle dorsiflexor, everter and inverter	Medial hamstring Tibialis posterior (difficult to obtain)
S1	Posterior thigh, calf, and heel	Sole, lateral foot and ankle, lateral two toes	Ankle plantarflexor, hamstring, gluteus maximus, toe flexor	Ankle joint
S2–4	Medial buttocks	Medial buttocks, perineal, perianal region	No extremity muscle involved unless S1–2 involved	Bulbocarvernosus, anal wink

EHL, extensor hallucis longus; TA, tibialis anterior.

- Supine SLR (Lasègue) and Bragard test, cross SLR and femoral stretch test (L3,4)
- Red flags: age >50 years old, previous history of (H/O) cancer, unexplained weight loss, and failure to improve after 1 month of treatment

Diagnosis
- Clinical diagnosis confirmed by correlating imaging study ± EMG test (confirm if positive)
  - MRI to confirm the presence of disc herniation, root impingement and R/O other structural pathologies
  - CT or CT myelogram if MRI is contraindicated
  - EMG test: useful to evaluate noncompressive radiculopathy (leptomeningeal metastasis, infectious radiculopathy, or diabetes amyotrophy), LS plexopathy, and other peripheral nerve disorders mimicking LS radiculopathy
- Differential diagnosis
  - Differential diagnosis of LS radiculopathy; etiologies (79)

ETIOLOGY	DIFFERENTIAL DIAGNOSIS
Degenerative (MC)	Intervertebral disc herniation Degenerative lumbar spondylosis
Neoplastic	Primary tumor Metastatic tumors (breast, lung, and prostate Ca: MC)

(continued)

ETIOLOGY	DIFFERENTIAL DIAGNOSIS
	Leptomeningeal metastasis (leukemia, lymphoma and breast Ca)
Infectious	Herpes zoster (HZ); usually single dermatome Spinal epidural abscess (SEA) HIV/AIDS-related polyradiculopathy Lyme disease; erythema migrans within the first two months
Inflammatory/ metabolic	Diabetic amyotrophy Ankylosing spondylitis Paget's disease Arachnoiditis Sarcoidosis
Developmental	Tethered cord syndrome; anorectal or inguinal pain In about one-third of cases, traumatic event preceding the onset of pain Dural ectasia
Others	Lumbar spinal cysts Hemorrhage

Ca, cancer; MC, most common.

○ Other mimickers of LS radiculopathy (80)

ETIOLOGY	INVOLVED STRUCTURE	DIFFERENTIAL DIAGNOSIS
Neurologic	Lower motor neuron Dz	Lumbar plexopathy • Suspect if sudden onset, without mechanical causes, preceding trauma/injury Herpes zoster • Characteristic skin lesion (although not always present) Peripheral mononeuropathy • Superior cluneal N: L1–2 • Lateral femoral cutaneous N: L2–3 • Sciatic neuropathy (piriformis syn.) • Peroneal (common/superficial/deep) nerve: L4–5 • Tibial N (soleal sling syndrome, tarsal tunnel syndrome): S1–2 • Sural N (S1)
	Upper motor neuron Dz	Multiple sclerosis Elevated intracranial pressure Syrinx
Musculo-skeletal (often concomitant)	Hip	Hip and pelvic bones and joint Dz • Stress fracture (if risk factors present)/inflammatory joint disease Soft-tissue mass Greater trochanteric pain • Focal tenderness, ± ITB syndrome Piriformis syndrome Iliopsoas bursitis Ischial bursitis
	Knee	ITB syndrome Pes anserine tendinobursitis • ± Infrapatellar branch of saphenous N irritation
	Foot and ankle	Plantar fasciitis/Baxter N entrapment (inf. calcaneal N)/interdigital neuritis
Rheumatologic Dz (Diffuse)		Myofascial pain syndrome Fibromyalgia Polymyalgia rheumatica Ankylosing spondylitis
Vascular		Abdominal aortic aneurysm Gluteal artery aneurysm • Buttock pain ± sciatica
Others		Catamenial sciatica (endometriosis) Nephrolithiasis

Dz, disease; N, nerve; inf., inferior; R/O, rule out; syn., syndrome; ITB, iliotibial band.

Treatment (81)
- Conservative treatment
  ○ Medrol Dosepack, IV glucocorticosteroid (usually during admission) if not contraindicated
  ○ PT: A limited course of structured therapy (eight sessions), insufficient data
    ▪ William flexion-based exercise, core muscle stabilization exercise, modality, stretching of hamstring, home exercise program, gradually increase aerobic endurance during exercise, spinal manipulation, traction
- Injection: transforaminal epidural steroid injection for 2 to 4 weeks of pain relief, but no evidence for 12 months, insufficient data for superiority of different injections
- Referral to surgery
  ○ Indications: failed conservative management or progressive neurological deficit
    ▪ Usually from 6 months to 1 year from an onset with failed conservative management: better outcome, level B
  ○ Outcome is better in patients with leg pain than with isolated back pain. Positive SLR test: better outcome predictor

Cauda Equina Syndrome (CES)

Introduction (39)
- Rare, 1% to 6% of all disc herniation undergoing surgery
- Etiologies
  ○ Herniated disk (MC), spinal stenosis, tumor, trauma/spinal fracture, epidural hematoma, or epidural abscess
  ○ Iatrogenic causes; spine surgery (0.1%–0.2%), durotomy, intradiscal annuloplasty, and the like

History and physical examination
- LBP (83%), radicular pain (90%), groin and perineal pain, and bilateral sciatica
- Lower extremity weakness, hyporeflexia (or areflexia), sensory deficits, perineal hypoesthesia or saddle anesthesia, and loss of bowel or bladder (required for clinical diagnosis) function
- Sensory examination: impaired pinprick in the perineal region (S2–4). Light touch and pressure usually preserved
- Rectal examination: tone (decreased) and impaired voluntary contraction
- Impaired bulbocavenous reflex; applying pressure to glans penis or clitoris and/or traction on the Foley catheter → normal response: contraction of the anal sphincter

Diagnosis
- Clinical diagnosis confirmed with imaging studies (urgent neuroimaging to evaluate structural lesion)
  ○ High index of suspicion in postoperative patient: increasing back and/or leg pain with difficulty voiding
- EMG if imaging findings are not conclusive
  ○ Typical pattern: polyradiculopathy involving anal sphincter muscles (normal sensory nerve conduction study [SNCS], possible abnormal motor nerve conduction study [MNCS] ± abnormal H reflex, abnormal needle EMG test of limb muscles)
  ○ External sphincter EMG
    ▪ Precautions: normal motor unit of external sphincter is of short duration and small amplitude, which has similar morphology to fibrillations
    ▪ Spontaneous activity on resting and increased motor units when coughing
- Urodynamic study: to follow-up (FU) progress, beneficial if done pre- and postoperatively

Treatment (13)
- Urgent surgical exploration and decompression, preferably within 24 hours (or 48 hours)
  - Surgical evaluation (medicolegal concern as well) ➔ if not candidate for surgery, treatment based on underlying etiologies (example: radiation oncology if metastatic cancer involved)
- Outcome
  - Sexual dysfunction; usually persistent
  - Factors related to poor outcome: pre-op chronic back pain, rectal dysfunction, and increasing age

Diabetic Radiculopathy and Radiculoplexus Neuropathy

Introduction (82)
- Nonmechanical (compressive) radiculopathy: much less common than mechanical (compressive) radiculopathy
- 1% in diabetic mellitus (in Rochester diabetic neuropathy study)
  - More common in middle age or older with DM type II
  - LS radiculoplexus neuropathy >thoracic and cervical and cranial nerve (CN III)
- Etiology
  - Ischemic injury caused by micro-vasculitis and altered immunity
    - Axonal atrophy with secondary segmental demyelination (axonal degeneration and empty nerve strand in pathology)
  - Metabolic derangement (in slower and more symmetric presentation)

History and physical examination
- Painful, rapidly evolving, asymmetrical lower limb weakness heralded by weight loss (mean: 30 lb)
  - Small group of patients presents without prominent pain
- Weakness persists for weeks to years; motor predominant, but sensory and autonomic as well
  - Proximal and not-length-dependent, asymmetric, and monophasic involvement

Diagnosis
- Clinical diagnosis confirmed by EMG with MRI to R/O mechanical causes of radiculopathy or plexopathy
- Electrodiagnosis (83)
  - Decreased amplitude in SNCS and MNCS with only mild slowing of CV, ASA, decreased recruitment, long duration, and high amplitude in multiple nerve roots and peripheral nerves
  - Paraspinal muscle usually involved
  - Distal diffuse peripheral neuropathy: not often involved
- Other test
  - Cerebrospinal fluid (CSF) protein: significantly elevated

Treatment
- Referral to neurology for intravenous immunoglobulin (IVIG) and/or prednisone ± cyclophosphamide
- Symptomatic management for neuropathic pain (TCA, gabapentin, often needs narcotics), PT, evaluation for bracing if indicated

Herpes Zoster Radiculopathy

Introduction (79)
- Epidemiology: incidence of herpes zoster: 3.6 per 1,000 person-years
  - 20% to 1/3 of patients older than 80 years with zoster develop postherpetic neuralgia
  - 5%: radiculopathy
    - Complete resolution of the motor deficit in 50% to 70%
- Zoster-associated limb paresis (study of $n = 49$) (84)
  - The mean age of onset: 71 years, male (~2/3) > female, and lower limb was affected in 55%
  - Etiology: radiculopathy (37%), plexopathy (41%), mononeuropathy (14%), and radiculoplexus neuropathy (8%)

History and physical examination
- Pain: single dermatomal distribution precedes the vesicular eruption
  - Rarely, without rash (known as zoster sine herpete)
  - Location: ophthalmic and thoracic dermatomes: MC
    - LS zoster accounts for ~20%
  - 10% to 15%: chronic pain, postherpetic neuralgia
    - Postherpetic neuralgia (92% at 1 month and 65% at 3 months) in group with motor paresis
- Weakness/paresis: 5% involving motor axon (zoster paresis)
  - Weakness: moderately diminished, 50% to 70% complete resolution, 50% for several months (~6 months) (85)

Diagnosis
- Clinical diagnosis confirmed by Tzanck test or direct fluorescent antibody testing or PCR and EMG (for Zoster-associated limb paresis, can't be ruled out by EMG)
- EMG: ASA in the abdominal, external oblique, and paraspinal muscles (86)
- MRI: may be better for plexopathy or mononeuropathy showing nerve enlargement, gadolinium enhancement, and T2 hyperintensity
  - Nerve enlargement, increased T2 signal intensity (SI), or enhancement in a majority (64%) of affected plexus and peripheral nerves

Treatment
- Antiviral within 72 hours of the development of the rash: valacyclovir 1,000 mg tid for 7 D
  - More rapid resolution of neuralgia symptom, shorter duration of postherpetic neuralgia (PHN) and smaller-pill burden
  - Corticosteroids with antiviral: may improve the acute pain, but not postherpetic neuralgia
- Pain control: amitriptyline or gabapentin/pregabalin, opioids and topical lidocaine patches
- Zoster vaccination: may be preventive

Lyme Radiculopathy

Introduction (87)
- Lyme caused by *Ixodes* ticks infected with the spirochete *Borrelia burgdorferi*
- Epidemiology
  - Geographic distribution (Northeast from Maryland to Maine, the Great Lakes of the Midwest, and Pacific Northwest)
  - Bimodal age distribution (children 5–9 years, and 55–59 years; 7–8/100,000), mostly occurs from June to August

History and physical examination
- Radiating back pain in dermatomal distribution: first 2 months of infection

- Usually occurs in conjunction with cranial neuropathies and lymphocytic meningitis
- Similar to the presentation of diabetic radiculopathy
- Erythema migrans in 50% to 90%, often flu-like illness

Diagnosis
- High index of suspicion confirmed by serologic test
- Serologic test: positive screening enzyme-linked immunosorbent assay (ELISA) then confirmed by Western blot
- Lumbar puncture: mildly elevated protein
- Differential diagnosis (Ddx): other peripheral nerve involvement from Lyme disease and other nonmechanical radiculopathy
  - LS plexopathy (also brachial), mononeuropathy, mononeuropathy multiplex, diffuse polyneuropathy
    - Diffuse polyneuropathy: MC peripheral nerve involvement in Lyme disease, in severe cases mimics Guillain-Barré syndrome in acute presentation
    - Common focal neuropathy: cranial neuropathy (C7; MC) and radiculoneuropathy

Management
- PO antibiotics: early disease, erythema migrans, doxycycline 100 mg bid, amoxicillin 500 mg tid or cefuroxime 500 mg bid for 21 days
- Admit to IV antibiotics (ceftriaxone, cefotaxime, and penicillin) for 12 to 28 days if meningitis or other central nervous system (CNS) involved
- Symptomatic management for pain, neurologic deficit if present

HIV Radiculopathy
Introduction (88)
- Polyradiculopathy: rare, 2% of all HIV-related neurology consultations, higher if CD 4 <100
  - Decreasing frequency with better HIV management; rare nowadays
- Etiology: CMV (MC)
  - Others: herpes simplex, lymphomatous meningitis, mycobacteria, cryptococci, and treponemal
- A poor prognosis, with minimal functional recovery after treatment and a median survival time of 2.7 months

History and physical examination
- Rapidly progressing CES with severe LBP, flaccid paraparesis and lower extremity areflexia (hyperreflexia rare, but possible if spinal cord involved)

Diagnosis
- Clinical suspicion confirmed by MRI, CSF analysis, and EMG
- Gadolinium-enhanced MRI of LS spine: first step, to R/O focal compressive lesion
  - Usually negative or meningeal enhancement
- Lumbar puncture for CSF analysis
  - Pleocytosis, with polymorphonuclear predominance and, in some patients, decreased glucose
  - A positive CSF polymerase chain reaction for cytomegalovirus
- Differential diagnosis: polyradiculopathy from syphilis, bacterial infection, tuberculosis, or lymphomatous polyradiculitis

- EMG: severe axonal polyradiculopathy with normal SNCS, decreased or absent compound motor action potential (CMAP) amplitude, or abnormal spontaneous activity (ASA) in needle EMG

Treatment
- Admit the patient and intravenous ganciclovir, foscarnet, or both for 3 to 6 weeks
- Rehabilitation after medically stabilized.

Leptomeningeal Metastasis/Meningeal Carcinomatosis
Introduction (89)
- Incidence: 5% to 15% in cancer patients, varies depending on type of primary tumors and stages
  - MC primary cancer: lung caner, leukemia (in the dura), lymphoma, breast cancer, and melanoma
- Severe morbidity and high mortality

Presentation
- Back pain (nonspecific), radicular pain, symptoms from cauda equina involvement (2%–3%)
  - Multifocal
- Other concomitant symptoms: cranial neuropathy (9%–22%, more common than radiculopathy/back pain: 1%–14%), headache (10%–31%), memory loss, seizures, and gait disturbances

Diagnosis
- High clinical suspicion (in patients with cancer) with MRI and confirmed by CSF analysis
  - Basic MRI: low sensitivity with 40% false negatives
    - T1-weighted, gadolinium-enhanced cranial and spinal cord MRI may identify or raise suspicion for leptomeningeal spread, and can be positive even if the cerebrospinal fluid is initially negative
  - Contrast enhancement of the meninges in a diffuse or nodular pattern
- CSF exam (to confirm): mildly increased cell count in 50%, elevated protein and low glucose in 25%
  - + cytologic exam in 1/2
  - 90% positive after three lumbar punctures

Management (90)
- Goal: palliative, stabilization, prevent further deterioration, and improve quality of life
- Referral to oncology, radiation oncology, and spine surgery
  - Radiotherapy and/or intra-CSF chemotherapy, shunting (ventriculoperitoneal to alleviate hydrocephalus)

Other Unusual Causes of Radiculopathy: Nerve Tumor (91)
Introduction
- MC peripheral nerve tumor: schwannoma (neurilemmoma)
- Very rare, 3% of all spinal tumors

History and physical examination
- Radicular leg pain ± back pain
- Neurological examination and provocative test: not specific

Diagnosis
- High index of suspicion with imaging study, confirmed by biopsy
- MRI: round mass in neural foramen with widening of foramen, hypo or isointense on T1, hyperintense on T2 with gadolinium enhancement
- Ddx: neurofibromatosis 1: increased neural foramen, inseparable from root (vs schwannoma separable)

Treatment
- Surgical referral for laminectomy, foraminotomy, and resection of mass

Epidural Liposis
Introduction (92)
- Very rare, <1% of spinal tumor, related to spinal dysraphism
  - Location of abnormal epidural fat deposits: thoracic >lumbar >cervical spine
- Risk factors of epidural lipomatosis: exogenous steroids (usually >6M) and obesity

History and physical examination
- Mostly asymptomatic, or LBP with radiation ± hyper/hypotrophy of calf or thigh muscle and abnormal neurologic examination (DTR)

Diagnosis
- High index of suspicion with imaging study
- MRI (diagnostic test of choice): bright signal Y sign (in T1 weighted image); thecal sac attached
- Serologic test: chemistry, lipid profile

Treatment
- Weight reduction and possible surgical referral in failed conservative treatment

Arachnoiditis
Introduction (93)
- Very rare, common location: lumbar spine (94)
- Etiology (95)
  - Contrast media (oil-based, in the past), epidural steroid injection, blood in CSF (subarachnoid hemorrhage), trauma (spinal surgery; extradural or repeated surgery or manipulation during surgery; very rare)
  - Infection: tuberculosis (rare in US), gonorrhea and syphilis and rarely, *Cryptococcus*

History and physical examination
- Back pain (often worse with activity) with/without leg pain (often bilateral), muscle spasm
  - Gradual onset: weeks to years
- Muscle atrophy, sensory dysfunction, hyporeflexia, and bowel/bladder/sexual dysfunction

Diagnosis
- High clinical suspicion with imaging study
- MRI of LS spine; sensitivity 92%, specificity 100%
  - Large conglomerations of adherent nerve roots centrally located within the thecal sac
  - An "empty sac" appearance with roots peripherally adherent to meninges
  - Soft tissue replacing the subarachnoid space
- CSF analysis: often limited

Treatment (96)
- Treat underlying pathologies and conservative symptomatic management
- Referral to intervention: intrathecal steroid (Depo-Medrol) injections, radiotherapy, surgical intervention (spinal cord stimulation, dorsal rhizotomy, dorsal root ganglionectomy and microsurgical lysis)
- Recurrent: common

Lumbar Spinal Stenosis
Introduction (97)
- Epidemiology
  - Incidence: 5/100,000, 4 times more common than cervical spinal stenosis, usually >50 years old
  - Location: L4–5 > L3–4 > L5–S1 and L1–2
- Anatomical classification
  - Central stenosis (with/without lateral stenosis)
  - Isolated lateral stenosis
    - Spondylolisthesis and defects (and callus) around the pars interarticularis ➔ lateral (mid zone) stenosis
  - Foraminal stenosis
- Etiology
  - Primary: idiopathic or achondrodysplasia
  - Secondary: much more common
    - Degenerative (spondylosis, spondylolisthesis, scoliosis): MC
    - Ossification of the PLL and ligament flavum
    - Metabolic or endocrine causes (epidural lipomatosis, acromegaly)
    - Infectious (discitis, osteomyelitis, and Pott's disease)
    - Neoplasm
    - Rheumatologic conditions (Paget's, spondylosis, ankylopoietica, and RA)
    - Posttraumatic or postoperative stenosis (fracture of vertebrae, laminectomy, and fusion or fibrosis)

History and physical examination
- LBP, usually from spondylosis rather than spinal stenosis
  - Relief of pain on sitting and bending forward (18)
- Claudication and sensation of "heavy leg"
  - Reduced arterial blood flow and venous congestion (compression of the nerve and secondary perfusion deficiency/vasa nervosum of the spinal roots)
  - Worsened by extension and standing (vertical load)
- Leg pain: radicular pattern usually
  - Lateral recess or foraminal stenosis
  - Autonomic dysregulation and impaired circulation
- Rare sphincter involvement (central position of sacral roots in cauda equina, relative protective in stenotic canal)
- Motor, sensory, and DTR: usually normal. SLR: usually negative

DIFFERENTIAL DIAGNOSIS OF CLAUDICATION		
	VASCULAR	NEUROGENIC
Walking distance	Fixed	Variable
Palliative factors	Standing	Sitting/bending
Provocative factors	Walking	Walking/standing
Stop walking	Immediate relief of symptoms (within seconds)	Some lingering symptoms (>30 seconds)
Walking uphill		Painless
Bicycle test	Painful	Negative
Pulses	Positive (painful) Absent/diminished (not always)	Present
Skin	Loss of hair, shiny	Normal
Weakness	Rarely	Occasionally
Back pain	Occasionally	Commonly
Pain character	Cramping-distal to proximal	Numbness, aching-proximal to distal
Atrophy	Uncommon	Occasionally

- Vascular claudication
  - If muscle is contracted (such as calf muscle during walking), blood supply demand can go up (by ~15 times)

Diagnosis
- Clinical diagnosis confirmed by imaging study ± EMG test
- Radiologic study
  - X-ray: be cautious, highly prevalent radiologic findings in elderly population
    - Midsagittal lumbar spinal canal <10mm: absolute stenosis, 10 to 12 mm: relative (Normal: 22–25 mm); unclear correlation with clinical presentation
    - Vertebral body: canal <0.82 (the Pavlov or Torg ratio); high false positive in athletes (bigger vertebral body)
  - MRI: often not correlating with clinical symptoms (worse than clinical picture)
    - High false positive (20% in asymptomatic subjects >60 years)
    - Trefoil canal shape predisposes to lateral recess stenosis rather than central stenosis
    - Lateral recess <2 mm (Physiologic: 3–5 mm), concept of reserve (occupancy of roots vs space) maybe more important
- Electrodiagnosis
  - For the differential diagnosis: distal polyneuropathy or concomitant peripheral nerve lesion
  - Normal SNCS and MNCS (usually normal except severely involved)
  - H reflex: usually involved bilaterally
  - Needle EMG
    - Mild membrane instability (fibrillations) at multiple limbs (more commonly distal) and paraspinal sites: can be patchy or negative
    - Paraspinal mapping (98)
      - Needling in 9 different directions, perpendicular to the skin, 45° angle to the skin surface (eight directions: cranial, cranial/lateral, lateral, lateral/caudal, caudal, caudal/medial, medial, and medial/cranial)
      - Abbreviated version: midline, cranial medial, and caudal medial
    - May be better correlated to clinical findings of spinal stenosis than MRI
    - Positive EMG findings may be associated with unsatisfactory outcomes (99)
- Differential diagnosis

DIFFERENTIAL DIAGNOSIS	
Vascular claudication	See Differential Diagnosis of Claudication table on this page
Radiculopathy (discogenic)	Preceding event (lifting, trauma, injury) and rather abrupt, frequently concomitant
Polyneuropathy	Distal stocking pattern irrespective of posture
Intraspinal synovial cyst	Mostly not symptomatic (incidental finding)
Tethered cord or spina bifida	Developmental (skin lesion or onset of age younger) or history of spine trauma or surgery
SI joint dysfunction	SI joint: back pain radiating to the buttock or thigh
Abdominal aortic aneurysm	High index of suspicion (may have abdominal pain)
Other nonmechanical radiculopathy	Red flags Neoplasia (meninges, bone or myelin or spinal root) Inflammatory/infectious (spondylodiscitis, arachnoiditis)
Somatization	Waddell sign

SI, sacroiliac.

Treatment
- Conservative management: multidisciplinary approach
  - Natural course: long-term clinical stability: common
    - Pain more than 5 years; 70% plateau, 15% exacerbation, and 15% spontaneously improved (100)
    - No worsening of symptoms over 2 years in conservative treatment group (73)
  - Therapeutic exercise: flexion/neutral based, stabilization exercise (paravertebral/core muscles), stretching (especially hip flexor as hip flexor tightness aggravates lumbar lordosis), manual therapy, and aerobic endurance exercise at home
- Epidural steroid/lidocaine or lidocaine injection: no significant difference (65)
- Surgery for spinal stenosis: better in first 2 to 3 years compared to the nonoperative group
  - Relatively poor prognostic factors: DM and depression (101)

BONE AND JOINT PATHOLOGY

Facet Arthropathy

Introduction (102)
- Facet pathology: contributory in 15% to 52% of patients with chronic LBP
  - Isolated facet joint pain: 4% of patients with chronic LBP
  - Unclear correlation with symptoms because of high prevalent asymptomatic pathologies

- Arthrosis in cadaveric study: 57% in 20 to 29 years old, 93% in 40 to 49, 100% in 60 years old

History and physical examination (103)
- LBP with/without referred pain (may be more specific on extension and standing)
- Usually normal motor, sensory, DTR, and facet loading test (pain on extension, not specific)

Diagnosis
- Clinical diagnosis confirmed by imaging (fluoroscopy)-guided local anesthetic block (see Figure 6.2)
  - Local anesthetic block to the facet joints or medial branches (short-acting local anesthetic or bupivacaine) (102)
  - Single block: 38% false positive rate (104) with second confirmatory injection (>50% relief)
- Imaging
  - X-ray: narrowing, irregularity of the facet joint space, sclerosis, subarticular bone erosions, subchondral cysts, joint space vacuum phenomenon, osteophyte formation, and hypertrophy of the articular process
  - Findings for disc degeneration (almost always)
  - CT or MRI (105): MRI to evaluate disc pathology, root and other lesions. Facet cyst; occasionally seen; unclear clinical correlation

Treatment
- Pharmacologic treatment: AAP, NSAID, short-term use of skeletal muscle relaxant, TCA, and gabapentin if concomitant positive sensory symptoms
- Therapeutic exercise/education for long-term (unclear evidence): core muscle stabilization exercise, correct posture and biomechanics, and education for aerobic endurance exercise
  - A few sessions of PT with myofascial release and manual therapy
- Radiofrequency denervation (67)
  - If use strict criteria (80 or 100% pain relief from branch block and double or triple block), may be longer duration of treatment effect

Degenerative Disc Disease

Introduction (106)
- Unclear correlation of symptoms and imaging findings: highly prevalent in asymptomatic population
- Degenerative changes of the disc, desiccation and fibrosis of the nucleus, mucinous degeneration and fissuring of the annulus, bulging of the annulus beyond the edges of the vertebral body ring apophyses with consecutive narrowing of the disc space, and defects and sclerosis of the cartilaginous end plates
- Etiology: mechanical, nutritional, and genetic variables
  - Discography and cardiovascular risk factors
  - Degenerative cascades: temporary dysfunction, unstable and stabilization

History and physical examination
- Ambiguous, bandlike LBP ± radiating down to the sacroiliac region, absent lower extremity claudication or radicular complaints (below the knee)
- Unremarkable physical examination, normal neurological examination, and provocative test
- Tenderness on the midline lumbar spine, limited ROM, worsening of pain on flexion and lessened with extension; not specific

Diagnosis (107)
- Diagnosis of exclusion: centralized back pain after other pathologies (spinal stenosis, facet arthropathy, herniated disc disease, SI joint pathology, vascular disease, etc.) are ruled out
- Differentiate the intraabdominal pathologies (renal stone, aortic aneurysm, pancreatic problems, and tumor) and check red flags
- Imaging (108)
  - X-ray: flexion/extension if concern for instability, spondylolisthesis
    - Instability and spondylolisthesis may be a favorable indicator for surgical stabilization
  - MRI: Modic changes (109); unclear correlation with clinical symptoms

Treatment
- Reassurance (improves usually within 3 months), aerobic endurance exercise, stop smoking, and symptomatic treatment for pain
- Physical therapy; core muscle strengthening, education of body biomechanics, manual therapy, back school (for back pain), McKenzie extension-based exercise, and LS corset (unclear efficacy)
- Surgical referral for fusion especially for level of spondylolisthesis in patients with disabling back pain after a failed conservative management

Spondylolisthesis

Introduction (110)
- Spondylolisthesis—a slip of one vertebral body over the one below
- Spondylolysis—a stress fracture/defect of the pars interarticularis (isthmus)
- Classification of spondylolisthesis (Wiltse)
  - Degenerative and isthmic spondylolisthesis; MC
  - Others: dysplastic (congenital abnormalities of the upper sacrum or the L5 arch), traumatic (fractures other than pars), pathologic

	DEGENERATIVE	ISTHMIC (SPONDYLOLYTIC)
Age at onset	>40 YO	About 10 YO
Location of lesion	L4–5 MC (>L3–4); L5 root Rarely greater than grade 1	L5–S1 MC (about 90%)
Presentation	Sx of spinal stenosis	Degree of slippage: no correlation with Sx
Pars interarticularis	Intact	Lysis
Central canal	Narrowed	Patent

(continued)

	DEGENERATIVE	ISTHMIC (SPONDYLOLYTIC)
Foraminal canal	Narrowed	Narrowed
Degree of slip	<30% of inferior vertebral body	No limit

YO, years old; MC, most common; Sx, symptom.

- Epidemiology
  ○ Degenerative spondylolisthesis: prevalence ~8% (Japan), >50 years old, female > male, African American >Whites (possibly secondary to increased ligamentous laxity)
    ▪ Listhesis progresses in 25% to 30%
  ○ Isthmic: 6% in young adults 12 to 25 years, more common with repetitive hyperextension activities (111)
    ▪ Increased in pediatric athletes with back pain (one of MC causes of pediatric back pain)
      – Sports involving repetitive flexion–extension of the trunk in combination with rotation
      – Divers: 83%, weightlifters: 45%, gymnasts: 38%, wrestlers: 33% football linemen: 24%

History and physical examination
- LBP ± radiating down to buttock or thigh
- Possible neurogenic claudication (spinal stenosis), radiculopathy (foraminal stenosis by anterior-posterior narrowing, can have concomitant vertical compression by disc disease), and rare bowel/bladder dysfunction in degenerative spondylolisthesis
  ○ Loss of lumbar lordosis, stooped posture (secondary hip flexion contracture/tightness), and spinal muscle atrophy
- ± Palpable step-off at the spinous process, lumbar hyperlordosis, frequently has limited spine ROM and tight hamstrings in isthmic spondylolisthesis
- Usually negative SLR and normal neurological examination

Diagnosis
- Clinical suspicion confirmed with imaging
- X-ray: standing AP and lateral x-rays of LS spine and pelvis, flexion/extension view (to evaluate the degree of motion of the adjacent segments)
  ○ >2 mm: instability with spondylolisthesis with persistent symptoms: indication for surgical referral
  ○ In 20%: unilateral, missed if oblique views from both sides are not done
  ○ Meyerding classification: grade 1: 0% to 25%, grade 2: 26% to 50%, grade 3: 51% to 75%, and grade 4: 76% to 100% (see Figure 6.7C)
- CT: pedicle size and orientation, facet morphology, R/O tumor (osteoblastoma)
- MRI: soft-tissue pathologies including synovial cysts, disc pathology, nerve root compression, ligament flavum hypertrophy, and other etiologies
  ○ Spina bifida occulta: may be common: up to 60% of patients with spondylolysis
- Consider EMG if the radicular symptoms or mild motor deficit present

Treatment
- Pain medication (NSAID) as needed and muscle relaxant for a short term
- One to two weeks of relative rest, activity restriction, rigid bracing (modified Boston) and abstinence from sports for 6 months for grade 1 and grade 2 slippages
- Physical therapy: stretching of hip flexor (stabilize the lumbopelvic movement to decrease psoas spasm), flexion-based exercise, core muscle strengthening, and aerobic conditioning)—stationary bicycle, modality, and education for home exercise program
- Epidural steroid injection for radicular symptoms, medial branch block (diagnostic), or injection to the pars interarticularis (right below the facet joint) for an axial back pain
- Surgery referral for intractable pain despite the conservative management
  ○ Decompression (rarely laminectomy only) with posterior and posterolateral, circumferential fusion (anterior, posterior lumbar interbody fusion, or transforaminal lumbar interbody fusion; transforaminal lumbar interbody fusion [TLIF])

Scoliosis

Introduction (11)
- Definition: increased lateral curvature >10° in AP standing x-ray
- Classification: idiopathic, congenital, related to other causes
- Idiopathic: infantile <3 years, juvenile: 3 to 9 years, adolescent: MC, and adult (after skeletal maturity)
- Prevalence: 2% in curve >10°, 0.2% >30°, female > male by 10 times
- Etiologies: multifactorial (genetic)

DEFORMITY	ETIOLOGIES
Idiopathic scoliosis	Unknown factors likely related to genetic susceptibility. Subtype classified by age of onset
Degenerative scoliosis and kyphosis	Consequence of advanced degenerative changes
Congenital scoliosis	Failure of formation such as wedge vertebra or hemivertebra Failure of segmentation: unilateral bar, block vertebra Mixed
Neuromuscular scoliosis	Neuropathic - Upper motor neuron Dz: cerebral palsy, spinocerebellar degeneration, Friedrich's ataxia, syringomyelia (spinal cord tumor or posttraumatic), myelomeningocele - Lower motor neuron Dz: poliomyelitis, spinal muscular atrophy, trauma, Charcot Marie Tooth Dz Myopathic - Myotonic dystrophy - Muscular dystrophy: Duchenne's, limb girdle, fascioscapulohumeral dystrophy - Congenital hypotonia or arthrogryposis
Posttraumatic deformity	Following a fracture with progressive vertebral collapse and angulation

(continued)

DEFORMITY	ETIOLOGIES
Post-infectious deformity	Following vertebral osteomyelitis/discitis with vertebral destruction following a tuberculosis infection (Pott disease)
Iatrogenic deformity	Consequence of previous interventions (ie, laminectomy)
Others	Neurofibromatosis Connective tissue; Marfan, Ehler-Danlos Osteochondrodystrophies: mucopolysaccharidosis Metabolic: Rickets, osteogenesis imperfecta, homocystinuria Tumor

Dz, disease

History and physical examination
- Asymptomatic (MC, incidental finding) or localized back pain on convex side and radicular pain on concave side
  ○ Upper back (scapular girdle) pain and pelvic/buttock pain: common
  ○ Respiratory symptoms in advanced scoliosis
  ○ Headache from neural axis malformation
- Physical examination
  ○ Inspection: waist asymmetry, shoulder (scapular) asymmetry, unilateral cavus foot, asymmetric calf girth, Adam's forward bend test (with scoliometer measuring inclination angle)
  ○ Neurological examination for neural axis malformation (112)
  ○ Tanner stage (growth potential)

Diagnosis
- Clinical suspicion confirmed by imaging study
- X-ray: standing posteroanterior (PA) (less radiation to breast) and lateral (Figure 6.7)
  ○ Orientation of film: right side goes to the right
  ○ Definition of scoliosis (Scoliosis Research Society)—x-ray done with knee and hip straight
  ○ Dextro (right)/levo (left): nomenclature for location of convexity of the main curvature
    ▪ >85% of adolescent idiopathic scoliosis is dextroscoliosis
    ▪ Levoscoliosis: more likely related to other pathologies
  ○ Frontal curve ≥10° (± rotation); measured using Cobb's angle
    ▪ Thoracolumbar curve and lumbar curve worse outcome than thoracic curve
  ○ Rotation
    1. Slight asymmetry
    2. One pedicle out of view
    3. Remaining pedicle near the center but not cross
    4. Remaining pedicle lateral to the center of vertebral body
  ○ Sagittal and coronal balance
  ○ Pelvis x-ray for Risser grade (ossification of the iliac apophysis; grades 1 to 4: 100% ossification, grade 5: fusion of ossified epiphysis to the iliac wing)
- MRI
  ○ Indications: scoliosis before 8 years, progression >1° per month, unusual curve (levoscoliosis), neurologic deficit and pain or presurgical evaluation
  ○ Comorbid conditions: diastematomyelia, syringomyelia, tethered cord, spinal tumor, and neurofibromatosis
- Evaluation for osteoporosis in adult degenerative scoliosis

Treatment
- Depending on likelihood of progression: initial angle (higher, more likely to progress) and skeletal maturity
  ○ Skeletal maturity: Risser stage on iliac crest, worsened for 15 months after menarche
  ○ Curves <20°: FU every 6 to 12 months until skeletal maturity, after maturity: no further evaluation
  ○ Curves 30° to 40° in skeletally mature patients: yearly standing PA radiographs for 2 to 3 years after skeletal maturity and then every 5 years throughout life
- Orthotic management
  ○ Bracing indications
    ▪ Skeletal immaturity
    ▪ Initial curve of 25° to 30° (flexible curve between 20° and 40°) and documented progression of 5° over a year
    ▪ Curves between T8–L2: best chance of correction with bracing
  ○ Milwaukee (CTLSO): apex higher than T7 (for 23 hours/day, 74% success rate (113)), Boston: lower than T7, better than Charleston (can wear night only, overcorrect the curve)
  ○ TLSO: apex should be T9 or lower
  ○ Derotational: Boston, Denver, nighttime wear brace
- Referral to surgery
  ○ Cobb's angle >45° in adolescent and >50° in adults (or 40° in thoracic and 30° in lumbar) or coronal balance >2.5 cm
  ○ Spinal instrumentation in neuromuscular disease: Cobb's angle >25°, forced VC >35% of normal, Duchene MD >35° (114)

Hyperkyphosis
T kyphosis >50° (normal: 20°–50°), L lordosis ≥80° (31°–79°: normal)

Classification and etiology

ELDERLY	ADOLESCENT
Vertebral fracture: MC, ~37%, 3.7–3.8° increase of kyphosis with each vertebral fracture Degenerative disc disease Postural change and aging (muscle weakness and intervertebral ligament weakness)	Scheuermann's disease (MC) Postural kyphosis: roundback deformity that often disappears with forward bending Congenital - Cormobidities: neurofibromatosis, osteogenesis imperfecta, Ehlers-Danlos syn, Marfan syn, cystic fibrosis etc. Kyphosis related to neuromuscular disease

syn., syndrome.

Compression Fracture (Osteoporotic)
Introduction (115)
- 700,000 per year, >20% in >50 years old, high in Caucasian women

- Actual incidence may be higher because only 1/4 to 1/3 of fractures become clinically evident
- Increase with age
- Increased risk of subsequent compression fracture by fivefold, other fragility fracture by two- to fourfold
- Common location: mid-thoracic (T7–8) or thoracolumbar transition zone (T12-L1)
  - Trabecular zone of minimal resistance

History and physical examination
- Asymptomatic: frequently incidental finding on x-ray
- New onset of LBP ± trauma, worsened by flexion ± radiation
- Chronic pain with kyphotic deformity ± breathing difficulties, deconditioning, insomnia, and depression
- Kyphosis, paraspinal muscle, or midline tenderness
  - If kyphosis deformity is progressing too fast, consider vertebral tumor

Diagnosis
- Clinical suspicion confirmed by imaging
  - Plain x-ray AP, lateral and flexion/extension of lumbar and thoracic spine
    - Serial x-ray q 1 year for progression of kyphosis; if the progression is too fast, evaluate for tumor
    - Limited in evaluation of compression fractures with an intact middle column and differentiation from a minimally displaced burst fracture (with associated middle-column involvement)
    - The PVBA on lateral view (Figure 6.7) (58)
      – The PVBA: the angle formed by either the superior or inferior end plate and the posterior vertebral body wall
      – Suspect burst fracture if an angle >100° for either the superior or inferior PVBA or a slight decrease in the height of the posterior wall relative to the vertebra above and below, loss of the biconcave contour, widening of the interpedicular distance
      – ≥20% of subtle burst fractures can be misdiagnosed on plain radiographs. CT: a better method for evaluating the middle column
  - CT or MRI
    - Decrease in height of ≥20% or >4 mm compared to the baseline height
    - Check retropulsion; if suspicious → CT or MRI
  - MRI (to determine chronological age of fracture and neural or ligamentous structure involvement)
    - Differential diagnosis: benign (osteoporotic) versus pathologic (tumor or infection)
      – If the disc is involved, likely infection
      – If not, then tumor or fracture. Fracture line is visible in fracture versus tumor (usually, the pedicle is involved earlier)
    - Useful adjunct for identifying the presence of posterior ligamentous injury
  - Bone density: spontaneous (without trauma) vertebral compression fracture; pathognomic for osteoporosis
- Differential diagnoses
  - Burst (bursting, dispersion) fracture
    - Anterior loss of height of the vertebral body and fragmentation of its posterior aspects (can displaced into the spinal canal) by vertical compression
    - Thoracolumbar transition; MC location
    - Often misdiagnosed as simple compression fracture with plain film (if wedging >20%, widening between the pedicles); laminar and articular process fracture often missed in plain films; CT or MRI recommended
    - Neurologic deficit in 50%
  - Chance fracture
    - A distraction of all three columns of the vertebrae by flexion or a lap seatbelt in a motor vehicle accident (MVA) or fall from a height
    - Thoracolumbar junction: MC location (~50%)
    - Lateral x-ray: distraction of spinous process, facets and vertebral body, AP x-ray may be normal → CT for details

Treatment (116)
- Nonoperative treatment: <40% anterior compression and <25 to 30° kyphosis
  - Good outcome, only ~4% had chronic disabling back pain (117)
- Pharmacologic
  - Narcotic pain medication with caution, NSAIDs (in recent fracture) with caution (theoretical inhibitory effect on bony healing), TCA, SSRI, gabapentin/pregabalin, tizanidine
  - Bisphosphonate, calcitonin, and teriparatide (recombinant parathyroid hormone)
- Physical therapy
  - Therapeutic exercise, aerobic exercise, gentle stretching (lying on supine or prone), spinal extensor-strengthening exercise (rather than abdominal flexion exercise), dynamic proprioceptive training, and functional exercise
  - Spinal proprioceptive extension exercise: dynamic program, spinal extensor strengthening exercise with weighted kypho-orthosis, postural and proprioceptive exercise (118)
  - Discourage lying supine on a soft mattress with multiple pillows (may accentuate the deformity)
- Bracing
  - Indication: thoracolumbar or lumbar compression fracture
    - No bracing indicated for stable fractures in the upper and middle thoracic spine because of the inherent stability of the rib cage
    - No significant difference in the outcome between early mobilization with or without a brace in patients with stable thoracolumbar injuries (119)
  - Duration: ≥3 months (up to 6 months), FU with standing lateral flexion and extension x-rays
    - Discontinue if no abnormal motion is seen through the fractured vertebra above and if the deformity has not progressed
  - Gradual cessation of bracing over a few weeks along with a muscle-strengthening program
  - Types of braces
    - Lumbar corset with moldable plastic posterior shell (ask patient to lie down on the back; may work although it can still be painful); for L1–3 level
    - Total-contact TLSO orthosis (custom): body jacket, cautious in patients with poor respiratory status
    - Posture training supports orthotic
    - Jewett/cruciform anterior spinal extension (3-point system; often difficult to wear, expensive, poor compliance) for young patients with fractures of the thoracolumbar junction

- Interventional spine procedure
  - Persistent pain despite conservative management without any posterior ligamentous injury
  - Vertebroplasty, balloon kyphoplasty (pain reduction, quality of life, function/mobility, but increase new fractures) (120)
  - Vertebroplasty versus sham; no difference in pain control or function from 1 week to 6 months FU (121)
  - Cages: KIVA™ (implant-based, structurally supportive implant) (122)
  - Lower fracture risk and extravasation of cement
- Surgery
  - Indication: + spinal instability and neurological compromise
    - If the posterior ligamentous structures are disrupted
      – Posterior column (ligament) compromise suspected if the anterior column is compressed ≥40% or if the kyphosis exceeds 25° to 30°
    - In those patients with abnormal motion at the level of injury, continued pain, or unacceptable progression of deformity
  - A posterior surgical approach using pedicle screw and rod fixation is preferred.
    - The goal is to restore coronal and sagittal alignment and to provide rigid fixation until a solid fusion is achieved.

Kümmell's Disease

Introduction (123)
- Failure of fracture healing process, delayed posttraumatic vertebral collapse, osteonecrosis, occurs weeks or months after an injury
- 10% (up to 1/3) of vertebral osteoporotic fracture, mainly in thoracolumbar zone

History and physical examination
- Persistent pain in the thoracolumbar junction (>6–8 weeks) with kyphotic thoracic spine ± neurologic deficit (usually later)

Diagnosis (124)
- Clinical suspicion with imaging study
- X-ray: flexion and extension views
  - Intravertebral vacuum, accentuated on extension view
  - Significant mobility through the fracture site is noted on flexion-extension views
- MRI ± contrast in ambiguous cases
  - The vacuum sign appears like a homogeneous fluid-filled cavity, decreased SI in T1 and hyperintense in T2 weighted images (initial gas replaced by fluid)
  - Gadolinium-enhanced sequences: absent enhancement of the crushed vertebral body initially and enhancement with successful treatment, indicating revascularization later
- Differential diagnoses: osteomyelitis and spinal malignancy

Treatment
- Referral for vertebral augmentation (stabilization of the pseudoarthrosis and elimination of motion) for relief of pain after treatment
- Referral to surgery if neurologically compromised or failed conservative management (decompress and restore sagittal balance)

Scheuermann's Disease

Introduction (125)
- Vertebral body wedging ≥5° of ≥3 consecutive vertebral bodies
- MC cause of kyphosis in adolescence, male ≥ female, 1% to 8% of general population (may be underreported)
- Normal range of kyphosis: 20° to 45°
- Unknown etiology. The mode of inheritance: multifactorial

History and physical examination
- Kyphosis of thoracic or thoracolumbar spine, usually appears before puberty
- Pain: mild if present, located in the apex usually (chronic back pain in untreated case) and fatigue
  - Often associated with tight hamstrings, gluteals, and lumbodorsal fascia
- Forward flexion of the trunk with inspection from the side: sharp angular deformity in Scheuermann's disease (disappears in postural kyphosis) (125)

Diagnosis
- Clinical diagnosis confirmed by imaging study
- X-ray: erect 36-inch PA view and lateral
  - Change in endplate/disc space, at least 3 or more
  - T-spine anterior wedging: 3 consecutive vertebrae
  - Irregular vertebral endplates
  - Schmorl's nodes and disc space narrowing
- MRI: evaluation of thoracic disc herniation or for presurgical planning

Treatment
- Conservative treatment (most often) when kyphotic angle <75° to 80°
  - Relative rest, lumbar stabilization and modalities for acute resolution of pain, periodic x-rays
  - Consider bracing (TLSO with anterior infraclavicular outriggers; initially >20 hours) in thoracic kyphosis >55° or >40° in thoracolumbar junction
  - Physical therapy: extension-based strengthening, core stabilization, aerobic endurance exercise, stretching of tight hamstring, gluteal, lumbodorsal fascia, and taping
- Surgery
  - Indications:
    - Symptomatic kyphotic deformity of 80° in the thoracic spine or 65° in the thoracolumbar spine not controlled by nonoperative treatment
    - Patients with significant sagittal imbalance secondary to the kyphotic deformity

Tumor of the Spine

Epidemiology
- Metastatic cancers >> primary tumor by 20 times
- Metastatic cancers
  - 20% to 85% of all patients with cancers
  - 5% to 10% of cancer patients develop spinal cord compression
- Location
  - Sites for metastasis: thoracic >> lumbar > cervical
- Higher risk of fracture: 40% of vertebral body involvement and location lower than T9
- Highest incidence in the middle age (40–65 years)

The common primary spinal bone tumors with their salient features (126,127)

	LOCATION	SYMPTOMS	PLAIN FILM AND CT	MRI
Hemangioma	T >L>C, VB MC benign lesion	Asymptomatic, occasionally painful	Plain film: Corduroy or fail bar CT: Polka dot sign	High SI on T1 and T2
Bone Island (Enostosis)	T >L, VB	Asymptomatic	Cortical bone density with spiculated margin	Low SI on T1 and T2
Osteochondroma	C (C2), PE	Mass-related nerve and cord compression	Continuity of marrow and cortex with underlying bone CT: cartilage cap	Cartilage cap with high SI on T2
Osteoid osteoma	L>T>C, PE	Unrelenting pain, worse at night, sensitive to aspirin	Radiolucent nidus with surrounding sclerosis, mineralization of nidus	Strong enhancement of nidus, surrounding low SI
Osteoblastoma	T>L, PE	Mild, dull localized pain	Expansile lesion with calcified matrix and soft-tissue mass >1.5 cm	
Aneurysmal bone cyst	T>L, PE >VB	Local pain	Expansile multiloculated lesion CT: fluid level	Cysts with fluid level
Giant cell tumor	S>C >T, VB, eccentric	Local pain	Expansile lytic lesion of VB	Low SI on T2
Eosinophilic granuloma	T>L >C, VB	Variable, sensitive to aspirin	Well-defined lytic lesion, may lead to vertebra plana (fracture)	Strong enhancement
Chordoma	Sacrococcygeal, VB, centrally located	Insidious local pain ± neurologic sym. based on location	Destructive lesion, may affect multiple vertebra, extend across the discs, amorphous calcification	
Chondrosarcoma	T, VB	Pain, palpable mass, neurologic Sx	CT: destructive bone lesion with ring and arc calcification	Ring and arc enhancement
Ewing's sarcoma	L>S, VB	Symptomatic	Permeative lesion with associated soft-tissue mass	
Multiple myeloma	T>L, VB	Local pain	Multiple lesions, lytic lesions, diffuse osteopenia, or vertebral collapse	Low SI on T1 and high SI on T2 "mini brain"

C; cervical, T: thoracic, L: lumbar, S: sacral, VB: vertebral body, PE: posterior element, SI: signal intensity

Presentation
- Spine pain in cancer patients: spinal metastasis until proven otherwise (in autopsy study, almost everyone has the metastasis)

Imaging study: malignant versus benign
- Radiologic characteristics

BENIGN	MALIGNANT
No cortical destruction Intravertebral vacuum phenomenon, multiple compression fractures Spared normal bone marrow SI of the vertebral body Focal concave collapse Retropulsion of bone fragments	Cortical bone lysis Expansive, convex posterior border Absence of normal bone marrow and abnormal signal intensity (SI) of the pedicle or posterior element Focal acute-angled collapse Other (vertebral) lesions accompanied, an encasing epidural mass or a focal paraspinal mass

Metastatic Tumors of the Spine

Introduction (128)
- Location of metastasis
  - Vertebral column: MC site for metastasis (30%–70%), vertebral body: MC site in the vertebral column (80%)
  - Lumbar spine more common than thoracic, but symptomatic: thoracic > lumbar > cervical (varies in different studies)
- Primary lesions
  - Solid tumors: breast (21%), lung (14%), prostate (7.5%), kidney (5%), gastrointestinal tract (5%)
  - Lymphoreticular malignancy and myeloma
- Classifications (129)
  - Extradural: 98% (dura: relative barrier)
    - Mechanisms of metastasis
      - Direct local extension to the extradural space
      - Retrograde spread through the valveless extradural venous channel (Batson plexus)
      - Arterial emboli with subsequent spread through cortical veins

∘ Intradural extramedullary and intramedullary: commonly from drop metastasis from intracranial lesions

History and physical examination (130)
- Back pain in the cancer patient: spinal metastasis until proven otherwise ± radicular pain if posterior column involved
  ∘ Referred pain: T12 to L1 level, SI joint and hip
- Neurological deficit (~50%)
  ∘ Sensory loss (70%–80%), and/or motor weakness (paraparesis or paraplegia) >60%
  ∘ Bowel and/or bladder difficulty in 14% to 77%
  ∘ Spinal cord compression: 8.5% to 20% of patients with vertebral column metastasis
    - 11% to 34% of patients are ambulatory at diagnosis

Diagnosis
- Clinical suspicion confirmed by imaging study and pathology
- Routine laboratory workup
- X-ray: low sensitivity, normal in 90% of patients with symptomatic disease
  ∘ Vertebral body collapse, pedicle erosion, osteoblastic and osteolytic lesions, and pathologic fractures
    - 30% to 40% of bone must be eroded to be visible
  ∘ Disc margin: usually spared (opposite to the infectious process)
- Contrast MRI
- CT-guided needle biopsy or open biopsy
- CSF cytology

Treatment
- Referral to spine surgery for possible surgical management, radiation oncology (radiation therapy), and medical oncology (primary tumor workup and chemo, bisphosphonate), and loading dose of steroid
- May need short-term inpatient rehabilitation and PT/OT referral
  ∘ Bracing for comfort (not effective for stability)
- Interventional spine management
  ∘ Epidural steroid injection and ablative therapies
  ∘ Vertebral augmentation
    - Vertebroplasty, balloon kyphoplasty (pain reduction, improve quality of life, function/mobility, but increase new fracture) (120)
    - Cages placement; KIVA™ (implant-based, structurally supportive implant) (122)
      – Lower fracture risk and extravasation of cement
  ∘ Percutaneous fusion
- Radiation treatment
  ∘ Conventional: pain improvement in 2/3, complete response in 1/3, no difference in single fraction versus multifraction schedule
    - Adverse effect: may cause bone marrow toxicity, fatigue, delay chemotherapy; not responsive in 1/3
  ∘ Stereotaxic radiotherapy: highly conformal, high dose, and few fractions
    - Advantages: higher rates of pain relief, earlier pain relief, limited toxicity, re-treat after full-dose external radiation

Multiple Myeloma
Introduction (131)
- Plasma-cell proliferation leading to lytic changes in bones (lytic lesions present in 90%)
- Epidemiology
  ∘ Incidence: 6/100,000, MC primary malignant tumor of bone, thoracic more than lumbar, vertebral body more involved than lumbar spine
  ∘ African American >Caucasian by ~2 times, male > female, 2/3 of patients above 55 years, median: 69 years
- Prognosis: ~50% survive in 5 years

History and physical examination
- Mechanical LBP, axial back pain ± radicular pain if posterior elements involved
- Symptoms and signs from renal disease or peripheral neuropathy. Nonspecific physical examination

Diagnosis
- Clinical suspicion with imaging, serologic test and biopsy
- X-ray: skeletal survey for diagnosis and staging (132)
  ∘ AP and lateral spine, lateral skull, AP ribs, humerus, pelvis, and femur
  ∘ Multiple, well-circumscribed, small lytic lesions. In some cases, structures can appear normal or osteopenic
  ∘ Less sensitive than CT or MRI because radiography requires that ~1/3 of the bone cortex be destroyed before lesions are detected
  ∘ Low-dose CT if there is bone pain and radiograph is negative.
- Labs: CBC (anemia), chemistry (increased Cr, lactate dehydrogenase (LDH), and β2 microglobulin), increased ESR, hypercalcemia, paraprotein in the serum and Bence-Jones protein in the urine, urine protein electrophoresis (UPEP) and serum protein electrophoresis (SPEP), immunofixation in urine and serum, and detection of free light chains in serum
- MRI: false negative up to 50% at initial stage
  ∘ Myeloma deposit: well-demarcated round focal low signal intensity in T1 and high intensity in T2 WI
  ∘ Post-contrast: marked enhancement
- Bone marrow boiopsy: abundance of malignant plasma cells

Treatment
- Referral to oncology, radiation oncology, and/or spine surgery: high-dose chemo, total-body radiation and bone marrow transplant

Chordoma
Introduction
- Slow-growing, low-grade malignant tumor arising from embryonic notochordal (spinal column precursor) remnants along the length of the neuraxis at developmentally active site
- Epidemiology: MC primary non-lymphoproliferative malignant tumor, 5th to 6th decade, male > female by 2 times
  ∘ Sacrum (50%), clivus (1/3), and C2 (axis)

History and physical examination
- Back pain of insidious onset ± radicular pain, neurologic involvement (bowel and bladder incontinence)

Diagnosis
- Clinical suspicion confirmed by imaging study
- X-ray: sacral lamina disappearance (50%) > intracranial at clivus
- MRI: heterogenous, lobular in appearance with predominant low to intermediate signal on T1-weighted images and very high in signal on T2-weighted images

Treatment
- Referral to spine surgery for resection (complete resection if S1 vertebrae are not involved) or radiofrequency ablation
  - Recurrence exceptionally high (66%), better prognosis in sacrococcygeal lesion due to possibility of complete resection

Tarlov Cyst

Introduction (133)
- Incidental finding in 1% to 5% of patients who had MRI of LS spine, more prevalent in younger patients
- Location: S2 and S3 (MC), at the junction of the dorsal root space between the perineurium and the endoneurium

History and physical examination
- Mostly asymptomatic: symptomatic in ~1% of cases
  - Nonspecific, low back, sacrococcygeal, perineal pain ± possible sciatica, weakness, claudication, and bowel/bladder/sexual dysfunction
  - Symptoms exacerbated by coughing, standing, and change in position (alter CSF pressure)
- Normal physical examination

Diagnosis
- Clinical suspicion confirmed by imaging study
- MRI: fluid-filled lesion (high SI on T2-weighted image), scalloping of the sacral vertebral body (VB) or posterior arch

Treatment
- No need for intervention in most cases (especially in asymptomatic cases). If no other lesion explaining patient's symptoms, then consider treatment
- No consensus for symptomatic cases: NSAID, oral steroid, PT, percutaneous aspiration, and direct microsurgical approach

Hemangioma

Introduction (127)
- MC primary spinal tumor, increase with age, 11% of spines at autopsy
- Thoracic (60%) > lumbar (29%), multiple in up to 30%
- Vertebral body, posterior element involvement is rare (more frequent in symptomatic cases)

History and physical examination
- Most cases: asymptomatic
- Symptomatic in <1%; mid-back (T3 to T9 level) pain secondary to bone, soft tissue, epidural extension, or due to pathologic fracture ± nerve/spinal cord compression (symptoms and signs)

Imaging
- X-ray: variably osteolytic, increased prominence of vertical striations due to reinforcement of the remaining vertebral cortical trabeculae "corduroy" pattern
- CT scan: spotted appearance (thickened trabeculae interspersed by low attenuating fat)
- MRI: increased SI in T1 and T2 images, interosseous lesion usually decreased in T1 and increased in T2

Treatment
- Referral to intervention only in symptomatic lesion; minimally invasive procedure with embolization, alcohol ablation, or radiotherapy
- Referral to surgery if cord or root is compressed

Vertebral Osteomyelitis

Introduction (134)
- Incidence: 2.4/100,000, increasing with age
- Location: lumbar spine: MC involved, >50%
- Mechanism: hematogenous seeding, direct inoculation at the time of spinal surgery, or contiguous spread from an infection in the adjacent soft tissue
- S. aureus: MC >E. coli, gram negative in immunocompromised

History and physical examination
- Back pain (86%), usually at the site of infection, not relieved by rest
  - Nonspecific: average delay between the onset and diagnosis: ~1.5 to 2 months
  - Severe lancinating and sharp back pain ➔ R/O epidural abscess
- Fever: invariable (35%–60%) and neurologic impairment in 1/3
- Tenderness on percussion <20%, neurological examination (root and spinal cord involvement depending on the level); usually normal initially

Diagnosis
- Clinical suspicion confirmed by imaging and serologic study
- Radiologic study
  - X-ray: low sensitive and specificity
    - Blurring of the vertebral endplate region ➔ disc space narrowing
  - MRI: high accuracy (90%), more sensitive than CT for the early detection of osteomyelitis
    - High T2 signal intensity within the disc, loss of the intranuclear cleft
    - The disc space and two adjacent vertebral bodies are involved (vs disc is spared in tumor/metastasis).
  - If MRI is contraindicated, consider CT or PET scan
    - CT-guided percutaneous biopsy
  - Difficult to differentiate from erosive osteochondrosis
- Serologic study
  - CBC: increased leukocyte or neutrophils >80%; not sensitive <50% of cases)
  - ESR and CRP (sensitivity: 98% and 100%); CRP is correlated with the clinical response
  - Blood culture (positive in 58%–78%), if + imaging and negative culture then biopsy warranted (or if polymicrobial, from intra-abdominal sepsis, then biopsy warranted)

PYOGENIC OSTEOMYELITIS	TUBERCULOUS OSTEOMYELITIS (POTT'S DISEASE)
	In history of exposure, or from endemic region
More common in lumbar spine	More common in thoracic spine (thoracolumbar junction)
Early involvement of intervertebral discs	Sparing or later involvement of discs
Spinal deformity: less common	Spinal deformity (gibbus): common
Small paraspinal abscess, less common	Large paraspinal abscess, common
Rapid progression, often severe pain	Slow progression, mild pain
High erythrocyte sedimentation rate (ESR)	ESR: may be normal
Subligamentous spreads uncommon	Subligamentous spread more common

ESR, erythrocyte sedimentation rate.
Source: From Ref. (132). Fast A, Goldsher D. *Navigating the Adult Spine: Bridging Clinical Practice and Neuroradiology.* New York: Demos; 2007: 186.

Treatment
- ER transfer, admit the patient, IV antibiotic for 4 to 6 weeks (ID consult)
- Spine surgery consult if not responsive to medical treatment, chronic osteomyelitis, neurological complications (signs of cord compression, spinal instability, or epidural abscess)
- After stabilized, needs early mobilization and outpatient PT
- If significant neurological sequelae present, consider short-term inpatient rehabilitation

Rheumatologic Diseases

Diffuse Idiopathic Skeletal Hyperostosis

Introduction (135)
- Ossification/calcification of ligament and enthesis in the axial skeleton (anterolateral spine)
- Prevalence: 2.7% to 27.3% (Caucasian >Asian, male > female, >50 years old)
- Thoracic spine (middle and lower part) MC involved
  - Extraspinal manifestations: iliac crests, ischial tuberosity, pubis, lateral acetabulum, greater/lesser trochanters, quad tendon insertion, medial/lateral epicondyles, foot: the plantar fascia attachment to calcaneus, plantar lig., Achilles tendon insertion, etc.
- Associated with hyperinsulinemia, obesity, hyperuricemia, dyslipidemia, hypertension (HTN), CAD, and prolonged use of isotretinol

History and physical examination (135)
- Stiffness and decreased range ± back pain (often not prominent)
  - ± Mechanical effect of ossification: spinal stenosis with ossification of lig. flavum, supra/infraspinatus ligament, dysphagia with cervical involvement
- Peripheral enthesopathy: stiffness, tenderness, not as painful as enthesopathy of spondyloarthritis

Diagnosis
- Clinical suspicion confirmed by imaging study
- Diagnosis: flowing ossification (anterior longitudinal ligament), two or three vertebrae (in thoracic), without degenerative disc disease, facet ankylosis, or SI joint erosion, fusion, and sclerosis
  - More in lower thoracic (7th–10th thoracic vertebrae), right side > left
  - SI joint: lower 2/3 is usually spared and facet joint usually spared
- Clinical manifestations compared with ankylosing spondylitis (AS) (136)

	DISH	AS
Age of onset	>50 years	<40 years
Kyphosis, limited spinal mobility, limited chest expansion	Frequent	Very frequent
Pain	Unusual	Very frequent
X-ray		
Hyperostosis	Very frequent (right side)	Frequent
SI Jt. involvement	Unusual except lig. obliteration	Very frequent
Facet Jt. obliteration	Absent	Very frequent
ALL ossification	Very frequent	Unusual
PLL ossification	Very frequent	Frequent
Syndesmophytes	Absent	Unusual
Enthesopathy	Without erosion (painful)	More with erosions >without (not painful)
HLA-B27	Very low (2%–8%)	50% (African American)-90% (European white)

ALL, anterior longitudinal ligament; Jt., joint; PLL, posterior longitudinal ligament; HLA, human leukocyte antigen; SI Jt: sacroiliac joint.

Treatment
- Conservative management: pain control (NSAID, AAP), core stabilization exercise, ROM/flexibility training, and standing-based lumbar extension exercise
- Surgical referral for removal of osteophytes in cases of severe dysphagia despite speech/swallow therapy

Ankylosing Spondylitis (47)

Introduction
- Inflammatory spine disease, usually in the form of sacroiliitis and spondylitis, which may lead to syndesmophyte formation and ankylosis
- Prevalence: 0.1% to 0.9%, higher in Asians, <40 years old (peak in 2nd–3rd decades)

- Increased risk of spinal cord injury and vertebral fracture
  ○ MC location: cervicothoracic junction (C5–7: 72%): more common than T or L spine
  ○ Likelihood of SCI: 11.4 times higher → imaging even with minor trauma
    ▪ Mechanism: slippage (53%)

History and physical examination
- Back pain (inflammatory, improves with exercise) and morning stiffness
  ○ Low-back and buttock pain/stiffness (SI joint: earlier involvement and most characteristic), neck and hip pain as well
  ○ Pain in the posterior heel and anterior knee from enthesopathy (25% involved)
- Examination of spinal mobility for a FU
  ○ Modified Schober index for lumbar mobility
  ○ Chest expansion for thoracic mobility: The difference to the nearest 0.1 cm between full expiration and full inspiration, measured at the nipples level
- Extraskeletal manifestations: uveitis (MC extra-articular manifestation), iritis, and aortitis (aortic regurgitation)
  ○ Vital capacity: inspiratory capacity: more significantly affected by reduced spinal mobility

Diagnosis
- Clinical diagnosis with imaging study
  ○ Modified NY criteria: sacroiliitis on x-ray + 1 of the following:
    ▪ H/O inflammatory back pain (<40 YO, >3months, improves with activity)
    ▪ Decreased ROM of spine
    ▪ Limited chest expansion
- Lab: negative RF, ANA, normal ESR, + HLA-B27
- Imaging study
  ○ X-ray: SI joint: erosion and pseudo-widening → fused SI joint, ossification of ALL and posterior facet, annular fibrosis, squaring, syndesmophytes (vertebral ossification and bridging), "bamboo spine"
  ○ MRI: inflammatory chondritis and subchondral osteitis (iliac and sacral surface: inferior 2/3): earlier fracture

Treatment (137)
- Therapeutic exercise to promote spine extension (prone lying with sleeping without a pillow), home therapy, and PT
- Indomethacin, sulfasalazine, methotrexate, TNF inhibitor (infliximab: effective on the musculoskeletal and GI complaints)
- Jewett brace; often poorly tolerated
- Engage in non-contact sports rather than contact sports

Paget's Disease

Introduction (138)
- Prevalence: 3% to 4%, primarily in Anglo-Saxons, family history present in 14% to 40%
- Etiology (unclear): genetic, environmental, and possibly viral (paramyxovirus)
- Location: predilection for axial skeleton and lumbar spine (58%), skull in 42%, thoracic spine in 45%, and cervical (14%)
- Pathophysiology
  ○ Increased bone resorption → mixed osteolytic-osteoblastic phase with deposition with ineffective mineralization
  ○ Thickened, highly vascularized fibrous tissue

History and physical examination
- Asymptomatic (>70%); for those with symptomatic back pain: 13% to 43% of patients with spine involvement
  ○ Local pain often with warmth, worse with rest
  ○ ± Spinal stenosis (2/3 have radiologic findings of spinal stenosis) and nerve compression
    ▪ Myelopathy and CES: rare
- MC neurologic manifestations: cranial nerve (CN) involvement (MC), hearing loss, and CNS involvement (138)

Diagnosis
- Clinical suspicion confirmed with imaging study
- X-ray: lytic lesion in early phase; mottled appearance in skull, tibia, pelvis, and vertebral body
- Increased bone turnover markers (alkaline phosphatase, and urine hydroxyproline)

Treatment
- Observation in asymptomatic patients
- Pharmacological treatment: bisphosphonate; first line treatment (alendronate, zoledronate)
  ○ Calcitonin in acute phase (inhibit osteoclastic activity) and calcium supplementation
- FU with bone marker or bone scan q3–6 months

MUSCLE AND LIGAMENT PATHOLOGY

Myofascial LBP

Introduction (139)
- Very common, up to 95% of people with chronic pain, coexisting with other pathologies
- Controversial diagnosis and assessment (often concomitant to other lumbar spine pathologies)
- MC location: quadratus lumborum and gluteus medius (140)

History and physical examination
- Localized back pain ± referred pain (typical referred pain zone in Figure 6.2)
- Palpation of trigger points (tender spots in a taut band) with predictable pain referral pattern, limited ROM (diagnostic criteria) ± local twitch response
- Normal motor, sensory examination, DTR, and provocative tests (SLR)
- Tightness of muscles (hamstrings, rectus femoris, and hip external rotators) common

Diagnosis
- Clinical diagnosis (± good response to trigger point injections); different criteria available
- X-ray and MRI: to evaluate the differential diagnosis (lumbar spine pathologies). Normal in isolated myofascial LBP (concomitant pathologies are very common)
- US: experimental (141); localization, elasticity of the tissues (elastogram) as well as to visualize twitch response
- Differential diagnosis (Ddx): fibromyalgia (can coexist as well) and other lumbar pathologies

Treatment
- Trigger point injection (dry needling ± lidocaine, and/or steroid initially) ± US guidance (deeper muscles such as quadratus lumborum or small hip external rotators)
- Pain medications as needed ± short-term muscle relaxants (no clear evidence)
- PT for manual therapy (myofascial release, deep pressure massage, osteopathic manipulation, spray and stretch using ethyl chloride), education for correct biomechanics, transcutaneous electrical nerve stimulation (TENS) unit
- Recommend/encourage gradual aerobic endurance exercise (fast walking or jogging) at home

Iliolumbar Ligament Sprain

Introduction (142)
- Anatomy (143)
  - L5 transverse process (anterior, inferior-lateral) to the upper part of the iliac crest (tuberosity)
  - Anterior (1-cm long, 0.5-cm wide) and posterior band (3–4 cm long, 0.5- to 1-cm wide, 2–3 mm thick)
  - Major stabilizer of the vertebral spine and the pelvis (144)
    - Limit anterior displacement of L5 on the sacrum during flexion and torsion
    - Three major lumbopelvic ligaments: iliolumbar, sacrotuberous, and sacrospinous ligaments
- Often attributed to the acute LBP on lifting or sudden slouching

History and physical examination
- LBP, medial/posterior to the ilium (lumbopelvic junction), attributed to slouching
- Worsening of pain on flexion and contralateral bending
  - Pain without significant axial force and with erector spinae muscle relaxed

Diagnosis
- Clinical diagnosis and US-guided lidocaine injection with small volume

Treatment (145)
- Physical therapy; not specific; flexibility (SI mobilization, stretching of hamstring, hip external rotator, rectus femoris), core stabilization, dynamic balance exercise, and aerobic endurance exercise
- US-guided steroid injection and prolotherapy (to the attachment site for the ilium)
  - Medial to lateral with longitudinal view; under erector spinae muscles (lateral to the transverse process)

CHEST WALL PAIN

BONE AND JOINT PATHOLOGY

Rib Fracture (Other than 1st Rib)

Incidence
- Epidemiology: prevalence is dramatically underreported, MC non-spine fracture in the elderly and MC fracture in older men (incidence: 2.5/1,000 person years) (146)
- Etiology
  - Stress fracture
    - Common in some athletes: golfer (beginner and amateur) and rower (elite), female > male
    - Minor trauma in patients with osteoporosis, Paget's disease, RA, coughing bouts in elderly
  - Direct trauma (fall, direct blow)
  - Pathologic fracture (metastatic lesion from lung, breast, prostate cancer)
- Location: posterolateral angles; common, due to serratus anterior and external oblique muscles (downward bending force), interdigitate or anterolateral (4th–8th ribs)
  - Floating (11 and 12th) ribs: avulsion of the attachments of external oblique muscles by opposing force of latissimus dorsi and external oblique muscles

History and physical examination
- Insidious onset of posterior thorax pain under the scapula. Pain may radiate in the distribution of the intercostal nerve
- LBP from 11th and 12th rib fractures
- Local tenderness and rarely crepitus

Diagnosis
- Clinical suspicion confirmed by imaging study
- X-ray (can be negative initially), ultrasound (discontinuity of the cortex; time-consuming), and bone scan

Treatment
- Rest from provocative activity for 4 to 6 weeks
- Return to sport in 10 weeks
- Gradual strengthening of serratus anterior and external oblique muscle
- Evaluation of osteoporosis and management

Slipping Rib Syndrome

Incidence (147)
- ~3% of new referrals to general medical/gastroenterology clinic
- Hypermobility of 8th to 10th ribs' costal cartilage: medial fibrous attachment inadequate or ruptured → cartilage slip superiorly and impinge on the intercostal nerve above (inferior rib slip under the superior rib)
- Referred as rib-tip, Cyriax's syndrome, clicking rib syndrome
- Female > male, unilateral, various sports using trunk

History and physical examination
- Pain under the rib cage (lower thoracic) or upper abdomen with muscle movements (Valsalva, respiratory movement, twisting, turning chest, or palpation)
  - Intermittent sharp stabbing pain for a few minutes or dull ache pain lasting as long as 5 days
- Hooking maneuver: lies on an unaffected side, hooks their fingers under the lower costal margin and pulls anteriorly, reproduces the pain with clicking

Diagnosis
- Clinical diagnosis: pain in the lower chest or upper abdomen, tender spot of the lower costal margin, and reproduction of the pain by palpation

Treatment
- Strapping of the rib and manual therapy such as costovertebral joint manipulation
- Local nerve block/intercostal nerve block or botulism toxin injection (to transverse abdominis, external oblique, rectus abdominis, and quadratus lumborum: case report)

Costochondritis

Incidence (148)
- 30% of chest pain in ER, 13% of musculoskeletal (MSK) chest pain (20% of chest pain) presented to primary care doctors
- Capsulitis without true joint pathologies, not likely degenerative
- Associated conditions: seronegative arthropathies, angina pain
- Location: 2nd to 5th costal cartilage

History and physical examination
- Anterior (upper) chest wall pain with tenderness localized to costochondral junction of 1 or more ribs without notable swelling, heat, and erythema
- Crowing rooster maneuver: abducted arm (90° to 100°) with examiner hyperabducting the arm from back (stretch anterior chest wall) → reproduction of pain
- Aggravated by movements of upper body, deep breathing, or exertional activity

Diagnosis
- Clinical diagnosis
- X-ray: normal. Bone scan (gallium scintigraphy), CT scan to R/O infections or neoplasms
- Possible diagnostic injection under US with 0.5 mL of lidocaine

Treatment
- Self-limiting usually within a year
- Stretching exercise, manual therapy, NSAID (often 2–3 months)
- US-guided steroid injection for pain control

Tietze's Syndrome

Introduction
- Uncommon, younger age group
- Painful nonsuppurative swelling of the cartilaginous articulation of the anterior chest wall
- 2nd and 3rd costochondral junctions
- Self-limiting

History and physical examination (149)

	TIETZE SYNDROME	COSTOCHONDRITIS
Nature of pain	Aching, sharp, initially stabbing later dull aching	Aching, sharp, pressure-like
Onset of pain	New vigorous physical activity (excessive coughing or vomiting, chest impact)	Repetitive physical activity, rarely at rest
Physical examination	Usually single and unilateral, 2nd and 3rd costochondral joints involved. Signs of inflammation present. ± Swelling (pain worse with swelling)	Multiple and unilateral >90%. 2nd-5th costochondral junctions. No signs of inflammation. No swelling

(continued)

Diagnosis
- Diagnosis of exclusion (R/O RA and pyogenic arthritis), negative imaging study (CT may show sclerosis of the sternal manubrium, partial calcification of the costal cartilage, and soft-tissue swelling)

Treatment
- Reassurance, NSAIDs, or acetaminophen for symptomatic pain control
- Steroid/lidocaine injection to the cartilage or intercostal nerve block in refractory patient

Bone Tumor

Sternum: primary tumor is rare; usually metastatic: plasma cell, myeloma, lymphoma, and chondrosarcoma

Rib: metastasis (primary lung tumor) > primary (osteochondroma [exostosis] at costochondral junction: MC) (150)

Costovertebral Joint Subluxation

Incidence (151)
- Common in some sports; rowing (19% of whole injuries) and butterfly swimming
- Etiology
  - Malalignment of the costovertebral joints and abnormal serratus anterior muscle contraction/strain

History and physical examination
- Upper back pain with referral to the lateral or anterior chest wall (common at 6th or 7th rib level)
- Worsening pain on lateral bending of the spine, deep inspiration, coughing, and sneezing
- Tenderness on the anterior portion of the 7th rib with pronounced kyphosis

Diagnosis
- Clinical diagnosis
- X-ray to R/O rib fracture or thoracic spine pathology

Treatment
- Manipulation: lie prone with arms elevated above the head and the head turned away from the painful side
  - Move rib cage (force on the rib downward, forward, and lateral directions) with audible and palpable click

NERVE PATHOLOGIES

Discogenic Thoracic Radiculopathy

Introduction (152)
- Rare, 0.15 to 4% of symptomatic disc herniations of the spine
- Male = female, peak in 3rd and 6th decades of life
- MC level of disc herniation: T11–12 (50%)

History and physical examination
- Radiating pain in the chest wall ± sensory symptoms (tingling, pins/needle sensation)
  - Dermatomal level: T4: nipple, T6: xyphoid, T10: umbilicus
  - Rarely LBP or shoulder pain
- Physical exam: not reliable, spine and paraspinal tenderness

Diagnosis
- Clinical suspicion supplemented by imaging study and EMG test
- MRI to evaluate mechanical causes of radiculopathy
- EMG to evaluate nonmechanical radiculopathy
  - Needle EMG of rectus abdominis as well as paraspinal muscles
- Differential diagnosis of thoracic radiculopathy with disc disease
  - Diabetic thoracic radiculopathy, herpes zoster intercostal neuralgia, intercostal strain, etc
  - Scheuermann's disease, osteomyelitis, achondroplasia, and epidural lipomatosis

Treatment
- Conservative treatment; usually successful (~75% return to previous functional level), NSAIDs, muscle relaxant, physical modalities, and spinal extension exercise
- Epidural steroid injection, or intercostal nerve block for pain control if not responsive to conservative management (153)
- Surgery: unremitting thoracic radicular pain by structural disease (failed conservative treatment) and/or progressive myelopathy
  - Anterior (transthoracic), posterior (pediclofacetectomy), and lateral (costotransversectomy and lateral extracavitary) approach

Diabetic Thoracic Radiculoneuropathy

Introduction (82)
- Rare, no epidemiologic study, but also underrecognized
- Consideration in radiculopathy without significant discal pathology or spondylosis

History and physical examination
- Band-like pain from thoracic spine region radiating toward the chest, often a feeling of tightness, "asleep" or "prickling" numbness with allodynia; clothing uncomfortable
- Flaccid outpouching of abdomen; weakness, focal area of anhidrosis

Diagnosis
- Clinical suspicion confirmed by needle EMG (fibrillation in thoracic paraspinal muscle or rectus abdominis muscle)
- MRI to evaluate disc disease or other spinal cord disease, especially with red flags (to R/O leptomeningeal metastasis)

Treatment
- Referral to neurology for immunotherapy IVIG ± prednisone, prednisone ± cyclosporine
- Pain medications for neuropathic pain, TENS, core muscle stabilization, chest PT, aerobic endurance exercise as necessary

Intercostal Neuritis

Introduction (154)
- Etiology: varicella zoster (MC), trauma (rib fracture), thoracotomy, lung cancer and primary tumor, or idiopathic

History and physical examination
- Chest wall pain of neuropathic pain characteristics

Diagnosis
- Clinical diagnosis with EMG study to R/O thoracic radiculopathy or other differential and nerve block

Treatment
- Pain control with NSAID, TCA, or gabapentin. TENS as needed
- US-guided nerve block

MUSCLE STRAIN

Intercostal Muscle Strain

Introduction (149)
- MC muscle strain (50%) in the chest wall followed by pectoralis muscle
- Anatomy: three incomplete thin layers of muscular and tendinous fibers: external, internal, and innermost layers
- Etiology: excessive exertion of untrained muscles with activities like painting a ceiling, chopping wood, or coughing or rowing
- Precordial catch syndrome: intercostal muscle spasm in the left parasternal area or near the cardiac apex, no local tenderness, relieved by correcting posture

History and physical examination
- Pain (localized) increased with deep inspiration, cough, and tenderness

Diagnosis
- Clinical diagnosis and imaging study to R/O rib fracture
- Differential diagnosis: intercostal neuralgia, thoracic radiculopathy, other causes of chest wall pain (eg, rib fracture)

Treatment
- Reassurance, local heat application/TENS, and analgesics
- Injection of lidocaine or steroid reserved for refractory cases
- US guidance to avoid injection to intercostal vessels and underlying lung

Abdominal Muscle Strain

Introduction (155)
- Anatomy
  - Internal, external, and transverse oblique abdominis muscle strain

MUSCLE	ORIGIN	INSERTION	INNERVATION	ACTION/FUNCTION
Internal oblique	Inguinal ligament, anterior 2/3 of the iliac crest, and thoraco-lumbar fascia	Course upward medially (in ventral) to the costal cartilages of the 9th, 10th, 11th, and 12th ribs and the linea alba	Ventral rami, T6–11, L1	Trunk side bending and rotation to the same side) Expiratory, act as an antagonist (opponent) to the action of diaphragm
External oblique	Lower 8 ribs, blending with the serratus anterior muscle and latissimus dorsi	Downward medially to the linea alba anteriorly and iliac crest inferiorly	T7–12 ventral rami	Trunk flexion and rotation to the opposite site Inspiratory (pull chest downward)
Transverse oblique	Lat 1/3 of inguinal ligament from the anterior 3/4 of the inner lip of the iliac crest, from the inner surfaces of the cartilages of the lower 6 ribs, interdigitating with the diaphragm, and from the lumbodorsal fascia	Aponeurosis/linea alba and the inguinal aponeurotic falx (the conjoint tendon)	T7–11, ilioinguinal and iliohypogastric N	Thoracic and pelvic stability

- Etiology
  - Direct trauma, strain, and repetitive overuse (trunk rotation)
  - Pitcher (in nondominant side, eccentric contraction of muscles during late cocking and acceleration phases)
  - Cricket bowlers, javelin throwers, rowers, swimmers, and ice hockey players

History and physical examination (149)
- Pain on the lower 4 rib cage or chest wall, increased by resisted side flexion to the affected side
- Local tenderness

Diagnosis (156)
- Clinical diagnosis supplemented by imaging study
- US: diagnosis and guidance for injection
  - Acute injury findings: hematoma, fluid between muscle layers, loss of normal architecture, gap in the insertion of the internal oblique to costal cartilages and ribs
  - Not sensitive to assess chronic injury and small tears
- MRI
  - Evaluate severity of the injury, neighboring structures (rib fracture), but can be limited due to motion artifact (from breathing)
  - Findings: hematoma, periosteal stripping, or stress injury to the ribs

Treatment
- Recovery: 2 to 10 weeks (4–6 weeks to return to play)
- Re-occurrence: common in the first 2 years
- Pain medications
- Steroid injection: limited evidence, quicker recovery and return to play
  - US to avoid injection into intercostal vessels and underlying lung

Others: Serratus Anterior Strain

Introduction
- Unknown epidemiology but under-recognized
- Increased incidence in a few sports such as rowing and weightlifting

History and physical examination
- Pain around the medial border of the scapula ± radiate to the anterior chest

Diagnosis
- Clinical diagnosis with typical pain on resisted scapular protraction
- Differential diagnosis: myofascial pain syndrome of rhomboids, scapulothoracic bursitis

Treatment
- Rest from activities, may take weeks, symptomatic pain control
- US-guided steroid injection to the muscle (may inject over the rib between intercostal space covered by the finger)

BUTTOCK PAIN

BONE AND JOINT PATHOLOGY

SI Joint Dysfunction

Introduction (160)
- Epidemiology: 13% to 30% of chronic LBP population (161)

- Etiology and risk factors
  - Axial loading and abrupt rotation ➔ capsular or synovial disruption
  - Leg length discrepancy (functional or anatomical), gait abnormality, prolonged vigorous exercise, scoliosis, and spinal fusion to the sacrum
  - Pregnancy
    - Increased weight gain, exaggerated lordotic posture, the mechanical trauma of parturition, and hormone induced ligament laxity

History and physical examination (38)
- Low back/buttock pain (midline or paramedian at the level of iliac crest) ± radiation to lower buttock and posterior thigh (occasionally below knee and anterior groin)
- Physical examination
  - ≥3 provocative tests; related to high positive predictive values (60%–87%) to SI joint injection
    - Tenderness on the sacral sulcus on prone position
    - Patrick test (FABER), Gaenslen's test, or Gillet's test
    - Distraction test, side-lying iliac compression test and prone sacrum compression test
  - Other tests; Fortin's finger (patient points the location of maximal pain to the SI dimple). Thigh thrust maneuver (supine with hip 90° flexion, examiner stabilizes the opposite ASIS and presses the knee (axial compression to the femur): positive if pain on the SI region

Diagnosis
- Clinical diagnosis confirmed by imaging-guided injection
- X-ray
  - AP and pelvic oblique views, modified Ferguson view
- CT/MRI to evaluate the differential diagnosis
- US for needle guidance, but intraarticular injection needs fluoroscope guidance to confirm
  - US guidance: may avoid intravascular injection

Treatment
- Address the underlying biomechanical problems: leg-length discrepancy (functional, pronation response) by heel lift or shoe lift
- Physical therapy, manual therapy
  - If restriction present, mobilization, stretch the hip rotator (piriformis; attached to sacrum), hamstrings, iliopsoas (muscle-controlling pelvic tilt)
  - Pelvic stabilization exercise (to control hyperactive ipsilateral gluteus muscles and contralateral latissimus muscles)
- Pelvic or sacral belt: decrease sagittal rotation, especially in pregnant woman
- Interventional management
  - Intra-articular steroid injection (162) using fluoroscopy or US (fluoroscopy has better accuracy than US, but clinical outcome similar)
    - US: detect periarticular blood vessels
  - Radiofrequency denervation of lateral branches of S1 to 3 (S4) or L5 posterior ramus
  - Evidence limited for short-term and long-term reliefs from intra-articular steroid injection and periarticular injection with steroid (163)
- Referral to surgery (fusion) if failed conservative management

Osteitis Condensans Ilii
Introduction (164)
- Prevalence: 0.9 to 2.5%, young female (<4th decade), common after pregnancy (but not exclusive)
- Sclerosis of ilium (at the SI joint), unknown pathophysiology, but not inflammatory

History and physical examination
- Axial/bilateral low back/buttock pain ± radiation of pain to the posterior thigh
- No sensory or motor symptoms and normal neurological signs
- FABER: positive and focal tenderness on contralateral SI joint

Diagnosis
- Clinical diagnosis confirmed by imaging study
- X-ray: well-defined triangular sclerosis with ossification affecting the iliac portion of the SI joint without narrowing of the joint space, bilateral and symmetric
  - Differential diagnosis from ankylosing spondylitis
- MRI: for other differential diagnosis (sacroiliitis, ankylosing spondylitis, metabolic bone disease)
- Negative inflammatory markers usually (HLA negative although ESR is variable)

Treatment
- Physical therapy, NSAID, image-guided steroid injections
- Surgical resection of osteitic bone if disabling pain despite other treatments

Coccygodynia
Introduction (165)
- Female > male by 5 times, mean age of onset: 40 years old
- Anatomy (166)
  - Coccyx: four bony segments. Site for attachment for gluteus maximus, coccygeal muscle, and anococcygeal ligament
  - Sacrococcygeal joint: either symphysis or true synovial joint
  - The ganglion impar: the lowest node in the paravertebral sympathetic chain, fusion of two sacral sympathetic trunks, located along the anterior aspect of the sacrococcygeal joint and coccyx
- Classification: traumatic (much more common) and idiopathic form (<1% of all nontraumatic vertebral column disorder)
- Etiology and risk factors
  - Trauma (a fall in a seated position; a direct blow to the coccyx), repetitive microtrauma (inadequate sitting position or activities (cycling or motor sports), or parturition
  - High body mass index

History and physical examination (167)
- Pain in the coccyx (pain localized just above the anus), usually provoked by sitting, walking, and defecation. Cycling: worse
- Pain/reproduction of symptoms with manual examination/mobilization

Diagnosis
- Clinical diagnosis aided by imaging and image-guided injection
- Imaging: x-ray (standard and dynamic sitting on hard stool: provocative), R/O fracture
- MRI: usually not necessary. Recommended if patient is not responsive to initial treatment or atypical presentation

- Differential diagnosis: epidermal inclusion cyst, levator ani syndrome, coccygeal bone disease (osteomyelitis, arthritis, lipoma, intraosseous chondroma, avascular necrosis [AVN]), radiculopathy or neurogenic tumor, meningeal cyst, chordoma, and paragangliomas

Treatment
- Avoidance of direct pressure, stool softener, padding (ring-shaped), and ice
- Manual mobilization (intra-rectal)
  - Sacrococcygeal mobilization can be achieved by pelvic floor muscle stretching and strengthening exercise
- Injection (to sacrococcygeal joint) and ganglion impar block/radiofrequency ablation through anococcygeal or sacrococcygeal ligaments using fluoroscopy or US (fluoroscopy is better than US) (168)
- Surgery referral for excision: rare, disabling pain despite all other treatments

TENDON AND BURSA PATHOLOGY

Piriformis Syndrome

Introduction (169)
- Prevalence: 5% to 35% (on different studies) of patients with low-back (buttock) pain and sciatica (170)
- Anatomy and biomechanics (Figure 6.9)
  - Sciatic nerve under (deeper) the piriformis in 83%, nerve passing through the muscle in 13%, and others
  - Hip rotator: external with hip extension (erect/stand) and internal rotator (and abductor) with hip 90° flexion
  - Abductor in supine, and weak hip flexor in walking
- Risk factors
  - Anatomical variation; split or hypertrophied piriformis muscle, split sciatic nerve
  - Piriformis muscle overloading (long-distance walking or running) with relative inflexibility of the other hip external rotators and adductors and weakness of the hip abductors
  - Gluteal trauma (often subtle), rarely after total hip arthroplasty and C section

History and physical examination
- Buttock pain (in the gluteal triangle) ± posterior hip and thigh pain
- Normal motor, sensory examination, DTR of lower extremities; negative SLR
- Provocative maneuver: Pace maneuver, Freiberg test, FADIR (flexion, adduction, and internal rotation) with reproduction of symptom

Diagnosis
- Clinical diagnosis with imaging and EMG to evaluate differential diagnosis
- EMG to evaluate LS radiculopathy, controversial for piriformis syndrome
  - Supportive finding for piriformis syndrome: the asymmetric latency of H reflex in functional posture (producing symptoms such as FADIR)
- MRI to evaluate lumbar pathology and other pelvic/SI pathologies
  - Asymmetric hypertrophy of the piriformis muscle and sciatic nerve; hyperintensity in MR neurography; 63% sensitivity and 93% specificity
- Differential diagnoses (often concomitant): LS radiculopathy, SI joint dysfunction, obturator internus syndrome, gluteal myofascial pain syndrome, etc

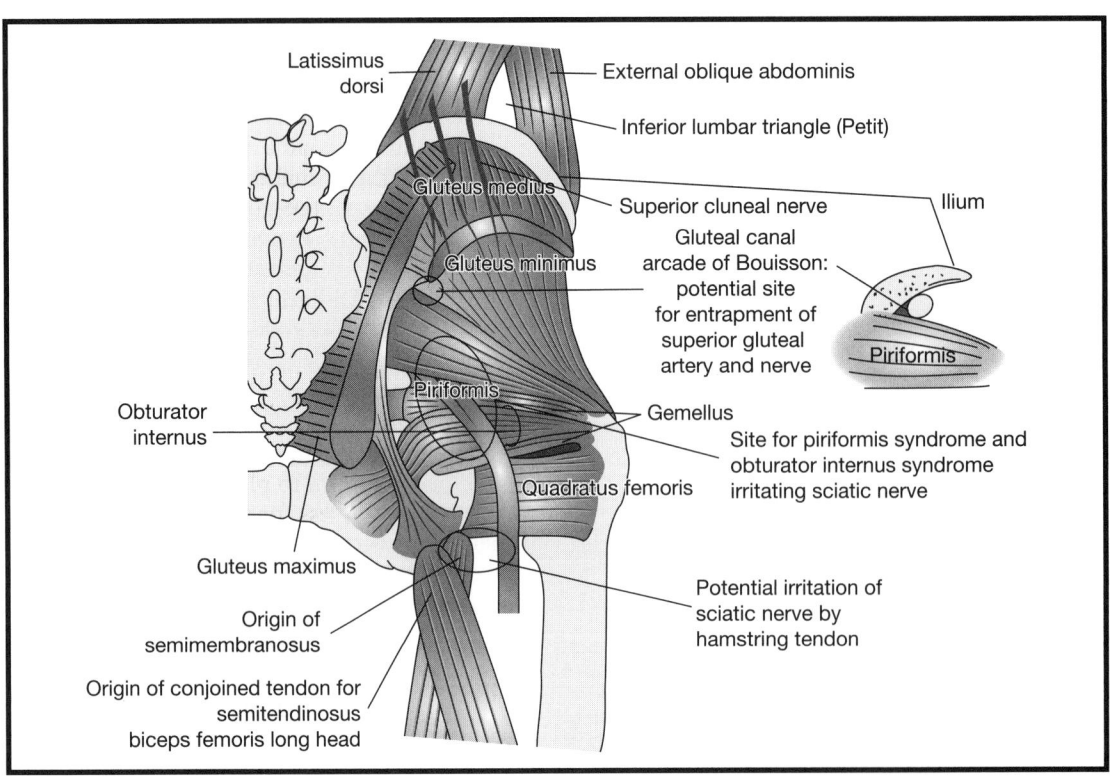

FIGURE 6.9
Piriformis muscle and tendon in the buttock with gluteal canal.

Treatment (171)
- PT: modality (US), stretching (internal/external rotation, hip adduction, iliopsoas and hamstring), isometric strengthening (then gradually to resistive), strengthening gluteal muscles, myofascial release (probably to the gluteus maximus rather than piriformis), then LS stabilization
- Injection
  - One finger palpates the tender muscle spot through the rectum (blind) and needle toward the finger, lateral to medial (be cautious of sciatic nerve)
  - US-guided: more accurate than fluoroscopy-guided injection
    - Identify sciatic nerve and accompanying gluteal artery using Doppler and avoid these structures
    - Initially steroid injection followed by Botox injection if there is muscle hypertrophy
    - Peri-sciatic injection (hydrodissection) if not responsive

Obturator Internus Syndrome
Introduction (172)
- Rare, but likely under-recognized (difficult to distinguish it from piriformis syndrome)
- Classification: strain, myofascial pain syndrome, muscle spasm, calcific tendinopathy, contusion, and bursitis
- Initial stage of SLR test: obturator internus muscles impinge on the sciatic nerve (but not the piriformis muscles) (173)

History and physical examination
- Buttock (gluteal triangle/mid-buttock, retro-trochanteric) pain
  - Pain with sitting can be attributed to either the obturator internus [OI] or the hamstring–ischial bursa complex
  - Symptoms of pudendal (perineal region) and sciatic nerve irritation (radiating leg pain)
- Tenderness in the interval between the piriformis muscle and the ischial tuberosity
- Provocative test: similar to piriformis, +FADIR, Freiberg sign, and PACE sign

Diagnosis
- Clinical diagnosis confirmed by image-guided injection
- MRI: usually normal
- Diagnostic US-guided injection although the injection can spill to the piriformis and nearby structures

Treatment
- PT for stretching, pelvic stabilization exercise, myofascial release and deep heating modality (US)
- US-guided injection (obturator internus and gluteus maximus or hydrodissection of sciatic nerve)
- Referral to surgical evaluation in disabling pain despite a conservative treatment

Proximal Hamstring Tendinopathy or Tear
Introduction (174)
- Epidemiology: less common than mid- or distal myotendinous lesion (8% to 25% of sports-related injuries), common in soccer (50% in one observational study), recurrent lesion >30%
- Conjoined tendon (semitendinosus and biceps long head; lateral: more commonly involved than semimembranosus (medially attached to ischial tuberosity)
- Mechanism of injury
  - Chronic microtrauma or single acute injury (forceful extension against resistance in basketball, sprinting, soccer, or waterskiing)

History and physical examination
- Ill-defined, deep buttock/posterior proximal thigh pain exacerbated by repetitive activity, such as long-distance running, and often aggravated by sitting (secondary to pain at avulsion site) ± sciatica (below knee)
- Ecchymosis (hematoma) in acute tear, stiff-legged gait (result of avoiding hip and knee flexion)
- Reproduction of pain with resisted hip extension (with knee extension, if knee flexed → more from gluteal muscle) or resisted knee flexion
- Puranen-Orava test: reproduction of symptoms with active stretching of the hamstring muscles in the standing position with the hip flexed at about 90°, the knee fully extended, and the foot on a support (such as a table) (175)

Diagnosis
- Clinical diagnosis confirmed by imaging study
- X-ray: usually negative, may show bony avulsion from the ischial tuberosity
- US and MRI (in doubtful case, to evaluate lumbosacral radiculopathy by MRI of LS spine)
  - MRI more sensitive than US (176)
    - US: unable to show bone marrow edema and discrete partial tears (detected by MRI <5 mm), calcification (US better than MRI) found in 5%
  - MC finding: peritendinitis, fluid or edema adjacent to the proximal hamstring origin
- EMG: if radiating leg pain or sensory and motor symptoms/signs present; to evaluate LS radiculopathy and possibly sciatic neuropathy in the thigh (rare)

Treatment (177)
- Conservative treatment in nondisplaced avulsion or partial tendon tear (single tendon involvement especially biceps femoris; less functional deficit)
  - Steroid injection (US-guided: medial to the sciatic N, avoid vascular structures by Doppler): approach; lateral to medial, pain relief (50% more than 1 month, 25% >6 months)
    - Temporary perineal numbness due to blocking of perineal branch from post-cutaneous nerve of thigh (on hamstring tendon)
  - Shock wave therapy (178): effective at 3 months (>70% in small study)
  - Platelet-rich plasma under US guidance (179): no benefit for early return to play by intramuscular injection (but study did not assess for injection at the attachment)
  - Return to exercise: 4 to 6 weeks
- Indication for surgical referral: tear of three tendons, significant retraction (>5 cm) (if <2 cm: nonoperative) (two tendons tear: surgery is controversial)

Ischiofemoral Impingement
Introduction (180)
- Impingement between the lesser trochanter and ischium usually involving quadratus femoris muscle
- Very rare, unknown prevalence, but under-recognized

- Etiology: idiopathic (or unknown) or intertrochanteric fracture, surgery (valgus producing intertrochanteric osteotomy), arthritis with femoral head migration, and enthesopathy of proximal hamstring tendon

History and physical examination (181)
- Pain and snapping in the buttock and/or groin ± radiation of pain distally
- Reproduced by a combination of extension, adduction, and external rotation of the hip

Diagnosis (182)
- Diagnosis of exclusion with imaging study
- MRI
  - Quadratus femoris edema without disruption of its fibers in T2-axial image
  - Decreased distance between the lesser trochanter and the ischial tuberosity (the ischiofemoral space): 13 ± 5 mm (vs 23 mm in control)
- Differential diagnoses
  - A snapping psoas tendon, LS radiculopathy, piriformis/obturator internus syndrome, hip OA, chronic hamstring injury, quadratus femoris tear, and adductor tendonitis

Treatment
- Physical therapy: pelvic mobilization, stretching/gradual strengthening of hip external rotator, hip adductor, strengthening of gluteal muscle, and deep-heating modality
- Injection: US-guided injection to the lesser trochanter or quadratus femoris
- Arthroscopic decompression/resection of quadratus femoris in disabling pain despite the conservative treatment

ISCHIOGLUTEAL BURSITIS

Introduction (183)
- Bursa (inconsistent) between the ischial tuberosity and gluteus maximus
- Weaver's bottom, rare, but under-recognized (17/768 MRI studies of hip region)
- Etiology
  - Prolonged sitting, tractor driving or road equipment machine driving, falling on buttocks, canoeing, horseback riding, wheelchair athletics
  - Cachexia and severe weight loss in cancer patients; reduction of subcutaneous fat in the buttock region → repetitive trauma of the bursa

History and physical examination
- Pain over the lower gluteal region (inferior to mod. gluteal triangle) and along the hamstring muscle ± occasional radiating pain

Diagnosis
- Clinical diagnosis with tenderness with diagnostic block (guided injection)
- Imaging; US and MRI (global view) (184)
- Differential diagnoses: abscess, hematoma, epidermoid cyst, dermoid cyst, hydatid cyst, gynecological tumor (in female), intra-cortical lesion of femur, or pelvis (tumor), and other causes of buttock pain

Treatment
- Avoid irritating positions, NSAIDs, and PT (to address tight hamstrings and SI mobility or general aerobic endurance exercise for deconditioning)
- Aspiration and injection of the bursa with steroid/lidocaine

Gluteal Aponeurotic Tear

Introduction (185)
- Unknown prevalence, under-recognized cause of posterolateral buttock pain
- Anatomy of aponeurosis: covering gluteus medius (anterior 2/3) from posterior lateral aspect of iliac crest to merge with ITB, just below the iliac crest
- Etiology
  - Trauma or degenerative
  - Fascial disruption with bulging or frank herniation of the underlying musculature
    - Gluteal muscle edema: reactive, muscle contusion, or myotendinous strain

History and physical examination
- Lateral hip and buttock pain: posterior or posterior/posterior-superior aspect of the greater trochanter
- Tenderness on the gluteus medius and maximus

Diagnosis
- Clinical suspicion confirmed by imaging study
- US: may see muscle herniation or effusion
- MRI: increased SI on T2 WI in gluteal muscles and fascia (aponeurosis)

Treatment
- PT for myofascial release, gradual gluteal strengthening exercise, ITB stretching, and deep-heating modality (as needed)
- Steroid injection to fascia with US guidance

NEUROPATHY

Sciatic Neuropathy

Introduction (186)
- 2nd MC neuropathy of the lower extremity
- MC location: hip (due to trauma and masses)
- Anatomy
  - L4 to S4, under the piriformis muscle, but in 10% to 30% (varied depending on studies), fibular branch either through or superficial to the piriformis muscle. Medial (tibial) and lateral division (peroneal; more commonly involved)
  - Location at lower buttock: halfway between the greater trochanter and ischial tuberosity; closer to the ischial tuberosity
  - Divides into common fibular and tibial branches about 6 cm above the popliteal fossa

History and physical examination
- Sensory (tingling, numbness in the posterior thigh, leg, ankle/foot) and motor symptoms (foot slapping, dragging, or frail leg rarely) depending on the severity of the involvement
- Buttock/posterior thigh pain radiating down to the leg/ankle/foot

- Physical examination to localize the lesion
  - Inspection: atrophy of calf, shin, foot intrinsic muscles in severe cases
  - Sensory examination: check dorsum (peroneal) and sole of foot (tibial), sparing medial leg (calf; saphenous), anterior thigh (femoral)
  - Motor examination: weakness in ankle dorsiflexor, plantarflexor, knee flexor, partial involvement of hip extensor (gluteal muscle spared → relatively normal hip extensor with knee flexion, normal hip abductor, hip flexor)
  - DTR: ankle (triceps surae) reflex involved with quadriceps reflex spared

Diagnosis
- Clinical suspicion confirmed by EMG
  - Fibular (peroneal) division of sciatic nerve: more commonly involved due to fascicular arrangement and tethering effect by fibular canal at fibular head
  - Sciatic nerve lesion can be mistaken as fibular N lesion
- NCS and needle EMG
  - Sensory NCS of sural and superficial peroneal nerves: abnormal usually
  - Motor NCS: normal or abnormal if severely involved
  - Abnormal H-reflex study: S1 radiculopathy/sciatic/tibial neuropathy of any duration and Achilles tendon lesion
  - EMG findings: abnormal tibial/peroneal nerve innervated muscles with normal superior/inferior gluteal and femoral nerve innervated muscles and paraspinal muscles
    - Biceps femoris short head (common peroneal nerve above the fibular head)
    - Biceps femoris long head (sciatic nerve)
- US or MRI for anatomic evaluation of sciatic nerve, evaluation of underlying etiologies and assistance in localization (187)

Treatment
- Symptomatic treatment addressing piriformis syndrome or structures irritating the sciatic nerve and medication for neuropathic pain (TCA, gabapentin, etc.)
- Evaluation of ankle foot orthotics (posterior leaf spring orthosis for dorsiflexion assist or semi/solid AFO to control knee partially (eg, knee hyperextension by controlling ankle plantarflexion weakness partially)
- Image-guided injection to control pain (perisciatic nerve injection with hydrodissection of the nerve from a surrounding soft tissue to improve mobility)
- Surgery in progressive lesion, underlying structural lesion, or disabling pain despite conservative management

Superior Cluneal Nerve Entrapment Syndrome

Introduction
- Under-recognized cause of neuropathic buttock pain; unknown prevalence
- Etiology
  - Entrapped between the iliac crest and rigid fibers of the thoracolumbar fascia
  - Posterior iliac crest bone graft or iatrogenic (gluteal muscle injection)
  - Anatomic variation: osteofibrous tunnels formed for medial branch

History and physical examination
- Buttock pain ± intermittent radiation to the lateral trochanter, rarely radiates distally
- Physical examination: tenderness on the posterior iliac crest (5–8 cm from the midline) with reproduction of pain (with radiation of pain down to greater trochanter), pain worse with trunk rotation on sitting (mobility of thoracolumbar junction: also positive for Maigne's syndrome), worsening pain on forward bending (rather than extension)

Diagnosis (24)
- Clinical diagnosis with diagnostic injection; modified Maigne's criteria
  - Unilateral LBP referred to the iliac crest and buttock with relief of symptoms by nerve block along the posterior iliac crest ~7 cm from the midline
  - 1 to 3 mL of 1% lidocaine at 5 to 8 cm lateral to midline L5 at the level of the iliac crest
    - 10 mL in the Maigne's criteria; may not be specific due to large volume
- Imaging: limited value; US may visualize the thickened nerve in the symptomatic side compared to the opposite
  - Focal enlargement: 2.3 ± 0.5 (symptomatic) versus 1.5 ± 0.3 mm (asymptomatic side)
- Differential diagnosis: thoracolumbar syndrome (Maigne's syndrome), lower lumbar facet arthropathy/disc disease, myofascial pain syndrome (gluteus medius, maximus, quadratus lumborum), iliolumbar ligament sprain, iliac crest contusion, gynecologic disorder, bony tumor, etc

Treatment
- PT: myofascial release of gluteus, quadratus lumborum, thoracodorsal fascia, SI joint mobilization, core muscle strengthening, manual therapy for thoracolumbar junction, and TENS as needed
- Steroid injection, alcohol block with/without US guidance and surgery for decompression if failed conservative management

MISCELLANEOUS PATHOLOGY

Superior Gluteal Arterial Disease: Steal, Stenosis, and Thrombosis

Introduction (188)
- Very rare, but under-recognized cause of buttock pain
- Etiology
  - Superior cluneal artery aneurysm (→ can cause superior gluteal nerve entrapment), arteriovenous (AV) malformation, or septic emboli (from infectious endocarditis or chronic septic sacroiliitis) (189)
  - Local entrapment by gluteal canal (osteo-fibro-muscular tunnel, supra-piriformis canal); bony crest of the greater sciatic notch and the arcade of Bouisson
  - Trauma or iatrogenic: hardware (eg, prosthesis of total hip arthroplasty)
- Anatomy: superficial and deep (superior and inferior) arteries
  - Supply gluteal muscle and superior gluteal nerve

History and physical examination
- Buttock claudication: pain after walking consistent distance, followed by quick improvement when stopping (within 15 to 30 seconds)
- Normal physical examinations usually (mild gluteal muscle weakness if superior gluteal nerve involved)

Diagnosis
- Clinical suspicion confirmed by imaging/vascular study
- MRI/magnetic resonance arthrography (MRA) to R/O other common differentials for buttock pain and vascular Doppler (can be negative)
- Selective angiography of aortoiliac artery (190)
- Differential diagnosis
  ○ Buttock claudication; 1.5% to 2% of aortoiliac lesion or AAA
  ○ Inferior gluteal artery aneurysm (191)
    - Extremely rare, after blunt or penetrating trauma
    - Gluteal pain ± pulsating mass, radiating leg pain (sciatic nerve irritation)
    - Clinical suspicion confirmed by imaging study (US → MRA and angiography for intervention)
  ○ Other pain generators for buttock pain

Treatment
- Referral to vascular surgery: angioplasty rather than stent
- Aerobic endurance exercise to the point of claudication, then gradual increase of the length of endurance exercise (to increase the threshold)

Gluteal Compartment Syndrome (192)

Introduction
- Incidence and prevalence: unknown, very rare
- Anatomy: three compartments
  ○ Gluteus maximus; superficial and deep fascia by the fascia lata of the thigh
  ○ Gluteus medius and minimus
  ○ Tensor fascia lata compartment
- Etiology: prolonged local pressure (drug/alcohol intoxication or surgical procedure), recent statin use, trauma, biopsy, or hematoma

History and physical examination
- Buttock pain ± sciatic nerve irritation/impairment (in 50%)
- Tenderness, swelling ± sensory/motor abnormalities of sciatic nerve

Diagnosis
- Clinical suspicion confirmed by increased CPK, and increased intra-compartmental pressure measurement (normal 30 to 45 mmHg)
- Imaging test (CT or MRI) for other differential diagnosis and metabolic panel and urinalysis for acute renal failure

Treatment
- Emergent referral to surgery for fasciotomy followed by PT (or brief inpatient rehabilitation)

REFERENCES

1. Deyo RA, Weinstein JN. Low back pain. *N Engl J Med.* 2001;344(5):363–370.
2. Baker RJ, Patel D. Lower back pain in the athlete: common conditions and treatment. *Prim Care.* 2005;32(1):201–229.
3. Trainor TJ, Wiesel SW. Epidemiology of back pain in the athlete. *Clin Sports Med.* 2002;21(1):93–103.
4. Williams FM, Sambrook PN. Neck and back pain and intervertebral disc degeneration: role of occupational factors. *Best Pract Res Clin Rheumatol.* 2011;25(1):69–79.
5. Costa-Black KM, Loisel P, Anema JR, Pransky G. Back pain and work. *Best Pract Res Clin Rheumatol.* 2010;24(2):227–240.
6. Jarvik JG, Deyo RA. Diagnostic evaluation of low back pain with emphasis on imaging. *Ann Intern Med.* 2002;137(7):586–597.
7. Franklyn-Miller A, Falvey E, McCrory P. The gluteal triangle: a clinical patho-anatomical approach to the diagnosis of gluteal pain in athletes. *Br J Sports Med.* 2009;43(6):460–466.
8. Deyo RA, Rainville J, Kent DL. What can the history and physical examination tell us about low back pain? *JAMA.* 1992;268(6):760–765.
9. Broder J, Snarski JT. Back pain in the elderly. *Clin Geriatr Med.* 2007;23(2):271–89, v.
10. Smith JS, Shaffrey CI, Fu KM, et al. Clinical and radiographic evaluation of the adult spinal deformity patient. *Neurosurg Clin N Am.* 2013;24(2):143–156.
11. El-Hawary R, Chukwunyerenwa C. Update on evaluation and treatment of scoliosis. *Pediatr Clin North Am.* 2014;61(6):1223–1241.
12. Wilson RK, Murinson BB. Sudden spasms following gradual lordosis–the stiff-person syndrome. *Nat Clin Pract Neurol.* 2006;2(8):455–9; quiz 460.
13. Gitelman A, Hishmeh S, Morelli BN, et al. Cauda equina syndrome: a comprehensive review. *Am J Orthop.* 2008;37(11):556–562.
14. Bartynski WS, Petropoulou KA. The MR imaging features and clinical correlates in low back pain-related syndromes. *Magn Reson Imaging Clin N Am.* 2007;15(2):137–54, v.
15. Troup JDG. Biomechanics of the lumbar spinal canal. *Clin Biomech.* 1986;1(1):31–43.
16. An HS, Butler JP. Lumbar spinal stenosis: historical perspectives, classification, and pathoanatomy. *Semin Spine Surg.* 1999;11:184.
17. Lee CK, Rauschning W, Glenn W. Lateral lumbar spinal canal stenosis: classification, pathologic anatomy and surgical decompression. *Spine (Phila Pa 1976).* 1988;13(3):313–20.
18. Suri P, Rainville J, Kalichman L, Katz JN. Does this older adult with lower extremity pain have the clinical syndrome of lumbar spinal stenosis? *JAMA.* 2010;304(23):2628–2636.
19. Rendina EA, Ciccone AM. The intercostal space. *Thorac Surg Clin.* 2007;17(4):491–501.
20. Magalhães JE, Januário AM, Lins OG. Intercostobrachial neuropathy due to axillary compression. *Muscle Nerve.* 2009;39(3):411–412.
21. Bierry G, Simeone FJ, Borg-Stein JP, et al. Sacrotuberous ligament: relationship to normal, torn, and retracted hamstring tendons on MR images. *Radiology.* 2014;271(1):162–171.
22. Apte G, Nelson P, Brismée JM, et al. Chronic female pelvic pain-part 1: clinical pathoanatomy and examination of the pelvic region. *Pain Pract.* 2012;12(2):88–110.
23. Laughlin RS, Dyck PJ. Electrodiagnostic testing in lumbosacral plexopathies. *Phys Med Rehabil Clin N Am.* 2013;24(1):93–105.
24. Tubbs RS, Levin MR, Loukas M, et al. Anatomy and landmarks for the superior and middle cluneal nerves: application to posterior iliac crest harvest and entrapment syndromes. *J Neurosurg Spine.* 2010;13(3):356–359.
25. Darnis B, Robert R, Labat JJ, et al. Perineal pain and inferior cluneal nerves: anatomy and surgery. *Surg Radiol Anat.* 2008;30(3):177–183.
26. Rofaeel A, Peng P, Louis I, Chan V. Feasibility of real-time ultrasound for pudendal nerve block in patients with chronic perineal pain. *Reg Anesth Pain Med.* 2008;33(2):139–145.
27. Labs JD, Williams GM, Manson PN, Hoopes JE. Superior gluteal artery steal syndrome. *Br J Plast Surg.* 1989;42(5):603–606.
28. Tucker KJ, Fels M, Walker SR, Hodges PW. Comparison of location, depth, quality, and intensity of experimentally induced pain in 6 low back muscles. *Clin J Pain.* 2014;30(9):800–808.

29. Wan Q, Lin C, Li X, et al. MRI assessment of paraspinal muscles in patients with acute and chronic unilateral low back pain. *Br J Radiol.* 2015;88(1053):20140546.
30. Kim CW, Siemionow K, Anderson DG, Phillips FM. The current state of minimally invasive spine surgery. *J Bone Joint Surg Am.* 2011;93(6):582–596.
31. Phillips S, Mercer S, Bogduk N. Anatomy and biomechanics of quadratus lumborum. *Proc Inst Mech Eng H.* 2008;222(2):151–159.
32. Bogduk N, Johnson G, Spalding D. The morphology and biomechanics of latissimus dorsi. *Clin Biomech (Bristol, Avon).* 1998;13(6):377–385.
33. Ferguson S. *Biomechanics of the Spine Spinal Disorders.* In: Boos N, Aebi M, eds. Springer, Berlin Heidelberg, Germany; 2008:41–66.
34. Crewe H, Campbell A, Elliott B, Alderson J. Lumbo-pelvic biomechanics and quadratus lumborum asymmetry in cricket fast bowlers. *Med Sci Sports Exerc.* 2013;45(4):778–783.
35. Glassman SD, Berven S, Bridwell K, et al. Correlation of radiographic parameters and clinical symptoms in adult scoliosis. *Spine.* 2005;30(6):682–688.
36. Fujiwara A, Lim TH, An HS, et al. The effect of disc degeneration and facet joint osteoarthritis on the segmental flexibility of the lumbar spine. *Spine.* 2000;25(23):3036–3044.
37. Denis F. Spinal instability as defined by the three-column spine concept in acute spinal trauma. *Clin Orthop Relat Res.* 1984(189):65–76.
38. Cohen SP. Sacroiliac joint pain: a comprehensive review of anatomy, diagnosis, and treatment. *Anesth Analg.* 2005;101(5):1440–1453.
39. Spector LR, Madigan L, Rhyne A, et al. Cauda equina syndrome. *J Am Acad Orthop Surg.* 2008;16(8):471–479.
40. Granata G, Padua L, Rossi F, et al. Electrophysiological study of the bulbocavernosus reflex: normative data. *Funct Neurol.* 2013;28(4):293–295.
41. Braddom RL, Chan L, Harrast MA. *Physical Medicine and Rehabilitation.* 4th ed. Philadelphia, PA: Saunders/Elsevier; 2011: xxiv, 1506.
42. Majlesi J, Togay H, Unalan H, Toprak S. The sensitivity and specificity of the Slump and the Straight Leg Raising tests in patients with lumbar disc herniation. *J Clin Rheumatol.* 2008;14(2):87–91.
43. van der Wurff P, Meyne W, Hagmeijer RH. Clinical tests of the sacroiliac joint. *Man Ther.* 2000;5(2):89–96.
44. Maslowski E, Sullivan W, Forster Harwood J, et al. The diagnostic validity of hip provocation maneuvers to detect intra-articular hip pathology. *PM R.* 2010;2(3):174–181.
45. van der Wurff P, Meyne W, Hagmeijer RH. Clinical tests of the sacroiliac joint. *Man Ther.* 2000;5(2):89–96.
46. Fishman LM, Dombi GW, Michaelsen C, et al. Piriformis syndrome: diagnosis, treatment, and outcome–a 10-year study. *Arch Phys Med Rehabil.* 2002;83(3):295–301.
47. Zochling J, Braun J. Assessments in ankylosing spondylitis. *Best Pract Res Clin Rheumatol.* 2007;21(4):699–712.
48. Wanders A, Landewé R, Dougados M, et al. Association between radiographic damage of the spine and spinal mobility for individual patients with ankylosing spondylitis: can assessment of spinal mobility be a proxy for radiographic evaluation? *Ann Rheum Dis.* 2005;64(7):988–994.
49. Bigos SJ; United States. Agency for Health Care Policy and Research. *Acute Low Back Problems in Adults. Clinical Practice Guideline.* Rockville, MD: U.S. Department of Health and Human Services, Public Health Service, Agency for Health Care Policy and Research; 1994: viii, 160.
50. Bratton RL. Assessment and management of acute low back pain. *Am Fam Physician.* 1999;60(8):2299–2308.
51. Waddell G, McCulloch JA, Kummel E, Venner RM. Nonorganic physical signs in low-back pain. *Spine.* 1980;5(2):117–125.
52. Fishbain DA, Cutler RB, Rosomoff HL, Rosomoff RS. Is there a relationship between nonorganic physical findings (Waddell signs) and secondary gain/malingering? *Clin J Pain.* 2004;20(6):399–408.
53. Gatchel RJ, Mayer TG. Psychological evaluation of the spine patient. *J Am Acad Orthop Surg.* 2008;16(2):107–112.
54. Bogduk N. Management of chronic low back pain. *Med J Aust.* 2004;180(2):79–83.
55. Longo UG, Loppini M, Denaro L, et al. Rating scales for low back pain. *Br Med Bull.* 2010;94:81–144.
56. Lønn JH, Glomsrød B, Soukup MG, et al. Active back school: prophylactic management for low back pain. A randomized, controlled, 1-year follow-up study. *Spine.* 1999;24(9):865–871.
57. Keynan O, Fisher CG, Vaccaro A, et al. Radiographic measurement parameters in thoracolumbar fractures: a systematic review and consensus statement of the spine trauma study group. *Spine.* 2006;31(5):E156–E165.
58. Chou R, Huffman LH; American Pain Society; American College of Physicians. Nonpharmacologic therapies for acute and chronic low back pain: a review of the evidence for an American Pain Society/American College of Physicians clinical practice guideline. *Ann Intern Med.* 2007;147(7):492–504.
59. Kent P, Mjøsund H, Petersen D. Does targeting manual therapy and/or exercise improve patient outcomes in nonspecific low back pain? A systematic review. *BMC Med.* 2010;8(1):1–15.
60. Standaert CJ, Herring SA. Expert opinion and controversies in musculoskeletal and sports medicine: core stabilization as a treatment for low back pain. *Arch Phys Med Rehabil.* 2007;88(12):1734–1736.
61. Lee TJ. Pharmacologic treatment for low back pain: one component of pain care. *Phys Med Rehabil Clin N Am.* 2010;21(4):793–800.
62. Duffy RL. Low back pain: an approach to diagnosis and management. *Prim Care.* 2010;37(4):729–741, vi.
63. Tong HC. Specificity of needle electromyography for lumbar radiculopathy in 55- to 79-yr-old subjects with low back pain and sciatica without stenosis. *Am J Phys Med Rehabil.* 2011;90(3):233–8; quiz 239.
64. Webster BS, Verma SK, Gatchel RJ. Relationship between early opioid prescribing for acute occupational low back pain and disability duration, medical costs, subsequent surgery and late opioid use. *Spine (Phila Pa 1976).* 2007;32(19):2127–2132.
65. Friedly JL, Comstock BA, Turner JA, et al. A randomized trial of epidural glucocorticoid injections for spinal stenosis. *N Engl J Med.* 2014;371(1):11–21.
66. Novak S, Nemeth WC. The basis for recommending repeating epidural steroid injections for radicular low back pain: a literature review. *Arch Phys Med Rehabil.* 2008;89(3):543–552.
67. Provenzano DA, Narouze S. Sonographically guided lumbar spine procedures. *J Ultrasound Med.* 2013;32(7):1109–1116.
68. Park Y, Lee JH, Park KD, et al. Ultrasound-guided vs. fluoroscopy-guided caudal epidural steroid injection for the treatment of unilateral lower lumbar radicular pain: a prospective, randomized, single-blind clinical study. *Am J Phys Med Rehabil.* 2013;92(7):575–586.
69. Doo AR, Kim JW, Lee JH, et al. A Comparison of Two Techniques for Ultrasound-guided Caudal Injection: The Influence of the Depth of the Inserted Needle on Caudal Block. *Korean J Pain.* 2015;28(2):122–128.
70. Bogduk N. Lumbar radiofrequency neurotomy. *Clin J Pain.* 2006;22(4):409.
71. Cohen SP, Hurley RW, Christo PJ, et al. Clinical predictors of success and failure for lumbar facet radiofrequency denervation. *Clin J Pain.* 2007;23(1):45–52.
72. Cohen SP, Huang JH, Brummett C. Facet joint pain--advances in patient selection and treatment. *Nat Rev Rheumatol.* 2013;9(2):101–116.
73. Weinstein JN, Tosteson TD, Lurie JD, et al.; SPORT Investigators. Surgical versus nonsurgical therapy for lumbar spinal stenosis. *N Engl J Med.* 2008;358(8):794–810.
74. Weinstein JN, Lurie JD, Tosteson TD, et al. Surgical versus nonsurgical treatment for lumbar degenerative spondylolisthesis. *N Engl J Med.* 2007;356(22):2257–2270.
75. Bogduk N, Andersson G. Is spinal surgery effective for back pain? *F1000 Med Rep.* 2009;1.
76. Peul WC, Bredenoord AL, Jacobs WC. Avoid surgery as first line treatment for non-specific low back pain. *BMJ.* 2014;349:g4214.
77. Chan CW, Peng P. Failed back surgery syndrome. *Pain Med.* 2011;12(4):577–606.
78. Shapiro CM. The failed back surgery syndrome: pitfalls surrounding evaluation and treatment. *Phys Med Rehabil Clin N Am.* 2014;25(2):319–340.
79. Tarulli AW, Raynor EM. Lumbosacral radiculopathy. *Neurol Clin.* 2007;25(2):387–405.
80. Lauder TD. *Musculoskeltal Disorders and Physical Examination Findings.* Rochester, MN: American Association of Electrodiagnostic Medicine; 1999.
81. Kreiner DS, Hwang SW, Easa JE, et al.; North American Spine Society. An evidence-based clinical guideline for the diagnosis and treatment of lumbar disc herniation with radiculopathy. *Spine J.* 2014;14(1):180–191.

82. Laughlin RS, Dyck PJB. Chapter 4 - Diabetic radiculoplexus neuropathies. In: Douglas WZ, Rayaz AM, eds. *Handbook of Clinical Neurology*. Amsterdam, the Netherlands; New York, NY: Elsevier; 2014:45–52.
83. Dyck PJ, Windebank AJ. Diabetic and nondiabetic lumbosacral radiculoplexus neuropathies: new insights into pathophysiology and treatment. *Muscle Nerve*. 2002;25(4):477–491.
84. Jones LK Jr, Reda H, Watson JC. Clinical, electrophysiologic, and imaging features of zoster-associated limb paresis. *Muscle Nerve*. 2014;50(2):177–185.
85. Yaszay B, Jablecki CK, Safran MR. Zoster paresis of the shoulder. Case report and review of the literature. *Clin Orthop Relat Res*. 2000;(377):112–118.
86. Santiago-Pérez S, Nevado-Estévez R, Pérez-Conde MC. Herpes zoster-induced abdominal wall paresis: neurophysiological examination in this unusual complication. *J Neurol Sci*. 2012;312(1–2):177–179.
87. Halperin JJ. Lyme disease and the peripheral nervous system. *Muscle Nerve*. 2003;28(2):133–143.
88. Robinson-Papp J, Simpson DM. Neuromuscular diseases associated with HIV-1 infection. *Muscle Nerve*. 2009;40(6):1043–1053.
89. Groves MD. Leptomeningeal disease. *Neurosurg Clin N Am*. 2011;22(1):67–78, vii.
90. Grewal J, Saria MG, Kesari S. Novel approaches to treating leptomeningeal metastases. *J Neurooncol*. 2012;106(2):225–234.
91. Karekezi C, Egu K, Djoubairou BO, et al. Unusual cause of non-discogenic sciatica: Foraminal lumbar root schwannoma. *Surg Neurol Int*. 2014;5(Suppl 4):S208–S210.
92. Qasho R, Ramundo OE, Maraglino C, et al. Epidural lipomatosis with lumbar radiculopathy in one obese patient. Case report and review of the literature. *Neurosurg Rev*. 1997;20(3):206–209.
93. Rice I, Wee MY, Thomson K. Obstetric epidurals and chronic adhesive arachnoiditis. *Br J Anaesth*. 2004;92(1):109–120.
94. Petty PG, Hudgson P, Hare WS. Symptomatic lumbar spinal arachnoiditis: fact or fallacy? *J Clin Neurosci*. 2000;7(5):395–399.
95. Rajpal S, Chanbusarakum K, Deshmukh PR. Upper cervical myelopathy due to arachnoiditis and spinal cord tethering from adjacent C-2 osteomyelitis. Case report and review of the literature. *J Neurosurg Spine*. 2007;6(1):64–67.
96. Dolan RA. Spinal adhesive arachnoiditis. *Surg Neurol*. 1993;39(6):479–484.
97. Siebert E, Prüss H, Klingebiel R, et al. Lumbar spinal stenosis: syndrome, diagnostics and treatment. *Nat Rev Neurol*. 2009;5(7):392–403.
98. Yagci I, Gunduz OH, Ekinci G, et al. The utility of lumbar paraspinal mapping in the diagnosis of lumbar spinal stenosis. *Am J Phys Med Rehabil*. 2009;88(10):843–851.
99. Amirjani N, Hudson AL, Butler JE, Gandevia SC. An algorithm for the safety of costal diaphragm electromyography derived from ultrasound. *Muscle Nerve*. 2012;46(6):856–860.
100. Johnsson KE, Rosen I, Uden A. The natural course of lumbar spinal stenosis. *Clin Orthop Relat Res*. 1992(279): 82–86.
101. McKillop AB, Carroll LJ, Battié MC. Depression as a prognostic factor of lumbar spinal stenosis: a systematic review. *Spine J*. 2014;14(5):837–846.
102. Binder DS, Nampiaparampil DE. The provocative lumbar facet joint. *Curr Rev Musculoskelet Med*. 2009;2(1):15–24.
103. Fukui S, Ohseto K, Shiotani M, et al. Distribution of referred pain from the lumbar zygapophyseal joints and dorsal rami. *Clin J Pain*. 1997;13(4):303–307.
104. Schwarzer AC, Aprill CN, Derby R, et al. The false-positive rate of uncontrolled diagnostic blocks of the lumbar zygapophysial joints. *Pain*. 1994;58(2):195–200.
105. Gellhorn AC, Katz JN, Suri P. Osteoarthritis of the spine: the facet joints. *Nat Rev Rheumatol*. 2013;9(4):216–224.
106. Madigan L, Vaccaro AR, Spector LR, Milam RA. Management of symptomatic lumbar degenerative disk disease. *J Am Acad Orthop Surg*. 2009;17(2):102–111.
107. Emch TM, Modic MT. Imaging of lumbar degenerative disk disease: history and current state. *Skeletal Radiol*. 2011;40(9):1175–1189.
108. Modic MT, Ross JS. Lumbar degenerative disk disease. *Radiology*. 2007;245(1):43–61.
109. Zhang YH, Zhao CQ, Jiang LS, et al. Modic changes: a systematic review of the literature. *Eur Spine J*. 2008;17(10):1289–1299.
110. Majid K, Fischgrund JS. Degenerative lumbar spondylolisthesis: trends in management. *J Am Acad Orthop Surg*. 2008;16(4):208–215.
111. Jones TR, Rao RD. Adult isthmic spondylolisthesis. *J Am Acad Orthop Surg*. 2009;17(10):609–617.
112. Akhtar OH, Rowe DE. Syringomyelia-associated scoliosis with and without the Chiari I malformation. *J Am Acad Orthop Surg*. 2008;16(7):407–417.
113. Arlet V, Reddi V. Adolescent idiopathic scoliosis. *Neurosurg Clin N Am*. 2007;18(2):255–259.
114. Cartwright MS, White DL, Demar S, et al. Median nerve changes following steroid injection for carpal tunnel syndrome. *Muscle Nerve*. 2011;44(1):25–29.
115. Prather H, Hunt D, Watson JO, Gilula LA. Conservative care for patients with osteoporotic vertebral compression fractures. *Phys Med Rehabil Clin N Am*. 2007;18(3):577–591, xi.
116. Wong CC, McGirt MJ. Vertebral compression fractures: a review of current management and multimodal therapy. *J Multidiscip Healthc*. 2013;6:205–214.
117. Hazel WA Jr, Jones RA, Morrey BF, Stauffer RN. Vertebral fractures without neurological deficit. A long-term follow-up study. *J Bone Joint Surg Am*. 1988;70(9):1319–1321.
118. Sinaki M. Exercise for patients with osteoporosis: management of vertebral compression fractures and trunk strengthening for fall prevention. *PM R*. 2012;4(11):882–888.
119. Schlickewei W, Schützhoff G, Kuner EH. [Early functional treatment of fractures of the lower thoracic and lumbar vertebrae with a 3-point brace]. *Unfallchirurg*. 1991;94(1):40–44.
120. Wardlaw D, Cummings SR, Van Meirhaeghe J, et al. Efficacy and safety of balloon kyphoplasty compared with non-surgical care for vertebral compression fracture (FREE): a randomised controlled trial. *Lancet*. 2009;373(9668):1016–1024.
121. Buchbinder R, Osborne RH, Ebeling PR, et al. A randomized trial of vertebroplasty for painful osteoporotic vertebral fractures. *N Engl J Med*. 2009;361(6):557–568.
122. Korovessis P, Vardakastanis K, Repantis T, Vitsas V. Balloon kyphoplasty versus KIVA vertebral augmentation–comparison of 2 techniques for osteoporotic vertebral body fractures: a prospective randomized study. *Spine*. 2013;38(4):292–299.
123. Freedman BA, Heller JG. Kummel disease: a not-so-rare complication of osteoporotic vertebral compression fractures. *J Am Board Fam Med*. 2009;22(1):75–78.
124. Pappou IP, Papadopoulos EC, Swanson AN, et al. Osteoporotic vertebral fractures and collapse with intravertebral vacuum sign (Kümmel's disease). *Orthopedics*. 2008;31(1):61–66.
125. Lowe TG. Scheuermann's kyphosis. *Neurosurg Clin N Am*. 2007;18(2):305–315.
126. Khan SHM, Schepper A. Primary tumors of the osseous spine. In: Goethem JM, Hauwe L, Parizel P, eds. *Spinal Imaging*. Springer: Berlin Heidelberg, Germany; 2007: 475–500.
127. Bernard SA, Brian PL, Flemming DJ. Primary osseous tumors of the spine. *Semin Musculoskelet Radiol*. 2013;17(2):203–220.
128. Andreula C, Murrone M, Algra PR. Metastatic disease of the spine. In: Goethem JWM, Hauwe L, Parizel PM, eds. *Spinal Imaging*. Springer: Berlin Heidelberg, Germany; 2007: 461–474.
129. Ecker RD, Endo T, Wetjen NM, Krauss WE. Diagnosis and treatment of vertebral column metastases. *Mayo Clin Proc*. 2005;80(9):1177–1186.
130. Selvaggi K, Abrahm J. Metastatic spinal cord compression: the hidden danger. *Nat Clin Pract Oncol*. 2006;3(8):458–461; quiz following 461.
131. Rollig C, Knop S, Bornhauser M. *Multiple myeloma*. Lancet. 2015;385(9983):2197–2208.
132. Fast A, Goldsher D. *Navigating the Adult Spine: Bridging Clinical Practice and Neuroradiology*. New York: Demos; 2007: 186.
133. Lucantoni C, Than KD, Wang AC, et al. Tarlov cysts: a controversial lesion of the sacral spine. *Neurosurg Focus*. 2011;31(6):E14.
134. Zimmerli W. Clinical practice. Vertebral osteomyelitis. *N Engl J Med*. 2010;362(11):1022–1029.
135. Sarzi-Puttini P, Atzeni F. New developments in our understanding of DISH (diffuse idiopathic skeletal hyperostosis). *Curr Opin Rheumatol*. 2004;16(3):287–292.
136. Olivieri I, D'Angelo S, Palazzi C, et al. Diffuse idiopathic skeletal hyperostosis: differentiation from ankylosing spondylitis. *Curr Rheumatol Rep*. 2009;11(5):321–328.
137. Valle-Onate R, Ward MM, Kerr GS. Physical therapy and surgery. *Am J Med Sci*. 2012;343(5):353–356.
138. Gruener G, Camacho P. Paget's disease of bone. *Handb Clin Neurol*. 2014;119:529–540.

139. Malanga GA, Cruz Colon EJ. Myofascial low back pain: a review. *Phys Med Rehabil Clin N Am.* 2010;21(4):711–724.
140. Simons, DG, Travell, JG, Simons, LS. *Travell & Simons' Myofascial Pain and Dysfunction: The Trigger Point Manual.* 2nd ed. Baltimore, MD: Williams & Wilkins; 1999: 1.
141. Rha DW, Shin JC, Kim YK, et al. Detecting local twitch responses of myofascial trigger points in the lower-back muscles using ultrasonography. *Arch Phys Med Rehabil.* 2011;92(10):1576–1580.e1.
142. Snijders CJ, Hermans PF, Niesing R, et al. The influence of slouching and lumbar support on iliolumbar ligaments, intervertebral discs and sacroiliac joints. *Clin Biomech (Bristol, Avon).* 2004;19(4):323–329.
143. Maigne JY, Maigne R. Trigger point of the posterior iliac crest: painful iliolumbar ligament insertion or cutaneous dorsal ramus pain? An anatomic study. *Arch Phys Med Rehabil.* 1991;72(10):734–737.
144. Sims JA, Moorman SJ. The role of the iliolumbar ligament in low back pain. *Med Hypotheses.* 1996;46(6):511–515.
145. Harmon D, Alexiev V. Sonoanatomy and injection technique of the iliolumbar ligament. *Pain Physician.* 2011;14(5):469–474.
146. Barrett-Connor E, Nielson CM, Orwoll E, Bauer DC, Cauley JA; Osteoporotic Fractures in Men Study Group. Epidemiology of rib fractures in older men: Osteoporotic Fractures in Men (MrOS) prospective cohort study. *BMJ.* 2010;340:c1069.
147. Pirali C, Santus G, Faletti S, De Grandis D. Botulinum toxin treatment for slipping rib syndrome: a case report. *Clin J Pain.* 2013;29(10):e1–e3.
148. Habib PA, Huang GS, Mendiola JA, Yu JS. Anterior chest pain: musculoskeletal considerations. *Emerg Radiol.* 2004;11(1):37–45.
149. Ayloo A, Cvengros T, Marella S. Evaluation and treatment of musculoskeletal chest pain. *Prim Care.* 2013;40(4):863–887, viii.
150. Guttentag AR, Salwen JK. Keep your eyes on the ribs: the spectrum of normal variants and diseases that involve the ribs. *Radiographics.* 1999;19(5):1125–1142.
151. Thomas PL. Thoracic back pain in rowers and butterfly swimmers–costo vertebral subluxation. *Br J Sports Med.* 1988;22(2):81.
152. O'Connor RC, Andary MT, Russo RB, DeLano M. Thoracic radiculopathy. *Phys Med Rehabil Clin N Am.* 2002;13(3):623–44, viii.
153. Baranto A, Börjesson M, Danielsson B, et al. Acute chest pain in a top soccer player due to thoracic disc herniation. *Spine.* 2009;34(10):E359–E362.
154. Santos PS, Resende LA, Fonseca RG, et al. Intercostal nerve mononeuropathy: study of 14 cases. *Arq Neuropsiquiatr.* 2005;63(3B):776–778.
155. Conte SA, Thompson MM, Marks MA, Dines JS. Abdominal muscle strains in professional baseball: 1991–2010. *Am J Sports Med.* 2012;40(3):650–656.
156. Stevens KJ, Crain JM, Akizuki KH, Beaulieu CF. Imaging and ultrasound-guided steroid injection of internal oblique muscle strains in baseball pitchers. *Am J Sports Med.* 2010;38(3):581–585.
157. Nelson P, Apte G, Justiz R 3rd, et al. Chronic female pelvic pain–part 2: differential diagnosis and management. *Pain Pract.* 2012;12(2):111–141.
158. Pool-Goudzwaard A, Hoek van Dijke G, Mulder P, et al. The iliolumbar ligament: its influence on stability of the sacroiliac joint. *Clin Biomech (Bristol, Avon).* 2003;18(2):99–105.
159. Johnson AW, Weiss CB Jr, Wheeler DL. Stress fractures of the femoral shaft in athletes–more common than expected. A new clinical test. *Am J Sports Med.* 1994;22(2):248–256.
160. Vanelderen P, Szadek K, Cohen SP, et al. 13. Sacroiliac joint pain. *Pain Pract.* 2010;10(5):470–478.
161. Slipman CW, Whyte WS 2nd, Chow DW, et al. Sacroiliac joint syndrome. *Pain Physician.* 2001;4(2):143–152.
162. Jee H, Lee JH, Park KD, et al. Ultrasound-guided versus fluoroscopy-guided sacroiliac joint intra-articular injections in the noninflammatory sacroiliac joint dysfunction: a prospective, randomized, single-blinded study. *Arch Phys Med Rehabil.* 2014;95(2):330–337.
163. Hansen H, Manchikanti L, Simopoulos TT, et al. A systematic evaluation of the therapeutic effectiveness of sacroiliac joint interventions. *Pain Physician.* 2012;15(3):E247–E278.
164. Mitra R. Osteitis condensans ilii. *Rheumatol Int.* 2010;30(3):293–296.
165. Patijn J, Janssen M, Hayek S, et al. 14. Coccygodynia. *Pain Pract.* 2010;10(6):554–559.
166. Patel R, Appannagari A, Whang PG. Coccydynia. *Curr Rev Musculoskelet Med.* 2008;1(3–4):223–226.
167. Wray CC, Easom S, Hoskinson J. Coccydynia. Aetiology and treatment. *J Bone Joint Surg Br.* 1991;73(2):335–338.
168. Datir A, Connell D. CT-guided injection for ganglion impar blockade: a radiological approach to the management of coccydynia. *Clin Radiol.* 2010;65(1):21–25.
169. Cassidy L, Walters A, Bubb K, et al. Piriformis syndrome: implications of anatomical variations, diagnostic techniques, and treatment options. *Surg Radiol Anat.* 2012;34(6):479–486.
170. Kean Chen C, Nizar AJ. Prevalence of piriformis syndrome in chronic low back pain patients. A clinical diagnosis with modified FAIR test. *Pain Pract.* 2013;13(4):276–281.
171. Miller TA, White KP, Ross DC. The diagnosis and management of Piriformis Syndrome: myths and facts. *Can J Neurol Sci.* 2012;39(5):577–583.
172. Smith J, Wisniewski SJ, Wempe MK, et al. Sonographically guided obturator internus injections: techniques and validation. *J Ultrasound Med.* 2012;31(10):1597–1608.
173. Meknas K, Christensen A, Johansen O. The internal obturator muscle may cause sciatic pain. *Pain.* 2003;104(1–2):375–380.
174. Zissen MH, Wallace G, Stevens KJ, et al. High hamstring tendinopathy: MRI and ultrasound imaging and therapeutic efficacy of percutaneous corticosteroid injection. *AJR Am J Roentgenol.* 2010;195(4):993–998.
175. Puranen J, Orava S. The hamstring syndrome. A new diagnosis of gluteal sciatic pain. *Am J Sports Med.* 1988;16(5):517–521.
176. Linklater JM, Hamilton B, Carmichael J, et al. Hamstring injuries: anatomy, imaging, and intervention. *Semin Musculoskelet Radiol.* 2010;14(2):131–161.
177. Cohen S, Bradley J. Acute proximal hamstring rupture. *J Am Acad Orthop Surg.* 2007;15(6):350–355.
178. Cacchio A, Rompe JD, Furia JP, et al. Shockwave therapy for the treatment of chronic proximal hamstring tendinopathy in professional athletes. *Am J Sports Med.* 2011;39(1):146–153.
179. Reurink G, Goudswaard GJ, Moen MH, et al.; Dutch Hamstring Injection Therapy (HIT) Study Investigators. Platelet-rich plasma injections in acute muscle injury. *N Engl J Med.* 2014;370(26):2546–2547.
180. Stafford GH, Villar RN. Ischiofemoral impingement. *J Bone Joint Surg Br.* 2011;93(10):1300–1302.
181. Ali AM, Whitwell D, Ostlere SJ. Case report: imaging and surgical treatment of a snapping hip due to ischiofemoral impingement. *Skeletal Radiol,* 2011;40(5):653–656.
182. Torriani M, Souto SC, Thomas BJ, Ouellette H, Bredella MA. Ischiofemoral impingement syndrome: an entity with hip pain and abnormalities of the quadratus femoris muscle. *AJR Am J Roentgenol.* 2009;193(1):186–190.
183. Van Mieghem IM, Boets A, Sciot R, Van Breuseghem I. Ischiogluteal bursitis: an uncommon type of bursitis. *Skeletal Radiol.* 2004;33(7):413–416.
184. Cho KH, Lee SM, Lee YH, et al. Non-infectious ischiogluteal bursitis: MRI findings. *Korean J Radiol.* 2004;5(4):280–286.
185. Huang BK, Campos JC, Michael Peschka PG, et al. Injury of the gluteal aponeurotic fascia and proximal iliotibial band: anatomy, pathologic conditions, and MR imaging. *Radiographics.* 2013;33(5):1437–1452.
186. Distad BJ, Weiss MD. Clinical and electrodiagnostic features of sciatic neuropathies. *Phys Med Rehabil Clin N Am.* 2013;24(1):107–120.
187. Lee SW, Thomas S, Drakes S, Kim DD. Ultrasonography of a sciatic nerve injury caused by a gunshot wound. *PM R.* 2014;6(7):662–663.
188. Berthelot JM, Pillet JC, Mitard D, et al. Buttock claudication disclosing a thrombosis of the superior left gluteal artery: Report of a case diagnosed by a selective arteriography of the iliac artery, and cured by per-cutaneous stenting. *Joint Bone Spine.* 2007;74(3):289–291.
189. Lowenthal RM, Taylor BV, Jones R, Beasley A. Severe persistent sciatic pain and weakness due to a gluteal artery pseudoaneurysm as a complication of bone marrow biopsy. *J Clin Neurosci.* 2006;13(3):384–385.
190. Batt M, Baque J, Bouillanne PJ, et al. Percutaneous angioplasty of the superior gluteal artery for buttock claudication: a report of seven cases and literature review. *J Vasc Surg.* 2006;43(5):987–991.
191. Aydin A, Lee CC, Schultz E, Ackerman J. Traumatic inferior gluteal artery pseudoaneurysm: case report and review of literature. *Am J Emerg Med.* 2007;25(4):488.e1–488.e3.
192. Berumen-Nafarrate E, Vega-Najera C, Leal-Contreras C, Leal-Berumen I. Gluteal compartment syndrome following an iliac bone marrow aspiration. *Case Rep Orthop.* 2013;2013:812172.

CHAPTER 7

Hip and Thigh

EPIDEMIOLOGY OF HIP PAIN

HIP PAIN IN THE GENERAL POPULATION

Prevalence
• ~3% of adult population has nonspecific hip pain

Osteoarthritis (OA)
• Most common (MC) cause of the hip pain in the elderly
• Symptomatic hip OA: increases with age, 2% to 10% in age >45 years (1)
• Similar in both genders (vs symptomatic knee OA, higher in female)

HIP PAIN IN CHILDREN

• Physis or apophysis injuries: MC cause
• Other common causes: fracture, subluxation/dislocation, infection, and avulsions

HIP PAIN IN ATHLETES (2,3)

Prevalence
• 2.5% of all sports-related injuries and 5% to 9% of injuries in high school athletes, 0.5% to 6.2% in professional athletes
• Higher prevalence of groin pain in some sports (eg, adult soccer players: 5%–18% and ice hockey)
  ○ Controversial in runners (4,5)

Risk factors
• Hip adductor muscle weakness, decreased hip range of motion (ROM), previous injuries, and muscle tightness in soccer players
• Activities: quick cutting, accelerations, decelerations, and directional changes
• Hip OA prevalence: higher in athletes (5.6% in athletes vs 2.8% in control subjects)
• Risk higher in elite soccer players (up to 14%), rugby players, javelin throwers, high jumpers, track and field sports participants, National Football League players (55.6% in survey) (6)

Other common problems
• Strain or sprain (especially adductor and gluteus), labral tear (often unclear correlation with clinical management), femoroacetabular impingement, and contusion

HIP PAIN AT WORK (1)

• Occupational workload correlated with hip pain in men, but not in women
• Relative risk is four to eight times higher in physically demanding job.

Higher-risk groups for hip OA
• Male farmers and construction workers, firefighters, food-processing workers, metal workers, and forestry workers
• Workers doing regular heavy lifting, kneeling, and crawling; limited evidence

DIFFERENTIAL DIAGNOSIS

DIFFERENTIAL DIAGNOSIS OF HIP PAIN BASED ON LOCATION (6,7)

Working definition for hip region: below iliac crest anteriorly (groin)/laterally (hip), posteriorly; thigh (below the buttock) (Flowcharts 7.1 and 7.2)

Surface anatomy (Figure 7.1)
• Groin triangle: anterior superior iliac spine (ASIS), pubic tubercle, and midline between the ASIS and superior pole of patella
  ○ Midline: femoral artery
• Femoral triangle: inguinal ligament, medial border of adductor longus (not brevis), and medial border of sartorius
  ○ Femoral vein (most medial), artery, and nerve (laterally), then iliopsoas (midline between femoral artery pulsation and ASIS)
  ○ Underneath of iliopsoas: hip joint at the level of inguinal ligament
  ○ Anterior recess (intracapsular) superficial to femoral neck

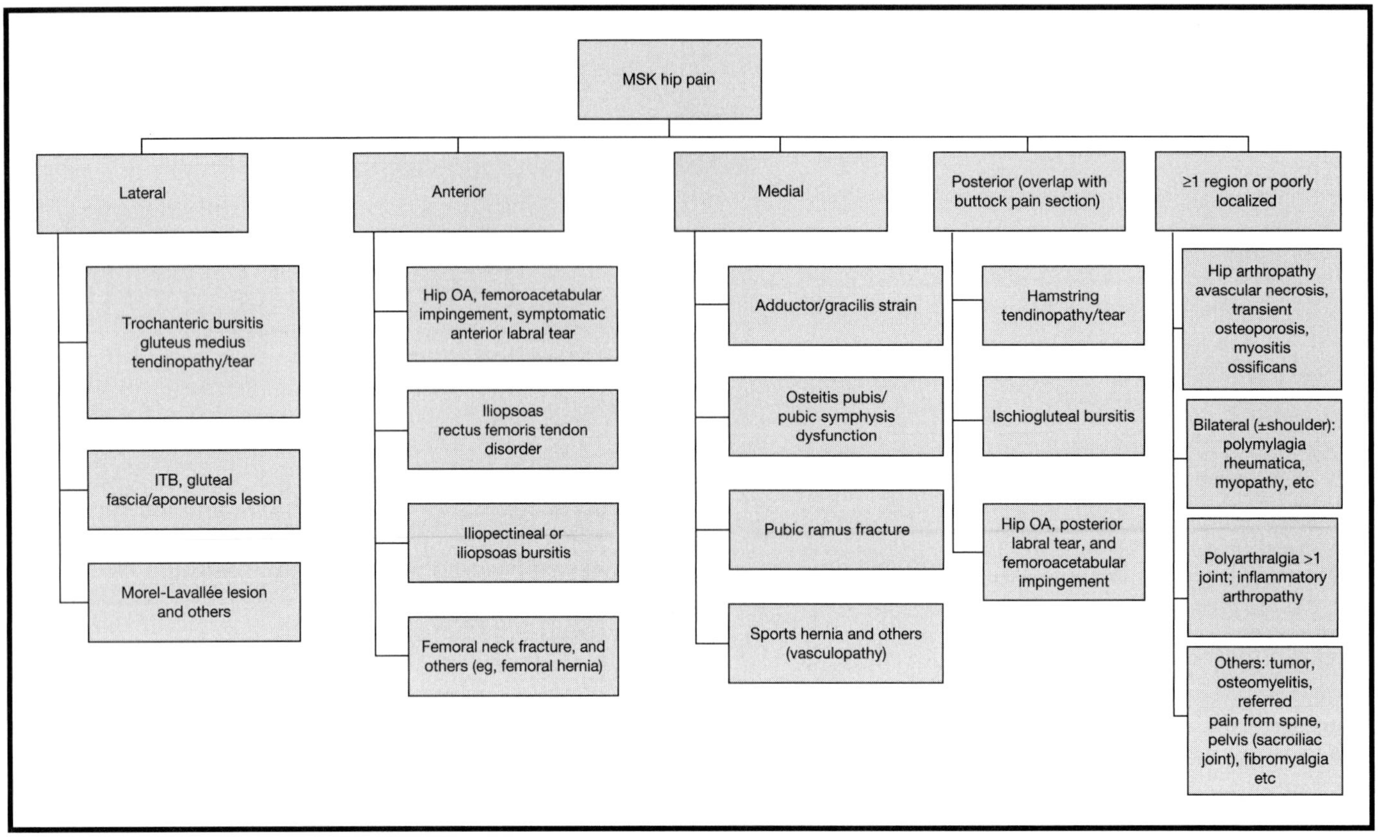

FLOWCHART 7.1
Differential diagnosis of musculoskeletal hip pain.

Fx, fracture; ITB, iliotibial band; MSK, musculoskeletal; OA, osteoarthritis.

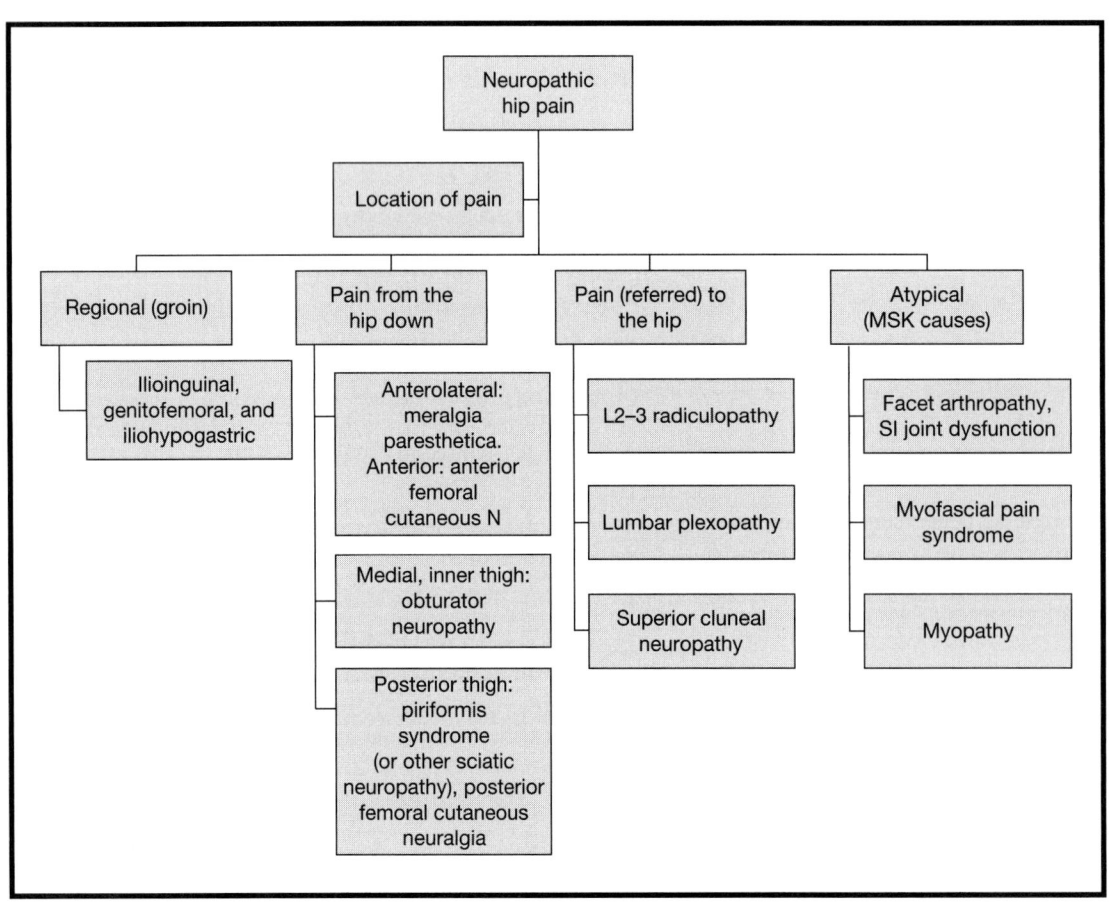

FLOWCHART 7.2
Differential diagnosis of neuropathic hip pain.

MSK, musculoskeletal; N, nerve; SI, sacroiliac.

Source: Adapted from Ref. (9). Martinoli C, Miguel-Perez M, Padua L, et al. Imaging of neuropathies about the hip. *Eur J Radiol*. 2013;82(1):17–26.

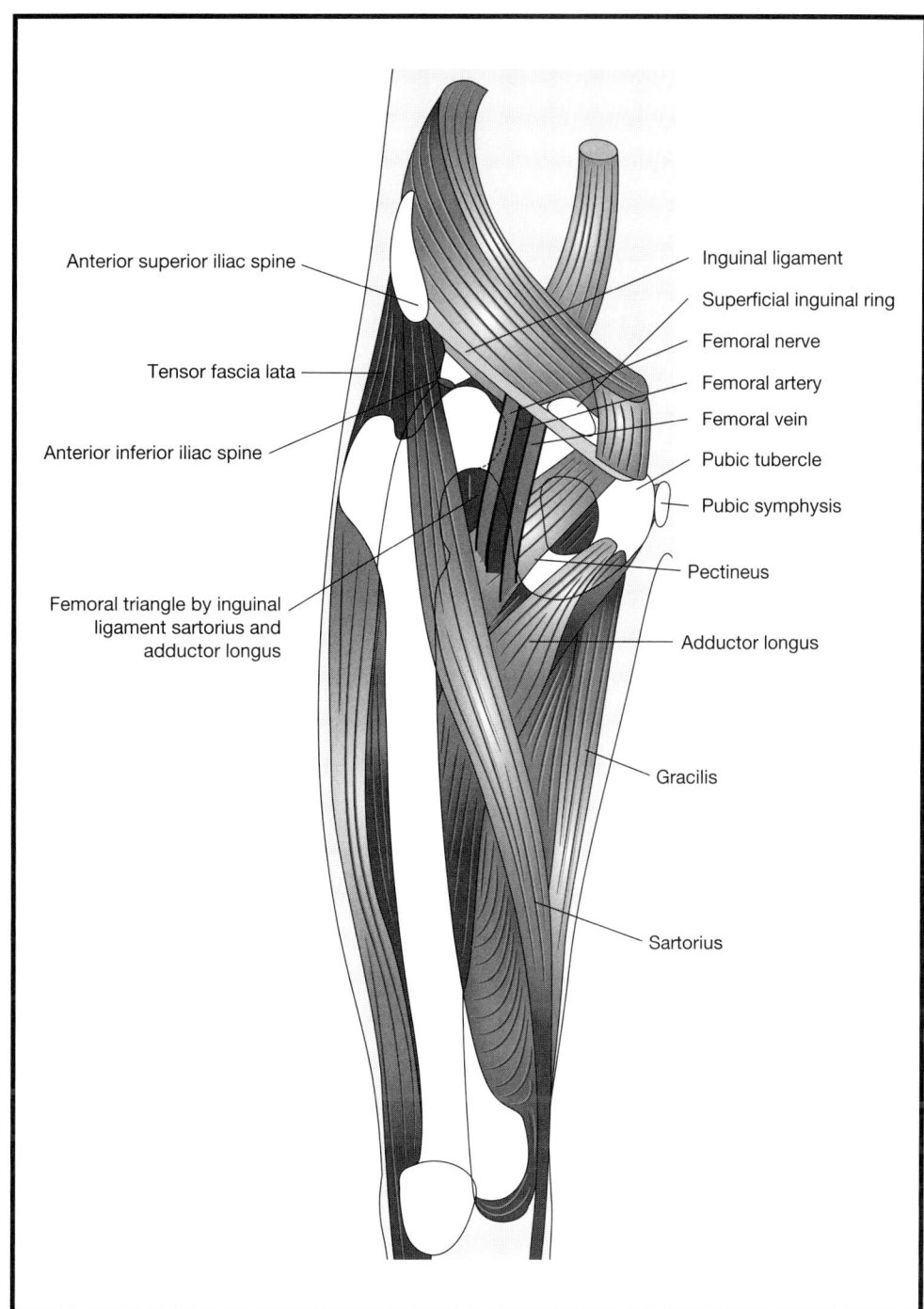

FIGURE 7.1
Surface anatomy of the hip and groin.
Source: Adapted from Ref. (8). Falvey EC, Franklyn-Miller A, McCrory PR. The groin triangle: a patho-anatomical approach to the diagnosis of chronic groin pain in athletes. *Br J Sports Med.* 2009;43(3):213–220.

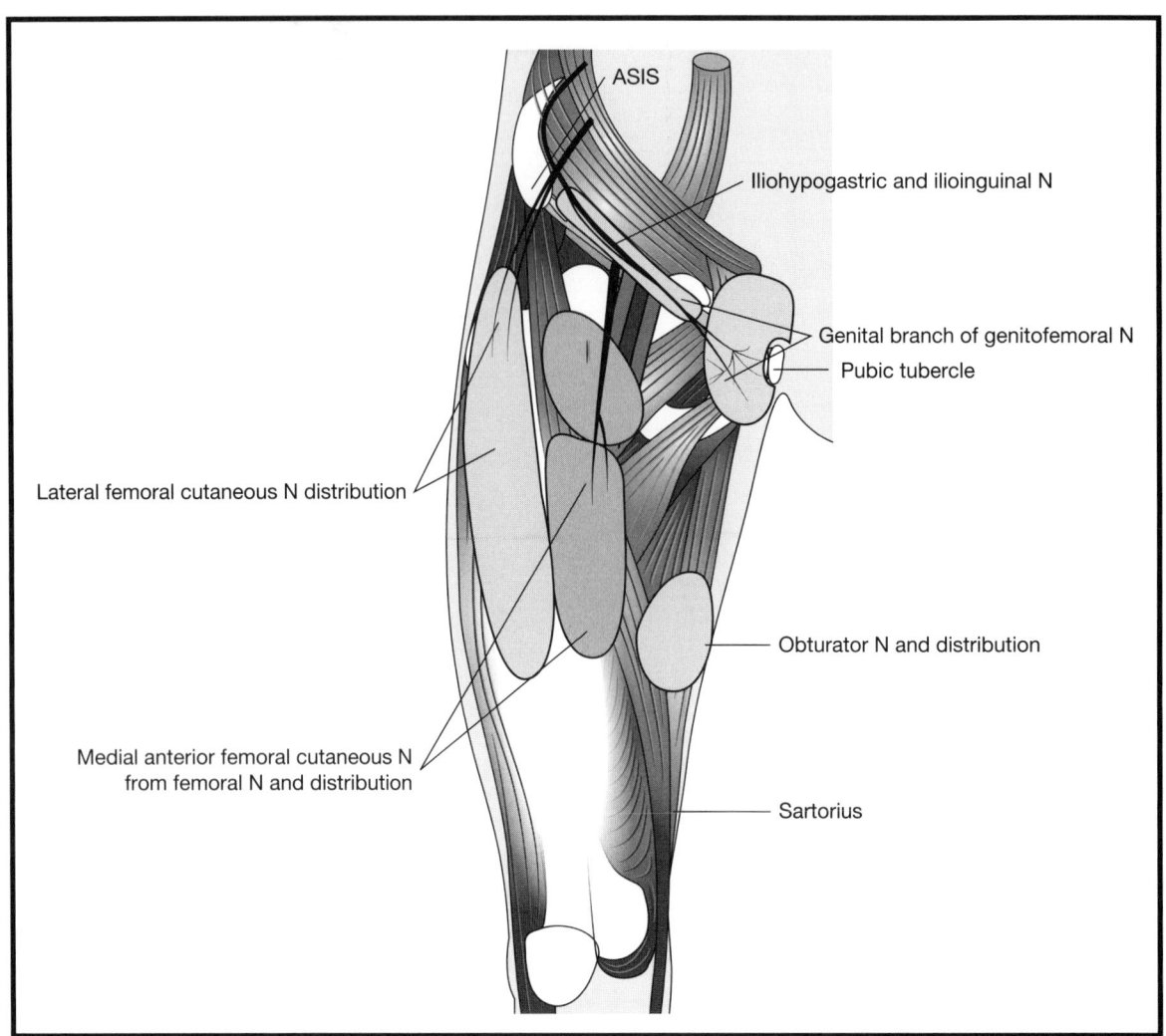

FIGURE 7.2
Nerve innervation in the groin area: border nerve (iliohypogastric, ilioinguinal, and genitofemoral nerves).
ASIS, anterior superior iliac spine; N, nerve.

LOCATION	STRUCTURES	PATHOLOGIES
Superior	Rectus abdominis	Rectus abdominis insertional tendinopathy • Pain from resisted sit-up, localized to insertion
	Conjoint tendon, external oblique aponeurosis	Sportsman's hernia
Lateral	Femoral neck	Femoral neck fracture: pain on internal rotation/hopping, progressive limitation of activity, minor trauma in osteoporotic elderly, or stress fracture (female athletic triad)
	Gluteus med, min, TFL, trochanteric bursa, ITB	Trochanteric bursitis, gluteus medius/minimus tendinopathy/tear, snapping ITB, and Morel-Lavallée lesion
	Lateral femoral cutaneous nerve	Meralgia paresthetica; local or minor trauma (belt or weight loss or gain, often without any preceding event)
Medial (pubic tubercle)	Pubic symphysis	Pubic bone stress injury (osteitis pubis), degenerative pubic symphysis • Pain with stair climbing, tenderness
	Pubic ramus	Inferior ramus injury: deep buttock pain, worse with hopping Stress fracture Rectus abdominis enthesopathy

(*continued*)

LOCATION	STRUCTURES	PATHOLOGIES
	Adductor/gracilis Obturator nerve	Adductor/gracilis avulsion/enthesopathy/tendinopathy at MT (musculotendinous) junction With/without obturator hernia (10)
	Vascular system	External iliac A endofibrosis • Thigh discomfort after high-intensity exercise (cyclist), exercise-induced weakness
	Ilioinguinal and genitofemoral nerve	Neuropathic pain on the groin ± inguinal hernia
In triangle	Iliopsoas tendon	Iliopsoas syndrome, iliopectineal bursitis
	Rectus femoris	Rectus femoris calcific tendonitis and musculotendinous junction tear
	Hip (femoroacetabular) joint	Hip OA Femoroacetabular impingement/labral pathology in younger adults Slipped femoral epiphysis in adolescents Avascular necrosis with medical comorbidities
	Others	Femoral hernia: painful lump-inferomedial to pubic tubercle, often not affected by exercise Genitofemoral and medial femoral cutaneous N lesion

ITB, iliotibial band; OA, osteoarthritis; TFL, tensor fascia lata.

Differential diagnosis of medial groin pain (11)

ADDUCTOR DYSFUNCTION	OSTEITIS PUBIS	SPORTS HERNIA
Tenderness localized to the adductor longus insertion (or 1–2 in. distal to insertion) Pain on passive stretch of the adductors Pain on adduction against resistance	Tenderness on palpation of the pubic symphysis	Local tenderness over the conjoined tendon, pubic tubercle, or midinguinal region Tender, dilated superficial inguinal ring Valsalva maneuver causes increasing pain with/without an inguinal bulge

Extrinsic causes of groin pain (12)
- Upper lumbar roots (L1–2), plexus pathologies, or superior cluneal neuropathy
- Myofascial pain referral pattern: quadratus lumborum or paraspinal muscles
- Vascular or ischemic pathologies: aneurysm, arterial pseudoaneurysm, or compartment syndrome
- Intra-abdominal disorders: appendicitis, diverticulosis, or inflammatory bowel disorders
- Genitourinary abnormalities: urinary tract infections, lymphadenitis, prostatitis, scrotal and testicular abnormalities (epididymitis), gynecological abnormalities/cysts, endometriosis, or nephrolithiasis

SNAPPING HIP (COXA SALTANS) (13)

Differential diagnosis based on the location
- External: more common
  - Friction or subluxation of the iliotibial band or gluteus maximus muscle on the greater trochanter with hip flexion
  - Friction of rectus femoris on iliopsoas tendon (14)
  - Pathologic (rare)
    - Iliotibial band impingement on a femoral osteochondroma
    - Venous hemangioma of the gluteus maximus muscle
- Internal
  - Iliopsoas tendon impingement on the iliopectineal eminence, anteroinferior iliac spine, and superior pubic ramus
    - Between the two components of a bifid psoas major tendon
  - Friction of the iliofemoral ligament on the femoral head
  - Pathologic
    - Iliopsoas tendon snapping on an anterior paralabral cyst or a protruding acetabular component of total hip arthroplasty (THA)
- Intra-articular: loose body, labral tear or redundant synovial fold, chondromatosis, joint instability, or ruptured ligamentous teres
- Posterior (underrecognized)
  - Subluxation of the tendon of the long head of the biceps femoris muscle
  - Ischiofemoral impingement with abnormalities of the quadratus femoris muscle

Prevalence: varies depending on population (up to 44% of ballet dancers), often not related to the pain

DIFFERENTIAL DIAGNOSIS OF GROIN MASS (15)

- Hernia (direct inguinal or indirect hernia) or lymphadenopathy (Figure 7.3)
- Iliopectineal or iliopsoas bursal effusion/ganglion cyst

In femoral triangle
- Neuroma, aneurysm, vein (deep vein thrombosis [DVT], saphena varix), lymphadenopathy, femoral hernia, skin and subcutaneous tissues (lipoma and sebaceous cyst), psoas abscess, hematoma, or bursal effusion
    - Saphena varix: reducible swelling (positional) in the groin below the inguinal ligament; differential diagnosis from femoral hernia

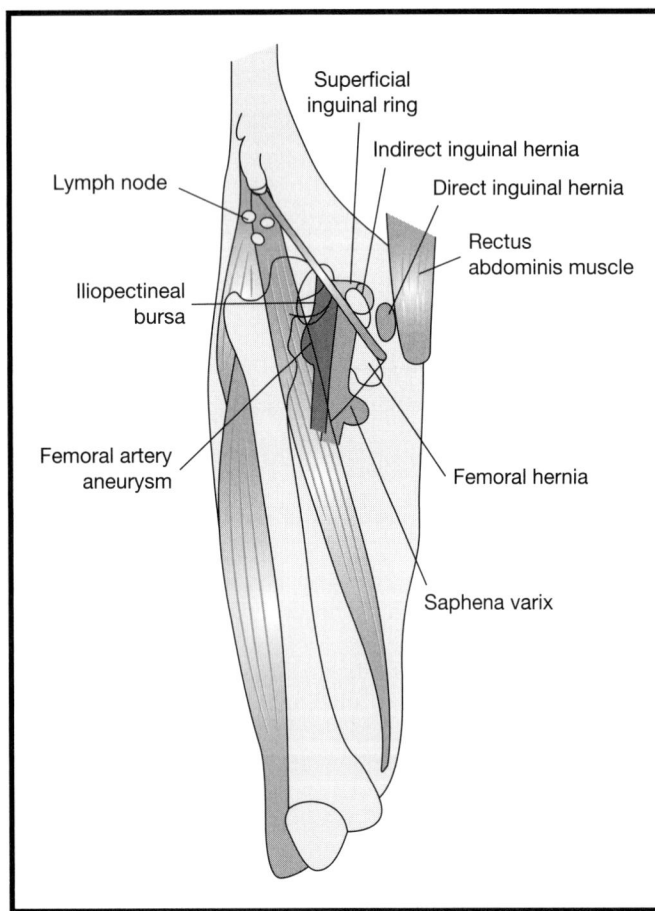

FIGURE 7.3
Mass in the groin region.

DIFFERENTIAL DIAGNOSIS OF HIP INSTABILITY

- Giving way ± clicking, locking, and catching

Atraumatic instability
- Hip pain elicited by position (hip OA)
- Developmental hip dysplasia
- Femoroacetabular impingement (± labral injury)
- Down syndrome, Ehlers-Danlos syndrome, Marfan syndrome
- Ligamentous laxity (idiopathic, congenital, acquired, iatrogenic) and generalized hypermobility of joints

Traumatic instability
- Fracture–dislocation of the acetabulum and femoral head
- Dislocation/subluxation of the hip (± osseous or labral injury)
- Repetitive microtrauma

ANATOMY

BONE AND JOINT

Hip Joint

Acetabulum (adult): angled forward about 15° (anteversion) and covers two-thirds of femoral head

Labrum
- Fibrocartilage, deepen the acetabular fossa → promoting hip joint congruency, increase acetabular volume by 20%
- Seal the articular cartilage surfaces and acetabulum
- Essentially avascular structure; blood vessels penetrate the labrum to a depth of only 0.5 mm
- Innervated by obturator nerve and branch to quadratus femoris (posteriorly)

Capsuloligamentous tension at the hip joint
- Maximum articular contact of the head of the femur
    - Femur in flexed, abducted, and laterally (externally) rotated position. Correction in Legg–Calvé–Perthes disease (LCPD) diagnosis used in congenital dislocation
- Minimal intra-articular pressure with the hip in moderate flexion, slight abduction, and minimal rotation; preferred position by patient with effusion (less pain) (16)

Cartilage on femoral head consists of type II collagen and a high concentration of hydrophilic glycosaminoglycans that trap water in the substance of the cartilage and accentuate the stress-shielding properties of the joint surface

Femur

Neck of femur
- Angled at 12° to 15° anterior to the long axis of the shaft (axial plane) (Figure 7.4)
    - Increased angle (anteversion) → internal rotation of femur
    - Decreased angle or posterior (increased retroversion) → external rotation; toe out (mild retroversion seen in slipped femoral epiphysis)
- Femoral neck–shaft angle: (coronal plane) normal, 120° to 135°; coxa vara <120°, coxa valga >135°
- Femoral neck is intracapsular (used as hip joint injection site) vs. greater and lesser trochanters are extracapsular

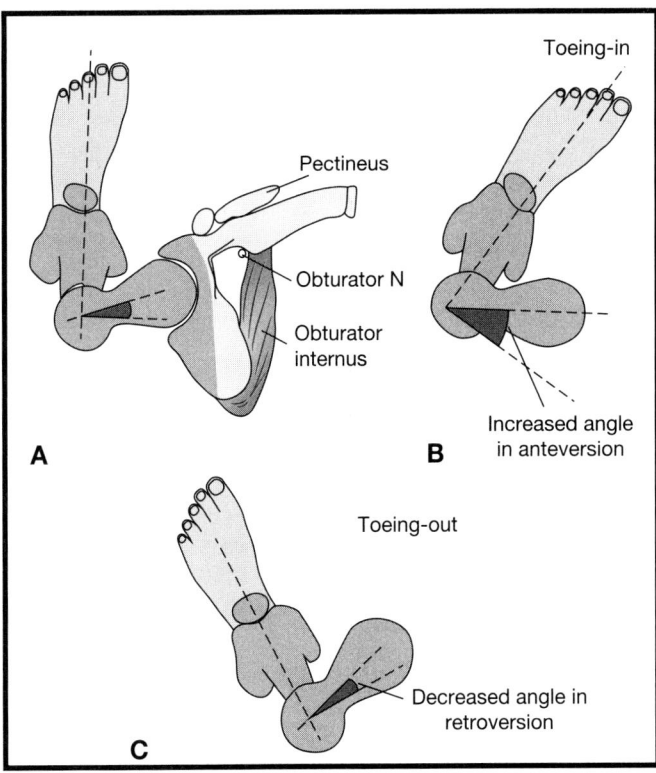

FIGURE 7.4
Alignment of *the* hip joint: (A) normal, (B) anteversion, (C) retroversion with position of foot (toeing).
N, nerve.

Blood supply to the femoral head and neck
- Retinacular branches of the medial (dominant posteriorly) and lateral circumflex arteries (anterior groin) from the profunda femoris; the lateral epiphyseal vessels (main)
- Obturator artery from ligament teres; variable in adults; 30%

Structural elements of the proximal femur
- Trabecular pattern: facilitate load transmission through the formation of three distinct arcades arranged at 60° orientations to manage the tensile and compressive forces experienced by the femoral head and neck
  ○ Medial trabecular system for the vertical compressive forces to the cortical bone
  ○ Lateral system will transmit shear forces of body weight and ground-reaction force to the cortical bone
    ▪ Lateral pattern: The lateral forces will go laterally and up into the pelvis
- The cortical structure of the femoral neck is thicker at the inferior margin as an adaptation to these loads

LIGAMENT

Anterior (Figure 7.5)
- Iliofemoral ligament: anterior inferior iliac spine to intertrochanteric line of the femur
  ○ Superior band: thickest and strongest; prevents hyperextension, and resists anterior translation
  ○ Medial (vertical) and lateral; Y ligament of Bigelow
    ▪ Restrict external rotation in both flexion and extension and internal rotation in flexion
- Pubofemoral ligament: inferiorly located; prevents excessive abduction
- Ligament teres: conduit for the secondary blood supply from the obturator artery and for nerves to travel along the ligament
  ○ In childhood, primary retinacular artery cannot travel through epiphysis

Posterior
- Ischiofemoral ligament: ischium to the neck of the femur, tightened by flexion

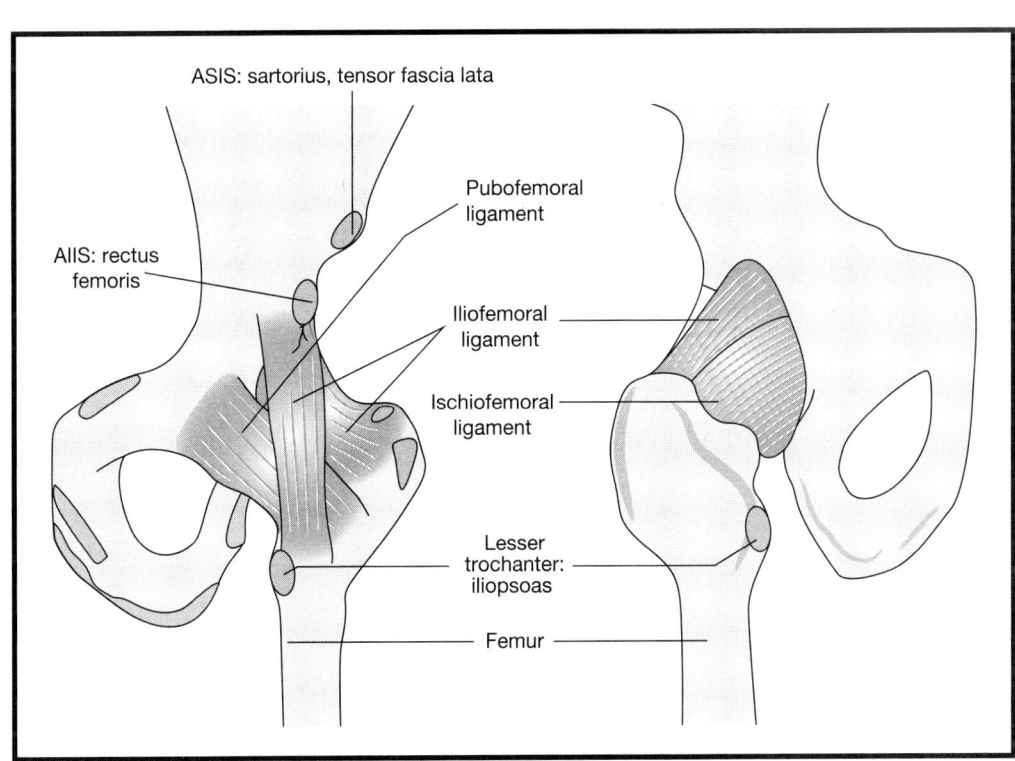

FIGURE 7.5
Ligaments in the hip joint.
ASIS, anterior superior iliac spine.

NERVE

Cutaneous nerves (see Figure 7.2)

CUTANEOUS NERVES	ROOT	INNERVATION	COURSE AND PATHOLOGIES
Lateral femoral cutaneous nerve	L2,3	Lateral thigh	Course under fascia iliaca (near ASIS), then perforates the fascia Meralgia paresthetica (MC)
Ilioinguinal and iliohypogastric nerve	L1	Lateral (ilioinguinal) and medial aspect (iliohypogastric) of the inguinal canal	Course between internal oblique abdominis and transverse abdominis Possible cause of persistent groin pain (neuropathic character)
Genitofemoral nerve	L1,2	Perforates the psoas fascia above the inguinal ligament and divides into genital and femoral branch	Course superficial to femoral nerve (lateral to the artery) Possible cause of persistent groin pain (neuropathic character)
Medial femoral cutaneous nerve	L2–4 Femoral nerve	Anterior medial thigh	Injury: very rare, usually iatrogenic or traumatic
Posterior femoral cutaneous nerve	S1–3 Sciatic nerve	Posterior thigh	Irritated by hamstring tendinopathy
Obturator nerve	L2–4	Distal medial thigh and knee, labrum of hip	Fascial entrapment at the entrance to adductor compartment

ASIS, anterior superior iliac spine; MC, most common.

Femoral nerve: L2–4, posterior division, runs between iliacus and psoas muscle → femoral nerve lateral to artery (vein medial to artery), but not contained in the femoral sheath, traverses midline of inguinal ligament
- Motor branches: sartorius, pectineus, and quadriceps
- Sensory branches: intermediate and medial femoral cutaneous nerves

Obturator nerve: L2–4, anterior division, formed within the psoas major muscle
- Runs over the pelvic brim → the obturator foramen (posterior to ramus), then between superior and inferior pubic ramus (posteior to anterior) → either anterior or posterior to obturator externus/adductor brevis (entrapment site)
- Anterior branch (more common pain generator): motor to adductor longus, brevis, and gracilis muscles and sensory fibers to the skin (distal two-thirds of the medial thigh) and fascia of the medial aspect of the mid-thigh, articular branch to the hip joint)
- Posterior branch: pierces and innervates the obturator externus → motor branch (adductor magnus) and sensory branch to knee joint (articular capsule, cruciate ligaments, and synovial membrane)

Sciatic nerve
- Runs between medial and lateral hamstring muscles
  - Lateral to the semimembranosus under the biceps femoris tendon at the level of the ischial tuberosity: chronic tendinopathy causes sciatic nerve irritation at this level (17)
- Tibial nerve: semimembranosus, semitendinosus, and biceps femoris long head
- Peroneal nerve: biceps femoris short head (only muscle innervated by peroneal nerve above the fibular head)

MUSCLE (FIGURE 7.6)

MUSCLE	ORIGIN	INSERTION	INNERVATION	ACTION	COMMENT
Hip Flexors					
Psoas major	T12–L5	Lesser trochanter	Lumbar root or plexus, L1, L2 (L3)	Flex hip	Covers lumbar plexus (not innervated by femoral nerve)
Psoas minor	T12–L1	Iliopubic eminence	L1–ventral ramus	Assists in hip flexion	Present in 50% of people

(continued)

MUSCLE	ORIGIN	INSERTION	INNERVATION	ACTION	COMMENT
Iliacus	Iliac fossa/lateral aspect of sacrum	Lesser trochanter	Femoral (L2–4)	Flex hip	Covers anterior ilium
Pectineus	Pectineal line of pubis	Pectineal line of femur	Femoral	Flex, adduct thigh (hip)	Part of femoral triangle floor
Sartorius	ASIS	Pes anserine	Femoral	Flex, ER hip	Avulsion fracture at ASIS
Hip Adductors					
Adductor magnus	1. Pubic ramus 2. Ischial tuberosity	Linea aspera, adductor tubercle	1. Obturator (L2–4) 2. Sciatic (L4–S3)	Adduct, flex/externally rotate thigh	
Adductor brevis	Pubic ramus	Pectineal line, linea aspera	Obturator	Adduct thigh	Deeper layer to pectineus
Adductor longus	Pubic ramus	Linea aspera	Obturator	Adduct thigh	Located medial to pectineus
Gracilis	Pubic ramus	Pes anserine (proximal medial tibia, inferior to sartorius insertion)	Obturator	Adduct thigh, flex/IR leg	
Hip Abductors					
Tensor fascia lata	Iliac crest, ASIS	Iliotibial band	Superior gluteal (L4–S1)	Abduct, flex, IR thigh	Commonly sampled muscle in needle EMG for L5 radiculopathy
Gluteus medius	Ilium between anterior and posterior gluteal lines	Posterior GT (anterior/medial portion to lateral facet, posterior portion to the posterosuperior facet)	Superior gluteal	Abduct, IR thigh	Trendelenburg gait with significant weakness Waddling gait if bilaterally involved
Gluteus minimus	Ilium between anterior and posterior gluteal lines	Anterior GT (anterior facet of greater trochanter) Hip joint capsule	Superior gluteal	Abduct, IR thigh	

ASIS, anterior superior iliac spine; EMG, electromyography; ER, external rotation; GT, greater trochanter; IR, internally rotate; US, ultrasound.

BIOMECHANICS

KINEMATIC AND KINETIC (18,19)

Hip joint movement
- Multiaxial ball-and-socket joint, mostly rotational movement, no detectable translational movement
- Depth of acetabulum deciding absolute limit of range (in addition to other factors)
- Retro and anteversion; angle between the posterior intercondyles (at the knee) and femoral neck (see Figure 7.4)
  ○ Affects rotation of the femur, knee, tibia → pronation or supination, location of patella on the intercondylar groove, and can cause leg-length discrepancy
- Muscles across the joint: gluteal muscle, iliopsoas, adductor, rectus femoris, and hip external rotator muscles; stability and tightness affect movement
  ○ Tight hip flexor with iliopsoas tightness (common in office workers, wheelchair ambulators)
  ○ Tight rectus femoris/iliopsoas (anterior tilting of the pelvis) versus hamstring (posterior tilting); affects the spine's sagittal alignment
  ○ Hip retroversion or hyperpronation; external rotation of the femur; shortened hip external rotator
- Extension reserve concept: the range of hip extension from the standing position: up to ~15°
  ○ Pelvic retroversion (to decrease the lumbar lordosis) → hip constantly extended and hamstring shortened in this position → mechanical disadvantage in shortened hamstring → affects the sagittal alignment of the spine

Hip joint motion in activities of daily living (ADLs) (20)
- Tying shoe with foot on floor 124° on the same side, 110° on the opposite side in sagittal plane
- Squatting 122°, sitting down and rising 104° in sagittal plane

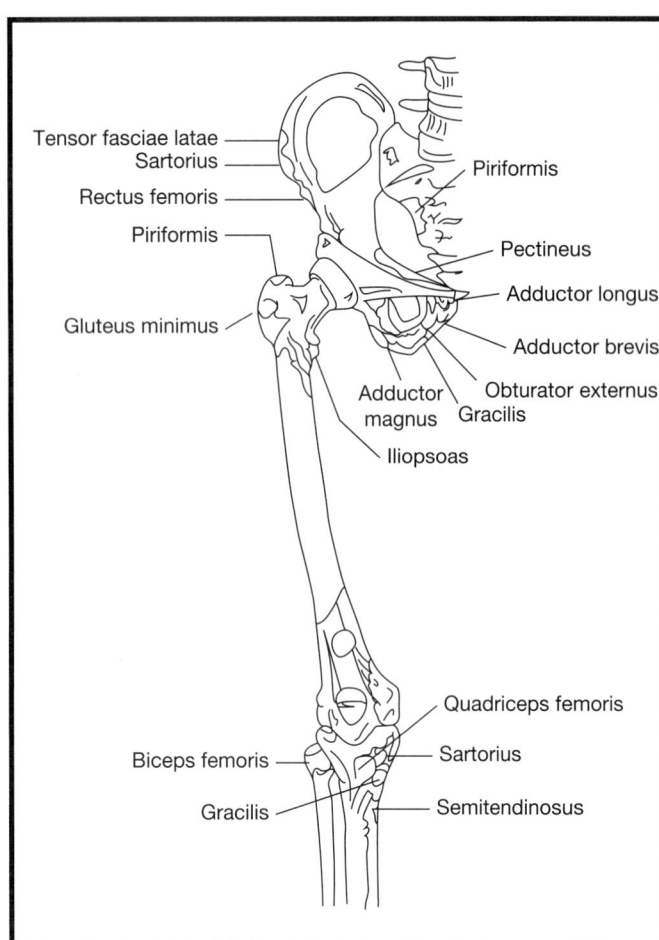

FIGURE 7.6
Muscles in the hip region.

- Ascending stairs versus descending: 67° versus 36° in sagittal plane
- Running: ~140° of flexion/extension range, but slow-paced jogging only requires 40°
- Jogging: propelled forward moment through hip flexion and knee extension rather than pushing off from ankle plantar flexion

Center of gravity (COG): within the pelvis, anterior to 2nd sacral vertebra, midline (medial to the hip joint)
- Fulcrum in the hip joint; hip abductor (short lever arm) counterbalancing body weight (opposite longer lever arm of the fulcrum)

Kinetics of the hip joint (at the center of femoral head)
- Joint reaction force (reflecting force on the joint): result of the need to balance the moment arms of the body weight and abductor tension
  ○ Bipedal stance: support two-thirds of the body weight (upper body and trunk); each hip supports one-third of the body weight
  ○ Unipedal stance: support five-sixths of body weight (2/3+ 6/1; one lower limb)
- Joint reaction force on the hip with different activity
  ○ Walking: 2.5 × body weight, jogging: 5 × body weight, some athletic activity (stumbling) >8 × body weight
  ○ Further increase in single stance during kicking, jumping, or cutting in
- Therapeutic implication: to decrease joint reaction force
  ○ Lever arm from the midline (center of mass to the hip joint; fulcrum)
  ○ Shift body weight over the affected hip or weak hip abductor
  ○ Decrease hip joint moment: (upper body weight + one lower leg weight) × lever arm (body weight)
    ▪ Trendelenburg and use of cane (shorten the lever arm for body weight by shifting the COG laterally)
      – Use of cane contralaterally; decreased muscle activity (EMG) of hip abductor by 40%

HIP STABILITY (21)

Stabilizers
- Bony stabilizer: acetabulum
  ○ 170° of femoral head coverage
  ○ Orientation: anterior tilt; anteversion ~20° → more posterior coverage; allowing more flexion than extension
  ○ Hip: most stable in full extension
- Soft tissue stabilizer
  ○ Labrum: extend acetabular coverage and ensure negative intra-articular pressure
  ○ Ligaments: iliofemoral, pubofemoral, ischiofemoral, and ligamentum teres (unclear function, free nerve ending, but hypertrophy can cause instability)
  ○ Iliopsoas and muscles around hip joint (gluteus, hip external rotator, etc); dynamic stabilizer

PHYSICAL EXAMINATION

INSPECTION

On standing: check the posture, leveled pelvis (posterior iliac crest), and exaggerated/diminished lumbar lordosis

Observation of gait: antalgic gait pattern (Trendelenburg, hip lurch, or slight hip flexion)

Pelvic tilt (lateral) and anterior (exaggerated lordosis) and posterior tilt (flat back)

Gross atrophy of quadriceps and hamstring muscles

Alignment of femur: coxa vara or valgum, ante-/retroversion (affecting direction of patellar facing)
- Coxa vara with genu valgum and anteversion (patellar or intercondylar groove facing medially)
- Ante-/retroversion; hip internal/external rotation on prone
  ○ Check foot angle (tibial torsion) and forefoot deformity (metatarsus adductus) in addition to hip anteversion for toeing in

Leg-length discrepancy (22)
- Compare the length of ASIS (or umbilicus) to medial malleolus and Galeazzi sign with hip and knee flexion; height

of the patella (can be affected by pelvic rotation; check the ASIS height)
- Causes: developmental hip dysplasia, previous fracture, dislocation, tumor, osteomyelitis, and functional discrepancies
- Up to half inch; well tolerated by the patient (therefore, no need for lift)

PALPATION

Anterior
- ASIS: start from lateral iliac crest and palpate the prominence anteriorly
- Femoral artery: midline between the pubic tubercle and ASIS
- Pubic symphysis palpation on supine (at the midline) for tenderness, gap, or overriding

Lateral
- Greater trochanter: lateral side, bony prominence on lateral or standing, a hand breadth below the ASIS

Posterior
- Ischial tuberosity: at the level of greater trochanter on 90° hip flexion

RANGE OF MOTION

MOTION	ROM (FUNCTIONAL)°	MOTION ON SUPINE	ROM (FUNCTIONAL)°	MOTION ON SUPINE WITH HIP FLEXION AT 90	ROM (FUNCTIONAL)°
Extension	0–30 (0–15) on prone	Abduction	45–50 (20–30)	External rotation	45–60 (15–40)
Flexion	125–135 (90–120)	Adduction	30–45 (20)	Internal rotation	40–45 (20–30)

ROM, range of motion.

Varies depending on the examination position, age, and gender: check for symmetricity

Flexion: tightness of hip flexor muscle/capsule; common in person sitting all day or in wheelchair

Hamstring-popliteal angle for hamstring tightness (hip 90° flexion, then extend the knee gradually)
- Useful to follow up the progression

SPECIAL EXAMINATION

NAME	DESCRIPTION	SENSITIVITY (SEN) AND SPECIFICITY (SPE) IN %
FABER (Patrick)	The patient lies supine and the examiner flexes, abducts, and externally rotates the hip (figure of 4) The examiner then stabilizes the pelvis by applying the pressure on the contralateral ASIS and applies pressure Positive with pain in the groin (hip pathology), buttock pain in the SI region (23)	Sen: ~70, Spe: up to 100 for positive response to SI joint injection
FADIR	The patient lies supine, the examiner flexes, adducts, and internally rotates the hip Positive if the pain is reproduced in the groin or in the buttock For femoroacetabular impingement (most sensitive test, sensitivity: 80%–90%) and piriformis syndrome (~80% sensitivity and specificity) (24)	
Log roll	The patient lies supine, and the examiner rolls the leg back and forth Positive with groin pain: suggests intra-articular hip problem	
Thomas test	To check for hip contracture. The patient bridges the knee to the chest (to decrease lumbar lordosis), and examiner measures the leg/thigh angle from the bed (positive if leg rises). Normal: 5°–20°. Check the contralateral side	
Modified Thomas test	To check for iliopsoas, rectus femoris, TFL/ITB complex tightness The patient is asked to sit on the end of a table, roll back to a supine position, and hold both knees to the chest. The patient holds the knee on the asymptomatic side close to the chest, and then the examiner slowly lowers the affected limb toward the floor Knee flexion less than 90° for rectus femoris tightness, external rotation for ITB tightness (25). Compare with the asymptomatic side	
Ely test	The patient lies prone while examiner flexes the knee Positive if the hip flexes (tightness of rectus femoris; hip flexion and knee extension)	

(continued)

NAME	DESCRIPTION	SENSITIVITY (SEN) AND SPECIFICITY (SPE) IN %
Ober test	The patient lies on the uninvolved side with the uninvolved hip and knee flexed to obliterate lumbar lordosis; abduct the involved hip maximally, extend ~20° with knee either flexed at 90° or extended (modified Ober test), and then let the thigh drop Positive if failure to adduct or if a catch is present	
Noble compression test	Pressure over the lateral femoral epicondyle while extending the knee from 90° of flexion Positive if pain is reproduced when the knee is flexed around 30° (26)	
Posterior hip impingement test	The patient lies supine (similar to Thomas test position), and the examiner places the patient's hip in extension and external rotation. Positive with discomfort or apprehension (27)	

ASIS, anterior superior iliac spine; FABER, flexion, abduction, external rotation; FADIR, flexion, adduction, and internal rotation; ITB, iliotibial band; SI, signal intensity; TFL, tensor fascia lata.

DIAGNOSTIC STUDIES

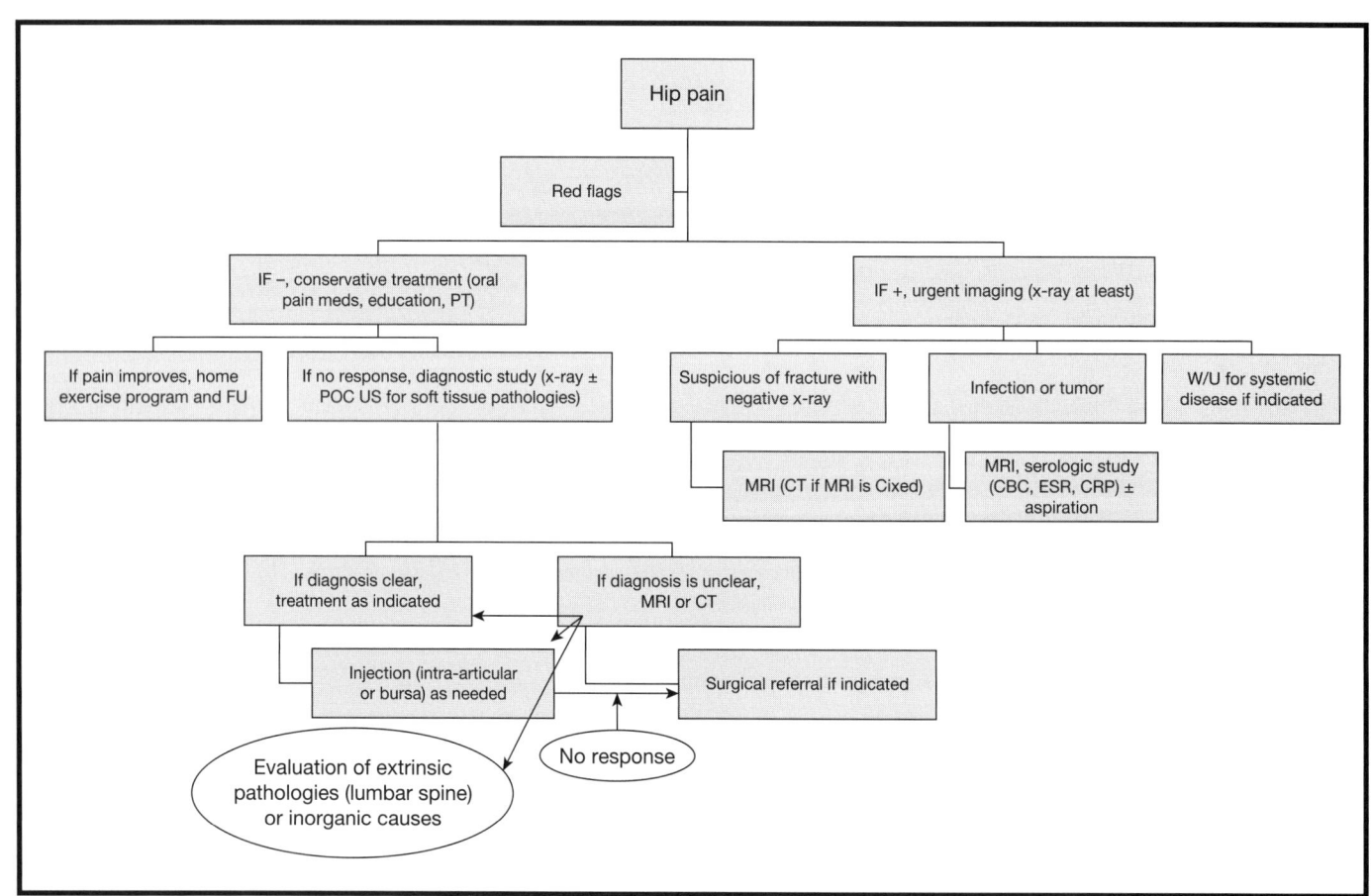

FLOWCHART 7.3

Diagnostic approach and management of hip pain.

AVN, avascular necrosis; CBC, complete blood count; CRP, C-reactive protein; ESR, erythrocyte sedimentation rate; FU, follow-up; PO, per os (oral); POC, point-of-care; PT, physical therapy; US, ultrasound; W/U, work up.

PLAIN RADIOGRAPHS (28)

Indications
- Chronic pain (>3 months): degenerative joint disease or inflammatory joint disease
- History of trauma or any red flags

Technique (29)
- Anteroposterior (AP): standing including pelvis (see Figure 7.7)
- Frog lateral view (abduct the hip): proximal femur, leg length, degenerative (better for osteophyte evaluation in femoral head than AP view), or dysplastic changes or bony lesion (30)
  - Cross table lateral (in trauma or acute pain, no need for hip abduction), Dunn view (to check femoral head spericity or femoral neck anteversion)
  - Other fractures: pelvic trauma (inlet/outlet view), acetabular fracture (Judet view)

Common findings
- Hip OA: osteophytes, joint space narrowing, sclerosis, and subchondral cyst formation
- Hip femoroacetabular impingement; pistol grip in cam type and cross-over (crossing of anterior and posterior wall outline medially rather than superiorly/laterally) in pincer type (common in asymptomatic young populations)
- Hip dysplasia: the center-edge angle, the femoral neck–shaft angle, and the vertical-center-anterior angle
  - Limited reliability
- Stress fracture: cortical thickening, possible lucent line in fatigue fracture, ill-defined linear sclerosis in insufficiency fracture. Plain radiograph is not sensitive

POINT-OF-CARE ULTRASONOGRAPHY (31,32,33)

Indications
- Tendon and muscle injuries, effusion or synovitis within the hip joint or adjacent bursa
  - Dynamic evaluation for snapping (especially external)
- Interventional: guidance for intra-articular hip joint injection (anterior recess or intracapsular) or bursal injection, or ultrasound (US)-guided nerve block (lateral femoral cutaneous nerve)

Setting
- Frequency: 12 MHz for superficial nervous structures; muscle: 8 to 12 MHz, and hip joint: 5 to 9 Hz
- Depth: depending on the patient's body habitus, 3 to 7 cm

Protocol
- Modified from the American Institute of Ultrasound in Medicine (AIUM) guidelines
- Anterior: oblique sagittal and transverse (with slight hip abduction)
  - Femoral head, neck, joint, capsule, labrum (part)
    - Joint effusion: distension >5 mm indicates >5 to 10 mL of fluid (2.7 mL in asymptomatic group)
    - Synovitis with increased vascularity, intra-articular loose body
    - Paralabral cyst
    - Cortical disruption in femoral neck
  - Tensor fascia lata, iliopsoas, rectus femoris (direct and reflected head), and sartorius
    - Enthesopathy (calcific tendinopathy), avulsion, tear
  - Bursa: iliopectineal and iliopsoas bursal effusion
  - Femoral nerve, saphenous or possibly anterior femoral cutaneous nerve
  - Dynamic view for snapping, anteriorly iliopsoas bursa (iliopectineal eminence)
- Medial: hip external rotation with 45° knee flexion, sagittal oblique
  - Adductor muscle (adductor longus, gracilis), pubic tubercle (osteitis pubis)/symphysis
- Lateral hip: lateral decubitus, transverse and longitudinal
  - Greater trochanter, gluteal tendon, and bursa
  - Snapping iliotibial band (ITB) (thickened TFL/ITB over the greater trochanter) during flexion and extension
  - Morel-Lavallée lesion (posttraumatic seroma)

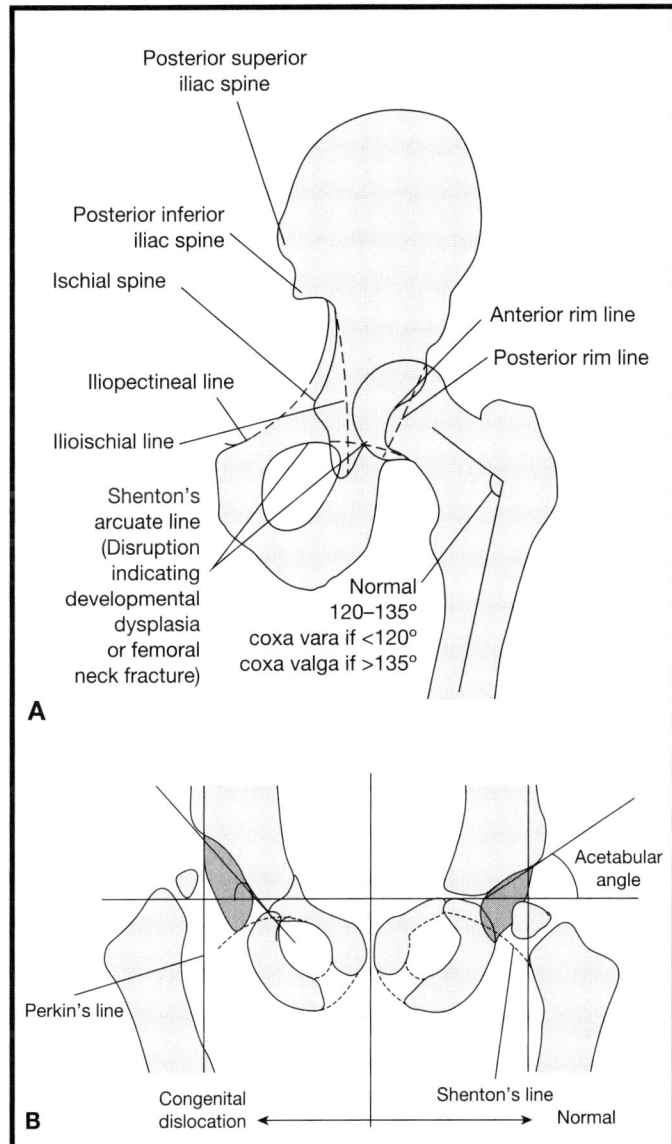

FIGURE 7.7
X-rays of (A) adult hip and (B) pediatric hip.

- Posterior: hip flexed (to tighten the hamstring) and extension to follow sciatic nerve
  - Hamstring tendon, ischial tuberosity, and ischiogluteal bursal space

MRI/MRA (34)

Indications
- Gold standard test for intraosseous and intra-articular (labral or ligament) abnormalities; better anatomic overview because of larger field of view than ultrasonography
  - Stress/insufficiency fracture when plain imaging is negative or to evaluate tumor/infection (if + red flags)
- More sensitive in deeper/proximal muscle pathologies (psoas and iliacus muscle) and tendon injury (hamstring and gluteal muscle) than US and may be more predictive of injury
- Evaluation of hernia (direct, indirect, and sports hernia), stress injury of symphysis pubis (osteitis pubis)
- Bursal effusion (iliopsoas bursa) in relation to hip joint capsule effusion

Technical considerations
- MR arthrography for intra-articular lesion (labral tear) better than MRI
  - Relatively low sensitivity and high specificity in cartilaginous pathologies (delamination tears)
- MRI of pelvis often required (for adductor strain, osteitis pubis, sports hernia, or posterior hip rotator muscles)

TREATMENT

NONOPERATIVE MANAGEMENT

Patient education
- Use cane on the contralateral side to decrease the workload of hip abductors (gluteal muscle) to decrease joint reaction force (35)
- Avoid irritation of superficial nerve (eg, lateral femoral cutaneous nerve) by clothing, tight belt, and so on
- Education of training errors or external factors
- Weight loss as well as good rest, nutrition in the athletic population (for energy balance, nutritional balance with calcium and vitamin D supplementation)
- Stay active
  - Exercise in a pool when available if in significant pain; well tolerated
  - Continue upper body exercise (eg, using upper body ergometer/bike)
- Use a high chair (avoid deep squatting) although ROM a few times a day is strongly recommended despite pain unless there is contraindication

Physical therapy (PT) and home exercise program
- Strengthening exercise of the gluteal and core muscles education
- Stretching
  - Hip external rotator; piriformis, obturator internus/gemelli muscles
  - Adductor, flexor, hip abductor (ITB band), hamstring, and knee extensor
  - Manual therapy technique can be utilized: counter strain, myofascial release, and so on
- Joint proprioceptive exercise and balance exercise
- Modalities: US (deep heating) or cold modalities usually provide temporary pain relief
- One session of PT occasionally for proper assistive device use education

Orthosis
- Bracing: articulated hip orthotic (abductor brace)
  - Rarely used in general outpatient clinic except postsurgical, such as hip arthroplasty or developmental hip dysplasia (for Pavlik abduction harness)
- Heel lift (up to 0.5-inch) or shoe lift for leg-length discrepancy; no intervention up to 0.5-inch difference; check and address pelvic malalignment (rotation)

Injection
- Soft tissue injection (bursa, tendon and ligament, etc)
  - Injectate: steroid (for bursitis), prolotherapy, and platelet-rich plasma (PRP) (chronic pain with tendon/ligament injury)
- Joint injection
  - Positive response to intra-articular injection; good indicator of the pain source from intra-articular pathologies (eg, labral injury as source of pain)
  - Steroid injection: either fluoroscopy guided (obese population) or US guided (36)
  - Viscosupplementation and PRP injection can be considered in patients who do not respond to steroid injection
- Nerve block (used with US guidance and/or nerve stimulator)
  - Lateral femoral cutaneous nerve for meralgia paresthetica: slightly distal to the ASIS, under/deeper to the fascia iliaca (vs femoral nerve, which is above/superficial to fascia iliaca) then over the fascia distally
  - Iliopsoas and ilioinguinal nerve between internal oblique and transverse abdominis near ASIS (cephalad-medial to ASIS)
  - Obturator nerve for medial thigh/groin pain; anterior division between adductor longus/brevis (or pectineus/adductor longus, a few cm distal to pubic symphysis with hip abduction position
  - Medial femoral cutaneous nerve for anterior thigh pain

SURGERY

Arthroscopy (37)

Indications
- Failed conservative treatment with persistent pain for femoroacetabular impingement, labral pathology (labral tear, capsular laxity)/snapping, other intra-articular pathologies; chondral lesion or loose bodies

Positions and approaches: supine or lateral position on a distraction table
- Portal placement: anterolateral portal (anterior superior to greater trochanter), anterior (bisection of the vertical line from ASIS and horizontal line from greater trochanter)

and posterolateral (2–3 cm posterior to greater trochanter) portals

Complications (38)
- Heterotopic ossification (MC reported), nerve injury (pudendal and sciatic or others) by traction, portal placement, or scuffing
- Iatrogenic chondrolabral injury, iatrogenic instability resulting in subluxation/dislocation, extravasation of fluid into the intra-abdominal cavity, femoral neck fracture, hematoma, thromboembolic disease

Total Hip Arthroplasty (THA) (39)

Indications
- Advanced OA or failed conservative treatment for disabling pain from OA

Surgical approaches (40)
- Direct anterior: less commonly done than other approaches, muscle sparing, earlier restoration of gait, low rate of dislocation
- Direct lateral: adequate exposure to proximal femur and acetabulum, low dislocation rate
- Posterior (posterolateral) approach: spare the abductor muscle, extensive exposure, posterior dislocation: more commonly done

Complications
- Pain
  ○ MC cause: aseptic loosing and infection
  ○ Extrinsic factors: heterotopic ossification, stress fractures, spinal pathology, vascular lesions, referred pain from the retroperitoneum and abdomen, and soft tissue inflammation such as tendinopathies or bursitis
- Wound infection: suspicious for infection if drainage more than 4 days (also can be fat necrosis)
  ○ Either immediate postoperative or delayed infection
  ○ Delayed infection: presents with pain usually, methicillin-resistant *Staphylococcus aureus* (MRSA) (MC cause)
    ▪ X-ray: radiolucency or new bone formation ➔ fine needle aspiration
    ▪ Urgent surgical referral (needs excision, temporary implant with local antibiotic therapy and intravenous [IV] antibiotic; then reimplant of new prosthetic)
- Dislocation depending on the surgical approach, abductor insufficiency, and fracture
- Heterotopic ossification
  ○ Persistent pain, swelling, and warmth for 2 to 3 weeks
  ○ Postoperative irradiation for prevention
- Peripheral nerve injury
  ○ Risk factors: revision surgery, limb lengthening, female gender, congenital hip dislocation, increased blood loss, and increased surgical time
  ○ Good prognosis. MC persistent complaints: dysesthetic pain
- DVT prophylaxis (up to 4 weeks) because it develops usually late in THA
  ○ Lower-molecular-weight heparin is better than Coumadin

Perioperative rehabilitation
- Preoperative exercise
  ○ About 12 weeks of aerobic exercise or resistance exercise
  ○ Supervised PT focusing on strengthening, ROM exercises, and functional training for 12 weeks
  ○ Joint protection technique and energy conservation principle
  ○ Psychological impairment intervention
- Postoperative exercise
  ○ Hip abductor strengthening, stair climbing exercise, and use of armchair (markedly reduce forces across the hip)
  ○ Exercise after THA
    ▪ Cycling is the least stressful. Diving, golfing, and bowling are acceptable sports after THA.
    ▪ Running, waterskiing, football, baseball, and basketball are discouraged
  ○ Crutches: reduce the lateral hip force by 30%
- Patient education and precaution
  ○ Dislocation
    ▪ Posterior approach: 6 weeks in uncomplicated and 12 weeks in complicated dislocation
    ▪ In high-risk patients: hip spica or hip abductor with knee ankle foot orthosis (KAFO; hip flexion stop at 80°, abduction 20°, and external rotation 10°)
  ○ Weight bearing usually cleared by surgeon. Generally, full weight bearing in all cemented or proximally fitting uncemented THA implants, unless there is the presence of a trochanteric osteotomy, fracture, bone grafting, significant acetabular or femoral bone loss, or other unusual occurrence
  ○ Driving after THA
    ▪ About 1 to 6 weeks after operation: left THA ➔ within 1 week of operation, and right THA ➔ 4 to 6 weeks postoperation
  ○ Leg-length discrepancy after THA
    ▪ Functional: pelvic obliquity from muscle imbalance, abductor contracture, tight capsular structures, knee flexion contracture, or spine abnormality
    ▪ Do not correct the discrepancy for 6 months after surgery

JOINT AND BONE PATHOLOGY

OA OF HIP

Introduction
- Epidemiology
  ○ Prevalence: 7% to 17% (varies depending on different studies); higher with increasing age
    ▪ Radiologic findings of hip OA: up to 27% (41)
  ○ Female > male, White and African American > Asian, unilateral (especially with history of [h/o] trauma) > bilateral (obesity) (42)
  ○ MC cause of chronic hip pain in elderly patients
- Risk factors
  ○ Age (>50 years), obesity, genetics, childhood hip disorder (hip dysplasia and slipped capital femoral epiphysis), femoroacetabular impingement, labral tears, and sequel of avascular necrosis
  ○ Sports with high loads or sudden irregular impacts; repetitive injuries are likely; soccer and track

- Running: equivocal, may be increased in the subgroup with biomechanical abnormalities (vs protective of cartilage)

History and physical examination
- Insidious pain in the groin (buttock; underrecognized) and morning stiffness (<1 hour)
- Decreased range ± pain, especially internal rotation
  - The position of the femoral condyle being deeper in the acetabulum with internal rotation
  - Capsular pattern of restricted ROM: first internal rotation loss followed by decrease in abduction and flexion

Diagnosis
- Clinical diagnosis supplemented by imaging study
- Differential diagnosis
  - Inflammatory arthropathy
    - Pain worse in the morning, prolonged stiffness, systemic involvement, enthesopathy, skin or bowel symptoms
    - Elevated erythrocyte sedimentation rate (ESR), C-reactive protein (CRP), white blood cells (WBC) in joint fluid; 2,500 to 50,000/mm^3
  - Femoroacetabular impingement, labral tear, or protrusio acetabuli
  - Avascular necrosis (especially with risk factors)
  - Septic arthritis (younger individuals, especially with risk factors, red flags)
  - Synovial chondromatosis, pigmented villonodular synovitis
  - H/O trauma: acetabular fracture or femur fracture (proximal femur)
  - Trochanteric tendinobursitis (snapping hip syndrome, adductor strain); often concomitant
  - Referred pain to hip (L2–3 radiculopathy/plexopathy, SI joint dysfunction or coccydynia)
- Imaging studies
  - X-ray (AP, frog leg lateral): joint line narrowing, osteophyte, subchondral sclerosis, and cyst
  - MRI: not necessary for diagnosis, but for differential diagnosis for intra-articular and intracortical lesion if atypical presentation or red flags present

Treatment
- Patient education (weight loss, cane use), pain medication (acetaminophen, nonsteroidal anti-inflammatory drug [NSAID]) → weak opioid (eg, tramadol if not responsive to NSAID or acetaminophen)
- Physical therapy (PT) (43,44)
  - Stretching of iliopsoas, rectus femoris, iliotibial band, and hamstring muscles; dynamic-balance exercise, and gluteal/quadriceps muscle strengthening
  - Adaptive equipment evaluation, avoid low-seat chair, and so on
  - Cane to decrease pull of hip abductor muscle (28,45)
- Injection
  - Corticosteroid: cautious about steroid-induced bone disease
  - Hyaluronic acid (46) under US or fluoroscopy guidance (47)
  - Consider platelet-rich plasma injection and prolotherapy if steroid and viscosupplementation fail
- Surgical referral (48)
  - Hip replacement: advanced OA after failed conservative treatment
  - Resurfacing: metal on ceramic rather than metal on metal
  - Minimally invasive versus conventional incision; no significant difference in outcomes

LABRAL TEAR

Introduction (49,50)
- The most common form of intra-articular pathology, often asymptomatic, may be related to early hip OA
- Anatomy of labrum: thin fibrocartilaginous structure; enhance the congruity and stability of the femoroacetabular joint
- Classification
  - Location: anterior (antero-superior more common) and posterior tear
  - Morphological: radial flap, radial fibrillated, longitudinal peripheral, and unstable tears
- Etiology
  - Femoroacetabular impingement, hip dysplasia, trauma/dislocation, capsular laxity, and joint degeneration
  - Increased incidence with developmental dysplasia of the hip and LCPD
  - Trauma and overuse: repetitive cutting, jumping, and twisting during sports
    - Anterior: hyperextension, pivoting injury, and external rotation: most symptomatic (golfer)
    - Posterior: axial loading in a flexed position

History and physical examination
- Often asymptomatic
- Groin pain (deep aching) ± painful clicking, transient locking and "giving way" of the hip
  - Pain with Buddha position
- Physical examination: provocative tests; low sensitivity
  - Pain with anterior impingement position (flexion, adduction, and internal rotation [FADIR]) or (flexion, abduction and external rotation [FABER] to extension, adduction, and internal rotation [IR])
  - Posterior impingement (hyperextension, abduction, and external rotation)

Diagnosis
- Clinical suspicion confirmed by imaging study or arthroscopy
- X-ray to rule out (R/O) OA, dysplasia, and loose body
- MRI/MR arthrogram
  - Normal labrum: a triangular structure of homogeneously low signal intensity (SI) on all pulse sequences
  - Typical findings: linear hyperintense T2 SI contacting the labral surface
  - Associated findings
    - Subchondral bone marrow edema and/or cystic changes
    - Osseous fragmentation at the superior acetabulum
    - Paralabral cyst: highly specific finding
- Differential diagnosis: similar to hip OA, avascular necrosis (AVN), stress fracture, referred pain from L2 to L3 radiculopathy, intra-abdominal or gynecologic disorder, or snapping hip syndrome

Treatment
- Nonoperative treatment: activity modification, NSAIDs/pain medication, gluteal muscle strengthening, dynamic-balance exercise, and cane or crutches

- Injection (51) for pain relief
  - Steroid: limited clinical benefit as therapeutic modality (average duration of benefit 10 days) in femoroacetabular impingement (FAI) with labral tear
  - Good indicator for response to surgical procedure
- Surgical referral for arthroscopic debridement if failed conservative management
- Return to play: 6 weeks (golf) to 12 weeks (baseball or soccer); intervention to bony abnormalities: longer

FEMOROACETABULAR IMPINGEMENT

Introduction (52)
- Hip joint damage because of abnormal mechanical contact of the acetabular rim and the proximal femur (head–neck junction)
  - May cause labral tears, cartilage lesions, and eventually premature OA
- Epidemiology: unknown incidence, high prevalence of asymptomatic morphologic abnormalities (15%–25%) (53)
  - Cam lesion: more common in young active males and pincer lesion: more common in middle-aged active women
- Classification based on the location of the morphologic abnormalities (see Figure 7.8)
  - Cam impingement: abnormality in the anterior femoral head–neck junction
    - Pistol-grip deformity: the prominence of the femoral head–neck junction can be seen as an overall decreased offset at the femoral head–neck junction
    - Often associated with anterior superior labral lesion: chondrolabral junction
  - Pincer impingement: retroverted acetabulum
    - Associated with posterior inferior labral lesion, intrasubstance labral tear
  - Mixed cam and pincer: MC

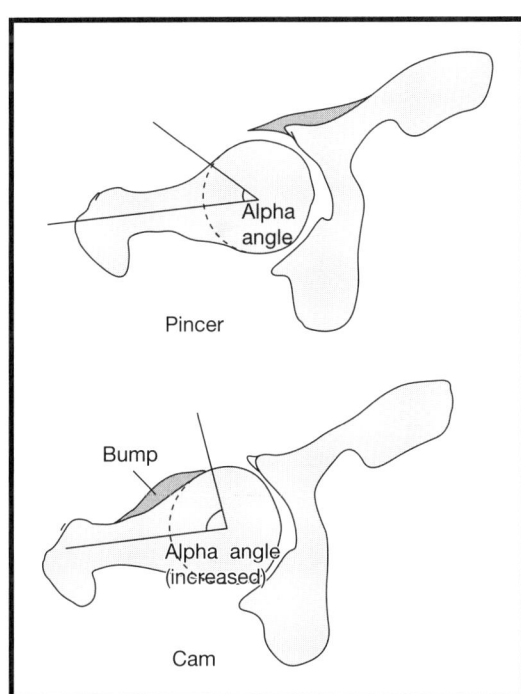

FIGURE 7.8
Femoroacetabular impingement: cam and pincer type.

- Risk factors
  - H/O slipped capital epiphysis, LCPD, osteonecrosis, and malunited femoral neck fracture (cam type)
  - Suprapysiologic flexion or rotational movements, repetitions, and forceful motions

History and physical examination
- History; similar to hip OA
  - Gradual onset of mild groin pain (less commonly buttock pain) with activities involving hip flexion (crouching, sitting) and weight bearing
    - Significant limping is unusual. If pain is significant, consider other etiologies
  - Stiffness or start-up pain and limited ROM (eg, "difficulty with tying shoe")
  - ± Symptoms from concomitant findings (labral tear)
- Physical examination
  - C sign: patient holds the hip when asked of the location of the pain (hip pathologies, not specific)
  - Limited flexion <90°, decreased passive external rotation more than internal rotation ± anterior impingement test, pain with FADIR (or internal/external rotation)

Diagnosis
- Clinical suspicion confirmed by imaging finding
- Differential diagnosis
  - Developmental dysplasia of the hip (eg, acetabular abnormality)
  - Decreased acetabular anteversion or coxa profunda (deep acetabular socket)
  - Acetabular protrusion (displacement of acetabulum and femoral head medially); primary or secondary (rheumatoid arthritis [RA], metabolic disease, or postsurgical)
  - Coxa vara
  - AVN, stress fracture (sacral), ischiofemoral impingement, plica lesion, synovial chondromatosis, and so on
- Imaging (54)
  - X-ray: AP and modified Dunn view (hip flexed 90° and abduction 20°)
    - Other lateral views: cross table lateral and false-profile view, often missing deformity
    - Acetabular retroversion
      – Center-edge angle: vertical line drawn through the center of the femoral head and a line drawn from the anterior edge of acetabulum to the center of femoral head; abnormal if >40° → more coverage of the anterior rim of the acetabulum compared with the posterior rim
      – Crossover sign; anterior rim over coverage (55)
    - Flattened head–neck junction, pistol grip deformity (cam) in AP and lateral view
  - MRI
    - The alpha angle (aspherical shape); cam impingement ≥55° (Figure 7.8)
      – Axial plane, between two lines from the center of the femoral head through the middle of the femoral neck and a line from the center of femoral head to where the contour of the femoral head–neck junction exceeds the radius of the femoral head
      – False positive: abnormality of the shape of the femoral head–neck junction such as a wide femoral neck,

osteophytes, or posterior displacement of the femoral head

Treatment
- Nonoperative management: activity modification, NSAID, exercise to prevent deconditioning
  - PT: increase passive range of motion (PROM) and stretching (may exacerbate symptoms), strengthening and neuromuscular training
- Injection: diagnostic (positive response is good indicator for intra-articular hip pathology and response to surgery) and symptom relief
- Surgery (48)
  - Open and arthroscopic procedure to debride the labrum, remove some of the femur (femoral osteoplasty) and/or acetabular osteotomy
  - Complications: peripheral nerve injury, trochanteric nonunion, osteonecrosis of the femoral head and femoral neck fracture
  - Postop: protected weight-bearing precautions for at least 4 to 6 weeks (56)
    - Return to full activity as early as 3 months. Premature return to activity: concern for femoral neck fracture

AVASCULAR NECROSIS OF HIP

Introduction (57)
- Epidemiology: ~15,000 cases per year, male ≥ female (equal or higher depending on different studies), peak incidence between 2nd and 5th decades, and 40% to 80% bilateral
- Etiology (58)
  - Risk factors: multifactorial, genetic, variation of vascular anatomy (absence or hypoplasia of the superior capsular artery), trauma, radiation, sickle cell disease (trait, caisson disease, myeloproliferative disease, etc), steroid (high dose, >20 mg/d, >2 g of prednisone within 2–3 months), alcohol, coagulation abnormalities, and smoking
  - Idiopathic: 10% to 20%

History and physical examination
- Insidious onset of groin pain with possible radiation to the buttock or knee
- Physical examination (not specific)
  - Pain with hip motion, particularly with internal rotation ± limited ROM

Diagnosis
- Clinical diagnosis (high index of suspicion) confirmed by imaging finding
- Differential diagnosis: similar to hip OA
- Imaging
  - Plain radiographs: the Arlet–Ficat staging

STAGES	FINDINGS
1	No radiographic finding
2	Subchondral sclerosis and cysts without overall changes in femoral head shape
3	Crescent sign: partial collapse of necrotic segment
4	Joint space narrowing; osteophytes, deformed femoral head

- Other criteria (Steinberg/University of Pennsylvania); further grading with A (mild) to C (severe)
  - MRI: sensitivity high as 88% to 100%, helpful in early stages and for differential diagnosis

Treatment (59)
- In early stages of the disease
  - Nonoperative treatment, including limited weight bearing and weight bearing with assistance to prevent head deformation and limit pain
  - Address underlying coagulation disorder with anticoagulation, bisphosphonates (to prevent resorption of necrotic bone), and statin (hyperlipidemia predispose to osteonecrosis) in patients taking steroids (52)
  - Optional surgical treatment: core decompression, 70% to 95% success rate for Stage I
- Referral to surgery in Stage II or III disease: bone grafting using vascularized fibula. Stage IV: THA

STRESS FRACTURE

Femoral Neck Stress Fracture

Introduction (60)
- Infrequent (5% of all stress fracture in athletes) but highly morbid condition
- Classification
  - Tension type: superior lateral cortex, distraction by weight-bearing axial force
    - Older population, high risk for nonunion and displacement
  - Compression type: inner aspect, weight-bearing cause compression, younger population
- High-complication rates 20% to 86%: complete fracture, malunion with impingement, nonunion, avascular necrosis, and arthritic change
- Anatomy
  - Femoral neck exposed to tensile (superior aspect) and compressive force (inferior aspect)
- Etiology and risk factors: an intense impact-loading training (young population) or osteoporosis (elderly)
  - History of a recent change in activity, duration, or frequency
  - Female, hormonal/menstrual disorder, poor nutrition (vitamin D and calcium deficiency), smoking, and other risk factors for osteoporosis
  - Biomechanical factors: leg-length discrepancy, coxa vara, pes cavus, worn-out shoe, and so on
  - Long-distance runners, ballet dancers, and military personnel
  - Training hours: if ≥8 hr/wk two times higher for stress fracture than ≤4 hr/wk in female athletes (61)

History and physical examination
- Gradual onset of activity-related groin pain, often pain at night
- Physical examination: not specific
  - Pain on extreme range (especially internal rotation), active straight leg raise, log rolling, and hopping
  - Usually not tender on palpation
  - Fulcrum test

- The patient is seated on the examination table with his lower legs dangling. The examiner places one of his arms under the symptomatic thigh (fulcrum). The arm moves toward the proximal thigh with other hand pushing down the knee. Test is positive if this reproduces pain or discomfort.
  ○ Hop test: reproduction of pain with one-legged hop

Diagnosis
- Clinical suspicion confirmed by imaging study
- Imaging
  ○ Plain x-ray: may be normal (can occur without cortical break), a visible fracture line, a visible break in the trabeculae, or callus formation
  ○ MRI: more sensitive and specific; study of choice when plain x-ray is normal in suspicious case and for differential diagnosis
- Differential diagnosis: other sources of groin pain

Treatment (62,63)
- Nonoperative treatment for medial side, nondisplaced fracture: 6 weeks weight-bearing restriction with crutches or limited weight bearing for 3 to 6 months
  ○ Bone scan at the end of the treatment (optional): to confirm healing
  ○ Address underlying etiologies: nutritional, footwear, training errors, and/or smoking cessation
- Referral to surgery for lateral side: because of poor healing (nonunion and AVN), displaced, or diastasis → open reduction internal fixation (ORIF)
- Return to play: asymptomatic full weight bearing, negative physical examination, and imaging study consistent with healed fracture

Pubic Ramus Stress Fracture

Introduction (64)
- Rare; stress fracture of the pelvis (~1%–2% of all stress fractures)
- Common in military recruits, and in female runners (in part to increase in female participation in marathon and partly because of anatomical configuration)
- Common location: inferior ramus because of tensile force (adductor magnus and gracilis pulling on the lateral aspect of the pubis ramus and ischium during hip extension) rather than compressive force

History and physical examination
- Groin pain worsening with weight bearing (not specific) and nonspecific physical examination

Diagnosis
- Clinical suspicion confirmed by imaging study
- Imaging study
  ○ X-ray: 2 to 4 weeks lag and 50% never show any changes in plain film
  ○ MRI rather than bone scan (poor specificity and poor anatomical detail; false positive up to ~30% because of high osteoblastic activity in the area, periosteitis, adductor tendonitis, and avulsion fracture)
- Differential diagnosis: periosteitis, adductor strain/tendonitis, and avulsion fracture

Treatment
- Protected weight bearing rather than non–weight bearing (not common)

Femoral Shaft Stress Fracture

Introduction (65)
- 3% to 20% of stress fracture (depending on studies and populations), underrecognized, athletes (proximal femur), and military recruits (distal femur)
- Common location: proximal one-third, posteromedial cortex by compressive force (medial side greater than lateral side)

History and physical examination
- Insidious onset of pain, often nonspecific, localized in the groin, thigh, or knee
- Specific tenderness: less likely given the overlying muscle bulk of the thigh
- Hop and fulcrum test reproducing pain

Diagnosis
- Clinical suspicion confirmed by imaging study
- X-ray (30%–70% positive) and MRI (especially to differentiate neoplasms)
- Comprehensive assessment of risk factors
- Differential diagnosis similar to femoral neck fracture

Treatment
- Relative rest with gradual return to play
  ○ Four phases, each lasting 3 weeks: at the end of the phase, hop and fulcrum test; if negative then advance
    - Walk with crutches, non–weight bearing in symptomatic side → normal walking, swimming, and exercise upper body and contralateral side → partial weight and run in straight line every other day → return to play
- Referral to surgery if displaced or persistent pain despite conservative treatment

OSTEITIS PUBIS

Introduction (66)
- Chronic, painful injury of pubic symphysis and parasymphyseal bone
- Common in athletes: 14% of groin pain in athletes (small study), male > female
- Etiology
  ○ Repetitive trauma, abnormal motion, and subtle pubic instability
    - Running, sprinting, soccer, football, and hockey
    - Repeated activities of cutting, kicking, and jumping
  ○ Iatrogenic: status post (s/p) urological and obstetrical procedures

History and physical examination
- Pain in the medial groin (midline) ± referred pain to the medial thigh, abdomen, or perineum
  ○ Pain on striding and pivoting
- Point tenderness over the pubic symphysis and painful range with passive abduction and resisted adduction

Diagnosis (67)
- Clinical diagnosis confirmed by imaging study

- Imaging study
  - X-ray: widening of symphysis, sclerosis, cyst, irregularity, and bone resorption
    - Flamingo view (stork view) for instability: AP with alternating unilateral lower-extremity weight bearing
      - Positive if symphysis widens >7 mm or superior ramus displaces >2 mm
  - MRI: bone edema (debate regarding clinical significance), secondary cleft sign (abnormal inferior extension of the cleft in the symphyseal fibrocartilage), and to differentiate other pathologies (68)
- Differential diagnosis
  - Adductor tendon dysfunction, injury to the prepubic aponeurotic complex, and sports hernia
  - Hip pathology (OA, femoroacetabular impingement), stress fracture, iliopsoas tendon dysfunction, referred pain from lumbar spine or SI joint, rarely direct inguinal hernia, and osteomyelitis

Treatment
- Nonoperative treatment: biomechanical assessment and improvement of mechanical imbalance and pain medication (NSAIDs) as needed
  - PT: water-based exercise initially (if available), stretching exercise of hip adductor, iliopsoas, isometric exercise of abdominal muscle, core, pelvis- and hip-stability exercises
  - Steroid injection (small volume), platelet-rich plasma injection, and prolotherapy
- Surgery is rarely needed
- Progressive return to sport: up to 3 months

AVULSION FRACTURE AND APOPHYSEAL INJURIES

Introduction (69)
- Peak incidence in adolescent/young athletes (14–25 years of age) by injury or displacement of unfused apophysis at the site of tendon attachment
- Etiologies
  - Apophyseal injuries: similar to musculotendinous junction injury in mature athletes
  - Inherent weakness in the unfused apophyseal growth plate
  - Forceful contraction of the muscle; usually associated with jumping, sprinting, or running
    - Football and soccer players, cheerleaders, and gymnasts
- Common locations of apophyseal injuries in adolescents
  - Ischium: hamstring, MC location of apophyseal avulsion injury in the pelvis
  - ASIS: sartorius and tensor fascia lata; can be confused with anterior inferior iliac spine (AIIS) avulsion fracture if avulsion fragment is retracted distally
  - AIIS: rectus femoris
  - Iliac crest apophysis: ossification between 15 to 18 years old, abdominal muscles, hip pointers, often bilateral, anterior third of the growth plate of the iliac crest
  - Symphysis pubis and inferior pubic ramus: adductor of the hip, associated with overuse injury of excessive twisting and turning of the abdomen and pelvis, athletic pubalgia
  - Lesser trochanter: iliopsoas, uncommon, adolescent soccer players before closure of the apophyseal growth plate (28,29)
- Location in adult avulsion injury
  - Adductor insertion avulsion syndrome: at the insertion of adductor longus and brevis (medial thigh), female athletes in track or long-distance running, military recruits
  - Abductor tendon avulsion syndrome: elderly >65 years of age, repetitive microtrauma from hyperadduction, falls; usually comes with gluteus tendinopathy or after THA
  - Lesser trochanter avulsion: often minimal (not excessive) amount of force in elderly

History and physical examination
- Pain (sudden onset and severe) at the location of avulsion, difficulty walking ± popping sensation, often not specific, aggravated by activity
- Tenderness and swelling, pain on stretching of the tendon or muscle involved
  - Reproduction of pain with contraction of the muscle involved

Diagnosis
- Clinical suspicion confirmed by imaging
- X-ray: often subtle if the displacement is minimal. In chronic cases: extensive callus or new bone production
- US and MRI if radiographs are indeterminate (minimally displaced or nondisplaced)
  - MRI: fluid or edema signal (increased T2 SI) in the growth plate
- Differential diagnosis: metastatic disease in adults with no significant trauma

Treatment
- Nonoperative management: rest, return to full weight bearing, and passive ROM exercise, great success with nonoperative management
  - In lesser trochanter avulsion in elderly: non–weight bearing with crutches initially for symptomatic treatment
- Return to play after full strength regained and full ROM without pain
- Surgery: ORIF in competitive athletes and if avulsed segment >2 cm in diameter. Timing of the surgery: controversial

HIP POINTER

Introduction (30)
- Iliac crest or surrounding soft tissue contusion, apophyseal injury of iliac crest
- Common injury in contact sports, football, hockey, and rugby
  - 11% of total hip injuries and 35% of total hip contusions in National Football League
  - MC cause: direct trauma
- Sequels: if untreated, it can lead to periostitis or the formation of new bone (exostosis)

History and physical examination
- Pain over the iliac crest or ASIS, difficulty walking ± fluctuating mass (hematoma) ± tingling/pins/needles with irritation of iliohypogastric, ilioinguinal, and lateral femoral cutaneous nerve
- A fluctuant mass over the area, resulting from hematoma

Diagnosis
- Clinical diagnosis ± confirmed by imaging study
- X-ray to R/O fracture or apophyseal avulsion in the skeletally immature patient

Treatment
- Rest, ice, compression and elevation (RICE), NSAIDs starting at 48 hours. Crutches if gait difficulty present
- If a large hematoma is present, consider immediate aspiration followed by ice and compression
- PT for ROM, stretching (TFL, sartorius, abdominal muscle, and iliopsoas), and strengthening
- Steroid injection to the iliac crest if the pain persists despite PT
- Return to play if full ROM and full strength achieved. Padding over the injured area to prevent recurrence or exacerbation

HIP DISLOCATION

Introduction (31)
- Etiology: severe injury from high-energy trauma; motor vehicle accident (MC causes), alpine skiing, football, and wrestling
- Posterior dislocation: MC, 80% to 85% (posteriorly directed force on flexed knee, dashboard injury)
- Complications
  - Acetabular and femoral head fracture, sciatic nerve injury: 10% to 20% (traction or direct trauma), ligaments injury and other associated fracture
  - Long-term complications: AVN (1%–17%), posttraumatic OA

History and physical examination
- Severe pain, decreased ROM with pain, and difficulty walking/impaired weight bearing
- Posterior: hip is held in flexion, adduction, and IR
- Anterior: hip is held in extension, abduction, and external rotation
- If this injury is suspected, a careful neurological and vascular exam is needed

Diagnosis
- Clinical diagnosis (high index of suspicion in children and adolescents in subtle cases), confirmed by imaging study
- AP pelvis and lateral view
- Investigation for concomitant avulsion of ligament teres, femoral neck fracture, and other lower extremity fracture, intra-abdominal/pelvic injuries, chest trauma, and head injury (concussion)

Treatment
- Urgent/emergent orthopedic consultation (referral to ER) is recommended
  - AVN of the femoral head is directly related to time from dislocation to reduction
  - A closed reduction should be attempted only after radiographs have been obtained

TUMOR OR TUMORLIKE LESION

Classification (32)
- Common osseous tumors
  - Primary osseous tumors of the pelvis in decreasing order of frequency; chondrosarcoma, Ewing sarcoma, osteosarcoma, and fibrosarcoma
  - Primary benign osseous tumors or pseudotumors of the proximal femur: fibrous dysplasia, solitary bone cyst (proximal humerus > proximal femur), aneurysmal bone cyst (proximal femur), and osteoid osteoma
    - Fibrous dysplasia (proximal femur 22%, pelvic 6%, mixed lysis and sclerosis, shepherd's crook deformity)
- Tumorlike lesions: trauma, infection, cysts, Langerhans cell histiocytosis, Paget disease (differential diagnosis with diffuse metastatic disease)

Common presentation
- Usually asymptomatic, rest pain or night pain, systemic symptoms, or palpable mass
- High index of suspicion with red flags
- Imaging study: x-ray (often insensitive), then MRI with/without contrast, especially for soft tissue tumors

Pediatric Tumors

Benign tumors: bone cysts, fibrous dysplasia
- Usually asymptomatic, but mechanical pain if it compromises the structural integrity of the bone
- Night pain and pain with weight bearing: benign aggressive neoplasms such as osteoid osteoma or chondroblastoma

Leukemia is the most common malignancy in childhood
- The hip can be the most frequent site of musculoskeletal (MSK) pain (33)
  - May present like infectious etiology (septic arthritis or osteomyelitis) initially
- Labs: elevated ESR with associated anemia, neutropenia, or thrombocytopenia
  - Often x-rays are normal, but MRI scans show the marrow replacement

BURSITIS AND TENDINOPATHY

LATERAL HIP

Trochanteric Bursitis (Greater Trochanteric Pain Syndrome) (34)

Introduction (70)
- Incidence: up to 5.6 per 1,000, may affect 10% to 25% of the population in industrialized societies
  - Female > male, peak incidence in 4th to 6th decades
  - One of the most common causes of lateral hip pain
- Risk factors: common in patients with leg-length discrepancy, pelvic obliquity, running on banked surfaces, low back pain, obesity, and knee pain
- Anatomy: three to four consistent bursas (Figure 7.9)
  - Subgluteus maximus (deep); "trochanteric bursa," largest (size: ~3 × 3 cm)
    - Deep to the fascia lata and gluteus maximus
  - Subgluteus medius bursa (between glut med and lateral facet)
  - Subgluteus minimus (between glut min and anterior facet

○ Sub ITB bursa (ITB and greater trochanter), piriformis bursa (posterior subgluteus medius bursa)

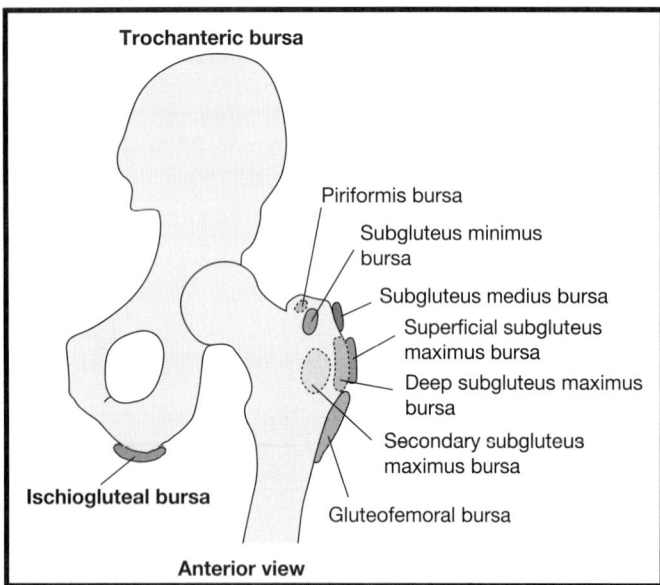

FIGURE 7.9
Trochanteric bursa and ischiogluteal bursa.

History and physical examination
- Lateral hip/buttock pain: pain on standing, by lying on the side (affected), and by abduction and external rotation
  ○ 50% of patients have radiating pain along the lateral aspect of the thigh to the knee
  ○ Gait disturbance with pain
- Point tenderness (posterolateral aspect of greater trochanter (GT); posterior facet) and pain on active resistant to abduction/external rotation

Diagnosis
- Clinical diagnosis ± image-guided injection (for confirmation)
- Imaging (x-ray, US, or MRI) (71,72)
  ○ X-ray: R/O hip or bony pathologies, secondary changes (cortical irregularity, calcification) from gluteal tendinopathy
  ○ US: bursal effusion (uncommon, up to 20% in some studies), gluteal tendinopathy (MC finding), thickened ITB and gluteal tears (rare) (73)
  ○ MRI: unresponsive to the initial treatment and equivocal US findings, intracortical and proximal pelvic pathologies
- Differential diagnosis
  ○ Gluteus medius tear or tendinosis
  ○ Lumbosacral (LS) radiculopathy, referred pain from facet joints, SI joint dysfunction (often concomitant)
  ○ Less common conditions: femoral head osteonecrosis, stress fracture, gluteal aponeurotic pain, or cluneal neuropathy

Treatment (74)
- Nonoperative treatment: mainstay of treatment
  ○ NSAID, activity modification, and/or cane
  ○ Therapy: stretching of ITB, hip external rotator, strengthening of gluteal, tensor fascia lata, hip external rotator, and modalities (ice, US)
  ○ Low-energy shock therapy (mixed results, temporary erythema, and skin irritation)
  ○ Steroid injection (using bony landmark): palpate the greater trochanter, needle down to the bone (posterolateral aspect of greater trochanter), then injection (on the bone, cautious of the depth, often needs a 3.5-inch needle)
    ▪ US-guided injection: subgluteus maximus bursa injection (on the posterior facet) more effective than subgluteus medius bursal injection (can inject both) (75)
- Referral to surgery: disabling pain with failed conservative treatment
  ○ Bursectomy, gluteus medius repair, ITB Z plasty or release, and trochanteric osteotomy

Gluteal Tendinopathy/Tear
Introduction (76)
- Underrecognized cause of lateral hip (greater trochanteric pain syndrome), buttock, and groin pain, up to ~15%
  ○ Gluteus medius partial tear > tendinosis and retracted tear (77)
  ○ Very common in patients diagnosed with trochanteric bursitis
- Female > male, mean age: 60 years
- Anatomy: anterior facet of greater trochanter: gluteus minimus tendon, lateral and superolateral facet: gluteus medius tendon, and posterior facet: subgluteus maximus muscle (with bursa)
- Etiologies
  ○ Chronic nontraumatic tear (MC): tension within ITB → friction to the gluteus medius and minimus
  ○ Iatrogenic abductor tendon avulsion after THA or others

History and physical examination
- Difficult to distinguish from trochanteric bursitis (often coexisting) → trochanteric tendinobursitis
- Often asymptomatic or lateral hip pain, can be resistant to treatment of bursitis
- Same examination findings as trochanteric bursitis (tenderness, Trendelenburg test; 72% sensitive, 76% specific for trochanteric tendinobursitis)
  ○ Weakness may be more prominent with large tar

Diagnosis
- Clinical diagnosis (high index of suspicion) confirmed by imaging study
- Imaging: US or MRI (71)
  ○ US: hypo or heterogenic echogenicity with tendon thickening, increased vascularity (uncommon), bald anterior facet (gluteus minimus tear/retraction), calcific tendinosis (better than MRI)
  ○ MRI: increased T2 SI, or focal tendon defect with fluid (high T2 SI) of the gluteus medius, either at the attachment to the bone or within the substance of the tendon; more reliable than US ± fluid in the trochanteric bursa

Treatment
- Nonoperative treatment: NSAIDs, activity modification, PT, and cane as needed
  ○ Steroid injection to trochanteric bursa to control pain, and PT (ITB/hip external rotator stretching, modality, and gradual strengthening of gluteal muscle)
  ○ Needling, prolotherapy, and platelet-rich plasma injection if pain persists despite steroid injection
- Surgical referral in disabling pain despite conservative management; ITB release, tendon reattachment

Tensor Fascia Lata Tendinopathy and Tear

Introduction (78)
- Common site for overuse tendinopathies of the hip (along with rectus femoris), high in sprinters
- Etiology and risk factors
  - Forceful extension of the hip
  - The gluteus medius/minimus tear (TFL hypertrophy observed) (79)

History and physical examination
- Lateral hip pain after or during activities
- Tenderness over ASIS and AIIS, reproduction of pain with resisted contraction (abduction and internal rotation of the femur)

Diagnosis
- Clinical diagnosis confirmed by imaging study
- US and MRI: increased thickness (compared with the asymptomatic side), heterogeneous echogenicity in US, and increased T2 SI in MRI

Treatment
- NSAIDs, rest, activity modification, and PT (pelvic mobilization exercise, stretching/flexibility, and gradual strengthening and dynamic-balance exercise)
- Injection for pain control, if significant

Morel-Lavallée Lesion

Introduction (80)
- Posttraumatic hemolymphatic collection related to shearing injury between the subcutaneous tissue and muscle
- Etiology
  - Trauma (shearing injury, tangential force to fascial plane), motor vehicle accident (MC cause)
  - Often with underlying fracture
- MC location: lateral to the greater trochanter (30%) above iliotibial tract of the fascia lata
  - Other areas: thigh, pelvis (~20%), or knee

History and physical examination
- Rapid development of pain and swelling (within hours or days, but can be months)
- Soft fluctuating mass with skin mobility ± decreased/altered cutaneous sensation

Diagnosis
- Clinical diagnosis confirmed by imaging (US or MRI)
  - US: nonspecific fluid collection, compressible with heterogeneous echogenicity (if <1 month) or anechoic (in chronic cases)
  - MRI: modality of choice to evaluate type, chronicity, differential diagnosis, or concomitant injury
- Differential diagnosis: soft tissue sarcoma (contrast enhancement in MRI) and bursitis (depending on location)

Treatment
- Compressive banding, aspiration with/without sclerosing agents (doxycycline, erythromycin, alcohol, etc)
- If persistent; incision and evacuation or open drainage and secondary closure

GROIN

Iliopsoas Tendinobursitis

Introduction (81)
- Iliopsoas bursa: the largest bursa located between femoral vessels (neurovascular structures) medially and iliopsoas tendon laterally (82) (Figure 7.10)
  - With distension; it extends to the lesser trochanter inferiorly and the iliac fossa superiorly

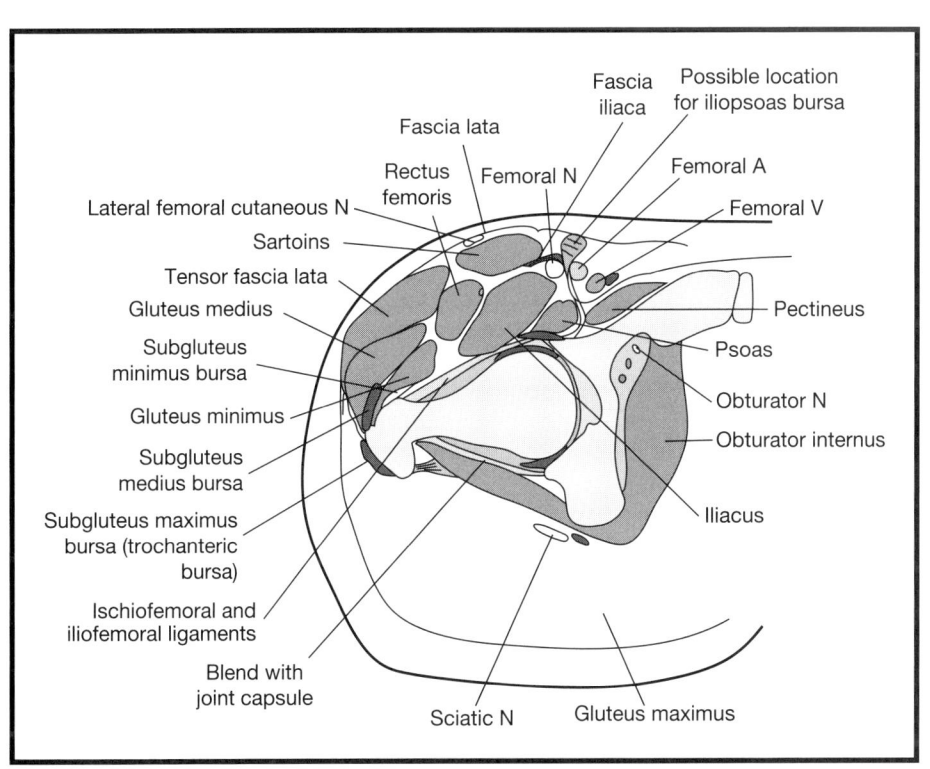

FIGURE 7.10
Cross sectional anatomy of the hip with the location of common bursae.
A, artery; N, nerve; V, vein.

○ Communicates with the hip joint; reservoir of hip effusion
- Etiology
  ○ Inflammatory or degenerative hip joint disease (RA, OA)
  ○ Trauma, repetitive overuse, and sports injuries (vigorous hip flexion and extension)
  ○ Uncommon causes: THA (up to 4.3% of pain after THA), synovial chondromatosis, AVN, and tuberculosis

History and physical examination
- Groin pain ± swelling (bulging mass) and snapping
  ○ Irritation of the iliopsoas over the iliopectineal eminence or femoral head
- Reproduction of snapping and pain on resisted hip flexion and/or passive hip extension

Diagnosis
- Clinical diagnosis (high index of suspicion) confirmed by imaging study
- Imaging study
  ○ X-ray: joint disease (RA and OA) and bony abnormalities; underlying and concomitant lesions
  ○ US (83)
    ▪ Static image (transverse and sagittal): usually normal. Possible thickened tendon and/or bursitis; compare with the opposite site.
    ▪ Dynamic maneuver (for snapping): from frog leg position (flexion, external rotation, and abduction) to full extension, adduction, and IR
    ▪ Diagnostic injection between iliopsoas tendon and acetabulum (lateral to medial approach on transverse view)
  ○ MRI for evaluation of hip joint/intra-articular pathologies. Indicated when the diagnosis is not clear
- Differential diagnosis
  ○ Paralabral cyst: smaller than bursal cyst, thick wall, noncompressible (because of mucoid content)
  ○ Other causes of groin pain (hip OA, symptomatic labral lesion, FAI, AVN, etc): often coexists

Treatment
- US-guided steroid injection to over the midportion of acetabulum with transverse imaging (under iliopsoas tendon), followed by PT (for stretching of iliopsoas and rectus femoris, pelvic mobilization exercise, gluteal and core muscle stabilization and modalities)
- Referral to surgery in refractory cases

Rectus Femoris Tendon Disorder

Introduction (84)
- Common in athletes (2nd MC after hamstring injury), especially soccer players (MC), football players, and martial arts participants
- Most susceptible among quadriceps because of superficial location, predominance of type II fibers, eccentric muscle action, and extension across two joints (85)
- Classification
  ○ Tear (partial more common than complete)
    ▪ Proximal tendon tear less common than myotendinous junction (MC; deep intramuscular myotendinous junction) or midsubstance of the muscle belly
    ▪ With/without AIIS avulsion
  ○ Tendinopathy and calcific tendinopathy (14): indirect head (around the capsular attachment); more common than direct head involvement
- Etiology for tear
  ○ Soccer (kicking a ball with the hip extended), martial arts, and sprinting

History and physical examination
- Groin pain ± snapping, mass (retracted muscle) in the upper thigh with rupture
- Pain on hip extension and pain reproduction on resisted hip flexion and stretching (Ely test)

Diagnosis
- Clinical diagnosis confirmed by imaging study
- Imaging study: x-ray and US
- MRI if US is not definite and symptoms persist despite initial treatment

Treatment
- NSAIDs, activity modification, and PT (stretching after modality, strengthening, and dynamic-balance exercise)
- Steroid injection (US guided), PRP injection, or US-guided barbotage of calcium after injection

Quadriceps Contusion

Introduction (86)
- Etiology: direct trauma usually by blunt object
- Location: deep in the muscle belly (compared with strain; located in superficial muscle)

History and physical examination
- Acute pain on thigh (often less symptomatic than strain) ± ecchymosis, tender lump (mass) on palpation
- Swelling, antalgic gait, and decreased ROM (decreased active knee flexion)

Diagnosis
- Clinical diagnosis confirmed by imaging study
- Imaging study (US, MRI) (85)
  ○ MRI: diffuse feathery appearance with increased SI on T2 weighted and STIR images (similar to 1st-degree myotendinous strain) ± intramuscular hematoma

Treatment
- Knee-hinged brace at 120° initially or compressive wrap (elastic) acutely to limit hematoma formation and ice
- Pain-free active ROM exercise after 24 hours with stretching of quadriceps and strengthening, lower-impact weight-bearing exercise, jogging, and stationary bike
- Up to 3 weeks off sports in severe cases

Hip Adductor Muscle Injury

Introduction
- Common muscle injury causing groin pain: 2% to 5%, peak incidence at 22 to 30 years of age
  ○ One of the main causes for athletic pubalgia with rectus abdominis injury and sports hernia

- MC location: adductor longus and gracilis at tendon origin, myotendinous junction > insertion
  ○ Adductor insertion avulsion syndrome (longus and brevis)
    ▪ Thigh splint (medial thigh), traction osteitis, almost always with ipsilateral rectus abdominis injury
    ▪ Often without osseous involvement
- Etiology and risk factor
  ○ MC involved sports: soccer (up to 23% in professional team), rugby, hockey; average 2 weeks' absence from sports
  ○ Tightness and decreased adductor strength, biomechanical abnormalities (excessive pronation and leg-length discrepancy)

History and physical examination
- Groin pain ± midthigh pain (in adductor insertion avulsion syndrome)
- Tenderness, pain on passive stretching and resisted adduction ± ecchymosis and swelling in acute tear

Diagnosis
- Clinical diagnosis ± imaging study confirmation
- US: useful if significant tear present
  ○ In acute tear: bell clapper, mixed appearance with hematoma, debris, and possibly damage of the fibrocartilage
  ○ In chronic tear: retracted tendon as a blunted hypoechoic mass with posterior attenuation
- MRI: secondary cleft sign on coronal STIR image (87)
  ○ Prolonged recovery in tear >50% of cross-sectional area, fluid collection and deep muscle, enthesis rather than musculotendinous junction
- Differential diagnosis: osteitis pubis, perhernia complex injury (sports hernia), or hip pathologies (often coexist)

Treatment
- Time for recovery: myotendinous junction: 1 to 2 weeks; avulsion: 1 to 3 months; insertion avulsion: 1 to 2 months
- Nonoperative management (11)
  ○ Brief rest, activity modification, PT: adductor stretching, strengthening, and pelvic stabilization exercise (12)
  ○ NSAIDs, pubic cleft (entheseal) injection, or tenotomy (inconsistent results)
  ○ PRP injection
- Surgery to partially release adductor longus tendon if persistent pain despite conservative management

Sport Hernia

Introduction (88)
- Occult hernia or tear of oblique aponeurosis without actual hernia
  ○ Common diagnosis in otherwise unexplained chronic activity-related groin pain in sports players
- Incidence and prevalence not studied; male > female
- Etiology
  ○ Weakness of the posterior inguinal wall ± periostitis of the insertion of the adductors and rectus abdominus on the os pubis
  ○ Repetitive hyperextension of the trunk; hyperabduction of the thigh; shear force across the symphysis pubis

History and physical examination
- Chronic groin pain, gradual, regional, unilateral ± radiation to perineum (scrotum in 30%), and upper medial thigh
  ○ Aggravated by resisted hip adduction and trunk flexion, cutting, and sprinting
- Tenderness at superficial inguinal ring (canal), pubic tubercle, and adductor origin (common finding)
- Pain with resisted adduction and tenderness along the adductors, tenderness over the symphysis pubis
- No palpable hernia (12)

Diagnosis
- Clinical diagnosis confirmed at surgery
- Differential diagnosis for groin pain
  ○ Adductor tendinopathy, iliopsoas tendinopathy, avulsion of lesser trochanter, hip OA, symptomatic labral lesion, FAI, and so on
  ○ Other underrecognized causes
    ▪ Gynecologic disorders, kidney disease, urinary tract infection, RA or ankylosing spondylitis, Reiter's syndrome, local bone infection (TB or osteomyelitis), or tumors
    ▪ Border nerve (genitofemoral, ilioinguinal) and obturator nerve entrapment neuropathy
- Routine imaging: not helpful (60), MRI to rule out other differentials

Treatment
- Rest from sport for 6 to 8 weeks, NSAIDs, gradual return to sport
  ○ PT: resistive adductor strengthening and stretching, in addition to core strengthening and agility training later
- Surgery (modified hernia repair; reinforcement of abdominal muscles or fascia near inguinal ligament) is reserved for failed conservative treatment

NEUROPATHY

LATERAL FEMORAL CUTANEOUS NERVE

Introduction (89)
- Incidence: 1 to 5 per 10,000, one of the most common entrapment neuropathies in the lower extremity
- Anatomy
  ○ From the ventral rami of the L2 and L3 spinal nerves
  ○ Course: inferior to the inguinal ligament on the anterior surface of the groin, deep to fascia lata, then divides into branches before piercing the fascia lata
- Etiology
  ○ Idiopathic (common)
  ○ Mechanical: obstructive sources from increased intraabdominal pressure such as pregnancy, obesity, pelvic tumors, braces/corsets, and pelvic crush injury
  ○ Surgical procedures and metabolic causes
- Common location: between the ASIS and the inguinal ligament to enter the thigh

History and physical examination
- Numbness, tingling, pain, or a burning sensation in the anterior lateral (down to distal one-third) thigh

- Tenderness with reproduction of pain, tingling, burning, and pins/needles sensation on the distribution of nerve (Valleix's phenomenon)

Diagnosis
- Clinical diagnosis ± confirmed by EMG (often technically difficult in obese patient) or imaging-guided nerve block
- EMG to evaluate other peripheral neuropathies (L2–3 radiculopathy or plexopathy), rarely muscle disease (90). Limited role in evaluation of border nerve (ilioinguinal, iliohypogastric nerve lesion) and anterior femoral cutaneous nerve

Treatment
- Weight reduction, avoidance of tight belt or garment, desensitization, or benign neglect
- Topical cream (lidocaine cream; may not be effective with difficult penetration in obese patients), or transcutaneous electrical nerve stimulation (TENS)
- US-guided diagnostic/therapeutic injection (preferred over electrical stimulation guidance), and radiofrequency ablation if responsive to injection temporarily

ANTERIOR FEMORAL CUTANEOUS NEURALGIA

Introduction (91)
- Very rare. Direct injury (penetration) or iatrogenic
- Anatomy: cutaneous branch of femoral nerve that innervates the anteromedial thigh
  - The intermediate femoral cutaneous nerve
  - The medial femoral cutaneous nerve (MFCN) → anterior and posterior branches
    - Posterior branch innervates the medial aspect of the leg just below the knee

History and physical examination
- Pain, tingling, burning, pins/needles sensation in the anteromedial aspect of the thigh
- Palpation: occasionally tenderness with reproduction of symptoms in the distribution of anterior femoral cutaneous nerve (AFCN)

Diagnosis
- Clinical diagnosis confirmed by US-guided injection or nerve conduction study
- Nerve conduction study; often limited with technical difficulty in obese patients and elderly population
  - To evaluate other differentials (same as LFCN/femoral neuropathy, lumbar plexopathy, L2–3 radiculopathy, and others)

Treatment
- Diagnostic and therapeutic injection
- Same as lateral femoral cutaneous nerve treatment

OBTURATOR NEUROPATHY

Introduction (92,93)
- Rare, but also underrecognized
- Etiology
  - Fascial entrapment at the entrance to adductor compartment
  - Osteitis pubis with secondary inflammatory changes
  - Iatrogenic, pelvic fracture, hemorrhage, or tumor compression

History and physical examination
- Deep aching pain in the groin and distal thigh
- Exacerbation of pain by extension or lateral leg movement (stretch the nerve with pectineal muscle)
- Howship–Romberg's sign: medial knee pain induced by forced hip abduction, extension, and IR
- Sensory symptoms may extend distally to the medial calf (numbness rare) ± motor weakness (adductor)

Diagnosis
- Clinical diagnosis, confirmed by EMG (negative if mild lesion or isolated sensory involvement) or imaging-guided nerve block (often not specific)
  - Indications for EMG: motor symptoms (weakness, atrophy); rule out other causes (lumbosacral plexopathy, radiculopathy), and/or imaging-guided nerve block
- Differential diagnosis: adductor muscle dysfunction, osteitis pubis, L2–3 radiculopathy, or plexopathy
- MRI for other differential diagnoses, may show denervated adductor muscle (increased T2 in acute and atrophy with fatty infiltration in chronic lesion)

Treatment
- US-guided steroid injection
  - Anterior branch between the pectineus and adductor longus, then distally between adductor longus and brevis
  - Posterior branch between the adductor brevis and magnus
- PT: stretching/strengthening adductor muscle, pelvic muscle stabilization exercise, and modality (TENS) as needed; aerobic endurance exercise
- Surgical referral for neurolysis or relief of the entrapment, or selective fascial release if not responsive to the conservative management

BORDER NERVE SYNDROME (ILIOINGUINAL, ILIOHYPOGASTRIC, AND GENITOFEMORAL NERVES)

Introduction (94,95)
- Very rare, but underrecognized
- Anatomy (see Figure 7.2)
  - Border nerve: supply cutaneous sensation between the abdomen and thigh (border)
  - Iliohypogastric nerve and ilioinguinal nerve (L1); subperitoneally in front of quadratus lumborum → pierce the transverse abdominis
    - Iliohypogastric nerve: motor branch to internal oblique, between internal and external oblique; innervates inguinal ring and skin over the lower part of the rectus abdominis
    - Ilioinguinal nerve: parallel and below iliohypogastric nerve; innervates superomedial aspect area of the thigh, skin over the penis and scrotum in the male, and mons pubis and labium major in the female
  - Genitofemoral nerve: L1,2; femoral nerve, follows external iliac artery and passes under the inguinal ligament, then penetrates fascia lata to supply skin to the femoral triangle and genital branch
- Etiology: idiopathic, iatrogenic (pfannenstiel incision, appendectomy, and inguinal herniorrhaphy, or trochar insertion)

History and physical examination
- Groin pain (pins/needles, burning sensation) ± radiating to the scrotum or testicle or labia majora and medial upper thigh
- Sensory symptoms (tingling, pins/needles, burning, numbness) in the distribution of individual nerves
- May have tenderness with reproduction of sensory symptoms (Valleix's phenomenon)

Diagnosis
- Clinical diagnosis confirmed by image-guided injection
- Differential diagnosis: gynecologic and intra-abdominal pathologies in addition to MSK etiologies for the groin pain

Treatment
- US-guided injection between the internal oblique and transverse abdominis at 1 to 2 inch medial/cephalad to ASIS
  - Radiofrequency ablation can be considered if recurrent injection is indicated
- Referral to surgery for neurolysis or spinal cord stimulator in patients with disabling pain despite the treatment discussed earlier

POSTERIOR FEMORAL CUTANEOUS NEUROPATHY

Introduction
- Very rare
- Sacral plexus, ventral rami of S1–3, course with sciatic nerve (greater sciatic foramen), under gluteus maximus
  - Branches of posterior femoral cutaneous nerve: pudendal nerve (perineum) and inferior cluneal nerve (lower part of buttock)
    - Innervate skin of the perineum, posterior thigh, and popliteal region of the knee
  - Accompanied by gluteal artery (useful for US localization)
- Etiology: hamstring tear, iatrogenic (injection, tourniquet, gluteal and thigh flap for breast reconstruction, THA) or idiopathic (venous loops)

History and physical examination
- Pain in the posterior thigh and buttock on sitting
- Tenderness at the inferior aspect of the ischial tuberosity adjacent to the hamstring insertion

Diagnosis
- Clinical suspicion confirmed by diagnostic block (imaging guided using small amount of local anesthetic, ~1 cc)
- Differential diagnoses: hamstring tendinopathy (often underlying problem), piriformis syndrome, facet arthropathy, L5–S1 radiculopathy, or pudendal neuropathy

Treatment (97)
- Diagnostic/therapeutic block, if the pain continues despite injection, then referral to surgery

OTHER PATHOLOGY

MYOSITIS OSSIFICANS

Introduction
- Rare, but common with repeated trauma, peak in 3rd decade, slightly more common in male
- Classification: congenital, idiopathic, or traumatic (MC)
- Traumatic myositis ossificans
  - Heterotrophic ossification of the soft tissues (mainly muscle) after direct trauma. Benign and self-limiting condition
  - MC location of traumatic myositis ossificans (MO): quadriceps femoris and brachialis
  - Etiology: exact mechanism unknown. Related to intramuscular hematoma by muscle contusion

History and physical examination
- Painful mass at the site of injury that restricts motion
- Often asymptomatic

Diagnosis (105)
- Clinical diagnosis confirmed by imaging study
- X-ray: intramuscular calcification at 2 to 4 weeks after injury
- US: useful in early stages before calcification in x-ray; heterogeneous hypoechoic soft tissue masses with focal hyperechoic center in early stage
- MRI for differential diagnosis, better for planned surgical excision
- Differential diagnosis: muscle abscess, rhadomyolysis, soft tissue sarcoma (synovial sarcoma and osteosarcoma), osteochondroma, focal myositis, and chronic avulsion injury

Treatment
- Restrict movement initially. Cold massage with gradual stretching to improve ROM, then strengthening and endurance exercise (if knee flexion >120°)
  - ROM exercise and local massage should be done with caution to avoid reinjury for up to 6 months after injury
- Early aspiration of the hematoma. No NSAIDs till 3 weeks postinjury to prevent further bleeding, then indomethacine and bisphosphonate
- Extracorporeal shock wave treatment for painful calcification
- Once a firm mass has formed, the muscle should be protected from further direct trauma
- Surgical excision: rarely indicated, if persistent pain for >1 year postinjury

TRANSIENT OSTEOPOROSIS

Introduction (99)
- Self-limited bone marrow edema, "bone marrow edema syndrome"
- Young and middle-aged men, rarely early postpartum (3 months)
- Location: hip > knee and ankle (only lower extremities)

History and physical examination
- Pain worse with weight bearing, limping, and difficulty walking, gradually subsides within 4 to 9 months, can recur
- Relatively normal ROM with mild pain at the extreme range

Diagnosis
- Clinical diagnosis confirmed by imaging study (MRI)
- Imaging study
  - X-ray normal in early stage, periarticular demineralization at 3 to 6 weeks from the onset of symptoms with normal joint margins, no erosion

○ MRI: imaging of choice; low SI in T1 and high SI in T2
- Serologic test: normal
- Differential diagnoses: regional migratory osteoporosis, reflex sympathetic dystrophy, osteonecrosis, neoplasm (metastatic cancer, multiple myeloma, leukemia, and lymphoma), and inflammatory arthropathy

Treatment
- Protected weight bearing (partial) for pain relief; symptoms and pathology resolve usually within 6 months
- Symptomatic pain control: NSAID, bisphosphonate (IV pamidronate), calcium supplementation, correct vitamin D if low
  ○ Oral bisphosphonate, especially if collagen type 1 metabolite (procollagen type 1 N-terminal propeptide) is elevated
- Intra-articular steroid injection discouraged because of concern for remineralization

PEDIATRIC HIP PATHOLOGY

Introduction
- Hip pathology relatively rare, but can cause lifelong disability if not treated
- Limp in older child or adolescent; hip rather than foot or knee pathology → strongly recommend hip imaging

Common hip pathologies depending on age group
- Newborn and infant: hip dislocation and septic arthritis
- Age 4 to 10 years: transient synovitis or Legg–Calvé–Perthes disease (LCPD)
- Age 10 to 15 years: slipped capital femoral epiphysis

Differential diagnoses of hip pain and limp by etiologies in children

TRAUMATIC/MECHANICAL (MOST COMMON)	INFLAMMATORY	VASCULAR	INFECTIOUS	NEOPLASTIC
Fractures Muscle injuries Contusions SCFE	Transient synovitis Juvenile RA Ankylosing spondylitis Reiter syndrome	LCP disease Osteonecrosis Hemoglobinopathy	Pyoarthrosis Osteomyelitis Pyomyositis Lyme disease	Benign aggressive tumors Malignant tumors Leukemia, lymphoma Benign tumor with impending fracture

LCP, Legg–Calvé–Perthes disease; RA, rheumatoid arthritis; SCFE, slipped capital femoral epiphysis.

History and physical examinations
- Pain history similar to adults: onset, location, aggravating and relieving factors
  ○ Red flags (eg, night and rest pain); urgent workup required
  ○ Knee pain equals hip pain, a maxim to consider in skeletally immature patient
    ▪ ~20% of patients with SCFE complain only of knee pain
  ○ Mechanism of injury in traumatic case
- Physical examination
  ○ Observational gait analysis: foot progression angle, pelvic and trunk balance
    ▪ Sitting or crawling: inability to sit comfortably; check spine pathology
    ▪ Ability to bear weight through the knees (crawling on the knee) indicates pathologies localized to legs or feet (rather than femur or hip pathologies)
  ○ Other inspection
    ▪ Thigh atrophy: long-standing hip (and/or knee) pathology or neuromuscular etiologies
  ○ ROM of hip: diminished or painful internal rotation
    ▪ Maximal intracapsular volume is possible with the hip in a position of flexion, abduction, and external rotation → pain on the opposite position (accommodate less intra-articular volume with extension, adduction, and inward rotation) suggests intra-articular pathology
    ▪ Log roll: internal/external rotation to assess side-to-side differences in hip rotation and guarding
  ○ Straight leg raise test with resistance: provoking hip pathology
  ○ Functional tests to observe side-to-side difference
    ▪ Squatting to the ground and rising
    ▪ Alternate single-leg hopping
  ○ Examination of other joints for swelling and skin examination for rashes can be helpful in identifying inflammatory or infectious causes of hip pain
  ○ Thorough palpation of the thigh is important to assess for any mass effect; the inguinal area should be palpated also for any mass or lymphadenopathy

Diagnostic workup (100)
- Clinical diagnosis confirmed by imaging study
- X-ray: AP of the pelvis on standing, lateral views
  ○ Indications: trauma, long-lasting symptoms, <1 year and >8 years; evaluate Perthes, SCFE, and osteomyelitis (or for FU) (see Figure 7.7)
- Pediatric US (101)
  ○ Normal hip: hypoechoic rounded femoral head over the hypoechoic triradiate cartilage in the acetabulum
  ○ Common indications and findings
    ▪ Development dysplasia of the hip; screening procedure in many countries at 4 to 6 weeks
    ▪ Dislocated hip anteriorly
    ▪ Irritable hip (transient synovitis), septic synovitis, Perthes disease, and slipped capital femoral epiphysis
      – Joint effusion distending the anterior recess of the hip joint ≥2 mm ± synovial thickening
      – US can be used for needle guidance
    ▪ Sporting injuries: apophyseal injury, tendinopathy, snapping of the iliopsoas tendon, insertional tendinopathy

- Laboratory study (102)
  - Complete blood count (CBC), erythrocyte sedimentation rate (ESR), C-reactive protein (CRP), rheumatoid factor, antinuclear antibody (ANA), and other rheumatoid panel
  - Lyme titer in endemic area, blood culture if infectious causes suspected

INDIVIDUAL CONDITIONS (103)

	DEVELOPMENTAL DISLOCATION OF THE HIP	LCPD	SLIPPED FEMORAL CAPITAL EPIPHYSIS
Characteristics	Previously known as congenital dislocation of the hip	Idiopathic avascular necrosis	Slipping or gliding of the femoral head or epiphysis in the growth plate
Risk factors	Breech (related to the oligohydramnios, congenital torticollis, chromosomal abnormalities), left > right	Idiopathic Related to Down syndrome	Idiopathic: MC Endocrine disease (hypothyroidism) and renal failure
Demographics at presentation	Newborn, infants, or older if not recognized Female > male by four times Incidence: 1–2/1,000	4–8 years old (less than 10 years old) 2–12 years old in some studies	Overweight boys Male (13–16) > female (11–13) Incidence 1/10,000
History and physical examination	Asymmetrical thigh creases, limited hip abduction Barlow dislocation, Ortolani relocation tests In older children → limitation of hip abduction: more reliable sign Metatarsus adductor	Limping (or painless limp), and limited ROM (similar to a transient synovitis) Painless loss of IR and adduction (FADIR) Thomas test +	Groin, thigh, medial knee pain (gradual) Increased pain on weight bearing Chronic slip, loss of hip IR Short leg in external rotation
Imaging study	US in 3–4 months of age	X-ray: Crescent's sign (subchondral fracture)	X-ray (AP, frog lat): widening of growth plate Lateral view (or abduction-external rotation view): posterior slippage of femoral epiphysis
Treatment	Craig Pavlik harness	Orthopedic referral Petrie casts, Toronto brace, Salter stirrup Abduction brace	Rest Surgery in unstable case (cannot walk even with crutches)

AP, anteroposterior; FADIR, flexion, adduction and internal rotation; IR, internal rotation; LCPD: Legg-Calvé-Perthes disease; MC, most common; ROM, range of motion; US, ultrasound.

TRANSIENT SYNOVITIS OR IRRITABLE HIP

Introduction (103)
- A self-limiting effusion of the hip in children, mainly between 4 and 10 years of age, MC cause of limping and hip pain in this age group
- Etiology: unknown, may be related to upper respiratory or gastrointestinal (GI) viral infection

History and physical examination
- Limping, limited abduction/rotation, and variable degrees of pain; no fever

Diagnosis
- Clinical diagnosis supplemented by US
- Normal serology and x-ray
- Repeat x-ray in 6 to 8 weeks or if symptoms persist >2 weeks to exclude Legg-Calvé-Perthes disease (LCPD)
- US: effusion usually disappears in 8 to 10 days
- Differential diagnosis: septic arthritis (aspiration and culture if strongly suspicious), LCPD

Treatment
- Rest for a few days and NSAIDs as needed
- Traction for a few days to decrease ROM and possibly to decrease intracapsular pressure

REFERENCES

1. Fransen M, Agaliotis M, Bridgett L, Mackey MG. Hip and knee pain: role of occupational factors. *Best Pract Res Clin Rheumatol*. 2011;25(1):81–101.
2. Tammareddi K, Morelli V, Reyes M Jr. The athlete's hip and groin. *Prim Care*. 2013;40(2):313–333.
3. Kelly BT, Maak TG, Larson CM, et al. Sports hip injuries: assessment and management. *Instr Course Lect*. 2013;62:515–531.

4. Ernst E. Jogging—for a healthy heart and worn-out hips? *J Intern Med*. 1990;228(4):295–297.
5. Hansen P, English M, Willick SE. Does running cause osteoarthritis in the hip or knee? *PM R*. 2012;4(5 Suppl):S117–S121.
6. Anderson K, Strickland SM, Warren R. Hip and groin injuries in athletes. *Am J Sports Med*. 2001;29(4):521–533.
7. DeAngelis NA, Busconi BD. Assessment and differential diagnosis of the painful hip. *Clin Orthop Relat Res*. 2003;(406):11–18.
8. Falvey EC, Franklyn-Miller A, McCrory PR. The groin triangle: a patho-anatomical approach to the diagnosis of chronic groin pain in athletes. *Br J Sports Med*. 2009;43(3):213–220.
9. Martinoli C, Miguel-Perez M, Padua L, et al. Imaging of neuropathies about the hip. *Eur J Radiol*. 2013;82(1):17–26.
10. de Bruijn KM, Franssen G, van Ginhoven TM. A stepwise approach to "groin pain": a common symptom, an uncommon cause. *BMJ Case Re*. 2013:1–2.
11. Schilders E, Dimitrakopoulou A, Cooke M, et al. Effectiveness of a selective partial adductor release for chronic adductor-related groin pain in professional athletes. *Am J Sports Med*. 2013;41(3):603–607.
12. Morelli V, Weaver V. Groin injuries and groin pain in athletes: part 1. *Prim Care*. 2005;32(1):163–183.
13. Bureau NJ. Sonographic evaluation of snapping hip syndrome. *J Ultrasound Med*. 2013;32(6):895–900.
14. Pierannunzii L, Tramontana F, Gallazzi M. Case report: calcific tendinitis of the rectus femoris: a rare cause of snapping hip. *Clin Orthop Relat Res*. 2010;468(10):2814–2818.
15. Shadbolt CL, Heinze SB, Dietrich RB. Imaging of groin masses: inguinal anatomy and pathologic conditions revisited. *Radiographics*. 2001;21 Spec No:S261–S271.
16. Schwarz N, Leixnering M, Hopf R, Jantsch S. Pressure-volume ratio in human cadaver hip joints. *Arch Orthop Trauma Surg*. 1988;107(5):322–325.
17. Saikku K, Vasenius J, Saar P. Entrapment of the proximal sciatic nerve by the hamstring tendons. *Acta Orthop Belg*. 2010;76(3):321–324.
18. Orchard JW, Fricker PA, Abud AT, Mason BR. Biomechanics of iliotibial band friction syndrome in runners. *Am J Sports Med*. 1996;24(3):375–379.
19. Bowman KF Jr, Fox J, Sekiya JK. A clinically relevant review of hip biomechanics. *Arthroscopy*. 2010;26(8):1118–1129.
20. Polkowski GG, Clohisy JC. Hip biomechanics. *Sports Med Arthrosc*. 2010;18(2):56–62.
21. Boykin RE, Anz AW, Bushnell BD, et al. Hip instability. *J Am Acad Orthop Surg*. 2011;19(6):340–349.
22. Gurney B. Leg length discrepancy. *Gait Posture*. 2002;15(2):195–206.
23. Stuber KJ. Specificity, sensitivity, and predictive values of clinical tests of the sacroiliac joint: a systematic review of the literature. *J Can Chiropr Assoc*. 2007;51(1):30–41.
24. Fishman LM, Dombi GW, Michaelsen C, et al. Piriformis syndrome: diagnosis, treatment, and outcome—a 10-year study. *Arch Phys Med Rehabil*. 2002;83(3):295–301.
25. Harvey D. Assessment of the flexibility of elite athletes using the modified Thomas test. *Br J Sports Med*. 1998;32(1):68–70.
26. Noble CA. Iliotibial band friction syndrome in runners. *Am J Sports Med*. 1980;8(4):232–234.
27. Leunig M, Beaulé PE, Ganz R. The concept of femoroacetabular impingement: current status and future perspectives. *Clin Orthop Relat Res*. 2009;467(3):616–622.
28. Theologis TN, Epps H, Latz K, Cole WG. Isolated fractures of the lesser trochanter in children. *Injury*. 1997;28(5–6):363–364.
29. Papacostas NC, Bowe CT, Shaffer Strout TD. Lesser trochanter avulsion fracture. *J Emerg Med*. 2013;45(2):256–257.
30. Hall M, Anderson J. Hip pointers. *Clin Sports Med*. 2013;32(2):325–330.
31. Yu JS. Hip and femur trauma. *Semin Musculoskelet Radiol*. 2000;4(2):205–220.
32. Bloem JL, Reidsma II. Bone and soft tissue tumors of hip and pelvis. *Eur J Radiol*. 2012;81(12):3793–3801.
33. Tuten HR, Gabos PG, Kumar SJ, Harter GD. The limping child: a manifestation of acute leukemia. *J Pediatr Orthop*. 1998;18(5):625–629.
34. Williams BS, Cohen SP. Greater trochanteric pain syndrome: a review of anatomy, diagnosis and treatment. *Anesth Analg*. 2009;108(5):1662–1670.
35. Brady LP. Hip pain. Don't throw away the cane. *Postgrad Med*. 1988;83(8):89–90, 95.
36. Smith J, Hurdle MF, Weingarten TN. Accuracy of sonographically guided intra-articular injections in the native adult hip. *J Ultrasound Med*. 2009;28(3):329–335.
37. Kelly BT, Williams RJ 3rd, Philippon MJ. Hip arthroscopy: current indications, treatment options, and management issues. *Am J Sports Med*. 2003;31(6):1020–1037.
38. Gupta A, Redmond JM, Hammarstedt JE, et al. Safety measures in hip arthroscopy and their efficacy in minimizing complications: a systematic review of the evidence. *Arthroscopy*. 2014;30(10):1342–1348.
39. Brander V, Stulberg SD. Rehabilitation after hip- and knee-joint replacement. An experience- and evidence-based approach to care. *Am J Phys Med Rehabil*. 2006;85(11 Suppl):S98–118; quiz S119.
40. Petis S, Howard JL, Lanting BL, Vasarhelyi EM. Surgical approach in primary total hip arthroplasty: anatomy, technique and clinical outcomes. *Can J Surg*. 2015;58(2):128–139.
41. Suri P, Morgenroth DC, Hunter DJ. Epidemiology of osteoarthritis and associated comorbidities. *PM R*. 2012;4(5 Suppl):S10–S19.
42. Zhang Y, Jordan JM. Epidemiology of osteoarthritis. *Clin Geriatr Med*. 2010;26(3):355–369.
43. Bennell KL, Egerton T, Martin J, et al. Effect of physical therapy on pain and function in patients with hip osteoarthritis: a randomized clinical trial. *JAMA*. 2014;311(19):1987–1997.
44. Uthman OA, van der Windt DA, Jordan JL, et al. Exercise for lower limb osteoarthritis: systematic review incorporating trial sequential analysis and network meta-analysis. *BMJ*. 2013;347:f5555.
45. Blount WP. Don't throw away the cane. 1956. *J Bone Joint Surg Am*. 2003;85-A(2):380.
46. Lieberman JR, Engstrom SM, Solovyova O, et al. Is intra-articular hyaluronic acid effective in treating osteoarthritis of the hip joint? *J Arthroplasty*. 2015;30(3):507–511.
47. Legré-Boyer V. Viscosupplementation: techniques, indications, results. *Orthop Traumatol Surg Res*. 2015;101(1 Suppl):S101–S108.
48. Gandhi R, Perruccio AV, Mahomed NN. Surgical management of hip osteoarthritis. *CMAJ*. 2014;186(5):347–355.
49. Bharam S. Labral tears, extra-articular injuries, and hip arthroscopy in the athlete. *Clin Sports Med*. 2006;25(2):279–292, ix.
50. McCarthy J, Noble P, Aluisio FV, et al. Anatomy, pathologic features, and treatment of acetabular labral tears. *Clin Orthop Relat Res*. 2003;(406):38–47.
51. Krych AJ, Griffith TB, Hudgens JL, et al. Limited therapeutic benefits of intra-articular cortisone injection for patients with femoroacetabular impingement and labral tear. *Knee Surg Sports Traumatol Arthrosc*. 2014;22(4):750–755.
52. Parvizi J, Leunig M, Ganz R. Femoroacetabular impingement. *J Am Acad Orthop Surg*. 2007;15(9):561–570.
53. Sink EL, Kim YJ. Femoroacetabular impingement: current clinical evidence. *J Pediatr Orthop*. 2012;32(Suppl 2):S166–S171.
54. Kassarjian A, Brisson M, Palmer WE. Femoroacetabular impingement. *Eur J Radiol*. 2007;63(1):29–35.
55. Standaert CJ, Manner PA, Herring SA. Expert opinion and controversies in musculoskeletal and sports medicine: femoroacetabular impingement. *Arch Phys Med Rehabil*. 2008;89(5):890–893.
56. Spencer-Gardner L, Eischen JJ, Levy BA, et al. A comprehensive five-phase rehabilitation programme after hip arthroscopy for femoroacetabular impingement. *Knee Surg Sports Traumatol Arthrosc*. 2014;22(4):848–859.
57. Parsons SJ, Steele N. Osteonecrosis of the femoral head: Part 1—Aetiology, pathogenesis, investigation, classification. *Current Orthopaedics*. 2007;21(6):457–463.
58. Malizos KN, Karantanas AH, Varitimidis SE, et al. Osteonecrosis of the femoral head: etiology, imaging and treatment. *Eur J Radiol*. 2007;63(1):16–28.
59. Parsons SJ, Steele N. Osteonecrosis of the femoral head: Part 2—Options for treatment. *Curr Orthop*. 2008;22(5):349–358.
60. McCormick F, Nwachukwu BU, Provencher MT. Stress fractures in runners. *Clin Sports Med*. 2012;31(2):291–306.
61. Chen Y-T, Tenforde AS, Fredericson M. Update on stress fractures in female athletes: epidemiology, treatment, and prevention. *Curr Rev Musculoskelet Med*. 2013;6(2):173–181.
62. Dugan SA, Weber KM. Stress fractures and rehabilitation. *Phys Med Rehabil Clin N Am*. 2007;18(3):401–416, viii.
63. Kaeding CC, Yu JR, Wright R, et al. Management and return to play of stress fractures. *Clin J Sport Med*. 2005;15(6):442–447.

64. Harrast MA, Colonno D. Stress fractures in runners. *Clin Sports Med.* 2010;29(3):399–416.
65. Ivkovic A., Bojanic I, Pecina M. Stress fractures of the femoral shaft in athletes: a new treatment algorithm. *Br J Sports Med.* 2006;40(6):518–520; discussion 520.
66. Hiti CJ, Stevens KJ, Jamati MK, et al. Athletic osteitis pubis. *Sports Med.* 2011;41(5):361–376.
67. Mullens FE, Zoga AC, Morrison WB, Meyers WC. Review of MRI technique and imaging findings in athletic pubalgia and the "sports hernia." *Eur J Radiol.* 2012;81(12):3780–3792.
68. Kunduracioglu B, Yilmaz C, Yorubulut M, Kudas S. Magnetic resonance findings of osteitis pubis. *J Magn Reson Imaging.* 2007;25(3):535–539.
69. Sanders TG, Zlatkin MB. Avulsion injuries of the pelvis. *Semin Musculoskelet Radiol.* 2008;12(1):42–53.
70. Rothschild B. Trochanteric area pain, the result of a quartet of bursal inflammation. *World J Orthop.* 2013;4(3):100–102.
71. Kong A, Van der Vliet A, Zadow S. MRI and US of gluteal tendinopathy in greater trochanteric pain syndrome. *Eur Radiol.* 2007;17(7):1772–1783.
72. Klauser AS, Martinoli C, Tagliafico A, et al. Greater trochanteric pain syndrome. *Semin Musculoskelet Radiol.* 2013;17(1):43–48.
73. Long SS, Surrey DE, Nazarian LN. Sonography of greater trochanteric pain syndrome and the rarity of primary bursitis. *Am J Roentgenol.* 2013;201(5):1083–1086.
74. Lustenberger DP, Ng VY, Best TM, Ellis TJ. Efficacy of treatment of trochanteric bursitis: a systematic review. *Clin J Sport Med.* 2011;21(5):447–453.
75. McEvoy JR, Lee KS, Blankenbaker DG, et al. Ultrasound-guided corticosteroid injections for treatment of greater trochanteric pain syndrome: greater trochanter bursa versus subgluteus medius bursa. *Am J Roentgenol.* 2013;201(2):W313–W317.
76. Lachiewicz PF. Abductor tendon tears of the hip: evaluation and management. *J Am Acad Orthop Surg.* 2011;19(7):385–391.
77. Kingzett-Taylor A, Tirman PF, Feller J, et al. Tendinosis and tears of gluteus medius and minimus muscles as a cause of hip pain: MR imaging findings. *AJR Am J Roentgenol.* 1999;173(4):1123–1126.
78. Asinger DA, el-Khoury GY. Tensor fascia lata muscle tear: evaluation by MRI. *Iowa Orthop J.* 1998;18:146–149.
79. Sutter R, Kalberer F, Binkert CA, et al. Abductor tendon tears are associated with hypertrophy of the tensor fasciae latae muscle. *Skeletal Radiol.* 2013;42(5):627–633.
80. Bonilla-Yoon I, Masih S, Patel DB, et al. The Morel-Lavallée lesion: pathophysiology, clinical presentation, imaging features, and treatment options. *Emerg Radiol.* 2014;21(1):35–43.
81. Nunley RM, Wilson JM, Gilula L, et al. Iliopsoas bursa injections can be beneficial for pain after total hip arthroplasty. *Clin Orthop Relat Res.* 2010;468(2):519–526.
82. Byrne PA, Rees JI, Williams BD. Iliopsoas bursitis-an unusual presentation of metastatic bone disease. *Br J Rheumatol.* 1996;35(3):285–288.
83. Blankenbaker DG, De Smet AA, Keene JS. Sonography of the iliopsoas tendon and injection of the iliopsoas bursa for diagnosis and management of the painful snapping hip. *Skeletal Radiol.* 2006;35(8):565–571.
84. Kassarjian A, Rodrigo RM, Santisteban JM. Current concepts in MRI of rectus femoris musculotendinous (myotendinous) and myofascial injuries in elite athletes. *Eur J Radiol.* 2012;81(12):3763–3771.
85. Bencardino JT, Rosenberg ZS, Brown RR, et al. Traumatic musculotendinous injuries of the knee: diagnosis with MR imaging. *Radiographics.* 2000;20(Spec No):S103–S120.
86. Laprade RF, Surowiec RK, Sochanska AN, et al. Epidemiology, identification, treatment and return to play of musculoskeletal-based ice hockey injuries. *Br J Sports Med.* 2014;48(1):4–10.
87. Brennan D, O'Connell MJ, Ryan M, et al. Secondary cleft sign as a marker of injury in athletes with groin pain: MR image appearance and interpretation. *Radiology.* 2005;235(1):162–167.
88. Caudill P, Nyland J, Smith C, et al. Sports hernias: a systematic literature review. *Br J Sports Med.* 2008;42(12):954–964.
89. Fowler IM, Tucker AA, Mendez RJ. Treatment of meralgia paresthetica with ultrasound-guided pulsed radiofrequency ablation of the lateral femoral cutaneous nerve. *Pain Pract.* 2012;12(5):394–398.
90. Seror P, Seror R. Meralgia paresthetica: clinical and electrophysiological diagnosis in 120 cases. *Muscle Nerve.* 2006;33(5):650–654.
91. Lo YL, Lee KT, Rikhraj IS. Isolated medial femoral cutaneous neuropathy. *Muscle Nerve.* 2004;30(6):812–813.
92. Tipton JS. Obturator neuropathy. *Curr Rev Musculoskelet Med.* 2008;1(3–4):234–237.
93. Bradshaw C, McCrory P, Bell S, Brukner P. Obturator nerve entrapment. A cause of groin pain in athletes. *Am J Sports Med.* 1997;25(3):402–408.
94. Peng PW, Tumber PS. Ultrasound-guided interventional procedures for patients with chronic pelvic pain—a description of techniques and review of literature. *Pain Physician.* 2008;11(2):215–224.
95. McDonald JS. Diagnosis and treatment issues of chronic pelvic pain. *World J Urol.* 2001;19(3):200–207.
96. Dellon AL. Pain with sitting related to injury of the posterior femoral cutaneous nerve. *Microsurgery.* 2015;35(6):463–468.
97. Topçu I, Aysel I. Ultrasound guided posterior femoral cutaneous nerve block. *Agri.* 2014;26(3):145–148.
98. Tyler P, Saifuddin A. The imaging of myositis ossificans. *Semin Musculoskelet Radiol.* 2010;14(2):201–216.
99. Korompilias AV, Karantanas AH, Lykissas MG, Beris AE. Transient osteoporosis. *J Am Acad Orthop Surg.* 2008;16(8):480–489.
100. Eich GF, Superti-Furga A, Umbricht FS, Willi UV. The painful hip: evaluation of criteria for clinical decision-making. *Eur J Pediatr.* 1999;158(11):923–928.
101. Martinoli C, Garello I, Marchetti A, et al. Hip ultrasound. *Eur J Radiol.* 2012;81(12):3824–3831.
102. Frick SL. Evaluation of the child who has hip pain. *Orthop Clin North Am.* 2006;37(2):133–40, v.
103. Fabry G. Clinical practice: the hip from birth to adolescence. *Eur J Pediatr.* 2010;169(2):143–148.

CHAPTER 8

Knee

EPIDEMIOLOGY OF KNEE PAIN

KNEE PAIN IN THE GENERAL POPULATION

Prevalence
- ~5% of adult population has nonspecific knee pain

Osteoarthritis (OA)
- Most common (MC) cause of chronic knee pain in people >50 years old
- Prevalence: 7% to 17% of people >45 years old from population-based studies (varies depending on the definition)
- More common in aged population: 20% of adult population, 25% of 56 to 84 years old (Sweden) (1,2)
- Higher in women, rural areas of developing countries

Other common causes
- Overexertion, minor trauma (contact with objects), and falls

KNEE PAIN IN ATHLETES

Anterior knee pain
- Occurs in 25% of athletes, 70% between 16 and 25 years old (3)

Knee injuries
- Second MC cause of lost playing time after ankle injuries in sports (4)

Knee ligament injuries
- MC sports injury leading to medical disability compensation
- Anterior cruciate ligament (ACL) injury: MC, 70% during athletic activity, female > male by 2 to 8 times, noncontact pivoting injury (eg, skiing, football, soccer, and basketball)
- Posterior cruciate ligament (PCL) injury from football (fall on flexed knee with plantar flexed foot)

Meniscal injury
- Noncontact cutting, deceleration, hyperflexion, or landing from a jump (eg, football, basketball, wrestling, skiing, baseball) (5)

Knee OA
- Higher prevalence in soccer players (7% vs 1.6% in control)

KNEE PAIN AT WORK (6)

Risk factors for chronic knee pain
- Exposure to loading of the joints, such as heavy lifting, kneeling, and crawling in obese patients
- Increased body weight correlates with knee pain in men and hip pain in women

Knee OA
- Odds ratio 2.2 for jobs requiring knee bending and at least medium level of physical activity (7)
- Relative risk two to three times higher in physically demanding jobs (shipyard workers, male farmers, male construction workers, firefighters, female janitors, and letter carriers)

DIFFERENTIAL DIAGNOSIS

MSK (MUSCULOSKELETAL) CAUSES OF KNEE PAIN BASED ON LOCATION (8) (FIGURE 8.1; FLOWCHART 8.1)

- Localization of pain is not discrete in intra-articular lesions, such as osteoarthritis (more discrete when irritating soft tissue and superficial tendons/ligaments).

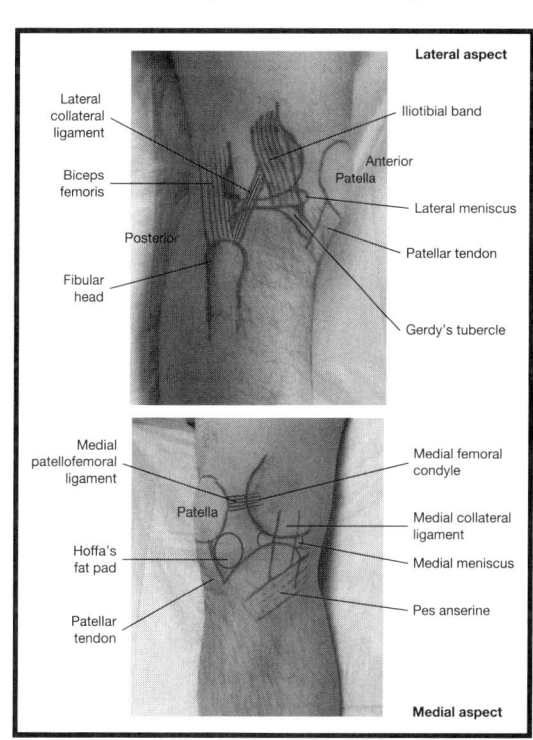

FIGURE 8.1
Surface anatomy of the knee.

```
                            ┌─────────────┐
                            │MSK knee pain│
                            └──────┬──────┘
                            ┌──────┴──────┐
                            │Location of pain│
                            └──────┬──────┘
    ┌───────────┬──────────┬──────┼──────┬──────────┬─────────────┐
┌───┴────┐ ┌────┴───┐ ┌────┴───┐ ┌┴──────┐ ┌────────┴────┐
│Anterior│ │ Medial │ │ Lateral│ │Posterior│ │Poorly localized│
└────────┘ └────────┘ └────────┘ └────────┘ └─────────────┘
```

Anterior:
- Patellofemoral syndrome (chondromalacia patellar, patellofemoral OA), patellar Fx/bipartite patella
- Quadriceps/patellar tendinopathy
- Infrapatellar/prepatellar bursitis
- Others: Hoffa's fat pad impingement, painful plica syndrome, patellofemoral ligament injury

Medial:
- Medial collateral ligament sprain/tear/bursitis
- Pes anserine tendinobursitis
- Acute medial meniscus tear/parameniscal cyst
- Medial femoral condyle lesion (osteochondritis dissecans, AVN); often poorly localized pain

Lateral:
- Iliotibial band syndrome
- Posterolateral corner strain/sprain (popliteus, biceps femoris, lateral collateral ligament injury)
- Acute lateral meniscus injury
- Tibiofibular joint/ligament dysfunction

Posterior:
- Baker's cyst rupture Popliteal cyst
- Hamstring tendinopathy
- Fabella syndrome
- Posterior horn of meniscus tear

Poorly localized:
- Osteoarthritis
- Referred pain from hip pathology
- Polyarthralgia >1 joint; inflammatory arthropathy
- Atypical neuropathic pain, fibromyalgia, etc.

FLOWCHART 8.1
Differential diagnosis of musculoskeletal knee pain.
AVN, avascular necrosis; Fx, fracture; MSK, musculoskeletal; OA, osteoarthritis.

REGION		DIFFERENTIAL DIAGNOSES
Anterior	Superior (at and proximal to patella)	Quadriceps tendinopathy/tear/enthesopathy Patellofemoral ligament (retinaculum) injury Painful medial plica syndrome in the medial patellofemoral space: pain with/without snapping Patellar fracture Indistinct localization • Patellofemoral syndrome/chondromalacia patellar/patellofemoral OA/synovitis; pain around the patella • Lateral patellofemoral overloading syndrome
	Inferior	Patellar tendinopathy and tear • Enthesopathy (adolescent): Sinding-Larsen-Johansson and Osgood-Schlatter syndrome Bursitis • Prepatellar: housemaid knee; on the inferior border of the patella • Infrapatellar (superficial and deep) bursitis (near tibial tuberosity) Indistinct localization • Hoffa's fat (infrapatellar) impingement syndrome/synovitis • Rarely fibroma of tendon sheath of the infrapatellar fat pad (9) • Anterior cruciate ligament cyst
Medial	Above joint line	Medial collateral ligament (MCL) sprain (MC on the femoral insertion) Distal adductor magnus tendinopathy (medial thigh pain: more common) Indistinct: osteochondritis dissecans, spontaneous osteonecrosis (more common in medial femoral condyle than lateral condyle)
	Joint line	MCL bursitis/sprain Medial meniscal tear, parameniscal cyst, and medial femorotibial OA
	Below joint line	Pes anserine tendinobursitis Indistinct localization • Infrapatellar branch of saphenous neuritis: typically neuropathic pain • Patellotibial ligament injury

(continued)

REGION		DIFFERENTIAL DIAGNOSES
Lateral	Proximal (near condyle)	Iliotibial band (ITB) syndrome (friction over the lateral condyle) Lateral collateral ligament sprain Popliteus tendinopathy; posterolateral
	Distal (at or below joint line)	Biceps femoris tendinopathy (insertional) ITB insertional enthesopathy (at lateral tibial tubercle) Indistinct localization • Lateral meniscal tear and lateral femorotibial OA • Tibiofibular joint arthralgia/ligament sprain
Posterior	Medial	Baker's cyst rupture: pain down to posteromedial calf (mimics deep vein thrombosis) Painful fabella syndrome: lateral gastrocnemius Indistinct localization • Posterior horn of meniscus tear • Popliteal aneurysm • Unruptured Baker's cyst or popliteal ganglia • Lymphadenopathy and tumor
Referred pain		Hip pathologies: 5% present with isolated knee symptoms, especially in younger age group • Slipped capital femoral epiphysis • Legg-Calves-Perthes disease Hip fracture, femoral shaft fracture (stress fracture)

MC, most common; OA, osteoarthritis

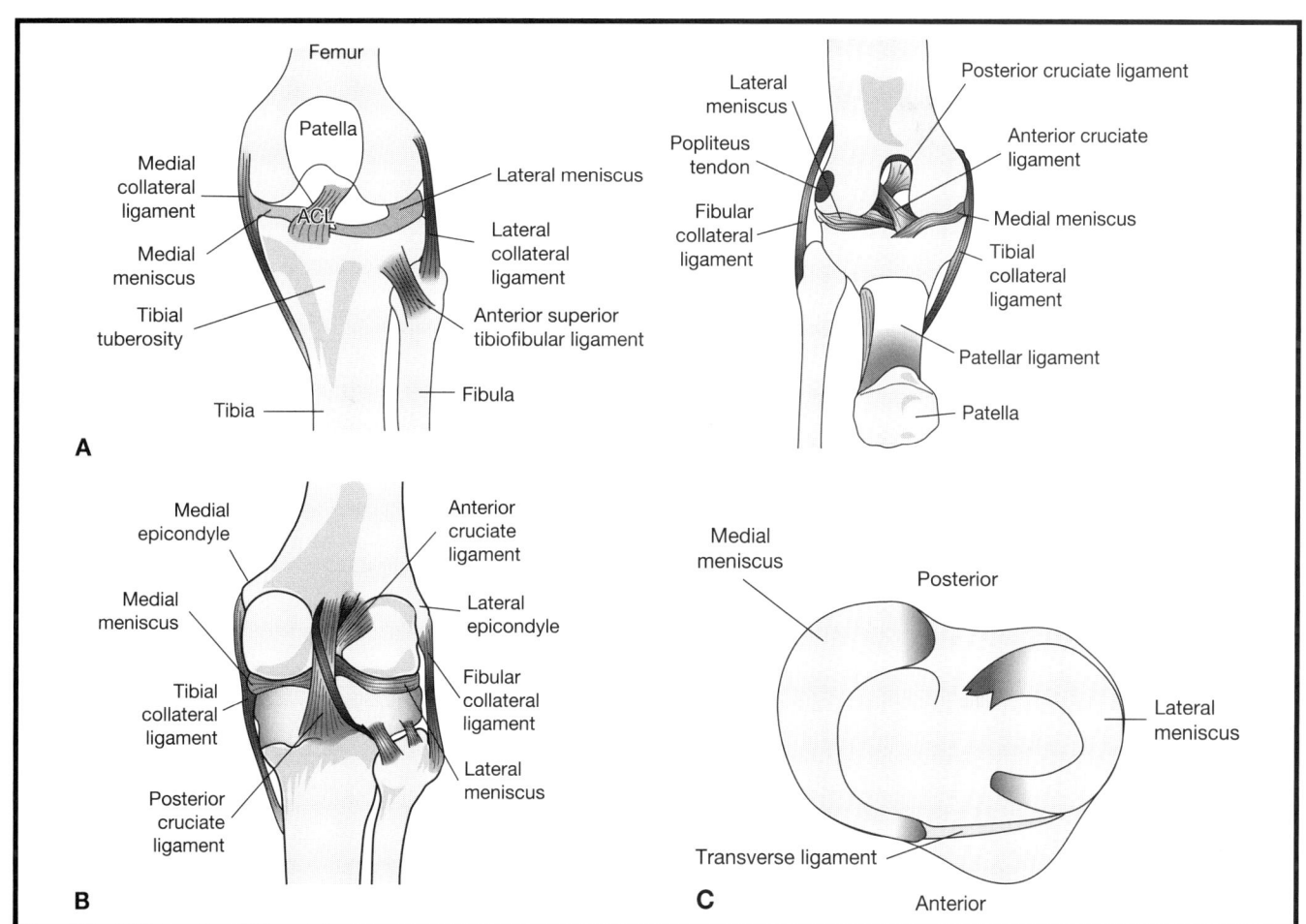

FIGURE 8.2
Bony and soft tissue anatomy (A) anterior aspect; (B) posterior aspect; (C) medial and lateral meniscus.

NEUROPATHIC CAUSES OF KNEE AND LEG PAIN (10) (FLOWCHART 8.2)

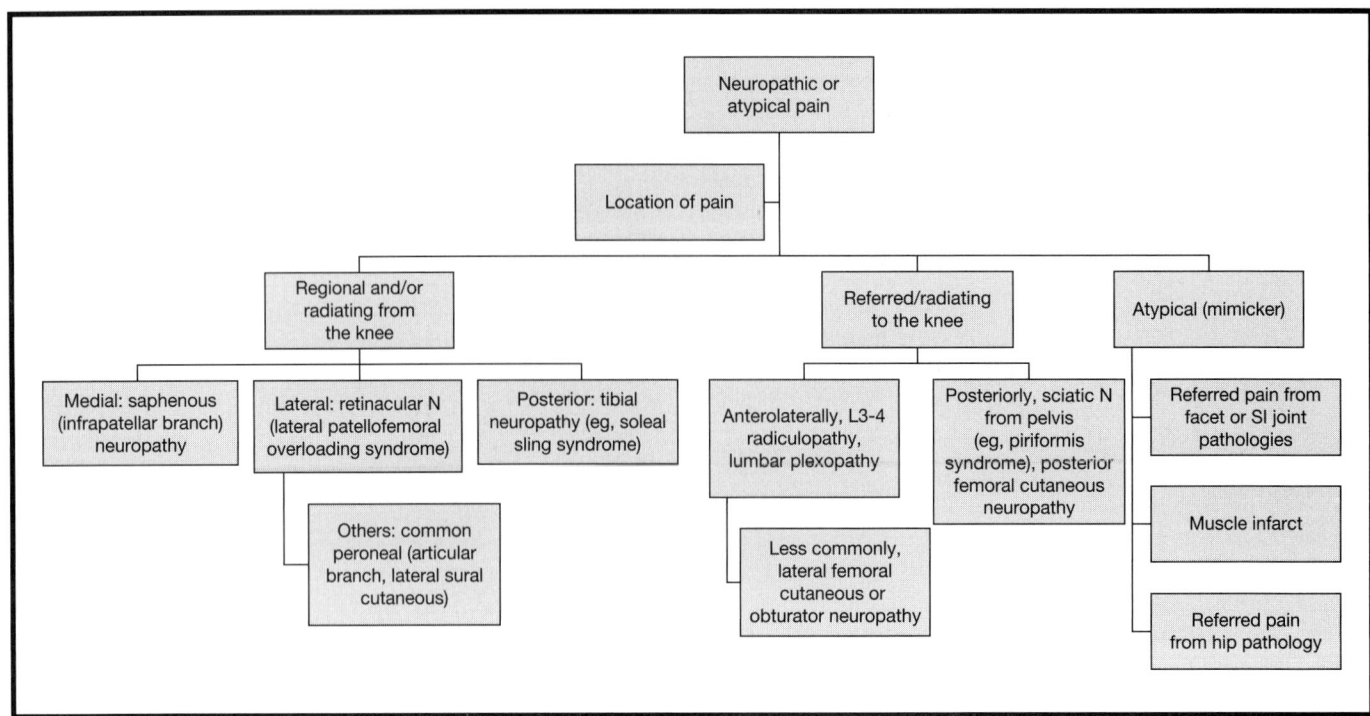

FLOWCHART 8.2

Differential diagnosis of neuropathic knee pain.

N, neuropathy; SI, sacroiliac.

REGION	PAIN LOCATION	DIFFERENTIAL DIAGNOSES
Medial	Localized knee pain	Saphenous N/infrapatellar branch neuralgia • Localized to knee if infrapatellar branch involved in isolation • Often concomitant with pes anserine tendinobursitis
	Pain radiating down to the knee	Less common than saphenous/infrapatellar neuropathy Medial femoral cutaneous N, N to vastus medialis lesion Anterior division of obturator neuropathy
Posterior	Knee pain radiating distally (tibial N)	Neuralgia of posterior articular branch of the tibial nerve • Trauma, iatrogenic, nerve tumor, intraneural ganglion cyst, and ossificans
	Pain radiating down to knee	Sciatic N irritation at the level of buttock and posterior hip Posterior femoral cutaneous neuropathy Facet arthropathy with referred pain Posterior division of the obturator nerve
Lateral	Localized knee pain	Retinacular branch from posterolateral genicular N • Patellofemoral syndrome or lateral patellofemoral overloading syndrome with lateral retinacular N irritation
	Knee pain radiating down to leg	Fibular N (sensory symptoms localized in the ankle and foot unless lateral sural cutaneous N involved) • Common peroneal neuropathy • Lateral sural cutaneous neuropathy (branch from common peroneal nerve)
	Pain down to knee	Lateral femoral cutaneous neuropathy (meralgia paresthetica) N to vastus lateralis, intermedius; unusual

N, nerve.

DIFFERENTIAL DIAGNOSIS OF KNEE SWELLING

Acute injury (hemarthrosis)

COMMON CAUSES	LESS COMMON CAUSES	MUST NOT BE MISSED
ACL tear/rupture Peripheral meniscal tear Tibial plateau fracture Patellar dislocation	Avulsion of ACL in children Osteochondral fracture	Knee dislocation Rupture of extensor mechanism

ACL, anterior cruciate ligament.

- Acute knee injury without significant swelling: central meniscal tear, medial collateral ligament (MCL) tear/rupture, PCL rupture, cartilage lesion, epiphyseal injury, or posterolateral corner injury

Knee swelling without significant trauma
- Osteoarthritis flare-up, inflammatory arthropathy (rheumatoid arthritis [RA], crystal-induced arthropathy, and other rheumatologic disease), and bursitis (suprapatellar, prepatellar, Baker's cyst), ganglion cyst or tumor (soft tissue or bony)

DIFFERENTIAL DIAGNOSIS OF SUBJECTIVE KNEE INSTABILITY (11,12)

MUSCULOSKELETAL CAUSES		
No trauma	Knee OA/chondromalacia patellar/patellofemoral syndrome	Effusion and pain Worse with descending stairs or standing from chair
	Meniscal degeneration/tear	Locking in bucket handle tear
	Intra-articular loose body	Osteochondritis dissecans
	Inflammatory joint disease (RA, crystal deposition disease/gout/pseudogout)	Effusion and stiffness
Trauma	Muscle and tendon tear	Localized pain
	Ligament (ACL/PCL and mediolateral collateral ligament injury)	Collateral ligament; mediolateral instability (more prominent) ACL/PCL: sagittal and rotational instability (more prominent) Indistinct pain
	Meniscal tear	Localized pain/tenderness ± swelling
NEUROLOGIC CAUSES		
Muscle weakness	Muscle disease, neuromuscular junction disease, femoral mononeuropathy, radiculopathy, motor neuron disease	Weakness > pain in muscle, neuromuscular and motor neuron disease Significant pain in radiculopathy/plexopathy typically
Spasticity	Upper motor neuron disease	Brain injury or spinal cord injury/disorder Spasticity with genu recurvatum with eventual incompetency of joint capsule
Sensory ataxia	Sensory neuropathy (peripheral neuropathy), neuronopathy (dorsal root ganglion), or myelopathy (dorsal column of spinal cord)	Numbness and loss of proprioception (foot and ankle equally or more involved)

ACL, anterior cruciate ligament; OA, osteoarthritis; PCL, posterior cruciate ligament; RA, rheumatoid arthritis.

DIFFERENTIAL DIAGNOSIS OF PAINFUL KNEE SNAPPING (13,14)

Lateral knee snapping: discoid lateral meniscus, biceps femoris tendon snapping, popliteus tendon snapping, and iliotibial band friction syndrome

Medial knee snapping: medial plicae, meniscal pathology, and subluxation of the gracilis and semitendinous tendons

Others: intra-articular loose body, fabella, congenital snapping knee, patellar dysplasia

ANATOMY

BONE AND JOINT (15)

Patellofemoral joint
- Patella: largest sesamoid bone, two facets with central ridge, lateral larger than medial (can be further divided into seven facets)
  - Medial facet: smaller and steeper angle (→ lateral subluxation and tilt of patella: more common). Thickest hyaline cartilage in our body

○ With aging, the patellofemoral (PF) joint is reduced to a cylindrical outline with reduced the bone-to-bone contact area
○ Complex arterial plexus supplies proximal two-thirds of the patella (16)
• Trochlea of the femur: concavity between the condyles
  ○ Lateral facet: larger, extends more proximally
  ○ Trochlear dysplasia: a loss of the normal concave anatomy and depth of the groove, creating a flat trochlea ➔ patellar instability and/or PF syndrome

Femoro-tibial joint: condylar articulation, incongruent shape (17)
• Allows transmission of body weight from the femur to the tibia while providing hinge-like sagittal rotation along with a small degree of tibial axial rotation
• Medial condyle: larger, increased curvature and projects further distally than lateral condyle
  ○ Femur slant medially (~6°)
  ○ Allows full flexion without contact between the posterior joint margins of the tibia and the femur
• Lateral condyle: more anterior than medial condyle
• Articular cartilaginous layer
  ○ Distributes reactive load over a wide area and helps contribute to cam shape of condyles, which maximizes the extensor lever arm
  ○ Type 2 collagen and an abundance of proteoglycan versus type 1 collagen mostly in meniscus

Proximal tibiofibular joint (12)
• Synovial joint, hyaline cartilage articulation, 10% to 12% communicates with the knee joint
• Oblique articulation varies; angle can affect stability
• Thicker capsule anteriorly
• Posterior proximal tibiofibular ligament reinforced by posterolateral corner structures of the knee; for example, biceps femoris and popliteus tendons

Other structures
• Capsule or capsular ligament (15)
  ○ Retinaculum: in the anterior third of capsule, the combined fascia, and aponeurotic sheet
    ▪ Medial patellofemoral ligament (MPFL): just proximal and posterior to the medial epicondyle and distal to the adductor tubercle ➔ the proximal and medial surface of the patella: important stabilizer against lateral subluxation/dislocation of the patella
  ○ Coronary ligament (meniscotibial ligament, deep layer of MCL): medial third, capsule between the tibia and the medial menisci (18)
  ○ Oblique popliteal ligament: (middle layer of MCL): thickened capsule by an expansion from the semimembranosus
• Synovial membrane and fluid
  ○ The largest synovium in the body, lining fibrous capsule, suprapatellar pouch, infrapatellar fat pad, cruciate ligament, and meniscus
  ○ Suprapatellar recess: up to 5 to 6 cm or above the patella; communicates with knee joint unless there is a complete plica
    ▪ Common location for intra-articular knee joint injection (supralateral approach)
  ○ Knee joint synovial fluid: less than 1 mL physiologically
  ○ Joint effusion (>15 mL) ➔ can inhibit quadriceps (vastus medialis more than rectus femoris, vastus lateralis)
  ○ Popliteal bursa and semimembranosus bursa may communicate with knee joint

Blood supply
• Popliteal artery (through adductor canal; anterior to posterior, medial and lateral genicular arteries: main suppliers), femoral artery (descending genicular artery, runs with saphenous nerve/infrapatellar branch), and anterior tibial artery (recurrent artery at the fibular neck)
  ○ Adductor canal: sartorius, vastus medialis, adductor magnus tendon/fascia, 3 to 10 cm above the superior pole of the patella
• Middle genicular artery: supplies the cruciate ligaments, synovial capsule, and the margin of the meniscus
• Inferior lateral genicular artery: under the lateral collateral ligament (LCL) near the meniscus; caution during lateral joint line injection or arthroscopy
• Inferior medial genicular artery: between the tibia and medial collateral ligament (MCL)

LIGAMENT AND MENISCUS

Intra-articular (Figure 8.2)
• Cruciate ligament (anterior and posterior cruciate ligament) (19)
  ○ Intra-articular and extrasynovial band of dense connective tissue
• Anterior cruciate ligament (ACL)
  ○ Lateral femoral condyle ➔ anterior portion of tibial eminence
  ○ Two bundles based on the location of the tibial insertion
    ▪ Anteromedial bundle: taut in flexion, resists anterior tibial translation in 60° to 90° of flexion, and resists rotatory subluxation
    ▪ Posterolateral bundle: taut in extension; resists anterior subluxation in full extension. More important restraint at knee in full extension
  ○ Function (20)
    ▪ Restraint to anterior translation of the tibia, internal rotation of tibia, and hyperextension of knee. Can cause rotational instability and limited knee full extension if impaired
    ▪ Secondary: resists varus and valgus force (can cause medial compartment overloading if impaired)
    ▪ Joint proprioception: repair does not improve proprioceptive deficit
      – Chronic ACL deficiency: medial compartment degenerative joint disease (DJD); increased risk regardless of ACL repair
    ▪ Functionally, hamstring analog: 25% of impaired function by ACL injury are compensated by hamstrings
      – Increased hamstring (biceps femoris) activity during midstance gait
  ○ Blood supply by middle genicular artery, innervated by posterior articular nerve
• Posterior cruciate ligament (PCL)
  ○ Posterolateral bundle: medial femoral condyle ➔ posterolateral to the tibia 1 cm distal to joint line, checking larger and less curved medial condyle
  ○ Stronger and thicker than ACL; more synovial tissue: better potential for healing than ACL
  ○ Anterolateral bundle: taut in flexion, posterolateral stability at 90° flexion and posteromedial: tight in extension

- Primary restraint to posterior translation of the tibia, stabilize in varus, and valgus stress
- Meniscus (21)
  - Fibrocartilaginous structure, type 1 collagen
  - Supplied by superior and inferior geniculate artery
    - Vascular in the outer 10% to 25% of the lateral and 10% to 30% of the medial meniscus
  - Collagen fibers in a circumferential pattern, much less proteoglycan (<1%)

MEDIAL MENISCUS	LATERAL MENISCUS
C shape; posterior horn is larger	Circular shape
Anchored to the tibial collateral ligament, coronary ligament (not in lateral meniscus)	Posteriorly anchored to the posterior/anterior meniscofemoral ligament (posterior horn to medial femoral condyle) and popliteus
More firmly attached to capsule	Less firmly attached to the capsule (separated posteriorly by popliteus tendon sheath)
Greater resistance to AP translation	Move further than medial meniscus (by ~2 times; less tear); popliteus pulls the meniscus backward during flexion
MC degenerative tear: posterior horn of the medial meniscus (posterior oblique fiber of MCL limit the movement)	

  - Function
    - Shock absorption and load transmission (to articular cartilage) in knee joint movement. Static loading by the tensile strength of the meniscal matrix (hoop tension). Distributes stress over a large area. Increase joint congruence
      – Fifty percent compressive force transmitted to the meniscus in extension → increased to 85% in 90° knee flexion
      – Increased OA in patients with meniscus injury
    - Contributes to joint stability, proprioception, and joint lubrication (distributes synovial fluid)
      – Primary stabilizer in ACL-deficient knee
    - Mobility
      – Lateral more mobile than medial meniscus
      – Anterior horn more mobile than posterior, lateral meniscus more mobile than medial (due to joint capsule and deep MCL), peripheral more mobile than central; firmly attached to intercondylar area of tibia
    - Varus alignment: potential risk factor for medial meniscal tear and extrusion

Extra-articular (22)
- MCL (23) (Figure 8.3)
  - Superficial MCL: one femoral and two tibial attachments (~1 and 6 cm from joint line)
    - Primary restraint to valgus laxity: higher load response at 90° knee flexion
    - MCL bursa under the superficial MCL
  - Deep MCL: meniscofemoral and meniscotibial ligaments
    - Secondary restraint to valgus loads: restraint against external rotation in 0 to 30° flexion
  - Posterior oblique ligament: fibrous extension of the semimembranosus that blends with and reinforces the joint capsule
    - Internal rotator and valgus stabilizer at between 0 and 30° flexion
  - Abundant blood supply; good potential for healing
- LCL (Figure 8.4)
  - Single layer, cord-like structure (vs band-like structure in MCL): ~7 cm in length, proximal/posterior to the popliteus origin on the femoral condyle to the fibular head
    - Primary static stabilizer to varus at knee from 0 to 30° of knee flexion
    - No direct attachment to the meniscus
    - Check rein to external rotation of the tibia and posterior tibial translation

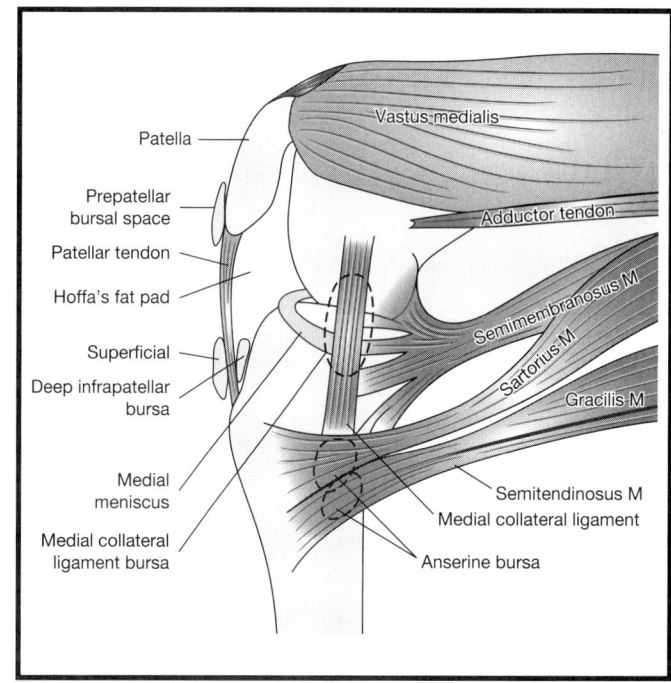

FIGURE 8.3
Extra-articular structures—the medial aspect of the knee.
M, muscle.

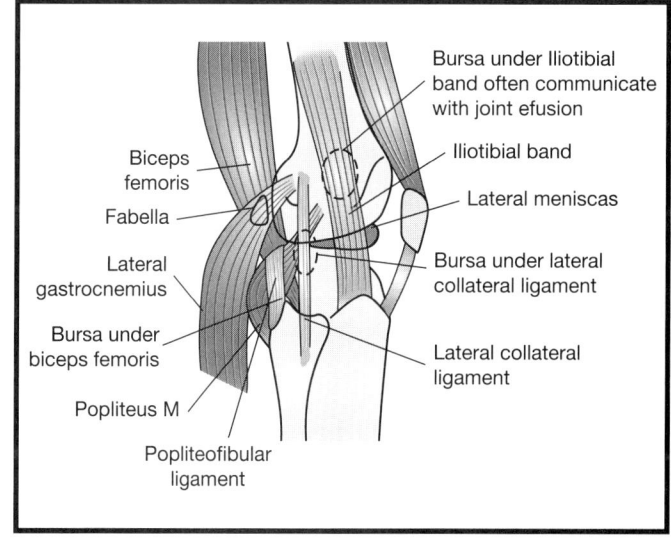

FIGURE 8.4
Extra-articular structures—the lateral aspect of the knee.
M, muscle.

- Arcuate ligament complex (posterolateral corner)
  - LCL, arcuate ligament (variable, fibular head to oblique popliteal ligament, and lateral gastrocnemius muscle), joint capsule, popliteus muscle, fabello fibular ligament (variable), lateral gastrocnemius
  - Popliteo fibular ligament, biceps femoris tendon, and iliotibial band (ITB): important stabilizer in posterolateral corner
  - Arcuate sign: avulsion of tip of the fibular head (LCL or biceps tendon rupture) → associated cruciate ligament injury (~90%)
  - Missed posterolateral corner injury → common cause of failed ACL reconstruction
- Popliteus muscle
  - Underneath the LCL (anterior/inferior to LCL) and inferior to (underneath) ITB when flexed. Intracapsular in the femoral insertion, and extrasynovial
  - Attached to the lateral meniscus (post horn)/fibular → allows the popliteus to withdraw the meniscus during knee flexion/stabilizes the meniscus and prevents medial entrapment of the meniscus when varus forces are applied
  - Flexes and internally rotates the tibia concentrically; eccentric contraction resists extension and external rotation → stability against external rotation. Unlocks the knee via externally rotating the femur on the tibia
    - Hyperpronation: risk factor for popliteal tendinopathy and symptom (from popliteal tendinopathy) worse with walking downhill and stair negotiation

NERVE

Innervation of the Knee (24) (Figure 8.5)

REGION	NERVES
Anteromedial	Infrapatellar branch of the saphenous N: well-recognized cause of anteromedial knee pain Other contributing nerves • The medial femoral cutaneous N: medial patellofemoral retinacular and articular cartilage • Nerve to the vastus medialis (medial retinacular branch) in the substance of the vastus medialis (in 90%) • Anterior branch of the obturator N

Lateral	Sciatic nerve
	• Superior lateral genicular nerve (8–10 cm above joint line from sciatic N) → lateral retinacular nerve
	  ○ Possible culprit of patellofemoral syndrome and lateral patellar overloading syndrome (25,26)
	Common peroneal N
	• Inferior lateral articular nerve: the lateral joint capsule and proximal tibiofibular joint
	  ○ From above the fibular head
	• Recurrent branch: from distal to the fibular head
	Small terminal branches
	• N to the vastus intermedius
	  ○ Articularis genu muscle and anterior superior aspect of the capsule
	• N to the vastus lateralis; no consistent branch to the capsule

(continued)

REGION	NERVES
Posterior	Posterior articular branch of the tibial N • One to five branches, branching 10–25 cm above the joint line Posterior division of the obturator N

N, nerve.

Local neuropathic pain (medial/lateral/posterior) can be secondary to the following
- Mononeuropathy (or 1–2 nerves): local injury/entrapment along the course
- Diffuse pain from local pathologies affecting the knee joint capsule complex (musculoskeletal etiology)
- Lesion at level of root or higher (rather than focal peripheral nerve lesion)

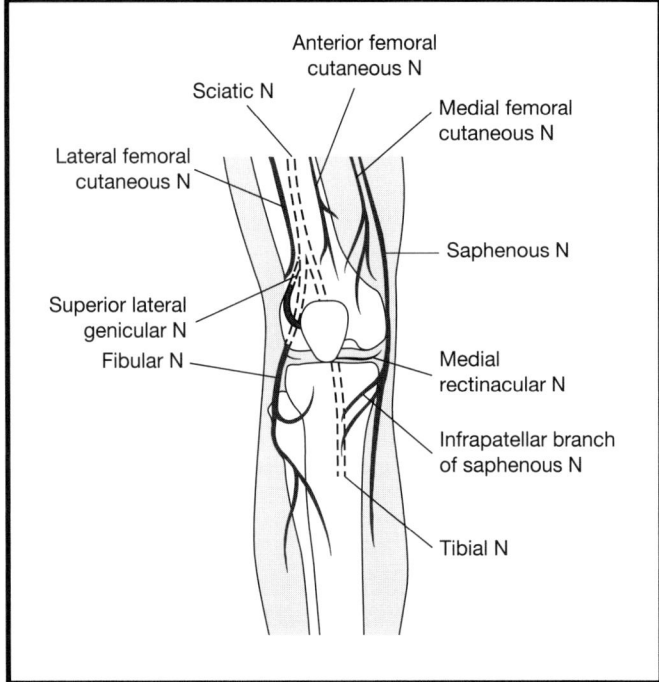

FIGURE 8.5
Nerve innervation of the knee.
N, nerve.

BIOMECHANICS

KINEMATIC AND KINETIC

Patellofemoral joint (15) (Figure 8.6)
- Zero to 20 degree knee flexion: accompanied by internal rotation of the tibia (by popliteus) and laterally directed quadriceps muscle vector → PF contact is made; the initial contact at the lateral facet of the patella → lateral PF joint and ITB pain at initial knee flexion
- Further flexion of knee moves patella anterior relative to center of rotation of the knee, which improves the mechanical advantage of the quadriceps mechanism

- Patella continues to move laterally at 90° of knee flexion, and lateral border of the patella provides the primary loading site
- Loading of PF joint
  - Increases with flexion (50% with 1°–15°, 300% in 60°, 800% of body weight in deep squatting)
  - Different activities: ~3 times higher in stair climbing, ~7 times higher in squatting. Maximal contact at 45° flexion
  - Q angle: angle of patellar ligament and pull of quadriceps (normal up to 10°–17°, female > male due to wider pelvis, genu valgum, femoral anteversion, abnormal if >20°)
    - Increased Q angle → increased lateral pull on patella

Tibiofemoral joint (27)
- Knee extension from flexion
  - Tibia externally rotates to accommodate the medial condyle (more anterior protruded medial condyle than lateral condyle in axial plane)
  - Tibia externally rotates 5° in the last 15° of extension
- Knee flexion from full extension preceded by the tibia internal rotation (if standing → closed kinetic chain, the femur externally rotates) by the popliteus muscle contraction
  - With knee flexion, the instant center of rotation on the femur moves posteriorly (posterior rollback), allows knee flexion without impingement
  - Relaxes tension of collateral ligaments sufficient to permit flexion
- Sagittal plane range 0° to 140°, other motions (transverse and frontal planes) limited by interlocking of the femoral condyles in extension; transverse plane motion: maximal at knee flexion (45° internal rotation, 30° external rotation)
- Knee range of motion (ROM) during functional activities
  - Level walking: 65° for swing phase, stairs 80°, sit to stand from low chair: 95°, and bath transfer 120° (in bath) to 130° (out of bath) (28)
  - Flexion of 110°: reasonable goal for activities for daily living (ADLs) otherwise compensated by other joints
- In osteoarthritis, greater femoral internal rotation, decreased tibial posterior translation → dysfunction of "screw home" motion during extension (17)
- Joint reaction force: three times during walking and four times with climbing

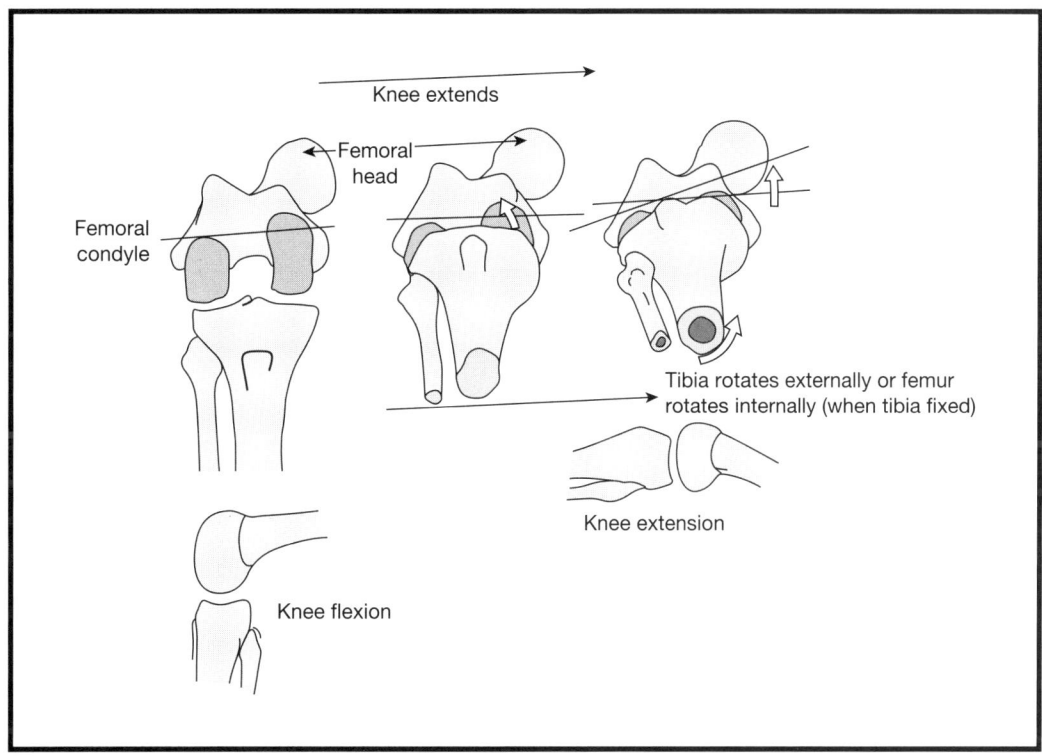

FIGURE 8.6
"Screw home" motion of knee (rotation of knee joint with flexion/extension movement).

Tibiofibular joint
- Dissipate torsional loads applied at ankle, absorption of lateral tibial bending movement, and transmission of 1/6 body weight
- Knee flexion and extension → fibular anterior-posterior motion
  - Knee extension: taut lateral collateral ligament (0°–30°) stabilizes tibiofibular joint. With knee flexion, proximal fibula moves anteriorly with relaxation of LCL (as well as biceps femoris); loose
- Affected by ankle movement: ankle dorsiflexion → external rotation of the fibula; forced ankle dorsiflexion → increase torsional load, predisposing higher risk of fracture or ligament sprain, dislocation

Knee joint in a closed kinetic chain (on standing and walking)
- Flexion and extension momentum depending on the center of mass and ground reaction force (GRF)

- If the GRF is posterior to the knee joint, flexion. If anterior, then extension momentum
- Response to foot and ankle biomechanics (pronation–supination)
  - Ankle dorsiflexed in standing (closed kinetic chain) → flexion momentum to knee versus ankle plantar flexion in standing → extension momentum
  - Pronation response (from foot and ankle conditions; eg, flat foot or functional leg length discrepancy) → tibia externally rotated (internal rotation moment proximally), genu valgum and slight knee flexion
    - Heel lift can affect GRF to decrease excessive extension momentum (pain in knee extension)
  - Adduction momentum diminished by medial heel/extended wedge
    - Increased adduction moment partly by increased medial quadriceps muscle hyperactivity
    - Medial wedge and extended wedge also can decrease tibia external rotation (pronation response)
    - Lateral wedge can decrease adductor moment by moving GRF closer to the knee center
- Response to hip biomechanics
  - Increased hip anteversion (increased angle from femoral neck axis and transcondylar line) → intercondylar groove rotates more internally and tibia also internally rotates → supination response occurs
  - Decreased hip anteversion or increased retroversion → intercondylar groove face laterally (external rotation) → pronation response occurs

Anterior cruciate ligament
- Biomechanics and clinical application
  - Gender differences in ACL injuries (29): female > male by three to six times (30), multifactorial
    - Over activation of quadriceps versus hamstring on landing and cutting
    - Posture: more upright during cutting (increased valgus of the knee and quadriceps activation)
      - More crouched position: may reduce the risk of ACL injuries
  - Jumping while fatigued: decreased hip flexion/knee flexion, decreased eccentric capacity, and increased knee valgus
- ACL-deficient knee
  - Compensation to avoid anterior displacement of the tibia during gait (during obstacle-crossing) → decrease knee extensor moment (effort)/prevent quadriceps contracture
    - Shift center of mass forward; increased anterior tilt of the pelvis and hip flexion
    - Increased peak hip extensor and ankle plantar flexor moments
  - Significant increases in the anterior tilt of the pelvis and flexion at both hips when the unaffected leading toe was above the obstacle
    - To prevent quadriceps contraction, patients may have to shift the center of body mass forward and thus cause greater pelvic anterior tilt and hip flexion, in both the swing limb and the stance limb, with normal leading toe clearance for safe obstacle crossing (31)

Biomechanics in knee OA
- Knee OA (medial tibiofemoral) associated with high external knee adduction moment, reflects compression of the medial compartment of the knee
  - Biomechanical intervention: to reduce the knee adduction moment, AposTherapy®, and foot inserts (32)
- Increased pelvic anterior tilt, swing-pelvic list, decreased standing knee abduction, as well as decreased standing hip flexor and knee extensor moments
- In severe bilateral medial knee OA: increased hip abduction, knee extension, and ankle plantar flexion
  - Training of the hip muscles and pelvic control are essential for patients with knee OA, especially in severe OA (33)

KNEE STABILITY

Tibofemoral joint stabilizers (29)
- Dynamic stabilizers: quadriceps, hamstring, gastrocnemius, and popliteus muscles
- Static stabilizers: joint capsule, lateral/medial meniscus, and ligaments (ACL, PCL, MCL, LCL, and another small ligament)
- Hamstring and ACL: resist anterior movement of tibia
- Quadriceps and PCL: resist posterior movement of tibia
- Posteromedial stabilizers: oblique ligament (semimembranosus), semitendinosus
- Anterolateral: ITB, retinaculum
- Posterolateral stabilizers: lateral collateral ligament, oblique trans-popliteal ligament (semimembranosus), arcuate ligament, fabellofibular ligament, and popliteus muscle
- Posterior: oblique trans-popliteal ligament, arcuate ligament, joint capsule, and popliteal muscle
- Medial and lateral knee-stabilizing structures by layer

MEDIAL	LATERAL
Layer I: sartorius and fascia Layer II: superficial MCL, posterior oblique ligament, semimembranosus M Layer III: deep MCL (meniscofemoral and meniscotibial), and capsule	Layer I: lateral fascia, ITB, and biceps femoris Layer II: patellofemoral retinaculum/ligament Layer III: • Superficial: lateral collateral ligament, fabellofibular ligament, • Deeper: popliteo fibular ligament, popliteus tendon and arcuate ligament (fibular to lateral condyle; reinforces the posterolateral capsule and covers the popliteus) and capsule

ITB, iliotibial band, MCL, medial collateral ligament; M, muscle.

Patellofemoral joint stabilizers (34)
- Medial: vastus medialis obliquus (VMO; primary dynamic restraint to lateral tracking of the patella), medial PF ligament (especially 0°–30° flexion) > patellotibial/meniscal ligament and retinaculum
- Lateral: vastus lateralis oblique > anterior fibers of ITB and lateral retinaculum

Tibiofibular joint stabilizers (12,35)
- Bony: angle of joint plane (from the coronal plane) and configuration variation of tibiofibular joint
- Ligaments and muscles: capsule (thicker in anterior), tibiofibular ligament; anterior (three bands), posterior (two

bands; weaker than anterior with reinforcement from posterolateral structures; LCL, arcuate ligament, fabellofibular ligament, popliteo fibular ligament, popliteus muscles), and biceps femoris muscle

PHYSICAL EXAMINATION

INSPECTION

Alignment of the lower extremities: genu valgum (X shaped), varum (diamond shaped), or recurvatum (hyperextended knee)
- Genu varum with medial joint pain, genu valgum with medial knee pain (MCL), and lateral knee joint line pain
  - Tibia vara (Blount disease: bowleg): multifactorial
    - Familial, physiologic genu varum (often symmetric)
    - Other skeletal dysplasia, metabolic disorder (renal osteodystrophy, vitamin D resistant rickets), posttraumatic, and postinfectious
- Genu recurvatum with infrapatellar pain (fat pad impingement) or posterior knee pain
- Ankle and foot: hyperpronation (genu valgum, hindfoot valgus), supination (genu varum, recurvatum, and equinovarus)
- Leg length discrepancy (pelvic obliquity, level of posterior iliac crest, and patellar)

Swelling: localized (bursal effusion, uncommon) or generalized (intra-articular) with bulging suprapatellar recess or prominent Hoffa's fat pad
- Bursal: prepatellar (can be subtle), superficial infrapatellar (between the patellar tendon insertion to tibial tuberosity, pes anserine (rare), Baker's cyst (posteromedial knee, loss of groove between the medial gastrocnemius and medial hamstring)
- Intra-articular: patient prefers slight knee flexion to accommodate the joint effusion

Symmetric muscle contours
- Rapid development of muscle atrophy may suggest neuromuscular lesion, although chronic musculoskeletal lesions cause disuse atrophy (gradual)

Erythema or wound; red flag for infectious etiology

PALPATION

Anterior
- Patella: superior base (superolateral for bipartite patella) and inferior apex
- Prepatellar bursal effusion (superficial, the inferior apex of the patella) or suprapatellar effusion (knee joint effusion)
- Tibial tuberosity; for prominence (especially in adolescent for Osgood-Schlatter disease)
- Quadriceps and patellar tendon (compare thickness and width with the asymptomatic side)

Medial
- Joint line (at the level of inferior border of the patella; medial meniscus and band-like MCL)
  - Palpate while rotating the leg; differential rotation between the two bones
  - Joint line tenderness for medial meniscus injury (sensitivity: 55%–80%; specificity: 29%–67%)
- Medial femoral condyle (tenderness on MCL insertion, PF ligament sprain, and rarely AVN), adductor tubercle (posterior aspect of the femoral condyle above medial epicondyle)
- Tibial condyle and pes anserine (about 6 cm inferior to the joint line, at the level of tibial tuberosity)
- Patellofemoral space: plica on the medial femoral condyle (band/string-like)

Lateral
- Joint line: lateral meniscus/coronary ligament, LCL
- Lateral femoral condyle (ITB friction, popliteal fossa [able to palpate]), attachment to LCL and popliteus (difficult to palpate)
- Lateral tibial plateau (Gerdy's tubercle): insertion of ITB; follow the ITB distally, laterally to the lateral border of the patellar tendon
- Head of fibular; LCL (toward femoral condyle), biceps tendon insertion; parallel to the femur, common peroneal nerve (around the inferior aspect of the fibular head, able to palpate in some cases)
- Tibiofibular joint; anterior to the fibular head

Posterior
- Popliteal artery, middle of bulge (formed by gastrocnemius muscle)
- Fabella on the lateral gastrocnemius (difficult to palpate)

RANGE OF MOTION

	RANGE OF MOTION (FUNCTIONAL)°		RANGE OF MOTION°
Extension	0 (5 of hyperextension)	External rotation	10
Flexion	130–140 (105–110)	Internal rotation	10

SPECIAL EXAMINATION (36)

NAME	DESCRIPTION	SENSITIVITY (SEN) AND SPECIFICITY (SPE) IN %
Joint Effusion		
Fluctuation test	Depress patella while maintaining thumb and index finger around the margin of the patella. Positive if synovial fluid fluctuation palpated	Generally insensitive in mild effusion, and in obese population
Ballotable patellar test	Slight tap on the patella → positive if floating of the patella felt	
Indentation test	Observe indentation next to the patellar tendon disappear as knee is flexed on supine patient Compare with the contralateral site	
Tightness of Muscles		
Ely test	To check rectus femoris tightness In prone position, flex the knee Positive if hip flexes as the examiner flexes the knee Sensitivity of ~50% and specificity of 90% for rectus femoris spasticity in cerebral palsy patients (37)	
Modified Thomas test	With contralateral hip in maximal flexion (knee to the chest) at the end of table, check the femur (hip flexion angle from horizontal for iliopsoas tightness), knee flexion (extend knee from 90° for rectus femoris tightness) and hip abduction (from midline for ITB tightness)	
Ober test	To check iliotibial band (especially tensor fascia lata) tightness With hip extended (TFL over the greater tuberosity) and knee flexed or straight (ITB more tight in modified Ober test), examiner releases knee support (drops the leg) Positive if failure to adduct or if a catch is present	
Cruciate Ligaments (38)		
Lachman test	With knee 15°–30° flexion and tibia slight external rotation (relax ITB), proximal aspect of the tibia is moved forward by examiner • Positive if there is mushy or soft end feel, indicating posterolateral band of ACL or posterolateral corner insufficiency • False negative if femur is not properly stabilized, blocked by meniscus lesion, or tibia is medially rotated • False positive: PCL tear, posterior oblique ligament, and arcuate-popliteus complex lesion • Sensitive, especially with general anesthesia ○ Grade 1: 5 mm displacement, grade 2: 5–10 mm, grade 3: >10 mm	Sen: 80–90's Spe: 90's
Pivot shift test	With the knee in full extension (should be relaxed), a valgus stress is placed on the tibia, while an axial load and internal rotation of tibia are simultaneously applied. The knee is then slowly flexed with these applied forces. During this motion, the lateral side of the tibia plateau subluxates to a greater extent than the medial side at 20°–30°. With further flexion, the lateral tibia reduces, producing the pivot shift (ITB becomes flexor of the knee (tibia moves posteriorly) from extensor of the knee (tibia moves anteriorly) as knee further flexes	Sen: 80–90's under anesthesia (~35%) Spe: 90–100
Anterior drawer test	Knee flexed 90° (relax hamstring) and hip 45° flexed, tibia is drawn forward (normal up to 6 mm) Positive in lesions of ACL (anteromedial band), posterolateral capsule, posteromedial capsule, MCL, ITB, posterior oblique ligament, and arcuate-popliteus complex	Sen: 22–90's (for acute injury; highest under anesthesia) Spe: 90's
Posterior drawer test	With knee flexed 90°, translate the tibia (press tibial tuberosity) posteriorly Positive if there is lack of end feel or excessive translation (compared to the other side) Positive in lesions of PCL, arcuate popliteus complex, posterior oblique ligament, and ACL	Sen: 51–90, Spe: 99
Posterior sag sign	Supine with hip flexed to 45° and knee 90° flexion Positive with tibia sagging	Sen: 79, Spe: 100

(continued)

NAME	DESCRIPTION	SENSITIVITY (SEN) AND SPECIFICITY (SPE) IN %
Collateral Ligaments		
Valgus stress test	To evaluate medial collateral ligament With knee flexion to 30° and full extension on supine, apply abduction (valgus) stress to distal tibia Measure medial gapping compared to the opposite site If full extension → stress posteromedial capsule or cruciate ligament	Sen: 80–90's
Varus stress test	To evaluate lateral collateral ligament (LCL) Knee flexion to 30° (for isolated LCL injury) and full extension on supine patient; then apply adduction (varus) stress to distal tibia. Measure lateral gapping Compare site-to-site difference Positive if laxity demonstrated with knee 30° flexion Laxity with full extension: LCL + cruciate ligament injury	Sen: 25
Dial test	Externally rotate the leg with patient prone with the knee positioned at 30° and then 90° of flexion. The degree of external rotation is measured by comparing the medial border of the foot with the axis of the femur. Positive if >10°–15° difference compared to the other side • An increase of external rotation only at 30° of knee flexion → an isolated posterolateral corner (PLC) injury • Increased external rotation only at 90° of flexion → posterior cruciate ligament • Increased external rotation at both 30° and 90° of knee flexion suggests a combined PCL and PLC injury	
Meniscus		
McMurray test	For medial meniscus evaluation: flexion/max external rotation of tibia /varus → then slowly extend the knee Lateral meniscus evaluation: flexion/internal rotation of tibia/valgus Or vice versa by Kim et al. (39) Positive if symptoms (painful snap or click) reproduced	Sen: 29–58 Spe: 77 to 90's
Appley grind test	Prone with knee 90°, rotate (internal/external) the leg with compression → more painful than with distraction: suggests meniscus lesion More painful with distraction: suggests ligament lesion	Sen: ~10, Spe: 80–90
Thessaly test	The patient rotates his or her knee and body, internally and externally on a single-leg stance, three times, with the knee flexed at 20°, first in the normal knee, and then in the symptomatic knee Positive if pain in the joint line reproduced	Sen: ~90, Spe: 96–97 (40)
Patellar Femoral Joint (41)		
Patellofemoral grind test (Clarke sign)	Supine with patella being pressed against superior pole by examiner while quadriceps contraction isometrically. Positive with pain with inability to contract quadriceps • Differential diagnosis from Hoffa's fat pad impingement: pain relieved with patellar distraction (to upward) in Hoffa's fat pad impingement	Sen: 39, Spe: 67 for chondromalacia patella (42)
Patellar tilt test	Patient supine with knee extension. The examiner puts downward pressure applied to the medial edge of the patella Positive if fails to raise (tilt) the lateral edge to at least a horizontal level indicating a tight lateral retinaculum	Sen: 43%, Spe: 92% (43)
Patellar glide test	Assessing side-to-side patellar mobility Positive if the examiner is unable to shift the patella medially >1/4 of its width indicating excessive tightness of the lateral retinaculum	
J sign	A sudden lateral movement of the patella as the knee nears full extension indicating excessive lateral forces acting on the patella as it exits the femoral trochlea Patellar pull test: positive if lateral patellar movement is bigger than superior migration during quadriceps contraction	
Apprehension test	Press/push medial aspect of the patella (to laterally directed force) with knee flexion 30° with quadriceps relaxed. Positive with apprehension or reproduction of pain	Sen: 7–39, Spe: 92 (43)

ACL, anterior cruciate ligament; ITB, iliotibial band; MCL, medial collateral ligament; PCL, posterior cruciate ligament; TFL, tensor fascia lata.

DIAGNOSTIC STUDIES

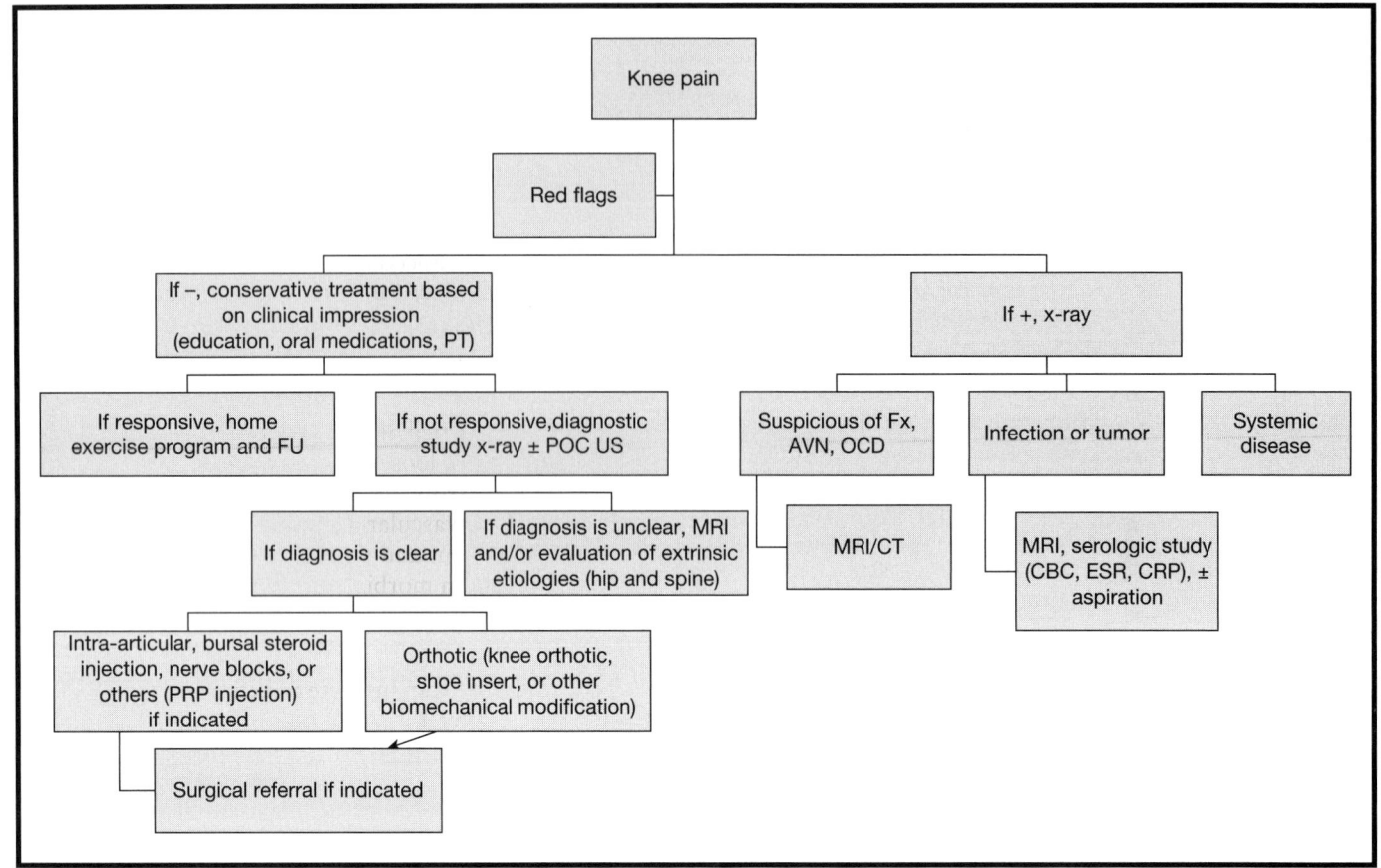

FLOWCHART 8.3

Diagnostic approach and management of the knee pain.

AVN, avascular necrosis; CBC, complete blood count; CRP, C-reactive protein; CT, computed tomography; ESR, erythrocyte sedimentation rate; FU, follow-up; OCD, osteochondritis dissecans; POC, point-of-care; PRP, platelet-rich plasma; PT, physical therapy.

PLAIN RADIOGRAPHS

Indications
- Chronic (≥3–6 months) nontraumatic knee pain or red flags (similar to the spine imaging)
- Traumatic knee injury
  ○ Ottawa or Pittsburgh rule (order x-ray selectively based on criteria) can improve sensitivity and specificity (44)
  ○ Ottawa knee rule
    ▪ Considering age, tenderness, and function
    ▪ Indication: age ≥55 years, tenderness at the head of the fibula, isolated tenderness of the patella, inability to flex to 90°, and inability to bear weight for four steps both immediately and after a period of observation on the sideline
    ▪ A sensitivity of 97% for identifying fractures, with a specificity of 27%
  ○ The Pittsburgh knee rules: an alternate set of decision guidelines
    ▪ Indications: blunt trauma/fall and ≥1 of the following factors
    ▪ (1) ≥50 years old and (2) inability to walk four steps in the emergency room (ER) or after a period of observation on the sideline
    ▪ A sensitivity of 99% and a specificity of 60%
  ○ Pediatric population has different sensitivity and specificity

Limitations
- Low capability to assess soft tissues (except tendon calcification), articular cartilage, intra-articular lesion or bursal effusion, meniscus or marrow

Specific views
- Routine: standing anteroposterior (AP), lateral, skyline view (PF joint)
- Standing AP: osteophytes and its size (for Kellgren stage for osteoarthritis), joint space narrowing, calcification in the soft tissue (or meniscus or articular cartilage) and coronal plane alignment (genu varum or valgum)
- Lateral: patella alta/baja, or effusion
  ○ Normal ratio of maximal length of the patella to the distance from the distal tip of the patella to tibial tuberosity is normally between 0.8 and 1.2; patella alta (proximal migration) is a ratio >1.2 and baja if <0.8 (Insall–Salvati ratio)
  ○ Measurement should be made at flexion from 20° to 70°
  ○ Differential diagnosis of patella alta: patellar tendon rupture (proximal 1/3, congenital elongation of the

patellar tendon, recurrent patellar subluxation, Osgood-Schlatter disease, and chondromalacia of the patella)
  ○ Differential diagnosis of patella baja: quadriceps dysfunction (poliomyelitis, myopathy, quadriceps rupture, fracture, and also seen with ACL repair and total knee arthroplasty [TKA] in 25%).
- Axilla view (skyline view, sunrise) for patellofemoral joint
  ○ Common indication: anterior knee pain
  ○ Merchant's view: modified sunrise (angle 30°–45°)
  ○ Tunnel view of the intercondylar notch
  ○ Sulcus angle (dysplasia) or tilting or the patella (laterally), subluxation/dislocation or osteophytes in patellofemoral OA
  ○ Consider it does not account for cartilage layer

POINT-OF-CARE ULTRASONOGRAPHY

Indications and findings
- Extra-articular soft tissue structure, effusion, and superficial joint structures (45)

REGION	COMMON FINDINGS
Anterior	Quadriceps tendon/muscle (enthesopathy, tear)
	Suprapatellar recess (for effusion, plica, synovitis [increased vascularity on Doppler], loose body)
	Patella (traction spur, bipartite, fracture, quadriceps enthesopathy, Sinding-Larsen-Johansson disease), prepatellar bursitis (above inferior pole of the patella)
	Patellar tendon (tendinopathy/tear), tibial tuberosity (osteophyte, Osgood-Schlatter disease), infrapatellar bursitis (superficial/deep; deep bursal effusion, physiologic <2 mm)
	Articular cartilage with hyperflexed knee: crystal deposition disease (inside and on the cartilage) or gout (double contour)
	Infrapatellar (Hoffa's fat pad): anterior cruciate ligament cyst or parameniscal cyst
Medial	Medial tibiofemoral joint with medial meniscus (osteophytes or joint space narrowing in OA, meniscal protrusion, cyst, peripheral tear)
	Medial collateral ligament (MCL): sprain, tear, MCL bursitis, MCL displacement by osteophyte or meniscus protrusion
	Pes anserine complex (thickened tendon, bursal effusion): bursa between MCL (deep) and anserine tendon (superficial)
	Saphenous N (for block and rarely neuroma) between vastus medialis and sartorius at the level of the adductor tubercle
Lateral	Iliotibial band: insertional enthesopathy, bursitis; bursal effusion usually communicating with knee joint effusion
	Femoral condyle: notch for popliteal tendon (tenosynovitis), lateral collateral ligament (LCL) sprain, tear, and bursitis
	Fibular head: biceps tendinopathy/tear/enthesopathy, LCL sprain with spur, avulsion
	Tibiofemoral joint (osteophytes), meniscus/lateral inferior geniculate artery
	Tibiofibular joint/ligament
	Peroneal nerve: ganglion, focal neuropathy with increased cross-sectional area (compared to the contralateral asymptomatic side)

(continued)

REGION	COMMON FINDINGS
Posterior	Sartorius, semimembranosus, semitendinosus, medial gastrocnemius: tear, tendinopathy, bursitis
	Semimembranosus-medial gastrocnemius bursal effusion (Baker's cyst)
	Tibial N: external compression by gastrocnemius, ganglion cyst, soleal sling ± focal enlargement (technically difficult to demonstrate)
	Tibial artery (aneurysm) and vein, biceps tendon, posterior cruciate ligament cyst
	Fabella on the lateral gastrocnemius

N, nerve; OA, osteoarthritis

Limitations
- Limited in intra-articular structures (ACL and PCL), inner portion of meniscus, loose body
- Intracortical (marrow) lesion: tumor, cyst, osteochondritis dissecans (OCD), avascular necrosis
- Operator dependent and variable measurement technique
- Deeper structure in morbidly obese patient

Protocols
- Based on the American Institute of Ultrasound in Medicine (AIUM); see Chapter 1

MRI

Indications
- Intra-articular lesion (ACL and PCL, meniscus, posterolateral corner structures) or loose body
  ○ Sensitivity and specificity for ACL: 82% and 94%; for PCL: 91% and 98%; and for meniscal lesion: 77% and 91%
- Intracortical lesion: avascular necrosis, OCD, tumor, or nondisplaced fracture
- Suspicion for infection and tumor: soft tissue or bone (intracortical lesion), or evaluation of mass
- Unclear diagnosis despite other imaging study
- Preoperative evaluation (not always necessary)

Common findings with systematic approach (46)
- Ligaments: low signal intensity (SI) in all sequences normally.
  ○ Common abnormal findings: abnormal SI and discontinuity of the structure
  ○ Cruciate ligament
    ▪ ACL (sagittal; primary plane to examine, axial and coronal); accuracy 90% to 95%, less accurate in depicting partial thickness tears and chronic ACL-deficient knee conditions
    ▪ PCL (primarily sagittal, rarely axial, and coronal)
    ▪ Cruciate cysts
  ○ Collateral ligament
    ▪ MCL tear → look for other accompanied lesions (ACL tear, medial meniscus or medial and posterior capsule, lateral femoral condyle, and tibia lesion)
- Meniscus
  ○ Normal: homogeneous low SI in all sequences
  ○ T1 or proton density: most sensitive for indentifying meniscal tears; T2: less sensitive but more specific
  ○ Grading system for abnormal meniscus

- Grade 1: globular foci of early mucinous degeneration, no clinical significance
- Grade 2: a linear horizontal area of increased SI that does not extend to an articular surface
- Grade 3: increased signal intensity to articular surface, indicating torn meniscus
- Chondromalacia patella: axial T2 images; cartilage loss and fissure
  - Poor correlation with symptoms
- OCD: more common in the medial condyle (non-weight-bearing lateral aspect)
- Popliteal mass: popliteal cyst, ganglion, aneurysms, or soft tissue masses

Limitations
- Cost and accessibility
- Also, it is often difficult to delineate symptomatic versus asymptomatic abnormalities
- MRI finding in OA (47)

	SIGNIFICANT CORRELATES	NOT SIGNIFICANT CORRELATES
Pain and function	Large joint effusion • Correlates with stiffness Patellofemoral osteophytes Large bone marrow lesion	Meniscus tear • Present in >60% of patients with Kellgren stage 2 or higher with/without symptom Baker's cyst
Prediction of symptoms change	Synovitis especially in the infrapatellar fat pad Weak correlation • Increased cartilage loss • Medial tibial cartilage damage (in patients with arthroscopic partial meniscectomy)	Effusion change

  - No significant difference in knee pain and function among OA patients with/without meniscal tear

MR AND CT ARTHROGRAPHY (48)

Indications for MR arthrography
- Assessment of the postoperative meniscus, the presence of chondral and osteochondral lesions, and the presence of intra-articular bodies

Indications for CT arthrography
- Suspected internal derangement in patients who are unable to undergo MRI

MANAGEMENT

NONOPERATIVE MANAGEMENT

Physical therapy
- Frequency: two to three per week for one to three months depending on the comorbidity
- Stretching of frequently tightened muscles (eg, iliopsoas, rectus femoris, ITB, and hamstrings)
  - Patellofemoral syndrome: rectus femoris, ITB
  - Pes anserine tendinobursitis: hamstring and adductor/gracilis
- ROM exercise for limited end range of flexion and terminal extension: easier after warm-up
- Strengthening of the frequently weak muscles with knee pathologies
  - Quadriceps and gluteal muscle strengthening for knee OA (49,50)
    - Hamstring and adductor muscle weakness; underrecognized
  - Closed kinetic chain (may be safer, mimic functional activities) to open kinetic chain
- Joint proprioceptive exercises/dynamic balance exercises: unstable board (wobble board), foam board, AposTherapy® (home-based exercise program using therapeutic shoe to enhance neuromuscular training and improve alignment/biomechanics)
- Modality (TENS, deep modality, or superficial modality): temporary pain relief
- Advance the sessions to the more functional or sport specific activity as progressive
- Home exercise program; transition to local gym (stationary bicycle, slow-speed treadmill, leg press, yoga class, etc)

Education for aerobic endurance exercise
- Education for common training errors (bicycle exercise with low seat height; adjust to minimize knee flexion if painful)
- Gradual increase in duration, intensity (often with resistance), and warm-up and cool-down phases, especially in patients with medical comorbidities

Injection
- Landmark-based injection: steroid injection in lean person or with significant amount of effusion
  - Intra-articular injections: different approaches available, using 27 G 1.5-inch needle
    - Suprapatellar (lateral vs medial); 1 inch diagonal from the upper patellar border (lateral preferred due to lack of muscle bulk)
    - Infrapatellar (go all the way to the cartilage layer; otherwise likely inject into the fat pad)
    - Midpatellar injection (medially); safe zone from infrapatellar branch of saphenous nerve:
      – Three-centimeter medial to the midpatellar medial margin and 1-cm medial to the medial margin of the inferior pole of the patella
- Ultrasound (US)-guided injection (51)
  - Improved accuracy of injection over anatomic guidance; may improve patient-reported clinical outcomes
  - Common indications: obese patient with minimal amount of effusion, significant osteophytes or joint space narrowing, injection of viscosupplementation (often more painful if not in the synovial cavity) and biologics, such as platelet-rich plasma
- Injectate
  - Intra-articular steroid injection; typical regimen: 40 mg of triamcinolone (or other long-acting) with 4 to 5 mL of 1% lidocaine ± after aspiration of effusion (if significant)

- Controversial in efficacy of repeated injection in OA (52), effective in pseudogout or as adjunct therapy for inflammatory arthritis
  ◦ Intra-articular viscosupplementation (53)
    ▪ Pain reduction in 5 to 13 weeks post injection period, can have effect at 6 months, no statistically significant effect on function (54)
    ▪ Increase viscoelastic properties of synovial fluid (improve lubrication) (55)
    ▪ Modest effect in knee OA, less likely effective in late-stage knee OA, and older than 65 years
    ▪ Contraindications: pregnancy, nursing, pediatric, bacteremia, or with infections
    ▪ Pseudoseptic reaction; can be decreased in accurate injection (imaging guidance)
      – Usually after second or third injection (sensitization with repeated treatment)
      – Less in 1% with sodium hyaluronate (Euflexxa®)
    ▪ No significant difference between the different formulas
    ▪ Superolateral injection approach recommended with aspiration of effusion
  ◦ Intra-articular platelet-rich plasma injection (PRP) (56)
    ▪ Indications: younger and middle-aged patients
    ▪ Pain reduction (limited evidence) and functional improvement (moderate evidence) compared to placebo in knee OA (57)
    ▪ PRP injections reduced pain more effectively than hyaluronic acid: moderate evidence (58)
    ▪ No significant difference between single and double spin (in preparation) prep in PRP
- Injection to the bursa: pes anserine, MCL bursal effusion, and popliteal bursa
- Nerve block: saphenous nerve, superolateral genicular nerve (lateral retinacular nerve) block under US guidance
- Intra-articular prolotherapy, with 10% dextrose and lidocaine (vs bacteriostatic water) (59)

Orthoses (60)
- McConnell taping and patellar taping
  ◦ Common indication: anterior knee pain (patellofemoral syndrome or patellar tendinopathy)
  ◦ Best way to predict the response is to try taping
- Foot orthotic (27)
  ◦ Heel lift to mitigate the excessive recurvatum with anterior knee pain (infrapatellar fat pad impingement with equinus or equinovarus)
  ◦ Medial knee pain with genu varum: lateral heel wedge (weak evidence) ± medial arch support or medial midfoot pad (61)
  ◦ Medial wedge (moderate quality of evidence) preferred
    ▪ Try in office if possible
  ◦ Overpronation with medial or lateral knee pain: heel lift ± medial heel wedge (with extension)
- Sport knee brace
  ◦ Prophylactic: lack of evidence for efficacy to prevent knee injury
  ◦ Postoperative knee orthotics (hinge with side upright) with dial lock after surgery (eg, ACL surgery): initial lock at extension, then progressively allow flexion
  ◦ Functional: may be used for athletes with unstable knee due to ligament injury
    ▪ For lateral subluxation of the patella, ACL-deficient knee: patellofemoral orthosis with patellar opening with horseshoe pad ± hinged metal upright (on the side)
    ▪ Not practical for the level of the loading to the knee during the athletic participation
- Patellar tracking knee orthotics (silicone patellar ring): for anterior knee pain (62,63)
- Chopart knee orthosis for patellar tendinopathy: encircle the patellar tendon
- Unloading knee orthoses by three-point leverage system
  ◦ Painful knee arthritis with varus (moderate evidence) or valgus alignment
  ◦ Limited in morbidly obese patient (slide down)
- Knee cage
  ◦ Three-point control system for minor to moderate genu recurvatum caused by ligamentous or capsular laxity
  ◦ Swedish knee cage: allows full knee flexion but prevents hyperextension
  ◦ Usually not enough control to knee recurvatum; may need solid ankle foot orthotic
    ▪ In pediatric population, may consider knee–ankle–foot orthosis (not functional in elderly population)
- Knee immobilizer
  ◦ Provide limited stability to knee in acute knee ligamentous (ACL, PCL) injury (comfort by decrease quadriceps muscle firing) and quadriceps/patellar tendon injury

SURGERY

Arthroscopic Knee Surgery

Indications
- In acute knee (cruciate ligament or meniscus) injury in high-performing athletes or young active persons: usually wait for 2 weeks to prevent arthrofibrosis
  ◦ Unclear benefit for sedentary population with unclear duration and mechanisms of injury
- Significant pain with functional impairment with failed conservative treatment

Individual surgery: see the specific disease section (beyond the scope of this book)

Postoperative care
- Usually immediately weight bearing; may be on knee immobilizer and dial lock knee orthosis and immediate referral to the physical therapist
- Outpatient follow-up
  ◦ Pain control if present
  ◦ Focus on the advancement of range restriction, review muscle-strengthening exercises (compliance), and endurance exercises (upper body, other limb)
  ◦ Evaluation of correct neuromuscular retraining, proprioceptive/balance exercises (early engagement recommended)
  ◦ Check possible complications, such as cutaneous nerve (saphenous) irritation/injury
  ◦ Review ADLs, and return to play and work

Total Knee Arthroplasty (64)

Common indications: severe knee osteoarthritis with pain despite conservative management (65)

Preoperative exercise
- Preoperative functional status affects the postoperative outcome
- ROM and active assistive exercise: leg cycle exercise, wall squats, lunges, and the like
  - Quadriceps strengthening (especially vastus medialis)
  - OA: disproportionate loss of isokinetic and isometric knee flexor and extensor strength
  - Efficacy of formal therapy session: equivocal

Postoperative rehabilitation protocol in the outpatient setting
- Typical course after the surgery: home discharge with home therapy versus short-term subacute rehab (~2 weeks) followed by home therapy or outpatient therapy
- Aggressive range of motion exercises with good pain control (initially)
  - Knee flexion contracture difficult to eliminate if existing >3 months
    - Manipulation under anesthesia: if knee flexion is <90° within 6 weeks of surgery
  - Knee flexion (60°–65° for walking, 105° for standing from chair)
  - Education: drop and dangle the leg (gravity-assisted knee flexion)
- Common problems at postoperative follow-up
  - Medial quadriceps insufficiency, inflexibility of the lateral retinacula, ITB, hamstring and gastrocs muscle, imbalance of hip internal and external rotators, and excessive foot pronation
  - Therapeutic exercise intervention
    - McConnell taping, proper shoe, and strengthening of the quadriceps via short arc exercises
    - Strengthening exercises: closed kinetic chain, concentric exercise to eccentric exercise
  - Return to work gradually in 3 to 6 weeks
- Pain management: short-term nonsteroidal anti-inflammatory drug (NSAID) ± opioids initially (long-acting narcotic with short-acting rescue; oxycodone/AAP or tramadol ± long acting)

INTRA-ARTICULAR STRUCTURES

BONE AND JOINT PATHOLOGY

Knee Osteoarthritis

Introduction (66)
- MC cause of knee pain
  - Prevalence of symptomatic OA ≥45 years old: 7% to 17%
  - Radiographic OA: more common, 19% to 28%
    - Increase with age ≥75 years old, 11% to 33% have symptomatic OA and 44% to 50% have radiographic signs of OA
- Etiology and risk factors for knee OA (67)
  - Excessive mechanical stress applied in the context of systematic susceptibility (55)
  - Occurrence
    - Age, sex, genetic, and malalignment (eg, varus and valgus malalignment)
    - Modifiable: physical activity, body mass index (BMI) (obesity), intense sport activities, quadriceps strength, bone density, previous injury, hormone replacement therapy (protective), vitamin D, and smoking
  - Progression
    - Age, BMI, vitamin D, hormone replacement therapy, malalignment, intense sport activities; similar to occurrence
    - Chronic joint effusion, synovitis, and subchondral bone edema (MRI scanning)

History and physical examination
- Knee pain; intermittent/chronic, poorly localized, morning stiffness (≤30 min), ± swelling (acute swelling in flare-up)
- Physical examination: effusion (bulging proximal to the patella or prominent Hoffa's fat pad), crepitus on ROM and joint line tenderness with palpable osteophytes
- Gait: antalgic gait (decreased stance phase of the affected limb → decreased swing phase in the contralateral leg) and decreased cadence
  - Decreased ankle plantar flexion and increase hip extension (help knee extensor weakness)

Diagnosis
- Clinical diagnosis supplemented with radiologic, serologic studies (American College of Rheumatology)
  - Osteoarthritis if 1, 2 or 1, 3, 5, 6 or 1, 4, 5, 6 are present
    1. Knee pain for most days of previous month
    2. Osteophytes at joint margins on radiographs
    3. Synovial fluid typical of osteoarthritis (laboratory)
    4. Age 40 years or older
    5. Crepitus on active joint motion
    6. Morning stiffness lasting 30 minutes or less
- X-ray
  - Standing AP, lateral, and axial view
  - Less sensitive/specific than physical examination
  - The Kellgren and Lawrence classification (too much emphasis on osteophyte, not linear relationship). Other scales (the OA Research Society International Grading Scale) available (68)

GRADE	KELLGREN AND LAWRENCE	AHLBÄCK CLASSIFICATION
0	Normal	
1	Doubtful narrowing of joint space and possible osteophytic lipping	Joint space narrowing (less than 3 mm)
2	Definite osteophytes and possible narrowing of joint space	Joint space obliteration
3	Moderate multiple osteophytes, definite narrowing of joint space, and some sclerosis and possible deformity of bone ends	Minor bone attrition (3–5 mm)

(continued)

GRADE	KELLGREN AND LAWRENCE	AHLBÄCK CLASSIFICATION
4	Large osteophytes, marked narrowing of joint space, severe sclerosis, and definite deformity of bone ends	Moderate bone attrition (5–10 mm)
5		Severe bone attrition (>10 mm)

- US (69,70)
  ○ Differential diagnosis for concomitant soft tissue disorders and early-stage evaluation, osteophytes (can detect smaller size than x-ray), calcification, effusion, synovial pathology (proliferation, increased Doppler blood flow)
  ○ Cartilage evaluation; evaluation of crystal deposition (pseudogout inside and at junction of the cartilage versus gout at junction; double contour) and early manifestation of cartilage loss and degeneration (transverse view suprapatellar/vertical with knee hyperflexion)
- MRI
  ○ Usually not necessary, differential diagnosis for atypical cases and early diagnosis
    ▪ Intracartilaginous signal changes, superficial erosions, diffuse cartilage thinning, and cartilage ulceration
  ○ Patients with red flags and other intracortical lesion mimicking OA (atypical presentation): OCD and avascular necrosis, or tumor or soft tissue lesion (often concomitant)
- Differential diagnosis; often concomitant
  ○ Pes anserine tendinobursitis (medial knee pain) and distal ITB friction syndrome or bicep femoris tendinopathy (lateral knee pain)
  ○ Inferior patellar branch of saphenous neuropathy: irritation/injury by osteophytes, injection or arthroscopic surgery. Patient complains of medial-anterior knee pain especially on flexion of knee
  ○ Osteonecrosis (spontaneous or avascular) or OCD
  ○ Hoffa's fat pad impingement syndrome (anterior knee pain, infrapatellar region)
  ○ Anterior tibiofibular ligament sprain/joint instability and popliteus tendinopathy/tenosynovitis (lateral knee pain)
  ○ Fabella (sesamoid in lateral gastrocnemius) syndrome (posterolateral knee pain)

Treatment (71)
- Education for self-management, weight reduction (if BMI >25, lose at least 5% of body weight), lower-impact aerobic fitness exercise, ROM exercises, strengthening exercise (maintenance after PT in poorly deconditioned person)
- Physical therapy (72)
  ○ Two to three/week for 4 to 12 weeks; tends to be shorter (driven by insurance) → focus on educational components
  ○ Strengthening exercise; level II (73)
    ▪ Quadriceps set; isometric strengthening exercise (quadriceps, hamstring) and gluteal muscle
    ▪ Straight leg raising (SLR) (particularly rectus femoris) and wall sits → isotonic exercise with increasing resistance, then to closed kinetic chain exercise (lunges)
  ○ Flexibility exercises (stretching of hamstring, ITB, and quadriceps)
  ○ Proprioception training: decreased proprioception puts knee in extension before loading response (maintain the knee in stable position)
    ▪ Tandem stance, single-leg stance on firm surface and on foam mat progressing to wobble board
- Orthoses (74)
  ○ Lateral wedge, especially in genu varum; if not working → medial arch support or medial midfoot posting or extended medial wedge (to decrease adduction moment)
  ○ Knee sleeve, patellar cutout, open popliteal fossa, a patellar reinforcement with C- or J-shaped cushion pad with/without buttress straps, and/or built-in lateral stays
  ○ Wrap-around knee orthosis with bilateral metal uprights: improve stability by enhancing proprioception; may decrease anterior knee pain from patellofemoral arthritis
  ○ Unloader; medial unloader for varus knee with medial knee pain
  ○ AposTherapy® (convex pod under the hindfoot (heel) and forefoot on the outsole platform of the shoe); calibration by physical therapy (PT)
- Oral medication: acetaminophen, NSAIDs, or topical capsaicin
  ○ Combination of glucosamine 1,500 mg and 1,200 mg of chondroitin sulfate/day may be effective in patients with moderate to severe knee pain (75)
- Injection
  ○ Corticosteroid injection; level II, B for short term
    ▪ If effusion present, aspiration (level II, B) and local steroid injection
  ○ Viscosupplementation injection (54,76)
    ▪ Good outcome in moderate knee joint effusion (requiring aspiration), a superolateral injection approach, and the radiographic findings of joint space loss in a single compartment and meniscal calcinosis
    ▪ Poor outcome in moderate to severe patellofemoral arthritis, and knee OA with Kellgren Lawrence grade IV
- Platelet-rich plasma injection; better than/equal to visco supplementation regarding pain reduction (56,77)
- Arthroscopic lavage or medical synovectomy: no strong evidence
- TKA if failed conservative treatment and disabling pain

Patellofemoral Syndrome

Introduction (78)
- Unclear definition: patellar maltracking, lateral patellofemoral overloading syndrome, also often used for chondromalacia patella (diagnosis either by MRI or pathology during arthroscopy) or mild patellofemoral osteoarthritis
- Incidence: MC cause of anterior knee pain
  ○ More common in some sports: 25% of injuries to the knee among runners (79)
- Anatomy
  ○ Pain generator in the patellofemoral space: subchondral bone, the synovium, medial patellofemoral ligament/retinaculum, nerve, muscle and Hoffa fat pad

- Etiology
  ○ Malalignment, blunt trauma, and overuse
  ○ Dysfunction of patellar stabilizers
    ▪ Medial side: vastus medialis oblique (often weak, delayed onset), patellofemoral ligament (primary stabilizer to the lateral subluxation), patellomeniscal ligament, and tight lateral retinaculum
    ▪ Lateral: iliotibial tract, lateral retinaculum, vastus lateralis, hamstring, and gastrocnemius in flexibility/tightness. Weakness of gluteus medius and hip external rotator
  ○ Femoral anteversion (with femoral internal rotation), weak hip external rotator, knee valgus, trochlear dysplasia, patella alta, laterally displaced tibial tuberosity, hyperpronation (80)

History and physical examination (81)
- Anterior knee pain, ill defined (achy or occasionally sharp), underneath/around the patella ± "giving way" or "buckling"
  ○ Worsening of pain with squatting, running, prolonged sitting, or ascending or descending steps
- Physical examination
  ○ Sitting: prominent infrapatellar fat pad or patella alta
  ○ Standing: rotation of patella (face medially or laterally indicating femoral anteversion/retroversion), increased Q angle (femur alignment versus patellar alignment, >16–20°; controversial clinical implication (82), recurvatum and leg length discrepancy
- Patellar mobility test
  ○ Lateral pull test (J sign) and patellar grind test (Clark)
  ○ Tightness of patellar tilting/retinaculum: if <10° to 15° with passive patellar tilting
  ○ Tenderness on the lateral patellofemoral space
- Kinetic chain: hyperpronation (hindfoot valgus, internal rotation of the tibia and femur), weak hip external rotator strength, and anteversion
- Functional test
  ○ Dynamic alignment: single-leg squat or step down with positive J sign

Diagnosis
- Clinical diagnosis supplemented by imaging study
- X-ray: AP, lateral, axial view ("skyline" view) for differential and underlying bony etiologies (Figure 8.7)
  ○ Lateral view for patellar patellaralta and baja
  ○ Axial/merchant view: sulcus angle: ~140° normally (correlates well with instability), congruence angle (line from central ridge (pointy bottom and midline sulcus vs sulcus bisecting line): –6° ± 11° (medial: –, lateral +) for measuring subluxation
    ▪ Patellar tilt angle: abnormal if >10°

Treatment
- Physical therapy to address abnormal patellofemoral tracking and alignment
  ○ Stretch tight hamstrings and ITB, ensure patellar mobility, and quadriceps muscle strengthening
  ○ Closed kinetic chain exercises initially (short arc extension; 0 to 30° flexion; minimal PF contact pressure), then open kinetic chain
    ▪ Closed kinetic chain exercises involving the gluteal musculatures tend to increase the external rotation of the femur and may decrease the Q angle during the gait cycle

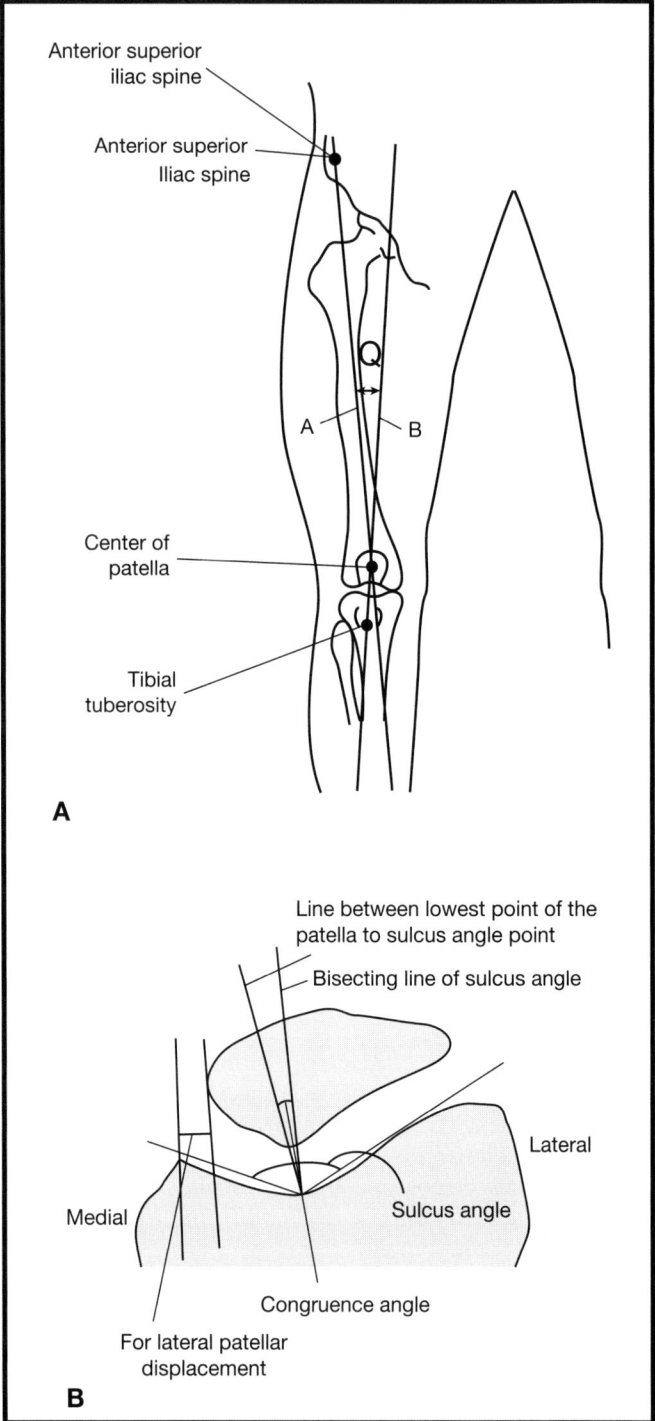

FIGURE 8.7
Commonly used angles for alignment in x-ray of knee
(A) Q angle; (B) congruence angle.

  ○ Proprioceptive exercise (standing on one leg, wobble board as progress) and education for biomechanics (sports specific)
  ○ Quad/gluteal strengthening: isolated vastus medialis oblique muscle-strengthening exercise often difficult
  ○ Hip internal rotation (external rotator strengthening) and anteversion
- Patellar bracing (with horseshoe padding), patellar, and McConnell taping for short-term pain relief

- Heel lift to mitigate subtalar joint pronation (secondary to tight heel cord) with stretching of gastrocnemius if present ± medial heel wedge AposTherapy®
- Referral to surgery if failed conservative management: lateral retinacular release for tight/overloading lateral patellofemoral syndrome (83)

Chondromalacia Patella

Introduction
- Softening or loss of the patellar cartilage
  - Possible cause of patellofemoral syndrome and possible precursor to degenerative joint disease in patellofemoral compartment of the knee
  - Unclear correlation of clinical symptoms or examination

History and physical examination
- Anterior knee pain (same as patellofemoral syndrome) if symptomatic

Diagnosis (84)
- Imaging diagnosis confirmed by arthroscopy
- MRI (axial T1 weighted image or fat suppressed proton density): partial thickness cartilage loss, fissure, and confirmed by arthroscopy
  - Poor correlation of MRI and arthroscopic findings with symptoms (85)

Treatment
- Same as patellofemoral syndrome

Patellar Instability; Subluxation and Dislocation

Introduction (86)
- Dislocation: 1/1,000 (incidence), more common in young (10–16 years), female > male
- First-time dislocation: low rate of subsequent dislocation, but two dislocations → 50% chance of redislocation
- Patellar instability; a cause of patellofemoral syndrome

History and physical examination
- Anterior knee (around the patellar) pain with intermittent "giving way" of the knee ± knee swelling (acute hemarthrosis in dislocation)
- Physical examination
  - Generalized ligament laxity; Beighton hypermobility score
  - "Miserable malalignment syndrome": femoral anteversion (femur internally rotated), genu varum, external tibial torsion/pronated foot (87)
  - Patellar tracking, tilt, mobility, apprehension with lateralization of the patella

Diagnosis
- Clinical diagnosis confirmed by imaging
- X-ray: AP, Rosenberg (posteroanterior [PA] 45° weight bearing), and Merchant view (45° flexion, vs skyline view with 115° flexion)
  - High rate of subluxation in asymptomatic knee
- MRI to evaluate articular cartilage, soft tissue evaluation (medial patellofemoral ligament injury; common in patellar attachment site (also can be evaluated by US) → increased risk of redislocation if compromised)

Treatment
- Dislocation: initial immobilization includes casting (full extension or in partial flexion), splinting, or bracing
  - Cast for 6 weeks lowers the risk for redislocation but results in higher rate of stiffness
  - Patient with patellar brace: three times the risk of redislocation
- Physical therapy: closed-chain strengthening of the quadriceps and gluteal musculature, patellar taping, and proprioceptive exercise
  - Patellar taping has been shown to control excessive patellar motion during therapy and serves to activate the vastus medialis oblique earlier than the vastus lateralis when climbing stairs
- Referral to surgical evaluation: failed conservative treatment or first-time dislocator with trochlear dysplasia and laxity or MRI-confirmed MPFL avulsion
  - Surgery versus conservative treatment: no significant difference in subjective outcome, recurrent instability, function, or activity scores

Bipartite Patella

Introduction (88)
- Failure of fusion in the secondary ossification center of the patella (2%–3% remain separated)
- Male > female (active young men) by 9 times, bilateral in 50%, MC within the superolateral pole (75% > lateral margin in 20%)

History and physical examination
- Usually incidental finding, painful (anterior knee pain on the patella) in ~2%, <20 years, active in sports
- Localized tenderness on the accessory segment (usually upper outer quadrant)

Diagnosis
- Clinical suspicion confirmed with imaging
- X-ray: weight-bearing skyline view (often incidental finding)
- MRI: may show bone marrow edema in the accessory fragment

Treatment
- Two to 4 weeks of rest, activity modification, NSAIDs, quadriceps muscle stretching, and patellar sleeve brace
- Knee immobilizing brace at 30° flexion for 1 to 2 weeks (to alleviate tension from vastus lateralis muscle)
- Referral to surgery if pain persists and unable to return to play in athletes after 6 months of conservative treatment

INFLAMMATORY ARTHROPATHY

Rheumatoid Arthritis (RA) of Knee

Introduction (89)
- 90% of patients with long-standing RA have knee joint symptoms, but concomitant osteoarthritis is also very common
  - 20% to 25% of RA patients develop advanced arthritis

- Knee: MC affected joint contributing to patient pain and overall disability
  - MC affected joints: wrist, metacarpophalangeal (MCP), and proximal interphalangeal (PIP), but patients complain of more problems in large joints, shoulder, hip, and knee
- Initially, symmetric synovitis (joint swelling, pain) → cartilage destruction, with subchondral bone and soft tissue change deformity (subchondral bone loss and ligament involvement)

History and physical examination
- Pain, swelling, stiffness, and deformity (later)
- Physical examination
  - Knee joint effusion (suprapatellar, parapatellar recess) and popliteal cyst (posteromedial) with occasional calf swelling (with ruptured cyst)
  - Valgus-flexion deformity of knee: more common than OA
    - Limited extension of knee: initially with large effusion, with hamstring tightness later
    - Valgus/flexion deformity → severe pronation of the subtalar joint and a planovalgus foot
  - Atrophic skin and fragile capillary with ecchymosis

Diagnosis
- Clinical diagnosis with imaging study (later stage) and serologic test (initial stage)
- X-ray: periarticular erosion and osteopenia (vs osteophytes, subchondral sclerosis, and joint space narrowing more common in OA)
- US: effusion, synovial proliferation with increased vascularity in addition to periarticular erosion, cartilage defect (less involved than OA)
- Serologic test: check RA of hand and wrist

Treatment
- Referral for rheumatology for immunomodulating treatment (check RA of the wrist and hand)
- PT: similar to knee OA although lacks evidence; just 4 to 8 sessions for education and home exercise program (for quadriceps and gluteal muscle strengthening)
- Intra-articular steroid or hyaluronate injection for synovitis in early stage as local adjunct treatment (90)
- Referral for surgery in advanced stages for TKA (91)
  - Rheumatology consultation for perioperative immunomodulator (eg, methotrexate and hydroxychloroquine continued, other medication held differently)
  - If the hip and knee are both involved, total hip arthroplasty before TKA
  - May affect/aggravate upper extremity during postoperative rehab course (wrist fusion can be considered)
  - Postoperatively, two to three times increased risk of infection, delayed surgical wound healing, but decreased risk of deep vein thrombosis (DVT) (than TKA from OA)

Calcium Pyrophosphate Dihydrate Crystal Deposition (CPPD) Disease and Pseudogout (92)

Introduction (93)
- Prevalence of CPPD from population based study: ~0.4%, prevalence of radiographic findings: 30% to 60% of by age 85 years
  - No consistent correlation between chondrocalcinosis and cartilage loss
- Idiopathic: MC, 20% to 25% present as pseudogout (acute inflammatory process); common presentation of CPPD disease
- Risk factors: associated with hyperparathyroidism, hemochromatosis (up to 40%–41%), hypophosphatasia, and the like
- Knee: most frequently involved joint by CPPD
  - Medial femorotibial joint > patellofemoral and lateral femorotibial joint

History and physical examination of pseudogout
- Knee pain (abrupt onset, unilateral); medial compartment ± swelling or minimal warmth
  - Occasionally triggered by trauma, infection, intra-articular injection, or surgery
- Knee effusion, tenderness on the joint line, mild deficit at the end range of knee flexion with pain

Diagnosis
- Clinical diagnosis confirmed by imaging study, no need for fluid analysis (unless to rule out [R/O] other inflammatory or infectious processes)
  - CPPD crystals under polarizing microscopy in the fluid: low sensitivity (but can differentiate urate crystal)
- Imaging study (92)
  - X-ray: low sensitivity (as low as ~40%), calcification in the meniscus, posterior hyaline cartilage, and even gastrocnemius tendon
  - US: hyperechoic punctuate lesion in the articular cartilage as well as inside the meniscus (94), and simple effusion

Treatment
- NSAIDs and intra-articular steroid injection ± aspiration. Colchicine may have some benefit
- PT similar to knee OA

OSTEOCHONDRITIS DISSECANS

Introduction (95)
- Focal subchondral bony lesion with risk for instability and disruption of adjacent articular cartilage. May result in premature osteoarthritis
- Incidence: 0.02% to 0.03%, peak in age 10 to 20 years: male > female by two to four times, higher in African Americans
- Knee: MC location, 75% of OCD, medial femoral condyle (85%) and lateral aspect in 51% to 74%
  - Bilateral in 15% to 40%
- Proposed etiologies: occult or repetitive microtrauma (higher in athletic population), genetic predisposition, inflammatory process, and vascular abnormalities

History and physical examination (96)
- Activity-related anterior or medial knee pain worsened by cutting and pivoting
  - Mimicking patellofemoral syndrome
- ROM: usually normal ± intermittent clicking, locking, and transient effusion ± tenderness above the joint line (on condyle)

Diagnosis
- Clinical suspicion diagnosed by imaging study
- X-ray (AP, lateral, and notch view): initial imaging modality
- MRI if x-ray is negative; sensitivity/specificity (92%–100%), classification based on MRI
  1. Compression of subchondral trabeculae with preservation of cartilage
  2. Incomplete detachment of osteochondral fragment
  3. Complete avulsion of an osteochondral fragment without dislocation
  4. Complete avulsion of an osteochondral fragment → loose body

Treatment (97)
- Nonoperative management
  ○ Observation with sports activity in asymptomatic: yearly x-ray or MRI
  ○ Stable symptomatic: return to play if no catching or locking, full ROM, normal strength, or no effusion
    ▪ Unloader knee brace
    ▪ Minimal displacement: 6 to 12 weeks non-weight-bearing activity and crutch
- Referral to surgical evaluation in unstable (buckling/giving away), persistent catching/locking or failed conservative treatment
  ○ Arthroscopy (gold standard for diagnosis), bone grafting with fixation or autologous chondrocyte implantation with bone grafting

SPONTANEOUS OSTEONECROSIS OF THE KNEE

Introduction (98,99)
- Classification
  ○ Primary/spontaneous: medial condyle (99%), common in female (>55 years)
    ▪ ~10% in >65 years old with medial joint line pain without significant x-ray findings (100)
  ○ Secondary: systemic steroid, alcoholism, hemoglobinopathy, lupus, and the like
    ▪ Presentation at younger age and bilateral involvement
- Slow progression to knee degenerative arthritis

History and physical examination
- Pain in the medial knee (acute, without apparent trauma), joint line tenderness (more on the medial femoral condyle) ± recurrent effusion, and restricted ROM (end range)
- Unilateral, similar to presentation of OCD, or can be bilateral in secondary osteonecrosis

Diagnosis
- Clinical suspicion confirmed by radiologic finding
- X-ray (AP, lateral, 30° flexion posteroanterior (PA) weight-bearing view): often negative
- MRI
  ○ High SI at the medial femoral condyle in T2-weighted images (WI), associated with a focal and low-signal intensity in the subchondral bone of the epiphysis on T1-WI in later stages
  ○ Less than or equal to 5 cm in AP diameter: unfavorable prognosis

Treatment
- Protected weight bearing, restriction of activity, NSAIDs, and possibly pulsed electromagnetic field (proposed as a treatment for femoral head necrosis)
- Vitamin D supplementation if low, ibandronate IV q 8 weeks twice, then repeat the test

PROXIMAL TIBIOFIBULAR SPRAIN AND INSTABILITY

Introduction (12,101)
- Anatomy of proximal tibiofibular joint: inherently stable by bony congruity, capsuloligamentous, and muscular support
- Uncommon/underrecognized cause of lateral knee pain in general population
  ○ Common in athletes in sports requiring violent twisting motions of the flexed knee, such as wrestling, parachute jumping, judo, gymnastics, skiing, rugby, football, soccer, track, baseball, basketball, racquetball, and roller skating
  ○ Subluxation common in preadolescent girl without trauma: resolves with skeletal maturity
- Anterolateral dislocation: MC type of dislocation
- Etiology
  ○ Trauma (fall, various sports), below-knee amputation, muscular dystrophy, congenital anomalies, and generalized ligamentous laxity
    ▪ A fall on the inverted foot with the knee flexed as the leg is violently adducted by the weight of the body
  ○ Simultaneous sudden contraction of the biceps femoris (hamstring) with knee flexion

History and physical examination
- Pain over the anterolateral aspect of the knee (anterior to the fibular head), mild to disabling pain, and inability to bear weight in severe cases; often lacks trauma, and frequently bilateral
  ○ In patients with transtibial (below-knee) amputation: anterior knee pain with ill-fitting socket
    ▪ Squeeze the distal part and distract the proximal tibiafibular joint with symptom reproduction
  ○ ± Sensory and motor dysfunction of peroneal nerves, especially with posterior dislocation
- Physical examination
  ○ Lateral fibular head prominence in anterior dislocation without knee effusion
  ○ Reproduction of pain on ankle dorsi/plantar flexion with knee flexed
    ▪ Worsening/reproduction of pain by squeezing ankle (distal tibiofibular joint) or distal shin to distract the proximal tibiofibular joint/ligament or by squeezing distal residual limb in below-knee amputation
  ○ Radulescu sign: prone and knee 90° flexion (relaxes lateral collateral ligament and biceps femoris tendon), and rotate internally with other hand to subluxate the fibular anteriorly → reproduction of symptoms

Diagnosis
- Clinical diagnosis confirmed by imaging study
- X-ray findings: compare with the other side
  ○ AP: the fibula is laterally displaced; the proximal interosseous space widened, greater overlap of the tibia and fibula
  ○ The lateral view: anteriorly displaced fibular head

○ Resnick's line (lateral tibial spine) over the midline of fibular head normally
  ▪ Anterior dislocation, fibular located in front of the line
• MRI for further evaluation and other differentials
• Differential diagnosis: lateral meniscal tear, cyst, ITB, popliteal tendinitis/posterolateral corner sprain, and ganglion

Treatment
• Stretching and strengthening of hamstring and gastrocnemius muscle ± calf strap 1 cm below the fibular head (cautious of fibular nerve irritation if too proximal to the head)
• US-guided injection (with small volume, 1 mL) for diagnosis (pain generator) and pain control
• Acute dislocation: closed reduction with knee flexed to 90°
• Referral to surgery in chronic pain and instability despite conservative treatment
  ○ Arthrodesis, open reduction/pinning, fibular head resection, and reconstruction

MENISCUS PATHOLOGY

Meniscal Injury

Introduction (102)
• Meniscal injury: 60 to 70/100,000, male > female by four times, one-third related to ACL injury
  ○ Medial meniscal tear: more common than lateral (with acute ACL tears, lateral > medial)
    ▪ Midportion and posterior horn, often longitudinal pattern
  ○ Commonly associated with tibial plateau and femoral shaft fracture/bruise
  ○ Mechanism of injury: twisting or hyperflexion
• Degenerative lesion: common in posterior horn of medial meniscus, fourth to sixth decade
  ○ Unclear correlation between knee pain and imaging finding
• Classification of tear (descriptive)
  ○ Vertical longitudinal tear: common, especially with ACL tears
  ○ Oblique tear
  ○ Horizontal: more common in elderly, often associated with meniscal cyst
  ○ Radial: decreased load bearing
  ○ Complex: increase after age 40 years, posterior horn or midbody with degenerative arthritis
  ○ Buckle handle tear: vertical tear displaced into the notch and mechanical block
  ○ Complete displaced vertical tear: mechanical block

History and physical examination
• Acute pain, swelling (in acute injury) ± locking/blocking or catching
• Physical examination
  ○ Effusion, limited extension, or mechanical block (displaced bucket handle tear)
  ○ Joint line tenderness: most accurate clinical examination of tear: 77% to 86%, 50% positive predictive value (PPV) (but not with combined ACL injury)
    ▪ Palpable joint line cyst related to the meniscus tears
  ○ McMurry test, Apley test, and Thessaly test
  ○ Squat test (Ege's test): repeated deep squat with the foot internally (lateral meniscus) and externally rotated (medial meniscus), positive if pain ± clicking, sensitivity: ~60%; specificity: 80% to 90%

Diagnosis
• Clinical suspicion/diagnosis confirmed by imaging study
• Differential diagnosis
  ○ Limited extension: severe effusion with pain, loose body, and osteochondral injury
  ○ Joint line tenderness: osteoarthritis, meniscal cyst (often with tear) and MCL bursitis
• Imaging
  ○ X-ray: merchant view (patellofemoral joint) with 45° knee flexion
    ▪ Joint space narrowing in posterior tibiofemoral joint with arthritis
  ○ US: limited role: only outer part; meniscal cyst, displacement, and joint effusion
  ○ MRI: 95% accuracy
    ▪ Grading: 0–3; 1 and 2: intrameniscal signal not extending to the edge; 3: linear signal extending to the surface of the meniscus
    ▪ Meniscal cyst: often related to tear
    ▪ "Double PCL" sign may indicate a bucket handle tear
    ▪ Unclear correlation with symptoms: increased signal in asymptomatic patients with negative physical examination (~10% in age <45 years, ~30% in age ≥45 years)

Treatment (103)
• Nonoperative treatment (104): maintain ROM and closed kinetic strengthening initially ± aspiration of effusion/injection for pain control
  ○ No significant difference in physical function between conservative management versus arthroscopic partial meniscectomy for meniscal tear and OA
  ○ Indications: degenerative tear, small (5–8 mm), longitudinal and stable (displacement <3 mm), stable partial tears, or shallow radial tears (<3 mm deep)
• Partial meniscectomy
  ○ Indications: white zone (inner third) tears, radial, oblique, flap tears, best result in acute case
• Meniscal repair (acute repair with ACL reconstruction; lower success rate for isolated repair) or transplantation (retear or extrusion are common)

Discoid Meniscus

Introduction (105)
• Common anatomical anomaly of hypertrophic and discoid-shaped meniscus from failure of central meniscal resorption
• "Popping knee syndrome"
• More common in lateral meniscus (incidence: 0.4%–17%) > medial (0.06%–0.3%), more common in Asians, bilateral in 20% to 25%
• Classification (Watanabe): type 1 (complete), type 2 (incomplete), type 3 (unstable)

○ Wrisberg variant: lack of posterior meniscotibial attachment causing hypermobile meniscus and thicker posterior meniscofemoral ligament ➔ snapping

History and physical examination
- Asymptomatic usually, but symptomatic if torn: pain, swelling, tenderness in joint line and limited ROM
- Snapping knee in children (especially near terminal knee extension, common in Wrisberg variant)
- Similar physical examination to meniscal lesion

Diagnosis
- Clinical suspicion confirmed by imaging study (MRI)
- X-ray: widened joint space, squaring of lateral condyle with cupping of lateral tibial plateau, hypoplastic lateral intercondylar spine
- MRI
  ○ Continuity between anterior and posterior horn on >2 sagittal slices, "bow-tie sign," thick and flat meniscus
  ○ A transverse meniscal diameter >15 or 16 mm, extending across entire lateral compartment
- Differential diagnosis (mechanical block)
  ○ Displaced meniscal tear, loose osteochondral fragments, and ACL tear

Treatment
- Observation in asymptomatic (snapping without pain or mechanical symptom) or minimally symptomatic
- Surgical referral indications similar to meniscal tear
  ○ Partial meniscectomy, saucerization, and/or repair in symptomatic tear in Wrisberg variant

LIGAMENT INJURY

ACL Injury
Introduction
- Epidemiology (106)
  ○ ACL rupture incidence: 1/3,000 in United States, female > male by four to five times (30)
  ○ Higher in pivoting sports: basketball, soccer, skiing, and the like
  ○ Common location: proximal interstitial or midsubstance
  ○ Concomitant with meniscal injury (lateral meniscus tear in up to 50% of acute ACL tears)
- Etiology and mechanism of injury: both high- and low-energy mechanism
  ○ Sport-related (80%), noncontact (70%), and pivoting: MC
    ▪ Noncontact pivot injury: sudden deceleration and rotation (sudden stop and pivot or cut in direction): valgus angulation at the knee with external rotation of the femur on the fixed tibia
    ▪ Hyperextension or valgus stress (landing a jump; awkward landing)
- Chronic ACL deficiency causes chondral injuries and complex meniscal tear, and possibly arthritis (controversial)

History and physical examination
- History: usually symptomatic and significant functional limitation in ~75%
  ○ Pain (tearing), popping (40%–70%), and swelling (hemarthrosis in 70% within hours) in acute injury
  ○ Instability, "gives way" especially during pivoting and cutting, and inability to return to sport
- Physical examination
  ○ Lachman test: most sensitive
  ○ Pivot shift test: pathognomic, highly specific, can be very uncomfortable
  ○ KT-1,000: quantify anterior knee laxity

Diagnosis
- Clinical diagnosis confirmed by imaging study
- Differential diagnosis in acute injury
  ○ Differential for traumatic effusion (± hemarthrosis)
    ▪ Patellar dislocation, PCL tear, fracture, meniscal tear, osteochondral injury, popliteal avulsion
- X-ray: usually normal
  ○ Segond's fracture: tibial plateau (lateral capsular) avulsion fracture (<5%): pathognomonic
  ○ Lateral notch symptom: lateral femoral condyle fracture
  ○ Chronic insufficiency/tear: OA in the middle age, loose body, osteophytes, and DJD
- MRI: ~85% sensitive, ~95% specific
  ○ Primary signs of injury: best seen at sagittal view: ill-defined mixed signal intensity (edema/hemorrhage), abnormal slope, discontinuity, nonvisualization of the ACL fibers on both sagittal and coronal planes, and avulsion of the anterior tibial spine
  ○ Indirect signs
    ▪ Bone contusion sign: lateral femoral condyle (mid 1/3) and posterior 1/3 (lateral) tibial plateau (pivot-shift injury)
      – Present in 50% to 80%. If no bone bruise, suspect either no ACL tear or chronic lesion
    ▪ Deep sulcus sign: lateral femoral condyle (>2 mm deep), Segond fracture, kissing contusions: anterior tibia and femur (hyperextension injury), anterior drawer sign: anterior translation of tibia relative to femur
    ▪ Buckling of PCL and acute hemarthrosis: nonspecific

Treatment
- Nonoperative treatment
  ○ Indications
    ▪ Copers: minimal giving way, good global rating of knee function/ADL, able to do single-leg hop
    ▪ Older individuals, sedentary lifestyle, willing to modify sports activity, participate in swimming, running, and cycling
    ▪ No significant difference in knee-related quality of life in ACL-deficient and ACL-reconstructed groups
    ▪ Return to play in nonelite competitive sports following ACL reconstruction (~40%): not necessarily higher than rehabilitation alone (107)
  ○ Cryotherapy initially, then heating modality, hamstring strengthening, full ROM, aggressive quadriceps strengthening exercise (significant predictor for postoperative function) (108,109)
  ○ Avoid high-risk activities: twisting, cutting, and deceleration maneuvers
    ▪ Straight running, weight training, and other activities can be performed
  ○ Functional braces: unclear benefit
  ○ Increased incidence of meniscal tears, articular injury, and degeneration

- Surgery: ACL reconstruction with graft, 3 to 4 (6) weeks after the injury to reduce arthrofibrosis
  - Indications: mechanical symptoms, instability or younger, more active, or professional athletes
  - Early surgery (do not wait for 3–4 weeks) if concomitant injury to posterolateral corner or other accompanied injuries (meniscus or cartilage)
  - Graft: bone-patellar tendon-bone graft (strong, possible anterior knee pain), hamstring autograft, or allograft
- Rehabilitation (108)
  - ACL repaired knee: follow surgeon's protocol and communicate with the surgeon
    - Graft fixation: 6 to 12 weeks
    - Return to play: ~6 (up to 12) months (graft resembles a native ACL in ~6 months)
    - Knee in full extension during ambulation for first 4 to 6 weeks to protect the extensor mechanism
      – Knee brace (Bledsoe knee brace, locked in full extension in first week; no clear evidence)
    - Early mobilization: weight bearing as tolerated (WBAT) with crutches immediately unless other concomitant injuries present
      – Neuromuscular electrical stimulation (E-stim), bike, wall slides, patellar mobilization, straight leg raise, gait training → ROM 0 to 90°, active quadriceps contraction with superior patellar glide
    - Three to 5 weeks: ROM, joint mobility, bike and StairMaster, closed kinetic chain exercise, balance and proprioceptive exercise
    - Late (6–8 weeks): increased intensity and duration, open kinetic chain exercise.
    - Transition (9–12 weeks): sport-specific, agility, functional training
    - Return to play: symmetric limb-to-limb function (vertical jump to check asymmetric landing: better than single-leg hopping), symmetric hamstring, and quadriceps strength (either clinical examination or using isokinetic measurement) (110)

PCL Injury

Introduction (111,112)
- Epidemiology: 5% to 20% (1%–44%) of all knee ligamentous injuries, underrecognized
  - Isolated PCL injury: rare (10% of ACL injury), 50% to 90% with other knee injuries (ACL/PLC together) or posterolateral rotatory instability
- Common location of tear: tibia in 75% > femoral and midsubstance
- Etiology and mechanism of injury
  - Motor vehicle accident: MC, dashboard injury (direct blow to the proximal tibia)
  - Fall on flexed knee with plantar flexed foot: less common in sports (low velocity, usually with partial tears) or hyperextension of the knee

History and physical examination
- Posterior knee pain (aggravated by stair climbing), instability (subtle and asymptomatic in isolated PCL tear), and swelling
- Physical examination
  - Inspection: posterior sagging of the tibia, + Godfrey's test (sagging of the tibia on knee 90° flexion and holding the tibia)
  - Quadriceps active test: the posterior sagging of the tibia reversed by quadriceps activation
  - Loss of the last 10 to 20° of knee flexion
  - Provocative test: posterior drawer test (may be more accurate). Dial test (PCL and PLC injury), KT-1,000 or 2,000 (instrument to quantify the laxity)
  - Neurovascular examination (dorsal pedal pulse), and motor/sensory examination (to evaluate concomitant peroneal nerve injury)

Diagnosis
- Clinical suspicion confirmed with imaging study
- X-ray, standing AP, and lateral
  - Bony avulsion fracture, arthritis changes, and stress radiographs (sagittal translation) with knee 90° flexion in chronic lesion
- MRI (accuracy 96% to 100%)
  - Complete tear: increased T2 signal intensity completely traversing the PCL (MC in the midsubstance) versus partial: incompletely traversing the PCL
  - Peel-off injury: an avulsion injury of the femoral insertion of the ligament with avulsion and posterior tibia (PCL insertion) avulsion
  - Secondary sign: bone marrow edema involving the anterior proximal tibia
  - Evaluate other ligamentous injuries (common)

Treatment
- Conservative management: partial/incomplete tear and isolated complete tear (posterior displacement only to medial femoral condyle)
  - Cylinder cast immobilization in acute stage (to prevent posterior sagging)
  - Quadriceps strengthening, cautious of resistive hamstring strengthening exercise
- Referral to surgery: complete tears (often MLI) and bony avulsion
  - PCL reconstruction (arthroscopic, single bundle, double bundle, tibial tunnel, "killer curve" tibial inlay) or high tibial osteotomy for chronic PCL deficiency

Posterolateral Corner (PLC) Injury (113,114)

Introduction (115)
- Isolated PLC injury: rare (<2% of knee ligament injuries), associated with ACL (~40%) and PCL injury (~80%)
  - Missed PLC injury: a common cause of failed ACL/PCL reconstruction
- Anatomy and biomechanics
  - PLC structures: LCL, popliteus tendon, popliteo fibular ligament, posterolateral capsule, variable arcuate ligament, and fabellofibular ligament
  - Static and dynamic stabilizer to excessive hyperextension, varus angulation, and tibial external rotation
    - Popliteus tendon, popliteo fibular ligament, and LCL: important static stabilizer
    - Dynamic stabilizer: popliteus muscle, ITB, biceps, and lateral gastrocnemius tendon
  - Stability at initial knee flexion (<45°) in weight-bearing activities

- Augment the contribution of PCL to tibiofemoral posterior stability at 30° of knee flexion
- Mechanism of injury
  - Force from anteromedial to posterolateral tibia (or vice versa), knee hyperextension, and severe tibial external rotation or varus blow with partially flexed knee
  - Chronic sprain/strain, knee recurvatum, and varus (in some spastic patients)

History and physical examination
- Posterolateral corner pain, tenderness at the fibular head or joint line on palpation
  - Secondary patellofemoral syndrome/pain in chronic PCL deficiency
- ± Instability in standing (knee full extension), difficulty with reciprocal stairs, pivoting, and cutting
- Special tests (114): check physical examination section
  - Dial (external rotation at 30° knee flexion), external rotation recurvatum, varus stress, reverse pivot shift, and standing apprehension tests
- Check vascular (posterior tibial/dorsal pedal pulse) and neurologic injury (common peroneal nerve: ~15%, and possible cutaneous branch; lateral sural cutaneous nerve irritation)
- Gait: hyperextended knee or varus thrust

Diagnosis
- Clinical suspicion confirmed by imaging study
- Imaging
  - X-ray: not sensitive, often subtle, fibular head or femoral condyle avulsion fracture, and lateral joint space widening
  - MRI: evaluate the integrity of the posterolateral components (avulsion vs midstance injuries), bone bruise of the medial femoral condyle and medial tibial plateau
    - Evaluate other associated injuries (meniscal and cruciate pathology)
  - Electromyography (EMG); R/O peroneal nerve injury
- Classification: different scales based on location of injury (Fanelli scale), instability (Hughston scale for varus instability) and x-ray (distance of joint line opening) on varus stress

Treatment
- Conservative management
  - Minimal laxity with partial injury: initial use of crutch and a hinged knee brace with full extension/protected weight bearing for 2 weeks, early mobilization, fibular head mobilization, taping of the fibular head (be cautious of peroneal nerve irritation), ROM and strengthening exercises (especially quadriceps initially, then lateral hamstring and gastrocnemius), neuromuscular control, and functional movement
  - Return to activity in 2 to 4 weeks
  - Posterior leaf spring orthosis if + foot slap
- Referral to surgery
  - Acute advanced cases, combined ligament injuries, bony avulsion, or functionally unstable despite rehab: PCL repair, open reduction and internal fixation (ORIF), or reconstruction
  - Postoperative mobilization: early motion in prone position, quadriceps strengthening, and avoidance of hamstring eccentric strengthening at the beginning

PLICA SYNDROME

Introduction (116)
- Plica: remnants of the compartment-separating membranes
- Painful impairment of knee function from thickened and inflamed synovial folds
- Epidemiology of painful plica syndrome: debate between overrated importance versus underrecognized
- Etiology
  - Intra-articular bleeding or synovitis secondary to a loose body, OCD, a torn meniscus, a subluxing patellar, or after arthroscopy
  - Trauma (blunt), twisting injury, activities involving repetitive flexion-extension of the knee, and increased activity level
- Classification: the suprapatellar, medial, and the infrapatellar more common than lateral (117) (Figure 8.8)
  - Medial plica: MC symptomatic, infrapatellar plica: MC observed during arthroscopy

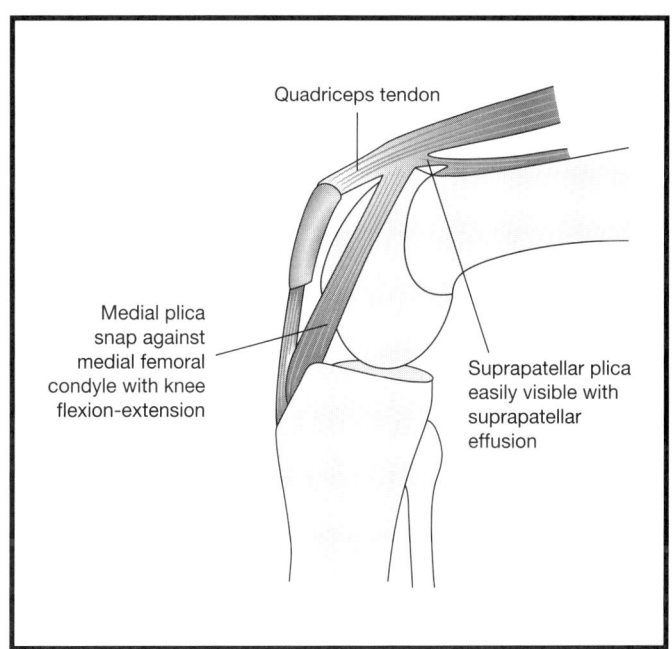

FIGURE 8.8
Plica of knee.
Source: Adapted from Ref. (116). Paczesny L, Kruczynski J. Medial plica syndrome of the knee: diagnosis with dynamic sonography. *Radiology.* 2009;251(2):439–446.

History and physical examination
- History
  - Pain over the area of plica: medial plica → intermittent dull pain between the patella and medial femoral condyle (proximal to the joint line)
  - Worsening pain by flexion (stairs; repeated flexion-extension, crouching, kneeling) and relieved by extension
  - ± Giving away, clicking, catching, pseudo locking, snapping, and tightness
- Physical examination
  - A palpable cord-like structure that pops and rolls on palpation with tenderness (on the medial patellofemoral space, more on the femoral condyle)

- Extension of the knee from 90° flexion, combined with internal rotation and medial gliding of the patella → popping between 60° and 45° of knee flexion
- Holding test: pain while the examiner flexes the knee with pushing the patella medially (by pinching the plica between the patella and femur)

Diagnosis
- Clinical diagnosis with imaging, imaging-guided injection, confirmed by arthroscopy
- Imaging
  - US of medial plica: thin hypoechoic band on the medial femoral condyle (between patellar-femoral joint space), dynamic view (knee flexion/extension) with palpation to locate, often difficult to visualize)
    - Suprapatellar plica with knee effusion (frequent finding with unclear clinical significance)
  - MRI to evaluate other intra-articular pathologies
- Differential diagnosis
  - Patellofermoral syndrome/patellar maltracking syndrome and patella bipartite
  - MCL tear, medial meniscus tear, DJD, OCD/loose body, or lipoma

Treatment
- Brief rest, modification of activities, and NSAIDs
- Quadriceps strengthening, stretching exercise, and patellar mobilization
- Intra-plical steroid injection using US
- Referral to arthroscopy if conservative management fails

EXTRA-ARTICULAR STRUCTURES (BURSA, TENDON, LIGAMENT PATHOLOGY)

MEDIAL KNEE PATHOLOGY

Pes Anserine Tendinobursitis

Introduction (118)
- Dysfunction of conjoined tendon of sartorius, gracilis, and semitendinosus (looks like goose [anserine] foot [pes]) and/or bursitis commonly between anserine tendons and MCL
- Common cause of medial knee pain, unclear prevalence in general population, underrecognized
  - ~20% of patients with symptomatic OA (119)
- Etiology and risk factors
  - Common with osteoarthritis, RA, obesity, and type 2 diabetes
  - Overuse of anserine tendon/muscle, knee flexor, and secondary internal rotation of tibia (resisting rotatory and valgus stress)

History and physical examination (120)
- Medial knee pain aggravated by climbing or descending stairs ± local swelling, and subjective instability
- Tenderness at the tendon insertion (1–2 in. distal to the medial joint line)
- Often common tightness of hamstring (semitendinosus), adductor (gracilis), and hip flexion (sartorius) and lower extremity kinetic chain (excessive pronation with tibial external rotation)

Diagnosis
- Clinical diagnosis confirmed by imaging study and/or diagnostic injection with a small volume of injectate
- US: abnormal finding (not sensitive) but an indicator of good response to injection
  - Increase in thickness of tendon at 2.5 to 5 cm below the knee joint line, loss of fibrillar pattern and anechoic fluid >2 mm, check contralateral asymptomatic side
  - Other findings: osteophytes at the medial joint line (common), joint effusion, MCL bursitis (under MCL), and popliteal cyst and the like
- MRI: usually not necessary; consider if not responsive to initial treatment and injection
  - Anserine bursal effusion: 5% in asymptomatic knee, 2.5% in symptomatic knee (from retrospective review of knee MRI)
  - To evaluate internal derangement/intracortical lesion or other concomitant lesion
- Differential diagnosis
  - Medial meniscal injury/cyst or MCL injury/bursitis, juxta-articular bone cysts, semimembranosus bursitis, ganglion cyst, and Baker's cyst; can coexist
  - Medial tibial plateau stress fracture: linear transverse sclerosis in x-ray

Treatment
- Hamstring/adductor/hip flexor stretching, biomechanical intervention (to mitigate excessive tibial external rotation; heel lift to mitigate pronate response or medial wedge/heel lift for genu valgum)
- Corticosteroid injection (to most tender point 2.5 to 5 cm below joint line) with/without US guidance (to space between the MCL and under anserine tendons; avoid the branch of genicular artery)

Medial Collateral Ligament (MCL) Sprain or Injury

Introduction (121)
- Incidence: MC injured ligament in the knee, 0.36/1,000 in male and 0.18/1,000 in female
- Etiology
  - Noncontact injury: valgus, external rotation, pivoting injury (MC)
  - Direct blow (to anterolateral knee, usually causing complete disruption of MCL) and knee dislocation
  - Overuse/repeated trauma
- Common location of injury/rupture: femoral insertion
  - Proximal tears having greater healing rates
  - Distal injuries tend to have excessive valgus laxity
- Commonly associated injuries: ACL tears more than meniscal tears

History and physical examination
- Medial knee pain ± swelling, side-to-side feeling of instability
- Tenderness on the medial femoral condyle or proximal tibia (rather than joint line) aggravated by valgus load at 20% to 30° knee flexion (± laxity)
- Valgus stress test and Swain test
  - Swain test: with knee flexed to 90°, the tibia is externally rotated. When the knee is externally rotating in flexion,

the collateral ligaments are tightened while the cruciate ligaments are relatively lax. Pain along the medial side of the joint indicates injury to the MCL complex

Diagnosis (122)
- Clinical diagnosis confirmed by imaging studies
- Imaging studies
  ○ X-ray: calcification in chronic cases, frequently in the proximal origin
    ▪ Stress radiograph: isolated injury of superior MCL: widening of joint line at 20° knee flexion > full extension. Complete (~1 cm with 20° flexion) more common than incomplete
    ▪ Pellegrini Stieda lesion: chronic MCL deficiency with calcification at the femoral insertion
  ○ US can evaluate dynamically similar to stress radiographs and hypoechoic swelling or discontinuity of the ligament
  ○ MRI can evaluate other intracortical lesions, combined intra-articular injury (ACL), and mild lesion (tissue edema and edema around the MCL)
- Differential diagnosis: medial compartment OA, meniscal lesion (worsening pain on varus or rotation), bursitis (MCL), pes anserine tendinobursitis, patellofemoral ligament sprain, or adductor magnus strain
- Grading

CLASSIFICATION	DEFINITION
Grade 1	Localized tenderness without instability
Grade 2	Localized tenderness and partially torn ligament (superficial or deep MCL)
Grade 3	Complete disruption with instability 1+: 3–5 mm laxity, 2+: 6–10 mm, 3+: >10 mm laxity (with valgus moment at 30° flexion)

MCL, medial collateral ligament.

Treatment (23)
- Nonoperative treatment: mainstay
  ○ Grades I and II: early controlled motion and protected weight bearing with hinged knee orthotics
    ▪ Immobilization ➔ reduction of collagen mass and increased collagen degradation
    ▪ ROM exercise, quadriceps, hamstring strengthening, joint proprioceptive exercise, and home exercise program
  ○ Return to play: grade I for ~10 days, grade II for 20 days, grade III for ~9 (4–10) weeks
    ▪ Grade III: a hinged knee brace for 6 weeks (protect valgus stress and external rotation)
- Operative treatment: ligament repair versus reconstruction
  ○ Relative indication: acute grade II injury (with avulsion, entrapment of the end, or multiligamentous injuries), and subacute injury with instability

MCL Bursitis (Voschell's Bursitis)

Introduction (123)
- Uncommon, but also underrecognized
- Anatomy of the MCL bursa
  ○ Constant bursa located between the deep (meniscofemoral/tibial ligament) and superficial layer (superficial and oblique) of the MCL
  ○ No intra-articular communication

History and physical examination
- Isolated medial joint line pain reproduced with valgus stress, tenderness, ± focal swelling
- Uncommon mechanical symptoms (catching and locking)

Diagnosis
- Clinical diagnosis confirmed by imaging
- Ultrasound: anechoic lesion under the superficial MCL, dynamic examination and guided injection, difficult to distinguish from meniscal cyst
- MRI to evaluate meniscal pathology or internal derangement
- Differential diagnosis: meniscal tear, cyst, MCL ligament tear, or tibial-semimembranosus bursa

Treatment
- Topical NSAIDs, or oral NSAIDs
- Injection under US guidance using a small volume (1 mL injectate)
- PT: modality, quad strengthening, and proprioceptive training to address faulty biomechanics (excessive pronation)

Medial Patellofemoral Ligament Dysfunction

Introduction (124)
- Uncommon but underrecognized cause of medial knee pain
- Anatomy and biomechanics
  ○ 5.5 cm in length and 0.3 to 3 cm in width from patella (medial upper) to femoral condyle (between medial epicondyle and adductor tubercle)
  ○ Patellar stabilizer (against lateral subluxation) in addition to vastus medialis (counterpart: lateral patellofemoral retinaculum and vastus lateralis); important in patellar stabilization with initial knee flexion
- Etiology (125)
  ○ Patellofemoral malalignment (often mild, valgus, or rotational deformity) and trochlear dysplasia
  ○ Patellar subluxation and dislocation

History and physical examination (34)
- Pain in the anteromedial knee (medial to the patella or at the medial femoral epicondyle), patellar subluxation in tear/insufficiency or retropatellar pain
- Patellar translation at 20° to 30° knee flexion if insufficiency exists
  ○ Positive J sign at the initial knee flexion (translation of the patella into the trochlear): exaggerated movement of the patella from lateral to medial

Diagnosis
- Clinical diagnosis confirmed by imaging
- Imaging: US (often hypoechoic due to anisotropy) or MRI (axial view and coronal view: avulsion at femoral site, effusion: very common)

Treatment
- Nonoperative treatment: VMO strengthening, a patella tracking knee brace, core stability exercise, strengthening of hip external rotator (functionally decrease Q angle)

LATERAL KNEE PATHOLOGY

Lateral Collateral Ligament (LCL)

Introduction (126)
- Isolated lateral collateral ligament injury: relatively rare
  - Sixteen percent of all knee ligament injuries involve LCL
  - Lateral ligamentous structures: more substantial and stronger, subject to greater forces during the normal gait cycle
  - Primary restraint to varus at 5 to 25° knee flexion
- Common etiologies: motor vehicle accident > sports-related injury
- Common location of tear: fibular (75%) > femoral attachment in 20% > midsubstance
- Concomitant pathologies: posterolateral corner injury and anterior/posterior cruciate ligament tears

History and physical examination (127)
- Pain along the lateral joint line ± instability (in chronic, near full extension), difficulty in cutting and pivoting
- Gait: hyperextension and varus thrust gait (or compensation to the other)
- Dial test for posterolateral laxity: increased tibial rotation with knee flexion at 30° or 90°: by >5 to 10°

Diagnosis
- Clinical diagnosis confirmed by imaging studies
  - Grading: 1 (minimal), 2 (partial), 3 (complete tear), or by lateral opening (0–5, 6–10, >10 mm)
- X-ray to R/O fibular head avulsion fracture and degenerative changes with chronic lateral instability or varus stress view
- MRI
  - Visible disruption, extensive surrounding soft tissue edema, or avulsion fracture or marrow edema involving the medial aspect of the fibular head

Treatment (126)
- Mild (grade 1): Rest, Ice, Compression, and Elevation (RICE), quad strengthening exercise, knee sleeve, or compression wrap (may decrease swelling)
- Grade II: hinged knee orthosis or knee immobilizer in extension and non-weight bearing for 2 weeks with crutch, then WBAT
- Referral to surgery for complete tear with other ligament injury present (posterolateral corner injury)
  - Arthroscopic evaluation of popliteus avulsion, meniscofemoral/tibial fibers of the lateral capsular ligament, and the lateral meniscus injury

Popliteus Tendinopathy

Introduction (128,129)
- Uncommon incidence, but underrecognized, higher in athletes with sports-related knee injury
  - One percent in retrospective knee MRI review, usually with posterolateral corner injury; isolated in 10%
  - Often concomitant with ACL injury or other posterolateral corner structure injury
- Anatomy
  - Three origins: lateral femoral condyle, fibula head, and lateral meniscus. Inserts to the proximal tibia above the soleal line
- Classification: tenosynovitis, tendonitis/acute calcific tendonitis, rupture, and avulsion
- MC location of injury at musculotendinous junction (>90%) (130)

History and physical examination (131)
- Posterolateral knee pain, worsened by downhill running ± joint swelling without gross instability (unless with concomitant ligament injury).
- Physical examination
  - Tenderness on the lateral condyle immediately posterior to the ITB, slightly above fibular collateral ligament, ± acute effusion (hemarthrosis) if tear presents
  - Garrick test: resisted internal rotation of the leg (tibia) with knee/hip flexion at 90°
  - Cross leg; figure of 4; provoke the pain

Diagnosis
- Clinical diagnosis and confirmed by imaging study
- Imaging study
  - US: limited evaluation of musculotendinous junction and muscle pathology; base of the popliteal fossa due to depth and turn
    - Femoral insertion: posterior to the ITB, on the groove for the popliteus
    - Tenosynovial effusion often difficult to distinguish from the intracapsular effusion
  - MRI: can evaluate other posterolateral corner structures
- Differential diagnosis
  - ITB syndrome, biceps femoris tendon, and lateral head of the gastrocnemius strain
  - Lateral meniscus injury
  - Posterolateral corner (including lateral collateral ligament) injury

Treatment
- PT: Eccentric quadriceps strengthening program, intervene underlying biomechanical problem (heel lift or medial wedge for overpronated foot and tight heel cord)
- Injection: ultrasound-guided injection (intracapsular)
- Referral to surgery if other posterolateral structures are involved (to prevent acute or chronic posterolateral instability) or failed conservative management

ANTERIOR KNEE PATHOLOGY

Quadriceps Tendinopathy and Tear

Introduction (132)
- Quadriceps rupture: peak incidence in athletes over 40 years old, quadriceps rupture > patellar tendon rupture

by ~3 times, male > female by ~8 times, unilateral, common in jumping sports (eg, basketball and volleyball) (133)
- Quadriceps tendinopathy less common than patellar tendinopathy
- Common location: 1–1.5 cm proximal to the patella
- Etiology and associated conditions
  ○ Calcific enthesopathy: seronegative spondyloarthropathy, diffuse idiopathic skeletal hyperostosis (DISH), renal failure, and hyperparathyroidism
  ○ Degeneration/fibromyxoid change

History and physical examination
- Anterior knee (suprapatellar) pain. "Pop" followed by pain and swelling in rupture
- Physical examination in patient with rupture
  ○ Palpable defect just above the patella, mass proximal to the rupture if retracted
  ○ Patella baja: distally moved patella compared to the other side
  ○ Impaired knee extension strength; if unable to extend against gravity (not pain limited), surgical referral

Diagnosis
- Clinical diagnosis confirmed by imaging study
- X-ray: patella baja, avulsion of the superior pole of the patella, calcification in the quad tendon
- US
  ○ Enthesopathy: calcification at the superior pole of the patella, increase thickness and hypoechogenicity of quadriceps tendon, tenderness with sono-palpation
    ▪ Increased vascularity (in Doppler); neovascularization: may be associated with greater pain
  ○ Rupture: anechoic/hypoechoic lesion (fluid or granulation tissue) filled gap with retracted tendon
- MRI to evaluate the internal derangement of knee

Treatment
- Partial tear/tendinopathy; conservative treatment especially if able to extend the knee, long leg cast for 4 to 6 weeks in significant tear
- Platelet-rich plasma injection (unclear evidence)
- Complete tear: referral for immediate repair (outcome linked to the time between injury and repair)

Patella Tendinopathy and Tear

Introduction (3,134)
- Jumper's knee; common in sports requiring repetitive jumping (basketball and volleyball); up to 20%
- Rupture: more common in athletes younger than 40 years old (than quad tendinopathy/rupture)
  ○ Increased in basketball, football, and soccer players
- Etiology and risk factor
  ○ Biomechanical: weight (high BMI), waist/hip ratio, leg length discrepancy, arch height, quadriceps/hamstring flexibility, vertical jump performance, and training volume
  ○ Postop in ACL reconstruction using patella tendon graft or tibial intramedullary nailing
  ○ Metabolic disorder, gout, or steroid injection

History and physical examination
- Anterior knee (near the patella) pain worse with walking, running, and jumping
- Bulging (swollen) patellar tendon (compared to asymptomatic side), tenderness on the inferior pole, patellar tendon, and possibly at tibial tuberosity
- Reproduction of pain on resisted knee extension
- Physical examination in patient with rupture
  ○ Patellar alta (proximally moved), palpable gap, inability to maintain active knee extension if ruptured
  ○ Effusion/hemarthrosis, ecchymosis, and difficulty in weight bearing in acute rupture

Diagnosis
- Clinical diagnosis confirmed by imaging study
- US
  ○ Tendinopathy: increased thickness of tendon in short axis, hypoechogenicity; often difficult to distinguish it from partial tear ± increased vascularity (neovascularization; may be associated with greater pain)
  ○ Tendinopathy and partial tear: more commonly involved in the deep central portion of the tendon and medial aspect of tendon
  ○ Rupture: discontinuity
- MRI to evaluate mild involvement, intracortical, intra-articular pathologies or for surgical planning
- Differential diagnosis (for anterior knee pain): prepatellar/infrapatellar bursitis, patellar fracture, patellofemoral syndrome, Hoffa's fat pad impingement, ITB insertional tendinopathy, osteoarthritis, and the like

Treatment
- Physical therapy for initial stretching of quad, especially rectus femoris, deep friction massage, isometric strengthening, and closed kinetic chain exercise to eccentric contraction exercise
- Patellar taping, Cho-Pat strap, and evaluation of foot orthosis to address biomechanical faults
- Platelet-rich plasma injection and US-guided percutaneous tenotomy (Tenex®) for tendinopathy (135)
- Long leg cast or knee brace in full extension for 4 to 6 weeks in tear
- Surgery for complete rupture, rerupture, rare stiffness, and weakness common

Patellar Sleeve (Avulsion) Fracture

Introduction (136)
- Very rare (<1% of pediatric fracture), high incidence in 8 to 12 years, important to recognize as a differential for other conditions
- MC location: the inferior pole of the patella
- Etiology and risk factor
  ○ Children with open growth plates, blow to the flexed knee and the simultaneous forceful eccentric contraction of the quadriceps

History and physical examination
- Knee pain (acute onset), swelling with inability to achieve terminal extension of knee
  ○ Distinguish between apophysitis by inability to perform the straight leg raising test in fracture
- Chronic case: anterior knee pain, quadriceps atrophy, and extension lag

Diagnosis
- Clinical diagnosis confirmed by imaging study
- Lateral x-ray: soft tissue swelling at the lower pole, small bony fragment, displacement of patella (alta more common than baja due to location of sleeve fracture)
- MRI: evaluate chondral injury and concomitant extensor mechanism injury
- Differential diagnosis: Sinding-Larsen-Johansson disease, patellar fracture/tendinopathy, and quadriceps tendon rupture

Treatment
- Long leg cylinder cast for 6 weeks for nondisplaced fracture with intact extensor mechanism
- Referral for surgery in patients with displaced fracture; internal fixation with plate, immediate mobilization, and early weight bearing (137)

Prepatellar Bursitis
Introduction (138)
- One of the MC knee bursitises. Septic bursitis is common (up to 20%)
- Located anteriorly between the patella and subcutaneous tissues
- Etiology
  - Overuse injury or chronic trauma, such as occupational or recreational kneeling or crawling (housemaid's knee, carpet-layer's knee, wrestlers)
    - MC reason for chronic bursitis: repeated microtrauma
  - Others: metabolic (eg, gout) and infectious in acute bursitis

History and physical examination
- Anterior knee (focal) pain, ± focal swelling, warmth, and erythema
- Tenderness ± bulging (often subtle) on inferior pole of the patella

Diagnosis
- Clinical diagnosis confirmed by imaging study
- US: acutely hypoechoic, or maybe echogenic; no septation and slightly thickened wall
  - Bursa can be collapsed even with slight pressure
- MRI: a focal fluid collection seen anterior to the patella; it may be heterogeneous or poorly defined
  - T2-weighted images: increased signal intensity from associated inflammation, hemorrhage, or even infection

Treatment
- Activity modification (avoid kneeling), NSAIDs, ice, or immobilization (knee immobilizer) for 1 week
- Aspiration for gram stain, culture, caution-giving steroid injection
- Rarely referral to surgery for bursal resection in failed conservative treatment

Infrapatellar Bursitis
Introduction (139)
- Unknown prevalence
  - Asymptomatic small bursal effusion in deep infrapatellar bursa is common
    - Often difficult to correlate with clinical symptoms
- Anatomy (140)
  - Superficial: just above the tibial attachment of the patellar tendon
  - Deep: between the patellar tendon and tibial tuberosity, slightly wider than patellar tendon (usually wider dimension in the lateral side than medial)
- Etiology and risk factor
  - During active stages of Osgood-Schlatter disease, or crystal deposition or rarely septic bursitis
    - May occur following patellectomy, and in infrapatellar contraction syndrome (141)
  - Acute or chronic injury (kneeling) in superficial bursitis

History and physical examination
- Anterior knee pain (above the patellar tendon, deeper to the patellar tendon insertion)
- Tenderness to palpation and occasional bulging at the side of the patellar tendon insertion to the tibial tuberosity

Diagnosis
- Clinical diagnosis confirmed by ultrasound ± diagnostic injection (with 0.5 to 1 mL of lidocaine)

Treatment
- Avoid aggravating activity, such as kneeling; perform gradual stretching of quadriceps tendon (rectus femoris) and gradual eccentric strengthening exercise of quadriceps tendon
- US-guided steroid injection

Hoffa's Fat Pad Impingement Syndrome
Introduction (142)
- Rare, but underrecognized, 1% to 6.8% of patients referred to specialized knee centers
- Anatomy: intra-articular and extrasynovial
  - Superior border: inferior pole of the patella and inferior border: proximal tibia and deep infrapatellar bursa
  - Anterior border: joint capsule and patellar tendon
  - Posterior border: synovium-lined joint cavity
- Etiology and risk factor
  - Eccentric load in jumping or running
  - Fat pad tethered after a trauma → patella and tibia impinges the fat pad with the knee hyperextension
- Concomitant with grade 1 chondromalacia patella in 85% (excessive loading patellofemoral joint to avoid knee hyperextension [locking])

History and physical examination
- Anterior knee pain, infrapatellar or retropatellar region, worsening pain on lying down than sitting
- Physical examination
  - Provocative test: application of pressure to the medial or lateral side of the patellar tendon of a flexed knee, which is passively extended while the pressure is maintained
    - Modified: reproduction of pain/symptom by passive extension of the knee by applying firm pressure over the proximal tibia with one hand while holding the heel in

the other hand (no direct palpation on the fat pad or patella)
- ± Prominent Hoffa's fat pad
- Check ligament laxity and pes cavus (promoting hyperextension moment to knee)

Diagnosis
- Diagnosis of exclusion; clinical suspicion confirmed by imaging study
- Differential diagnosis (often concomitant) (143)
  - Anterior horn of medial meniscus tear, infrapatellar plica syndrome (144,145)
  - Patellar tendon-lateral femoral condyle friction syndrome
    - Inflammatory changes of the fat pad between the patellar tendon and the lateral femoral condyle, secondary to patellar maltracking; patellar alignment abnormalities, including patella alta
- MRI (146)
  - In the acute setting, increased T2 signal intensity in fat pad and mass effect (bowing of the patellar tendon) and a small joint effusion may be present
  - Chronically, fibrosis and hemosiderin deposition may occur → decreased signal intensity on T1 and T2 images

Treatment
- Rehabilitation: pillow under the knee with lying supine (to avoid full knee extension but do stretching exercise at least 2 to 3 times daily), stretching of rectus femoris, and taping to push the patella proximally
  - Heel lift (mitigate knee extension momentum) in pes cavus
  - Patellar tracking hinged knee orthosis with terminal extension stop (20°–30°)
- Arthroscopic resection of fat pad if conservative management failed (147)

Osgood–Schlatter Disease

Introduction (148)
- A traction apophysitis of the tibial tubercle that develops during the adolescent growth spurt
  - Creates increased tensile forces at the tendon insertion, causing avulsion fractures
- Epidemiology
  - Preteen or early teen boy (12–15 years) > girl (8–12 years), 20% in adolescents active in sports (vs 5% in non-athletes), bilateral up to 25% to 50%
- Etiology and risk factor
  - Skeletal growth faster than the elongation of the muscle tendon units → relative tightness of the soft tissues
  - Patella alta

History and physical examination
- Pain localized to the tibial tubercle aggravated by kneeling, eccentric quadriceps activity. Symptom begins with growth spurt
- Tenderness on the tibial tubercle, protuberance at the tibial tubercle, and tightness of rectus femoris

Diagnosis
- Clinical diagnosis confirmed by imaging study
- X-ray: irregularity and fragmentation of the tibial tuberosity
- US: similar findings as x-ray ± infrapatellar bursal effusion

Treatment
- Temporary suspension of sports activities; NSAIDs, knee padding, and ice
- Temporary immobilization in severe case with hinged knee orthosis or knee immobilizer with crutch if not responding to treatment
  - Twelve to 18 months for physiologic epiphysiodesis (improve spontaneously)
- Gentle progressive quad stretch and pain-free quad strengthening
- Referral to surgery: rare, refractory cases, persistent symptoms in skeletally mature patients

Sinding-Larsen-Johansson Disease

Introduction
- Traction apophysitis of the inferior pole of the patella by persistent traction at immature inferior patellar pole due to dissimilar growth plate
- Active adolescents between 10 and 14 years and more common in boys

History and physical examination
- Activity-related pain in the anterior knee (interior pole of the patella) with running and jumping
- Tenderness with occasional swelling over the inferior pole

Diagnosis
- Clinical diagnosis confirmed with imaging study
- Imaging (x-ray and US): calcification and ossification, osseous fragmentation with possible avulsion and fracture. Increased vascularity in the inferior pole of the patella on Doppler US

Treatment
- Spontaneous resolution in 3 to 12 months, rest and conservative management (gradual stretching and strengthening)
- Consider dry needling or platelet-rich plasma for persistent pain despite conservative treatment
- Surgical referral in rare refractory cases for debridement

POSTERIOR KNEE PATHOLOGY

Popliteal Cyst (Baker's Cyst)

Introduction (138)
- MC cyst in the knee
  - Prevalence of Baker's cyst in patients who had MRI: 5% to 38%, increasing with age
  - Unclear correlation with pain
- Anatomy
  - Located between the semimembranosus and medial gastrocnemius or separately under semimembranosus (larger bursa) and medial gastrocnemius
  - Communication with knee joint >50% (cadaveric study)

- Etiology/mechanism
  ○ Knee joint effusion → weakness of posterior joint capsule; weaker in posteromedial aspect (often with tear of the posterior horn of the meniscus attached to the capsule) → slit like communication with escaped fluid in the popliteal region
  ○ Associated findings: internal derangement (81%), joint effusion (77%), and degenerative arthropathy (69%)
    ▪ Tears of the posterior horn of the medial meniscus: MC derangement, >60%

History and physical examination
- Asymptomatic usually, a bulging mass or subtle swelling, symptomatic (popliteal or vague pain) with internal derangement or cyst rupture or dissection (with upper calf pain mimicking DVT)
  ○ Proximal dissection can rarely cause irritation/compression of the sciatic nerve

Diagnosis
- Clinical suspicion confirmed by imaging study
- US: anechoic cyst in the posterior medial knee
  ○ Identify neck and base of the cyst (to differentiate other popliteal cyst and ganglion cyst)
  ○ Small cyst: differentiate the anisotropy of medial gastroc tendon and semimembranosus tendon; also consider scanning on the dependent position (fluid may drain into the knee joint in prone position)
- MRI to evaluate intra-articular pathology or derangement
- Differential diagnosis
  ○ Ganglion cyst and tumors (lipoma, xanthoma, vascular tumor, fibrosarcoma, and others)
  ○ Popliteal aneurysm/pseudoaneurysm, and popliteal artery entrapment syndrome (calf claudication)
  ○ Deep vein thrombosis
- No treatment required if asymptomatic

Treatment
- If symptomatic, aspiration, and corticosteroid injection ± compression with elastic bandage
- Referral to arthroscopy (intra-articular pathology evaluation and closure of the posteromedial capsule) or open surgery if conservative management fails

Fabella Syndrome

Introduction (149)
- Fabella: sesamoid bone in the lateral gastrocnemius tendon, 10% to 30% in ≥12 years old
- Etiology of painful fabella syndrome
  ○ Chondromalacia common in adolescent age 15 to 17 years, osteoarthritis and isolated fabello-femoral degeneration in older adults

History and physical examination
- Pain in the posterolateral aspect of the knee, accentuated by extension of knee ± peroneal nerve dysfunction

Diagnosis
- Clinical diagnosis ± imaging study and diagnostic injection
- X-ray; often unremarkable other than fabella
- MRI: minimal osteocartilaginous lesions in chondromalacia, articular cartilage change and sclerosis (anterior facet) in arthritis

Treatment
- Diagnostic and therapeutic injection (US-guided injection of 1 mL into the fabella-posterior femoral condyle articulation)
- NSAIDs, stretching of gastrocnemius muscle and hamstring muscle
- Referral for surgical resection if nonoperative management fails

Popliteal Artery Aneurysm

Introduction (150)
- MC peripheral arterial aneurysm (less common than abdominal aortic aneurysm [AAA]), often bilateral (50%–70%), male >> female, peak incidence in sixth to seventh decades
  ○ Thirty to 50 percent of popliteal artery aneurysm (PAA) patients have AAA
- Classification: true aneurysm (all layers of the arterial wall dilated, diameter >0.7 cm) and pseudoaneurysm (partial defect in the arterial wall due to trauma or infection)
  ○ Popliteal artery occlusion: 30% to 50% of patients with complete knee dislocation
  ○ Rarely associated with connective tissue disease (Marfan or Ehlers Danlos syndrome)
  ○ Spontaneous relocation of knee dislocation (causing pseudoaneurysm); often unrecognized by the patient
- Complication of untreated aneurysm: 18% to 31%, occlusion, thrombosis, rupture, and the like

History and physical examination
- Asymptomatic (45%) ± popliteal mass
- Symptoms of ischemia: claudication (lower extremity ischemia), rest pain (burning pain with recumbent position or elevation with relief by sitting and standing), severe ischemia associated with thrombosis or embolization
- Palpable distal pulse does not R/O the popliteal artery lesion

Diagnosis
- High index of suspicion confirmed by vascular imaging study
- US, magnetic resonance angiography (MRA) (delineate the aneurysmal sac and mural thrombosis), or angiography (especially if thrombosed or traumatic cases)
- US to differentiate other popliteal mass (such as Baker's cyst, ganglion cyst, etc)
- Evaluate AAA (considering high rate of concurrent lesions)

Treatment
- Referral to vascular surgery for possible repair or thrombolytic treatment for acute thrombosis
- Aerobic endurance exercise (graded) for claudication

NEUROPATHY

SAPHENOUS NEUROPATHY; GONALGIA PARESTHETICA

Introduction (151)
- Anatomy (152)

- A branch of femoral nerve, L4
- In thigh: course in the subsartorial or Hunter's canal with femoral vessel (in the same sheath)
  - Pierces the subsartorial fascia approximately 10 cm proximal to the medial femoral condyle (adductor canal, fascia between the vastus medialis and adductor magnus)
- Distal to adductor canal: divide into infrapatellar branch (pierce the sartorius muscle subcutaneously, then two branches between the apex of the patella and tibial tubercle) and sartorial branch (between the sartorius and gracilis muscle) (153)
- Unknown incidence: but likely underrecognized
- Etiology
  - Iatrogenic: knee surgery (154), knee injection
  - Trauma, compression (surfer's neuropathy), kneeling, subluxation/dislocation of patella or knee
  - Pes anserinus bursitis
  - Idiopathic

History and physical examination
- Pain (typically electric, burning, tingling, pins/needles, not uncommonly dull and achy) in the medial knee, distal thigh ± radiation of pain distally (medial leg/calf) and occasionally proximally
- Aggravating symptoms by walking, sitting, or climbing stairs
- Tenderness at the subsartorial fascia (between sartorius and vastus medialis 7 to 10 cm above the medial joint line) reproducing symptoms in the medial knee ± referred pain (Valleix's phenomenon)
  - Nerve stretch test (reproduction of symptoms with valgus stress, tibial external rotation, and flexion/extension)

Diagnosis
- Clinical diagnosis confirmed by diagnostic block, and EMG to evaluate differentials
- Imaging study
  - X-ray to evaluate concomitant knee OA; rarely spur/osteophyte can irritate the nerve
  - US as screening for soft tissue mass and imaging guidance for diagnostic block
  - MRI for underlying etiologies; spur, ganglion cyst, lipoma, neurilemma, and the like
- Differential diagnoses: L3–4 radiculopathy, lumbar plexopathy, diabetic amyotrophy, muscle infarct, and mononeuritis multiplex/peripheral neuropathy and musculoskeletal conditions (anserine tendinobursitis, meniscal lesion, MCL sprain, medial compartmental OA often concomitant)

Treatment
- US- or stimulator-guided injection initially with steroid/lidocaine or lidocaine/bupivacaine; then consider pulse radiofrequency
- Biomechanical intervention to decrease stretching by decreasing hyperpronation (hindfoot eversion or valgus/tibial external rotation moment)
- Referral to neurectomy for disabling pain despite the conservative management

PERONEAL NEUROPATHY

Introduction (155)
- Anatomy
  - Course: L4–S2, sciatic nerve ➔ common peroneal nerve (in sciatic nerve) innervating short head of biceps femoris before bifurcating ➔ lateral sural cutaneous nerve branches out at proximal to fibular head
  - Common peroneal nerve passing around the fibular neck in an exposed fibro-osseous tunnel bordered superficially by the peroneus longus tendon ➔ bifurcates into recurrent articular branch, deep and superficial branches
  - Deep peroneal nerve: more anterior and closer to the fibular, pierces the anterior intermuscular septum and travels with the tibial A and vein between tibialis anterior [TA] and extensor digitorum longus [EDL] and EDL/extensor hallucis longus (EHL) distally
- MC mononeuropathy in the lower extremity: very unusual cause of neuropathic knee pain
- Etiology
  - External compression and direct trauma
    - ~25% of individuals, common peroneal nerve travels within a tighter tunnel between biceps femoris and lateral gastrocnemius
      - Entrapment by gastrocnemius muscle hernia, biceps femoris, or lateral gastrocnemius muscle hypertrophy, aberrant muscle
    - Direct compression on the exposed fibro-osseous tunnel/fibrous bands of the peroneus longus muscle; tight plaster casts, synovial cysts or ganglions, habitual leg crossing, after significant weight loss (slimmer's paralysis), and prolonged squatting (strawberry picker's palsy)
    - Prolonged immobilization (Saturday night palsy or anesthesia), lithotomy position during childbirth, knee surgery, or osteophytes
    - Fibular head fracture, crush injury, proximal tibiofibular joint (anterolateral direction) or temporary knee dislocation (can be underrecognized)
    - Tumor, osteochondromas, synovial or meniscal cysts, arterial or venous aneurysms, intraneural and extraneural ganglia, nerve tumor
  - Stretch injury
    - Ankle sprain (similar mechanism to Maisonneuve fracture; proximal fibular fracture with ankle syndesmosis injury) or excessive ankle inversion (inversion sprain)
    - Repetitive inversion and pronation (runners, cyclists, machine operators)
  - Idiopathic

History and physical examination
- History
  - Sensory (numbness, tingling in dorsum of the foot) and motor symptoms (foot slapping or dragging)
  - Pain over the lateral upper calf (lateral sural cutaneous nerve) and dorsum of the foot (superficial peroneal nerve)
  - Less commonly, anterolateral knee pain (para-patellar region) from recurrent branch involvement (156)
- Physical examination
  - Tinel sign with reproducing pain and paresthesia in the anterolateral aspect of the leg
  - Motor weakness (ankle dorsiflexor, evertor; main deficit; impaired heel walk or heel lift 5 or 10 times in mild case),

- Ankle plantar flexor and knee flexor can be slightly weak (due to peroneus longus: first ray plantar flexor and biceps femoris short head by common peroneal nerve)
- Check ankle flexor/hip extensor (to R/O sciatic nerve) and hip abduction (to R/O lumbar plexus or root lesion)
◦ Sensory: first web space (deep peroneal), dorsal aspect of foot/ankle (superficial peroneal), lateral calf (lateral sural cutaneous nerve)

Diagnosis
- Clinical diagnosis confirmed by EMG test
- NCS and needle EMG
  ◦ Nerve conduction study (NCS)
    - Superficial peroneal sensory nerve conduction study (SNCS) recording at ankle (lateral one-fourth between medial malleolus-lateral malleolus with stimulation at 12 cm proximal)
      – If normal, isolated deep peroneal neuropathy, pathology only involving myelin segment or preganglionic lesion (eg, L5 radiculopathy)
    - Sural SNCS: R/O sciatic nerve lesion or distal peripheral polyneuropathy
    - Motor NCS: deep peroneal recording at extensor digitorum brevis as well as tibialis anterior (if ankle dorsiflexion is weak) across the fibular head (proximal and distal to evaluate focal demyelination lesion)
    - Needle EMG: tibialis anterior (L4/5, deep peroneal), peroneus longus (superficial peroneal, L5/S1), biceps femoris short head (common peroneal proximal to fibular head, L5-S2), medial gastroc (tibial, S1/2), tibialis posterior (tibial, L5), tensor fascia lata (superior gluteal, L4-S1), lumbar paraspinal muscle (lower) for differential diagnosis of sciatic neuropathy, LS plexopathy or LS radiculopathy
  ◦ US to evaluate underlying causes (soft tissue mass; ganglion cyst, lipoma, etc)
  ◦ MRI to find the underlying causes, and MRI also can evaluate muscle denervation (increased T2 signal intensity) and fatty infiltration/atrophy (by US too)

Treatment
- Education: avoid leg cross and other causes with shoe/running technique modification, and gastrocnemius/biceps femoris stretching)
- Orthotics
  ◦ Heel lift for foot slapping, and lateral heel wedge to decrease peroneal overloading
  ◦ Significant motor symptoms; orthosis (ankle-foot orthotics, likely dorsiflexion assist, such as posterior leaf spring orthosis)
- US-guided lidocaine block (1–2 mL) for diagnosis and hydrodissection around the peroneal nerve (using normal saline)
- Referral for surgery (fascial release): pain or sensory symptoms without significant axonal damage (157)

REFERENCES

1. Turkiewicz A, Gerhardsson de Verdier M, et al. Prevalence of knee pain and knee OA in southern Sweden and the proportion that seeks medical care. *Rheumatology (Oxford)*. 2015;54(5):827–835.
2. Norvell DC, Czerniecki JM, Reiber GE, et al. The prevalence of knee pain and symptomatic knee osteoarthritis among veteran traumatic amputees and nonamputees. *Arch Phys Med Rehabil*. 2005;86(3):487–493.
3. Hiemstra LA, Kerslake S, Irving C. Anterior knee pain in the athlete. *Clin Sports Med*. 2014;33(3):437–459.
4. O'Connor FG. *Sports medicine just the facts*. New York, NY: McGraw-Hill; 2005.
5. Baker BE, Peckham AC, Pupparo F, Sanborn JC. Review of meniscal injury and associated sports. *Am J Sports Med*. 1985;13(1):1–4.
6. Fransen M, Agaliotis M, Bridgett L, Mackey MG. Hip and knee pain: role of occupational factors. *Best Pract Res Clin Rheumatol*. 2011;25(1):81–101.
7. Felson DT, Hannan MT, Naimark A, et al. Occupational physical demands, knee bending, and knee osteoarthritis: results from the Framingham Study. *J Rheumatol*. 1991;18(10):1587–1592.
8. Saavedra MÁ, Navarro-Zarza JE, Villaseñor-Ovies P, et al. Clinical anatomy of the knee. *Reumatol Clin*. 2012;8 Suppl 2:39–45.
9. Okada J, Shinozaki T, Hirato J, et al. Fibroma of tendon sheath of the infrapatellar fat pad in the knee. *Clin Imaging*. 2009;33(5):406–408.
10. Damarey B, Demondion X, Wavreille G, et al. Imaging of the nerves of the knee region. *Eur J Radiol*. 2013;82(1):27–37.
11. Blalock D, Miller A, Tilley M, Wang J. Joint instability and osteoarthritis. *Clin Med Insights Arthritis Musculoskelet Disord*. 2015;8:15–23.
12. Sekiya JK, Kuhn JE. Instability of the proximal tibiofibular joint. *J Am Acad Orthop Surg*. 2003;11(2):120–128.
13. Vavalle G, Capozzi M. Symptomatic snapping knee from biceps femoris tendon subluxation: an unusual case of lateral pain in a marathon runner. *J Orthop Traumatol*. 2010;11(4):263–266.
14. Guillin R, Marchand AJ, Roux A, et al. Imaging of snapping phenomena. *Br J Radiol*. 2012;85(1018):1343–1353.
15. Flandry F, Hommel G. Normal anatomy and biomechanics of the knee. *Sports Med Arthrosc*. 2011;19(2):82–92.
16. Kirschner MH, Menck J, Nerlich A, et al. The arterial blood supply of the human patella. Its clinical importance for the operating technique in vascularized knee joint transplantations. *Surg Radiol Anat*. 1997;19(6):345–351.
17. Vincent KR, Conrad BP, Fregly BJ, Vincent HK. The pathophysiology of osteoarthritis: a mechanical perspective on the knee joint. *PM R*. 2012;4(5 Suppl):S3–S9.
18. El-Khoury GY, Usta HY, Berger RA. Meniscotibial (coronary) ligament tears. *Skeletal Radiol*. 1984;11(3):191–196.
19. Bicer EK, Lustig S, Servien E, et al. Current knowledge in the anatomy of the human anterior cruciate ligament. *Knee Surg Sports Traumatol Arthrosc*. 2010;18(8):1075–1084.
20. Ingersoll CD, Grindstaff TL, Pietrosimone BG, Hart JM. Neuromuscular consequences of anterior cruciate ligament injury. *Clin Sports Med*. 2008;27(3):383–404, vii.
21. Wenger A, Wirth W, Hudelmaier M, et al. Meniscus body position, size, and shape in persons with and persons without radiographic knee osteoarthritis: quantitative analyses of knee magnetic resonance images from the osteoarthritis initiative. *Arthritis Rheum*. 2013;65(7):1804–1811.
22. Miller TT. Imaging of the medial and lateral ligaments of the knee. *Semin Musculoskelet Radiol*. 2009;13(4):340–352.
23. Miyamoto RG, Bosco JA, Sherman OH. Treatment of medial collateral ligament injuries. *J Am Acad Orthop Surg*. 2009;17(3):152–161.
24. Horner G, Dellon AL. Innervation of the human knee joint and implications for surgery. *Clin Orthop Relat Res*. 1994;(301):221–6.
25. Huberti HH, Hayes WC. Patellofemoral contact pressures. The influence of q-angle and tendofemoral contact. *J Bone Joint Surg Am*. 1984;66(5):715–724.
26. Huberti HH, Hayes WC. Contact pressures in chondromalacia patellae and the effects of capsular reconstructive procedures. *J Orthop Res*. 1988;6(4):499–508.
27. Nakajima K, Kakihana W, Nakagawa T, et al. Addition of an arch support improves the biomechanical effect of a laterally wedged insole. *Gait Posture*. 2009;29(2):208–213.
28. Rowe PJ, Myles CM, Walker C, Nutton R. Knee joint kinematics in gait and other functional activities measured using flexible electrogoniometry: how much knee motion is sufficient for normal daily life? *Gait Posture*. 2000;12(2):143–155.
29. Giugliano DN, Solomon JL. ACL tears in female athletes. *Phys Med Rehabil Clin N Am*. 2007;18(3):417–38, viii.

30. Hewett TE, Myer GD, Ford KR. Anterior cruciate ligament injuries in female athletes: Part 1, mechanisms and risk factors. *Am J Sports Med.* 2006;34(2):299–311.
31. Lu TW, Chang CF. Biomechanics of human movement and its clinical applications. *Kaohsiung J Med Sci.* 2012;28(2 Suppl):S13–S25.
32. Reeves ND, Bowling FL. Conservative biomechanical strategies for knee osteoarthritis. *Nat Rev Rheumatol.* 2011;7(2):113–122.
33. Lu TW, Chen HL, Wang TM. Obstacle crossing in older adults with medial compartment knee osteoarthritis. *Gait Posture.* 2007;26(4):553–559.
34. Luhmann SJ, Schoenecker PL, Dobbs MB, Eric Gordon J. Adolescent patellofemoral pain: implicating the medial patellofemoral ligament as the main pain generator. *J Child Orthop.* 2008;2(4):269–277.
35. Bozkurt M, Yilmaz E, Atlihan D, et al. The proximal tibiofibular joint: an anatomic study. *Clin Orthop Relat Res.* 2003;(406):136–40.
36. Malanga GA, Andrus S, Nadler SF, McLean J. Physical examination of the knee: a review of the original test description and scientific validity of common orthopedic tests. *Arch Phys Med Rehabil.* 2003;84(4):592–603.
37. Marks MC, Alexander J, Sutherland DH, Chambers HG. Clinical utility of the Duncan-Ely test for rectus femoris dysfunction during the swing phase of gait. *Dev Med Child Neurol.* 2003;45(11):763–768.
38. Kopkow C, Freiberg A, Kirschner S, et al. Physical examination tests for the diagnosis of posterior cruciate ligament rupture: a systematic review. *J Orthop Sports Phys Ther.* 2013;43(11):804–813.
39. Kim SJ, Min BH, Han DY. Paradoxical phenomena of the McMurray test. An arthroscopic investigation. *Am J Sports Med.* 1996;24(1):83–87.
40. Comley, L. Chiropractic management of greater occipital neuralgia. *Clinical Chiropractic.* 2003;6(3–4):120–128.
41. Fredericson M, Yoon K. Physical examination and patellofemoral pain syndrome. *Am J Phys Med Rehabil.* 2006;85(3):234–243.
42. Doberstein ST, Romeyn RL, Reineke DM. The diagnostic value of the Clarke sign in assessing chondromalacia patella. *J Athl Train.* 2008;43(2):190–196.
43. Haim A, Yaniv M, Dekel S, Amir H. Patellofemoral pain syndrome: validity of clinical and radiological features. *Clin Orthop Relat Res.* 2006;451:223–228.
44. Hollingworth W, Dixon AK, Jenner JR. 18 Imaging for knee and shoulder problems. In: Medina LS, Blackmore CC, Applegate K, eds. *Evidence-Based Imaging.* New York, NY: Springer; 2011:309–326.
45. Özçakar L, Kara M, Chang KV, et al. EURO-MUSCULUS/USPRM. Basic scanning protocols for knee. *Eur J Phys Rehabil Med.* 2015;51(5):641–646.
46. Sanders TG, Miller MD. A systematic approach to magnetic resonance imaging interpretation of sports medicine injuries of the knee. *Am J Sports Med.* 2005;33(1):131–148.
47. Hill CL, Hunter DJ, Niu J, et al. Synovitis detected on magnetic resonance imaging and its relation to pain and cartilage loss in knee osteoarthritis. *Ann Rheum Dis.* 2007;66(12):1599–1603.
48. Kalke RJ, Di Primio GA, Schweitzer ME. MR and CT arthrography of the knee. *Semin Musculoskelet Radiol.* 2012;16(1):57–68.
49. Juhl C, Christensen R, Roos EM, et al. Impact of exercise type and dose on pain and disability in knee osteoarthritis: a systematic review and meta-regression analysis of randomized controlled trials. *Arthritis Rheumatol.* 2014;66(3):622–636.
50. Uthman OA, van der Windt DA, Jordan JL, et al. Exercise for lower limb osteoarthritis: systematic review incorporating trial sequential analysis and network meta-analysis. *BMJ.* 2013;347:f5555.
51. Berkoff DJ, Miller LE, Block JE. Clinical utility of ultrasound guidance for intra-articular knee injections: a review. *Clin Interv Aging.* 2012;7:89–95.
52. Henriksen M, Christensen R, Klokker L, et al. Evaluation of the benefit of corticosteroid injection before exercise therapy in patients with osteoarthritis of the knee: a randomized clinical trial. *JAMA Intern Med.* 2015;175(6):923–930.
53. Bellamy N, Campbell J, Robinson V, et al. Viscosupplementation for the treatment of osteoarthritis of the knee. *Cochrane Database Syst Rev.* 2006;(2):CD005321.
54. Rutjes AW, Jüni P, da Costa BR, et al. Viscosupplementation for osteoarthritis of the knee: a systematic review and meta-analysis. *Ann Intern Med.* 2012;157(3):180–191.
55. Hunter DJ. Viscosupplementation for osteoarthritis of the knee. *N Engl J Med.* 2015;372(11):1040–1047.
56. Laudy AB, Bakker EW, Rekers M, Moen MH. Efficacy of platelet-rich plasma injections in osteoarthritis of the knee: a systematic review and meta-analysis. *Br J Sports Med.* 2015;49(10):657–672.
57. Patel S, Dhillon MS, Aggarwal S, et al. Treatment with platelet-rich plasma is more effective than placebo for knee osteoarthritis: a prospective, double-blind, randomized trial. *Am J Sports Med.* 2013;41(2):356–364.
58. Vaquerizo V, Plasencia MÁ, Arribas I, et al. Comparison of intra-articular injections of plasma rich in growth factors (PRGF-Endoret) versus Durolane hyaluronic acid in the treatment of patients with symptomatic osteoarthritis: a randomized controlled trial. *Arthroscopy.* 2013;29(10):1635–1643.
59. Rabago D, Slattengren A, Zgierska A. Prolotherapy in primary care practice. *Prim Care.* 2010;37(1):65–80.
60. Duivenvoorden T, Brouwer RW, Van raaij TM, et al. Braces and orthoses for treating osteoarthritis of the knee. *Cochrane Database Syst Rev.* 2015;(3):CD004020.
61. Nakajima M, Ono N, Kojima T, Kusunose K. Ulnar entrapment neuropathy along the medial intermuscular septum in the midarm. *Muscle Nerve.* 2009;39(5):707–710.
62. Yeung EW, Yeung SS. A systematic review of interventions to prevent lower limb soft tissue running injuries. *Br J Sports Med.* 2001;35(6):383–389.
63. Yeung SS, Yeung EW, Gillespie LD. Interventions for preventing lower limb soft-tissue running injuries. *Cochrane Database Syst Rev.* 2011;(7):CD001256.
64. Brander V, Stulberg SD. Rehabilitation after hip- and knee-joint replacement. An experience- and evidence-based approach to care. *Am J Phys Med Rehabil.* 2006;85(11 Suppl):S98–118; quiz S119.
65. Carr AJ, Robertsson O, Graves S, et al. Knee replacement. *Lancet.* 2012;379(9823):1331–1340.
66. Suri P, Morgenroth DC, Hunter DJ. Epidemiology of osteoarthritis and associated comorbidities. *PM R.* 2012;4(5 Suppl):S10–S19.
67. Bijlsma JW, Berenbaum F, Lafeber FP. Osteoarthritis: an update with relevance for clinical practice. *Lancet.* 2011;377(9783):2115–2126.
68. Hunter DJ, Guermazi A. Imaging techniques in osteoarthritis. *PM R.* 2012;4(5 Suppl):S68–S74.
69. Saarakkala S, Waris P, Waris V, et al. Diagnostic performance of knee ultrasonography for detecting degenerative changes of articular cartilage. *Osteoarthr Cartil.* 2012;20(5):376–381.
70. Malas FÜ, Kara M, Kaymak B, Akıncı A, Özçakar L. Ultrasonographic evaluation in symptomatic knee osteoarthritis: clinical and radiological correlation. *Int J Rheum Dis.* 2014;17(5):536–540.
71. Richmond J, Hunter D, Irrgang J, et al.; American Academy of Orthopaedic Surgeons. Treatment of osteoarthritis of the knee (non-arthroplasty). *J Am Acad Orthop Surg.* 2009;17(9):591–600.
72. Sisto SA, Malanga G. Osteoarthritis and therapeutic exercise. *Am J Phys Med Rehabil.* 2006;85(11 Suppl):S69–78; quiz S79.
73. Vincent KR, Vincent HK. Resistance exercise for knee osteoarthritis. *PM R.* 2012;4(5 Suppl):S45–S52.
74. Segal NA. Bracing and orthoses: a review of efficacy and mechanical effects for tibiofemoral osteoarthritis. *PM R.* 2012;4(5 Suppl):S89–S96.
75. Clegg DO, Reda DJ, Harris CL, et al. Glucosamine, chondroitin sulfate, and the two in combination for painful knee osteoarthritis. *N Engl J Med.* 2006;354(8):795–808.
76. Cianflocco AJ. Viscosupplementation in patients with osteoarthritis of the knee. *Postgrad Med.* 2013;125(1):97–105.
77. Lai LP, Stitik TP, Foye PM, et al. Use of Platelet-Rich Plasma in Intra-Articular Knee Injections for Osteoarthritis: A Systematic Review. *PM R.* 2015;7(6):637–648.
78. Fulkerson JP. Diagnosis and treatment of patients with patellofemoral pain. *Am J Sports Med.* 2002;30(3):447–456.
79. Taunton JE, Ryan MB, Clement DB, et al. A retrospective case-control analysis of 2002 running injuries. *Br J Sports Med.* 2002;36(2):95–101.
80. Insall JN. *Surgery of the knee.* New York, NY: Churchill Livingstone; 1984:xiv, 828 p., 4 p. of plates.
81. Collado H, Fredericson M. Patellofemoral pain syndrome. *Clin Sports Med.* 2010;29(3):379–398.
82. Post WR. Clinical evaluation of patients with patellofemoral disorders. *Arthroscopy.* 1999;15(8):841–851.
83. Clifton R, Ng CY, Nutton RW. What is the role of lateral retinacular release?. *J Bone Joint Surg Br.* 2010;92(1):1–6.

84. Pihlajamäki HK, Kuikka PI, Leppänen VV, et al. Reliability of clinical findings and magnetic resonance imaging for the diagnosis of chondromalacia patellae. *J Bone Joint Surg Am*. 2010;92(4):927–934.
85. Thomas S, Rupiper D, Stacy GS. Imaging of the patellofemoral joint. *Clin Sports Med*. 2014;33(3):413–436.
86. Koh JL, Stewart C. Patellar instability. *Clin Sports Med*. 2014;33(3):461–476.
87. Bruce WD, Stevens PM. Surgical correction of miserable malalignment syndrome. *J Pediatr Orthop*. 2004;24(4):392–396.
88. Hong E, Kraft MC. Evaluating anterior knee pain. *Med Clin North Am*. 2014;98(4):697–717, xi.
89. Sculco TP. The knee joint in rheumatoid arthritis. *Rheum Dis Clin North Am*. 1998;24(1):143–156.
90. Cheng OT, Souzdalnitski D, Vrooman B, Cheng J. Evidence-based knee injections for the management of arthritis. *Pain Med*. 2012;13(6):740–753.
91. Danoff JR, Moss G, Liabaud B, Geller JA. Total knee arthroplasty considerations in rheumatoid arthritis. *Autoimmune Dis*. 2013;2013:185340.
92. Bencardino JT, Hassankhani A. Calcium pyrophosphate dihydrate crystal deposition disease. *Semin Musculoskelet Radiol*. 2003;7(3):175–185.
93. Rosenthal AK. Update in calcium deposition diseases. *Curr Opin Rheumatol*. 2007;19(2):158–162.
94. Gutierrez M, Di Geso L, Filippucci E, Grassi W. Calcium pyrophosphate crystals detected by ultrasound in patients without radiographic evidence of cartilage calcifications. *J Rheumatol*. 2010;37(12):2602–2603.
95. Grimm NL, Weiss JM, Kessler JI, Aoki SK. Osteochondritis dissecans of the knee: pathoanatomy, epidemiology, and diagnosis. *Clin Sports Med*. 2014;33(2):181–188.
96. Grimm N, Tisano B, Carey J. Three osteochondritis dissecans lesions in one knee: a case report. *Clin Orthop Relat Res*. Apr 2013;471(4):1186–1190.
97. Carey JL, Grimm NL. Treatment algorithm for osteochondritis dissecans of the knee. *Orthop Clin North Am*. 2015;46(1):141–146.
98. Marcheggiani Muccioli GM, Grassi A, Setti S, et al. Conservative treatment of spontaneous osteonecrosis of the knee in the early stage: pulsed electromagnetic fields therapy. *Eur J Radiol*. 2013;82(3):530–537.
99. Breer S, Oheim R, Krause M, et al. Spontaneous osteonecrosis of the knee (SONK). *Knee Surg Sports Traumatol Arthrosc*. 2013;21(2):340–345.
100. Pape D, Seil R, Fritsch E, et al. Prevalence of spontaneous osteonecrosis of the medial femoral condyle in elderly patients. *Knee Surg Sports Traumatol Arthrosc*. 2002;10(4):233–240.
101. Turco VJ, Spinella AJ. Anterolateral dislocation of the head of the fibula in sports. *Am J Sports Med*. 1985;13(4):209–215.
102. Greis PE, Bardana DD, Holmstrom MC, Burks RT. Meniscal injury: I. Basic science and evaluation. *J Am Acad Orthop Surg*. 2002;10(3):168–176.
103. Greis PE, Holmstrom MC, Bardana DD, Burks RT. Meniscal injury: II. Management. *J Am Acad Orthop Surg*. 2002;10(3):177–187.
104. Katz JN, Brophy RH, Chaisson CE, et al. Surgery versus physical therapy for a meniscal tear and osteoarthritis. *N Engl J Med*. 2013;368(18):1675–1684.
105. Sun Y, Jiang Q. Review of discoid meniscus. *Orthop Surg*. 2011;3(4):219–223.
106. Micheo W, Hernández L, Seda C. Evaluation, management, rehabilitation, and prevention of anterior cruciate ligament injury: current concepts. *PM R*. 2010;2(10):935–944.
107. Filbay SR, Culvenor AG, Ackerman IN, et al. Quality of life in anterior cruciate ligament-deficient individuals: a systematic review and meta-analysis. *Br J Sports Med*. 2015;49(16):1033–1041.
108. van Grinsven S, van Cingel RE, Holla CJ, van Loon CJ. Evidence-based rehabilitation following anterior cruciate ligament reconstruction. *Knee Surg Sports Traumatol Arthrosc*. 2010;18(8):1128–1144.
109. Kruse LM, Gray B, Wright RW. Rehabilitation after anterior cruciate ligament reconstruction: a systematic review. *J Bone Joint Surg Am*. 2012;94(19):1737–1748.
110. Hewett TE, Di Stasi SL, Myer GD. Current concepts for injury prevention in athletes after anterior cruciate ligament reconstruction. *Am J Sports Med*. 2013;41(1):216–224.
111. Lee YS, Jung YB. Posterior cruciate ligament: focus on conflicting issues. *Clin Orthop Surg*. 2013;5(4):256–262.
112. Wind WM Jr, Bergfeld JA, Parker RD. Evaluation and treatment of posterior cruciate ligament injuries: revisited. *Am J Sports Med*. 2004;32(7):1765–1775.
113. Levy BA, Stuart MJ, Whelan DB. Posterolateral instability of the knee: evaluation, treatment, results. *Sports Med Arthrosc*. 2010;18(4):254–262.
114. Lunden JB, Bzdusek PJ, Monson JK, et al. Current concepts in the recognition and treatment of posterolateral corner injuries of the knee. *J Orthop Sports Phys Ther*. 2010;40(8):502–516.
115. Ranawat A, Baker CL 3rd, Henry S, Harner CD. Posterolateral corner injury of the knee: evaluation and management. *J Am Acad Orthop Surg*. 2008;16(9):506–518.
116. Paczesny L, Kruczynski J. Medial plica syndrome of the knee: diagnosis with dynamic sonography. *Radiology*. 2009;251(2):439–446.
117. Kent M, Khanduja V. Synovial plicae around the knee. *Knee*. 2010;17(2):97–102.
118. Rennie WJ, Saifuddin A. Pes anserine bursitis: incidence in symptomatic knees and clinical presentation. *Skeletal Radiol*. 2005;34(7):395–398.
119. Uysal F, Akbal A, Gökmen F, et al. Prevalence of pes anserine bursitis in symptomatic osteoarthritis patients: an ultrasonographic prospective study. *Clin Rheumatol*. 2015;34(3):529–533.
120. Yoon HS, Kim SE, Suh YR, et al. Correlation between ultrasonographic findings and the response to corticosteroid injection in pes anserinus tendinobursitis syndrome in knee osteoarthritis patients. *J Korean Med Sci*. 2005;20(1):109–112.
121. Wijdicks CA, Griffith CJ, Johansen S, et al. Injuries to the medial collateral ligament and associated medial structures of the knee. *J Bone Joint Surg Am*. 2010;92(5):1266–1280.
122. Marchant MH Jr, Tibor LM, Sekiya JK, et al. Management of medial-sided knee injuries, part 1: medial collateral ligament. *Am J Sports Med*. 2011;39(5):1102–1113.
123. Jose J, Schallert E, Lesniak B. Sonographically guided therapeutic injection for primary medial (tibial) collateral bursitis. *J Ultrasound Med*. 2011;30(2):257–261.
124. Bicos J, Fulkerson JP, Amis A. Current concepts review: the medial patellofemoral ligament. *Am J Sports Med*. 2007;35(3):484–492.
125. Hensler D, Sillanpaa PJ, Schoettle PB. Medial patellofemoral ligament: anatomy, injury and treatment in the adolescent knee. *Curr Opin Pediatr*. 2014;26(1):70–78.
126. Quarles JD, Hosey RG. Medial and lateral collateral injuries: prognosis and treatment. *Prim Care*. 2004;31(4):957–75, ix.
127. Bahk MS, Cosgarea AJ. Physical examination and imaging of the lateral collateral ligament and posterolateral corner of the knee. *Sports Med Arthrosc*. 2006;14(1):12–19.
128. Olson WR, Rechkemmer L. Popliteus tendinitis. *J Am Podiatr Med Assoc*. 1993;83(9):537–540.
129. Blake SM, Treble NJ. Popliteus tendon tenosynovitis. *Br J Sports Med*. 2005;39(12):e42; discussion e42.
130. Brown TR, Quinn SF, Wensel JP, et al. Diagnosis of popliteus injuries with MR imaging. *Skeletal Radiol*. 1995;24(7):511–514.
131. Guha AR, Gorgees KA, Walker DI. Popliteus tendon rupture: a case report and review of the literature. *Br J Sports Med*. 2003;37(4):358–360.
132. Pfirrmann CW, Jost B, Pirkl C, et al. Quadriceps tendinosis and patellar tendinosis in professional beach volleyball players: sonographic findings in correlation with clinical symptoms. *Eur Radiol*. 2008;18(8):1703–1709.
133. Perfitt JS, Petrie MJ, Blundell CM, Davies MB. Acute quadriceps tendon rupture: a pragmatic approach to diagnostic imaging. *Eur J Orthop Surg Traumatol*. 2014;24(7):1237–1241.
134. Duri ZA, Aichroth PM, Wilkins R, Jones J. Patellar tendonitis and anterior knee pain. *Am J Knee Surg*. 1999;12(2):99–108.
135. Nanos KN, Malanga GA. Treatment of Patellar Tendinopathy Refractory to Surgical Management Using Percutaneous Ultrasonic Tenotomy and Platelet-Rich Plasma Injection: A Case Presentation. *PM R*. 2015;7(12):1300–1305.
136. Kimball MJ, Kumar NS, Jakoi AM, Tom JA. Subacute superior patellar pole sleeve fracture. *Am J Orthop*. 2014;43(1):29–32.
137. Kastelec M, Veselko M. Inferior patellar pole avulsion fractures: osteosynthesis compared with pole resection. *J Bone Joint Surg Am*. 2004;86-A(4):696–701.

138. Beaman FD, Peterson JJ. MR imaging of cysts, ganglia, and bursae about the knee. *Magn Reson Imaging Clin N Am*. 2007;15(1):39–52.
139. Resnick D, Kang HS, Pretterklieber ML. *Internal derangements of joints*. 2nd ed. Philadelphia, PA: Saunders/Elsevier; 2007.
140. Dye SF, Campagna-Pinto D, Dye CC, et al. Soft-tissue anatomy anterior to the human patella. *J Bone Joint Surg Am*. 2003;85-A(6):1012–1017.
141. Paulos LE, Wnorowski DC, Greenwald AE. Infrapatellar contracture syndrome. Diagnosis, treatment, and long-term followup. *Am J Sports Med*. 1994;22(4):440–449.
142. Kumar D, Alvand A, Beacon JP. Impingement of infrapatellar fat pad (Hoffa's disease): results of high-portal arthroscopic resection. *Arthroscopy*. 2007;23(11):1180–1186.e1.
143. Nouri H, Ben Hmida F, Ouertatani M, et al. Tumour-like lesions of the infrapatellar fat pad. *Knee Surg Sports Traumatol Arthrosc*. 2010;18(10):1391–1394.
144. Coleman HM, Simmons EH, Barrington TW. Torsion of the infrapatellar fat pad. *J Bone Joint Surg Br*. 1964;46:740–743.
145. Comert RB, Aydingoz U, Atay OA, et al. Vascular malformation in the infrapatellar (Hoffa's) fat pad. *Knee*. 2004;11(2):137–140.
146. Jacobson JA, Lenchik L, Ruhoy MK, et al. MR imaging of the infrapatellar fat pad of Hoffa. *Radiographics*. 1997;17(3):675–691.
147. O'Keeffe SA, Hogan BA, Eustace SJ, Kavanagh EC. Overuse injuries of the knee. *Magn Reson Imaging Clin N Am*. 2009;17(4):725–39, vii.
148. Launay F. Sports-related overuse injuries in children. *Orthop Traumatol Surg Res*. 2015;101(1 Suppl):S139–S147.
149. Ehara S. Potentially symptomatic fabella: MR imaging review. *Jpn J Radiol*. 2014;32(1):1–5.
150. Wright LB, Matchett WJ, Cruz CP, et al. Popliteal artery disease: diagnosis and treatment. *Radiographics*. 2004;24(2):467–479.
151. Worth RM, Kettelkamp DB, Defalque RJ, Duane KU. Saphenous nerve entrapment. A cause of medial knee pain. *Am J Sports Med*. 1984;12(1):80–81.
152. Le Corroller T, Lagier A, Pirro N, Champsaur P. Anatomical study of the infrapatellar branch of the saphenous nerve using ultrasonography. *Muscle Nerve*. 2011;44(1):50–54.
153. Morganti CM, McFarland EG, Cosgarea AJ. Saphenous neuritis: a poorly understood cause of medial knee pain. *J Am Acad Orthop Surg*. 2002;10(2):130–137.
154. Kachar SM, Williams KM, Finn HA. Neuroma of the infrapatellar branch of the saphenous nerve a cause of reversible knee stiffness after total knee arthroplasty. *J Arthroplasty*. 2008;23(6):927–930.
155. Donovan A, Rosenberg ZS, Cavalcanti CF. MR imaging of entrapment neuropathies of the lower extremity. Part 2. The knee, leg, ankle, and foot. *Radiographics*. 2010;30(4):1001–1019.
156. Rousseau E. The anterior recurrent peroneal nerve entrapment syndrome: a patellar tendinopathy differential diagnosis case report. *Man Ther*. 2013;18(6):611–614.
157. Møller BN, Kadin S. Entrapment of the common peroneal nerve. *Am J Sports Med*. 1987;15(1):90–91.

CHAPTER 9

Leg

EPIDEMIOLOGY OF LEG PAIN

LEG PAIN IN THE GENERAL POPULATION (1)

Leg discomfort
- Common complaints in elderly population (up to two-thirds in some studies)
- Varying characterization by patients: cramps, heaviness, shooting pains etc.

Associated conditions
- Often related to knee pain, radiating neuropathic pain (sciatic pain), and referred pain from other locations

LEG PAIN IN ATHLETES

Prevalence
- Common, up to 80% of athletes experience chronic leg pain at some point (2)
- Lower leg overuse injuries comprise 10% of all overuse injuries in athletes; higher in older athletes and with weight-bearing sports

Common causes
- Chronic exertional compartment syndrome (CECS; most common cause of exercise-induced anterior leg pain)
- Medial tibial stress syndrome (MTSS; shin splint)—5% of all athletic injuries, and stress fracture of tibia and fibula (less than half of all musculoskeletal injuries)

DIFFERENTIAL DIAGNOSIS

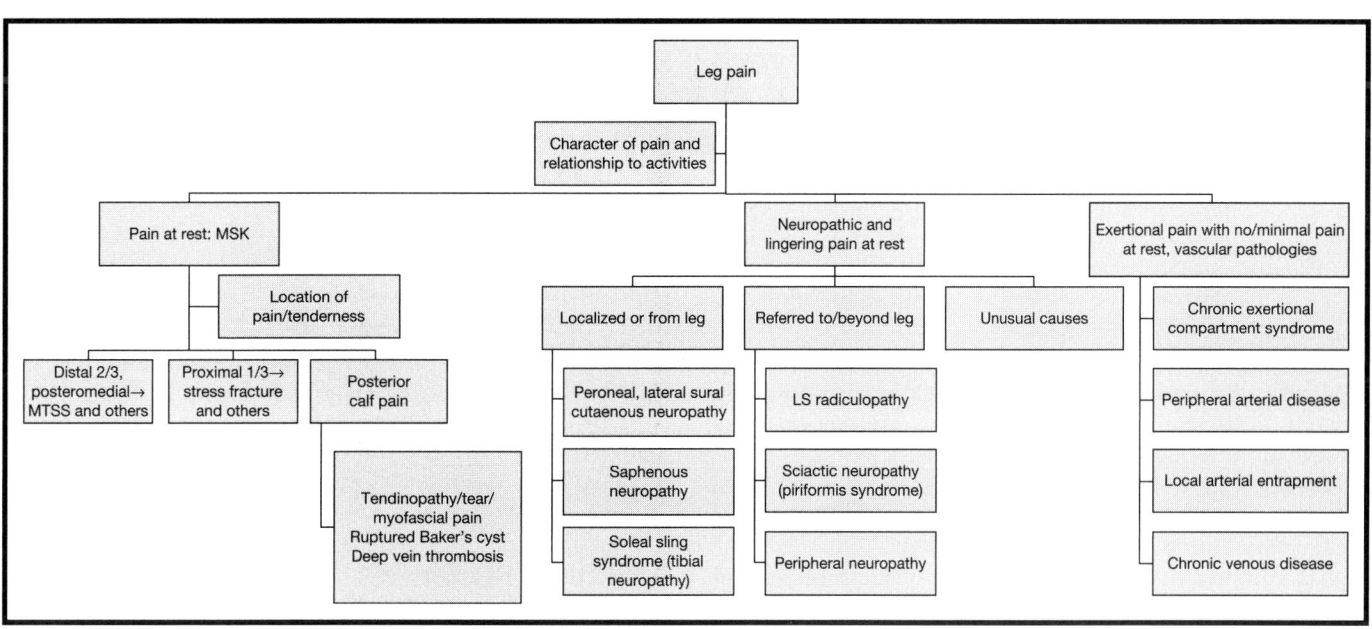

FLOWCHART 9.1
Differential diagnosis of leg pain.
LS, lumbosacral; MSK, musculoskeletal; MTSS, medial tibial stress syndrome.

DIFFERENTIAL DIAGNOSES BASED ON LOCATION OF PAIN (FLOWCHART 9.1)

POSTERIOR LEG (CALF) PAIN	ANTERIOR LEG (SHIN/TIBIA) PAIN
Muscle and tendon • Medial gastrocnemius tear (tennis leg) • Achilles tightness/tendinopathy • Myofascial pain syndrome • Compartment syndrome (deep posterior) • Muscle infarct: diabetic muscle infarct Nerve • Referred to leg: spinal stenosis (neurogenic claudication), radiculopathy (L5–S1 roots), sciatic neuropathy (piriformis syndrome) • Local nerve compression (tibial nerve entrapment; soleal sling syndrome) Vessels • Artery: arterial insufficiency (femoral or popliteal arteries), entrapment of arteries (popliteal or external iliac arteries) • Vein: DVT, postphlebitic syndrome Others • Ruptured Baker's cyst • Tumor, infection (cellulitis), or fracture	Bone • Stress fracture • Tumor, infection (osteomyelitis) Muscles and tendons • Chronic compartment syndrome (the anterior compartment) • Fascial defect/herniation (with/without superficial peroneal N irritation) Nerves • Referred to leg: radiculopathy (L4–L5 roots), saphenous neuropathy • Peripheral nerve entrapment (lateral sural cutaneous, superficial peroneal nerves) Vessels (more common etiology in posterior leg pain than anterior leg) • DVT • Entrapment of arteries (popliteal or external iliac arteries)

DVT, deep vein thrombosis; N, nerve.

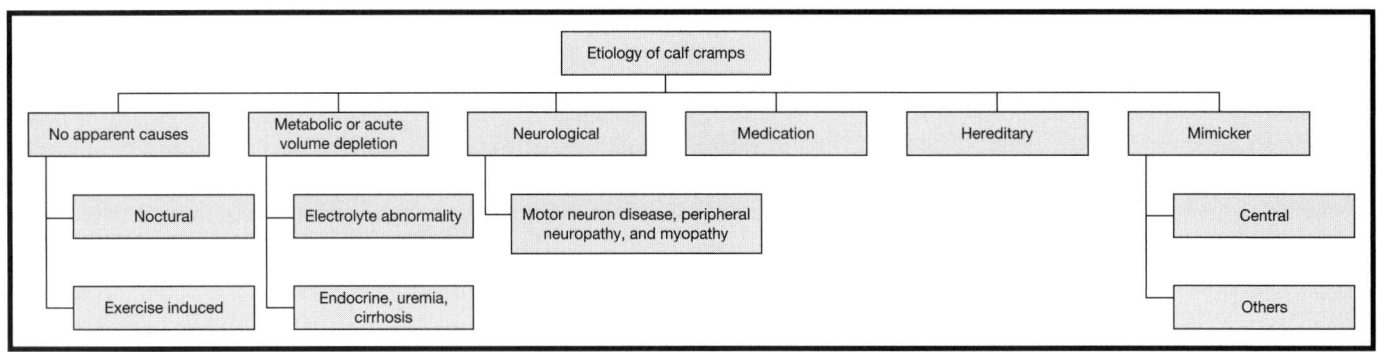

FLOWCHART 9.2
Underlying causes of calf cramps.

DIFFERENTIAL DIAGNOSIS OF CALF PAIN AND CRAMPS (FLOWCHART 9.2)

- Calf cramps (3)
  ○ Definition of cramps: sudden involuntary, painful contractions of skeletal muscles
  ○ Occurs in 30% to 95% of the general population
- Muscle strain, ischemic or neuropathic claudication, restless leg syndrome, Parkinson's disease, multiple sclerosis, dystonias, and nocturnal myoclonus (4)
- Paraphysiologic (occasional cramps that occur in otherwise healthy patients); seen during sports activity or during pregnancy
  ○ Cramps during exercise (recurrent)
    ▪ Common causes: serum deficit of magnesium and on medications
    ▪ Other causes of cramps: diabetes mellitus, hypothyroidism, vascular disorders, metabolic myopathy, radiculoneuropathy
- Metabolic: uremia (dialysis), hypothyroidism, hypovolemic hyponatremia (excess perspiration or "heat cramps," diarrhea, vomiting, diuretic therapy), hypomagnesemia, hypocalcemia, hypoadrenalism, cirrhosis
- Neurologic
  ○ Peripheral nervous system: motor neuron disease, acute poliomyelitis, radiculopathy, peripheral neuropathies and syndromes associated with antibodies to voltage-gated K^+ channels (eg, neuromyotonia) (5)
- Muscle disease: inflammatory myopathies, metabolic, mitochondrial, endocrine myopathy, dystrophinopathies, and myotonia
- Medications/toxins/supplements: inhaled long-acting β2 agonist, K^+ sparing and thiazide diuretics, cimetidine, statin medications, lithium, alcohol, Ca^{2+} channel blockers, creatine, and oral contraceptives

DIFFERENTIAL DIAGNOSIS OF LEG SWELLING (6)

Unilateral
- Acute (<72 hours): deep vein thrombosis (DVT; MC), ruptured Baker's cyst, compartment syndrome, ruptured medial head of gastrocnemius
- Chronic: venous insufficiency (MC), secondary lymphedema (tumor, radiation, surgery, infection), pelvic tumor/mass, or reflex sympathetic dystrophy

Bilateral
- Acute: acute worsening of systemic cause (heart failure or renal disease)
- Chronic: venous insufficiency, pulmonary hypertension, heart failure, idiopathic edema, lymphedema, drugs, premenstrual edema, pregnancy, lipedema, renal disease, and liver disease

DIFFERENTIAL DIAGNOSIS OF ATROPHY AND PSEUDOHYPERTROPHY

Ipsilateral calf atrophy (7)
- S1 radiculopathy, tethered cord or meningomyelocele, chronic sciatic neuropathy/tibial neuropathy, motor neuron disease (amyotrophic lateral sclerosis [ALS], progressive muscular atrophy, Kennedy disease), peripheral neuropathy (multifocal motor neuropathy, diabetic amyotrophy), myopathy (Miyoshi, inclusion body myositis), benign focal amyotrophy, and so on.

Peroneal pseudohypertrophy
- Hereditary sensory motor neuropathy (Charcot Marie Tooth), spinal muscular atrophy, muscular dystrophy (Duchenne or Becker type), and myopathies

DIFFERENTIAL DIAGNOSIS OF COMMON TIBIAL DEFORMITY

Tibial torsion
- Medial or lateral tibial torsion (rotation)
- Medial (intoeing): femoral anteversion, metatarsus adductus, or foot deformity
- Lateral tibial rotation: normal developmental finding during childhood

Bowing leg
- Anterolateral bowing: frequently associated with dysplasia of the tibia leading to pathologic fractures and pseudoarthrosis, although a benign form also exists
  - Neurofibromatosis type 1 present in ~50% of patients with anterolateral bowing
- Posteromedial bowing: usually benign
- Anteromedial bowing: associated with fibular hemimelia (congenital fibular aplasia or hypoplasia)

OTHER HISTORY TO ASK

- Onset: acute (vascular, trauma > inflammatory) versus gradual (musculoskeletal, nerve entrapment)
- Associated precipitating or aggravating activities
- Details of training regimen: any recent change in type/intensity of training, distance of running, or sports activity (lower extremity weight bearing activity, or jumping sports)
  - Abrupt increase in activity can lead to overuse or stress injury
- Duration of pain/timing of pain and relief after the cessation of the activity
  - Time until pain resolution is faster in vascular etiologies compared to neuropathic and musculoskeletal etiologies, in which pain is often persistent or presents after the inciting activity
- Female athletic triads: inadequate nutritional status, amenorrhea or oligomenorrhea, osteoporosis, and excessively thin/lean (8)
- Claudication

	VASCULAR CLAUDICATION	NEUROGENIC CLAUDICATION
Triggered/aggravated by	Increased vascular demand/inadequate vascular supply	Lumbar extension/lateral flexion
Relieved by	Rest	Lumbar flexion
Effect of walking on pain	Pain occurs after fixed amount of exertion	Pain after variable amount of exertion
Effect of resting on pain	Immediate relief of pain after stop	Continued lingering pain

ANATOMY

CROSS-SECTIONAL ANATOMY

Bony and cross-sectional anatomy of the leg (9) (see Figure 1.5B)

BONES

Tibia
- Main weight-bearing structure, stress reaction to the loading
- The tibial plateau, tibial tubercle, tibial eminence, proximal tibia, tibial shaft (narrowest at junction of middle and distal third), and tibial plafond distally
- Superficial location of the bone (subcutaneous in the anterior–medial aspect): predispose to open fracture

Fibular
- Not directly involved in transmission of weight

Superior and inferior tibiofibular joint
- (See Chapters 8 and 10; knee and ankle) with interosseous membrane to bind tibia and fibula

MUSCLES

MUSCLE	ORIGIN	INSERTION	INNERVATION	ACTION	COMMENT
Ankle Dorsiflexors					
Tibialis anterior	Lateral condyle, upper 2/3 of tibia, interosseus membrane (IOM)	Medial cuneiform and 1st MT	Deep peroneal L4, L5	Inversion at subtalar and transverse tarsal joints (Jt.)	L4 innervated muscle below knee
Extensor digitorum longus (EDL)	Lateral condyle of the tibia, proximal 3/4 of fibular and IOM	Mid and distal phalanges of toes 2–5 via extensor expansion	Deep peroneal L5, S1	Extends lateral four toes, dorsiflex the ankle synergistically with other anterior compartment muscle	
Extensor hallacus longus (EHL)	Anteromedial fibular and IOM	Dostal phalange of big toe	Deep peroneal L5 >S1	Extends the hallux, dorsiflex the foot. Contribute to inversion	
Peroneus tertius	Shaft of fibula and interosseous membrane	Base of 5th metatarsal	Deep peroneal L5, S1	Dorsiflexes foot; evertion of foot at subtalar and transverse tarsal joints	
Peroneus brevis	Distal fibula	5th metatarsal	Superficial peroneal L5, S1	Eversion	
Ankle Plantar Flexors					
Peroneus longus	Fibular head and upper fibula	Medial cuneiform and 1st metatarsal	Superficial peroneal L5, S1	Eversion. First ray of foot plantar flexion	Transverse arch support
Gastrocnemius	Medial/lateral condyle of femur	Calcaneus	Tibial Lateral (L5, S1) Medial (S1, S2)	Knee flexion and ankle plantar flexion	Hindfoot invertor Evertor in pronated foot
Soleus	Proximal tibia, fibula and IOM	Calcaneus	Tibial S1, S2	Ankle plantar flexion without knee flexion	
Plantaris	Above the lateral condyle (supracondylar ridge)	Calcaneus (medial to the Achilles tendon)	Tibial S1, S2	Assist in knee flexion and ankle plantar flexor	Used for Achilles tendon graft
Popliteus	Lateral condyle of femur	Shaft of tibia	Tibial, L5–S1	Flexes leg; unlocks full extension of knee by laterally rotating femur on tibia (with standing)	
Tibialis posterior	Shafts of tibia and fibula and interosseous membrane	The navicular tuberosity, all cuneiforms, the cuboid, the bases of the 2nd to 4th metatarsals	L5 >S1	Plantar flexes foot; inverts foot at subtalar and transverse tarsal joints	Supports medial longitudinal arch of foot, MC cause of acquired flatfoot
Flexor hallucis longus (FHL)	Mid third of fibular, IOM	Distal phalange of the big toe	Tibial L5, S1	Flex big toe. Weak ankle plantar flexor	Active contributor to the longitudinal foot arch during toe off and tip toe movement
Flexor digitorum longus (FDL)	Posterior tibia	Distal phalanges of the 2nd to 5th toe	Tibial L5, S1	Flex lateral 4 toes. Contribute to stabilize the heads of the metatarsals on standing and walking	

Jt., joint; MC, most common; MT, metatarsal.

PHYSICAL EXAMINATION

INSPECTION

Atrophy, edema, deformity, erythema/ecchymosis, wound, hyperpigmentation, and the like
- Deformity: usually developmental but also occurs secondary to posttraumatic sequelae
  - Medial tibial torsion: check femoral anteversion, and foot/ankle inspection
- Edema
  - Hyperpigmentation in the medial ankle (hemosiderin deposition) and pitting edema: venous insufficiency
  - Kaposi–Stemmer sign: inability to pinch a fold of skin on the dorsum of the second toe; lymphedema
- Ecchymosis, focal swelling (hematoma), or mild depression/palpable deficits in muscles occurs with massive muscle tear (MC)

PALPATION

Tibial crest and muscles (anterior, lateral, and posterior)

Evaluate for masses (eg, lipoma, muscle herniation, or bony protuberance or mass)

	MTSS	STRESS FRACTURE	EXERTIONAL COMPARTMENT SYNDROME
Palpation tenderness	Diffuse (distal)	Focal, proximal two third	±
Edema/warmth	Negative	±	Negative
Percussion pain	Negative	Positive	Negative
Distant percussion pain	Negative	Positive	Negative
Neurovascular examination	Normal	Normal	±
Painful ROM	±	±	Negative

MTSS, medial tibial stress syndrome; ROM, range of motion.
Source: From Ref. (10). Kortebein PM, Kaufman KR, Basford JR, Stuart MJ. Medial tibial stress syndrome. *Med Sci Sports Exerc.* 2000;32(3 Suppl):S27–S33.

Palpate arterial pulses with knee in extension and flexion (arterial entrapment syndrome)
- Absence of both dorsal pedal and posterior tibial pulses strongly suggests peripheral arterial disease (PAD), whereas presence of either pulse suggests PAD is less likely

NEUROLOGICAL EXAMINATION

Motor examination
- Check ankle dorsiflexion, plantar flexion, eversion, inversion, and knee flexion (gastrocnemius)

Sensory examination
- Evaluate both dermatomal and peripheral nerve distributions
- Peripheral nerve distributions
  - Proximal lateral calf: lateral sural cutaneous nerve, branches from common peroneal nerve
  - Proximal medial leg: saphenous nerve
  - Distal anterior: superficial peroneal nerve
  - Distal posterior: sural nerve

Palpate over areas of scarring or percuss over common entrapment site to check reproduction of paresthesia or pain in the distribution of peripheral nerves (Tinel sign or Valleix's phenomenon)

Evaluate sensory symptoms in relation to the inciting activity

EVALUATION OF FOOT FOR PES PLANUS (OVERPRONATION) AND PES CAVUS (WITH SUPINATION)

Overpronation
- Evaluate hindfoot valgus, tibial internal rotation, tight Achilles tendon (gastrocnemius), and genu valgum
- Frequently encountered in Achilles tendinopathy, MTSS, tibialis posterior tendon dysfunction

Oversupination
- Evaluate hindfoot varus, tibial external rotation, and genu varum
- Frequently encountered in overloading of lateral compartment (peroneus longus and brevis) or proximal tibiofibular joint dysfunction and creates risk of stress related bony injury

DIAGNOSTIC STUDIES

PLAIN RADIOGRAPHS

- Generally the first diagnostic imaging modality used for lower leg pain (11) (Flowchart 9.3)
- Specific for fractures if fracture line or displaced fracture is present

Limitations
- Insensitive for early-stress–related bony injuries: may need to repeat in 2 weeks or MRI if suspicious

Bone scan
- Sensitive for early bony injury but is not specific

MRI

- Imaging modality of choice for leg pain
- Fat-suppressed fluid-sensitive sequences (T2-weighted, proton density): best for detecting edema
- T1-weighted images: used for better depiction of anatomy, muscle atrophy, fatty infiltration
- Marrow edema: intermediate or low signal intensity in T1-weighted and high signal intensity on fat-suppressed fluid-sensitive sequences
- Muscle edema (eg, in compartment syndrome): high signal intensity on T2-weighted sequences

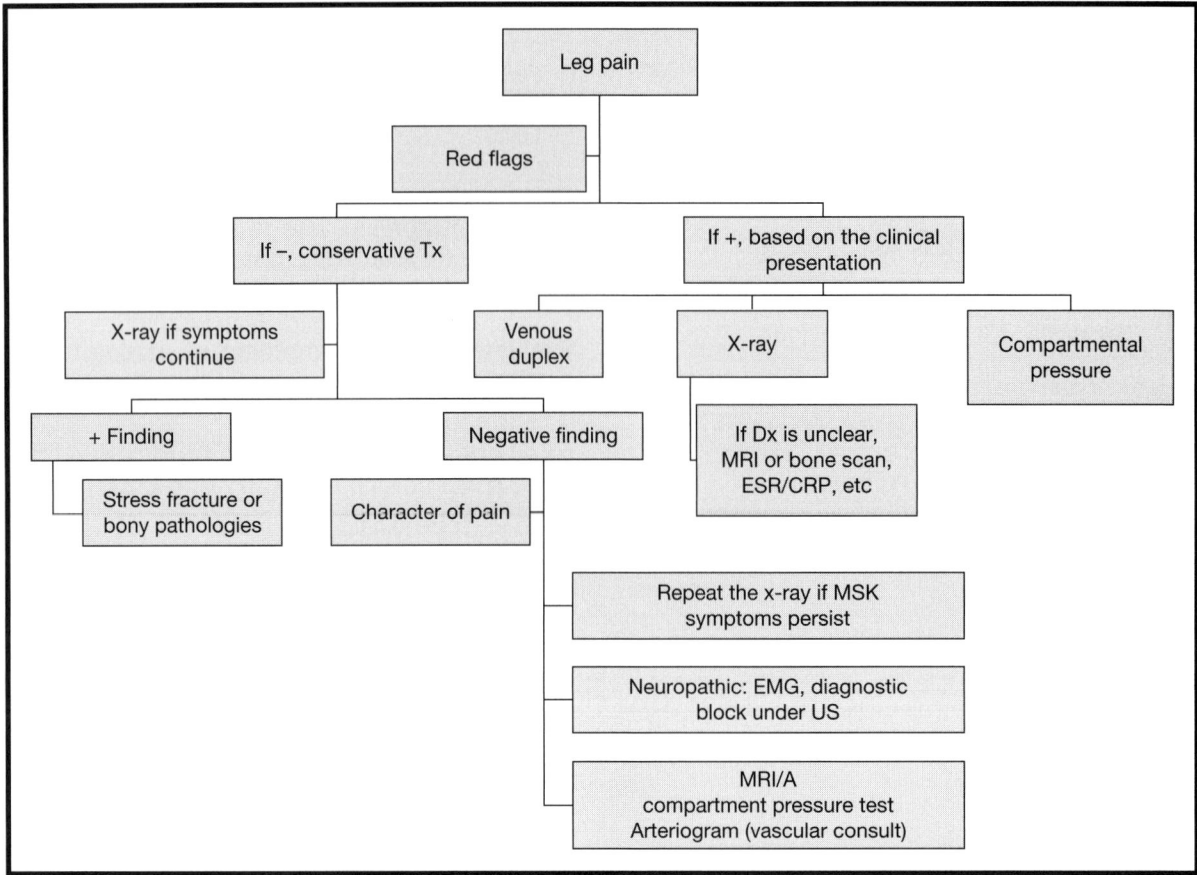

FLOWCHART 9.3
Diagnostic workup for leg pain in an outpatient clinic.
CRP, C-reactive protein; Dx, diagnosis; EMG, electromyography; ESR, erythrocyte sedimentation rate; Tx, treatment; US, ultrasound.
Source: Adapted from Ref. (12). Edwards PH, Jr, Wright ML, Hartman JF. A practical approach for the differential diagnosis of chronic leg pain in the athlete. *Am J Sports Med.* 2005;33(8):1241–1249.

POINT-OF-CARE ULTRASONOGRAPHY (US)

Indications
- Diagnostic evaluation of acute tendon or muscle injury or tear, tendinosis; anatomical evaluation of nerve trunk
- Needle guidance for injections

Advantages
- Allows for dynamic maneuvers/evaluation, such as evaluation of muscle/tendon impingement (rotator cuff), tendon instability, or muscle herniation (occurs upto 40% in CECS)

Limitations
- Operator dependant, inadequate penetration/resolution of deep structures
- Intracortical (marrow) lesion: tumor, cyst, osteochondritis dissecans, avascular necrosis

CT SCAN

- Useful in differentiating stress reactions from stress fracture versus other bony abnormalities
- Able to detect osseus cortical findings as osteopenia, resorption cavities, and striations
- Limitations: insensitive in the early stages of bony stress injury (normal). Unable to detect cancellous bone marrow edema or bone bruise

VASCULAR STUDY AND OTHER TESTS

Venous studies: venous duplex to rule out DVT

Arterial studies: ankle brachial index (ABI), duplex US, and angiography (CT or MR angiography) used to evaluate PAD
- ABI: systolic blood pressure (SBP) in ankle divided by SBP in arm, correlates well with findings on angiography. ABI values ≤0.9; PAD >1.4; noncompressible/calcified vessels

Compartment pressure study: gold standard for CECS

TREATMENT

NONOPERATIVE MANAGEMENT

General guidelines
- Initial relative rest (from prolonged lower extremities weight bearing or any symptom provocation activities and/or decreasing activity duration depending on the condition) with use of modalities (eg, therapeutic US) as needed, and gradual return to exercise as symptoms improve

- Maintain upper extremity endurance exercise during period of recovery
- Water based exercise often useful for maintaining limited weight bearing
- Cross-training can be considered after initial rest period
• Clarify weight-bearing status (on specific condition, based on follow-up imaging)
• Identify biomechanical culprit in overuse injury
- Intervene faulty biomechanics, for example, pes planus (hindfoot eversion), hyperpronation, tight Achilles cord (gastrocnemius), pes cavus (hindfoot inversion) with appropriate foot orthotics: heel lift, medial or lateral heel wedge
- Footwear education: for example, roomier (wider and longer) shoe with higher toe box
  ▪ Clarify utility and proper fit of anti-supinator and anti-pronator shoe options; patient often confused.
  ▪ For example, anti-pronator (medial hindfoot reinforcement) shoes will aggravate pain from peroneal tendinopathy due to resultant varus positioning of hindfoot

Therapeutic exercises
• Stretching of gastrocnemius (Achilles stretching with neutral subtalar placement), hamstring (knee extension and flexion), flexor hallucis longus (FHL), and flexor digitorum longus (FDL; stretch with toe dorsiflexion)
• Evaluation of proximal (knee and hip) and distal segment (foot and ankle) deformity: assessment of biomechanics and address it
• Aerobic endurance exercise (upper body ergometer) to avoid deconditioning

Oral medication
• First line: acetaminophen, nonsteroidal anti-inflammatory drugs (NSAIDs), and/or short duration of muscle relaxant
• Second line: weak opioid medications

Orthotic
• Check foot and ankle orthoses part

Injection
• Trigger point injection with lidocaine ± steroid injection used for myofascial pain syndrome and fascial tear
• Cutaneous nerve block (sural, saphenous nerve, and superficial peroneal nerve) used most often for focal entrapment neuropathy or neuroma
- Can be used as an adjunct treatment for complex regional pain syndrome (superficial peroneal nerve and posterior tibial nerve blocks) or diffuse pain syndrome
• Botox for exertional compartment syndrome (13)

MUSCULOSKELETAL PATHOLOGY

MEDIAL TIBIAL STRESS SYNDROME

Introduction (10)
• Commonly used definition: pain and tenderness along the posteromedial border of the tibia resulting from exercise (14)
- Traction induced periostitis of tibia secondary to dysfunction of the tibialis posterior, FDL, and medial soleus
- Excess tibial stress results in remodeling of the tibial cortex with resultant osteopenia
• Common in physically active population; 4% to 35% depending on the studies

Etiology and risk factors (15)
• Increased hindfoot (calcaneal) eversion and pes planus (tibialis posterior dysfunction results in a biomechanical disadvantage)
• Weakness or inflexibility/tightness of the calf muscle (gastrocnemius) results in impaired biomechanics and diminished shock absorption capability

History and physical examination
• Intermittent or continuous pain on the medial side of the lower leg
- Described as dull or intense and is exacerbated by repetitive weight-bearing activity
• Tenderness over the distal two-thirds of the posterior medial tibial crest
• Reproduction of tibial pain/symptoms on provocative maneuvers (not specific)
- Passive ankle dorsiflexion and active ankle plantar flexion against resistance
- Bilateral or unilateral standing toe raises and jumping

Diagnosis
• Clinically diagnosed with imaging study to rule out other etiologies
• Imaging studies
- X-ray to rule out stress fracture (may have to repeat in 1–2 weeks)
- Bone scan: may be positive in MTSS and stress fractures
- MRI: equivocal in MTSS. Positive in stress fracture and chronic compartment syndrome
• Compartmental pressure testing for evaluation for chronic compartment syndrome

Treatment (14)
• Ice, NSAIDs, activity modification, tibialis posterior strengthening, closed kinetic chain functional exercise, and graded running program of interval training with increasing duration and intensity
• Custom made foot insole can be considered in pes planus (16,17)
• Extracorporeal shockwave therapy has been shown to result in a faster return to running (18)

CHRONIC EXERTIONAL COMPARTMENT SYNDROME (CECS)

Introduction (19)
• Reversible ischemia occurring secondary to a noncompliant osseofascial compartment that is unaccommodating to the expansion of muscle volume that occurs with exercise
• Location: most commonly in anterior compartment (45%), followed by deep posterior (40%), lateral (10%), and superficial posterior (5%)
- Occurs bilaterally in 75% to 90% of cases

- Female > male and mean age of presentation: 20 years old
- Etiology and risk factors (20)
  - Aberrant biomechanics (rear foot landing or overpronation)
  - Anabolic steroid and creatine use
  - Training errors with excessive eccentric exercise

History and physical examination
- Recurrent exercise-induced leg discomfort occurring at a well defined and reproducible point in the run or training time (gradual onset of discomfort)
  - Characterized as tight, cramp-like, or squeezing pain
  - Relief of pain with discontinuation of inciting activity
- Often accompanied by nerve irritation (superficial peroneal nerve in the anterolateral compartment, tibial nerve in the deep posterior compartment)
- Physical examination: muscle firmness and tenderness to palpation and pain with passive stretching of the muscle
- Foot overpronation or possible weakness of involved muscle (not striking)
- Muscle herniation (through facial defects) may be noted on examination in 40% to 60% of cases (commonly in anterior compartment)

Diagnosis
- Clinical suspicion confirmed by intracompartmental pressure measurement criteria as noted in the following. Application of these criteria with a history suggestive of CECS: <5% false-positive rate in the diagnosis of CECS (21)
  - Pressure value interpretation by Stryker intracompartmental pressure monitor:
    - 0 to 8 mmHg: normal; 30 to 50 mmHg: equivocal; >50 mmHg: surgical emergency
  - Three criteria by Pedowitz et al. (22)
    - Pre-exercise resting intracompartmental pressure: ≥15 mmHg
    - 1-minute postexercise pressure: ≥30 mmHg
    - 5-minute postexercise pressure: ≥20 mmHg
  - Intracompartmental pressure increase >10 mmHg from baseline pressure with exercise
- Differential diagnosis
  - Stress fracture: commonly coexist (up to 30%)
  - MTSS, periosteitis or tenosynovitis/tendonitis
  - Nerve entrapment, lumbosacral (LS) radiculopathy, or neurogenic claudication
  - DVT, vascular claudication, or popliteal artery entrapment
  - Infection, myopathy, or tumor

Treatment
- Conservative treatments
  - Limit activities to the level of minimal symptom, NSAIDs, soft tissue release, stretching and strengthening, and foot orthotic (for overpronation)
  - Forefoot running (23), gradual increase (no greater than 10%/wk) in duration and intensity
  - Heel lift and medial wedge if significant Achilles tightness present or pes planus
  - Botox injection (13); good pain relief and mild weakness without functional decline
- Surgical fasciotomy: indicated for persistent symptoms despite 6 to 12 weeks of conservative treatment
  - Endoscopic release site should be distal from location where superficial peroneal perforates the fascia (7–10 cm above ankle)
  - Success rate greater than 80% for anterior/lateral and 50% for posterior compartment fasciotomies
  - Complications occur in about 10% of surgeries
    - Females are generally less responsive to fasciotomy compared to males
  - Postoperatively, return to activity as soon as possible is recommended with no limitation of activity

STRESS FRACTURE (OF TIBIA)

Introduction (24)
- Most common location of stress fracture is the tibia (50% of stress fracture in athletes). Posteromedial tibia is the most common location within tibia
  - Anteromedial tibial stress fractures result from tension type stress and have a high risk for nonunion. Posteromedial tibial stress fractures present like shin splints
  - High risk of delayed healing and nonunion
- Risk factors: young and healthy adults who participate in activities that involve significant amounts of walking, running, or jumping such as seen in certain sports (most commonly in running, though also seen in dancers and basketball and soccer players) and military recruits, impaired bone mineralization

History and physical examination
- Little discomfort even in the setting of nonunion
- Gradually progressive (weeks to months) anterior leg pain or vague discomfort that occurs with activities
- Localized tenderness, swelling, and palpable callus
  - Percussion of the bone away from the site of the fracture may produce the pain

Diagnosis
- Clinical suspicion (suggestive history and examination) confirmed by imaging study
- X-ray: negative for first 2 to 3 weeks. Findings suggestive of stress fractures include evidence of a periosteal reaction, cortical thickening, sclerosis, or a true fracture line
  - "Dreaded black line" refers to a transverse fracture line in the anterior tibial shaft
- MRI: grading of tibial stress injuries (25)
  - Grade 1: periosteal edema on fat-suppressed T2 images (shin splints)
  - Grade 2: grade 1 + marrow edema on fat-suppressed T2 images
  - Grade 3: grade 2 + marrow edema on T1 images
  - Grade 4: grade 3 + clearly visible fracture line
- Differential diagnosis
  - MTSS: relief of symptoms with rest or daily ambulation, pain is nonfocal, shorter time course to symptom onset, rarely cause proximal tibial pain
  - Stress reaction, muscle strain, and neoplasm
  - CECS

Treatment
- 6 to 8 weeks of non–weight bearing
  - Radiologic union at 3 months and return to play at 4 months (pain and tenderness has to be resolved)

- Typical return-to-running program for a non-elite athlete after the initial period of rest with uncomplicated stress fracture (24)
  - a: Runs on softer surfaces during the initial return-to-running phase
  - b: Nonimpact activity on off days, which can be the same form of cross-training that the athlete was performing before resuming running
  - c: Gradual increase in distance and intensity depending on the runner's goals over 4 to 6 weeks.
    - 1st week: a for 5 minutes → b → 10 minutes → b → 15 minutes → b × 2 days
    - 2nd week: a for 15 minutes → b → 20 minutes → b → 25 minutes → b × 2 days
    - 3rd week: for 25 minutes → 30 minutes → b → 30 minutes → 35 minutes → 40 minutes → b →
    - 4th week: 45 minutes → c
- Anterior tibial fracture may need surgical referral for intramedullary nailing given risk for nonunion
- For improvement of bone mineralization: vitamin D supplementation, improved nutritional intake, and smoking cessation

MEDIAL GASTROCNEMIUS TEAR

Introduction (26,27)
- Medial gastrocnemius tears are a common location of muscle tears in the leg
- "Tennis leg": leg pain caused by tear of the medial gastrocnemius (MC), followed by, in order of decreasing incidence, soleus tear, both gastrocnemius and soleus tears, tears of both heads of gastrocnemius and lastly, plantaris tear
  - Isolated tear of the lateral head of the gastrocnemius occurs in ~15% of cases involving gastrocnemius tears.
- Peak incidence in middle age men

Etiology and mechanism of injury
- Ankle dorsiflexion while the knee is extended, short/abrupt sprints, climbing stairs, sudden forceful eccentric contraction of the muscle (eg, lunging forward by pushing off of leg while in a crouched position as seen commonly in tennis)

History and physical examination
- Sudden intense calf pain, as if the calf has been kicked or struck by a ball or racket followed by swelling, cramping, and discolorization or ecchymosis within 24 hours
- Visible depression of the musculature in distal leg and proximal migration of muscle bulk

Diagnosis
- Clinical diagnosis confirmed by imaging study
- US
  - Common findings
    - Disruption of the normal fiber alignment at the musculotendinous junction
    - Hematoma and fluid collection between the gastrocnemius and soleus muscles
  - Longitudinal views are obtained to evaluate the size and extent of muscle retraction and transverse scans are used to evaluate the degree of tear (partial vs complete tear)
- MRI: helps to further characterize the lesion, distinguish hemorrhage versus hematoma at musculotendinous junction, and evaluate for any concurrent bony pathology (ie, stress fracture and intracortical structure abnormalities)
- Differential diagnosis: ruptured Baker's cyst, hematoma without muscle tear, DVT, plantaris, or Achilles tendon tear and intracortical lesion of the bone

Treatment
- First employ the RICE method
  - *R*est until able to walk without a limp
  - *I*ce, *C*ompression, and *E*levation until swelling subsides
- Initially, also beneficial to use gentle stretch, massage, and cryotherapy
- Pain medications (acetaminophen, NSAIDs) can be used as needed
- One- to two-centimeter heel lift (to decrease calf stretch) initially and/or Unna boot for 2 weeks can help with pain.
  - Three-dimensional (3D) walking boot and crutches can be used in severe strains.
- Progress to eccentric strengthening, heel raises/dropping exercise, proprioception exercises and closed kinetic chain exercises with core and general conditioning
- Running, jumping, and cutting activity can be initiated in 6 to 12 weeks
- Prognosis: benign prognosis with no significant difference in strength compared to the contralateral leg after about 2 years

PLANTARIS TENDON AND SOLEUS MUSCLE TEAR

Introduction (27)
- Rare; even existence of plantaris tendon tear has been disputed in the past
- Plantaris tears occur at the musculotendinous junction (mid-calf level), similar to the gastrocnemius
- Soleus tears occur when the ankle is passively dorsiflexed while the knee is flexed (eg, position of foot landing while uphill running). Tears can occur throughout the extent of the muscle

History and physical examination
- Patients complain of painful weight bearing
- Inspection shows swelling (less than what is seen with other muscle tears) ± ecchymosis
- Pain can be elicited with active dorsiflexion of affected ankle and point tenderness is noted on palpation
- Often difficult to distinguish from gastrocnemius or proximal Achilles tendon injury

Diagnosis
- Clinical suspicion based on history and exam confirmed by imaging study
- US and MRI evidence of fluid between the gastrocnemius and soleus

Treatment
- Similar to the gastrocnemius tendon tear

NEUROPATHY

See the Neuropathy section in Chapter 8 (pages 360–361)

SUPERFICIAL PERONEAL NEUROPATHY

Introduction (28,29)
- Rare, may be underrecognized
- Anatomy: arises from the common peroneal nerve at the neck of the fibula and runs in the lateral leg compartment; 7 to 10 cm above the lateral malleolus, the superficial peroneal nerve pierces the deep fascia and becomes subcutaneous
- Etiology
  - Fascial entrapment at the fascial opening
  - Ankle sprain: inversion and plantar flexion of the foot results in tethering effect of the nerve
  - CECS (in 10% of CECS) with or without muscle herniation
  - Compression from healed midshaft fibular fracture, lipoma, or ganglion cyst (intraneural ganglion) (30)

History and physical examination
- Localized pain ± radiation of pain proximally (anterolateral leg) and distally (dorsum of the foot)
- Subtle weakness with foot eversion and first ray plantar flexion if entrapment occurs proximally at the level of proximal fibula

Diagnosis
- Clinical diagnosis based on history and examination confirmed electrodiagnostically with electromyography (EMG) and nerve conduction studies (NCS); however, results may be normal with mild lesions
- US-guided diagnostic nerve block can also be used if needed to help with diagnosis
- US and MRI are used for visualization of any compressive structural lesions (eg, lipoma, muscle herniation, ganglion cyst [extrinsic or intraneural], or, rarely, nerve tumor)

Treatment (31)
- Diagnostic and therapeutic injection
- Roomier shoe, skipped lace, and lateral wedge (± heel lift) to alleviate symptoms (symptoms are aggravated by hindfoot inversion, which causes peroneal nerve stretching)
- Surgery can be considered for failed conservative management

TIBIAL NEUROPATHY—SOLEAL SLING SYNDROME

Introduction (32)
- Rare but underrecognized cause of tibial nerve entrapment by soleal sling
- The soleal sling is the fibrous sling at the origin of the soleus muscle, which lies between the tibia and fibula, about 9 cm distal to the popliteal crease
  - The soleal sling is the outlet of the deep compartment
- Entrapment of the tibial nerve at the proximal soleal sling can be the cause of "failed" surgical decompression through release at the more distal tarsal tunnel

Etiology of proximal tibial neuropathy (33)
- Soleal sling syndrome
  - Idiopathic (by hypertrophied soleal sling) or secondary soleal sling syndrome from CECS and outlet trauma
- Other proximal tibial neuropathy
  - Popliteus muscle strain/hypertrophy, gastrocnemius hypertrophy, or anomalous band between gastrocnemius heads
  - Baker's cyst, extraneural ganglion cyst, popliteal venous or artery aneurysm
  - Tumor
- Intrinsic compression: nerve tumor, intraneural ganglion cyst
- Iatrogenic: surgery and injections

History and physical examination
- Tingling, and numbness in the plantar aspect of the foot ± pain and tightness in the calf
- Palpation over area of soleal sling (~9 cm below the popliteal crease) elicits pain, reproduction of symptoms, and Tinel's sign

Diagnosis
- Diagnosis is made by high clinical suspicion based on history and exam along with confirmatory findings on imaging and electrodiagnostic studies
  - EMG: often negative, to evaluate other differential diagnosis
- MRI (MR neurography) and possible US-guided diagnostic injection
- Differential diagnosis: L5–S1 radiculopathy, tarsal tunnel syndrome, sciatic neuropathy (piriformis syndrome or mononeuritis)

Treatment
- Trial of steroid injections for diagnostic and therapeutic purpose and Botox injections to the deep posterior compartment under US guidance
- Possible surgical release for cases of failed conservative management

SAPHENOUS NEURITIS

See the Neuropathy section in Chapter 8 (pages 360–361)

LATERAL SURAL CUTANEOUS NEUROPATHY

Introduction
- Very rare, but also underrecognized
- Etiology
  - Entrapment most commonly occurs where the lateral sural cutaneous nerve perforates the deep fascia near the fibular head or may also occur near the biceps femoris muscle (34)
  - Mononeuritis (especially in patients with diabetes mellitus)

History and physical examination
- Lateral calf pain of neuropathic character
- Tenderness and reproduction of pain or paresthesias in the distribution of the nerve with palpation

Diagnosis
- Clinical diagnosis confirmed by EMG, specifically nerve conduction study of the lateral sural cutaneous nerve (often technically difficult) and/or diagnostic nerve block under US guidance

○ Nerve conductions study setup (lateral sural cutaneous nerve): stimulation at 2 cm medial and 4 cm proximal to the fibular head with recording electrode placed 12 cm distal to fibular head
• Differential diagnosis: L5 radiculopathy, sciatic neuropathy, or lateral retinacular neuralgia
• US and MRI are used to evaluate any structural lesions

Treatment
• Transcutaneous electrical nerve stimulation (TENS), topical lidocaine gel and capsaicin gel (if able to tolerate), and desensitization
• US-guided injection and referral to surgery if only temporary responsiveness to injection

VASCULAR PATHOLOGY

ARTERIAL DISEASE

Peripheral Arterial Disease

Introduction (35)
• Prevalence of PAD: 11% to 16% in the populations aged 55 years or older
• Underrecognized by patients and physicians
• Risk factors include: smoking, diabetes > older age > male sex, hypertension, dyslipidemia, hyperhomocysteinemia, race (more common in blacks and other non-white Americans compared to white Americans), and renal insufficiency (36)
• Significant morbidity and mortality
  ○ Acute limb ischemia (ALI): a high mortality rate and significant risk of limb loss; considered a medical emergency
  ○ Chronic limb ischemia: may result in limb amputation within 6 months if left untreated
    ▪ Occurs in less than 5% to 10% of patients with PAD
    ▪ Patients with diabetes are at risk for developing chronic limb ischemia

History and physical examination
• Intermittent claudication (reproducible pain in the lower limbs during exercise relieved by rest), atypical leg pain
  ○ Deconditioning and a decline in function can occur without any pain symptoms: decreased walking velocity, distance, and balance
• Critical limb ischemia: pain in extremity occurs at rest
  ○ Foot pain at rest: worse while supine and improves when the limb is placed in a dependent position
  ○ Nonpositional chronic resting limb pain, ulcers, or gangrene may also be seen
• ALI
  ○ Signs/symptoms of ALI include the five "P's": pain, pallor, paresthesia, pulselessness, and poikilothermia
  ○ May be a form of chronic limb ischemia but is more commonly related to an acute event such as embolism or local thrombosis
• Physical examination
  ○ Skin discoloration (red or dusky purple), pallor, hair loss, cool skin, atrophic nail changes
  ○ Diminished pulses in femoral artery, popliteal artery (if too strong; suspect aneurysm) and/or posterior tibial artery
    ▪ Examination of pulse from the posterior tibial artery is more specific than examination of the dorsalis pedis artery (continuation of the anterior tibial artery)
  ○ Painful ulcers on the toes or lateral malleolus with surrounding cellulitis or gangrene

Diagnosis
• Clinical diagnosis confirmed by vascular study
  ○ ABI: ratio of the SBP in the ankle to SBP in the arm
    ▪ Good screening test for PAD
    ▪ Abnormal if less than 0.9
      – 0.7 to 0.89: mild PAD
      – 0.4 to 0.69: moderate PAD
      – <0.4: severe PAD
  ○ Other noninvasive tests: pulse volume recordings with Doppler, arterial duplex, computed tomography angiography (CTA) or magnetic resonance angiography (MRA) (particularly useful for tibial vessels)
  ○ Digital subtraction arteriography (invasive): the gold standard arterial imaging with improved spatial resolution over CTA and MRA
• Differential diagnosis
  ○ Spinal stenosis, osteoarthritis, peripheral neuropathy, and venous claudication

Treatment
• Nonoperative management
  ○ Antiplatelet agents: aspirin 75 to 325 mg daily, clopidogrel 75 mg daily, cilostazol (phosphodiesterase type 3 inhibitor)
  ○ Statin to lower low density lipoprotein (LDL) <100 mg/dL (can consider target LDL <70 mg/dL if multiple risk factors for PAD are present)
  ○ BP control with use of angiotensin-converting enzyme (ACE) inhibitors (or angiotensin receptor blockers)
  ○ Treatment of diabetes to achieve hemoglobin A_{1C} goal of less than 7.0%
  ○ Smoking cessation, diet control (low fat, sodium, and/or carbohydrates), weight loss, and meticulous foot care
  ○ Exercise training, preferably supervised
    ▪ 30 to 45 minutes of exercise, three times weekly for at least 12 weeks found to increase maximum walking time, pain free walking distance, and maximum walking distance (level 1A evidence)
• Vascular surgery referral: endovascular revascularization in selected cases and surgical revascularization in selected cases

Popliteal Artery Entrapment Syndrome

Introduction (37)
• Uncommon cause of claudication
• Prevalence: occurs in 3.3% of cases of atypical claudication (38), though may be underrecognized
  ○ Peak incidence seen in younger, otherwise healthy populations
• Anatomic entrapment: male > female, mean age: 43 years, sedentary, severe claudication
• Functional entrapment (overuse injection): female > male, mean age: 24 years, physically active (39)

- A common location of entrapment is under the medial head of gastrocnemius (40)

History and physical examination
- Calf pain with exercise, occurs bilaterally in about one-fourth to two-thirds of cases
  - Anterior and posterior leg pain
- Ischemic skin changes: rare
- Numbness and tingling of the foot and paresthesias in the tibial nerve distribution
- Diminished pulse in ankle passive dorsiflexion or active plantar flexion

Diagnosis
- Clinical diagnosis based on history and physical examination confirmed by vascular study
- Dynamic stenosis of the artery: ABI
  - ABI: normal at rest and decreased at one minute exercise
  - Worsening of ABI with knee extension and ankle dorsiflexion (passive) or active ankle plantar flexion
- Duplex US, pulse volume recording, plethysmography, angiography (gold standard, however also invasive), CT angiography, or MRA
- Differential diagnosis: CECS

Treatment
- Referral to vascular surgery for bypass or thromboendarterectomy
  - Bypass surgery is more effective than thromboendarterectomy

Arterial Endofibrosis (of External Iliac Artery [EIA])

Introduction (41)
- Uncommon
- Can cause arterial stenosis in young people without atherosclerosis or inflammatory lesions
- Unknown incidence, underrecognized, 85% unilateral
  - External iliac endofibrosis occurs in one-fifth of competitive cyclists or athletes in other endurance sports that require repetitive hip flexion (cross-country skiing, speed skating, and running)
- MC location: EIA
  - The EIA travels along anterior portion of the psoas muscle (anterior to the hip axis) and provides perforating branches to the psoas
  - Repeated hip flexion and psoas muscle hypertrophy causes EIA to take a serpentine course. EIA then becomes kinked, which results in intimal hyperplasia and arterial stenosis

History and physical examination
- Pain, cramping, tightness, distension, or weakness with near maximal exercise effort; absent in submaximal exercise
  - Unilateral, involves more than three compartments in the lower limb (distal to the stenosis) with resolution of symptoms within 5 minutes of cessation of exercise
  - Worsening of pain with the position
- Physical examination: normal at rest other than bruit (femoral bruits are normal after exercise)

Diagnosis
- Clinical suspicion confirmed by vascular study and imaging study
- Pre- and postexercise ABI
  - Normal pre-exercise ABI (0.9–1.2) with significantly decreased postexercise: ABI ≤0.66 after 1 minute of exercise: 90% sensitivity and 87% specificity
- Ankle SBP difference of 23 mmHg or 1-minute ABI difference >0.18
- Duplex US, MRA, or CT angiography can help identify location and degree of stenosis and may show endofibrotic lesions, arterial kinking, and external compression

Treatment
- Education regarding modification of activity
  - With cycling: more upright posture, avoid the pulling up on the pedals
- Referral to vascular surgery if symptoms persist

Cystic Adventitial Disease

Introduction (41)
- A rare cause of calf claudication, male > female by five times
- Generally occurs in individuals between the ages of 20 to 50 years who have no risk factors for atherosclerotic disease (40)
- Location: large arteries near joints; popliteal artery most commonly affected
- Etiology
  - Repeated minor trauma forming cystic structures in the popliteal artery wall
  - Others (embryological, synovial theory, and others)

History and physical examination
- Intermittent claudication ± rapid progression; rarely rest pain, normal or reduced pulse
- Obliteration of the pulse with rapid flexion of the knee (Ishikawa sign)

Diagnosis
- Clinical suspicion confirmed by vascular study
- ABI (with pulse volume recording) and arterial Doppler flow will show findings of arterial stenosis with surrounding cysts
- CT, MRI, and MRA can differentiate from pseudoaneurysm

Treatment
- Conservative: can resolve by itself, avoid vigorous, repetitive contraction of the calf muscles
- Referral for vascular surgery for angioplasty and grafting with veins

VENOUS DISEASE

Deep Vein Thrombosis

Introduction (42)
- 8% to 15% of calf DVT's progress and extends to popliteal and femoral veins in untreated groups

- Risk factors: immobility, history of DVT, recent/ongoing cancer, trauma to the deep vein (surgery, fracture, or other trauma), pregnancy in 6 weeks postpartum, central venous catheter, >60 years, hormone therapy or birth control pills, smoking, obesity, and inherited coagulation disorders
- Clot usually lysed within 3 to 6 months

History and physical examination
- Pain, heaviness, cramps, and swelling in the lower extremity, particularly in the calf
  - Typically progresses over several days ± sudden blue-red or cyanotic discoloration (uncommon)
- Low grade fever, increased heart rate, calf tenderness
- Homans' sign (pain with the dorsiflexion of the ankle): high negative predictive value, low positive predictive value

Diagnosis
- Clinical suspicion confirmed by vascular study (venous duplex)
- D-dimer: used to rule out DVT
  - If negative D-dimer with unlikely clinical presentation, no need for US study (43)

Treatment (44)
- Send the patient to emergency room (ER), and referral to vascular surgery
- Evaluation for any underlying causes and anticoagulation for 3 months for first episode of DVT (but duration varies depending on the comorbidities)
- Early ambulation (does not increase recurrent DVT or fatal pulmonary embolism)
- Compressive stocking (30–40 mmHg ankle pressure) within 2 weeks for 2 years to prevent postphlebitic syndrome

Chronic Venous Insufficiency (CVI)

Introduction (45)
- Prevalence of symptomatic CVI is about 1% with equal incidence among males and females
  - Prevalence of varicose veins: 5% to 30% in adult populations. Female > male by three times
- Risk factors: age, female sex, history of prior DVT, family history of varicose veins, obesity, pregnancy, phlebitis, and previous leg trauma
- Etiology and pathophysiology
  - Congenital (present since birth), primary (undetermined cause), and secondary (post-thrombotic and traumatic)
  - Reflux (in axial and perforating veins), obstruction (acute and chronic), and combination (valvular dysfunction and thrombosis)

History and physical examination
- Dilated veins, swelling, ± leg pain (calf pain, spasm)
- Spectrum of symptoms from telangiectases in mild cases to skin fibrosis and venous ulceration in advanced cases
- Varicose veins, hyperpigmentation (hemosiderosis in medial lower third of shin), stasis dermatitis, atrophic blanche, lipodermatosclerosis, pitting edema, brawny discoloration (long standing)
- Tourniquet (or Trendelenburg) test
  - The patient lies down to empty the lower extremity veins. The upright posture is resumed after applying a tourniquet or using manual compression at various levels
  - In the presence of superficial disease, the varicose veins will remain collapsed with compression placed cephalad to the point of reflux
  - With deep (or combined) venous insufficiency, the varicose veins will still be apparent despite the use of the tourniquet or manual compression

Diagnosis
- Clinical diagnosis with noninvasive vascular study
- Venous duplex imaging (presence of reflux by provocation test) and phlebography/venography
- Differential diagnosis: DVT, heart failure, nephrosis, liver/endocrine disease, medication side effects (calcium channel blocker etc)

Treatment (46)
- Compressive therapy
  - Unna boot placement initially
  - Graded compressive garment, commonly knee length, with pressure of 30 to 40 mmHg at the ankle, though pressure gradients from 20 to 30 mmHg to 40 to 50 mmHg can be used depending on the severity
  - ProFore (nonadhesive) dressing
- Calf and foot muscle exercise
- Pharmacological treatment: coumarins (alpha-benzopyrenes), flavonoids, saponoidises (not approved in the United States)
- Referral to surgery (ablation, stripping, valve reconstruction, or stenting)

Effort Thrombosis

Introduction (41)
- A rare cause of DVT after strenuous activity (Paget–Schroetter syndrome)
- Etiology and risk factors
  - Runners, skiers, and soccer players and after performing martial arts
- Post-thrombotic syndrome (PTS): up to 50%

History and physical examination
- Unilateral swelling in the lower limb after exertion
- Pain with flexion or extension of the knee and hip, and a positive Homans' sign
  - Rarely ulceration

Diagnosis
- Clinical suspicion confirmed by imaging study
- Imaging studies: duplex ultrasonography, impedance plethysmography, and venography
  - Extensive thrombosis in the posterior tibial, popliteal, and femoral vein distributions.

Treatment
- Emergency room evaluation for hospitalization or referral to hematology
  - Intravenous followed by oral anticoagulation and evaluation for an underlying hypercoagulable state

- Catheter-directed venous thrombolysis, particularly for ileofemoral venous clots, reduces the risk of PTS when the thrombosis is less than 14 days old
- Compression garment therapy, with pressures of at least 20 to 30 mmHg, should be used as part of the routine treatment for DVT to reduce PTS
- Return to play

TIMELINE	ACTIVITIES
Weeks 1–3	Gradual return to activities of daily living
Week 4	Non-weight-bearing exercise (eg, swimming)
Week 5	Non-impact-loading exercise (eg, cycling)
Week 6	Start impact-loading exercise (eg, return-to-running program) Restricted to activities with low risk of trauma until anticoagulation medications have been discontinued

OTHER PATHOLOGY

RESTLESS LEGS SYNDROME

Introduction (47)
- During rest, primarily at night, patients note discomfort and an urge to move their legs. Relieved by movement
  - Willis–Ekbom disease
- Prevalence is ~5% (1%–29% depending on studies) of the population, often familial
- Risk factors
  - Pregnancy (last trimester), iron deficiency, neuropathy, spinal cord lesion, end-stage renal disease (ESRD), and medications
  - Possibly Parkinson's disease and essential tremor

History and physical examination (48)
- Discomfort "creepy-crawly, jittery, throbbing, tight, tearing, electrical current," not positional
- Painful in up to 40%
- Duration can last up to hours

Diagnosis
- Clinical diagnosis; essential criteria
  - Urge to move limbs ± sensory complaints, worsens at rest, at night, improves with activity
- Initial evaluation: check labs, including serum feritin, iron, and chemistry (renal failure), as well as NCS/EMG
- Differential diagnosis: akathisia, muscle cramps (nocturnal leg cramps), arthritis, peripheral neuropathy

Treatment (49)
- Dopaminergic agonist (pramipexole, ropinirole, rotigotine)
- Gabapentin, opioid medication, benzodiazepine (little data to support), and iron supplementation (unclear evidence)
- Nonpharmacological management; behavioral modification (sleep hygiene)/cognitive behavioral treatment, and lifestyle changes (50)

STATIN MYOPATHY

Introduction (51)
- A spectrum of conditions: myalgia, myositis, rhabdomyolysis
- Statin-related myalgia ± myopathy: 5% to 10% of statin users, myopathy: 1.5% to 5% of statin users
- Leg: most commonly affected site
- Risk factors
  - History of myopathy, family history, high dose therapy, increased age, and female sex
  - Concomitant medications with fibrates and cytochrome P450 inhibitor (amiodarone, cyclosporine, protease inhibitors, macrolide Abx, and calcium channel blocker)

History and physical examination
- Pain in the calves and thighs (average 1 month after statins initiation, but up to 6–12 months), can last 2 months after cessation
- Myalgia often described as heaviness, stiffness, or cramping ± tenderness, swelling, mild weakness

Diagnosis
- Clinical diagnosis confirmed by laboratory finding
- Lab: creatinine kinase (CK), serum creatinine (elevated in rhabdomyolysis), and thyroid-stimulating hormone (TSH)
  - Myopathy: CK ≥10 times the upper limit of normal, rhabdomyolysis ≥50 times the upper limit of normal (food and drug administration criteria)
- Work up for myopathy: muscle biopsy for autoimmune myopathy (52)
- Common differential diagnoses: viral illness, hypothyroidism, polymyositis, and polymyalgia rheumatica

Treatment (53)
- Observation, reduce excessive physical work; if CK increased >3 to 10 times the upper limit of normal, consider stopping statin, reducing dose, using alternative statin (pravastatin 10 mg or atorvastatin 10 mg), changing dose regimen to every other day or adding coenzyme Q or vitamin D (limited evidence)
- When initiating statin medication initially, avoid excessive exercise

REFERENCES

1. Berger D. Leg discomfort: beyond the joints. *Med Clin North Am.* 2014;98(3):429–444.
2. Burrus MT, Werner BC, Starman JS, et al. Chronic leg pain in athletes. *Am J Sports Med.* 2015;43(6):1538–1547.
3. Maquirriain J, Merello M. The athlete with muscular cramps: clinical approach. *J Am Acad Orthop Surg.* 2007;15(7):425–431.
4. Butler JV, Mulkerrin EC, O'Keeffe ST. Nocturnal leg cramps in older people. *Postgrad Med J.* 2002;78(924):596–598.
5. Miller TM, Layzer RB. Muscle cramps. *Muscle Nerve.* 2005;32(4):431–442.
6. Ely JW, Osheroff JA, Chambliss ML, Ebell MH. Approach to leg edema of unclear etiology. *J Am Board Fam Med.* 2006;19(2):148–160.
7. Felice KJ, Whitaker CH, Grunnet ML. Benign calf amyotrophy: clinicopathologic study of 8 patients. *Arch Neurol.* 2003;60(10):1415–1420.
8. Nattiv A, Loucks AB, Manore MM, et al. American College of Sports Medicine position stand. The female athlete triad. *Med Sci Sports Exerc.* 2007;39(10):1867–1882.

9. Khatri VP, Asensio JA. *Operative Surgery Manual*. Philadelphia, PA: Saunders; 2003: xvii, p. 332.
10. Kortebein PM, Kaufman KR, Basford JR, Stuart MJ. Medial tibial stress syndrome. *Med Sci Sports Exerc*. 2000;32(3 Suppl): S27–S33.
11. Bresler M, Mar W, Toman J. Diagnostic imaging in the evaluation of leg pain in athletes. *Clin Sports Med*. 2012;31(2):217–245.
12. Edwards PH, Jr, Wright ML, Hartman JF. A practical approach for the differential diagnosis of chronic leg pain in the athlete. *Am J Sports Med*. 2005;33(8):1241–1249.
13. Isner-Horobeti ME, Dufour SP, Blaes C, Lecocq J. Intramuscular pressure before and after botulinum toxin in chronic exertional compartment syndrome of the leg: a preliminary study. *Am J Sports Med*. 2013;41(11):2558–2566.
14. Winters M, Eskes M, Weir A, et al. Treatment of medial tibial stress syndrome: a systematic review. *Sports Med*. 2013;43(12): 1315–1333.
15. Rathleff MS, Samani A, Olesen CG, et al. Inverse relationship between the complexity of midfoot kinematics and muscle activation in patients with medial tibial stress syndrome. *J Electromyogr Kinesiol*. 2011;21(4):638–644.
16. Yeung SS, Yeung EW, Gillespie LD. Interventions for preventing lower limb soft-tissue running injuries. *Cochrane Database Syst Rev*. 2011(7):CD001256.
17. Cho JC, Haun DW, Kettner NW. Sonographic evaluation of the greater occipital nerve in unilateral occipital neuralgia. *J Ultrasound Med*. 2012;31(1):37–42.
18. Moen MH, Rayer S, Schipper M, et al. Shockwave treatment for medial tibial stress syndrome in athletes; a prospective controlled study. *Br J Sports Med*. 2012;46(4):253–257.
19. Wilder RP, Magrum E. Exertional compartment syndrome. *Clin Sports Med*. 2010;29(3):429–435.
20. Tucker AK. Chronic exertional compartment syndrome of the leg. *Curr Rev Musculoskelet Med*. 2010;3(1–4):32–37.
21. Tiidus PM. Is intramuscular pressure a valid diagnostic criterion for chronic exertional compartment syndrome? *Clin J Sport Med*. 2014;24(1):87–88.
22. Pedowitz RA, Hargens AR, Mubarak SJ, Gershuni DH. Modified criteria for the objective diagnosis of chronic compartment syndrome of the leg. *Am J Sports Med*. 1990;18(1):35–40.
23. Diebal AR, Gregory R, Alitz C, Gerber JP. Effects of forefoot running on chronic exertional compartment syndrome: a case series. *Int J Sports Phys Ther*. 2011;6(4):312–321.
24. Harrast MA, Colonno D. Stress fractures in runners. *Clin Sports Med*. 2010;29(3):399–416.
25. Fredericson M, Bergman AG, Hoffman KL, Dillingham MS. Tibial stress reaction in runners. Correlation of clinical symptoms and scintigraphy with a new magnetic resonance imaging grading system. *Am J Sports Med*. 1995;23(4):472–481.
26. Russell AS, Crowther S. Tennis leg–a new variant of an old syndrome. *Clin Rheumatol*. 2011;30(6):855–857.
27. Campbell JT. Posterior calf injury. *Foot Ankle Clin*. 2009;14(4): 761–771.
28. Daghino W, Pasquali M, Faletti C. Superficial peroneal nerve entrapment in a young athlete: the diagnostic contribution of magnetic resonance imaging. *J Foot Ankle Surg*. 1997;36(3):170–172.
29. Styf J. Entrapment of the superficial peroneal nerve. Diagnosis and results of decompression. *J Bone Joint Surg Br*. 1989;71(1): 131–135.
30. Spinner RJ, Amrami KK. Superficial peroneal intraneural ganglion cyst originating from the inferior tibiofibular joint: the latest chapter in the book. *J Foot Ankle Surg*. 2010;49(6):575–578.
31. Styf J, Morberg P. The superficial peroneal tunnel syndrome. Results of treatment by decompression. *J Bone Joint Surg Br*. 1997;79(5):801–803.
32. Chhabra A, Williams EH, Subhawong TK, et al. MR neurography findings of soleal sling entrapment. *Am J Roentgenol*. 2011;196(3):W290–W297.
33. Williams EH, Rosson GD, Hagan RR, et al. Soleal sling syndrome (proximal tibial nerve compression): results of surgical decompression. *Plast Reconstr Surg*. 2012;129(2):454–462.
34. Khalil NM, Nicotra A, Kaplan C, O'Neill KS. Entrapment of the lateral cutaneous nerve of the calf. *BMJ Case Rep*. 2013;2013.
35. Salameh MJ, Ratchford EV. Update on peripheral arterial disease and claudication rehabilitation. *Phys Med Rehabil Clin N Am*. 2009;20(4):627–656.
36. Norgren L, Hiatt WR, Dormandy JA, et al. Inter-Society Consensus for the Management of Peripheral Arterial Disease (TASC II). *J Vasc Surg*. 2007;45 Suppl S:S5–67.
37. Turnipseed WD. Popliteal entrapment syndrome. *J Vasc Surg*. 2002;35(5):910–915.
38. Turnipseed WD. Popliteal entrapment in runners. *Clin Sports Med*. 2012;31(2):321–328.
39. Turnipseed WD. Functional popliteal artery entrapment syndrome: A poorly understood and often missed diagnosis that is frequently mistreated. *J Vasc Surg*. 2009;49(5):1189–1195.
40. Elias DA, White LM, Rubenstein JD, et al. Clinical evaluation and MR imaging features of popliteal artery entrapment and cystic adventitial disease. *Am J Roentgenol*. 2003;180(3):627–632.
41. Rajasekaran S, Kvinlaug K, Finnoff JT. Exertional leg pain in the athlete. *PM R*. 2012;4(12):985–1000.
42. Bauersachs RM. Clinical presentation of deep vein thrombosis and pulmonary embolism. *Best Pract Res Clin Haematol*. 2012;25(3):243–251.
43. Wells PS, Anderson DR, Rodger M, et al. Evaluation of D-dimer in the diagnosis of suspected deep-vein thrombosis. *N Engl J Med*. 2003;349(13):1227–1235.
44. Masuda EM, Kistner RL, Musikasinthorn C, et al. The controversy of managing calf vein thrombosis. *J Vasc Surg*. 2012;55(2):550–561.
45. Eberhardt RT, Raffetto JD. Chronic venous insufficiency. *Circulation*. 2005;111(18):2398–2409.
46. Hamdan A. Management of varicose veins and venous insufficiency. *JAMA*. 2012;308(24):2612–2621.
47. Ondo WG. Restless legs syndrome. *Neurol Clin*. 2009;27(3):779–99, vii.
48. Chokroverty S. Differential diagnoses of restless legs syndrome/ Willis-Ekbom disease: mimics and comorbidities. *Sleep Med Clin*. 2015;10(3):249–62, xii.
49. Sharon D. Restless legs syndrome and sleep related movement disorders. *Sleep Med Clin*. 2015;10(3):xvii–xviii.
50. Sharon D. Nonpharmacologic management of restless legs syndrome (Willis-Ekbom Disease): myths or science. *Sleep Med Clin*. 2015;10(3):263–78, xiii.
51. Joy TR, Hegele RA. Narrative review: statin-related myopathy. *Ann Intern Med*. 2009;150(12):858–868.
52. Argov Z. Statins and the neuromuscular system: a neurologist's perspective. *Eur J Neurol*. 2015;22(1):31–36.
53. Lasker SS, Chowdhury TA. Myalgia while taking statins. *BMJ*. 2012;345:e5348.

CHAPTER 10

Ankle and Foot

EPIDEMIOLOGY OF ANKLE AND FOOT PAIN

FOOT AND ANKLE PAIN IN THE GENERAL POPULATION (1)

Prevalence
- 20% to 42% in people >65 years (2)
- Significant foot pain is more common in obese females and older people (especially individuals 65–74 years old [YO])

Risk factors
- Relationship between shoes and foot pain
  - Rare in population not wearing shoes. More common in females wearing tighter shoes (3)
- Foot pain can be related to poor functional performance, walking, stair negotiation, and history of multiple falls

FOOT AND ANKLE PAIN IN ATHLETES (4)

Prevalence
- Ankle: most commonly (MC) injured joint among athletes (up to 30%); ankle sprain (75%–85%) (5)
- Common in soccer, basketball (>40%), football (>10%, lateral sprain: MC), long-distance runners (overuse), young dancers, and gymnasts (fracture and fatigue fracture)

Adolescent athletes
- Growth-related problems (coalitions and accessory ossicles), overuse injuries (apophysitis and osteochondrosis), stress fractures, and epiphyseal fractures

FOOT AND ANKLE PAIN AT WORK (6)

Prevalence
- 10% of total workplace injury, median of 5 days off

Common causes
- Direct trauma, secondary to slip, trip/fall, or shoe-related problem
- Related to environment (construction zone, type of floor, etc), type of footwear, long periods of standing
- Ankle: sprains and strains: MC (>70%) followed by fractures (15%) and bruises (contusion, 5%)
- Foot: bruises > fractures > sprains and strains > cuts and punctures
- Toes: fractures > bruises

DIFFERENTIAL DIAGNOSIS

MUSCULOSKELETAL (MSK) CAUSES OF FOOT AND ANKLE PAIN BASED ON LOCATION (FLOWCHART 10.1)

Classification of foot regions (Figure 10.1)
- Forefoot: metatarsal (MT) and phalanges

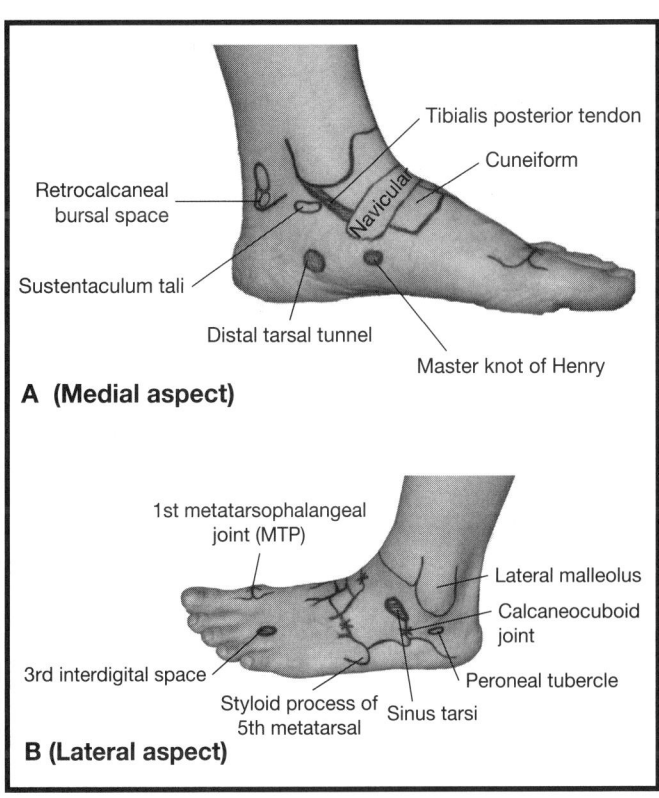

FIGURE 10.1
Surface anatomy of the foot and ankle.
Source: Courtesy of Dr. Mooyeon Oh Park.

(continued)

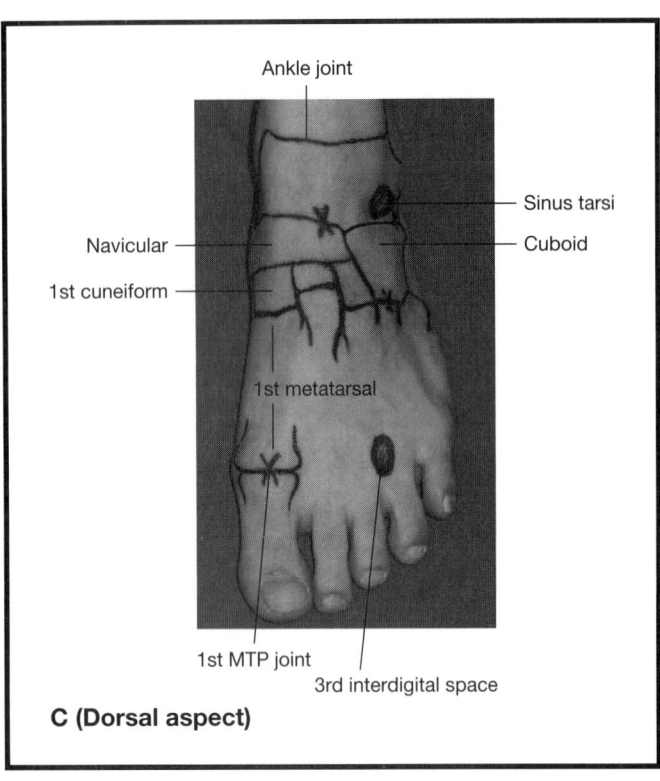

- Midfoot: cuneiform, cuboid, tarsometatarsal (TMT) (Lisfranc) joint, and cuneiform-navicular joint
- Hindfoot: talus, calcaneus, subtalar, and midtarsal joint (Chopart joint: talonavicular and calcaneocuboid joints) (7)
- Ankle joint: tibiotalar joint and tibiofibular syndesmosis

FIGURE 10.1 *(continued)*

Foot pain

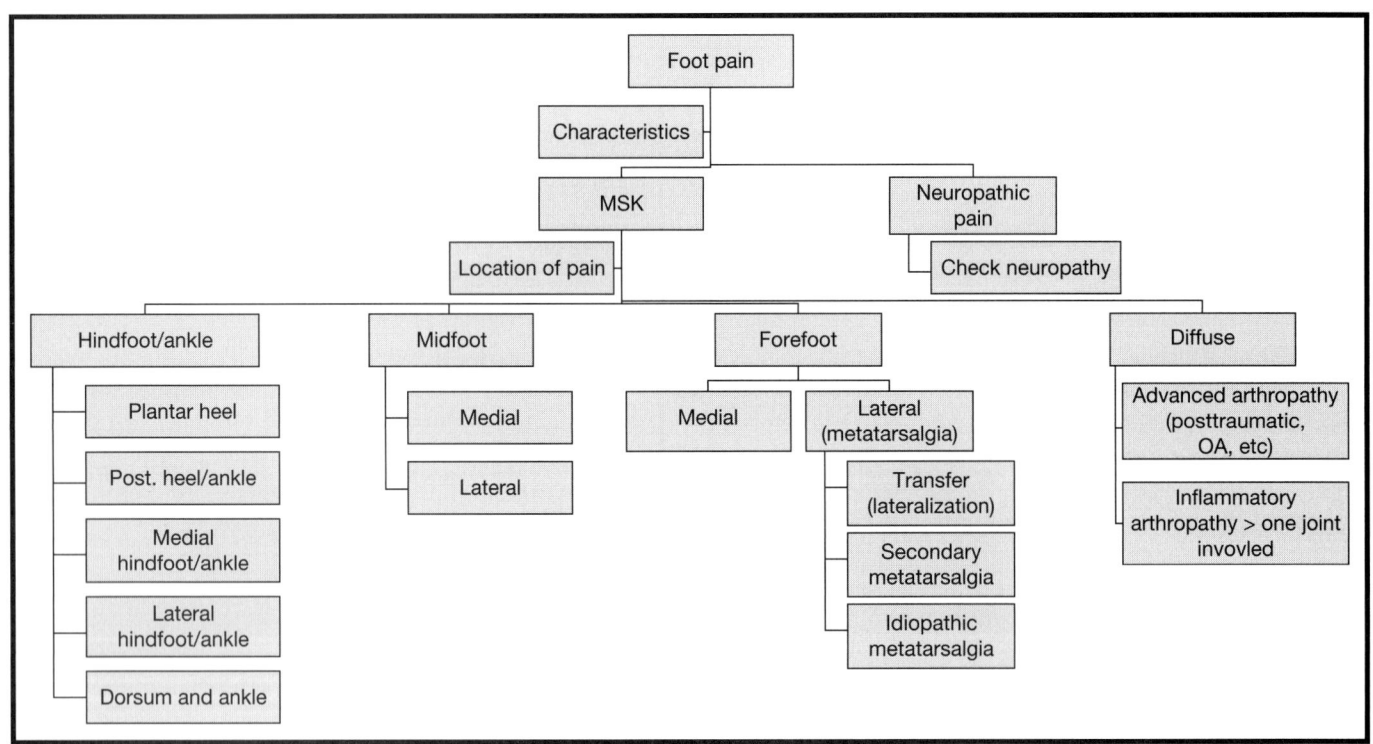

FLOWCHART 10.1
Classification of foot and ankle pain.
MSK, musculoskeletal; post., posterior.

DIFFERENTIAL DIAGNOSIS OF MSK HINDFOOT AND ANKLE PAIN

REGION	ANATOMIC STRUCTURE	PATHOLOGIES
Plantar heel	Fat pad	Fat-pad atrophy: middle age, rare in young adult ± H/O steroid injection
	Plantar fascia	Plantar fasciitis: MC cause of plantar heel pain. Pain at the fascial insertion to medial calcaneal tuberosity Plantar fibromatosis: distal to the insertion, palpable nodule
	Calcaneus	Stress fracture: vague pain, H/O osteoporosis, diabetes mellitus (DM), or recent change in activity
	Peroneus longus tendon	Tendinopathy/tear: Lateral plantar heel to medial midfoot, deep, ± H/O inversion sprain
Posterior heel/ankle	Achilles tendon	Non-insertional tendinopathy/tear: MC cause of the posterior heel pain (4 times more than insertional) Insertional Achilles tendinopathy (2nd MC)
	Os trigonum	Os trigonum syndrome: deep posterolateral pain ± H/O minor ankle trauma or repetitive trauma
	Flexor hallucis longus tendon	Tendinopathy/tenosynovitis: posterior medial ankle/hindfoot pain, ± H/O ankle sprain or overuse (ballet)
	Bursa	Retrocalcaneal/superficial calcaneal bursitis: often irritated from shoe (heel counter) ± bulging. Patient prefers open back shoes (clogs, slippers, flip flops)
	Joint	Posterior ankle/subtalar joint effusion/synovitis or loose body. Worsening pain on tip toe walking
Dorsum and ankle	Tibiofibular lig. (syndesmosis)	High ankle sprain: persistent pain after sprain (eversion and dorsiflexion) ± instability
	Soft tissue	Anterolateral impingement syndrome: gradual onset of pain after injury Pain on ankle dorsiflexion (late stance phase of gait)
	Talar dome	Osteochondritis dissecans: chronic pain after ankle sprain. Pain is typically not localized
	Midtarsal joint	Talonavicular and calcaneocuboid joint/ligament sprain or arthritis
Medial ankle/hindfoot	Tibialis posterior (TP) tendon	Tendinopathy, tear, and tenosynovitis • Pain between medial malleolus and navicular tuberosity, acquired pes planus
	Deltoid ligament	H/O eversion sprain, significant pain, often difficult weight bearing initially, and ecchymosis
	Talonavicular joint	Arthritis: tarsal coalition or foot alignment issues (pes planus, cavus)
Lateral ankle/hindfoot	Lateral ligament	Sprain: MC cause of ankle pain (especially, anterior talofibular ligament) • Common with pes cavus (hindfoot inversion), and H/O previous injury
	Peroneal tendon	Tendinopathy, tear (brevis: more common), tenosynovitis, and subluxation • Pain on the behind/distal to the lateral malleolus (posterolateral) ± intermittent snapping, usually after inversion injury
	Sinus tarsi	Sinus-tarsi syndrome: common cause of persistent pain after ankle sprain
	Calcaneocubiod joint	Arthritis Sprain common in dancing, underrecognized cause of sinus-tarsi pain

DM, diabetes mellitus; H/O, history of; lig., ligament; MC, most common; TP, tibialis posterior.

DIFFERENTIAL DIAGNOSIS OF MSK MIDFOOT PAIN

REGION	ANATOMIC STRUCTURE	PATHOLOGIES
Lateral	Cuboid-4th metatarsal bone	Arthritis, subluxation (cuboid subluxation, often reduced by the patient), and sprain
	Os peroneum	Painful Os peroneal syndrome
Medial	Navicular	Kohler disease (navicular osteochondrosis) or Müller–Weiss syndrome (navicular osteonecrosis) Painful accessory navicular syndrome
	Naviculocuneiform arthritis	Often associated with 1st ray insufficiency (hypermobile 1st ray)
	FHL or FDL (at master knot of Henry)	Tendinopathy or tethering • Rare cause of medial arch pain

FDL, flexor digitorum longus; FHL, flexor hallucis longus.

DIFFERENTIAL DIAGNOSIS OF MSK FOREFOOT PAIN

REGION	ANATOMIC STRUCTURE	PATHOLOGIES
1st ray	1st metatarsophalangeal (MTP) joint	Gout: MC cause of acute disabling foot pain, 1st MTP joint; MC location for gout Hallux rigidus/limitus: pain on the dorsum of 1st MTP joint initially Hallux valgus with bursitis: pain on the medial side
	Sesamoid	Sesamoiditis, sesamoid fracture/necrosis: plantar aspect of the MTP joint
2nd ray	2nd MTP joint	Subluxation or dislocation. Pain can be worsened by tight shoe ± crossing over/overlying toes
	2nd metatarsal bone	Stress fracture Change in amount of weight-bearing activity; common in athletes (with nutritional imbalance), and osteoporosis Freiberg disease (osteonecrosis of 2nd metatarsal head): adolescent female
Lesser toes	Bursa	Intermetatarsal bursitis ± irritation of interdigital N Taylor's bunion (Bunionette deformity) on the lateral side of 5th metatarsal head
	MTP joints and soft tissues	MTP joint arthritis/synovitis (highly involved in inflammatory arthropathy; underrecognized) Lateral overloading syndrome: often H/O medial arch support (excessive)

MC, most common; MTP, metatarsophalangeal; N, nerve.

NEUROPATHIC CAUSES OF FOOT AND ANKLE PAIN BASED ON LOCATION (FLOWCHART 10.2)

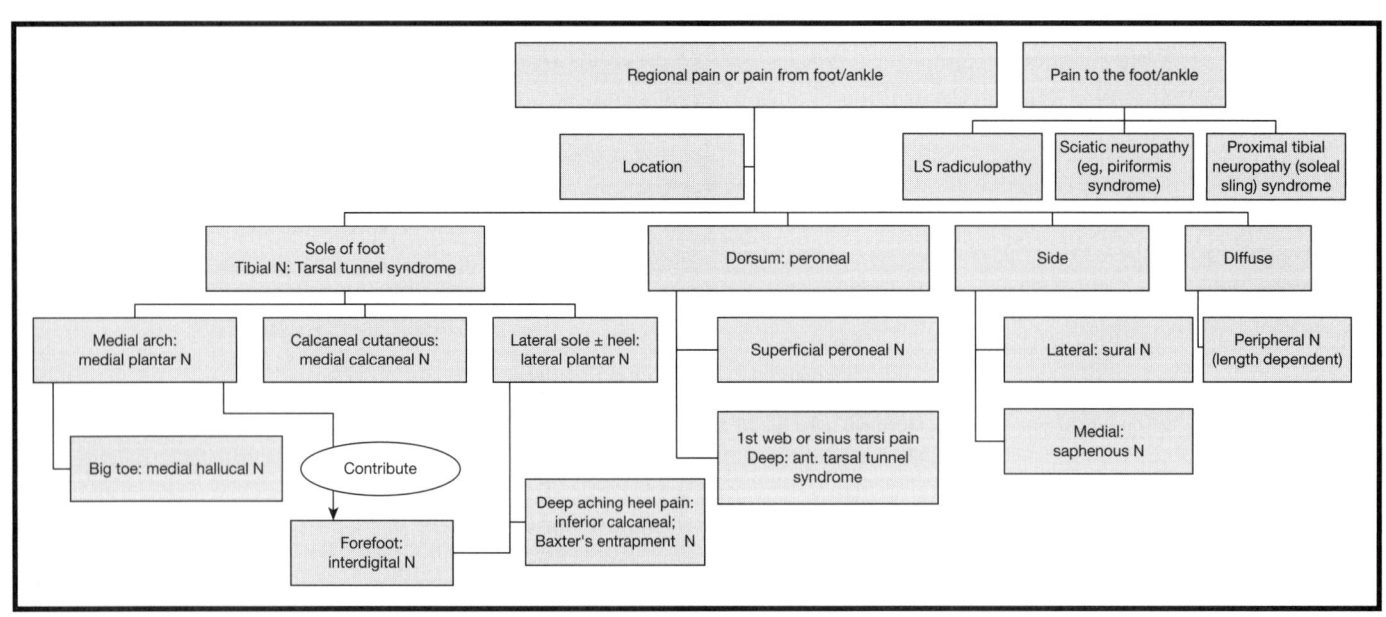

FLOWCHART 10.2

Differential diagnosis of neuropathic causes of foot and ankle pain.

Ant., anterior; LS, lumbosacral; N, neuropathy.

REGION	DIFFERENTIAL DIAGNOSES	NOTES
Heel	Baxter's (inferior calcaneal N) entrapment neuropathy	Deep, aching (because of periosteum innervation), and tingling Underrecognized cause of chronic recalcitrant heel pain. Aggravated by hindfoot valgus
	Medial calcaneal entrapment neuropathy	A rare cause of burning, pins/needles pain in the heel
Dorsal	Superficial peroneal neuropathy	Worse at night (weight of blanket plantarflex the ankle with stretching of superficial peroneal nerve) and aggravated by tight shoe H/O inversion ankle sprain
	Deep peroneal neuropathy	Underrecognized cause of sinus-tarsi pain by compression of the lateral branch of deep peroneal N to extensor digitorum brevis
Sole	Tarsal tunnel syndrome	Neuropathic pain on the sole of the foot, often aggravated by hindfoot eversion, pronation Distal tarsal tunnel syndrome: involving a branch similar to presentation of isolated inferior calcaneal, medial calcaneal, or medial plantar neuropathy
	Peripheral neuropathy	Large fiber-mediated symptoms (unsteadiness) and small fiber symptoms (burning, pins/needles sensation), symmetric.
Medial	Medial plantar N (jogger's foot)	Medial arch pain with radiating pain distally and proximally
	Hallucal neuropathy	Numbness, tingling, pins/needles pain in the big toe with pain radiation proximally (Valleix's phenomenon)
Lateral forefoot	Interdigital neuritis	Pain radiating distally but occasionally radiating proximally, with numbness
Regional or Diffuse	Peripheral neuropathy/small fiber neuropathy, or erythromelalgia Complex regional pain syndrome: often focal neuropathy misinterpreted as generalized pain Herpes neuralgia; can precede the skin lesions	

N, nerve; H/O, history of.

OTHER CAUSES OF SEVERE (DISABLING) FOOT PAIN

- Compartment syndrome: history of trauma or injury
- Acute ischemia: with history of vascular disease, rest pain, pain relieved by dependent position
- Drug-seeking behavior

COMMON CAUSES OF PES CAVUS (HIGH ARCH FOOT)

CATEGORIES	CAUSES
Neuromuscular (progressive) Muscle disease Peripheral nerves and root Anterior horn cell Dx Long tract and central nervous Dx	Muscular dystrophy Charcot-Marie-Tooth disease/peripheral neuropathy (common) Polio, spinal dysraphism (can involve root only), diastematomyelia, syringomyelia, spinal cord tumor, spinal muscular atrophy Cerebral palsy, Friedreich's ataxia, Roussy-Lévy syn., primary cerebellar disorder
Congenital (lifelong)	Idiopathic, residual of clubfoot (equino-cavovarus), arthrogryposis, and fibular hemimelia
Traumatic	Residuals of compartment syndrome, crush inj. to lower ext. severe burn, malunion of foot Fx. Talar neck fracture

Dx, diagnosis; ext., extreme; Fx, fracture; inj., injury; syn., syndrome.

DIFFERENTIAL DIAGNOSIS OF PES PLANUS (FLAT FOOT, NORMAL UP TO 6 YEARS)

CATEGORIES	CAUSES
Congenital	Congenital vertical talus: congenital rigid flat foot • Associated with neuromuscular disease (arthrogryposis, meningocele) Tarsal coalition: severe osteophyte in the talonavicular joint (common)
Muscle weakness	TP dysfunction (insufficiency): MC cause of acquired flat foot
Ligament laxity	Hypermobile flat foot
Hyperpronated foot	Dropping of the talar head ± spring ligament injury/insufficiency Femoral int. rotation, coxa vara, and medial tibial torsion
Trauma and others	Calcaneal fracture Charcot neuroarthropathy (long-standing DM: MC cause)

DM, diabetes mellitus; MC, most common, TP, tibialis posterior.

DIFFERENTIAL DIAGNOSIS OF ANKLE EQUINUS

Muscular
- Normal aging, immobility, upper motor neuron syndrome, deconditioning, DM, Achilles enthesopathy/tendinopathy/tear, and the like

Osseous (pseudoequinus): anterior tibiotalar exostosis, distal tibiofibular osseous bridging

DIFFERENTIAL DIAGNOSIS OF ANKLE INSTABILITY

Recurrent ankle sprain (MC cause), occurs in 10% to 30% of recurrent ankle sprain

Mechanical causes: arthrokinetic restriction, synovial, and degenerative pathologies
- Loose bodies, osteochondral injuries, chondromalacia, osteophytes/painful ossicles, synovitis/adhesion, impingement, and peroneal tendon pathology

Functional causes: proprioception, neuromuscular, impaired postural control, and strength deficit

DIFFERENTIAL DIAGNOSIS OF SNAPPING ANKLE (8)

Lateral (behind the lateral malleolus, MC)
- Peroneal tendon subluxation with retinacular injury, more common than extensor digitorum longus (EDL) with inferior retinaculum injury
  - Static MRI: not sensitive → better evaluated by dynamic ultrasound (US) with passive ankle dorsi/plantarflexion with eversion

Medial
- TP subluxation and dislocation or tibialis anterior (TA) snapping

LATERALIZATION OF PAIN

Pain on the lateral forefoot, midfoot, hindfoot, and lateral calf due to compensatory mechanism (avoid weight bearing on the medial side)

Common underlying medial foot pathologies
- Hallux rigidus/limitus (with/without gout or degenerative joint disease (DJD) of MTP joint)
- 1st ray insufficiency (with medial cuneiform-metatarsal joint arthropathy)
- 2nd MTP joint arthralgia/subluxation
- Plantar fasciitis
- Posterior tibialis tendon dysfunction
- Ambitious arch syndrome from medial arch support (or foot orthotics)

DIFFERENTIAL DIAGNOSIS OF NEUROPATHIC ANKLE AND FOOT PAIN

Length-dependent neuropathy: stocking pattern, distal symptoms more severe than proximal

Focal/regional pain

Plantar	More than one part of foot (regional or diffuse) involved • Tarsal tunnel syndrome (proximal) • Distal peripheral neuropathy • Lumbosacral radiculopathy
	Medial • Distal tarsal tunnel syndrome involving the medial plantar nerve • Medial plantar neuropathy (jogger's foot) • Medial hallucal nerve lesion (at MTP joint area) Lateral • Morton's interdigital neuritis • Distal tarsal tunnel syndrome involving the lateral plantar nerve • Lateral plantar neuropathy; neurilemma, iatrogenic, etc Heel • Medial calcaneal nerve: posterior heel/cutaneous burning, pins/needles sensation • Baxter's nerve (1st branch of the lateral plantar nerve); deep aching pain in the heel
Dorsum	Medial • Superficial peroneal neuropathy (where it perforates the crural fascia above the ankle, rarely at the level of the knee) • Anterior tarsal tunnel syndrome involving deep peroneal neuropathy • Hallux rigidus/limitus with dorsal osteophytes irritating the deep and superficial peroneal nerves/medial dorsal branch, or the medial dorsal hallucal nerve • Saphenous N lesion (at the knee or leg) • L5 radiculopathy Lateral • Deep peroneal N (branch to EDB, sinus-tarsi syndrome) • Superficial peroneal N (perforating the crural fascia or distally at navicular junction) • Sural neuralgia • S1 radiculopathy

EDB, extensor digitorum brevis; N, nerve.

ANATOMY

BONE AND JOINT

Ankle joint
- Talus
  - Talar dome: wider anteriorly
    - Ankle dorsiflexion engages anterior part into the mortise → fits more securely (stable) and can cause pain in syndesmosis injury (widen tibiofibular space)
    - Plantar flexion of ankle (narrower posterior dome) → unstable (more common position in ankle sprain)
  - Axis of talus to the 1st web space (in relation to impingement)
    - Bony impingement
      - Dorsiflexion → anteromedial impingement
      - Plantarflexion → Posterolateral impingement
    - If impingement location is at anterolateral or posteromedial of the ankle → suspect soft tissue (ligament and scar tissue) impingement
  - Direct blood supply retrograde fashion in talus (because of limited soft-tissue attachments) → vulnerable to osteonecrosis

(continued)

- Ankle joint axis: medial 8° higher (lower in lateral side) in coronal plane, the lateral malleolus is 20° to 30° posterior compared to the medial malleolus (axial plane)
  - Ankle dorsiflexion ➔ slight abduction of forefoot due to tilting
  - Ankle joint x-ray (mortise view): internally rotate the leg by 20°
- Ankle stabilizers: bony (mortise with wide anterior talar dome), ligaments, muscles across the ankle joint
  - Ankle dorsiflexion blocks (stabilizes) the movement in the ankle mortise, and tightens the Achilles tendon and locks the subtalar joint

Subtalar joint (Figure 10.2)
- Between talus and calcaneus with three articular facets: anterior, middle, and posterior facets
  - Multiple configurations in joint articulations and orientations
- Triplanar mechanism (movement similar to 45° oblique hinge)
  - Axis: 42° (posterior–inferior to anterior–superior in sagittal plane) and 16° (posterolateral to anteromedial in axial plane)
  - Pronation: dorsiflex in sagittal plane with forefoot abduction in axial plane and hindfoot eversion in coronal plane
  - Supination: the opposite of pronation when the foot responds to the demands of uneven terrain
- Stabilizers (9)
  - Bony configuration of facets: anterior, middle, and posterior facets
  - Muscles across the subtalar joint
  - Ligamentous stabilizers
    - Major stabilizers: interosseous talocalcaneal ligament (most important), cervical ligament, and lateral talocalcaneal ligament
    - Posterior, anterior, medial, and lateral capsular thickening ➔ eversion/inversion control
    - Anterior part: cervical ligament; floor of sinus tarsi to talar neck ➔ primarily limits inversion
    - Lateral talocalcaneal ligament limits inversion, medial talocalcaneal limits eversion
    - Calcaneofibular ligament: lateral stability to the ankle and subtalar joint
    - Bifurcate ligament

Midtarsal joint (Chopart or transverse tarsal joint)
- Calcaneocuboid and talonavicular joint
  - 20° adduction and 10° abduction
  - Stability
    - Congruence of the calcaneocuboid joint
    - Subtalar joint motion (supination ➔ calcaneocuboid and talonavicular joint axes are not parallel ➔ close-packed position; midtarsal joint locking)

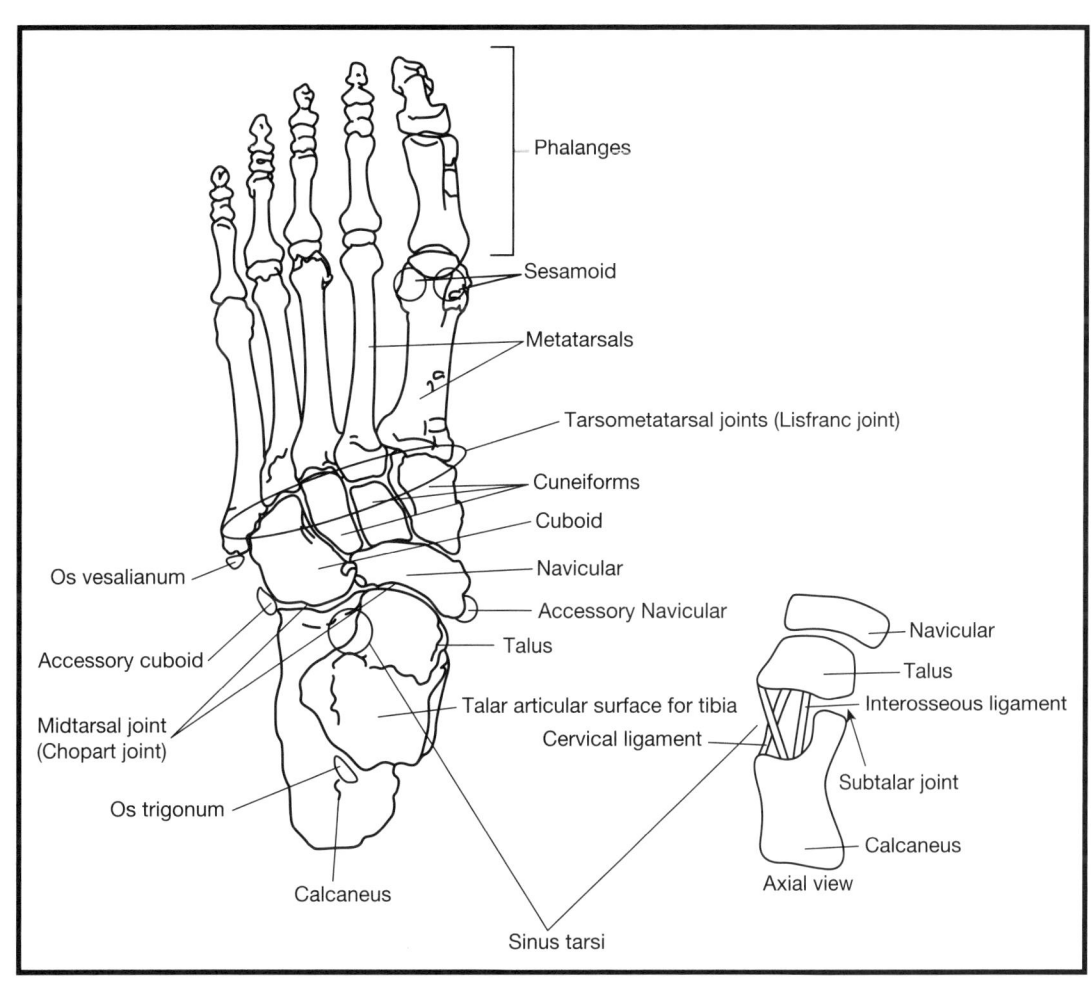

FIGURE 10.2
Bony anatomy of foot with location of accessory bone (ossicles).

- Ligaments
  - Bifurcate ligament (calcaneocuboid, calcaneonavicular) in the dorsum
  - Wedge-shaped labra within calcaneocuboid joint
  - Spring ligament (calcaneonavicular) in the medial/plantar aspect
  - Plantar calcaneocuboid ligament

TMT joint: referred as midfoot joint or Lisfranc joint
- Cuneiform-metatarsal and cuboid-metatarsal joints
- Medial column (1st ray, medial cuneiform–1st metatarsal (MT)), middle (2nd and 3rd ray, intermediate, lateral cuneiform-metatarsal) and lateral column (cuboid-4th and 5th MT)
  - Medial cuneiform-metatarsal (1st TMT) joint: reciprocal saddle joint similar to 1st carpometacarpal (CMC) joint in hand
  - Mobile lateral column: 20° flexion/extension versus rigid medial column; cuneiform-2nd MT (<4°)
- Stabilizers of TMT joint
  - Osseous, ligamentous (1st cuneometatarsal ligament; large dorsal and broader but inconsistent plantar, inconsistent interosseous, and absent intermetatarsal ligament), and muscles (peroneus longus and flexor hallucis longus against dorsal instability)
    - If stabilizer is dysfunctional → 1st ray hypermobility with compensation mechanism to increase stability with stiffening strategy
      - Reduced range of motion (ROM) of the 1st MT during walking
      - Disproportionate increase in 1st MT and calcaneal eversion ROM
  - Osseous stability
    - Lisfranc joint: Roman arch configuration, apex at the 2nd MT (transverse arch)
    - Base of 2nd metatarsal (longer than other metatarsals) in keystone shape; inherent stability
      - Stress fracture more common in 2nd metatarsal bone
      - Can be related to intractable plantar keratosis underneath
- Cuneiform-metatarsal; less mobile versus cuboid-metatarsal; more mobile
  - Stability of cuboid-4th metatarsal joint
    - Dorsal and plantar cuboideometatarsal ligaments
    - Wedge-shaped fibroadipose labra within cuboid metatarsal joints
    - 4th metatarsal cuboid sprain → subluxation/instability

1st MTP joint
- Stabilizers (inherently unstable joint)
  - Static: collateral ligaments, capsule, and plantar fascia
  - Dynamic: peroneus longus and intrinsic muscle of the foot insert to the base of the proximal phalanx, augmented by extrinsic muscles (EHL and FHL)

LIGAMENT

Ankle ligaments (10)
- Lateral ankle ligaments: anterior/posterior talofibular, and calcaneofibular ligaments
  - Anterior talofibular ligament (ATFL)
    - Two bands, anteromedial, 1 cm proximal to tip of fibula to talar body
    - Posterolateral to anteromedial course: resist anterior translation and internal rotation of talus
    - Thinnest of all lateral ligaments: MC injured ligament, not pivotal in gross stability
- Deltoid ligament
  - Superficial: tibiocalcaneal (to sustentaculum tali), tibionavicular, superficial tibiotalar/tibiospring ligament
    - Holds calcaneus and navicular against the talus and reinforces the action of the spring ligament on which the head of the talus rests
  - Deep: deep anterior and posterior tibiotalar ligament (strongest)
  - Constant: tibiospring, tibionavicular ligament, and deep anterior/posterior tibiotalar ligament

Syndesmosis
- Anterior-inferior tibiofibular ligament (accessory ligament: Basset ligament), post-inferior tibiofibular ligament (the strongest), inferior transverse tibiofibular ligament (form a labrum/fibrocartilagenous), and interosseous tibiofibular ligament
- Important ankle mortise stabilizer

Spring ligament (11)
- Composed of inferior (more rigid) and superomedial (more elastic, injured MC) calcaneonavicular ligament
- Functions
  - Articular sling around the head of the talus (sling around the head of the talus like acetabulum (with navicular and calcaneus)
    - Functional spring–ligament complex including anterior portion of superficial deltoid ligament and posterior tibialis tendon (PTT)
  - Major supporter of medial arch and head of the talus
  - Control talocalcaneonavicular joint

Liscfranc ligament (12,13)
- Ligaments at TMT joint
  - Plantar and dorsal ligaments: longitudinal, oblique (tarsal to metatarsal bone), and transverse (between metatarsals)
    - The plantar ligaments are stronger than the dorsal ligaments, which may account for the dorsal direction of dislocations of TMT joints
  - Interosseous ligaments
    - The Lisfranc ligament (medial interosseous ligament)
      - Located between the medial cuneiform and the base of the second metatarsal
      - The largest of the interosseus ligaments and strongest in providing the most stability, followed by the plantar and dorsal ligaments, respectively
    - Absent between the bases of the first and second metatarsals and between medial and middle cuneiforms

RETINACULUM (14)

Flexor retinaculum
- Medial side, roof of tarsal tunnel

Extensor retinaculum
- Dorsum of the foot and ankle
- Superior (above the ankle joint) and inferior (at ankle joint and tarsal bone) extensor retinaculum
- Inferior extensor retinaculum

○ Inferior (inferomedial) band: roof of anterior tarsal tunnel (deep peroneal nerve entrapment site; anterior tarsal tunnel syndrome [TOS])
○ Lateral portion (stem, frondiform ligament): forms ligament like roots located in the sinus tarsi (15)

Peroneal retinaculum
• Superior: sheath covering peroneal tendons in retromalleolar groove, can be injured during inversion injury causing instability or lateral ankle snapping
• Inferior: from lateral rim of the sinus tarsi to a point of attachment below the trochlea of the calcaneus. If injured → underrecognized source of pain

NERVE (16)

Tibial nerve (main motor nerve to intrinsic foot muscles and sole of the foot), peroneal nerve (dorsum of foot and extensor digitorum brevis and peroneus tertius), saphenous nerve (medial), and sural nerve (lateral side of ankle and foot)

Tibial nerve branches (17) (Figure 10.3)
• Medial plantar nerve: 1st lumbrical, abductor halluces, and FHB; cutaneous sensation of medial plantar sole. Continues to be the medial hallucal nerve (with other nerve contribution)
• Lateral plantar nerve: 4th interosseous; quadratus plantae, flexor digiti minimi brevis, adductor hallucis, 2nd to 4th lumbricals, and lateral plantar sole
• Interdigital nerves: sensory branches from medial and lateral plantar nerves
 ○ Third interdigital nerve is formed by contribution from both medial and lateral plantar nerves
• Inferior calcaneal nerve (Baxter's nerve, or 1st branch of lateral plantar nerve)
 ○ 40% direct branch from the tibial nerve
 ○ Flexor digitorum brevis, abductor digiti quinti pedis (ADQP), periosteum medical calcaneus (sensory afferent); no cutaneous innervation

Peroneal nerve (Figure 10.3)
• Common peroneal nerve passing around the fibular neck in an exposed fibro-osseous tunnel bordered superficially

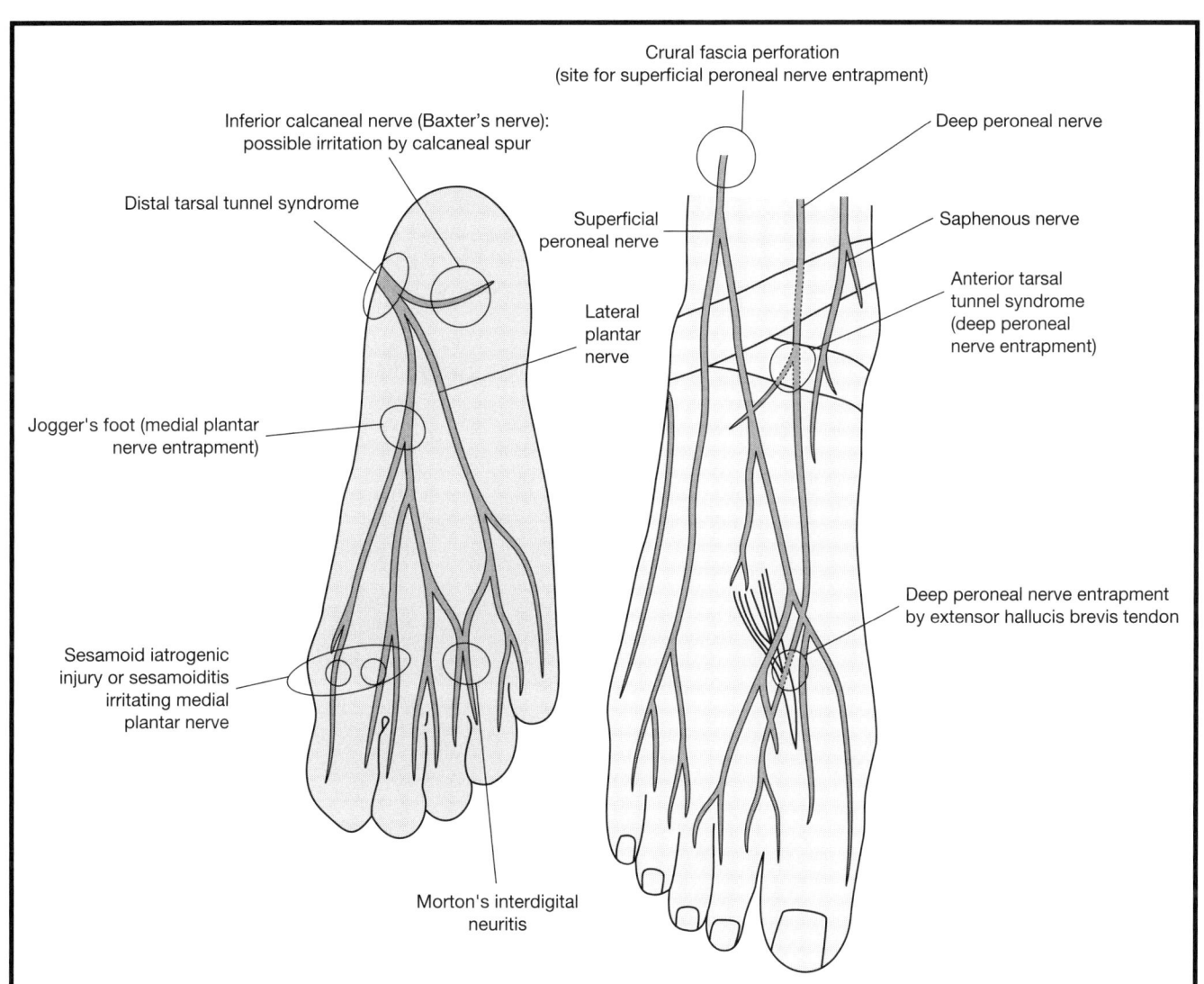

FIGURE 10.3
Nerve innervation of the foot and ankle.

by the peroneus longus tendon → bifurcates into recurrent articular branch, and deep and superficial branch in the lateral leg compartment
- Superficial peroneal nerve
  ○ Superficial peroneal nerve pierces the deep fascia and becomes subcutaneous 7 to 10 cm above the ankle
  ○ Major innervation of cutaneous sensation in the dorsum of the foot except the 1st web space
- Deep peroneal nerve
  ○ First-web space cutaneous sensation and afferent sensation from periosteum of sinus tarsi
  ○ After bifurcating, the deep peroneal nerve enters anterior compartment under peroneus longus, piercing the intermuscular septum between the lateral and anterior compartment (potential entrapment site)
  ○ Deep to EDL to the anterior interosseous membrane (anterior compartment), reaching the anterior tibial artery in the proximal one-third of the leg
  ○ At the ankle, it divides into the lateral branch to extensor digitorum brevis (EDB) muscle, sinus tarsi, lateral tarsal joints, and medial terminal branches (lateral to the dorsalis pedis artery)
- Anatomy of anterior tarsal tunnel
  ○ Roof: inferomedial border of the inferior extensor retinaculum, floor: talonavicular joint capsule

Big-toe innervation
- Medial hallucal nerve; extension of medial plantar nerve
- Deep peroneal nerve (1st web space)
- Superficial peroneal nerve (medial dorsal branch)
- Saphenous nerve (controversial)

MUSCLE

MUSCLE	ORIGIN	INSERTION	INNERVATION	ACTION	COMMENT
Muscles on the Dorsum of Foot					
Extensor digitorum brevis	Calcaneus	Four tendons into the proximal phalanx to 2nd, 3rd, and 4th toes Big toe (called extensor hallucis brevis)	Deep peroneal nerve (N) L5, S1	Extends toes	Isolated involvement in anterior tarsal tunnel syndrome (rare) Muscle belly: One finger breadth distal from sinus tarsi, recording site for NCS
Muscles of the Sole of the Foot (First Layer)					
Abductor hallucis	Medial tubercle of calcaneus; flexor retinaculum	Medial side, base of proximal phalanx of big toe	Medial plantar N, S1-2	Flexes, abducts big toe; supports medial arch	Roof of distal tarsal tunnel
Flexor digitorum brevis	Medial tubercle of calcaneum	Middle phalanx of four lateral toes	Medial plantar nerve versus 1st branch of the lateral plantar N, S1-2	Flexes lateral four toes; supports medial and lateral longitudinal arches	Immediately under plantar fascia
Abductor digiti minimi	Medial and lateral tubercles of calcaneum	Lateral base of proximal phalanx, 5th toe	1st branch of the lateral plantar nerve, S2-3	flexes, abducts 5th toe; supports lateral longitudinal arch	Denervated in Baxter's N (1st branch of lateral plantar N) entrapment
Muscles of the Sole of Foot (Second Layer)					
Quadratus plantae	Medial and lateral sides of calcaneum	Flexor digitorum longus tendon	Lateral plantar nerve, S2-3	Aids long flexor tendon to flex lateral four toes	Baxter's N course superficial to quadratus plantae (deep to AH and flexor digitorum brevis)
Flexor digitorum longus (FDL) tendon	Shaft of tibia	Base of distal phalanx of lateral four toes	Tibial N, S1-2	Flexes distal phalanges of lateral four toes; plantar flexes foot; supports longitudinal arch	Master knot of Henry (cross of FDL and flexor hallucis longus tendons)

(continued)

MUSCLE	ORIGIN	INSERTION	INNERVATION	ACTION	COMMENT
Lumbricals	Tendons of flexor digitorum longus	Dorsal extensor expansion of lateral four toes	1st lumbrical from medial plantar; other lumbricals from lateral plantar N, S2-3	Extends toes at interphalangeal joints	
Flexor hallucis longus	Shaft of fibula	Base of distal phalanx of big toe	Tibial N, S2-3	Flexes distal phalanx of big toe; plantar flexes foot; supports medial longitudinal arch	Passes in the groove between talar processes and under sustentaculum tali
Muscles of Sole of Foot (Third Layer)					
Flexor hallucis brevis (FHB)	Cuboid, lateral cuneiform; TP insertion	Medial and lateral sides of base of proximal phalanx of big toe	Medial plantar N, S2-3	Flexes MTP joint of big toe; supports medial longitudinal arch	Needle EMG for medial plantar N Middle/inferior border of 1st metatarsal shaft
Adductor hallucis (oblique head)	Bases of 2nd, 3rd, and 4th metatarsal bones	Lateral side of base of proximal phalanx of big toe	Lateral plantar N, S2-3	Flexes big toe, supports transverse arch	
Adductor hallucis (transverse head)	Plantar ligaments				
Flexor digiti minimi brevis	Base of 5th metatarsal bone	Lateral side of base of proximal phalanx of big toe	Lateral plantar nerve, S2-3	Flexes little toe	Needle EMG site for lateral plantar N (at the middle/inferior aspect of 5th metatarsal bone)
Muscles of Sole of Foot (Fourth Layer)					
Dorsal interossei (DI)	Adjacent sides of metatarsal bones	Bases of phalanges and dorsal expansion of corresponding toes	Lateral plantar N, S2-3	Abduct toes with 2nd toe as reference; flex MTP joints; extend interphalangeal (IP) joint	4th DI: site for lateral plantar N needle EMG
Plantar interossei	3rd, 4th, and 5th metatarsal bones	Bases of phalanges and dorsal expansion of corresponding toes	Lateral plantar N, S2-3	Adduct toes with 2nd toe as reference; flex MTP joints; extend IP joints	No 2nd metatarsal insertion→ unopposed lumbricals action on the 2nd metatarsal bone
Peroneus longus tendon and tibialis posterior tendon	Check leg muscles (TP; L5, S1 and peroneus longus L5, S1)				

DI, dorsal interossei; EMG, electromyography; FDL, flexor digitorum longus; FHB, flexor hallucis brevis; N, nerve.
[a]S1–2 unless indicated.

BIOMECHANICS

KINETIC AND KINEMATIC (18)

Ankle joint: approximately 5 times the body weight (BW) loading during walking

Ground reaction force (GRF) during stance phase: typical muscle pattern (first peak; initial heel strike, 2nd peak: heel rise and heel off), lower during midstance

Compensation mechanism (19,20)
- In a closed chain system (eg, standing or stance phase of gait), each segment is interrelated and interdependent (eg, pronation and supination response)
- Loss of mobility at any one joint → a complex series of compensations that affect all the other articulations of the foot, ankle, and lower extremity
- Tight Achilles cord (gastrocnemius) increases loading on the forefoot
  - Decreased ankle dorsiflexion (during stance phase) compensated by neighboring (subtalar, midtarsal, knee) joints with pronation response usually
  - Navicular drop/in rolling (as the compensation response) can cause other problems
- Rationale for orthotic or footwear: mitigating painful or abnormal degrees of compensation by accommodating loss of mobility in addition to decreasing painful ROM

ANKLE AND FOOT IN GAIT (21)

Ankle joint (19)
- To advance in the mid- to terminal stance of gait, 10° dorsiflexion is ideally required
  - In equinus state/deformity, other functional ankle joints compensate for the decreased ankle (tibiotalar) joint motion; sagittal compensation
  - Functional ankle joints are other neighboring joints that substitute or compensate for an ankle joint motion
    - Subtalar joint (talocalcaneal) compensation with other components of pronation response kicks during dorsiflexion → forefoot abduction, navicular drop (in rolling), and hindfoot eversion
    - Midtarsal (transverse tarsal) joint
    - Knee joint (knee recurvatum compensate/or secondary to tight Achilles cord)
      – Can cause posterior knee pain or infrapatellar fat-pad impingement
    - Shoe (*rocker bottom simulating* dorsiflexion). Solid ankle cushion heel (SACH) simulating a plantarflexion
  - Gait changes with ankle osteoarthritis (OA) (22)
    - Lower walking speed, lower ankle and hindfoot ROM, lower peak-ankle plantarflexion moment and lower peak-ankle power, lower peak-muscle activation of the calf muscles during walking

Subtalar joint
- Subtalar eversion and tibial-talar internal rotation during initial heel strike
  - Dissipates the GRF from an axial to a rotational vector at heel strike

Midfoot and forefoot
- The weight-bearing cross-lateral oblique (toe break line: weight bearing, shorter lever) to medial oblique (mobile, longer lever from calcaneus to big toe)
- Midfoot joint
  - Compensation mechanism to increase stability if midfoot stability compromised: stiffening strategy
    - Reduced ROM of the 1st metatarsal bone during walking
    - Disproportionate increase in 1st MT and calcaneal eversion ROM in more challenging activities (eg, stair descent)
- Loss of dorsiflexion of the first metatarsal phalangeal joint (MTPJ); hallux limitus/rigidus → limiting the transition from midstance to propulsion in the gait cycle referred to as "sagittal plane blocking"
  - Picking up the foot early (steppage), rolling-off the medial aspect of the foot abruptly, and shortening the stride on the involved side (limp)
  - Late and excessive supination, overloading the lateral metatarsals (or causing lateral side foot and lateral leg pain from peroneal overloading)

Pronation and supination response

	PRONATION	SUPINATION
Forefoot Midfoot/ hindfoot	Forefoot abduction Midfoot dorsiflexion Talonavicular and calcaneocuboid joint are parallel → Flexible, adaptive to irregular surface (initial stance phase) Navicular dropping Talus: medially deviated, plantarflexed Calcaneal eversion (normal up to 5°–10°)	Forefoot adduction Midfoot plantarflexion Talonavicular and calcaneocuboid joint intersect → Stiff, lever arm for push up (late stance phase) Calcaneal inversion
Common foot pattern/ deformity	Flat foot (forefoot varus/hindfoot valgus)	Cavus foot (forefoot valgus and hindfoot varus)
Proximal segment	Tibial/femur internal rotation (on standing; closed kinetic chain)	Tibia/femur external rotation
Common pathologies	Posterior tibialis tendon insufficiency Navicular pain, calcaneocuboid joint pain	Peroneus tendinopathy Midtarsal joint pain

FOOT ALIGNMENT AND DEFORMITY (23)

Arches of the foot
- Longitudinal arch (24,25)
  - Lever for transmission of plantarflexion force of Achilles tendon (not in other primate)
  - Medial arch and lateral arch (often neglected, calcaneus, cuboid, 4th and 5th metatarsals, important in Charcot neuroarthropathy progression)

- Beam (plantar ligament) and truss mechanism and windlass mechanism (plantar aponeurosis)
- Apex of the arch located at the transverse tarsal (midtarsal) joint medially and laterally (at cuboid)
- Key dynamic stabilizers: TP and gastroc-soleus muscle
- Transverse arch
  - Three metatarsocuneiform and two metatarsocuboid joints
  - Roman arch by the wedge-shaped bone (apex at intermediate cuneiform)
  - Dynamic stabilizers: TP and peroneus longus

Neutrally aligned feet: lower frequencies of intrinsic muscle atrophy, bony prominences, and toe deformities

Pes cavus (high arch foot) (26)
- Selective muscle weakness → imbalance of muscles → flexible deformity initially with fixed deformity later
  - Hereditary sensory motor neuropathy (CMT): peroneus brevis and TA primarily affected
    – Unopposed pull of posterior tibialis tendon (with fascia of abductor hallucis shortened) and tight Achilles cord → hindfoot varus
    – Unopposed pull of peroneus longus (PL) (plantarflexion of 1st MT; forefoot supinatus)
    – Achilles cord; hindfoot adductor (varus), EHL recruited as secondary ankle dorsiflexor
  - Foot intrinsic muscle weakness in peripheral neuropathy → unexposed extrinsic muscles such as EDL and FDL
    – Unopposed EDL: hyperextend the lesser MTP joint and flexion deformity of interphalangeal joint, forefoot equines → further shorten plantar fascia—cock-up hallux deformity
- Foot pain and deformity related to pes cavus (27)
  - Prolonged MTP joint plantarflexion (forefoot supinatus/varus) in cavus foot
    ▪ By putting the lateral forefoot on the ground, forefoot tilt laterally (forefoot varus) followed by hindfoot inversion; forefoot-driven hindfoot varus
    ▪ Limited lateral forefoot weight bearing on walking (forefoot already in varus) and functional hallux rigidus (MTP joint dorsiflexion) → Overusing toe break with pain during walking; at the end of stance phase or MTP joint subluxation
  - Ankle/subtalar arthropathy, midfoot arthropathy (asymmetric articular buttress)
  - Overload in the lateral aspect of the foot: peroneal tendinopathy, stress fracture on the metatarsal, and hindfoot varus (inversion): lateral ankle sprain
  - MTP joint overloading → MTP subluxation, high arch (plantar fasciitis)
  - Tight/short plantar fascia; plantar fasciitis

Pes planus (flat foot)
- Principal mechanical contributors: contracture of the triceps surae, attenuation of the ligamentous supports, and PTT dysfunction (25)
- Common foot pain conditions related to pes planus (28)
  - Leg pain (EDL overuse as it becomes major ankle dorsiflexor rather than TA with subtalar axis changes)
  - Plantar fasciitis with excessive traction to the plantar fascia
  - Functional hallux rigidus: as the foot rolls inward, the medial column (navicular, medial cuneiform, and first metatarsal) of the foot is elevated or dorsiflexed. Hallux valgus
  - TP dysfunction (etiology as well as result)
  - Arthralgia: ankle, subtalar, and talonavicular joint pain, later, calcaneocuboid joint pain by increased stress and asymmetry of forces transmitted through the ankle and subtalar joints

PHYSICAL EXAMINATION

INSPECTION (29)

Medial longitudinal arch
- From medial side inspection: look for congruence, flat in pes planus, and high arch (acute angle) in pes cavus

Hindfoot and midfoot
- Talonavicular joint area (observation from behind): concave (cavus) or convex (bulge: planus)
- Lateral aspect: convex (bulge) in pes cavus and concave below the lateral malleolus in pes planus
- Posterior aspect: calcaneus inversion (medial) in pes cavus and eversion in pes planus

Forefoot
- Alignment: abduction (lateral; too many toes sign) in pes planus or adduction in pes cavus (on axial plane)
  - With subtalar neutral, valgus in pes cavus and varus in pes planus (coronal plane)
- Forefoot deformities: hallux valgus, varus, toes (claw, hammer toes similar principles to finger deformity), joint enlargement/osteophytes, gout, OA, hallux rigidus/limitus
  - Toe deformity: claw, hammer toes similar principles to finger deformity
- Overlying toe, widening of 2nd web space, 2nd MTP subluxation (medially)
  - Often deformity is subtle
- Too-many-toes sign (≥2 toes laterally, from observation from behind) observed in forefoot abduction (pes planus and with posterior tibialis dysfunction)

Excessive callus
- Metatarsal heads (at MTP joint) common with Achilles tightness and pes cavus (1st ray plantarflexion), callus under the lesser toes common with 1st ray insufficiency (with pinch callus in phalange)
- Baby-like skin (indicating limited weight bearing) common with 1st ray insufficiency

Inspection of shoes
- Size; tight shoes (especially with forefoot pain), and worn-out pattern (laterally worn out in pes cavus, medially worn out in pes planus)

Foot posture index for pes cavus and planus (29)
- To semiquantify the degree of pronation or supination; useful in follow-up
  - Normal: 0 to 5, highly pronated: ≥10, highly supinated ≤−5

- Each component has −2 (supination) to +2 (pronation)
- Lateral malleolar curvature (concave), calcaneal position in coronal plane (eversion), prominence in the region of the talonavicular joint, congruence of medial longitudinal arch, and abduction of the forefoot
- Palpation for talar head
- Inspection for other foot deformities: equinus, varus, equinovarus, equinovalgus, and calcaneovalgus
- Have patient undress to evaluate the proximal segments
- Calf for atrophy or pseudohypertrophy, knee and hip alignment, and back for spinal deformity

PALPATION (SEE FIGURE 10.1)

Medial side
- Bony landmark
  - Medial malleolus, TP (on medial malleolus)
  - Navicular tuberosity: prominent bone 1- to 1.5-finger breadth distally/inferiorly (obliquely)
    - Talonavicular joint: proximal to navicular tuberosity
    - Naviculocuneiform: distal to navicular tuberosity
  - Cuneiform-1st MT joint: gap with metatarsal bone movement with shifting distal metatarsal bone (like seesawing a log)
  - Sustentaculum tali: one-finger breadth below and slightly distal to the medial malleolus (between medial malleolus and navicular tuberosity)
    - Calcaneal attachment site for calcaneonavicular ligament (spring ligament)
- Tendon
  - TP (between the medial malleolus and navicular tuberosity, visible with mild resisted hindfoot inversion and forefoot adduction)
  - Flexor digitorum longus (FDL) superficial to sustentaculum tali, and FHL is below the sustentaculum tali (not palpable)
  - Groove behind the medial malleolus: TP, FDL, vein, artery, nerves, and FHL (anterior to posterior)

Lateral side
- Lateral malleolus: ATFL attached at the tip
  - Tenderness on the anterior fibular tip in sprain
- Peroneal tubercle: inferior (1–1.5 cm below) and slightly distal to the lateral malleolus; bony crest between peroneus longus (below) and brevis (above); prominent in males, pes cavus, and osteoma formation
  - Peroneal tendon: visible with resisted eversion
- Cuboid: groove for peroneus longus
  - Calcaneocuboid joint: immediately distal to the sinus tarsi
  - Cuboid-4th metatarsal joint; mobile (compared to cuneiform-metatarsal joints): move the distal part of metatarsal bone while palpating the cuboid-4th metatarsal joint
- 5th MT (styloid process); gives attachment to peroneus brevis

Dorsum
- Ankle joint: about 1 cm above the bisecting line of the medial and lateral malleolus
- Talar head: bisecting line between the medial malleolus and navicular tuberosity, immediately proximal to the talonavicular joint prominent on eversion → more prominent in pes planus
  - Talonavicular joint; N spot; common location for spur or ganglion cyst, can irritate the superficial/deep peroneal nerve
- Sinus tarsi: depression at distal/medial (perpendicular to the foot axis) to the lateral malleolus
  - Common location of subtalar joint pain
- TA (easily visible with slight inversion and dorsiflexion), extensor hallucis longus (lateral to TA), dorsalis pedis artery, and deep peroneal nerve (not palpable) laterally

Plantar
- Medial calcaneal tuberosity: attachment site of plantar fascia
- Master knot of Henry: medial plantar nerve entrapment site at crossing of FHL and FDL (under the naviculocuneiform joint); difficult to palpate
- Sesamoids (move with flexion/extension of big toe as these are embedded in FHB, differential with MTP joint in tenderness)

RANGE OF MOTION

ANKLE	ROM (FUNCTIONAL)°	SUBTALAR	ROM (FUNCTIONAL)°	1ST MTP	ROM °	FOREFOOT	ROM °
Dorsiflexion	20 (10)	Inversion	35 (5–10)	Dorsiflexion	45	Adduction	20
Plantarflexion	45–50 (20)	Eversion	25 (5–10)	Plantarflexion	80	Abduction	10

MTP, metatarsophalangeal; ROM, range of motion.

Ankle joint motion
- Place subtalar joint in neutral, move the calcaneus and measure the angle between fibular shaft and lateral aspect of the sole
- Subtalar neutral with congruent talonavicular or calcaneocuboid joint: removes subtalar/midtarsal joint compensation. Compensation usually occurs with over-pronation response with navicular lateral deviation or drop
- Silfverskiold test: check ankle dorsiflexion (for Achilles cord tightness) while extending flexed knee (differentiate gastrocnemius component from soleus)
  - Gastrocnemius: two joints muscle (across the knee, therefore, ankle plantarflexion tightness worse as knee extends) (30)
- Equinus: inability to dorsiflex the ankle ≥10° (31)
  - Equinus state: <10°, equinus deformity <5° of dorsiflexion
  - Inspection for other deformities (varus, valgus, and toe deformities)

Subtalar joint motion
- Subtalar motion: 25° inversion/supination and 10° of eversion/pronation (2:1 ratio of inversion to eversion)

- Subtalar neutral: anatomical neutral position for physical examination
  ◦ Often used conceptually for balanced position in deformity (correction to anatomically neutral position can aggravate symptoms in a patient with long-standing deformity)
- With patient in a prone position, the bisected line of the heel is compared with the bisected line of the lower leg while the calcaneus is being inverted and everted
  ◦ Normal ROM is a 2:1 (20°:10°) relationship of inversion to eversion
  ◦ Check rigidity as it affects the decision for treatment (correction versus accommodation)

Check the forefoot (MTP joint) sitting and standing (MTP dorsiflexion with tethering effect from tight FHL)

Check for hypermobility: Beighton scale ≥4/9 (1 point for each side; 5th MCP hyperextension >90°, passive apposition of the thumb to forearm, elbow hyperextension >10°, knee hyperextension >10°, and trunk forward flexion to place the palm of the hand at rest on the floor; see Figure 1.2)
- Benign joint hypermobility syndrome; major criteria:
  ◦ Beighton scale ≥4, arthralgia >3 months in four joints (revised Brighton Criteria) (32)

SPECIAL TESTS (see following table)

NAME	DESCRIPTION	SENSITIVITY (SEN) AND SPECIFICITY (SPE) IN %
Ankle Sprain		
Inversion/eversion stress test (talar tilt test)	With ankle plantarflexion at 20° and knee flexion at 90°, heel is held from below by one hand while the other hand holds the lower leg Push the calcaneus and talus into eversion while the other hand grips the lower leg laterally and pushes medially for deltoid ligament injury and the opposite (inversion for anterior talofibular and calcaneofibular lig. injury) Positive if pain and laxity found during maneuver	Sen: 71–96, Spe: 33–84 (within 48 hours), higher in 4–7 days (33)
Anterior drawer test	Examiner stabilizes the distal tibia with one hand, while grasping the heel with the other hand. Apply an anteriorly directed force to the heel. This test should be performed bilaterally to compare for differences in anterior translation Positive if pain or increased joint laxity ± a dimple or if >3 mm translation Limited in patients with ligament laxity or guarding with pain	Sen: 80, Spe: 74
Anterolateral drawer test	Isolated testing of ATFL. Anterior drawer test with slight medial rotation of the forefoot. Slight medial rotation isolates resistance of anterior translation by tibionavicular lig. With ankle plantarflexed, it can isolate CFL	
Syndesmosis Injury		
Squeeze test	With proximal calf squeeze (distract/widen the distal part), the patient reports pain in the ankle. Less reliable than passive ankle dorsiflexion test • Passive ankle dorsiflexion test; widen mortise (stretch the syndesmosis) as anterior talar dome is wider	
Cross leg test	With crossing the symptomatic leg, the patient reports pain (in the ankle) and symptom reproduction • Weight of foot externally rotate the leg by gravity → widen the mortise	
External rotation stress test	Similar principle to cross leg test with widening the mortise by abducting forefoot	
Other Heel Examination		
Calcaneal squeeze test	Mediolateral compression simultaneously by thenar eminence causing pain Positive in calcaneal fracture and Sever's disease (apophysitis) • Heel propping test: stand with examiner holding the fat pad with hypothenar eminence → relief of pain indicating fat-pad atrophy	Sen: 97, Spe: 100 for Sever's disease
Coleman's block test	To evaluate the midfoot flexibility of forefoot-driven (PL-driven) cavovarus Place wooden block (1 or 1/2 inch) under the lateral border of the foot (4th and 5th MT) to reverse forefoot supinatus (varus) • If hindfoot varus is supple, hindfoot varus correctable, Figure 10.4 • If hindfoot varus is fixed → hindfoot varus not corrected (34,35)	

(continued)

NAME	DESCRIPTION	SENSITIVITY (SEN) AND SPECIFICITY (SPE) IN %
Tibialis Posterior (TP) Dysfunction		
Heel rise test	Normally, the patient inverts the hindfoot as they lift heels, positive if failed to do on double heel rise test Single heel rise test if the double heel rise test is intact (36)	
Metatarsal rise test	The patient stands, fully loading both feet. The shin of the affected side is taken with one hand and externally rotated. By doing this, the heel is passively brought into a varus position because of the mechanical coupling between the tibia and calcaneum (supination response). The head of the first metatarsal remains on the ground in normal function of the tendon but is lifted in dysfunction (37)	
Morton's Interdigital Neuritis (38)		
Lateral squeeze test	Squeeze the metatarsal shaft from the sides → positive if it reproduces the pain (lateral forefoot) Often false positive if pressed on the MTP joint (pain source can be from MTP joint pathology)	
Mulder's click	Squeezing the forefoot (metatarsal shaft) from the sides. Positive (for neuroma) if a palpable (not necessarily audible) clicking is appreciated	
Compression test	Compress the nerve from the plantar aspect (distal to the MTP joint) with MTP dorsiflexion (therefore, exposing the interdigital N plantarly). Positive if reproducing the symptom	
Pinch test	Pinch from the plantar and dorsum of interdigital space. Positive if reproducing the symptom	
First Ray Insufficiency		
Drawer sign	Shift 1st metatarsal head compared to the 2nd MT head. Positive if ≥8 to 10 mm of dorsal displacement occurs	
Achilles Tendon Rupture		
Matles test	In the prone position, with the foot over the end of the table, the patient is asked to flex the knee to 90°. The position of the foot is observed throughout the arc, and the foot is slightly plantarflexed normally. Positive if the foot falls into neutral or the slightest dorsiflexed position	Sen: 88, Spe: 85
Thompson test	When squeezing the calf of the affected leg, normally the ankle will be slightly plantarflexed. Positive if no motion of the foot occurs	Sen: 96, Spe: 93

ATFL, anterior talofibular ligament; CFL, calcaneofibular ligament; lig., ligament; N, nerve; Sen., sensitivity; Spe., specificity; TP, tibialis posterior.

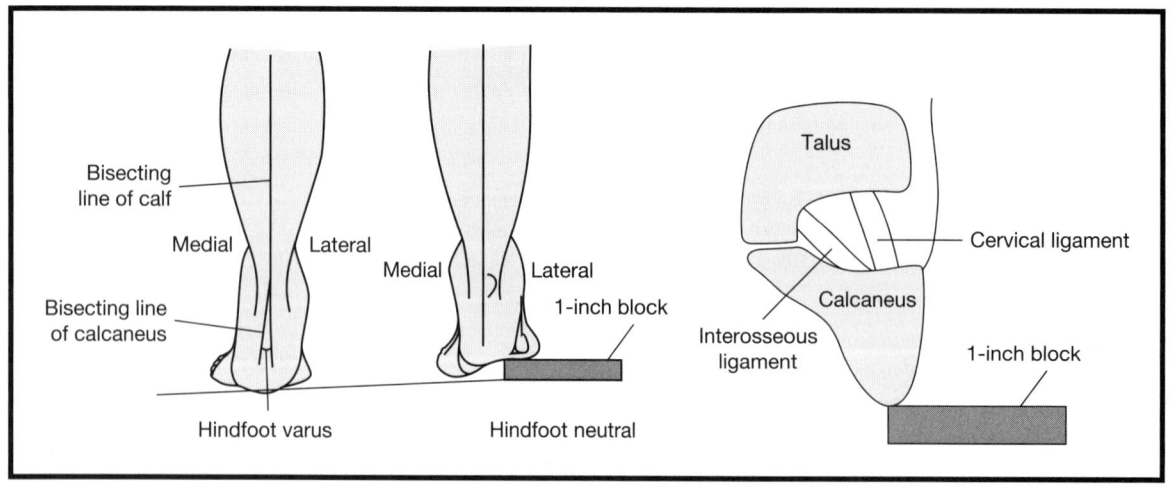

FIGURE 10.4
Coleman's block test

Evaluation for instability (39)
- Ankle and subtalar instability; difficult to distinguish clinically (9)
- Evaluate cavus deformity (hindfoot varus, 1st ray plantarflexion), generalized ligamentous laxity (Beighton score), hindfoot varus (inspection and Coleman block test), and ankle ligaments injury
- Subtalar instability test: calcaneus inversion test with ankle dorsiflexion (stabilizing the ankle joint)
- Midtarsal joint examination by abduction/adduction stress test

DIAGNOSTIC STUDIES

PLAIN RADIOGRAPHS (40) (FLOWCHART 10.3)

Indications
- History of trauma: rule out (R/O) fracture or dislocation
  - The Ottawa ankle rules: (41) x-ray is only required in the ankle pain with one of the following:
    - Tenderness along the distal 6 cm of the medial, lateral malleolus, the base of 5th MT or navicular bone
    - Inability to bear weight for four steps at the time of the injury
    - High sensitivity (useful in ruling out), high false positive and overall reduction of radiographs by 30% to 40%
- Chronic pain, swelling, and decreased ROM
- Deformity

Limitations
- Low capability to assess soft tissues (except tendon calcification), articular cartilage, intra-articular or intracortical lesion, or bursal effusion
- X-ray underestimates the disease

Individual views
- Routine
  - Anteroposterior (AP), standing lateral, medial/lateral oblique (for lateral and medial structures)
  - Ankle: AP, lateral, mortise view
  - Ankle x-ray analysis
    - 3 to 4 mm in width, medial clear space 3 to 4 mm and lateral clear space 5 mm
    - Tibiofibular syndesmosis should have slight overlap
    - Soft-tissue swelling: ankle effusion, pre-Achilles triangle, or Kager fat pad
    - Osteochondritis dissecans: involves talus, tibial plafond, and navicular: often negative in x-ray
- Standing AP
  - Pes planus: talocalcaneal angle >35°, increased angle of talus and 1st MT, heel valgus, talonavicular uncoverage

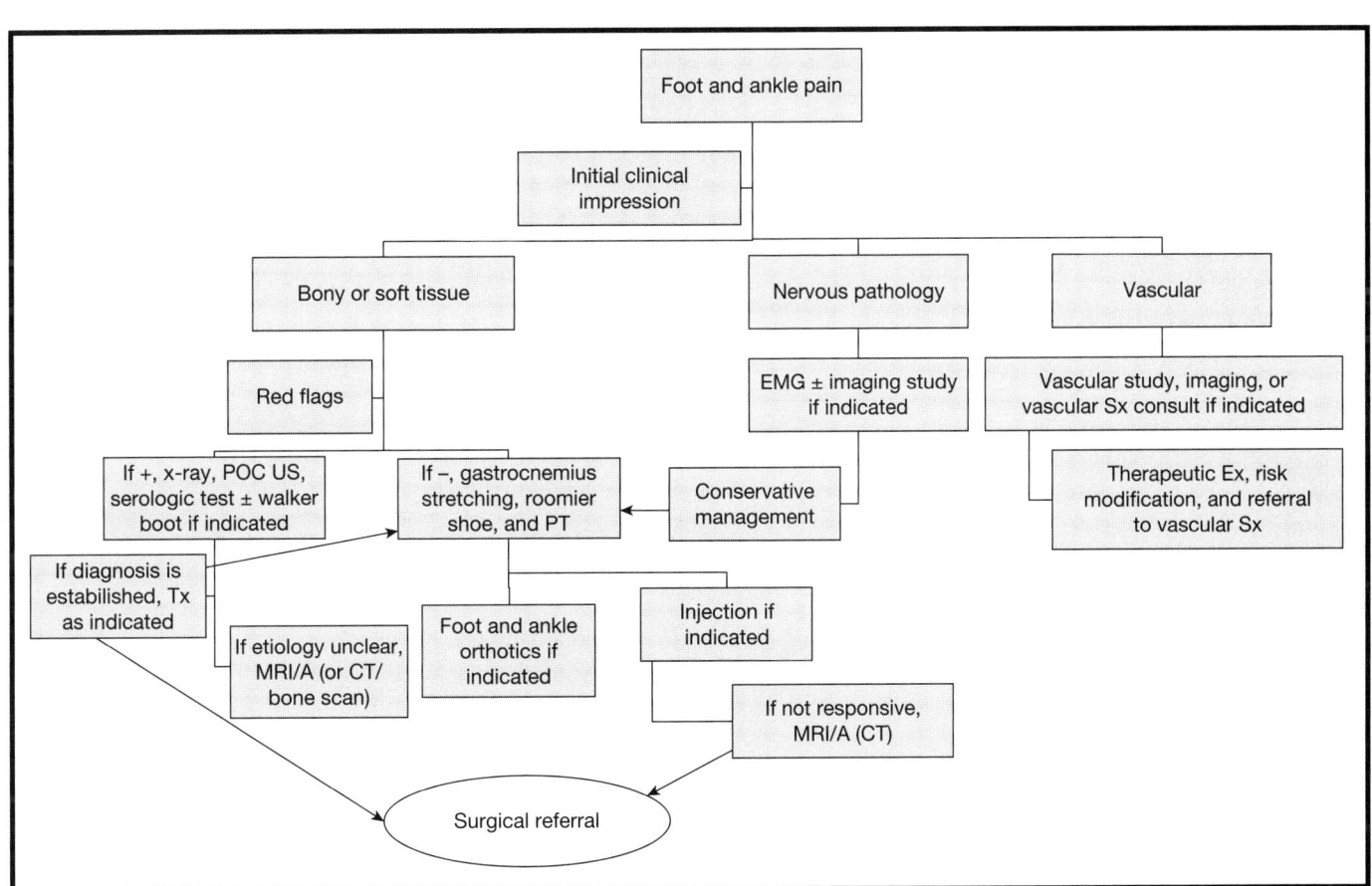

FLOWCHART 10.3
Diagnostic approach and management plan for foot and ankle pain in outpatient clinic.
EMG, electromyography; Ex, exercise; POC, point-of-care; PT, physical therapy; Sx, surgery; Tx, treatment; US, ultrasound.

- Pes cavus: negative talus-1st metatarsal angle, decreased talocalcaneal angle, and metatarsus abduction
- Lateral weight-bearing view (42) (Figure 10.5)
  - Meary's angle (A)
    - Angle between long axis of the talus and long axis of the 1st metatarsal: collapse of longitudinal arch may occur at the talonavicular (TN), naviculocuneiform (NC), or cuneiform-metatarsal (CM) joints. >4° convex downward = pes planus, >4° convex upward = pes cavus. Angle of 15° to 30° considered moderate, and greater than 30° is severe
  - Calcaneal pitch line (B)
    - Normal 17° to 32°. Decreased calcaneal pitch = pes planus. Increased pitch = pes cavus
  - Böhler angle
    - Angle between two lines drawn from the top of the anterior tuberosity to posterior facet and from the top of the posterior tuberosity of the calcaneus to posterior facet on the lateral radiograph
    - Normal: 20° to 40°. Less than 20° can be seen in calcaneal fracture. However, a normal Böhler angle does not exclude a calcaneal fracture
  - Hibbs' angle: angle of intersection of the lines along the axes of the calcaneus and the first metatarsal bones
    - Normal >150°, less than 150°: pes cavus
  - Findings for coalition: calcaneonavicular coalition (anteater nose sign; tubular prolongation of the superior calcaneus overlaps the navicular) and talocalcaneal coalition (complete C-sign; posterior ring around the talus and sustentaculum tali)
- Oblique view
- Others: Harris Beath view for body of calcaneus, middle facet of subtalar joint (Broden's view), and sustentaculum tali (43)

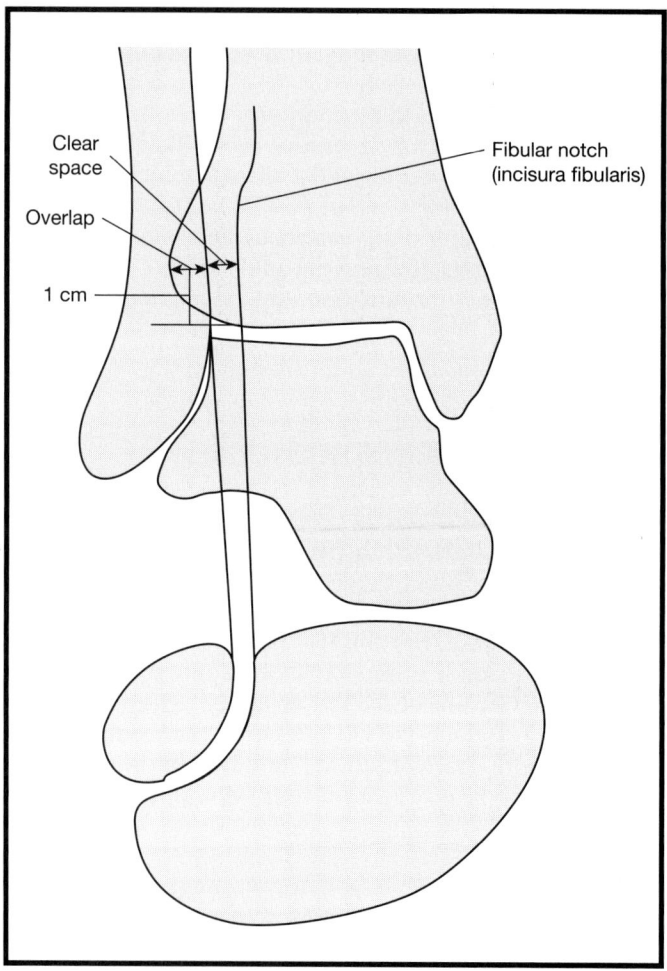

FIGURE 10.5 *(continued)*

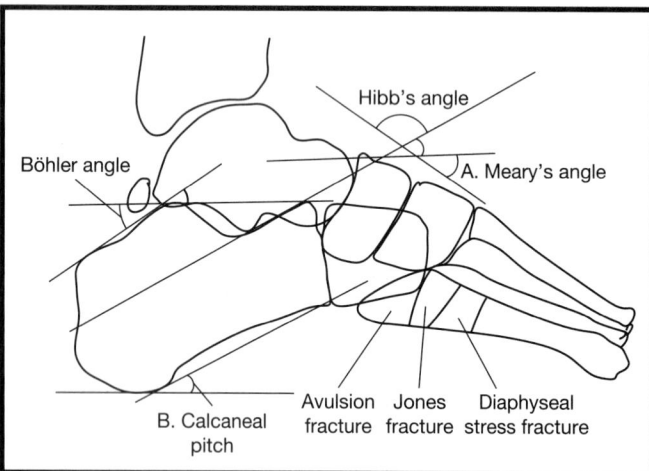

FIGURE 10.5
X-ray measurements in foot and ankle disorders.

(continued)

POINT-OF-CARE ULTRASONOGRAPHY (44)

Ankle and Hindfoot (45)

Indications and findings
- Joint evaluation (46)
  - Ankle (talocrural) joint; anterior recess evaluation with ankle plantarflexion
    - Joint effusion: US can detect about 2 mL of effusion (vs 1 mL by MRI)
      - Differential diagnosis: synovitis, osteoarthritis flare up, intra-articular bodies (limited), and simple effusion versus complex effusion (limited)
  - Subtalar joint (posterior, lateral, and medial), and midtarsal (talonavicular and calcaneocuboid) joint effusion, osteophytes, bulging ligament, and capsule/soft tissue
  - Ganglion cyst in periarticular region; often communicate with the joint

Tendon evaluation
- Medial: TP and FDL (at the sustentaculum tali). Posterior: Achilles tendon/FHL. Lateral: peroneus longus and brevis (peroneal tubercle)
- The distal end of the TP tendon usually becomes thickened as it nears its attachment to the medial border of navicular bone and may also appear hypoechoic due to anisotropy
- Lateral: peroneus longus, brevis, and hyperechoic superior and inferior peroneal retinacula above tendons
  - Peroneus longus superficial to brevis in the retromalleolar groove
  - Peroneus brevis above peroneal tubercle and longus below peroneal tubercle
  - Dynamic view for subluxation (with peroneal retinaculum tear)
- A small or even moderate amount of fluid in the posterior peri-articular tendons may be a normal finding or may reflect fluid communicating from an ankle joint effusion
- Sesamoid bones and accessory ossicles: often confused with tendon or tendon sheath calcification. Also a smooth margin and an absence of surrounding edema/fluid should help distinguish them from an acute tendon or ligamentous avulsion injury

Ligament and other soft-tissue evaluation
- Lateral ankle ligaments
  - ATFL: the ligament course parallel to the sole, distal to the tip of the fibula
    - Often hypoechoic due to anisotropy
    - Dynamic maneuver to check for full thickness tear (hindfoot inversion or forefoot adduction)
  - Calcaneofibular ligament; courses under peroneal tendon, slightly tilt the distal part of the probe posterior (10°–20°), forced dorsiflexion or inversion → taut ligament; better image
    - Dynamic maneuver with ankle inversion → peroneus tendon pushed up by intact calcaneofibular ligament (CFL), but if torn, no bowstring effect
- Medial ankle ligaments
  - Deltoid ligament: under the medial tendons (TP and FDL)
    - Anterior, posterior tibiotalar, tibionavicular, and tibiocalcaneal ligaments
    - Often difficult to probe parallel to the structure
- Challenge: acute ligament tear is less well-defined as hemorrhage may be echogenic, masking the tear in the ligament. Tears may, therefore, be better seen on delayed scanning (2–3 days)
- Plantar fascia
  - Fasciitis: asymmetric, thickened fascia with hypoechoic appearance
  - Plantar fascia thickness is measured on transverse scan

Imaging for instability: subluxation of tendon or ligament tear with dynamic maneuver

Forefoot (47) and Midfoot

Joint and bone evaluation
- 1st MTP joint for arthropathy (inflammatory or DJD), 2nd MTP subluxation (medially subluxation → overlying toes), and sesamoid pathology on the plantar aspect (of 1st MTP)
- Joint effusion ± synovitis, crystal deposition (cartilage-soft-tissue junction in gout), and tophaceous form in late stage of gout
- 2nd metatarsal bone: stress fracture (common site: periosteal reaction, elevated periosteum with hypoechoic band, cortical interruption, and hypervascularity) and metatarsal head pathology (Freiberg disease)

Tendon
- Anterior tibialis inserts on cuneiform and 1st metatarsal bone (check for tear, tendinopathy, and enthesopathy)
- Flexor/extensor hallucis longus tendon (check for tenosynovitis, tendinopathy, and enthesopathy) and FHB (sesamoids)

Bursa and nerve
- Interdigital bursitis (adventitial: compressible), ganglion cyst (usually not compressible), and interdigital neuroma (MC in 3rd interdigital space, not compressible, and displaced upward by dorsally directed force)

MRI (48)

Indications
- Evaluation of soft-tissue lesions, intra-articular lesions (eg, osteochondritis dissecans), intracortical, and preoperative surgical evaluation

Common findings
- Bony and joint pathologies: stress fractures, synovial pathologies (synovial chondromatosis, pigmented villonodular synovitis), and gout (tophaceous form: a late manifestation)
- Cystic lesions: ganglia (MC soft-tissue masses), synovial cysts, and bursitis
- Noncystic lesions: Morton's neuroma, lipoma, giant cell tumor of tendon sheath, plantar fibromatosis, and rheumatoid nodules
- Neoplasms: fibromatosis and giant cell tumor of tendon sheath: MC benign tumors.
  - MC malignant tumors: synovial sarcoma, malignant fibrous histiocytoma (undifferentiated pleomorphic sarcoma), and leiomyosarcoma

CT SCAN

- Indication: when MRI is contraindicated, and for complex or intra-articular fracture, and preoperative planning

TREATMENT

NONOPERATIVE MANAGEMENT

Physical therapy for therapeutic exercise (49)
- Stretching of gastrocnemius, flexor hallucis, digitorum longus, EDL, and plantar fascia (not stretched together with Achilles tendon usually as it can lead to rupture of plantar fascia)
  - Stretching gastrocnemius muscle
    - Tight gastrocnemius: highly prevalent
    - Extremely effective for non-insertional tendinopathy but only one-third responsive in insertional tendinopathy

- Precaution: subtalar joint should be neutral (or slightly inverted; forefoot shouldn't be abducted, which is a common error)
  - Precaution in patient with diabetes → caution for midfoot fracture in Charcot neuroarthropathy
  ○ Stretch the proximal hip internal/external rotator and hamstring (affects pronation and supination response; however, often difficult to stretch)
- Strengthening
  ○ Strengthen peroneus longus, brevis muscles in ankle inversion sprain (especially in eccentric mode) and instability (inversion type)
  ○ Eccentric strengthening exercise of gastrocsoleus (heel slowly lowered to floor [neutral in insertional tendinopathy]) or the edge of a step (to ankle dorsiflexion in noninsertional Achilles tendinopathy)
  ○ Posterior tibialis muscle strengthening: unclear role in PTT. Isometric and/or eccentric strengthening exercise
  ○ Address the proximal and foot intrinsic muscles (short foot exercise) (50)
- Therapy for instability (51)
  ○ Neuromuscular training: balance, restore posture control, and active stability in addition to strengthening and stretching exercise
  ○ Wobble board activity, hop to stabilization exercise, single-limb stance balance exercise with different surface
  ○ Education for taping (try taping during session), and air stirup (improve proprioceptive feedback)

Oral medications
- Acetaminophen (AAP), nonsteroidal anti-inflammatory drug (NSAID), and short course of muscle relaxant and short course of methylprednisone
- Weak opioid medications if the above medication is not effective or contraindicated
  ○ Follow analgesic ladder
- Neuropathic pain medication as needed

Common injections
- Ankle joint injection
  ○ Distal to proximal, using 27 G, 1.5-inch needle unless needed for aspiration, ankle plantarflexion, medial to the tibialis anterior tendon
  ○ Cautious of the deep/superficial peroneal nerve (SPN) and dorsalis pedis artery
- Subtalar joint injection
  ○ Different approaches available (52)
    - Medial: on top of sustentaculum tali (with slight ankle eversion), lateral: under the peroneal tendon and posteriorly
  ○ Usually requiring imaging guidance like US
- Sinus-tarsi injection: for sinus-tarsi pain secondary to ligamentous, retinacular, and possibly subtalar joint arthropathy
- Morton's interdigital nerve injection to nerve–bursal complex
  ○ Cautious of the plantar fat pad (dorsal approach, needs US guidance, not beyond the nerve–bursal complex)
- Retrocalcaneal bursal injection
  ○ Immediately underneath the Achilles tendon above the calcaneus, cautious of sural nerve and Achilles tendon (27 G 1.5-inch needle if no aspiration indicated)
- Plantar fascia injection
  ○ Posterolateral; cautious of fat-pad injection (causing fat-pad atrophy, approach through the dorsal skin), US guidance and using 27 G, 1.5-inch needle
  ○ Other approach: medial (cautious of tibial nerve, branches from tibial nerve, artery)
  ○ Baxter's nerve injection (or blocking tibial nerve at the distal tarsal tunnel)
- Other joint injection; midtarsal (talonavicular, calcaneocuboid joint) and MTP joint (gout) using imaging guidance, ≤1 mL of injectate volume
- Platelet plasma injection (53) for plantar fascia, Achilles tendon, and intra-articular injection
- Nerve block
  ○ Tarsal tunnel steroid injection for neuropathic pain in the sole of the foot
    - Pulsed radiofrequency for tarsal tunnel syndrome (TOS) (54)
  ○ Superficial peroneal nerve block at the location of entrapment (using US guidance) and deep peroneal nerve injection next to the dorsal pedal artery
  ○ Motor branch block (with alcohol, phenol) (55,56), botulism toxin injection for spastic muscle (tibial nerve motor point block to gastrocnemius) followed by casting or ankle foot orthosis (AFO) after injection

Foot Orthosis (57)

Taping application (58)
- Indications: plantar fasciitis, plantar fat-pad atrophy, Achilles tendinopathy, 2nd MTP subluxation, midfoot arthritis or toe fracture, and others
- Classification of taping
  ○ Nonelastic (cotton, cotton polyester blends, and Leukotape)
    - Optimal joint support, limiting abnormal or excessive ROM, or possibly improving alignment
    - Leukotape: a high tensile strength, rayon-backed tape with aggressive zinc-oxide adhesive
      – Contains natural latex rubber, which may cause skin reactions and is specified for use over cover-roll stretch bandage (hypoallergenic, translucent, and permeable to air and exudates)
  ○ Elastic sports tapes
    - Often used in combination with nonelastic tapes
    - Easily conform to angular body parts and joints and can be used when circling soft tissues that require room for expansion
    - Made of 100% porous cotton fibers, which allow for evaporation and quicker drying
    - Can be stretched up to 30% to 40% of its resting length longitudinally
    - Wear time: up to 3 to 4 days

Commonly used taping

TAPING	MECHANISM	INDICATIONS
Budin taping	Figure of 8 tape across the 2nd toe to the mid- and hindfoot	2nd MTP subluxation/ overlying toe
Buddy taping	Decrease free movement of phalange	Fracture of the toe or subluxation of toe (2nd toe to 3rd if 2nd toe is medially subluxed)

(continued)

TAPING	MECHANISM	INDICATIONS
Modified low-Dye taping	Support longitudinal (plantar fascia) and transverse arch Contain the fat pad Provide extra layer; attachment site for padding	Plantar fasciitis Fat-pad dysfunction PTT dysfunction (trial before orthoses) Midfoot arthritis (tape covering the dorsum, for trial)
Achilles taping	Limit ankle dorsiflexion or improve proprioceptive awareness	Achilles tendinopathy

MTP, metatarsophalangeal; PTT, posterior tibialis tendon.

- Unna boot
  - Semirigid dressing with zinc, glycine ± calamine: edema control, improve venous return without restriction of the physical activity
  - Indications
    - Ankle sprain, PTT and peroneal tendon dysfunction (tendinopathy, tenosynovitis, partial tear) ± padding, rheumatoid arthritis (RA) flare up or other arthropathy
    - Venous insufficiency
    - Subacute or chronic pain with vasomotor instability (complex regional pain syndrome [CRPS])
    - Two to three layers or more overlap (especially if resting and limiting motion are required)
- General principle for orthotic prescription
  - Identify the underlying biomechanical problem → intervention directed toward abnormal biomechanics (often accommodating some deformity or limiting progression rather than correction)
  - Trial of off-the-shelf orthotics if available: the best way to predict a response and compliance
    - Premade available (if trial successful, then may consider custom-made)
    - Can be made (cut) from felt-pad material
  - Require roomier shoe (to accommodate room for orthotic, otherwise not successful)

Commonly used foot inserts (Figure 10.6)

FOOT INSERTS	BIOMECHANICS	INDICATIONS AND NOTES
Heel lift	Prevent abnormal sagittal plane compensation of tight Achilles cord Decrease toe break, tension for plantar fascia and flexor muscles Modification available (with U-shaped relief) ± other orthotics - Three layers of felt pad (office-made) - ¼-inch bottom; shortest layer - ¼-inch U-shape: medium length layer - ⅛-inch top: longest layer	Pes cavus Heel spur (heel lift with relief), plantar fasciitis, peroneal tendon irritation by heel counter (pseudo-peroneal tendinopathy), winter heel/Haglund's deformity, FHL tendinitis (with carbon plate) Leg length discrepancy (heel lift should not be more than 1-cm thickness) Foot slapping (weak ankle dorsiflexion weakness) Always recommend gastrocnemius stretching (education and a few sessions of PTs) as heel lift promotes Achilles tightness
Medial wedge ± extension	Mitigate flexible hindfoot eversion; ± navicular padding/relief Thomas heel and Barton's wedge	PTT dysfunction, medial ankle sprain (eversion) Knee pain with genu valgum (often with heel lift) Forefoot varus (heel lift with medial extension to forefoot) 1st ray plantarflexion in cavus (Barton's wedge ± heel lift)
1st ray posting	Increase contact of the 1st ray weight-bearing surface; therefore, reduce lateral overloading	1st ray insufficiency with the lateral forefoot or lateral foot overloading syndrome
Lateral wedge	Mitigate flexible hindfoot inversion (varus)	Lateral ankle sprain, pes cavus, sinus-tarsi syndrome Often with medial forefoot wedge (post) or lateral wedge (pillow for peroneal overloading syndrome) Flexible pes cavus (with extension to the lateral forefoot; if subtalar joint is flexible on Coleman block test) Medial knee pain with genu varum
Cuboid pad	Mitigate the downward instability of cuboid	Cuboid subluxation (± carbon plate) Cuboid-4th MT subluxation and arthropathy (± carbon plate)
Metatarsal pad	Restore transverse arch and mitigate the plantarflexion of metatarsal head (MTP hyperextension); distribute weight bearing more proximally The bulk of the pad should sit proximal to the metatarsal heads	Metatarsalgia, MTP subluxation (± Budin splint), Morton's neuritis, intermetatarsal bursitis, and metatarsal stress fracture (with carbon plate) Pes cavus with forefoot overloading
Interdigital spacer	Widen the interdigital space and decreased subluxing force temporarily	2nd MTP subluxation Hallux valgus

MTP, metatarsophalangeal joint.

- Other over-the-counter and office-made orthotics
  ○ Dorsal donut pad (to relieve the irritation of cutaneous nerves such as superficial peroneal and deep peroneal nerves)
  ○ 1/8-inch plastazote insert acts as an "additional fat pad" under the insole with/without hole (eg, pressure relief for sesamoiditis)
  ○ Carbon plate: limit joint mobility in the foot, contoured (slight plantarflexion on the midfoot and forefoot), used with rocker-bottom shoe
    ▪ Common indications: midtarsal and midfoot arthritis, hallux rigidus, stress fracture, cuboid subluxation, and the like
    ▪ Can be fabricated (Arch rival®) with lateral flare and 1st MTP depression (for 1st-ray plantar flexion) or custom-made
  ○ Pneumatic ankle brace and anklet (laced): may not provide sufficient control of the subtalar complex, although it may offer some edema control and sensory feedback
  ○ Catalogs available on the Internet

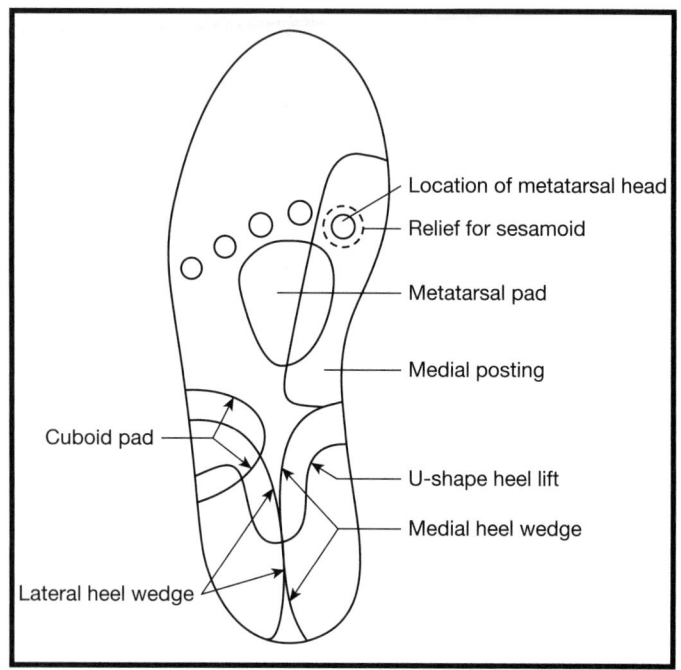

FIGURE 10.6
Location of foot inserts.

Commonly prescribed foot and ankle orthoses

ORTHOSIS	MECHANISM	COMMON INDICATIONS AND PROBLEMS

Custom-made foot orthosis (insole)	Conform to the plantar contour and accommodate the deformity (combination of other inserts; heel lift, medial extension/posting, metatarsal pad, etc)
	• Requires roomier shoe
	• Four layers
	  ○ Plastazote; closed cell form of polyethylene
	  ○ PPT® (polyurethane foam); open cell, not heat moldable
	  ○ Spenco (on the top): closed cell expanded rubber, ~¼-inch thickness
	  ○ Cork (hard material)
		More successful after trial of in-office orthotic (felt pad or heel lift) for metatarsalgia, 1st-ray insufficiency, sesamoiditis etc.
		Problems
		• Medial arch pain with ambitious medial arch support
		  ○ With aging, medial arch of patient can further collapse
		  ○ May cause the medial plantar N irritation (Jogger's foot) and lateral overloading syndrome (due to tilting)
		• May cause functional hallux rigidus because the foot orthosis elevates the metatarsal bone with forefoot adduct
		• 2D orthosis or arch support: minimally effective in ≥ stage 2 PTT dysfunction

University of California Biomechanics Laboratory (UCBL) orthosis	3-point control system • One point on the medial side (on sustentaculum tali) → elevation of the anteromedial calcaneus → upward thrust against the sustentaculum tali to prevent medial in-rolling • Two points on the lateral side: 5th MT (lateral shaft) and calcaneus Longitudinal arch support (maintains the optimal position of the calcaneus relative to the talus) Control excessive pronation by controlling the calcaneus eversion to keep the subtalar joint in a neutral position	Indications: posterior tibialis dysfunction with/without pes planus Problems • Discomfort wearing it and fitting inside the shoe • Forefoot covers two-thirds or half of metatarsal head (lateral wall), if higher → may not fit the shoe • Long-lateral walls (control forefoot abduction) Precautions • Better tolerated by the patient if not too rigid (5/32-inch copolymer or polypropylene) • Naviculocuneiform relief by Gillet posting: under the medial arch to dampen the medial rolling • Cupping the heel • Avoid aggressive arch support

(continued)

ORTHOSIS	MECHANISM	COMMON INDICATIONS AND PROBLEMS
Supramalleolar orthotic (SMO)	Mitigate forefoot abduction by long lateral extension and forefoot varus by posting inside Holds calcaneus Soft interface medially Medial posting (Gillet posting) outside the medial wall to dampen medial in-rolling Heel lift under the SMO to accommodate the ankle equinus U-shape relief (Haglund modification) for posterior heel pain with Haglund deformity	Indications: PTT dysfunction, painful pes planus, Haglund deformity Problems and precautions • Thickness: slightly thinner than 5/32-inch polypropylene or co-polymer (maybe too soft) • Aggressive medial arch support causes medial hindfoot (navicular tuberosity) pain → Gillet posting (medial posting) to accommodate/allow some pronation with padding or relief at navicular tuberosity • Medial arch: can be added later (preferred over arch support built in the SMO, which is difficult to modify)
Dynamic AFO	Articulation/posterior support: provides additional stiffness to resist dorsiflexion torque while allowing some ankle dorsiflexion to occur	Indication: pediatric hypermobile flat foot
Arizona (lace up leather) AFO	Ankle support while fitting in many shoes Dampens the effect of deforming force of gastrocsoleus and mitigating ankle dorsiflexion Diminishes the dorsiflexion moment on the midfoot structure and retains normal anatomic rocking motions	Indication: PTT dysfunction, ankle, subtalar, and midtarsal arthritis • Soft, short, ankle set at slight plantarflexion is better tolerated (especially with tight Achilles cord). Soft material (co-polymer) is better tolerated
Cam walker (walking boot)	Similar to cast	Indications: nondisplaced stress fracture, osteochondritis dissecans, tendinopathy/tear with significant pain, severe ankle sprain, Charcot neuroarthropathy • Advantage: allows observation of wound, convenient • Disadvantage: cannot control edema, wall weight bearing is not possible, and poor patient compliance

AFO, ankle foot orthotic; lat., lateral; N, nerve; PTT, posterior tibialis tendon; SMO, supramalleolar orthotic; UCBL, California Biomechanics Laboratory.

- Pain using AFO
  ○ Common location of pain: medial hindfoot near the navicular tuberosity
  ○ Common cause: the ankle angle of AFO set neutrally or slightly dorsiflexed in patients with tight Achilles cord → compensation at subtalar joint to accommodate this (put the heel down to the ground) with pronation response including navicular dropping → medial hindfoot irritation against AFO
  ○ Recognize the tight heel cord when casting, or accommodate by putting heel lift on heel of AFO

Shoes (59)
- Diabetic shoes; traditional
  ○ Triple depth (extra-depth), three-layer insoles, steel shank (less common because too heavy), medial reinforcement (buttress), and Thomas heel (medial heel extension)
  ○ Modified rocker; location of rocker can change the pressure. Forefoot rocker may increase midfoot or hindfoot pressure
  ○ In-shoe relief can be added for pressure relief
  ○ If not available, roomier walking sneakers are good alternatives
- Shoes ideal for foot pain
  ○ Roomier shoes: especially for forefoot pain, consider the space for possibly adding inserts
  ○ Generally, rigid heel counter, straight-shaped last, dual density midsole, flexible forefoot are ideal characteristics
  ○ Modification or custom-designed shoes: available in some shoe repair shops or supplied by pedorthotist (usually expensive)
    ▪ Thomas heel extension (especially for obese patients), medial buttress modification for support, steel shank
    ▪ Rocker: restoring the motion in the foot and ankle and off-loading the plantar pressure; more effect on forefoot (rocker mechanism requires steady/stiff midsole; otherwise, it can collapse)
    ▪ Toe spring can work as a rocker with carbon plate
    ▪ Cushion heel: simulates plantarflexion
- Pronation control versus supination-control shoes
  ○ Pronation-control shoes: usually for pes planus, medial-side firmer/reinforcement, straight last
    ▪ Advertised as motion control
    ▪ If used in patients with pes cavus (medial hindfoot reinforcement similar medial wedge), lateral overloading can occur by lateral tilting or sliding
  ○ Supination control: lateral side thicker/reinforcement, curved last
    ▪ Most of running sneakers
- Shoes for pes cavus
  ○ Extra-depth, roomier shoe (accommodate high arch and possible orthotics), split last (if possible; however, more expensive)
  ○ Running shoes: anti-supinator and lateral flare (reinforcement on the lateral side to address a lateral overloading)

- Shoes for pes planus
  - Flexible flat foot without symptoms
  - Bracing or taping if causing pain or secondary problems (roomier shoe required): heel lift, medial heel wedge, foot/ankle orthotic (University of California Biomechanics Laboratory [UCBL], supramalleolar orthotic [SMO])
- Common problems with shoes and foot orthotics
  - Tight shoes: MC culprit (for >50% of forefoot pain)
    - Check width and toe box height (room) and heel counter (lateral heel counter often irritating lateral malleolus mimicking peroneal tendinopathy). Achilles notch (especially for posterior heel pain)
    - Too-firm midsole; masked by soft insole. Take the insole out and press the bottom of the shoe to check firmness of the midsole
  - Different types of heeled shoes for different foot phenotypes
    - Low-heeled shoe with pes cavus; overstretching plantar fascia and overloading forefoot (therefore, better with heeled shoe)
    - The high-heeled gait: slower gait speed, shorter stride length, and increased knee-flexion moment at heel strike and during the stance phase. Smaller knee flexion and hip flexion during the swing phase (60,61)
  - Ambitious arch syndrome: pain under the medial arch when using with foot orthosis
    - Fat-pad atrophy with aging causes digging of foot orthotics irritating medial plantar structures (eg, medial plantar nerve, plantar fascia, FHL, etc)
    - Lateral posting (in-office to try); if relieving pain/discomfort → lower the medial arch support (gliding off), decrease subtalar joint compensation (by heel lift); less navicular digging
  - Lateral overloading syndrome: lack of lateral support (flare), foot sliding laterally with constant peroneal muscle overactivity
  - Forefoot pain: orthosis often does not accommodate the forefoot cavus (forefoot plantarflexion), or orthosis not accommodating 1st-ray plantarflexion resulting in pain at the MTP joint
    - If the shoe is not roomy enough, orthosis can cause or worsen pain (especially at the forefoot)

SURGERY

Ankle arthroscopy
- Common indications: failed conservative treatment for osteochondritis dissecans, ankle impingement syndrome, symptomatic loose body, and persistent painful synovitis

Ankle arthrodesis
- Common indications: failed conservative treatment for painful arthritis (traumatic, avascular necrosis (AVN), OA, instability, inflammatory, and infectious), neuropathic arthropathy, tumor-failed open reduction and internal fixation (ORIF), or arthroplasty
- Position: neutral dorsiflexion, 5°–10° external rotation and 5° hindfoot valgus
- Complication: nonunion, arthritis in the neighboring joints (subtalar, midtarsal joints) and iatrogenic nerve injury

Total ankle arthroplasty
- Indications: end-stage ankle OA (alternative to ankle arthrodesis), usually better for older patients, not obese, without significant ankle alignment issues
- Two to three components (talar, tibia components ± polyethylene mobile-bearing meniscus)
- 10 years of survival of prosthetic component: 70% to 90%, but no high level of evidence of benefit over arthrodesis
- Complications: delayed wound healing (MC), wound complication, nerve damages (superficial, deep peroneal up to ~20%), intraoperative fracture, loosening of components, and osteolysis

Surgery for deformity
- Surgical procedure for pes cavus or cavovarus
  - Soft-tissue procedure
    - Indication: flexible deformity after failed conservative management
    - Plantar fascia release, Achilles tendon lengthening, or extensor tendon resection
    - EHL transfer to 1st MTP neck (Jones procedure for symptomatic claw toes), peroneus longus to brevis transfer, transfer of TP to dorsum of the foot
    - Split anterior tibialis tendon transfer (SPLATT) for hindfoot varus; lateral half of the AT tendon attached to the cuboid
  - Bony procedure
    - Indication: rigid deformity failing conservative management
    - Calcaneal osteotomy (valgus producing), interphalangeal fusion with 1st metatarsal osteotomies and midfoot osteotomies
    - Triple arthrodesis; becoming less common
- Surgery for equinus
  - Musculotendinous lengthening of the gastrocnemius-soleus muscle unit (medial gastrocnemius preferred; gastrocnemius recession)
  - Percutaneous lengthening of the Achilles tendon (Z-plasty)
  - Posterior ankle capsular release

Instability: referral to surgery if not responsive to conservative management; anatomic repair or tenodesis stabilization (62)
- Reconstructive tenodesis for generalized ligament laxity and heavy athletes (eg, football linemen)
- Anatomic repair: MC done
  - Direct sutures, transosseous anchoring suture, refixation with small screws
  - Minimizes the loss of ROM
  - Brostrom technique: midsubstance imbrication and suture of the lateral ankle ligaments
  - Gould augmentation: augmentation of the Brostrom repair with mobilized lateral portion of the extensor retinaculum
- Reconstruction using a tendon transfer and tenodesis (Chrisman-Snook, Evans reconstruction)
  - Watson-Jones procedure: peroneus brevis graft tenodesis to fibula and talus.
  - Evans procedure: peroneus brevis graft tenodesis to fibula. ROM and eversion strength may be compromised
  - Chrisman-Snook procedure: split peroneus brevis graft tenodesis to fibula and calcaneus
  - Subtalar stiffness: common complication

ANKLE AND HINDFOOT

LIGAMENT, TENDON, AND BURSA PATHOLOGY

Ankle Sprain

Introduction (63)
- Incidence: 2 per 1,000 people per year in the United States
  - MC MSK injury in athletes, ~25% of all sports-related injuries
- Risk factors

INTRINSIC	EXTRINSIC
Generalized ligamentous laxity, lateral lig. instability (previous injury) Lateral ankle sprain with pes cavus (hindfoot varus/inversion) Muscular exhaustion (weak peroneal muscle) and neurological deficits Gender (male <40, female >40 YO), age (15–19 YO) and race (more in Black and White races than in Hispanic race) (64)	Unsuitable footwear High heel, worn-out shoes (laterally for lateral ankle sprain) Sports: frequent contact with other players, repetitive running, jumping, and sharp cutting

lig., ligament; YO, years old.

- Classification
  - Lateral ankle ligaments by inversion: ~75%, ATFL: MC-involved
    - Injury mechanism: inversion with plantarflexion with ankle mortise loose, less stable
    - Stretching of superficial peroneal nerves (neurapraxic lesion) and peroneal tendon
  - Syndesmosis injury and deltoid ligament injury; less common, but more significant morbidity
    - Injury mechanism: forced dorsiflexion with abduction and external rotation
    - Can occur with lateral ankle fracture, proximal fibular fracture (Maisonneuve fracture), TP tendon injury, and saphenous neuralgia

History and physical examination
- Pain, swelling, ± ecchymosis (suggesting tear of the ligament) on the lateral or medial ankle (and/or the foot) "pop," "snap," and "click," inability to play, "give out," or inability to bear weight
- Physical examination
  - Effusion (unable to see contour of the malleolus)
  - Palpation—systematic way
    - Tip of malleolus (fibular insertion in ATFL and medial malleolus), calcaneal insertion in CFL (inferior to the peroneal tendon), sustentaculum tali
    - 5th metatarsal bone (styloid process) and navicular
  - Provocative tests
    - Inversion/eversion stress test (talar tilt test) and anterior drawer test
    - Anteromedial rotatory drawer test
      – Isolated testing of ATFL (otherwise tibionavicular ligament resist anterior translation in anterior drawer test), ankle plantarflexion (to isolate CFL)
    - Test for syndesmosis injury (provoke the syndesmosis by widening tibiofibular joint)
  - Functional tests: walking, single-leg standing and hopping

GRADE	ANATOMIC LESION	HISTORICAL FINDINGS	EXAMINATION FINDINGS
I	Stretching of the ATFL	Subacute pain and swelling Able to continue athletic activity	Mild swelling, tenderness. Ankle is stable
II	Partial tearing of the ATFL	Acute pain and swelling, inability to continue athletic activity, painful gait	Moderate swelling, tenderness. Ankle is stable
III	Complete rupture of the ATFL	Associated "pop," acute severe pain and swelling, inability to walk	Severe swelling, tenderness, unstable ankle

ATFL, anterior talofibular ligament.

Diagnosis
- Clinical diagnosis confirmed by an imaging study
- X-ray if satisfying Ottawa ankle rules
  - AP, lateral, oblique with weight bearing, mortise view, and two views of entire tibia/fibula
    - Normally, a tibiofibular overlap >6 mm or >42% of the width of the fibula on the AP view, or >1 mm on the mortise view. The overlap is measured 1 cm proximal to the plafond (see Figure 10.5)
    - Proximal segment (tibia/fibula) evaluation R/O Maisonneuve fracture; proximal fibular fracture
  - Stress radiography: problem with a significant variability in normal values
- US (65)
  - Direct ligament evaluation (lateral ATFL, cortical irregularity, avulsion fracture). Limited evaluation of deltoid ligament and syndesmosis injury
  - Dynamic maneuver with inversion, anterior drawer, rotatory movement, and eversion
  - Effusion in tibiotalar joint: 100% positive predictive value with history of ligament injury
  - Evaluation of tendons (peroneal tendon in inversion and flexor tendon (TP, FDL, and FHL) in eversion type injury)
- CT and MRI if persistent symptoms despite normal x-ray or for preoperative planning (66)
  - CT is able to detect minor (2–3 mm) syndesmotic diastasis
  - MRI: indicated for persistent pain despite initial conservative management, atypical presentation, or for differential diagnosis
- Differential diagnosis (67)
  - Tarsal fracture
    - Osteochondritis dissecans of talus and lateral process fracture
    - Posterior process fracture

- Lateral tubercle: differential diagnosis with Os trigonum and FHL tenosynovitis
 - Medial tubercle: differential diagnosis with deltoid ligament sprain
- Calcaneal fracture; may repeat x-ray in 1 to 2 weeks (for stress fracture)
- Bifurcate ligament injury (calcaneonavicular and calcaneocuboid ligament) or midtarsal ligament injury
- Sinus-tarsi syndrome: pain that is slightly distal to the lateral malleolus tip
- Cuboid subluxation: lateral midfoot pain, or pain on weight bearing or walking

Treatment (68)
- Physical therapy (69)
  - Initial phase
    - One to two days of rest, ice, and elevation, and full weight bearing; early mobilization (better outcome)
    - Week 2 to 4: ROM exercise, active exercise, manual therapy or kinetotherapy, tilt or balance board exercise (proprioceptive training)
  - Late phase: week 5 to 8, increase weight-bearing exercise
  - Final functional phase: week 9
    - Sport activity: jumping, turning, and twisting ± external support
    - Isokinetic strength training of the peroneal muscles
- Bracing
  - Cam walker or short leg cast for an initial short period in high grade sprain to facilitate rapid decrease of pain and swelling
  - Unna boot
  - Air stirrup pneumatic splint or taping
    - Function bracing versus casting: functional bracing is better in short term, no difference in long term
- Check foot wear; replace worn-out shoe (laterally worn-out shoe in lateral ankle sprain)
- Prevention (70)
  - "The FIFA 11+"
    - Core stabilization, eccentric training of thigh muscles, proprioceptive training, and dynamic stabilization
    - Plyometrics with straight leg alignment: reflex joint stabilization
  - Proprioceptive or neuromuscular training
    - Perturbation training: improves muscle reaction time of peroneus muscle
  - Endurance training: improves muscle fatigue (causing reflex inhibition of motor neuron pool)
  - Taping: Increases sensory feedback
  - Double upright ankle brace for prevention in female volleyball players (71)
- Treatment for syndesmosis injury (72)
  - Stable syndesmotic sprain: prolonged immobilization in a walking boot (~8 weeks)
  - PT with focus on TP strengthening for medial stability
  - Unstable syndesmotic injury → surgical referral (for syndesmosis widening)
- Surgery
  - No clear superiority of surgery over conservative management for most ankle sprains
  - Indications (73)
    - Patients with chronic, symptomatic ankle laxity
      - Rupture of medial and lateral ankle ligaments with instability and talar tilt of >30°
    - Acute instability of syndesmosis (with/without malleolar fracture) for syndesmosis screw
    - Osteochondral fracture of the talus
    - Massive hematoma requiring immediate decompression
  - Primary repair or reconstruction using tendon transfer and tenodesis

Ankle Impingement Syndrome

Introduction (74)
- Incidence: not studied, underrecognized.
  - Common in athletes (soccer, basketball, dancing, and rugby) and walking uphill
- Classification
  - Anterior impingement: between talus and tibia
    - Hypertrophy of a triangular soft-tissue synovial fold, subsynovial fat, and collagen tissue
  - Posterior impingement: between the posterior process of the calcaneus and the tibia
- Etiology or risk factor
  - Trauma (MC cause), overuse, degenerative changes, and anomalous muscles (eg, low-lying FHL muscle belly) (74)
  - Anterior impingement
    - Talotibial osteophytes
    - Lateral ankle ligament (superior portion of ATFL) and syndesmosis injury
  - Posterior impingement
    - Periarticular ganglion cyst commonly originates from medial tibiotalar or subtalar joints
    - Forced plantarflexion or push-off activities (dance, kicking sports, walking, or running downhill and wearing high heels)

History and physical examination (75)
- Pain in the ankle, hindfoot depending on the location and position (impingement position) ± decreased ROM, mechanical locking reproducing pain ± instability
  - Anterior impingement: anterior ankle (between malleolus, medial or lateral or both) aggravated by ankle dorsiflexion. Posterior impingement: the opposite (75)
- Impingement sign for anterolateral impingement: Ankle plantarflexion and thumb pressure over the lateral gutter (anterior recess medial to the lateral malleolus) then gentle ankle dorsiflexion → reproducing pain by impingement (76)
- Pain with passive ankle plantarflexion
  - Posteromedial ankle pain with passive movement of big toe → suspect FHL lesion

Diagnosis (77)
- Clinical diagnosis with imaging studies to find the etiologies and for other differentials
- X-ray: osteophytes (oblique view for talar osteophytes) and loose bodies (not sensitive)
- US for further soft-tissue evaluation; synovitis, ganglion cyst, capsular bulging (thickening), osteophytes with dynamic maneuver, and Doppler (78)
- MRI for further characterization of the deeper structures, accessory ligaments, and evaluation of intra-articular abnormalities (talar osteochondritis/loose body), and the like (79)

Management
- NSAIDs for a short period of time, activity modification (avoid plantarflexion in posterior impingement), heel lift

(in anterior impingement with roomier shoes), and walking boot initially if the pain is significant
- Injection: diagnostic as well as therapeutic (intra-articular injection improves impingement but is less effective in extraarticular causes)
- Referral for arthroscopic debridement for persistent pain with failed conservative management (80)

Sinus-Tarsi Syndrome

Introduction (81)
- Unknown incidence, but rare (vague definition → diagnosis of exclusion), or overutilized diagnosis
- Etiology
  ○ Ligament injury (sprain) with scarring on the ligament, inflammatory disease (RA) with hypertrophy/pinching of the synovial membrane, deposits of hemosiderin, and posttraumatic fibrotic changes of soft tissues
  ○ Hypertrophy of the soft tissue (fat, synovial tissue, scar tissue, etc) → impingement of the neural plexus and lateral branch of deep peroneal nerve (afferent sensory fibers from the sinus tarsi)
- Commonly involved structures in sinus-tarsi syndrome (82)

Superficial	Lateral root of the inferior-extensor retinaculum Lateral talocalcaneal ligament Calcaneofibular ligament
Intermediate	Intermediate root of the inferior-extensor retinaculum Cervical ligament • Injured by inversion with dorsiflexion • Secondary inversion stabilizer of the subtalar Jt
Deep	Medial root of the inferior extensor retinaculum Interosseous talocalcaneal ligament • Injured by inversion with plantarflexion • Partial Inj.: MC finding in arthroscopic surgery

Inj., injury; Jt, joint; MC, most common.

History and physical examination
- Lateral hindfoot pain (over the dimple, 1 inch distal/slightly medial to lateral malleolus), often deep aching/dull pain
- Tenderness on the sinus tarsi ± swelling (rarely retrocalcaneal bursal effusion) and feeling of instability

Diagnosis
- Clinical diagnosis: diagnosis of exclusion, with relief of pain after a local anesthetic injection
- Imaging (83)
  ○ X-ray to R/O other causes (occult fractures or subtalar arthritis)
  ○ MRI findings: nonspecific inflammation (increased T2 signal intensity) in the sinus tarsi, fat alterations, chronic synovitis and synovial thickening, interosseous talocalcaneal ligament, cervical ligament tears, or soft-tissue mass (MC: ganglion cyst)
- Differential diagnosis: ankle, subtalar, and midtarsal (calcaneocuboid, calcaneonavicular) arthropathy, or ligament sprain (especially lateral ankle sprain)

Treatment
- Local anesthetic (± steroid) injection for diagnostic or therapeutic purposes
- PT: strengthening of peroneus muscle and joint proprioceptive exercise/dynamic balance exercise
- Wedges (medial: more commonly used than lateral, try in office) or heel lift → consider UCBL or SMO if partially responsive to wedge or heel lift
- Referral to arthroscopic surgery if not responsive to nonoperative treatment

Subtalar Sprain and Instability

Introduction (84)
- Underrecognized due to difficulty separating it from ankle sprain/instability
  ○ Subtalar instability: 10% of lateral ankle instability
  ○ Isolated injury is less common
- Etiology and mechanism of injury
  ○ Similar to lateral ankle sprain; supination of dorsiflexed ankle
    ▪ Acute/recurrent inversion injury, rolling over, stepping off a curb, or running across the street
  ○ Indoor cutting and jumping athletes at risk

History and physical examination; similar to ankle inversion strain (9)
- Pain on the lateral hindfoot (sinus tarsi) and instability "give way," stiffness and swelling
- Physical examination
  ○ Lateral ecchymosis in acute injury, swelling, and tenderness
  ○ Subtalar instability test: inversion and internal rotation stress while holding the foot in 10° of dorsiflexion. The heel and foot are held rigid followed by an adduction stress applied to the forefoot. Positive if the examiner felt a medial shift of the calcaneus under the talus

Diagnosis
- Clinical diagnosis confirmed by imaging
- Imaging
  ○ X-ray: AP, lateral, and mortise view
    ▪ Subtalar view: Harris-Beath view, Broden view, and anterior drawer stress view
  ○ US for instability: fibulo-trochlear (peroneal tubercle) length ratio (abnormal if >1.6)
    ▪ Measured in a neutral position and under an inversion stress position (85)

Treatment (86)
- Taping, proprioceptive training, peroneal strengthening, and Achilles stretching
- Bracing and strapping: lateral heel wedge, high top sneaker, Unna boot, anklet, and SMO (if Unna boot improves the symptoms)
- Referral to surgery for persistent symptoms despite conservative treatment

Plantar Fasciitis

Introduction (87)
- Self-limiting, fibrofatty degeneration of the plantar fascial origin with micro tears in the fascia and collagen necrosis

- Prevalence: 1 in 10 persons c/o plantar heel pain at some time, 80% of heel pain from plantar fasciitis, male = female, peak incidence in 40 to 60 (70) years old
  - 1/3 bilateral, 10% of injuries in runners and 11% to 15% of all foot pain symptoms
- Anatomy
  - Thickening of deep fascia, three aponeurosis; central (medial calcaneal tuberosity to proximal phalanx), lateral, and medial
  - Origin at the medial process of the calcaneal tuberosity → fans out distally to form digital bands inserting into bones, ligaments, and dermis of the forefoot and toes
  - Proximal and medial portion: thickest (up to 4 mm) and most conspicuous
- Risk factors
  - Obesity and enthesopathy (often bilateral)
  - Decreased subtalar motion: pes cavus or pes planus; biomechanical disadvantage
    - Shortened in pes cavus, overpronation of the foot, and tight Achilles cord
  - Sudden increase in activities, hard sole, low heel, or tight footwear

History and physical examination
- Plantar heel (medial fore-quadrant portion) pain, rarely lateral plantar heel
  - Pain worse with first few steps, then gradual improvement, then worsens by the end of the day
- Physical examination
  - Tenderness in medial tuberosity of calcaneus (medial-distal 1/4 of the plantar heel) or along the proximal plantar fascia, aggravated by MTP extension (taut fascia by windlass mechanism)
  - Tight heel cord (therapeutic implication to stretch Achilles cord as well as heel lift with cup) and Silfverskiold test for tight gastrocsoleus
  - Tinel test at the distal tarsal tunnel (Baxter's neuropathy reproducing symptoms), calcaneal squeeze test (for calcaneal bony pathology/enthesopathy), heel fat-pad propping test (or modified low-Dye taping)

Diagnosis
- Clinical diagnosis confirmed by an imaging study
- Imaging studies
  - US
    - Typical finding: hypoechogenic swelling (thickness >5 mm on transverse image); compare it with the other asymptomatic site
    - Can evaluate fat pad: 6 to 7 mm (varies individually depending on age)
  - X-ray for other differential diagnosis
    - Heel spurs: slightly higher incidence in patients with plantar fasciitis, no correlation with symptoms; however, it can irritate Baxter's nerve (inferior calcaneal nerve or 1st branch of lateral plantar nerve)
  - MRI; if not resolving after 4 to 6 months of nonsurgical treatment, R/O other causes of heel pain
- Electromyography (EMG) R/O Baxter's entrapment neuropathy; same as TOS protocol (see TOS)
  - Abnormal findings in the ADQP (denervation potential) with otherwise normal study (normal medial and lateral plantar nerve study)
- Differential diagnosis
  - Baxter's entrapment neuropathy (and TOS, medial calcaneal neuropathy)
  - Fat-pad atrophy and plantar fascia rupture
  - Calcaneal fracture (stress fracture, bone contusion) and subtalar arthritis
  - Insertional Achilles tendinopathy, enthesopathy, peroneus longus tendon dysfunction at the cuboid groove
  - Rare causes: infection (osteomyelitis, subtalar pyoarthrosis), neoplasm, plantar vein thrombosis, and arterial insufficiency

Treatment (88)
- Nonoperative treatment: 85% to 90% success, try at least 12 months
- Physical therapy
  - Plantar stretching (use cold bottle) then gastroc-soleus stretching (with subtalar joint neutral), hamstring stretching, deep tissue mobilization, Graston technique (using stainless steel instrument), active release technique, foot intrinsic muscle strengthening (short foot exercise), modalities: ice preferred or US
  - Iontophoresis; using 5% acetic acid >0.4% dexamethasone
- Foot orthotics: off-the-shelf heel insert, heel lift can be made from a felt pad in the office with three layers (Bottom: U-shape 1/4-inch, longer middle layer 1/4-inch, top: 1/8-inch longest layer)
  - Heel lift especially for cavus foot, heel cup ± U-shape relief or medial channel relief
  - Prefabricated silicone insert: 3/4-inch thick
  - Custom-foot orthotics with heel lift and other modifications integrated
- Night splint (5° dorsiflexion or neutral) for 1 to 3 months, cast boot for 4 weeks in severe pain cases
- Modified low-Dye taping (figure of 8), or calcaneal taping with education
- Injection for subacute phase
  - Corticosteroid injection for short-term relief
    - Adverse effects: plantar fascial rupture and fat-pad atrophy
    - US guidance not to infiltrate steroid into the fat pad
  - Platelet-rich plasma (PRP) injection; more effective than steroid injection in chronic recalcitrant cases (89)
- Extracorporeal shock-wave therapy; high level of evidence, used for chronic recalcitrant cases
- Surgery in recalcitrant pain despite conservative management: partial release, open procedure if 1st branch of lateral plantar nerve entrapment is of concern

Plantar Fibromatosis

Introduction (90)
- Single or multiple tender nodules adherent to the plantar fascia
- Relatively rare, male > female: 2:1, peak in individuals 30 to 50 years of age, bilateral in 10% to 50% of cases

- Risk factor: epileptics, diabetics, and alcoholics with liver disease
- Associated with adhesive capsulitis and Dupuytren's disease (up to 65%)

History and physical examination
- Medial arch (plantar aspect, midfoot) pain with local pressure ± swelling, and difficulty walking
- Palpable nodule, less than 2 cm in diameter ± tenderness distal to the insertion of plantar fascia

Diagnosis
- Clinical diagnosis confirmed by an imaging study
- US: fusiform nodular thickening, middle 1/3 of plantar fascia, most nodules are superficial, uniform hypoechoic lesion without internal cystic lesion or calcific deposits (91)
- MRI: lower signal intensity in T1 and lower or increased T2 signal intensity depending on cellularity (92)
- Differential diagnoses: fibrosarcoma, extra-abdominal desmoid tumor, giant cell tumor of tendon sheath, and the like

Treatment
- Local steroid injection into the nodule (under US guidance)
- 1/8-inch Plastazote with punch-out relief → If responsive, custom-made insole with relief
- Others: irradiation, ECSW, and surgery (local excision) if recalcitrant

Achilles (Noninsertional) Tendinopathy

Introduction (93)
- Epidemiology
  - Incidence: ~2/1,000 (94)
  - Common in athletes (11% of runners, 9% in dancers), but 1/3 of patients are nonathletes
- Anatomy
  - No tendon sheath but has paratendon; dorsal, medial, and lateral to the tendon (not under)
  - Superficial to deep; paratendon/mesotendon/epitenon/endotenon surrounding fascicles
  - Sensory innervation by sural nerve, blood supply at musculotendinous junction distally
  - The conjoined tendon rotates 90° as it progresses distally, and the medial fibers become most posterior at the insertion (rotation more marked at 5–6 cm to insertion)
- Etiology: unclear (95)
  - Overuse stresses (overpronation especially), poor gastrocsoleus flexibility, muscle fatigue, low flexibility shoes, and poorly designed shoes (heel tabs)
  - Poor vascularity (2–6 cm proximal to insertion), genetics, endocrine, or metabolic factor

History and physical examination (96)
- Pain 2 to 6 cm proximal to the tendon insertion and morning stiffness
  - Worsening pain in the beginning and at the end of training
- Tenderness, thickening (loss of the lateral border of tendon), nodule, crepitation, and warmth
  - Moving tenderness in tendinopathy versus the same location in paratendinopathy with an ankle ROM
- Silfverskiold test for tight gastrocnemius

Diagnosis
- Clinical diagnosis confirmed by an imaging study
- Imaging studies
  - US
    - In the short axis, fusiform thickening, >6 mm in the anterior–posterior dimension
    - Disruption or subtle change in the fibrillar pattern (thickening, fragmentation, and disappearance of specular echoes)
    - Proximal 2/3 of tendon and medial fibers are more commonly involved
  - MRI: consider in surgical planning or in atypical cases for other differentials
  - X-ray for other differentials
- Differential diagnosis (often coexist)
  - Achilles tendon tear (partial), plantaris tendon tear, insertional Achilles tendinopathy, retrocalcaneal bursitis, and precalcaneal bursitis
  - FHL, TP, and peroneus longus/brevis tendinopathy/tenosynovitis/tear
  - Posterior impingement syndrome, and ankle/subtalar arthritis

Treatment (97)
- Tylenol, or NSAIDs initially, or glycerol trinitrate patch consider if not responsive to others
- Physical therapy for stretching (especially gastrocnemius) and eccentric contraction exercise (heel-drop exercise)
  - Heel-drop exercise: heel rise with asymptomatic ankle, then down (eccentric contraction) with symptomatic ankle for 6 to 12 weeks, then maintain exercise for 6 to 12 months, responsive up to 90%
- Injection
  - Steroid injection (to retrocalcaneal bursal space or paratenon, not into the tendon)
  - Sclerosing injection (with polidocanol into the local neovessel using US guidance), or platelet-rich plasma injection
- Surgical referral if failed conservative treatment

Achilles Tendon Tear

Introduction (98)
- The most frequently ruptured tendon (incidence of Achilles tendon rupture: 7/100,000)
  - Male > female, left > right
- Etiology and risk factor
  - Sports activity (>75%–80%)
  - Overuse, corticosteroid injection, fluoroquinolone antibiotic, prior rupture of the other side, and hyperthermia

History and physical examination
- Pain in acute injury, "being kicked" with inability to bear weight, weakness, and stiffness (weakness often subtle due to other intact ankle plantar flexor)
  - Chronic tear: often underrecognized, pain without significant functional deficit
- Physical examination: diffuse edema and ecchymosis acutely
  - Palpable gap (can be masked by significant swelling), Thompson test and the Matles test

Diagnosis
- Clinical diagnosis confirmed by an imaging study (US and MRI)

- Ultrasonography
  - Partial thickness tear: increased thickness (10–15 mm in AP diameter) with hypo/anechoic lesion
  - Acute tendon rupture: tendon ends abut without intervening gap. Paratendon often intact (hyperechogenic)
  - Complete tear: fat herniation into the tendon gap and increased visualization of the plantaris tendon
  - Gentle passive dorsiflexion can assist visualization of the gap

Treatment (99)
- Surgery versus nonoperative (with early ROM protocol): no significant difference (including risk of rupture).
  - Surgical patients return to work faster and nonsurgical patients have less complications (100)
- Cast (hanging equinus cast) for 10 days → 3D boot (Cam Walker) in 20° plantarflexion for 10 days to 2 weeks, then neutral (at 4 weeks) with crutches, weight bearing as tolerated at 6 weeks → wean-off crutches at 8 weeks
  - Daily active plantarflexion exercise as early as 10 days following an injury

Insertional Achilles Tendinopathy

Introduction (101)
- 5% to 20% of Achilles tendinopathies: more common in older, less athletic, and overweight individuals
- Etiology and risk factor
  - Mucoid degeneration, necrosis, hemorrhage, and calcification
    - Anterior portion of Achilles tendon insertion (more common); "stress-shielded" → intratendinous bone formation through endochondral ossification
  - Tight Achilles tendon, hyperpronation, pes cavus (hindfoot varus), and obesity

History and physical examination (102)
- Posterior heel pain at the calcaneal tuberosity ± morning stiffness
  - ± Recent history of training change or poor warming up
  - Worsening pain after activity (stair climbing, running on hard surface, or heel running)
- Calcaneal exostosis (bony enlargement), midline tenderness at calcaneal tuberosity (can be slightly medial as well as lateral), thickening or nodularity of the Achilles insertion
- Tight Achilles cord with subtalar neutral position and positive Silfverskiold test for gastrocnemius tightness

Diagnosis
- Clinical diagnosis confirmed by an imaging study
- US: initial imaging choice; calcification, heterogenic echogenicity at insertion ± increased vascularity ± signs of noninsertional Achilles tendinopathy
- X-ray: "fishhook" like osteophyte, ossification at the insertion of the Achilles tendon
- Deferential diagnosis
  - Bursitis (retrocalcaneal, superficial calcaneal bursitis): often concomitant
  - Medial calcaneal neuritis
  - Tendonitis of TP, FHL, or PL/PB

Treatment
- Nonoperative management
  - Rest, ice initially, modification of training, heel lift, and orthosis
  - Eccentric training without ankle dorsiflexion; only 1/3 responsive
    - Ankle dorsiflexion: decreased blood flow in power Doppler (possible mechanism of improvement in stretching; decrease neovascularization). Heel drop exercise (not beyond the neutral dorsiflexion angle)
  - Sclerosing therapy
  - Extracorporeal shock wave (low energy shock wave) therapy
- Surgery (excision, resection, debridement, and reattachment) if conservative management fails

Sever's Disease

Introduction (103)
- Traction/apophysitis of Achilles tendon insertion on the posterior calcaneus in active adolescents
- MC in boys 10 to 12 years, girls 8 to 10 years, active in sports
- Risk factor
  - Overweight, pes planus/cavus, physically active, high-impact sports (track, soccer, gymnastics, ballet, or tennis), and improper footwear

History and physical examination
- Posterior heel pain (localized to posterior calcaneal tuberosity) when running and walking
- Tender on deep pressure
- A positive calcaneal squeeze test is the most reliable finding

Diagnosis
- Clinical diagnosis confirmed by an imaging study
- US findings similar to an insertional Achilles tendinopathy
- X-ray: R/O other differentials (fracture or neoplasm)
  - Findings: sclerosis and fragmentation (however, can be common in asymptomatic adolescents)

Treatment
- Rest (usually a week-off from running) followed by stretching (gastrocnemius and hamstring)
- Heel lift, pad or heel cup for 2 months after symptoms improve (bilaterally to avoid leg length discrepancy), cast or walking boot if the pain persists (2–3 weeks)
- Return to sports in 2 to 8 weeks

Retrocalcaneal Bursitis

Introduction
- Prevalence unknown, but underrecognized
- Haglund's syndrome: retrocalcaneal bursitis in the setting of abnormal bony protuberance of the posterosuperior border of the calcaneus (104)

History and physical examination
- Pain and swelling (anterior/deep to the Achilles tendon)
- Tenderness on the posterolateral aspect of the posterior calcaneal tuberosity, not in the midline (suggesting Achilles insertional tendinopathy), ballottement of the bursa on either side of Achilles tendon ± warm to palpation

Diagnosis

- Clinical diagnosis confirmed by an imaging study to differentiate pathologies in neighboring structures
- US
  - More than 3-mm depth of hypoechoic fluid in any plane is abnormal and consistent with bursitis (105)
    - Subtalar or ankle joint effusion, FHL/peroneal tenosynovial effusion to be evaluated
  - Evaluate intrinsic Achilles pathology and insertional Achilles tendinopathy (frequently concomitant)
- X-ray: to draw parallel pitch lines (inferior line: medial tuberosity to the anterior calcaneal tubercle) to confirm the presence of exostosis
- Differential diagnosis
  - Superficial (subcutaneous/adventitial) bursitis: female > male (shoe-related), not common in athletes, often concomitant
  - Other differentials similar to insertional Achilles tendinopathy

Treatment

- Roomier shoes, heel lift (often decrease friction and irritation from a heel counter), U-shape pad for exostosis (Haglund's deformity), custom insole (or SMO) with relief
- Injection: not more than 1 mL, usually under US guidance, landmark: between Achilles tendon and calcaneal tuberosity
- Surgery: open versus endoscopic removal with sufficient resection of the bone (106)

Tibialis Posterior (TP) Tendon Dysfunction

Introduction (107)

- Epidemiology (108)
  - Common in two age groups; 30s with inflammatory disease and 50s with overuse disease
  - Prevalence in elderly women; up to 10% (109)
  - TP tenosynovitis: 13% to 64% in patients with RA (110)
- Anatomy and biomechanics
  - Invert and plantar flexes the foot (↔ peroneus brevis: antagonist)
    - TP is 2 times bigger in cross-sectional area
  - Most active in midstance (to heel off), primarily preventing the foot from everting past the neutral position (hindfoot stabilizer; assist supination) with locking both calcaneocuboid and talonavicular joints → creating a rigid lever for forward propulsion of the foot
  - Short excursion → even a 1-cm elongation leads to ineffective action (vicious cycle with pronated foot)
- Etiology and risk factor; multifactorial
  - Degenerative, inflammatory, or microtraumatic causes
    - Hypovascularity as vulnerable area for degeneration: 4 cm proximal to the insertion of the tendon, which is about 14 mm in length. However, most pathologies are slightly distal to this region
  - Obese females, age (>40 years), hypertension, DM, and seronegative arthropathy
  - A remote trauma history in >50%; stepping awkwardly off a curve (may be due to recall bias)
  - Accessory navicular (14% in adult population but only 0.1% symptomatic); unclear relationship

History and physical examination (111)

- Insidious onset of pain at the medial-hindfoot/ankle ± mild swelling
  - Pain generators: TP and medial mid-/hindfoot ligaments secondarily; spring (calcaneonavicular), deltoid, and long plantar (calcaneocuboid) ligaments
  - Pain in the lateral hind-/midfoot due to impingement of calcaneus on fibula or calcaneocuboid arthritis (from overloading/impingement) or ankle arthritis in advanced cases
- Physical examination
  - Swelling, pes planus, hindfoot valgus, forefoot abduction with too-many-toes sign
    - Check foot wear for medial side wear
  - Tenderness on the TP tendon between the medial malleolus and navicular
  - Tight Achilles cord with positive Silfverskiold test (for tight gastrocnemius)
  - TP muscle strength examination with the foot in maximal passive eversion and plantarflexion; prevents substitution for an anterior tibialis tendon
  - 1st metatarsal rise sign (37), double heel- and single-heel rise tests (check physical examination section)
- Classification based on the history and physical examination

STAGE	1	2	3	4
Pathology	Tenosynovitis or degeneration or both	Elongation and degeneration		
Pain	Medial	Medial or lateral or both		
Deformity	No deformity	Flexible planovalgus, hindfoot with equinus	Fixed irreducible planovalgus	
Too-many-toes sign	Negative	Positive		
Single heel rise	Hindfoot inversion	No or weak hindfoot inversion	Unable, no inversion of hindfoot	
Ankle arthritis	Not present			Present

Source: From Ref. (107). Pomeroy GC, Pike RH, Beals TC, Manoli A 2nd. Acquired flatfoot in adults due to dysfunction of the posterior tibial tendon. *J Bone Joint Surg Am*. 1999;81(8):1173–1182.

Diagnosis
- Clinical diagnosis confirmed by an imaging study
- Imaging studies
  - US: tenosynovial effusion, increased thickness (compared to the asymptomatic side), increased vascularity by Doppler, or tear
    - Short axis: better than long axis to image longitudinal split tears
    - False negative
      - Hypoechoic debris and granulation tissue filling the tendinous bed with a thinned and degenerated tendon
      - Patent FDL tendon often mistaken as intact PTT (in ruptured cases)
    - False positive
      - Subtle intratendinous vessels in inflammatory conditions mimic a tendon fissuration; color Doppler can identify the vessels (not always visualized clearly)
      - Normal effusion (up to 1–2 mm) between medial malleolus and navicular bone
  - X-ray: negative in early stage
    - Findings: talonavicular sagging on lateral view, talonavicular uncoverage (abduction) on standing AP, lateral tilt of the talus (failure of deltoid ligament in advanced stage) on ankle mortise view
  - MRI: tenosynovitis (increased T2 signal), tendon tear, and/or other joint, intracortical bony lesion, and neighboring ligaments evaluation
- Differential diagnosis
  - Medial hindfoot pain (often coexisting); talonavicular joint disease, deltoid ligament or spring ligament sprain, painful accessory navicular, bony navicular disease (stress fracture, Müller–Weiss, and Kohler disease) (112)
  - Other causes of pes planus (eg, ligament laxity, tarsal coalition, etc)

Treatment
- Unna boot for 1 to 2 weeks, 2 to 3 times (Cam walker can be alternative but often poorly tolerated), heel lift and/or medial wedge, extended wedge (medial posting) in forefoot varus (chronic case)
- Roomier shoes (walking sneakers), straight last, pronation control with medial buttress (reinforcement)
- Orthotics: UCBL, SMO, dynamic AFO, and Arizona AFO (in the order of increasing restriction) considering the activity, body habitus, and aesthetic preference
  - 2D orthosis or arch support is minimally effective in ≥stage 2
- Surgery if failed conservative treatment
  - Tenosynovectomy, medial calcaneal osteotomy, gastroc/Achilles lengthening, FDL transfer, triple arthrodesis, deltoid ligament reconstruction, and lateral column lengthening

Tibialis Anterior (TA) Tendinopathy and Tear
Introduction (113)
- Rare, male > female, peak incidence in 50s to 70s
- Etiology and risk factor
  - Trauma (forced plantarflexion and eversion) or spontaneous rupture usually occurs with degenerative process
    - Avascular zone: 0.5 to 3 cm from the insertion point under the inferior extensor retinaculum (may be more vulnerable to degeneration)
  - DM, steroid, RA, SLE, psoriasis, renal insufficiency, hyperparathyroidism, and gout

History and physical examination
- Asymptomatic ± pain at the dorsum of the ankle and foot (hindfoot/midfoot)
- Palpable defect on palpation ± tenderness
- Weakness (often subtle), foot slap (foot drop: rare unless other dorsiflexors such as EHL and EDL are compromised), and overpronation in standing and walking

Diagnosis (114)
- Clinical suspicion confirmed by an imaging study
- US: discontinuation of the tendon with hypoechoic swelling (retraction) at the proximal end
  - Dynamic maneuver (ankle dorsi/plantarflexion) with an anechoic gap
- MRI: similar to US, better in evaluation of extent of the defect, often difficult to distinguish a partial tear from tendinopathy as both have thickened and increased intrasubstance signals
- Differential diagnosis: peroneal neuropathy, compartment syndrome, lumbar radiculopathy, neoplasm, and insertional tendinopathy of TA

Treatment
- Casting in acute tear (for 6 weeks), heel lift, or AFOs (posterior leaf spring orthotic)
- Referral for surgery in acute rupture or highly active person/athlete

Peroneal Tendon Dysfunction (115)
Introduction (116)
- Under-recognized cause of lateral hindfoot pain
  - More common in pes cavus (hindfoot inversion) and ankle instability
  - Common in some sports: skiing, basketball, ice skating, soccer, rugby, and gymnastics
  - Peroneal subluxation: 0.3% to 0.5% of traumatic events to the ankle
- Classification: tendonitis/tenosynovitis, subluxation/dislocation and tear/rupture
  - Peroneus brevis splits (tear): MC, 11% to 26% of peroneal tendon pathologies (117)
- Etiology
  - Mechanism of injury: a sudden, forceful, passive dorsiflexion of the inverted foot combined with reflex contraction of the peroneal tendons, more common in pes cavus
  - Intrinsic anatomic variability
    - Tendinopathy: avascular zone in the peroneal tendon (PB/PL at the turn around the lateral malleolus, PL around the cuboid)
    - Subluxation: shape of the groove in lateral malleolus; flat groove or convex surfaces (instead of concave), 30% of the people lack the fibrocartilaginous ridge
    - Os peroneum: 20% of population; may be associated with peroneus longus tear (unclear)

History and physical examination
- Lateral ankle pain (retromalleolar groove or lateral hindfoot), ± swelling, snapping/clicking (one tendon over the other/popping), instability, and subjective weakness

○ History of inversion ankle injury: often missing
- Hindfoot varus, tenderness on the retromalleolar region, and between the lateral malleolus and cuboid
- Pain/apprehension with ankle eversion and pain on resisted ankle eversion or forced inversion and 1st-ray plantarflexion; often palpable snapping with subluxation or dislocation
- Dislocated tendon: swelling and tenderness anterior and/or superior to the lateral malleolus

Diagnosis
- Clinical diagnosis confirmed by an imaging study
- Imaging studies
  ○ X-ray
    ▪ Fracture of posterolateral fibular tip (lateral malleolus), fracture of the styloid process of 5th metatarsal or Maisonneuve fracture, or other differentials
    ▪ Fleck sign in oblique view: small fleck of bone detached from the outer aspect of the tip of the fibula; pathognomic for avulsion of the superior peroneal retinaculum
  ○ US
    ▪ Tenosynovial effusion in the retromalleolar groove (small effusion is normal when it is immediately distal to the lateral malleolus), thickened tendon with hypoechoic, heterogenic echogenicity (compare with the asymptomatic site), bisected peroneus brevis (split tear)
    ▪ Dynamic study for subluxation/dislocation over the lateral malleolus and intrasheath subluxation
  ○ MRI (118): circumferential fluid in the tendon sheath >3 mm, highly specific for tenosynovitis
- Differential diagnosis
  ○ Lateral malleolar fracture, 5th metatarsal avulsion fracture (peroneus brevis), os peroneum fracture (119), cuboid avulsion fracture, cuboid subluxation, and calcaneal fracture
  ○ Pseudo tendinopathy: pain on the inferior border of the lateral malleolus, where the top line of the shoe quarter abuts the lateral malleolus
    ▪ Use heel lift to decrease irritation between the malleolus and top line of the heel counter

Treatment
- Nonoperative management: acute injury
  ○ Short leg cast with ankle plantarflexion and inversion for 6 weeks (alternatively Cam walker; less ideal) with crutches; NWB for 2 weeks and then PT in acute subluxation or dislocation
  ○ Unna boot with U-shaped felt pad (around the malleolus) to decrease a dead space for tenosynovitis and tendinopathy
  ○ Lateral heel wedge/heel lift, NSAIDs and PT for gradual strengthening (eccentric) and proprioceptive/balance exercise
- Surgery
  ○ Indication: high-level athletes/highly active persons or recurrent, failed conservative treatment
  ○ Tenosynovectomy (120,121)
  ○ For tear: repair and tubularization of the tendon in simple tear or tenodesis with reconstruction in complex tear
  ○ Acute repair of retinaculum, deepening of the fibular groove versus groove deepening with soft-tissue transfer and/or osteotomy in chronic/recurrent dislocation

FHL Tendon Dysfunction
Introduction
- Rare but underrecognized, chronic injury more common than acute
- Etiology and risk factor
  ○ Hyperextension against resistance (similar to Achilles tendon injury), and pushing off the forefoot planted during heel raise
  ○ Dancers (pointe position), gymnasts, and runners
- Common location (122)
  ○ Stenotic tenosynovitis at posterior ankle or within the fibroosseous tunnel between the medial and lateral posterior talar processes
  ○ Midfoot at the knot of Henry, forefoot under MTP joint, and avulsion/tear of the plantar aspect of the distal phalanx of the hallux

History and physical examination
- Posteromedial ankle pain and snapping (1st interphalangeal joint flexion/extension with ankle dorsiflexion)
- Tenderness posterior to the medial malleolus, triggering/snapping, or crepitus
- Pain on resisted flexion of the great toe

Diagnosis
- Clinical diagnosis confirmed by an imaging study
- Imaging studies
  ○ US: tenosynovial effusion proximal to the fibroosseous tunnel (medial to the Achilles tendon) and tendinopathy distally (near MTP); check for ankle/subtalar effusion (often communicating with tenosynovium of FHL)
  ○ X-ray: os trigonum (common), avulsion injury at the insertion site of the tendon, or to evaluate other bony pathologies
  ○ MRI for other intracortical or intra-articular pathologies; can evaluate intratendinous signal change (in mild cases)
- Differential diagnosis (often concomitant)
  ○ Posterior ankle impingement: posterolateral pain with passive ankle plantarflexion
  ○ Achilles tendinopathy
  ○ TP tendinopathy
  ○ OA of the ankle and subtalar joint, and OCD of the talus

Treatment
- Nonoperative treatment: relative rest, Cam walker in severe pain, modalities and gradual eccentric strengthening exercise
- US-guided injection for painful tenosynovitis
- Surgery (if not responsive to conservative management): release of the fibroosseous tunnel, tenosynovectomy, and repair

BONE AND JOINT

Ankle Arthritis (123)
Introduction (22)
- Relatively rare compared to the other joints as the ankle is one of the most arthritis-resistant joints

- Etiology
  - Posttraumatic: MC, >2/3 of ankle arthritis, incidence varies depending on fracture type
    - More common with cartilaginous and ligamentous insufficiency or abnormal alignment
    - High in cases of osteochondral fractures of the talus (20%–50%) and tibia fractures
  - Idiopathic (primary) osteoarthritis <10%
  - Others: inflammatory (RA, gout), hemochromatosis, septic, or neuropathic (Charcot) arthropathy
- Concomitant MSK pathologies secondary to or contributing to ankle arthritis
  - Neighboring joint pathologies: subtalar and midtarsal joint (talonavicular) DJDs
  - Coexisting other soft-tissue pathologies with/secondary to deformity and by compensatory mechanisms

History and physical examination
- Pain (worse with weight bearing) at the medial/lateral gutter (around the bimalleolar line), and stiffness
- Varus deformity more common than valgus, effusion (often subtle) and decreased ROM (subtle, other than decreased ankle dorsiflexion with tight Achilles tendon and alignment issues)

Diagnosis
- Clinical diagnosis supplemented with imaging findings
- Imaging study
  - X-ray (weight-bearing AP, lateral, oblique, and mortise views)
    - Common findings: loss of joint space, subchondral sclerosis and cysts, eburnation, and deformity
  - US: to evaluate effusion, synovial hypertrophy, and concomitant soft-tissue pathologies

Treatment (124)
- Nonoperative treatment
  - NSAIDs, acetaminophen, nutritional supplementation: glucosamine and chondroitin
  - Injections
    - Viscosupplementation (using US guidance): limited evidence but promising (125)
    - Steroid injection: a benefit up to 16 to 24 weeks after injection; diagnostic value as well
    - Platelet-rich plasma injection: limited evidence
  - Orthotics
    - High-top boot with lateral stabilization along with a rocker sole (requires stiff midsole), cushion heel (decreased ankle motion in transition from heel strike to push off), heel lift inside (decreased ankle ROM; but can promote tight Achilles), and wedges
    - Arizona (lace-up leather) AFO
    - Supramalleolar orthotic (less bulky than Arizona, but also provides less control)
    - Lace-up anklet (off-the-shelf): when there is no ankle instability
- Surgery (126)
  - Indication: failed conservative treatment with disabling pain
  - Arthrodesis, arthroplasty (limited in severe deformity, instability, and highly active people), and others (debridement, distraction arthroplasty, and malleolar osteotomy)

Subtalar Arthritis

Introduction (127)
- Unknown prevalence; rare, but also underrecognized
- Etiology
  - Traumatic: calcaneal intra-articular fracture (MC), talar fracture, or subtalar dislocation
  - Osteoarthritis, inflammatory arthropathy, and neuropathic arthropathy (Charcot)
  - PTT dysfunction with pes planus

History and physical examination
- Pain in the lateral ankle and sinus tarsi, stiffness ± swelling and deformity (rearfoot varus or valgus)
- Tenderness, fullness in the sinus tarsi, decreased subtalar joint range with pain and crepitus ± subtalar instability

Diagnosis
- Clinical diagnosis supplemented by an imaging study
- X-ray: weight-bearing AP, mortise view
  - Harris-Beath view (axial calcaneal), Broden view (visualizes the posterior facet of the talocalcaneal joint), and Canale view (visualizes the sinus tarsi)
  - Common findings: nonuniform space narrowing of joint, subchondral sclerosis, and osteophyte formation
- MRI to evaluate periarticular structures (eg, cartilaginous and ligamentous structures)

Treatment
- NSAIDs, high top sneakers, orthotics same as ankle arthritis
- Injection
  - Steroid injection (for symptomatic relief), viscosupplementation to sinus tarsi (128)
  - US guidance for injections: medial, lateral, and posterior approaches available
- Referral to surgery if not responsive to conservative treatment: fusion at 5° to 10° of valgus (for optimal function) (129)

Rheumatoid Arthritis

Introduction (130)
- 90% of RA patients c/o foot and ankle-related symptoms. In 20%, symptoms begin in the foot
  - Increase with duration of RA (8% <5 years, 25% >5 years)
- Location: forefoot (MC/earlier involvement, MTP joint) in 50 to 60% > hindfoot > ankle (last and least, 8%)
  - Common forefoot pathologies: dislocation of MTP joint, hallux valgus, compensatory varus of 5th toe, fat-pad migration, and claw toes
  - Hindfoot and midfoot (131)
    - Tendinopathy, tenosynovitis, and tear in TP (MC), PL and TA
    - Retrocalcaneal bursitis/superficial calcaneal bursitis (adventitial)
    - Pes planovalgus (MC deformity), PTT dysfunction, deltoid ligament, fibular fracture, and lateral column shortening
    - Synovitis and arthritis of joints; talonavicular (MC), calcaneocuboid, and subtalar joint (up to 60%)
    - Entrapment neuropathy: TOS
    - Plantar fasciitis/fat-pad atrophy
    - RA nodules: adjacent or under Achilles tendon

History and physical examination (132)
- Pain, stiffness, swelling, warmth (often not specific), and/or deformity (in advanced)
- Overlying toes (dislocation of MTP joint, especially 2nd), hallux valgus, claw toes, and subcutaneous rheumatoid nodules (up to 20%)
- Hindfoot valgus (>varus) and planus, tight Achilles (especially gastrocnemius), effusion in the ankle and midtarsal joint, tenderness on the TP tendon (between navicular and medial malleolus)

Diagnosis (133)
- Clinical diagnosis (American college of Rheumatology [ACR] criteria)—check RA of hand and wrist
- Imaging studies: x-ray (for erosive disorder), US (early diagnosis: synovitis in MTP joints, joint erosions, and tenosynovitis), and MRI (gold standard, R/O other differential diagnosis)

Treatment (134)
- Referral to rheumatology (start DMARD)
- Orthotics (metatarsal pad, foot orthotics, SMO, more effective for rear foot pain not for forefoot pain)
- PT (limited; a few sessions for gastrocnemius stretching, strengthening (isometric and gradual strengthening), balance/proprioceptive exercise, and exercise in the pool
- Intra-articular or periarticular steroid injections for localized symptoms
- Referral for surgery if failed to respond to conservative treatment: synovectomy, arthrodesis, or total arthroplasty (135)

Osteochondritis Dissecans of Talus

Introduction (136)
- Incidence: 0.09%, prevalence: 2/100,000 person/year, most frequent in 2nd decade of life
  - Talus: 3rd most frequently involved area of OCD after knee and elbow joints
- Etiology: unclear
  - Trauma (malleolus fracture: MC cause), recurrent sprain (2%–6% of ankle sprain, inversion, and dorsiflexion), bilateral in 10%
  - Ischemia (failure or anastomosis in the epiphyseal cartilage) or genetic
- Location: medial (post-med, frequently ischemia-related) more common than anterolateral

History and physical examination
- Ankle pain, intermittent swelling ± mechanical symptom (popping and catching) and instability
- Tenderness/pain behind medial malleolus with dorsiflexion or anterolateral aspect of ankle with plantarflexion, ± effusion

Diagnosis
- Clinical suspicion confirmed by an imaging study
- X-ray
  - Mortise view: not sensitive nor specific, often normal
  - Hawkin's sign (137)
    - A subchondral radiolucent band in the talar dome, visible at 6 to 8 weeks after the trauma in the AP view and seldom found in lateral radiographs
    - Favorable prognosis and its presence rules out the development of AVN
- MRI; if suspicious despite normal x-ray
  - MRI classification
    - (a) articular cartilage damage, (b) cartilage injury with underlying fracture ± edema, (c) detached osteochondral fragment but undisplaced, (d) displaced fragment, and (e) subchondral cyst formation

Treatment
- In acute lesions: 6 to 8 weeks of immobilization in a non-weight-bearing cast → progressive weight bearing
  - Lateral process; 16% to 17% of BW, partial weight bearing for 6 weeks then full weight bearing (138)
- Pain related to the lesion: hyaluronic acid or platelet-rich plasma into the tibiotalar (ankle) joint
  - PRP may be better than hyaluronic acid (139)
- Surgery: within 12 months
  - Loose body removal ± simulation of fibrocartilage growth, securing osteochondral lesion, and stimulating development of hyaline cartilage through OC graft
  - Postoperative rehabilitation: peroneal strengthening, ROM and proprioceptive training

Tarsal Coalition

Introduction (140)
- Aberrant union between two or more tarsal bones; osseous or nonosseous (cartilaginous or fibrous)
- Prevalence: ≤1% (as high as 12.7% in a cadaveric study, underrecognized), bilateral in ≥50% of cases, and male ≥ female
  - Talocalcaneal and calcaneonavicular (anterior process of the calcaneus): MC type
- Etiology
  - Congenital (genetic) more common than acquired (trauma, surgery, arthritis, infection, and neoplasm)

History and physical examination
- Asymptomatic or pain during 2nd decade of life, stiffness, and deformity (pes plano-valgus/flat foot)
  - Activity-related hindfoot and ankle pain
- Rigid valgus hindfoot and forefoot abduction (less commonly equinovarus), ±dorsal navicular spur (bird beak)
- Loss of subtalar and midtarsal joint motion with tenderness

Diagnosis
- Clinical suspicion confirmed by an imaging study
- X-ray: AP, lateral, and oblique
  - Lateral: Anteater nose sign (elongated anterior process of the calcaneus, talar beaking: upward projected osteophyte)
  - 45° oblique for calcaneonavicular coalition: elongated lateral navicular and hypoplasia of the lateral talar head and C sign
- CT: evaluate size and extent of coalition
- MRI: evaluate fibrous or cartilaginous coalition and possible other pathologies
- Differential diagnosis (often concomitant)
  - Ligament strain, sinus-tarsi syndrome or ankle, subtalar, midtarsal arthrosis, and tendinopathy (TP and peroneal tendons)

Treatment
- NSAIDs, medial wedge/heel lift, cast or walker boot for 3 to 6 weeks in severe cases
- Consider UCBL or SMO depending on the response to initial immobilization
- Surgery if not responsive to conservative treatment; surgical resection, interposition of EDB/fat graft, subtalar, or triple (subtalar and midtarsal joints) arthrodesis (in advanced cases)

Painful Accessory Bone (Os) (see Figure 10.2)

Painful Os Trigonum Syndrome

Introduction (141)
- Accessory ossicle (secondary ossification center that is separate from the normal adjacent bone) of posterolateral tubercle of the talus
- Prevalence of Os trigonum: 10% to 25%, usually unilateral
- More common in ballet dancers, gymnasts, and ice skaters
- Common cause of bony posterior impingement syndrome: mechanical impingement of the posterior talus/Os trigonum between the posterior tibia and the calcaneous when the foot is in plantarflexion

History and physical examination
- Pain in the posterolateral ankle that is reproducible on palpation and active plantarflexion
- Tenderness on the anteromedial aspect of the Achilles tendon. Pain with great toe dorsi and plantarflexion (FHL irritating Os trigonum)

Diagnosis
- Clinical diagnoses with an imaging study
- X-ray: lateral view with ankle plantarflexion as an ossicle located posterior to the calcaneus
- MRI: edema in the os trigonum and surrounding structures, evaluate other neighboring structures
- Differential diagnosis
  - Fracture of the posterior talar process (Shepherd's fracture), FHL, Peroneus and PTT tendinitis/tenosynovitis, insertional Achilles tendinopathy, and retrocalcaneal bursitis

Treatment
- Nonoperative treatment: avoid plantarflexion as much as possible. Soft heel (rear) can help (similar to SACH foot function, mitigate plantarflexion) and CAM walker in severe cases
- Injection of small-volume injectate under image guidance: diagnostic as well as therapeutic
- Referral to surgery for early resection in competitive athletes

Painful Accessory Navicular

Introduction (142)
- Prevalence of accessory navicular: 2% to 14%, common in adolescent female athletes, and majority are asymptomatic
- Clinical implication
  - No causal relationship between pes planus and accessory navicular
  - The degree of PTT weakness corresponds to the severity of the injury

History and physical examination
- Medial arch pain (the accessory navicular hitting/rubbing against narrow shoes) ± twisting injury, partial or complete disruption of the synchondrosis
- Tenderness on the navicular tuberosity (medial and plantar aspect)

Diagnosis
- Clinical suspicion confirmed by an imaging study
- X-ray: 45° eversion oblique view and internal oblique view
- US and MRI to evaluate soft tissues (such as lesion in the posterior tibialis tendon) (143)

Type 1	A sesamoid bone may be within the PTT: anatomically separate from the navicular bone, present in about 30% of cases, 2–3 mm in size, ovoid in shape, rarely symptomatic
Type 2	An accessory ossification center (ossicle) Symptomatic, present in 50%–60% of cases, 8–12 mm in size, triangular in shape • 2a: PTT line of pull and talar process → tension: more risk for avulsion • 2b: Acute angle, more inferiorly → more shearing force → arthritic changes
Type 3	Cornuate or gorilliform navicular Results from bony fusion of the accessory ossification center (type 2) with the tuberosity

PTT, posterior tibialis tendon.

Treatment
- Roomier shoes (straight last, medial reinforcement), heel lift, navicular pillow, U-shaped felt pad, heel lift, and CAM walker initially if pain is severe and then UCBL and SMO
- Referral to surgery for failed conservative management; excision

Painful Os Peroneum

Introduction (144)
- Prevalence of Os peroneum: 9% to 20%, bilateral in 60%, and bipartite in 30%
- Sesamoid bone in the peroneus longus tendon near the cuboid
- Etiology
  - Acute fracture of os peroneum or acute diastasis of multipartite os peroneum
  - Chronic os peroneus fracture with stenosing tenosynovitis
  - Hypertrophied peroneal tubercle with peroneus longus entrapment
  - Common mechanism of injury: direct trauma, or supination or inversion injury

History and physical examination
- Pain in the lateral hind/midfoot, tenderness along the peroneal tendon distal to the fibula ± paresthesias along the course of the sural nerve distal to the lateral wall of the calcaneus
- Worsening symptoms or pain with resisted plantar flexion of the 1st ray and resisted eversion. Mild weakness with pain on eversion

Diagnosis
- Clinical suspicion confirmed by an imaging study
- X-ray shows migration of the os peroneum, the presence of a multipartite os peroneum, and/or an enlarged peroneal tubercle. Contralateral foot x-ray to compare
- US to evaluate peroneal tendon: tendinopathy, tenosynovial effusion, and cortical disruption of os peroneum (119)
- MRI for intracortical bony abnormality and other differential diagnosis

Treatment
- Nonsurgical treatment (only 20% response); NSAIDs, Felt relief pad, and Plastazote
- In failed conservative management, surgical referral including excision of the os peroneum with débridement and repair of the tendon and tenodesis

Fracture

Calcaneal Fracture

Introduction (145)
- 60% of tarsal bone injury, male (80%–90%) > female, and high complication rate (up to 40%)
- Classification
  - Intra-articular (oblique shear ➜ ≥2 segments); more common than extraarticular (better outcome, avulsion injury of anterior process by bifurcate ligament, sustentaculum tali, calcaneal tuberosity with Achilles tendon avulsion)
  - Stress fracture: second MC after metatarsal stress fracture in the foot
    - Fatigue stress versus insufficiency
- Mechanism of injury
  - Fall from a height or motor vehicle accident (MVA) (MC)
  - Stress fracture: extensive contraction of gastrocnemius; jumping, running, or prolonged standing
- Associated injuries: extension to the calcaneocuboid joint (63%), vertebral injury (10%), and contralateral calcaneal injury (10%)
- Complications (delayed onset)
  - Subtalar arthritis, peroneal nerve irritation and peroneal tendonitis, FHL injury, compartment syndrome with claw toes, malunion (limited ankle dorsiflexion), and flat foot

History and physical examination
- Pain in the hindfoot (posterior calcaneal body), ecchymosis, and swelling in acute injury
- Short and widened heel with varus deformity, pes planus, tenderness with medial to lateral compression (calcaneal squeeze), and tight Achilles tendon (gastrocnemius; Silfverskiold test)
- Subtalar mobility; similar to Coleman's block test: medial or lateral wedge trial under the heel and check for forefoot valgus
  - Check whether it is flexible or fixed (give medial vs lateral extension wedge accordingly)

Diagnosis
- X-ray: AP, lateral, oblique, Broden and Harris-Beath view
  - Stress fracture: not visible in x-ray for first 10 to 14 days; sclerotic line between the tuberosity and postarticular surface, perpendicular to the long axis of the calcaneus, rare periosteal reaction
  - Böhler angle (see Figure 10.5): normally 20 to 40°, flattening in fracture
  - Angle of Gissane: intersection of the lines along the downslope of the posterior facet and the upslope of the anterior process in lateral view
    - Normally 130° to 145°; increase in calcaneal fracture except stress fracture (usually normal)
- CT (gold standard), and MRI (for stress fracture or uncertain diagnosis and to evaluate neighboring structures)

Treatment (146)
- Stress fracture: cast immobilization and NWB for 6 weeks
  - Typically heals in 4 to 6 weeks after injury, then advance to crutches with weight bearing as tolerated
  - Alternatives: body compression dressing, definitive casting within 7 days, NWB for 2 to 3 days, ice and elevation, and active ROM of foot as early as possible
- Cast immobilization for 10 to 12 weeks for small (<1 cm) extraarticular, minimally displaced (<2 mm) fracture
- Surgical referral in cases of intra-articular fracture (including subtalar joint), displaced fracture, decreased Böhler angle
  - Closed reduction with percutaneous pinning, ORIF, and primary subtalar arthrodesis
- Pain with history of calcaneal fracture: try heel lift and/or heel wedge (medial or lateral depending on deformity and flexibility), Unna boot, and orthotics. Surgical referral if not responsive to conservative management

Talus Fracture

Introduction (147)
- 2nd MC fracture after calcaneal fracture in the foot
- Talar neck: MC site > talar body and lateral process
- MC mechanism of injury: high energy, forced dorsiflexion with axial load (for neck fracture)
- Complications after talus fracture with/without surgery: osteonecrosis, posttraumatic arthritis (subtalar > ankle, talonavicular), varus deformity (with limited eversion), mal- or nonunion, and infection

History and physical examination
- Severe pain in the hindfoot and ankle, usually unable to bear weight
- Tenderness on posteromedial ankle in posterior process fracture often misdiagnosed as ankle sprain (or avulsion fracture with ankle sprain)
  - Big toe flexion and extension ➜ pain within the posterior aspect of the hindfoot (pain in Os trigonum and FHL tendon dysfunction)

Diagnosis
- Clinical suspicion confirmed by an imaging study
- X-ray (AP, lateral, and Canale view), if unclear CT scan (also for preoperative evaluation)

Treatment
- For talar neck: ER for reduction with short leg cast for 8 to 12 weeks, NWB in the first 6 weeks for nondisplaced fractures. Other nondisplaced talar fractures: short leg cast for 6 weeks
- Ortho consult: talar neck or other displaced fractures ➜ open reduction and internal rotation

Navicular Stress Fracture

Introduction (148)
- Prevalence: underrecognized, ~1% up to 30% of all stress fractures (depending on different studies), male > female
  - More common in track and field athletes (less common in long-distance runners)
- High risk (of complication) fracture
- Etiology and risk factors
  - Compression between the talus and cuneiforms during heel strike → force on the central third of the bone and decreased vascular supply in central portion of navicular bone
  - More common in pes cavus, short 1st metatarsal, metatarsus adductus, limited subtalar or ankle motion, and medial narrowing of the TN joint

History and physical examination
- Pain in the navicular tuberosity (or medial midfoot), worse with weight bearing activity
- Tenderness on the navicular tuberosity and dorsal "N" spot
- Reproduction of pain by hopping on the affected leg with the foot in an equinus position (tiptoes)

Diagnosis
- High clinical suspicion confirmed by an imaging study
- Plain radiograph can be normal up to 3 to 6 weeks
- MRI, CT scan, or bone scan when clinical suspicion with negative x-ray
- Differential diagnosis
  - Müller–Weiss syndrome: idiopathic osteonecrosis of the navicular in adults
  - Kohler disease: osteochondrosis of the navicular in children
  - PTT dysfunction or midfoot arthritis

Treatment
- Non-weight-bearing with cast until the fracture is healed (6 weeks for fracture involving only dorsal cortex) → start weight bearing if pain resolves. Up to 8 months to return to play
- If not responsive, then referral to surgery: screw fixation ± bone grafting with postoperative cast for 8 weeks
  - 3 to 5 months to return to full activity with conservative management
- Manage underlying problems; vitamin D/calcium, bisphosphonate as necessary, roomier shoes/rigid midsole, double socks ± heel lift

Navicular Osteonecrosis (Müller–Weiss Disease)

Introduction (149,150)
- Adult onset osteonecrosis, middle-aged females in their 50s, frequently bilateral, and underrecognized
- Etiology
  - Delayed ossification of navicular with compression of the lateral aspect of the navicular bone, mechanical overload (subtalar supination), trauma, and osteochondritis
  - Congenital dysplasia

History and physical examination
- Dorsal-medial aspect of mid- and hindfoot pain, usually asymmetric ± triggered by minor trauma
- Hindfoot varus or pes planovarus (with forefoot valgus). Tenderness on the navicular bone

Diagnosis
- Clinical suspicion confirmed by x-ray and CT/MRI
  - Begin in the lateral aspect, comma-like shape with subsequent superior protrusion of the fragments (151)
  - Initially, there is a minimal change in x-ray, edema in MRI then dorsal angulation, compression, splitting of navicular, reduction of space between the talar head and cuneiforms, and complete extrusion of navicular (152)
- Differential diagnosis: Kohler disease, navicular stress fracture, and other etiologies for pes planus

Treatment
- Roomy shoes, pain medications as needed, relative rest, navicular pad with relief, heel lift, and SMO
- Referral for surgical evaluation if not responsive to a conservative treatment: internal fixation of the navicular, arthrodesis of the talo-naviculocuneiform joints, and open/arthroscopic triple arthrodesis

Kohler's Disease (153)

Introduction
- Childhood osteonecrosis/osteochondrosis of navicular bone, presents between ages 4 to 7 years (2–9 years), male > female, and bilateral in 25%

History and physical examination
- Midfoot pain (dorsomedial) ± swelling, warmth, and redness
- Focal tenderness over the navicular bone, antalgic gait (weight bearing on the lateral side)

Diagnosis
- Clinical suspicion confirmed by x-ray
- Common findings: navicular sclerosis, fragmentation, and flattening (although can be found in normal asymptomatic patient)

Treatment
- No need for treatment (self-limiting), casting if symptomatic (may provide early resolution of pain). Weight-bearing status does not affect outcome

Charcot Foot (Neuroarthropathy) (154)

Introduction (155,156)
- Prevalence: 0.1% to 0.4% in DM, 7.5% to 30% in DM with peripheral neuropathy
  - True prevalence; unknown/maybe higher due to under-recognition
- Etiology and risk factors
  - Neurotraumatic (autonomic dysfunction with increased blood flow through AV shunting) and neurovascular (peripheral vascular disease: unclear role). May be related to increased inflammatory cytokines

○ Risk factors: diabetes, DM neuropathy, alcoholism, leprosy, meningocele, tabes dorsalis/syphilis, and syringomyelia
• Poor prognosis and high mortality

History and physical examination
• Asymptomatic, swelling ± pain, or painless deformity (flat foot, rocker-bottom deformity)
• Erythema (decrease with elevation) and increased warmth of the involved foot and ankle (~2°C higher than contralateral asymptomatic side)
• ± Crepitus, palpable loose body, large osteophyte, excessive callus formation (head of 1st, 2nd, 5th metatarsals, posterior calcaneus), blisters, and foot ulceration
• Natural history (modified Eichenholz stages)
  ○ Stage 0: clinical signs of inflammation (localized warmth, swelling, and redness)
  ○ Stage 1 (development-fragmentation): erythema, increased warmth, and marked swelling
  ○ Stage 2 (coalescence): decreased erythema, decreased warmth, and decreased swelling
  ○ Stage 3 (reconstruction-consolidation): marked decrease or absence of warmth, swelling and redness, and fixed deformity

Diagnosis
• Clinical diagnosis, high clinical suspicion confirmed by an imaging study
• X-ray: initially negative, pronated oblique view (for lateral forefoot)
  ○ Findings: 5Ds: joint distension, dislocation, debris, disorganization, and increased density
    ▪ Disruption of articular surfaces (irregularity, narrowing, or obliteration of joint spaces; mimics osteoarthritis), metaphysical and epiphyseal fragmentation, bone resorption, osteopenia, and dislocation of joints
  ○ Findings based on modified Eichenholz stages
    ▪ Stage 0: no findings
    ▪ Stage 1: bony debris, fragmentation of subchondral bone, periarticular fracture, subluxation, and/or dislocation
    ▪ Stage 2: absorption of fine debris, new bone formation, coalescence of fragments, fusion of joints (ankylosis), and/or sclerosis of bone ends
    ▪ Stage 3: new bone formation, decreased sclerosis, and/or residual deformity
• MRI
  ○ To evaluate soft-tissue swelling, abscess, or other subtle bony pathologies
    ▪ Nondisplaced fracture and increased marrow edema in the initial stage with negative plain x-ray
  ○ Often difficult to differentiate osteomyelitis from neuroarthropathy
    ▪ Findings favoring osteomyelitis: sinus tract, fluid collection, and fat and bone marrow infiltration, contrast enhancement of bone and adjacent soft tissue, "ghost sign": visible on contrast enhanced T1-weighted series compared with native T1-weighted series
• Bone scan with indium 111 white blood scintigraphy, and US
• Anatomic classification (by Sanders and Frykberg) (157)

TYPE/PATTERN	LOCATION OF INVOLVEMENT	X-RAY FINDINGS
1. Forefoot; 15%	MTP joints and distal to the MTP joints Plantar ulceration	Osteopenia, osteolysis, juxtaarticular cortical bone defects, subluxation, and destruction on radiographs
2. TMT joints; 40% (27%–60%)	MC-involved site in DM Charcot foot Plantar ulceration at the apex of deformity Collapse of midfoot with resultant rocker-bottom deformity	Subluxation, fracture dislocation, dorsal prominence of metatarsal base, fragmentation later
3. Naviculocuneiform, talonavicular and calcaneocuboid joints; 30%	Usually naviculocuneiform and navicular bone ± ulceration at the apex of the deformity	Osteolysis of naviculocuneiform Jt. with fragmentation with osseous debris both dorsally and plantarly
4. Ankle and subtalar joints; 10%	Involves ankle Jt. ± the subtalar Jt. and medial/lateral malleolar fracture → severe structural deformity with instability	Malleolar fractures, erosion of bone and cartilage with collapse of Jt., loose bodies in ankle, extensive destruction and lateral dislocation of ankle
5. Calcaneus; 5%	Rarely involved alone Avulsion Fx of the posterior tubercle (Achilles attachment) is common	Osteolytic change and avulsion Fx of the posterior tubercle ± Osteolysis at the naviculocuneiform Jt.

DM, diabetes; Fx, fracture; Jt., joint; MTP, metatarsophalangeal.

• Differential diagnosis (158)
  ○ Septic arthropathy, osteomyelitis, and cellulitis
    ▪ Osteomyelitis: occurs at pressure points and areas of ulceration along bony protuberances (at metatarsal heads and at interphalangeal joints in the forefoot)
    ▪ Osteomyelitis is very likely if there is ulcer and sinus tract formation (down to the bone)
  ○ Osteoarthritis, calcium pyrophosphate dihydrate (CPPD) crystal deposition disease, gout, RA, osteonecrosis, or stress fracture
  ○ Deep vein thrombosis or rarely alkaptonuria (black urine, skin pigmentation, and early onset polyarthritis)

Treatment
• Nonoperative treatment
  ○ Off-loading: non–weight bearing and protected weight bearing for 2 to 4 months (up to 6 months)

- Total contact cast/walking cast; check for ischemia, step to pattern to minimize forefoot pressure, change q 2 weeks
- CAM walker; able to observe wound. Disadvantage: inability to control the edema. Limitation: wall weight bearing not possible
  ○ Patellar-tendon weight bearing double upright with plastic shell AFO (Charcot-restrained orthotic walker [CROW]) after total contact cast application
  ○ Custom-made shoe once consolidated
- Referral to surgery
  ○ Indications: open wound, infection, and severe deformity (if unable to cast)
  ○ Types: Achilles lengthening, resection of bony prominence, deformity correction, arthrodesis, or amputation

FOREFOOT, MIDFOOT, AND TOES

COMMON MEDIAL FOREFOOT AND TOE PATHOLOGIES

Hallux Valgus

Introduction (159)
- Prevalence: ~20% in adults, MC foot problem (usually asymptomatic), female > male, peak incidence in >65 years
- Etiology (160)
  ○ Intrinsic factor: genetic predisposition (metatarsal morphology or varus), ligament laxity, pes planus, tight Achilles tendon/functional hallux limitus, 1st ray insufficiency, age, and female gender
    - Pes planus and tight Achilles cord: increased loading under 1st MTP head from everted calcaneus, flexible forefoot valgus, plantarflexed 1st ray → 1st MTP joint dorsiflexion with 1st ray hypermobility
  ○ Extrinsic factor: high-heeled narrow shoes, excessive weight bearing
    - High heel: hallux into the valgus → incompetent medial capsule, flexor tendon sublux laterally; pronatory effect → worsens/accelerates the condition
    - Occupation and excessive walking and weight bearing: unlikely to be notable factors
- Foot pain related to hallux valgus
  ○ Adventitial bursitis over the prominence at MTP joint (MC cause of pain)
  ○ Compression of hallucal nerve, impingement of the hallux on the 2nd toe
  ○ 2nd MTP dysfunction (weight bearing moved to 2nd MTP)

History and physical examination
- Pain over medial/dorsal eminence at MTP joint in 70%: aggravated by wearing shoes (especially tight or high-heeled shoes)
- Symptomatic callus on the 2nd MT and 2nd toe with hammer deformity

Diagnosis
- Clinical diagnosis confirmed by an imaging study
- Imaging study
  ○ X-ray: AP, lateral oblique, and lateral and axial projections (to evaluate sesamoid)
    - Hallux valgus angle: long axis of 1st MT and proximal phalanx (>15°); lateral displacement of sesamoid(s), and degenerative changes
- Differential diagnosis (and/or concomitant lesions)
  ○ Inflammatory arthropathy, generalized ligament laxity, and neuromuscular disease (pes cavus and planus)

Treatment
- Address the unrealistic shoe issues
  ○ Recommend wide/high toe box and soft-sole shoe
  ○ Modification of the existing shoe by ball and socket stretcher
- Achilles stretching with gastrocnemius stretching ± night splints
- Off-the-shelf orthotics
  ○ Toe spacer temporarily/intermittently (prolonged use → valgus progression of the 2nd toe), bunion pad/post, metatarsal bar (weight bearing to the lesser metatarsals), medial arch support (decreased pronatory force)
  ○ Foot insert with elastic strap to hold the hallux
- Referral to surgery when there is pain and distress from deformity despite a conservative management
  ○ Metatarsal osteotomy (Chevron), congruency of 1st MTPJ (modified McBride), arthrodesis at 1st TMT joint (for instability), fusion (Lapidus; 1st TMT fusion with modified McBride), resection arthroplasty (proximal phalanx (Keller) resection)
  ○ Complications: recurrence, AVN, metatarsalgia (weight-bearing transfer), hallux varus, cock-up toe deformity (FHL injury, common in Keller resection), and nerve injury (hallucal nerve)

Hallux Limitus and Rigidus

Introduction (161)
- Stiffness of MTP joint often associated with arthritis or altered biomechanics
  ○ Hallux rigidus is the end stage of hallux limitus
- Prevalence: 1 in 45 in >50 years old (2nd MC forefoot disorder after hallux valgus), female > male, often bilateral
- Etiology (162)
  ○ Primary: idiopathic; chondral defect in the dorsal metatarsal head
  ○ Secondary
    - Traumatic (MC): single isolated or chronic repeated microtrauma
    - Excessive pronation with tight heel cord or iatrogenic (high arch support, which elevates metatarsal head)
    - Inflammatory arthropathy
    - Collapsed medial arch from Charcot neuroarthropathy, tethering of the FHL tendon, or a rarely deep posterior compartment syndrome

History and physical examination
- Medial forefoot/arch pain with walking then, later constant at advanced stage (just before toe off; requiring MTP dorsiflexion)
  ○ Deep pain in the joint aggravated when walking barefoot and with raising the toes
  ○ ± Burning pain in the dorsum of the medial forefoot (by irritation of superficial/deep peroneal nerve by osteophytes)

○ ± Diffuse pain at the medial midfoot/hindfoot or the lateral side by lateralization
○ Shoe-fitting problem and over-stretched lateral counter or excessive wear pattern on the lateral outsole (secondary to lateralization to decrease medial forefoot weight bearing)
• Physical examination
  ○ Metatarsus primus elevatus (elevation of 1st ray, normal up to 5 mm); often a subtle finding
  ○ Tenderness on the MTP joint with dorsal or dorsolateral osteophytes
  ○ Decreased MTP joint dorsiflexion with weight bearing (<12°) and non–weight bearing (<50°)
    ▪ Functional hallux limitus: limited dorsiflexion with weight bearing only
    ▪ Limited/painful dorsiflexion as well as plantarflexion (due to irritation of the medial dorsal cutaneous branch of the SPN)
  ○ Gait: weight bearing on the lateral side of the foot leading to peroneus tendinitis with laterally worn-out sneaker

Diagnosis
• Clinical diagnosis supplemented by imaging findings
• Classification
  ○ Grade 0: dorsiflexion (DF) 40° to 60°, negative radiologic finding
  ○ Grade 1: DF 30° to 40°, minimal osteophytes
  ○ Grade 2: DF 10° to 30°, early DJD + osteophytes
  ○ Grade 3: DF 10° or less, DJD + osteophytes
  ○ Grade 4: pain at mid-range, ankylosis, and end stage DJD
• Differential diagnosis or concomitant (underlying mechanism) lesions
  ○ Inflammatory arthropathy (such as gout and RA), or osteoarthritis
• Imaging study
  ○ X-ray of the foot (standing AP, lateral and oblique)
    ▪ Joint space narrowing (asymmetric loss of cartilage), osteophytes, subchondral cysts in advancing cases, increased sclerosis and bony proliferation at the joint margins, and loose bodies around the joint
    ▪ Metatarsus adductus

Treatment
• Nonoperative management: successful in 60% to 75% for stages 0 to 2 (162)
  ○ Roomier shoes (high toe box, stiff soled with rocker-bottom shoes)
    ▪ Eliminate mechanical irritation of the nerve between dorsal osteophytes and shoe
    ▪ Donut-shaped padding on the dorsum of the MTP joint for relief
  ○ Addressing iatrogenic causes/faults (eg, excessive medial arch support, causing functional hallux rigidus)
  ○ Orthotic management; more successful in early stages; less likely to be successful if dorsiflexion <10° (163)
    ▪ Carbon plate (prefabricated) with metatarsal pad and medial posting (if excessive, then it can make it worse), DonJoy Arch Rival®, Vasyli Dananberg insole® (plug on the MTP joint area; can be unplugged for relief)
    ▪ Reverse Morton's extension with cutoff to accommodate for plantarflexed metatarsal

○ Intra-articular steroid injection in mid- to moderate grades: up to 6 months of improvement (164)
○ Home-exercise program: biking and swimming (water-based exercise)
• Surgical management; if failed, conservative management with structural or advanced stages
  ○ Stage 2: cheilectomy (removal of bone spur), stage 3: osteotomy, and stage 4: arthrodesis or implant arthroplasty

Gout

Introduction (165)
• Prevalence: ~3.9%, ~8.3 million in the United States, male > female by 3 to 4 times (decreasing disparity with age due to loss of uricosuric effect of estrogen decrease), and peak incidence in 40 to 60 years
• Location: peripheral joints in the lower extremity (1st MTP, podagra; MC) > tarsal joint, ankle, and knee
  ○ MC location in upper extremity: olecranon bursa (166)
• Risk factor
  ○ Thiazide diuretics, cyclosporin, low-dose aspirin (<1 g/d); can cause hyperuricemia
  ○ Associated factors
    ▪ Insulin resistance, metabolic syndrome, obesity, CHF, and organ transplantation
    ▪ Increased intake of purines, meat and seafood, ethanol, soft drinks, fructose, coffee, dairy products, and vitamin C

History and physical examination
• Rapid development of severe pain (usually within 24 hours), erythema, and swelling; 82% chance of gout (167)
  ○ The first phase: intermittent acute attacks with spontaneous resolution in 7 to 10 days
  ○ The second phase: chronic tophaceous gout; polyarticular attacks with crystal depositions in soft tissue and joints (untreated gout for 20 years or more)
• Tenderness (moderate to severe) and decreased ROM ± erythema, swelling, and tophi (common in Achilles tendon, olecranon, ear helix, and eyelid)

Diagnosis
• Clinical diagnosis confirmed by joint aspiration (crystal analysis)
• Imaging study
  ○ X-ray often negative: punched out periarticular erosion with sclerotic overhanging borders and soft-tissue crystal deposition
• Joint aspiration (US guidance for small joints)
  ○ Synovial fluid or tophus aspiration with identification of negatively birefringent monosodium urate crystals under polarizing microscopy
  ○ Joint aspiration with Gram staining and culture for septic arthritis
• US: synovial effusion, double contour (urate crystal deposits on the articular cartilage)
• MRI (168)
  ○ Indicated for patients who are not responsive to treatment or if diagnosis is unclear
  ○ MRI with contrast more sensitive than US in detecting occult destructive findings such as bone marrow edema, synovial pannus, soft-tissue tophi, and edema

- Differential diagnosis: other crystal induced arthritis, septic joint, RA, OA, and the like

Treatment
- Acute attack
  - Colchicine 1.2 mg followed by 0.6 mg 1 hour later, then 0.6 mg bid
  - NSAIDs; naproxen or indomethacin (50mg tid, no difference in results compared to colchicine), or COX-2 inhibitor
  - Intra-articular steroid injection for 1 to 2 inflamed large joints if not tolerating PO NSAIDs
    - 30 G needle under US guidance into the synovium
  - After the acute symptoms subside, consider UA-lowering treatment such as low-dose colchicine or allopurinol (xanthine oxidase inhibitor) for 6 months

Sesamoid Disorders of the Hallux

Introduction (169)
- Anatomy and biomechanics
  - Two sesamoids (tibial and fibular) embedded in FHB
  - Absorb weight-bearing forces, decrease friction, protect the FHB tendons, and increase the moment of FHB
  - Elevate the first metatarsal head, which functions to dissipate the forces on the metatarsal head
- Prevalence of painful sesamoid disorders: unknown, but underrecognized
- Etiology
  - Fracture acutely by hyperextension and axial loading, stress fracture, bipartite sesamoid, chondromalacia, osteochondritis/osteonecrosis, and FHB tendonitis
  - Bilateral sesamoiditis often related to Reiter disease, psoriatic arthritis, and seronegative RA

History and physical examination
- Unilateral, insidious pain on weight bearing and terminal stance phase
  - Tibial sesamoid (medial and plantar) more symptomatic than fibular sesamoid (lateral and plantar)
  - Significant hallux valgus or varus and pes cavus (with metatarsal plantarflexion) or pes planus
  - Direct palpation on resisted plantarflexion of big toe (FHB activation)
  - Tenderness shifts distally with dorsiflexion of the 1st MTP joint as the sesamoids are embedded in the FHB tendon)
  - Tightness of the flexor hallucis muscle

Diagnosis
- Clinical diagnosis with an imaging study to evaluate other differential diagnosis
  - X-ray AP, lateral, oblique, and axial sesamoid view (bilateral)
    - Acute fracture (bilateral: unusual), presence of bipartite or multipartite sesamoid (usually symmetric), diastasis, fragmentation, proximal retraction, or medial or lateral translation
  - US study with similar findings, MTP joint and FHB and longus tendon evaluation
- Differential diagnosis
  - Turf toe (plantar plate injury), synovitis, or arthritis

Treatment
- Short leg cast with toe extension in acute fracture
- 1/8-inch Plastazote with punch-out hole and shaving keratotic lesion (referral to podiatry)
- Referral to surgery if failed a conservative treatment; partial or complete sesamoidectomy or bone grafting
  - Complications of sesamoidectomy: cock-up deformity, hallux valgus (tibial sesamoid excision), or hallux varus (fibular sesamoid resection)

Turf Toe

Introduction (43)
- Sprain of plantar capsule/plate of 1st MTP joint (including sesamoid complex injury as well)
- Common in contact sports and athletes who practice/compete on rigid surfaces; 83% in football players
- Anatomy of plantar plate
  - A fibrocartilaginous thickening of the MTP joint capsule
    - Stabilize and resist hyperextension of the MTP joint and absorb compressive loads
    - Assist in the windlass mechanism due its attachment to the plantar fascia
- Mechanism of injury and risk factor
  - Hyperextension injury with concomitant axial load applied to the heel as well as hyperflexion
  - The hardness of the artificial turf, increased surface friction, and shoe stiffness (using softer soled shoe)

History and physical examination
- Pain at plantar aspect of the MTP joint ± redness and swelling
- Tender plantar aspect of MTP joint, ecchymosis (grade 2–3) acutely, painful ROM and pain with weight bearing (grade 2), or inability to bear weight (grade 3)
- Hammer toes, angulation and subluxation of MTP joint

Diagnosis
- Clinical diagnosis confirmed by an imaging study
- Grading: grade 1 sprain: a stretch injury; grade 2: a partial tear; grade 3 sprain: a complete tear of the capsuloligamentous complex with disruption of the plantar plate from the metatarsal neck
- Imaging (AP, lateral, and oblique bilateral): capsular avulsion, sesamoid fracture, or proximally migrated sesamoid (in rupture)
- MRI if abnormal x-ray or advanced degree of injury

Treatment
- Rest, Ice, Compression, and Elevation (RICE), stiff-soled shoe, walking boot (CAM walker), gradual return to play when pain-free MTP joint ROM to 60° or in 4 weeks (walking, running, cutting, and then sport specific exercise)
- Surgical referral if grade 3 injury, loose fragment present, or failed conservative management

Hypermobile First-Ray Syndrome

Introduction (170)
- Hypermobile 1st metatarsal-cuneiform joint causing pain and dysfunction (symptomatic hallux valgus, medial midtarsal arthritis, and 2nd MTP joint pain) in the forefoot

- No report of prevalence, but underrecognized
- Biomechanics
  ○ First ray (1st ray): rigid lever during the heel rise (171)
    ▪ Double amount of weight supported in the 1st ray when standing or walking on the tiptoes
    ▪ Incorrect ground contact of first toe (excessive movement of MTP) ➔ rotation and loss of strength
  ○ Shortness, hypermobility or elevation of the first metatarsal
    – Dorsiflexed 1st metatarsal ➔ restrict proximal phalanx ➔ compression and degeneration of 1st MTP ➔ hallux rigidus
    – Affect more stable 1st MT-cuneiform joint (dorsiflexed) ➔ develop dorsal osteophytes (TMT arthritis)

History and physical examination (172)
- Pain under the metatarsal heads (as well as arch pain), a dorsal bunion and pinch callus on the big toe (by flexing)
- Soft skin under the 1st ray (suggestive of minimal weight bearing) and pinch callus on the distal phalange and exuberant callus on the lateral forefoot
- Drawer sign: >8 to 10 mm of dorsal displacement of the 1st metatarsal head compared to the 2nd metatarsal head
- Tenderness on the cuneiform-metatarsal joint with crepitus

Diagnosis
- Clinical diagnosis supplemented by imaging findings
- X-ray: >5 mm separation between the 5th metatarsal and inferior border of sesamoids on a standing lateral view

Treatment
- Medial posting (forefoot), 1/4 inch thick (all the way forward to toe)
  ○ Increase the contact ➔ restore weight-bearing function
  ○ Fill the gap lateral to the medial posting
- Heel lift or medial heel wedge, carbon plate to decrease joint movement of the mid-/forefoot
- Referral to surgery if failed conservative treatment: arthrodesis of the 1st TMT joint with dorsal tissue repair

2nd MTP Joint Disorder and Subluxation

Introduction (173)
- Common 2nd MTP joint pathologies: sprain/injury (plantar plate), synovitis/capsulitis, subluxation/dislocation
  ○ 2nd MTP is the most frequent site for symptomatic MTP synovitis, female > male
- Etiology of 2nd MTP instability
  ○ Idiopathic (MC cause)
  ○ Risk factor
    ▪ Excessive length of 2nd metatarsal (Morton's foot); increased pressure with chronic deterioration of the plantar aspect of the capsule
    ▪ Hallux valgus, excessive pronation and 1st ray insufficiency
    ▪ Pes cavus
  ○ Trauma, synovitis, or inflammatory arthritis
  ○ The capsular tear usually arises from the base of the proximal phalanx

History and physical examination (174)
- Ill-defined pain in the forefoot often similar to interdigital neuritis, and fullness
  ○ Concomitant Morton's interdigital neuritis: common (~20%)
  ○ Pain aggravated by walking barefoot on hard surface (may suggest capsulitis or plantar plate injury)
- Exuberant calluses in the lateral aspect (lateral overloading), baby-like skin in the 1st ray (suggestive of the 1st-ray insufficiency)
- Separation/overlying toe deformity (dorsomedial deviation of the 2nd toe: MC)
  ○ Deterioration of plantar aspect of capsule ➔ hyperextension and deterioration of fibular collateral ligament ➔ medial deviation
  ○ Hammer toe
- MTP drawer test; apply displacement force in dorsal direction to the proximal phalanx ➔ ≥2 mm or 50% joint displacement with pain (modified Lachman test)
- Painful MTP dorsiflexion (plantar aspect)

Diagnosis
- Clinical diagnosis confirmed by an imaging study
- X-ray: weight-bearing AP and lateral
  ○ Narrowing of joint line with even complete disappearance of the joint line, clear overlapping of the base of the phalanx and the metatarsal head
  ○ Oblique views confirm the malposition of the phalangeal base
- MRI if diagnosis is unclear and to quantify the extent of plantar plate or ligamentous disruption
- Differential diagnosis
  ○ Morton's neuritis, Freiberg's infarction, degenerative disease, and inflammatory arthropathy

Management
- RICE, NSAID, roomier shoes (rocker sole with stiff insole or carbon plate), and socks (mitten)
- Orthotics and taping
  ○ Metatarsal pad/bar (reduces the plantar pressure), Budin splint, and heel lift
  ○ Taping: plantarflexion strapping of the 2nd toes (figure of 8)
- Steroid injection: cautious for dislocation or worsening instability, and extraarticular injection (for bursal sac)
- Surgical referral if not responsive to nonoperative treatment: synovectomy, osteotomy, plantar plate repair ± tendon transfer (FDL to EDL) or capsular release

Metatarsal Stress Fracture (March Fracture)

Introduction
- 10% to 20% of stress fractures among athletes, low risk for complications
- MC location: 2nd or 3rd metatarsal shaft (2nd >3rd)
  ○ 5th metatarsal: MC location of overall metatarsal fractures (rare location for stress fractures but high risk for associated complications)
- Etiology and risk factors
  ○ Abrupt increase in duration, intensity, or frequency of physical activity, and impaired energy balance and inadequate nutritional support

History and physical examination
- Pain, swelling, worsens with weight bearing (often lacking the typical history of increased physical activity)
- Edema (pitting), tenderness, and limited ROM with pain

Diagnosis
- Clinical suspicion confirmed by an imaging study
- X-ray: AP, lateral, and oblique
  - Usually negative in first 2 weeks. Subtle periosteal bone formation can be seen initially, followed by a visible callus after a few weeks
- MRI: not all stress reactions in MRI correlate with symptoms (~40% in a study of 21 asymptomatic runners)
- US (47)
  - Cortical interruption (hypoechoic lesion)
  - Periosteal reaction: hyperechoic band along the cortex, periosteal hemorrhage (hyperechoic periosteum is elevated from the cortex by a hypoechoic band)
  - Increased blood flow in the soft tissue
- Bone scan: abnormal findings can be seen in 6 to 72 hours

Treatment
- Nondisplaced metatarsal shaft fracture: hard sole postoperative shoe, CAM walker or short-leg cast for 4 to 6 weeks, or carbon plate with rocker-bottom shoe ± metatarsal pad with crutch walking. Gradual return to play
  - Modalities: US and E-stimulation; may enhance the healing rate (equivocal evidence)
- In young females, check weight, menstrual cycle, and bone density, and optimize the nutritional status by increasing energy intake and decreasing energy expenditure (female athlete triad)
  - Vitamin D and calcium supplementation
  - Check BMD: provide bisphosphonates if necessary
- Referral to surgery for displaced fracture (especially 1st metatarsal) and open fracture
  - Percutaneous versus open reduction and fixation

Freiberg Disease

Introduction (175)
- Cartilage degeneration of lesser metatarsal heads
  - Ischemia or bone necrosis within the head of the metatarsal → collapse of articular surface and subchondral bone
- Uncommon, unknown prevalence/incidence, female > male, between 12 and 15 years, can be bilateral
- Common location: 2nd MT head (~70%) >3rd MT head (~30%), rarely 4th and 5th
- Risk factor: greater length of 2nd metatarsal in relation to 1st and 3rd and genetic predisposition

History and physical examination (159)
- Pain, swelling ± ecchymosis on the dorsum of the foot
  - Pain aggravated by weight bearing and activity

Diagnosis
- Clinical diagnosis confirmed by imaging
- X-ray: normal in early stages. Later changes: sclerosis, flattened metatarsal head with signs of osteoarthritis in proximal phalanges (defect usually located in the upper half of the articular surface)
- Differential diagnosis
  - Stress fracture, juvenile RA, intermetatarsal bursitis, and overuse injury

Treatment
- Non–weight bearing for 3 to 6 weeks, rest, and pain medication as needed (aspirin is contraindicated in children younger than 12 years old)
- CAM walker, metatarsal pad, and carbon plate
- Surgery referral if failed conservative treatment: MTP arthrotomy with removal of loose bodies, wedge osteotomy, and partial MT head resection

Metatarsalgia
Classification

SECONDARY METATARSALGIA (176,177)	IATROGENIC METATARSALGIA
Interdigital neuritis (Morton's), peripheral neuropathy, tarsal tunnel syndrome (rare)	Malalignment of metatarsal osteotomies or metatarsal head resection
Trauma (sprain, turf toe)	Failed hallux valgus surgery
Inflammatory arthropathy; RA	Failed MTP fusion, osteotomies
Metabolic disease: gout	Failed shortening of 2nd ray
MTP joint arthritis	
Freiberg disease	

MTP, metatarsophalangeal; RA, rheumatoid arthritis.

Lateralization of Foot (Medial) Pain
- Pain from compensatory mechanisms of primary pain source at the medial side of the foot

Causes
- Arthropathy in the 1st MTP joint (gout and hallux rigidus/limitus)
- Medial arch over-support (aging foot on the previous-made arch support)
- 1st ray insufficiency with/without 1st cuneiform metatarsal arthritis
- Plantar fasciitis

Common conditions
- Peroneal tendinopathy (behind lateral malleolus and lateral calf/proximal tibiofibular joint)
- Metatarsalgia (intermetatarsal bursitis, cuboid-metatarsal arthralgia)

TOE DEFORMITY AND FRACTURE

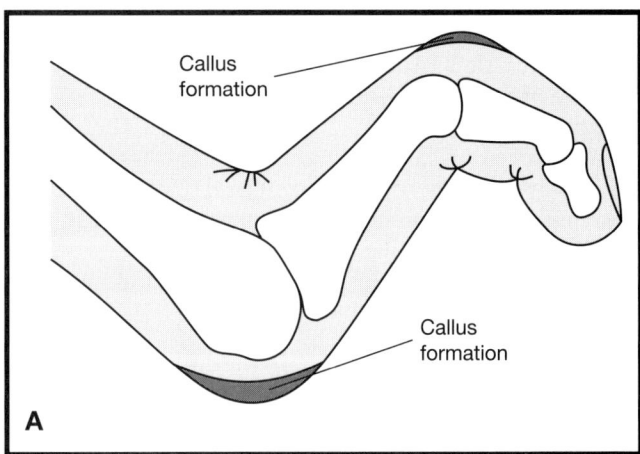

FIGURE 10.7
Common toe deformities: (A) claw and (B) hammer toe.

(continued)

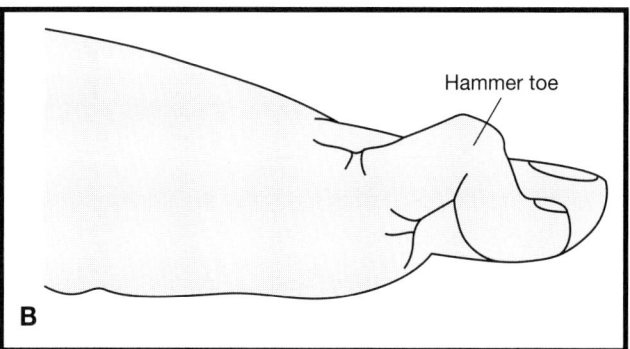

FIGURE 10.7 *(continued)*

Claw Toe (174)
Introduction
- MTP hyperextension with flexed IP joints
  - Drifting of the fibrofatty pad, metatarsal head plantarflexion
- Etiology
  - Insufficiency of MTP capsule (MC cause: synovitis with instability), inflammatory arthropathy, which can be isolated
  - Deep posterior compartment syndrome in the calf or other causes of FDL contracture or tethering
  - Neuromuscular dysfunction and cavus foot
  - Weak intrinsic foot muscles (lumbricals and interosseous) → long-toe extensor (extend MTP) and secondary pull from long-toe flexor (IP flexion) by tenodesis

History and physical examination (Figure 10.7)
- Pain, callosity over PIP dorsally, and MTP plantarly → callus and metatarsalgia
- Mid- and hindfoot examination for cavus deformity, hindfoot varus, and Achilles tightness
- Flexible type if the claw toe deformity corrects as the ankle is plantarflexed

Diagnosis
- Clinical diagnosis
- Imaging study or EMG to evaluate for underlying etiology

Treatment
- Roomier shoes (toe box) with soft-leather upper
- Toe crest, soft insole (1/8-inch Plastazote), and metatarsal pad
- Persistent pain or distress from deformity despite the conservative management → surgical referral to correct the deformity (extensor tenotomy, lengthening tendon transfer, capsulotomy, and osteotomy)

Hammer Toe (178)
Introduction
- A plantarflexion deformity at the PIP joint of the lesser toes
- MC deformity of the lesser toes with 2nd toe being MC location (longer toe), more common in older women
  - Mallet toe: flexion contracture of the DIP (Hammer toe is 9X more common than mallet toe)
- Etiology and risk factor
  - Forefoot overloading and overpull of EDL
  - Tight footwear (related to symptom aggravation)

History and physical examination (Figure 10.7)
- Pain on dorsum of PIP joints (increased pressure/contact with footwear), often associated with callus formation
- Flexible hammertoes initially then rigid contracture as it progresses
  - Flexible deformity correct as the ankle is plantarflexed or metatarsal head pushed dorsally (plantarflex the MTP)
- Inspection: PIP flexion ± MTP extension during standing

Diagnosis
- Clinical diagnosis

Treatment
- Roomier shoes, toe sleeve or padding, stretching of tight heel cord (gastrocnemius)
- Referral to surgery if persistent pain and distress from deformity despite conservative management
  - Postoperative immediate ambulation on the heel (stiff soled postoperative shoes)

Tailor's Bunion (Bunionette Deformity)
Introduction (179)
- Lateral prominence of the 5th metatarsal head with/without bursitis
- Female > male by 2 to 4 times, often bilateral
- Etiology and risk factors
  - Abnormal transverse metatarsal ligament (spray foot), constrictive footwear, pes planus, inflammatory arthropathy, and iatrogenic (from surgery)

History and physical examination
- Painful deformity (bursa, callus, even ulceration) of the lateral aspect of the forefoot, associated with tight footwear
- Widened forefoot, erythema or swelling in 5th bunion, pes planus (forefoot abduction), often painless ROM

Diagnosis
- Clinical diagnosis supplemented with imaging
- X-ray: dorsoplantar, lateral, and oblique
  - The 4th–5th metatarsal bisecting line angle: the normal 4th–5th intermetatarsal angle is <6.5° to 8° (in symptomatic bunionette: ~10°)

Treatment
- Wider shoes or shoes altered to accommodate the deformity (cutouts or stretching), or padding with relief
- Referral to surgery for symptomatic deformity with failed conservative treatment
  - Lateral condylectomy or osteotomy

5th Metatarsal Fracture (Including Jones Fracture)
Introduction (180)
- 5th metatarsal fracture: MC site for metatarsal fractures
- Common location: diaphysial (junction with metaphysic) fracture, typically extending to 4th to 5th intermetatarsal facet

- Mechanism of injury
  - Pivoting or cutting maneuver (forefoot adduction, MC for Jones fracture)
  - Hindfoot inversion (inversion ankle sprain, for avulsion fracture)

History and physical examination
- Pain, swelling on the lateral forefoot, difficulty walking/standing
- Tenderness (styloid process or slightly distal to it), edema, limited ROM of MTP joint with pain and difficulty weight bearing

Diagnosis
- Clinical diagnosis confirmed with radiographs
- Imaging x-ray
  - Avulsion fracture (usually perpendicular to the long axis of the shaft)
    - Normal apophysis oriented parallel to the shaft
    - Os vesalianum can be confused with true fractures; distinguished from fractures by their smooth border and often found in the opposite site
  - In delayed or nonunion cases: medullary canal is obliterated, lateral cortex is thickened and sclerotic, and fracture lines are sclerotic
  - Stress fracture: initially negative
    - Typical findings: longitudinal cortical hypertrophy, narrowing of the medullary canal, and periosteal reaction

- Classification of 5th metatarsal fractures
  - Zone 1: avulsion fracture, at the insertion of the peroneus brevis tendon and the lateral plantar aponeurosis
  - Zone 2: Jones fracture; metaphyseal–diaphyseal junction, which is a vascular watershed area (prone to nonunion, up to 25%), transverse fracture
  - Zone 3: proximal 1.5 cm of the diaphysis, stress or fatigue fracture (see Figure 10.8)

Treatment (181)
- Zone 1 fracture: symptomatic treatment; WBAT in a hard sole postoperative shoe, CAM walker or short-leg walking cast. Heals in 6 to 8 weeks. Return to play up to 6 months
- Nondisplaced Jones (type 2) fracture and acute diaphysial stress fracture: NWB in short leg cast for 6 to 8 weeks. Complete healing up to 6 months
- Referral to surgery for screw fixation
  - Indications: Jones fracture in active persons/athletes, articular step off (>2–3 mm), fragments >30%, or symptomatic nonunion
  - Failures and complications related to screw technique occur in 20 to 30% of operated cases
  - Running and sports ability after operative treatment: returns in 2 to 3 months with successful screw or tension band treatment
    - If bone grafting is used, the final healing time is several months longer

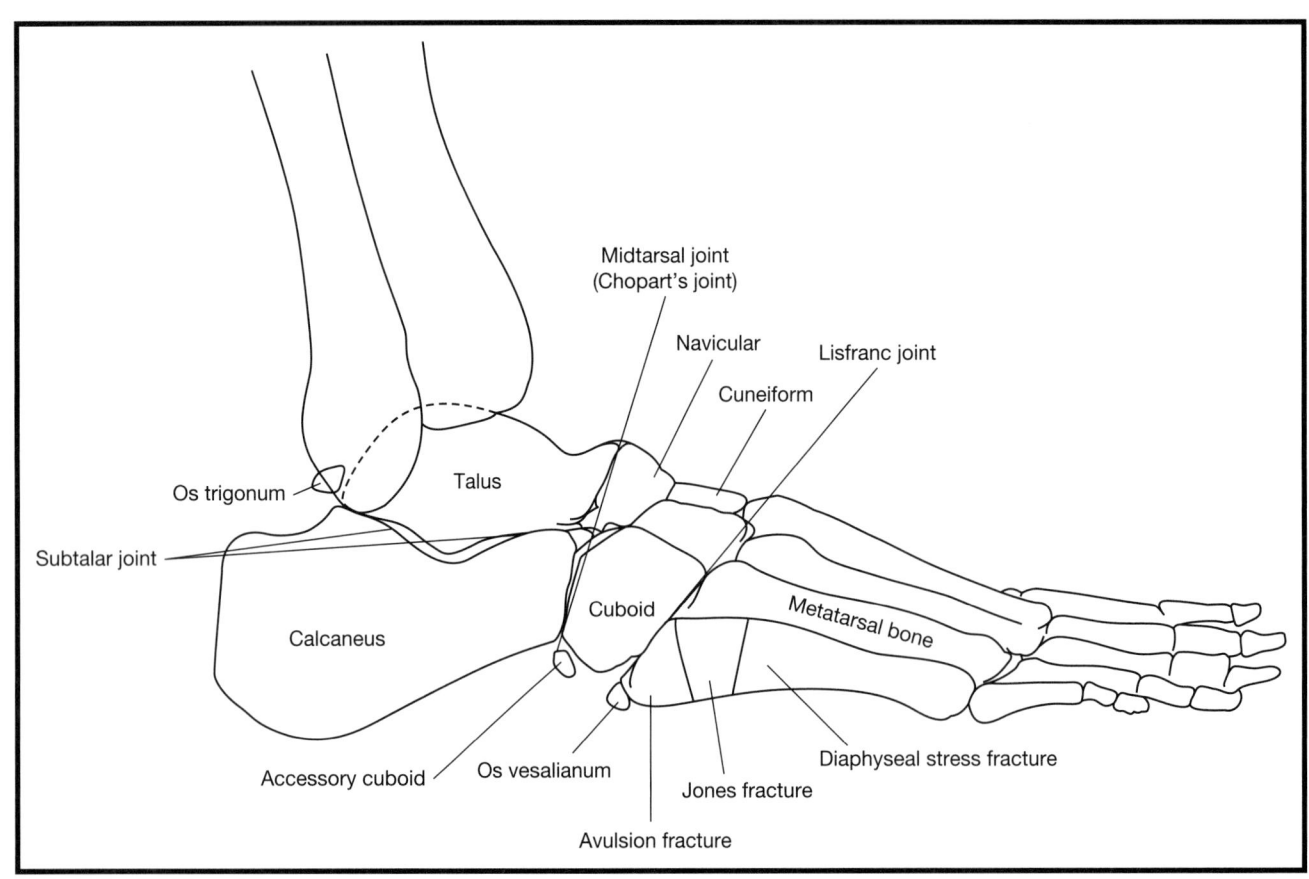

FIGURE 10.8
Location of fifth metatarsal fracture.

Toe Fracture

Introduction (182)
- One of the most commonly encountered fractures in the outpatient clinic
- Lesser toe fractures: 4 times more common than big toe, nondisplaced or minimally displaced are the MC types
- Mechanism of injury
  - Axial force (stubbed toe) or a crushing injury and interphalangeal joint hyperextension (spiral and avulsion fracture)

History and physical examination
- Throbbing pain (worse with dependent position), ecchymosis, and swelling
- Subungual hematoma and/or visible deformity (dislocation)
- Delayed capillary refill if there is vascular compromise
- Sharp pain with axial force: likely fracture rather than contusion

Diagnosis
- Clinical suspicion confirmed with imaging
- X-ray: AP, lateral, and oblique

Treatment
- Splinting with buddy tape and rigid soled shoe
- Surgical referral
  - Indication: big toe fracture-dislocation, displaced intra-articular fractures, unstable displaced fractures, children with big toe fractures involving the physis

COMMON SKIN LESION (183)

	CALLUS AND CORNS	PLANTAR WART
Features	Mechanically induced hyperkeratosis Corn: inverted callus Localized to high friction areas Skin lines pass through the lesion No punctuate hemorrhages at the base Maximum pain with direct pressure	Human papilloma virus–induced hyperplasia of the stratum spinosum Skin lines pass around the lesion. Cauliflower-like surface Central core punctuate hemorrhages at the base Maximal pain with side to side squeezing May observe satellite lesions
Tx	Roomier shoe Callus reduction by scalpel and corn enucleation Pressure off by felt pad (U-shaped or donut shaped pad)	Referral to podiatry Salicylic acid more effective than cryotherapy Intralesional injection of bleomycin Other topical preparation

Tx, treatment.

COMMON MIDFOOT PATHOLOGIES

Midfoot Arthritis

Introduction (7)
- Midfoot joint includes naviculo-cuneiform-metatarsal and cuboid-metatarsal joints
  - Talonavicular or calcaneocuboid (midtarsal) joints are included in hindfoot more often than midfoot (depending on the classification system)
- Etiology: primary, inflammatory (including gout), and posttraumatic
  - 1st ray hypermobility, hypoplastic 1st metatarsal (short), and long 2nd MT joint
  - Midfoot arthropathy secondary to acquired flatfoot (184)
    - Incompetent medial column and dysfunctional PTT → prevent full inversion during midstance → overloading to midfoot rather than metatarsal head (MTP joint)
  - Tight Achilles cord with incompetent medial ray → overload of the more stable midfoot joint (2nd cuneiform-MT >3rd cuneiform-MT joint then 1st ray)
    - Dorsal collapse of transverse arch → TMT spur

History and physical examination
- Midfoot pain, worsened by level walking or activities require heel rise, difficulty wearing shoes with pain
- Tenderness on palpation, dorsal bony spurs, abnormal foot posture (pes planus), and tight heel cord (Silfverskiold test)

Diagnosis
- Clinical diagnosis confirmed by imaging
- X-ray: standing AP, lateral, internal (medial) oblique (lateral column)
  - Lateral weight-bearing view
    - Pronated foot position: lower medial cuneiform height and talus–1st MT angle (convex downward, Meary's line); apex deformity at midfoot
    - Sagging of the medial column at naviculocuneiform and talonavicular joint
- Diagnostic injection: often leaks into the adjacent joint up to 20% of the time; decreased specificity

Treatment
- Nonoperative treatment
  - NSAIDs as needed
  - Low-dye taping and carbon plate → if patient responds well, consider UCBL or SMO
    - If pain is in the lateral side of the midfoot (4th MT-cuboid pain), then add cuboid pad
  - Stiff-soled shoes and rocker-bottom shoes
    - Carbon fiber plate: reduce plantar pressure and contact time of midfoot
  - Hyaluronic acid or cortisone injection using imaging (US) guidance
- Surgical referral if not responsive to conservative management
  - Arthrodesis of the medial and middle columns

Cuboid Subluxation

Introduction (185)
- 4% in athletic foot injuries (up to 17% in ballet dancers)
- Mechanism of injury and risk factors
  ○ Plantarflexion-inversion injury of the ankle ➔ peroneus longus (with eccentric contraction) pulls the medial side of the cuboid downward, displacing the lateral side of cuboid dorsally
    ▪ Plantar and medial side subluxation (common pattern)
    ▪ ± Sprain of dorsal calcaneocuboid and cuboid-metatarsal ligaments
  ○ More common in pronated foot (increased moment arm of peroneus longus)

History and physical examination
- Lateral (mid) foot pain ± inability to walk through gait (pain and instability in push off)
- Lingering pain with downward pressure on the cuboid
- Tenderness over 4th MT–cuboid joint ± instability
- Provocation maneuvers
  ○ Cuboid squeeze test (dorsally directed compression on cuboid from sole): cuboid whip ➔ relief of pain
  ○ Midtarsal adduction test: the midtarsal joint is manipulated passively in the transverse plane while the calcaneus is stabilized (compress the medial aspect of calcaneocuboid joint). Positive with reproduction of symptoms

Diagnosis
- Clinical diagnosis supplemented by imaging
- Weight-bearing X-ray: midtarsal joint alignment (calcaneocuboid joint incongruity; increased gap, deviation, and jamming)
- Differential diagnosis
  ○ Lateral ankle sprain, sinus-tarsi syndrome, midtarsal arthropathy/synovitis (calcaneocuboid), fractures (lateral process of the talus, anterior process of the calcaneus), plantar fasciitis (rarely involving lateral side), peroneus longus tendinopathy, or painful os peroneum

Treatment (186)
- Manual reduction (mobilization): cuboid whip and squeeze (Figure 10.9)
  ○ Thumb placed on the plantar surface of the cuboid (pushing up) during forefoot plantarflexion from dorsiflexion
  ○ With forefoot adduction, apply pressure to cuboid upward direction (reposition inferiorly subluxed cuboid)
- 1/8-inch- to 1/4-inch-thick felt pad under the cuboid with carbon plate (contoured carbon plate with Spenco cover) or UCBL or SMO (pronation control and midfoot stabilization)
- Avoid vigorous exercise a day or two after reduction
- Taping: medial (proximal to the 1st MT head) to lateral and around the cuboid (figure of 8) then another tape (reverse from the lateral)

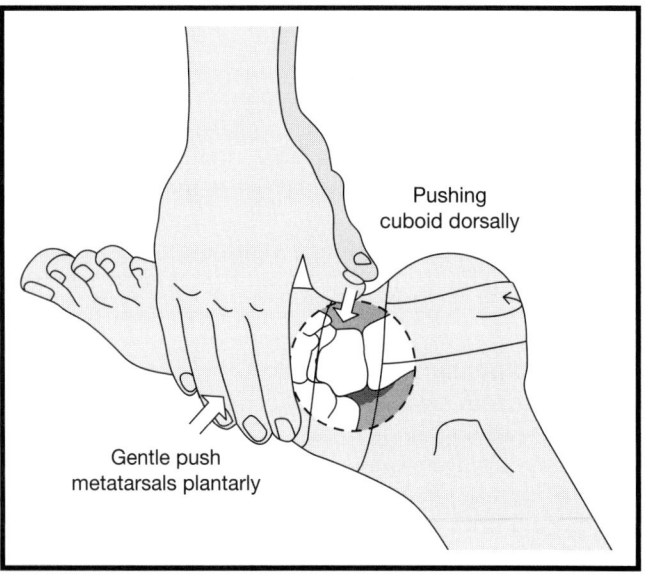

FIGURE 10.9
Cuboid whip and taping for cuboid subluxation.
Source: Adapted from Ref. (186). Marshall P, Hamilton WG. Cuboid subluxation in ballet dancers. *Am J Sports Med*. 1992;20(2):169–175.

Lisfranc (TMT) Joint Injury

Introduction (13,43)
- Incidence of Lisfranc sprain: 4% of football players, fracture: 1 in 55,000 annually
- Etiology
  ○ High-velocity injury: MVA and fall from height
  ○ Low-velocity injury: axial load to plantarflexed or slightly rotated foot followed by forceful abduction (windsurfer and equestrian accident) and twisting movement (football, basketball, and running)

History and physical examination
- Midfoot pain, swelling ± inability to bear weight
- Ecchymosis initially (delayed on the plantar aspect) and tenderness
- Pain on passive pronation and abduction test with fixed hindfoot
- Instability test: dorsally directed force to the forefoot ➔ TMT joint subluxation if unstable

Diagnosis
- Clinical diagnosis confirmed by an imaging study
- X-ray: comparison (bilateral) standing AP (50% false negative in non-weight-bearing x-ray), 30° oblique and lateral (dorsal displacement of proximal metatarsal)
  ○ Grading system (by Nunley and Vertullo): stage 1: no widening of 1st and 2nd ray; stage 2: widening 2 to 5 mm; stage 3: widening 2 to 5 mm with loss of longitudinal arch height
  ○ Check associated injury/fracture: the base of 2nd metatarsal and cuboid by nut cracker effect

- CT and MRI to evaluate plantar ligament bundle → stable midfoot if not injured

Treatment (187)
- Nonoperative treatment: <2 to 5 mm between 1st and 2nd MTs; cast immobilization for 6 weeks if painful, then removable boot for additional 4 weeks followed by custom-molded orthotics and protected weight bearing
  ○ Repeat x-ray in 2 weeks, ROM in 6 to 8 weeks, progressive weight bearing in 3 months
- Referral to surgery if displacement >2 mm or with associated fracture
  ○ Percutaneous screw, ORIF, or arthrodesis
  ○ Postop: NWB cast or boot for 8 weeks, PWB 8 to 12 weeks; then FWB with orthosis after 3 months
  ○ Complications: posttraumatic arthritis and nonunion

NEUROPATHY

TARSAL TUNNEL SYNDROME (TIBIAL NERVE ENTRAPMENT NEUROPATHY AT ANKLE)

Introduction (188)
- Anatomy (189)
  ○ Tarsal tunnel: posterior to medial malleolus, formed by the flexor retinaculum or lancinate ligament
  ○ Four nerves: medial, lateral plantar nerve, medial calcaneal nerve, and Baxter's nerve (1st branch of lateral plantar nerve, inferior calcaneal nerve, often direct branch from tibial nerve)
  ○ Tibial nerve usually divides to the medial/lateral plantar nerves (>90%) in 1 to 2 cm proximal to the imaginary line above the medial malleolus to the calcaneus
- Distal tarsal tunnel
  ○ Under the upper edge of the abductor hallucis muscle, which can irritate the terminal branch of the tibial nerve, medial/lateral plantar, inferior and medial calcaneal nerves
- Etiology
  ○ Hypermobile subtalar joint (hindfoot eversion, hyperpronation): tibial nerve can be entrapped by a prominence of the posteromedial talus
  ○ Ganglion cyst from subtalar joint or tendon sheath, lipoma, accessory muscles, tenosynovitis, varicose vein, bone spicule (history of fracture of calcaneus), and foreign body

History and physical examination
- Pain (pins and needles, burning) in the medial hindfoot/ankle with radiation (proximally and distally), tingling, and numbness on the sole of the foot
- Physical examination
  ○ Tenderness posteromedial to the medial malleolus, a positive Tinel's sign, rarely bulging of the tarsal tunnel, and intrinsic muscle atrophy/unsteadiness
  ○ Provocative test: dorsiflexion–eversion test: maximum dorsiflexion and eversion of the calcaneus with toe dorsiflexion for 5 to 10 seconds: positive if reproduction of the pain +/− numbness (190)

Diagnosis
- Clinical diagnosis confirmed by EMG and imaging for underlying etiologies
- Electrodiagnosis to confirm and to differentiate other peripheral nerve pathologies
  ○ Nerve conduction study
    ▪ Sensory nerve conduction study (SNCS)
      − Sural or SPN (R/O diffuse sensory peripheral neuropathy), normal in TOS
      − Orthodromic mixed nerve conduction study recording at the tibial nerve (above the tarsal tunnel) with stimulation at medial plantar nerve (between 1st and 2nd MT shafts) or lateral plantar nerve (between 4th and 5th metatarsals), at 14 cm distal to the recording site
    ▪ Motor nerve conduction study (MNCS)
      − Medial plantar nerve: abductor hallucis, and FHB (midline of 1st MT shaft)
      − Lateral plantar nerve (flexor digiti quinti); midline of 5th MT, and 1st branch of lateral plantar nerve (ADQP); midline between the lateral malleolus and plantar sole
      − Deep peroneal nerve: R/O peripheral neuropathy or severe L5–S1 radiculopathy, normal in TOS
    ▪ H reflex (S1 radiculopathy, mild peripheral neuropathy, or sciatic/tibial nerve lesion), normal in TOS
    ▪ Needle EMG: medial plantar (FHB), lateral plantar nerve (4th dorsal interosseous in 4th interdigital web space or FDM), and Baxter's nerve (ADQP)
      − Other muscles for differential diagnosis; medial gastrocnemius (proximal tibial nerve), EDB or TA (deep peroneal nerve), gluteus medius (superior gluteal nerve), and/or paraspinal muscles
- Differential diagnosis
  ○ Isolated entrapment syndrome of the branch (Baxter's nerve, medial, lateral plantar nerve, medial calcaneal nerve), soleal sling syndrome (proximal tibial nerve), sciatic nerve lesion, S1 radiculopathy, peripheral neuropathy, and the like
  ○ MSK causes (often coexist): plantar fasciitis, fibromatosis, TP and FHL tendonitis/tenosynovitis, arthropathy of talonavicular, naviculocuneiform, cunneiform-1st metatarsal joint, or 1st MTP joint, and sesamoiditis
- MRI or US (better than CT): evaluate for space-occupying lesion, ganglion cyst (from the subtalar joint), lipoma, aberrant muscle, tenosynovitis, and neurilemma

Treatment
- Medial heel wedge/heel lift: to decrease the hyperpronation with calcaneal eversion, which stretches the tibial nerve
- Heel lift with relief, custom-made insole with medial channel relief (at the cork layer filled with gel elastomer)
- Aspiration and injection of the ganglion cyst
- Steroid injection into the tarsal tunnel under US guidance
- Surgery: release of the laciniate ligament and removal of the mass

BAXTER'S NEUROPATHY (INFERIOR CALCANEAL NEUROPATHY, 1ST BRANCH OF LATERAL PLANTAR NEUROPATHY)

Introduction
- Anatomy
  - Inferior calcaneal nerve; ~45% separate branch directly from the tibial nerve (instead of branching from lateral plantar N)
  - Under the upper edge of the abductor hallucis, the branch is given off posteriorly → travels under the AH muscle with the lateral plantar nerve → deeper to the abductor hallucis/fascia and over the quadratus plantae, under the flexor digitorum brevis muscle and the medial edge of the plantar fascia
  - Provides sensory innervation to the periosteum of the medial calcaneal tuberosity and innervates abductor digiti quinti muscle
- Accounts for 20% of chronic heel pain cases (191); underrecognized
- Etiology
  - Entrapment at AH and quadratus plantae (soft spot) and irritation by distal plantar fasciitis (in front of the heel spur)
  - Iatrogenic after injection, or nerve sheath tumor

History and physical examination
- Chronic heel pain, often worse with running
  - Medial plantar heel pain ± proximal radiation into the medial region of ankle and foot, and distal radiation into the lateral plantar aspect of the foot
  - Constant pain at rest as well as with activity although it can be worse in the morning (venous engorgement adding to the compression)
  - Numbness is unusual unless other nerve lesion co-exists
- Physical examination
  - Tenderness on the soft spot (medial aspect of the heel, not the plantar aspect, medial border of AH muscle) reproducing the symptoms and radiation of pain proximally and distally
  - Sensory examination of the sole (lateral plantar nerve vs. medial plantar nerve); should be normal
  - Normal motor examination except ADQP atrophy (difficult to recognize and examine) and deep tendon reflexes typically

Diagnosis
- Clinical diagnosis confirmed by EMG or an imaging study
- MRI: atrophy, increased T2 SI with fatty infiltration in the abductor digiti quinti pedis (ADQP) muscle
- EMG: same as tarsal tunnel syndrome: isolated finding in the ADQP; NCS comparison to the opposite site and needle EMG examination
  - NCS of medial calcaneal nerve (192)
    - Recording: distal 1/3 of the line from midpoint of navicular tuberosity and medial malleolus apex to the calcaneal apex
    - Stimulation: tibial nerve above the flexor retinaculum
- Differential diagnosis
  - Plantar fasciitis and calcaneal fracture
  - Neurologic conditions similar to the tarsal tunnel syndrome

Treatment
- Felt-pad relief or off-the-shelf foot insert with relief for the Baxter's nerve (medial aspect of the heel and soft spot)
- Total contact insert with the posteromedial nerve relief channel (filled with a viscoelastic polymer)
  - 2/3 of patients get better
- Stretching of plantar fascia and gastrocnemius muscle
- NSAIDs for a short term and possible US-guided injection
- Surgery if failed conservative management

JOGGER'S FOOT (MEDIAL PLANTAR NEUROPATHY)

Introduction (193)
- Medial plantar neuropathy at the level of the Master knot of Henry
  - Medial plantar nerve runs along the plantar surface of the FDL and through the Master knot of Henry (crossing of flexor pollicis longus and FDL tendon)
- Unknown incidence, rare, but underrecognized
- Risk factor
  - Forefoot abduction, heel valgus, or hyperpronation
  - Arch support (ambitious medial arch support irritating the nerve) with aging foot (further collapsing arch) and tight shoes

History and physical examination
- History: medial arch pain, numbness, or tingling sensation distally as well as proximally
- Physical examination
  - Tenderness under navicular bone (or naviculocuneiform joint)
- Differential palpation with plantar fascia, FHL tendon and nerve

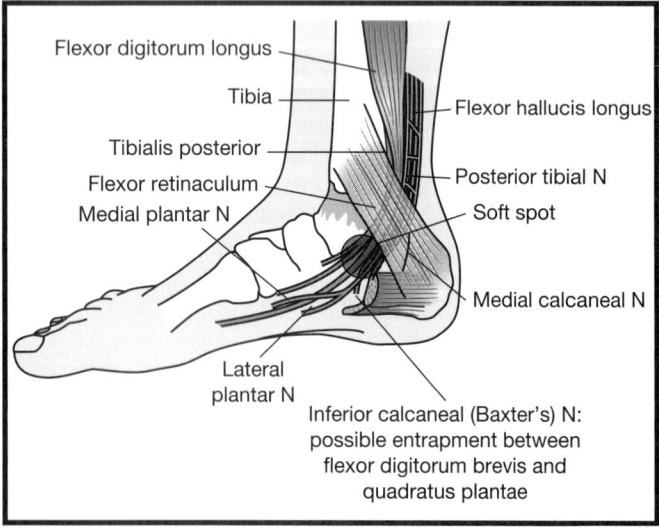

FIGURE 10.10
Location of tarsal tunnel (under the flexor retinaculum) and distal tarsal tunnel syndrome (the soft spot).

a./v., artery/vein; N, nerve.

Source: Adapted from Ref. (188). Gould JS. Tarsal tunnel syndrome. *Foot Ankle Clin.* 2011;16(2):275–286.

- Identify the plantar fascia (by windlass mechanism), plantarflex the MTP joint, then pinch and push the plantar fascia to laterally, FHL tendon, again push it laterally then palpate the nerve (often difficult to palpate)

Diagnosis
- Clinical diagnosis with high suspicion
- NCS and needle EMG: same as the Tarsal tunnel protocol; normal lateral plantar nerve, Baxter's nerve and abductor hallucis muscle
  - Abnormal medial plantar orthodromic study, MNCS and needle EMG in FHB muscle (sparing abductor hallucis muscle)
- US and MRI for soft-tissue mass at the Master knot of Henry (tethering lesion)
- Differential diagnosis same as tarsal tunnel syndrome

Management
- U-shaped (or donut-shaped) felt pad for relief of tender point
- Remove iatrogenic cause (remove/grind off excessive medial arch support)
- Roomier shoes and extra socks
- Surgical referral if not responsive to conservative treatment.

MORTON'S INTERDIGITAL NEURALGIA

Introduction (194)
- Common cause of lateral forefoot pain, mean age: 55 years old, female > male by 4 to 15 times
- Epineural/perineural fibrosis of interdigital nerve distal to the transverse metatarsal ligament (at the level of the metatarsal head)
- MC location: 3rd interdigital nerve
  - Communicating branch of 3rd (medial plantar) and 4th (lateral plantar) digital nerves (~25% in a cadaver study)
  - 2nd and 3rd interdigital space is narrower than 4th space
  - Relative fixed cuneiform-metatarsal (1–3) versus mobile 4th and 5th MT-cuboid; transit point
- Etiology and risk factors
  - Idiopathic or rarely secondary to MTP ganglion, plantar lipoma, MTP joint instability, or thickened transverse metatarsal ligament
  - Fashion shoes: narrow toe box, high-heel, and tight-heel cord: more pressure to the forefoot and MTP dorsiflexion (stretch interdigital nerve)

History and physical examination
- Plantar forefoot pain distal to the metatarsal heads (often diffuse forefoot pain) ± radiation distally (45%) and proximally, often unilateral (15% bilateral). Numbness is relatively rare (<5%)
- Tenderness at plantar surface of distal intermetatarsal space (95%) and palpable mass (~10%) (195)
- Mulder's click: palpable (± audible) clicking sensation is appreciated by the examiner's hand by squeezing the forefoot
- Lateral squeeze test (squeeze metatarsal shafts, not head), pinch test (plantar and dorsal pinch), and compression test (from plantar aspect with MTP dorsiflexion to expose)

Diagnosis
- Clinical diagnosis confirmed by an imaging study
- US (196) if not responsive to initial treatment
  - Usually negative in interdigital neuralgia (without structural change) (194)
  - Can be more sensitive than MRI
  - Typical finding of interdigital neuroma: oval hypoechoic mass in the intermetatarsal space in cases of neuroma. Can be found in asymptomatic population
- EMG: limited role (197), orthodromic conduction study recording from the tibial nerve at the ankle with stimulation of interdigital nerve using ring electrode between toes

Treatment (198)
- Nonoperative management: relieves symptoms in more than 50% of cases
  - Roomier shoes (longer, wider, and higher toe box), metatarsal pad (proximal to the metatarsal head), possibly carbon plate to address MTPJ synovitis or instability if present
  - Injection: corticosteroid (avoid larger volume or multiple injection) (199) and alcohol sclerosing therapy (30% ethyl alcohol) (200)
    - US guidance to bursal–nerve complex, not to the plantar fat pad
- Surgery if failed conservative treatment
  - Failed surgery: often with true neuroma
    - Due to recurrence, trauma, incorrect diagnosis or other coexisting lesion (tarsal tunnel syndrome), or inadequate short dorsal incision

ANTERIOR TARSAL TUNNEL SYNDROME (DEEP PERONEAL NERVE ENTRAPMENT NEUROPATHY)

Introduction (201)
- Neuropathy of distal portion of deep peroneal nerve with sensory deficit, paresthesia and possibly pain
- Etiology
  - Entrapment at anterior tarsal tunnel
    - Inferior edge of the inferomedial band of inferior extensor retinaculum
    - Dorsal osteophyte of the talonavicular joint (N spot), ganglion cyst, fracture, subluxation, and rarely tumor
  - Repetitive compressive trauma from tight-shoe straps or high-heel shoes (stretched with high heels and even with sleep when ankle is plantarflexed): MC (202)
    - Biomechanics: rigid forefoot valgus with plantarflexed 1st ray (with subtalar supination and midtarsal inversion)

History and physical examination
- Pain on the dorsum of the foot (radiating down to the 1st web space); often vague, poorly localized, burning, and worse at night time
  - Sinus-tarsi pain (lateral hindfoot); deep aching (cutaneous pins/needle or burning; uncommon)
  - Paresthesia in the 1st web space
- Knee evaluation: tibiofibular joint instability, reproduction by fibular mobilization with proximal irritation of the deep peroneal nerve
- Pes cavus with tight shoes, inspection for mass on the dorsum, check for EDB atrophy

- Tinel's sign at N spot (talonavicular joint) but often present at naviculocuneiform or cuneiform and 2nd MT/1st MT
- Ankle (forefoot) plantarflexion aggravates the symptoms (by stretching and compression between TNJ and retinaculum)

Diagnosis
- Clinical diagnosis with high suspicion, an imaging study to evaluate for underlying causes ± diagnostic nerve block
- X-ray for TN osteophyte/fracture, MSK US for soft-tissue mass (ganglion cyst, lipoma), US for guided injection for diagnosis and therapeutic purpose
- NCS and needle EMG: limited
  - Deep peronal SNCS recording at the ankle stimulating at 1st web space using ring electrode or slightly proximally on 1st interdigital nerve. MNCS recording at EDB with stimulation at the ankle and distal/proximal to fibular head
- Differential diagnosis
  - Deep peroneal entrapment neuropathy at other locations
    - Proximal calf (entering lateral and anterior compartment)
    - Superior extensor retinaculum (~5 cm above the ankle joint)
    - Under the tendon of extensor hallucis brevis (distally)
  - Other peripheral nerve disorders: superficial peroneal neuropathy, interdigital neuritis, L5 radiculopathy, peripheral neuropathy, and tarsal tunnel syndrome
  - Others: ankle impingement syndrome, midfoot arthritis, gout, ankle sprain or fracture, peripheral arterial disease

Treatment
- Roomier shoes (remove external pressure), skipped lace (avoid irritation from the tongue of the shoe), donut-shaped felt pad (to relieve the irritation from shoe) with double socks
- Diagnostic and therapeutic injection (US guided)
  - Nerve block proximal to the joint; differentiate nerve as pain generator from other local structures (such as joint and ligament)
  - Limitation: at the ankle level, superficial and deep peroneal nerves are near (even saphenous nerve); can block all three nerves by overflow of medication

SUPERFICIAL PERONEAL NERVE ENTRAPMENT SYNDROME

Introduction (203)
- Epidemiology
  - Unknown prevalence, but common in ankle injury (inversion sprain and ankle fracture (15% injured SPN) (204)
- Etiology
  - Direct trauma to nerve (25%): MC cause
  - Traction injury with ankle inversion sprain, fibular fracture, and ankle fusion
  - Muscle herniation and chronic exertional compartment syndrome (even after fasciectomy)
  - Lipoma or rarely nerve tumor
  - High-riding boots, and tight laces

History and physical examination (205)
- Distal anterolateral lower leg and dorsal foot pain (neuropathic pain character)
  - Often aggravated by physical activity and relieved by rest
- Tenderness at the opening of the crural fascia: nerve pierce crural fascia (7–10 cm from ankle joint) reproducing symptoms with referred pain proximally and distally (Valleix's phenomenon)
- Palpation of nerve: with the toes in plantarflexion (also aggravates the symptoms); difficult in obese patients or if ankle is swollen
- Three provocative maneuvers; positive with finding of pain and paresthesia over distribution of the SPN in two out of the three provocative maneuvers
  - Pressure over entrapment site while patient actively dorsiflexes and everts his ankle against resistance
  - Examiner passively plantarflexes and inverts the ankle
  - Percussion over the course of the nerve, while maintaining passive stretch with an ankle inversion

Diagnosis
- Clinical diagnosis confirmed by EMG test and/or diagnostic block
- EMG test: SPN antidromic and orthodromic study (recording above the ankle with stimulation at the distal branches, inching technique if possible)—often negative
- Diagnostic and therapeutic injections to the SPN at the potential entrapment site under US guidance

Treatment
- Lateral wedge and Unna boot (relative immobilization allowing physical therapy, reducing edema and soothing effect)
- Steroid injection (US guided) into the fascial perforating spot, botulism toxin injection to the leg muscle (anterior compartment) where the SPN perforates the crural fascia
- Skipped lace technique, donut-shaped felt pad and double socks, shields (under the tongue of the shoe)
- Education for desensitization, trial of TENS, gradual stretching, and strengthening exercise (gradual)
- Referral to surgery if not responsive to conservative management
  - Decompression and nerve release at the peroneal tunnel, fasciectomy in exertional compartment syndrome, release of extensor retinaculum (leave the superior portion intact)
  - No significant improvement in 20% of cases

SAPHENOUS MONONEUROPATHY

Introduction
- Anatomy: runs with greater saphenous vein anteriorly to the medial malleolus, then to the medial midfoot (navicular or naviculocuneiform) or even distal to the big toe in some cases
- Etiology
  - Iatrogenic (graft, injection), ganglion cyst in the medial ankle (medial to the TA), and hyperpronation

History and physical examination
- Medial leg (calf), ankle and medial midfoot pain; burning, pins/needles sensation and tingling
- Worsens by ankle dorsiflexion and eversion, and partially relieved by inversion

Diagnosis
- High clinical suspicion confirmed by NCS (if abnormal in the symptomatic side compare to the normal contralaterally; often limited; often unobtainable in both legs) or imaging-guided diagnostic injection
- Differential diagnosis: painful accessory navicular, TP tendinopathy (can be concomitant), midfoot arthritis, medial plantar neuropathy, and tarsal tunnel syndrome

Treatment
- Medial heel wedge and heel lift to decrease hyperpronation and hindfoot eversion
- Imaging-guided nerve block

SURAL MONONEUROPATHY

Introduction (206)
- Isolated lesion: very rare
- Etiology
  ○ Iatrogenic: Achilles tendon repair, grafting from the sural nerve with neuroma formation, calcaneal fracture treated with instrumentation, possible sural nerve entrapment in the scar
  ○ Others: Achilles or peroneal tendon pathology, Baker's cyst, tumors, osteochondroma, ganglia (intraneural or compression by ganglion), fibrosis after ankle sprain or other trauma (fractures of 5th metatarsal base, talus, calcaneus, cuboid), and irritation by myositis ossificans

History and physical examination
- Pain, burning, paresthesia along sural nerve distribution (lateral side of ankle/foot and can extend to 5th metatarsal head ± lateral/posterior calf pain)
- Tinel sign at the entrapment site with radiating pain distally or proximally (Valleix's phenomenon)
- Symptoms aggravated by ankle dorsiflexion and inversion (stretching the sural nerve)

Diagnosis
- Clinical suspicion confirmed by NCS study (often negative) ± diagnostic and therapeutic injection under US guidance
- US or MRI to evaluate possible underlying structural lesion

Treatment
- Address biomechanics: lateral wedge if hindfoot varus (inversion) can aggravate the symptoms
- Steroid injection or block with lidocaine/bupivacaine

MEDIAL HALLUCAL NEUROPATHY

Introduction (207)
- Joplin's neuroma/neuralgia (hallucal nerve): entrapment, injury, or neuroma of plantar proper digital nerve to the hallux
- Unknown prevalence, rare, but underrecognized
- Anatomy
  ○ Crosses the proximal pole of the medial (tibial) sesamoid (under the 1st MTP joint), then courses distally to innervate the medial and plantar aspects of the great toe
- Etiology
  ○ Entrapment as it exits the distal abductor hallucis muscle (~1.5 cm proximal to cuneiform-1st MT joint) (208)
  ○ Iatrogenic: after medial sesamoidectomy and capsular closure of the first MTP joint
  ○ Hallux valgus → prominent tibial sesamoid pressing on the nerve or after hallux valgus surgery
  ○ Chronic compression (tight footwear, sports requiring repetitive pivoting impact and motion of 1st MTPJ)

History and physical examination
- Pain, numbness, pins/needles, and tingling in the big toe and 1st ray
- Tenderness at the entrapment site with pain radiating distally and proximally (Valleix's phenomenon)

Diagnosis
- Clinical diagnosis with imaging-guided lidocaine block (often limited specificity due to diffusion of medication)
- Differential diagnosis (often coexisting): sesamoiditis (AVN, fracture, etc), MTP arthralgia (gout, osteoarthritis, etc.), tarsal tunnel syndrome/jogger's foot/proximal nerve lesion

Treatment
- Proper shoe with stiff sole (to prevent the forefoot/toe crease bending)
  ○ Prolonged use of shoes with flexion of the crease → can impinge the medial hallucal nerve
  ○ If the patient responds, then consider carbon plate
- Bunion relief on the shoe (using ball and socket stretcher or by shoemaker)
- Injection with US guidance for pain control

REFERENCES

1. Menz HB, Gill TK, Taylor AW, Hill CL. Age and gender differences in disabling foot pain using different definitions of the Manchester Foot Pain and Disability Index. *BMC Musculoskelet Disord*. 2011;12:243.
2. Thomas MJ, Roddy E, Zhang W, et al. The population prevalence of foot and ankle pain in middle and old age: a systematic review. *Pain*. 2011;152(12):2870–2880.
3. Bálint GP, Korda J, Hangody L, Bálint PV. Regional musculoskeletal conditions: foot and ankle disorders. *Best Pract Res Clin Rheumatol*. 2003;17(1):87–111.
4. Malanga GA, Ramirez-Del Toro JA. Common injuries of the foot and ankle in the child and adolescent athlete. *Phys Med Rehabil Clin N Am*. 2008;19(2):347–71, ix.
5. Pommering TL, Kluchurosky L, Hall SL. Ankle and foot injuries in pediatric and adult athletes. *Prim Care*. 2005;32(1):133–161.
6. Conti SF, Silverman L. Epidemiology of foot and ankle injuries in the workplace. *Foot Ankle Clin*. 2002;7(2):273–290.
7. Patel A, Rao S, Nawoczenski D, et al. Midfoot arthritis. *J Am Acad Orthop Surg*. 2010;18(7):417–425.
8. Guillin R, Marchand AJ, Roux A, et al. Imaging of snapping phenomena. *Br J Radiol*. 2012;85(1018):1343–1353.
9. Barg A, Tochigi Y, Amendola A, et al. Subtalar instability: diagnosis and treatment. *Foot Ankle Int*. 2012;33(2):151–160.
10. Golanó P, Vega J, de Leeuw PA, et al. Anatomy of the ankle ligaments: a pictorial essay. *Knee Surg Sports Traumatol Arthrosc*. 2010;18(5):557–569.
11. Mansour R, Teh J, Sharp RJ, Ostlere S. Ultrasound assessment of the spring ligament complex. *Eur Radiol*. 2008;18(11):2670–2675.
12. Early JS, Bucholz RW. Lisfranc injuries and their management. *Curr Orthop*. 1996;10(3):169–173.
13. DeOrio M, Erickson M, Usuelli FG, Easley M. Lisfranc injuries in sport. *Foot Ankle Clin*. 2009;14(2):169–186.
14. Demondion X, Canella C, Moraux A, et al. Retinacular disorders of the ankle and foot. *Semin Musculoskelet Radiol*. 2010;14(3):281–291.
15. Lektrakul N, Chung CB, Lai Ym, et al. Tarsal sinus: arthrographic, MR imaging, MR arthrographic, and pathologic findings in cadavers

and retrospective study data in patients with sinus tarsi syndrome. *Radiology.* 2001;219(3):802–810.
16. Glazebrook MA, Paletz JL. Treatment of posttraumatic injuries to the nerves in the foot and ankle. *Foot Ankle Clin.* 2006;11(1):183–90, x.
17. del Toro DR, Park TA. *Needle EMG Examination of the Foot.* AANEM Workshop, San Francisco, CA; 2011.
18. Mayich DJ, Novak A, Vena D, et al. Gait analysis in orthopedic foot and ankle surgery–topical review, part 1: principles and uses of gait analysis. *Foot Ankle Int.* 2014;35(1):80–90.
19. Caselli MA, George DH. Foot deformities: biomechanical and pathomechanical changes associated with aging, Part I. *Clin Podiatr Med Surg.* 2003;20(3):487–509, ix.
20. Barton T, Lintz F, Winson I. Biomechanical changes associated with the osteoarthritic, arthrodesed, and prosthetic ankle joint. *Foot Ankle Surg.* 2011;17(2):52–57.
21. Snedeker JG, Wirth SH, Espinosa N. Biomechanics of the normal and arthritic ankle joint. *Foot Ankle Clin.* 2012;17(4):517–528.
22. Nüesch C, Barg A, Pagenstert GI, Valderrabano V. Biomechanics of asymmetric ankle osteoarthritis and its joint-preserving surgery. *Foot Ankle Clin.* 2013;18(3):427–436.
23. Ledoux WR, Shofer JB, Ahroni JH, et al. Biomechanical differences among pes cavus, neutrally aligned, and pes planus feet in subjects with diabetes. *Foot Ankle Int.* 2003;24(11):845–850.
24. Kogler GF, Solomonidis SE, Paul JP. Biomechanics of longitudinal arch support mechanisms in foot orthoses and their effect on plantar aponeurosis strain. *Clin Biomech (Bristol, Avon).* 1996;11(5):243–252.
25. Richie DH Jr. Biomechanics and clinical analysis of the adult acquired flatfoot. *Clin Podiatr Med Surg.* 2007;24(4):617–44, vii.
26. Marks RM. Midfoot and forefoot issues cavovarus foot: assessment and treatment issues. *Foot Ankle Clin.* 2008;13(2):229–41, vi.
27. Whitney KA. Foot deformities, biomechanical and pathomechanical changes associated with aging including orthotic considerations, Part II. *Clin Podiatr Med Surg.* 2003;20(3):511–26, x.
28. Lee MS, Vanore JV, Thomas JL, et al.; Clinical Practice Guideline Adult Flatfoot Panel. Diagnosis and treatment of adult flatfoot. *J Foot Ankle Surg.* 2005;44(2):78–113.
29. Redmond AC, Crane YZ, Menz HB. Normative values for the foot Posture Index. *J Foot Ankle Res.* 2008;1(6);1–9.
30. DiGiovanni CW, Kuo R, Tejwani N, et al. Isolated gastrocnemius tightness. *J Bone Joint Surg Am.* 2002;84-A(6):962–970.
31. Frykberg RG, Bowen J, Hall J, et al. Prevalence of equinus in diabetic versus nondiabetic patients. *J Am Podiatr Med Assoc.* 2012;102(2):84–88.
32. Simpson MR. Benign joint hypermobility syndrome: evaluation, diagnosis, and management. *J Am Osteopath Assoc.* 2006;106(9):531–536.
33. van Rensburg CJ. *Approach to and management of acute ankle ligamentous injuries. Contin Med Educ.* 2009;22(3):112–115.
34. Perera A, Guha A. Clinical and radiographic evaluation of the cavus foot: surgical implications. *Foot Ankle Clin.* 2013;18(4):619–628.
35. Abbasian A, Pomeroy G. The idiopathic cavus foot-not so subtle after all. *Foot Ankle Clin.* 2013;18(4):629–642.
36. Houck JR, Neville C, Tome J, Flemister AS. Foot kinematics during a bilateral heel rise test in participants with stage II posterior tibial tendon dysfunction. *J Orthop Sports Phys Ther.* 2009;39(8):593–603.
37. Hintermann B, Gächter A. The first metatarsal rise sign: a simple, sensitive sign of tibialis posterior tendon dysfunction. *Foot Ankle Int.* 1996;17(4):236–241.
38. Cloke D, Greiss M. *The digital nerve stretch test: A sensitive indicator of Morton's neuroma and neuritis. Foot Ankle Surg.* 2006;12(4):201–203.
39. Watson AD. Ankle instability and impingement. *Foot Ankle Clin.* 2007;12(1):177–195.
40. Kouloris G, Morrison WB. Foot and ankle disorders: radiographic signs. *Semin Roentgenol.* 2005;40(4):358–379.
41. Heyworth J. Ottawa ankle rules for the injured ankle. *BMJ.* 2003;326(7386):405–406.
42. Alexander IJ, Johnson KA. Assessment and management of pes cavus in Charcot-Marie-tooth disease. *Clin Orthop Relat Res.* 1989(246):273–281.
43. Mullen JE, O'Malley MJ. Sprains–residual instability of subtalar, Lisfranc joints, and turf toe. *Clin Sports Med.* 2004;23(1):97–121.
44. Ansede G, Lee JC, Healy JC. Musculoskeletal sonography of the normal foot. *Skeletal Radiol.* 2010;39(3):225–242.
45. Fessell DP, Jacobson JA. Ultrasound of the hindfoot and midfoot. *Radiol Clin North Am.* 2008;46(6):1027–43, vi.
46. Rogers CJ, Cianca J. Musculoskeletal ultrasound of the ankle and foot. *Phys Med Rehabil Clin N Am.* 2010;21(3):549–557.
47. Gregg JM, Schneider T, Marks P. MR imaging and ultrasound of metatarsalgia–the lesser metatarsals. *Radiol Clin North Am.* 2008;46(6):1061–78, vi.
48. Bancroft LW, Peterson JJ, Kransdorf MJ. Imaging of soft tissue lesions of the foot and ankle. *Radiol Clin North Am.* 2008;46(6):1093–103, vii.
49. Woodburn J, Turner DE. Chapter 13—Podiatry, biomechanics and the rheumatology foot. In Dziedzic K, Hammond A, eds. *Rheumatology.* Edinburgh, Scotland: Churchill Livingstone; 2010:171–184.
50. McKeon PO, Hertel J, Bramble D, Davis I. The foot core system: a new paradigm for understanding intrinsic foot muscle function. *Br J Sports Med.* 2015;49(5):290.
51. Maffulli N, Ferran NA. Management of acute and chronic ankle instability. *J Am Acad Orthop Surg.* 2008;16(10):608–615.
52. Smith J, Finnoff JT, Henning PT, Turner NS. Accuracy of sonographically guided posterior subtalar joint injections: comparison of 3 techniques. *J Ultrasound Med.* 2009;28(11):1549–1557.
53. Vannini F, Di Matteo B, Filardo G, et al. Platelet-rich plasma for foot and ankle pathologies: a systematic review. *Foot Ankle Surg.* 2014;20(1):2–9.
54. Chon JY, Hahn YJ, Sung CH, et al. Pulsed radiofrequency under ultrasound guidance for the tarsal tunnel syndrome: two case reports. *J Anesth.* 2014;28(6):924–927.
55. Jang SH, Ahn SH, Park SM, et al. Alcohol neurolysis of tibial nerve motor branches to the gastrocnemius muscle to treat ankle spasticity in patients with hemiplegic stroke. *Arch Phys Med Rehabil.* 2004;85(3):506–508.
56. Kocabas H, Salli A, Demir AH, Ozerbil OM. Comparison of phenol and alcohol neurolysis of tibial nerve motor branches to the gastrocnemius muscle for treatment of spastic foot after stroke: a randomized controlled pilot study. *Eur J Phys Rehabil Med.* 2010;46(1):5–10.
57. Riskowski J, Dufour AB, Hannan MT. Arthritis, foot pain and shoe wear: current musculoskeletal research on feet. *Curr Opin Rheumatol.* 2011;23(2):148–155.
58. Ewalt KL. Bandaging and taping considerations for the dancer. *J Dance Med Sci.* 2010;14(3):103–113.
59. Janisse DJ, Janisse E. Shoe modification and the use of orthoses in the treatment of foot and ankle pathology. *J Am Acad Orthop Surg.* 2008;16(3):152–158.
60. Opila-Correia KA. Kinematics of high-heeled gait. *Arch Phys Med Rehabil.* 1990;71(5):304–309.
61. Opila-Correia KA. Kinematics of high-heeled gait with consideration for age and experience of wearers. *Arch Phys Med Rehabil.* 1990;71(11):905–909.
62. Czajka CM, Tran E, Cai AN, DiPreta JA. Ankle sprains and instability. *Med Clin North Am.* 2014;98(2):313–329.
63. Hintermann B, Knupp M, Pagenstert GI. Deltoid ligament injuries: diagnosis and management. *Foot Ankle Clin.* 2006;11(3):625–637.
64. Waterman BR, Owens BD, Davey S, et al. The epidemiology of ankle sprains in the United States. *J Bone Joint Surg Am.* 2010;92(13):2279–2284.
65. Hsu CC, Tsai WC, Chen CP, et al. Ultrasonographic examination for inversion ankle sprains associated with osseous injuries. *Am J Phys Med Rehabil.* 2006;85(10):785–792.
66. Endele D, Jung C, Bauer G, Mauch F. Value of MRI in diagnosing injuries after ankle sprains in children. *Foot Ankle Int.* 2012;33(11):1063–1068.
67. Mansour R, Jibri Z, Kamath S, et al. Persistent ankle pain following a sprain: a review of imaging. *Emerg Radiol.* 2011;18(3):211–225.
68. Karlsson J, Sancone M. Management of acute ligament injuries of the ankle. *Foot Ankle Clin.* 2006;11(3):521–530.
69. DiGiovanni BF, Partal G, Baumhauer JF. *Acute ankle injury and chronic lateral instability in the athlete. Clin Sports Med.* 2004;23(1):1–19, v.
70. Ergen E, Ulkar B. Proprioception and ankle injuries in soccer. *Clin Sports Med.* 2008;27(1):195–217, x.
71. Pedowitz DI, Reddy S, Parekh SG, et al. Prophylactic bracing decreases ankle injuries in collegiate female volleyball players. *Am J Sports Med.* 2008;36(2):324–327.
72. Mak MF, Gartner L, Pearce CJ. Management of syndesmosis injuries in the elite athlete. *Foot Ankle Clin.* 2013;18(2):195–214.

73. Kerkhoffs GM, Van Dijk CN. Acute lateral ankle ligament ruptures in the athlete: the role of surgery. *Foot Ankle Clin.* 2013;18(2): 215–218.
74. Schaffler GJ, Tirman PF, Stoller DW, et al. Impingement syndrome of the ankle following supination external rotation trauma: MR imaging findings with arthroscopic correlation. *Eur Radiol.* 2003;13(6):1357–1362.
75. Tol JL, van Dijk CN. Anterior ankle impingement. *Foot Ankle Clin.* 2006;11(2):297–310, vi.
76. Molloy S, Solan MC, Bendall SP. Synovial impingement in the ankle. A new physical sign. *J Bone Joint Surg Br.* 2003;85(3):330–333.
77. Robinson P. Impingement syndromes of the ankle. *Eur Radiol.* 2007;17(12):3056–3065.
78. Pesquer L, Guillo S, Meyer P, Hauger O. US in ankle impingement syndrome. *J Ultrasound.* 2014;17(2):89–97.
79. Cerezal L, Abascal F, Canga A, et al. MR imaging of ankle impingement syndromes. *AJR Am J Roentgenol.* 2003;181(2):551–559.
80. Coull R, Raffiq T, James LE, Stephens MM. Open treatment of anterior impingement of the ankle. *J Bone Joint Surg Br.* 2003;85(4):550–553.
81. Wukich DK, Tuason DA. Diagnosis and treatment of chronic ankle pain. *Instr Course Lect.* 2011;60:335–350.
82. Harper MC. The lateral ligamentous support of the subtalar joint. *Foot Ankle.* 1991;11(6):354–358.
83. Lee KB, Bai LB, Park JG, Song EK, Lee JJ. Efficacy of MRI versus arthroscopy for evaluation of sinus tarsi syndrome. *Foot Ankle Int.* 2008;29(11):1111–1116.
84. Zwipp H, Rammelt S, Grass R. Ligamentous injuries about the ankle and subtalar joints. *Clin Podiatr Med Surg.* 2002;19(2):195–229, v.
85. Waldecker U, Blatter G. Sonographic measurement of instability of the subtalar joint. *Foot Ankle Int.* 2001;22(1):42–46.
86. Thermann H, Zwipp H, Tscherne H. Treatment algorithm of chronic ankle and subtalar instability. *Foot Ankle Int.* 1997;18(3):163–169.
87. Neufeld SK, Cerrato R. Plantar fasciitis: evaluation and treatment. *J Am Acad Orthop Surg.* 2008;16(6):338–346.
88. Toomey EP. Plantar heel pain. *Foot Ankle Clin.* 2009;14(2):229–245.
89. Monto RR. Platelet-rich plasma efficacy versus corticosteroid injection treatment for chronic severe plantar fasciitis. *Foot Ankle Int.* 2014;35(4):313–318.
90. Veith NT, Tschernig T, Histing T, Madry H. Plantar fibromatosis–topical review. *Foot Ankle Int.* 2013;34(12):1742–1746.
91. Martinoli C, Bianchi S. *Ultrasound of the Musculoskeletal System.* Berlin, Heidelberg, Germany: Springer; 2007:773–834.
92. Woertler K. Soft tissue masses in the foot and ankle: characteristics on MR Imaging. *Semin Musculoskelet Radiol.* 2005;9(3):227–242.
93. Kader D, et al. *Achilles tendinopathy tendon injuries.* In Maffulli N, Renström P, Leadbetter W, eds. London: Springer; 2005:201–208.
94. de Jonge S, van den Berg C, de Vos RJ, et al. Incidence of midportion Achilles tendinopathy in the general population. *Br J Sports Med.* 2011;45(13):1026–1028.
95. Kader D, Saxena A, Movin T, Maffulli N. Achilles tendinopathy: some aspects of basic science and clinical management. *Br J Sports Med.* 2002;36(4):239–249.
96. Schepsis AA, Jones H, Haas AL. Achilles tendon disorders in athletes. *Am J Sports Med.* 2002;30(2):287–305.
97. Alfredson H, Cook J. A treatment algorithm for managing Achilles tendinopathy: new treatment options. *Br J Sports Med.* 2007;41(4):211–216.
98. Longo UG, Petrillo S, Maffulli N, Denaro V. Acute achilles tendon rupture in athletes. *Foot Ankle Clin.* 2013;18(2):319–338.
99. Twaddle BC, Poon P. Early motion for Achilles tendon ruptures: is surgery important? A randomized, prospective study. *Am J Sports Med.* 2007;35(12):2033–2038.
100. Soroceanu A, Sidhwa F, Aarabi S, et al. Surgical versus nonsurgical treatment of acute Achilles tendon rupture: a meta-analysis of randomized trials. *J Bone Joint Surg Am.* 2012;94(23):2136–2143.
101. Krishna Sayana M, Maffulli N. Insertional Achilles tendinopathy. *Foot Ankle Clin.* 2005;10(2):309–320.
102. Irwin TA. Current concepts review: insertional achilles tendinopathy. *Foot Ankle Int.* 2010;31(10):933–939.
103. Hendrix CL. Calcaneal apophysitis (Sever disease). *Clin Podiatr Med Surg.* 2005;22(1):55–62, vi.
104. Sofka CM, Adler RS, Positano R, et al. Haglund's syndrome: diagnosis and treatment using sonography. *HSS J.* 2006;2(1):27–29.
105. Ozgocmen S, Kiris A, Kocakoc E, et al. Evaluation of metacarpophalangeal joint synovitis in rheumatoid arthritis by power Doppler technique: relationship between synovial vascularization and periarticular bone mineral density. *Joint Bone Spine.* 2004;71(5):384–388.
106. Wiegerinck JI, Kok AC, van Dijk CN. Surgical treatment of chronic retrocalcaneal bursitis. *Arthroscopy.* 2012;28(2):283–293.
107. Pomeroy GC, Pike RH, Beals TC, Manoli A 2nd. Acquired flatfoot in adults due to dysfunction of the posterior tibial tendon. *J Bone Joint Surg Am.* 1999;81(8):1173–1182.
108. Trnka HJ. Dysfunction of the tendon of tibialis posterior. *J Bone Joint Surg Br.* 2004;86(7):939–946.
109. Kohls-Gatzoulis J, Angel JC, Singh D, et al. Tibialis posterior dysfunction: a common and treatable cause of adult acquired flatfoot. *BMJ.* 2004;329(7478):1328–1333.
110. Barn R, Turner DE, Rafferty D, et al. Tibialis posterior tenosynovitis and associated pes plano valgus in rheumatoid arthritis: electromyography, multisegment foot kinematics, and ultrasound features. *Arthritis Care Res (Hoboken).* 2013;65(4):495–502.
111. Deland JT. Adult-acquired flatfoot deformity. *J Am Acad Orthop Surg.* 2008;16(7):399–406.
112. Ribbans WJ, Garde A. Tibialis posterior tendon and deltoid and spring ligament injuries in the elite athlete. *Foot Ankle Clin.* 2013;18(2):255–291.
113. Anagnostakos K, Bachelier F, Fürst OA, Kelm J. Rupture of the anterior tibial tendon: three clinical cases, anatomical study, and literature review. *Foot Ankle Int.* 2006;27(5):330–339.
114. Gallo RA, Kolman BH, Daffner RH, et al. MRI of tibialis anterior tendon rupture. *Skeletal Radiol.* 2004;33(2):102–106.
115. Roth JA, Taylor WC, Whalen J. Peroneal tendon subluxation: the other lateral ankle injury. *Br J Sports Med.* 2010;44(14):1047–1053.
116. Heckman DS, Gluck GS, Parekh SG. Tendon disorders of the foot and ankle, part 1: peroneal tendon disorders. *Am J Sports Med.* 2009;37(3):614–625.
117. Slater HK. Acute peroneal tendon tears. *Foot Ankle Clin.* 2007;12(4):659–74, vii.
118. Kijowski R, De Smet A, Mukharjee R. Magnetic resonance imaging findings in patients with peroneal tendinopathy and peroneal tenosynovitis. *Skeletal Radiol.* 2007;36(2):105–114.
119. Oh SJ, Kim YH, Kim SK, Kim MW. Painful os peroneum syndrome presenting as lateral plantar foot pain. *Ann Rehabil Med.* 2012;36(1):163–166.
120. Cerrato RA, Myerson MS. Peroneal tendon tears, surgical management and its complications. *Foot Ankle Clin.* 2009;14(2):299–312.
121. Guillo S, Calder JD. Treatment of recurring peroneal tendon subluxation in athletes: endoscopic repair of the retinaculum. *Foot Ankle Clin.* 2013;18(2):293–300.
122. Baan H, Drossaers-Bakkers WK, Dubbeldam R, et al. Flexor Hallucis Longus tendon rupture in RA-patients is associated with MTP 1 damage and pes planus. *BMC Musculoskelet Disord.* 2007; 8:110.
123. Daniels T, Thomas R. Etiology and biomechanics of ankle arthritis. *Foot Ankle Clin.* 2008;13(3):341–352, vii.
124. Schmid T, Krause FG. Conservative treatment of asymmetric ankle osteoarthritis. *Foot Ankle Clin.* 2013;18(3):437–448.
125. Lucas Y, Hernandez J, Darcel V, et al. Viscosupplementation of the ankle: A prospective study with an average follow-up of 45.5 months. *Orthop Traumatol Surg Res.* 2013;99(5):593–599.
126. Wiewiorski M, Barg A, Valderrabano V. Chondral and osteochondral reconstruction of local ankle degeneration. *Foot Ankle Clin.* 2013;18(3):543–554.
127. Andersen LB, Stauff MP, Juliano PJ. Combined subtalar and ankle arthritis. *Foot Ankle Clin.* 2007;12(1):57–73.
128. Mei-Dan O, Carmont M, Laver L, et al. Intra-articular injections of hyaluronic acid in osteoarthritis of the subtalar joint: a pilot study. *J Foot Ankle Surg.* 2013;52(2):172–176.
129. Lopez R, Singh T, Banga S, Hasan N. Subtalar joint arthrodesis. *Clin Podiatr Med Surg.* 2012;29(1):67–75.
130. Lorenzo M. Rheumatoid arthritis. *Foot Ankle Clin.* 2007;12(3):525–37, vii.
131. Aronow MS, Hakim-Zargar M. Management of hindfoot disease in rheumatoid arthritis. *Foot Ankle Clin.* 2007;12(3):455–74, vi.

132. Nelissen RGHH. The lower limb in the rheumatoid arthritis patient.: Focus on the hind, mid and forefoot and the ankle. *Curr Orthop.* 2007;21(5):340–343.
133. Mann RA, Horton GA. Management of the foot and ankle in rheumatoid arthritis. *Rheum Dis Clin North Am.* 1996;22(3):457–476.
134. Loveday DT, Jackson GE, Geary NP. The rheumatoid foot and ankle: current evidence. *Foot Ankle Surg.* 2012;18(2):94–102.
135. Stevens BW, Anderson JG, Bohay DR. Hallux metatarsophalangeal joint fusion for the rheumatoid forefoot. *Foot Ankle Clin.* 2007;12(3):395–404, v.
136. Zanon G, DI Vico G, Marullo M. Osteochondritis dissecans of the talus. *Joints.* 2014;2(3):115–123.
137. Tezval M, Dumont C, Stürmer KM. Prognostic reliability of the Hawkins sign in fractures of the talus. *J Orthop Trauma.* 2007;21(8):538–543.
138. von Knoch F, Reckord U, von Knoch M, Sommer C. Fracture of the lateral process of the talus in snowboarders. *J Bone Joint Surg Br.* 2007;89(6):772–777.
139. Mei-Dan O, Carmont MR, Laver L, et al. Platelet-rich plasma or hyaluronate in the management of osteochondral lesions of the talus. *Am J Sports Med.* 2012;40(3):534–541.
140. Zaw H, Calder JD. Tarsal coalitions. *Foot Ankle Clin.* 2010;15(2):349–364.
141. Nault ML, Kocher MS, Micheli LJ. Os trigonum syndrome. *J Am Acad Orthop Surg.* 2014;22(9):545–553.
142. Leonard ZC, Fortin PT. Adolescent accessory navicular. *Foot Ankle Clin.* 2010;15(2):337–347.
143. Chuang YW, Tsai WS, Chen KH, Hsu HC. Clinical use of high-resolution ultrasonography for the diagnosis of type II accessory navicular bone. *Am J Phys Med Rehabil.* 2012;91(2):177–181.
144. Philbin TM, Landis GS, Smith B. Peroneal tendon injuries. *J Am Acad Orthop Surg.* 2009;17(5):306–317.
145. Barei DP, Bellabarba C, Sangeorzan BJ, Benirschke SK. Fractures of the calcaneus. *Orthop Clin North Am.* 2002;33(1):263–85, x.
146. Stockenhuber N, Wildburger R, Szyszkowitz R. Fractures of the os calcis. *Curr Orthop.* 1996;10(4):230–238.
147. Summers NJ, Murdoch MM. Fractures of the talus: a comprehensive review. *Clin Podiatr Med Surg.* 2012;29(2):187–203, vii.
148. Jones MH, Amendola AS. Navicular stress fractures. *Clin Sports Med.* 2006;25(1):151–8, x.
149. Doyle T, Napier RJ, Wong-Chung J. Recognition and management of Müller-Weiss disease. *Foot Ankle Int.* 2012;33(4):275–281.
150. Maceira E, Rochera R. Müller-Weiss disease: clinical and biomechanical features. *Foot Ankle Clin.* 2004;9(1):105–125.
151. Rosenberg ZS, Beltran J, Bencardino JT. From the RSNA Refresher Courses. Radiological Society of North America. MR imaging of the ankle and foot. *Radiographics.* 2000;20 Spec No:S153–S179.
152. Mohiuddin T, Jennison T, Damany D. Müller-Weiss disease - review of current knowledge. *Foot Ankle Surg.* 2014;20(2):79–84.
153. DiGiovanni CW, Patel A, Calfee R, Nickisch F. Osteonecrosis in the foot. *J Am Acad Orthop Surg.* 2007;15(4):208–217.
154. Rajbhandari SM, Jenkins RC, Davies C, Tesfaye S. Charcot neuroarthropathy in diabetes mellitus. *Diabetologia.* 2002;45(8):1085–1096.
155. Trepman E, Nihal A, Pinzur MS. Current topics review: Charcot neuroarthropathy of the foot and ankle. *Foot Ankle Int.* 2005;26(1):46–63.
156. Wukich DK, Sung W. Charcot arthropathy of the foot and ankle: modern concepts and management review. *J Diabetes Complicat.* 2009;23(6):409–426.
157. Rogers LC, Frykberg RG, Armstrong DG, et al. The Charcot foot in diabetes. *Diabetes Care.* 2011;34(9):2123–2129.
158. Stanley JC, Collier AM. Charcot osteo-arthropathy. *Curr Orthop.* 2008;22(6):428–433.
159. Frowen P, O'Donnell M, Lorimer D, Burrow G. *Neale's Disorders of the Foot.* 8th ed. Amsterdam, the Netherlands; New York, NY: Elsevier; 2010.
160. Perera AM, Mason L, Stephens MM. The pathogenesis of hallux valgus. *J Bone Joint Surg Am.* 2011;93(17):1650–1661.
161. Coughlin MJ, Shurnas PS. Hallux rigidus. *J Bone Joint Surg Am.* 2004;86-A Suppl 1(Pt 2):119–130.
162. Shurnas PS. Hallux rigidus: etiology, biomechanics, and nonoperative treatment. *Foot Ankle Clin.* 2009;14(1):1–8.
163. Sammarco VJ, Nichols R. Orthotic management for disorders of the hallux. *Foot Ankle Clin.* 2005;10(1):191–209.
164. Solan MC, Calder JD, Bendall SP. Manipulation and injection for hallux rigidus. Is it worthwhile? *J Bone Joint Surg Br.* 2001;83(5):706–708.
165. Neogi T. Clinical practice. Gout. *N Engl J Med.* 2011;364(5):443–452.
166. Perez-Ruiz F, Castillo E, Chinchilla SP, Herrero-Beites AM. Clinical manifestations and diagnosis of gout. *Rheum Dis Clin North Am.* 2014;40(2):193–206.
167. Zhang W, Doherty M, Bardin T, et al.; EULAR Standing Committee for International Clinical Studies Including Therapeutics. EULAR evidence based recommendations for gout. Part II: Management. Report of a task force of the EULAR Standing Committee for International Clinical Studies Including Therapeutics (ESCISIT). *Ann Rheum Dis.* 2006;65(10):1312–1324.
168. Carter JD, Kedar RP, Anderson SR, et al. An analysis of MRI and ultrasound imaging in patients with gout who have normal plain radiographs. *Rheumatology (Oxford).* 2009;48(11):1442–1446.
169. Cohen BE. Hallux sesamoid disorders. *Foot Ankle Clin.* 2009;14(1):91–104.
170. Wukich DK, Donley BG, Sferra JJ. Hypermobility of the first tarsometatarsal joint. *Foot Ankle Clin.* 2005;10(1):157–166.
171. Greisberg JK. Hallux valgus and first ray mobility. A prospective study. *J Bone Joint Surg Am.* 2008;90(5):1166; author reply 1166–1166; author reply 1167.
172. Meyer JM, Tomeno B, Burdet A. Metatarsalgia due to insufficient support by the first ray. *Int Orthop.* 1981;5(3):193–201.
173. Mainard D. *The second ray syndrome. Eur J Orthoped Surg Traumatol.* 1997;7:159–164.
174. Coughlin MJ. Lesser toe abnormalities. *Instr Course Lect.* 2003;52:421–444.
175. Talusan PG, Diaz-Collado PJ, Reach JS, Jr. Freiberg's infraction: diagnosis and treatment. *Foot Ankle Spec.* 2014;7(1):52–56.
176. Espinosa N, Maceira E, Myerson MS. Current concept review: metatarsalgia. *Foot Ankle Int.* 2008;29(8):871–879.
177. Espinosa N, Brodsky JW, Maceira E. Metatarsalgia. *J Am Acad Orthop Surg.* 2010;18(8):474–485.
178. Smith BW, Coughlin MJ. Disorders of the lesser toes. *Sports Med Arthrosc.* 2009;17(3):167–174.
179. Cohen BE, Nicholson CW. Bunionette deformity. *J Am Acad Orthop Surg.* 2007;15(5):300–307.
180. Fetzer GB, Wright RW. Metatarsal shaft fractures and fractures of the proximal fifth metatarsal. *Clin Sports Med.* 2006;25(1):139–50, x.
181. Thevendran G, Deol RS, Calder JD. Fifth metatarsal fractures in the athlete: evidence for management. *Foot Ankle Clin.* 2013;18(2):237–254.
182. Hatch RL, Hacking S. Evaluation and management of toe fractures. *Am Fam Physician.* 2003;68(12):2413–2418.
183. Bae JM, Kang H, Kim HO, Park YM. Differential diagnosis of plantar wart from corn, callus and healed wart with the aid of dermoscopy. *Br J Dermatol.* 2009;160(1):220–222.
184. Gentchos CE, Anderson JG, Bohay DR. Management of the rigid arthritic flatfoot in the adults: alternatives to triple arthrodesis. *Foot Ankle Clin.* 2012;17(2):323–335.
185. Durall CJ. Examination and treatment of cuboid syndrome: a literature review. *Sports Health.* 2011;3(6):514–519.
186. Marshall P, Hamilton WG. Cuboid subluxation in ballet dancers. *Am J Sports Med.* 1992;20(2):169–175.
187. Eleftheriou KI, Rosenfeld PF. Lisfranc injury in the athlete: evidence supporting management from sprain to fracture dislocation. *Foot Ankle Clin.* 2013;18(2):219–236.
188. Gould JS. Tarsal tunnel syndrome. *Foot Ankle Clin.* 2011;16(2):275–286.
189. Franson J, Baravarian B. Tarsal tunnel syndrome: a compression neuropathy involving four distinct tunnels. *Clin Podiatr Med Surg.* 2006;23(3):597–609.
190. Bland JD. Treatment of carpal tunnel syndrome. *Muscle Nerve.* 2007;36(2):167–171.
191. Presley JC, Maida E, Pawlina W, et al. Sonographic visualization of the first branch of the lateral plantar nerve (baxter nerve): technique and validation using perineural injections in a cadaveric model. *J Ultrasound Med.* 2013;32(9):1643–1652.
192. Seo JH, Oh SJ. Near-nerve needle sensory conduction study of the medial calcaneal nerve: New method and report of four cases of medial calcaneal neuropathy. *Muscle Nerve.* 2002;26(5):654–658.

193. Rask MR. Medial plantar neurapraxia (jogger's foot): report of 3 cases. *Clin Orthop Relat Res.* 1978(134):193–195.
194. Peters PG, Adams SB Jr, Schon LC. Interdigital neuralgia. *Foot Ankle Clin.* 2011;16(2):305–315.
195. Coughlin MJ, Mann RA, Saltzman CL. *Surgery of the foot and ankle.* 8th ed. Philadelphia, PA: Mosby; 2007.
196. Xu Z, Duan X, Yu X, et al. The accuracy of ultrasonography and magnetic resonance imaging for the diagnosis of Morton's neuroma: a systematic review. *Clin Radiol.* 2015;70(4):351–358.
197. Aydinlar EI, Uzun M, Beksac B, et al. Simple electrodiagnostic method for Morton neuroma. *Muscle Nerve.* 2014;49(2):193–197.
198. Adams SB Jr, Peters PG, Schon LC. Persistent or recurrent interdigital neuromas. *Foot Ankle Clin.* 2011;16(2):317–325.
199. Fanucci E, Masala S, Fabiano S, et al. Treatment of intermetatarsal Morton's neuroma with alcohol injection under US guide: 10-month follow-up. *Eur Radiol.* 2004;14(3):514–518.
200. Hughes RJ, Ali K, Jones H, et al. Treatment of Morton's neuroma with alcohol injection under sonographic guidance: follow-up of 101 cases. *AJR Am J Roentgenol.* 2007;188(6):1535–1539.
201. DiDomenico LA, Masternick EB. Anterior tarsal tunnel syndrome. *Clin Podiatr Med Surg.* 2006;23(3):611–620.
202. Akyüz G, Us O, Türan B, et al. Anterior tarsal tunnel syndrome. *Electromyogr Clin Neurophysiol.* 2000;40(2):123–128.
203. Styf J. Entrapment of the superficial peroneal nerve. Diagnosis and results of decompression. *J Bone Joint Surg Br.* 1989;71(1):131–135.
204. Redfern DJ, Sauvé PS, Sakellariou A. Investigation of incidence of superficial peroneal nerve injury following ankle fracture. *Foot Ankle Int.* 2003;24(10):771–774.
205. Styf J, Morberg P. The superficial peroneal tunnel syndrome. Results of treatment by decompression. *J Bone Joint Surg Br.* 1997;79(5):801–803.
206. Beltran LS, Bencardino J, Ghazikhanian V, Beltran J. Entrapment neuropathies III: lower limb. *Semin Musculoskelet Radiol.* 2010;14(5):501–511.
207. Still GP, Fowler MB. Joplin's neuroma or compression neuropathy of the plantar proper digital nerve to the hallux: clinicopathologic study of three cases. *J Foot Ankle Surg.* 1998;37(6):524–530.
208. Phisitkul P, Sripongsai R, Chaichankul C, Femino JE. Anatomy of the plantarmedial hallucal nerve in relation to the medial approach of the first metatarsophalangeal joint. *Foot Ankle Int.* 2009;30(6):558–561.

CHAPTER 11

Other Pain Syndromes

EPIDEMIOLOGY

EPIDEMIOLOGY OF WIDESPREAD PAIN

Definition
- ≥4 anatomic sites (with bilateral counting one) for 3 months or longer although not universally accepted

Prevalence
- Up to ~10% by survey in adult population
- Fibromyalgia (FM): most common (MC) cause of widespread pain (up to 3%), varies by geography (1)
- Female > male, bell-shaped curve in age prevalence (highest between 60 and 69 years)

Risk factors
- Depressive symptoms, psychiatric disorder, and sociocultural factors (more important than regional pain syndrome) in addition to mechanical factors (2)

EPIDEMIOLOGY OF CANCER PAIN

Prevalence
- Varies widely due to lack of standardization in definition and heterogeneity of classification
- High prevalence of pain in several cancers (up to 90%): head and neck, prostate, uterine, genitourinary, breast, and pancreatic (International Association for the Study of Pain)

EPIDEMIOLOGY OF COMMON NEUROPATHIC PAIN CONDITIONS (3)

Prevalence
- In general population: ≥1.5%
- Chronic pain with neuropathic pain character: ~7%
- Peak in age 50 to 64 years old (YO)

CONDITIONS	INCIDENCE	PREVALENCE IN PATIENT POPULATION
Painful diabetic neuropathy	15.3/100,000	15%
HIV-related painful neuropathy	11–40/100,000	7%–27%

(continued)

CONDITIONS	INCIDENCE	PREVALENCE IN PATIENT POPULATION
Postherpetic neuralgia		35%
AIDS-related painful neuropathy		50%
Trigeminal neuralgia	5–8/10,000,00	
Phantom limb pain		53%–85%
Central poststroke pain		8%–11%
Multiple sclerosis-related neuropathic pain		23%
Spinal cord injury-related neuropathic pain		40%–70%

DIFFERENTIAL DIAGNOSIS

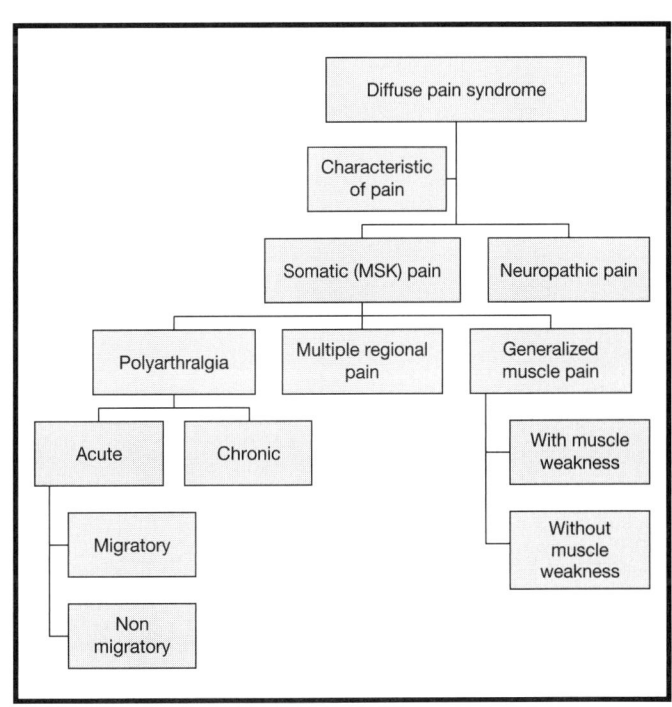

FLOWCHART 11.1
Classification of diffuse pain syndrome.

GENERALIZED MUSCULOSKELETAL PAIN (FLOWCHART 11.1)

Differential diagnosis of polyarthralgia
- Acute polyarthralgia
  - Acute migratory polyarthritis: Neisserial (gonorrhea) infection, reactive or postinfectious arthritis (acute rheumatic fever, Reiter's syndrome, poststreptococcal arthritis), early stage of Lyme disease, viral infection (rubella, mumps, Epstein–Barr virus [EBV]), serum sickness (occasionally), and acute leukemia
  - Acute nonmigratory polyarthritis: rheumatoid arthritis (RA), polyarticular juvenile RA, serum sickness, systemic lupus erythematosus (SLE), acute phase of seronegative spondyloarthropathies (psoriatic arthritis, Reiter's syndrome, ankylosing spondylitis (AS), enteropathic arthritis), crystal-induced disease, sarcoidosis, vasculitis, hematologic disorders (leukemia, sickle cell, lymphoma), serum sickness, viral arthritis (HIV, EBV)
- Chronic polyarthralgia
  - RA, polyarticular juvenile RA, SLE, sarcoid arthritis, connective tissue disease or overlap syndrome, and the like

Differential diagnosis of generalized myalgia (4)
- Without muscle weakness (or mild weakness with pain)
  - Polymyalgia rheumatica (PMR)
  - FM
  - Myalgia in collagen-vascular disease and myalgia in infection or fever
  - Muscle pain-fasciculation syndrome
  - Steroid withdrawal, hypothyroidism
  - Parkinsonism
  - Fabry's disease
- With muscle weakness
  - Inflammatory muscle disease (polymyositis, dermatomyositis, etc.)
  - Infection
    - Trichinosis, toxoplasmosis, poliomyelitis, West Nile virus infection, viral syndrome
    - Secondary to bacterial toxin, for example, toxic shock syndrome
  - Toxic and metabolic disorders
    - Hypophosphatemia, potassium deficiency, total parenteral nutrition (essential fatty acid deficiency)
    - Acute alcoholic myopathy
    - Necrotic myopathy secondary to malignancy
    - Hypothyroid myopathy
    - Carnitine palmitoyltransferase 2 deficiency (autosomal recessive, most common inherited disorder of lipid metabolism affecting skeletal muscles)
  - Medications (lipid-lowering agent, ± weakness)
  - Amyloidosis
  - Osteomalacia, hyperparathyroidism

DIFFERENTIAL DIAGNOSIS OF DIFFUSE NEUROPATHIC PAIN (FLOWCHART 11.2)

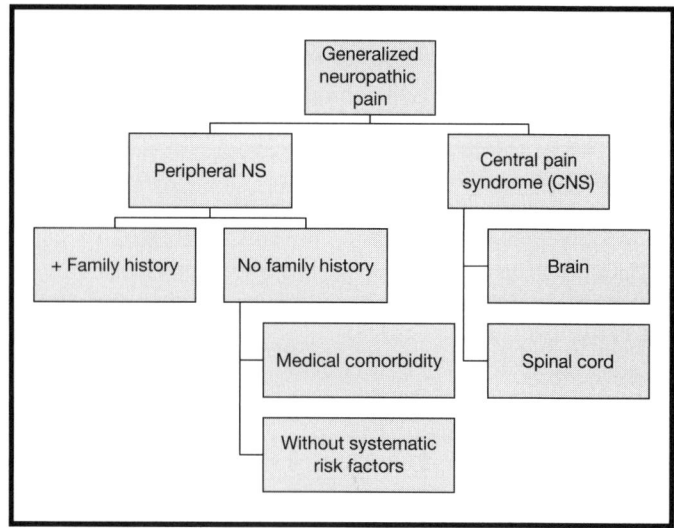

FLOWCHART 11.2

Classification of diffuse neuropathic pain.

Source: Adapted from Ref. (5). Baron R, Binder A, Wasner G. Neuropathic pain: diagnosis, pathophysiological mechanisms, and treatment. *Lancet Neurol.* 2010;9(8):807–819.

LOCATION OF INVOLVEMENT	COMMON DIAGNOSIS	NOTES
Peripheral nervous system	Diabetes mellitus PN	Heterogeneous, but length-dependent neuropathy "dying back" is MC pattern
	HIV PN (6)	Heterogeneous, distal symmetric (MC), HAART related
	Alcohol	
	Plasmacytoma	Monoclonal gammopathy, POEMS (polyneuropathy, organomegaly, endocrinopathy, M protein, and skin changes)
	Hypothyroidism	
	Neuroborreliosis (7)	
	Vitamin B deficiency	
	Toxic neuropathies	Arsenic, thallium, chloramphenicol, metronidazole, nitrofurantoin, isoniazid, vinca alkaloids, taxoids, gold, etc.

(continued)

LOCATION OF INVOLVEMENT	COMMON DIAGNOSIS	NOTES	
		Based on family history	
		Significant family history	CMT type 2B, 5, hereditary sensory and autonomic PN type 1, type 1B
		With/without family history	Amyloid neuropathy
			Fabry's disease; α-galactosidase deficiency, burning pain in palms and soles, anhidrosis
Central nervous system	Brain (especially the thalamus and brainstem)		Poststroke (ischemic, hemorrhage, and vascular malformation)
			Tumor, infection, epilepsy, and Parkinson's disease
	Spinal cord		Spinal cord injury, infarct, tumor, myelopathy (compressive from spinal stenosis, HIV, postischemic, postradiation), and syringomyelia • Below and at the level of spinal cord injury • Different presentation depending on the involvement (focal, multifocal and diffuse, also spine and brain) Multiple sclerosis or other central demyelinating disease
Others	Complex regional pain syndromes type I and II (reflex sympathetic dystrophy, causalgia)		I: After trauma (no nerve lesion)
			II: After peripheral nerve injury

CMT2B, Charcot–Marie–Tooth disease type 2B; HAART, highly active antiretroviral therapy; MC, most common; PN, peripheral neuropathy.

PHYSICAL EXAMINATION

EXAMINATION FOR NEUROPATHIC PAIN (3)

	DEFINITION	EXAMINATION	SUBJECTIVE COMPLAINTS AND CLINICAL IMPLICATIONS
Negative Symptoms			
Hypoesthesia	Reduced sensation to non-painful stimuli	Examination with brush, cotton swab, or gauze	Numbness, reduced perception
Hypoalgesia	Reduced sensation to painful stimuli	Pin prick sensation	Numbness, reduced perception
Thermal hypoesthesia	Reduced sensation to cold or warm	10°C metal roller, glass with water, coolants, or 45°C metal roller glass with water	Reduced perception
Spontaneous Pain			
Paresthesia	Nonpainful sensation	Grade intensity (0–10) area in cm^2	Ant crawling
Paroxysmal pain	Shooting electrical attack for seconds	Number of episode intensity, threshold for evocation	
Superficial pain	Painful ongoing sensation	Grade intensity (0–10) area in cm^2	Often burning
Evoked Pain			
Mechanical static/dynamic allodynia	Pain from nonpainful static pressure/moving stimuli	Pressure (static)/brush cotton swab or gauze (dynamic)	Dull pain (static) in affected area/sharp burning superficial (dynamic) in affected area

(continued)

	DEFINITION	EXAMINATION	SUBJECTIVE COMPLAINTS AND CLINICAL IMPLICATIONS
Mechanical punctuate hyperalgesia	Pain from nonpainful stinging sensation	Pin prick sensation (using safety pin)	Sharp superficial pain spreading into unaffected skin areas Sensitized A delta nociceptors
Heat and cold hyperalgesia	Pain from nonpainful heat or cold stimuli	20°C or 40°C subject (cold or warm water or metal roller) with control; touch skin with objects of skin temperature	Cold hyperalgesia • Traumatic nerve injury, trench foot syndrome, CRPS, oxaliplatin-induced PN, central poststroke pain Heat hyperalgesia: sensitized c fibers
Mechanical deep somatic hyperalgesia	Pain from nonpainful pressure on deep somatic tissue	Manual light pressure at joints or muscle	Deep pain at joints or muscles CRPS

CRPS, complex regional pain syndrome; PN, peripheral neuropathy.

DIAGNOSTIC STUDIES

SEROLOGIC TESTS (8)

- Basic serologic workup: complete blood count (CBC), basic metabolic panel, erythrocyte sedimentation rate (ESR), C-reactive protein (CRP), thyroid function test
- Rheumatologic workup (see Chapter 1, Other Workup section)
- Serologic test for peripheral neuropathy: glucose, serum B12, serum protein electrophoresis (SPEP; immunofixation)
  - Genetic test: Charcot–Marie–Tooth disease type 1A (CMT 1A; PMP 22 duplication)/hereditary neuropathy with liability to pressure palsies (PMP 22 deletion), Cx 32, GJB 1 mutation (CMT X linked), GQ1b (Miller Fisher variant of Guillain–Barré syndrome [GBS]), and GM1Ab (multifocal motor neuropathy)

ELECTRODIAGNOSIS (9)

- Evaluation of large diameter nerve fiber
  - Large fiber-mediated symptoms: numbness, proprioceptive loss (ataxia), or tingling
  - Limited in small fiber neuropathy (without large fiber involvement)
    - Small fiber mediated symptoms: pins and needles, burning sensation → consider small fiber study such as epidermal nerve fibers density in skin biopsy or autonomic nervous system study
  - Radiculopathy involving motor (subclinical and clinical) segment and axonal involvement
    - Pure sensory radiculopathy (preganglionic lesion) or focal demyelination lesion: negative in electromyography (EMG) test → somatosensory evoked potential study may show abnormality
- Nerve conduction studies (NCS) and needle EMG
  - Sensory NCS: sural, superficial peroneal ± medial plantar (may be more sensitive for distal peripheral neuropathy), ulnar, radial, and median nerve
  - Motor NCS: posterior tibial, deep peroneal, ulnar, and median, with F waves (can be more sensitive)
  - H reflex to evaluate S1 root, sciatic, tibial nerve, or multifocal lesion (eg, demyelinating neuropathy)
  - Needle EMG study: motor nerve involvement (axonal involvement, limited in focal demyelinating lesion) and muscle pathology
- Interpretation
  - Findings suggestive of demyelinating lesion: conduction block, delayed distal latency, and F wave latency (>125% of upper limits of normal), decreased conduction velocity <70% of lower limits of normal)
  - Findings suggestive of axonal lesion
    - Reduced amplitude or unobtainable action potentials in nerve conduction study
      - Sensory nerve action potential effected more than compound motor action potential (CMAP); CMAP amplitude is less affected due to compensation mechanism with terminal sprouting
      - Cautious of conduction block (can be misinterpreted as axonal lesion if stimulation is at proximal to the lesion)
    - Abnormal spontaneous activity and neuropathic motor units (decreased recruitment and increased duration of motor unit action potential) in needle EMG
  - Mixed pattern

OTHER DIAGNOSTIC TESTS

- Workup for autonomic (or small fiber) neuropathy; only available in selective centers
  - Three main tests for sudomotor response (sympathetic cholinergic efferent); the quantitative sudomotor axon reflex test (QSART), the thermoregulatory sweat test (TST), and sympathetic skin response
- Nerve biopsy: rule out vasculitis, sarcoidosis, chronic inflammatory demyelinating polyneuropathy (CIDP), infectious disease (eg, leprosy), tumor, and amyloidosis

IMAGING TESTS

- Anatomic diagnosis and possible underlying structural evaluation
- Evaluation of central nervous system (spinal cord and brain): MRI of cervical, lumbar, and thoracic spine and brain

GENERALIZED MUSCULOSKELETAL PAIN

FIBROMYALGIA

Introduction (10)
- Epidemiology: most common cause of generalized musculoskeletal pain in women between the ages of 20 and 55 years
  - Prevalence: 2% (up to 8% in some studies), increases with age, female > male by 2 times or more
- Etiology and risk factors
  - Unknown etiology; not associated with tissue inflammation
    - Muscle pathology is secondary to pain and inactivity rather than primary cause
  - Many physical and/or emotional stressors may trigger or aggravate symptoms
  - A disorder of pain regulation (central sensitization); altered pain processing
  - Oxidative stress and mitochondrial dysfunction or neurohormonal perturbation
  - Others: sleep abnormalities, autonomic system dysfunction, and altered immune system
- Prognosis
  - Little change in the patient's symptoms (pain and fatigue) after an average follow-up of 14 years
  - Two-thirds of patients work full-time

History and physical examination
- History
  - Chronic, generalized pain involving both sides of the body and above and below the waist
    - Pain may initially be localized, often in the neck and shoulders
    - ± Swelling (without history of synovitis) and paresthesia
  - Fatigue
  - Sleep disturbances
    - Waking frequently during the early morning and having difficulty getting back to sleep
  - Cognitive disturbances
    - Difficulty with attention and doing tasks that require rapid thought changes
  - Mood disturbances: depression and/or anxiety in 30% to 50%
  - Headache: >50%, migraine and muscular (tension) types
  - Irritable bowel syndrome, pelvic pain, and bladder symptoms of frequency and urgency
  - Others: ocular dryness, multiple chemical sensitivity, palpitations, dyspnea, vulvodynia, dysmenorrhea, sexual dysfunction, weight fluctuations, night sweats, dysphagia, dysgeusia, and orthostatic intolerance
- Physical examination
  - Multiple tender areas of muscles and tendons (not required for the diagnosis)
    - ≥11/18 tender points, both above and below the waist, and affecting both the right and left sides of the body (sensitivity >85%, specificity >85%; Figure 11.1)
    - The amount of pressure: ≥4 kg/cm² (enough to whiten the nail bed of the examiner's finger tip)
    - Control locations: over the thumb, the mid forearm, or the forehead (less tender generally)
  - Joint examination: for signs of synovitis and tenderness over the joint line
  - Normal neurological examination (can have concomitant problem or minor abnormalities)

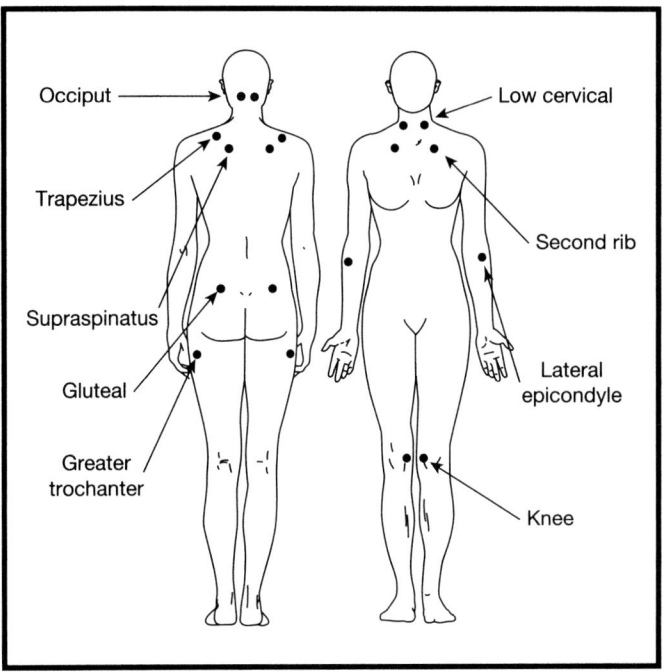

FIGURE 11.1
Tender points in fibromyalgia.

Diagnosis
- Clinical diagnosis (diagnosis of exclusion) using diagnostic criteria (11)
  - Widespread pain index (WPI) ≥7 and symptom severity (SS) scale score ≥5 or WPI 3–6 and SS scale score ≥9. Duration of symptoms ≥3 months
  - WPI: involvement of pain or tenderness during past 7 days, 0–19
    - Neck, jaw left/right (L/R), shoulder girdle L/R, upper arm L/R, lower arm L/R, chest, abdomen, upper back, lower back, hip (buttock, trochanter) L/R, upper leg L/R, lower leg L/R
  - SS scale
    - The SS scale score: the sum of the severity of the three symptoms (fatigue, waking un-refreshed, cognitive symptoms, 0–3 each) plus the extent (severity) of somatic symptoms in general (0–3)
      - No symptoms (0); few, intermittent, mild symptoms (1); a moderate number of symptoms (2); continuous, severe, and life disturbing (3)
    - For each of the three symptoms just noted, indicate the level of severity over the past week using the following scale (total score: 0–12)
- Laboratory tests; unremarkable
  - CBC, ESR, CRP, BMP, TSH (antinuclear antibody [ANA], RF only if significant clinical suspicion of inflammatory, systemic rheumatic disease, otherwise very poor predictive value; CPK if any suspicion of inflammatory muscle disease)

- 10% to 15% of FM patients have + ANA; also + in 5% to 10% of healthy women
- Differential diagnosis (often concomitant)

DIAGNOSIS	CHARACTERISTICS
Functional somatic syndromes	Irritable bowel syndrome (12), chronic fatigue syndrome (CFS), temporomandibular dysfunction, vulvodynia, and irritable bladder
Noninflammatory musculoskeletal disorders: multiple osteoarthritis or lumbar spinal stenosis	More localized pain + Evidence of structural abnormalities on physical examination and imaging studies
RA or lupus	Symmetrical polyarthritis, systemic features (dermatitis, nephritis), elevated ESR, CRP, abnormal serologic findings (RF, anti-DNA antibodies)
Ankylosing spondylitis	Abnormal spinal motion and radiologic features
Polymyalgia rheumatica	Elderly, elevated ESR, stiffness > pain, responds well and quickly to steroids
Myositis/myopathy	Muscle weakness, elevated muscle enzymes, normal/nonspecific muscle biopsy findings
Myofascial pain syndrome	More focal pain, (+) trigger points with taut bands ± referred pain
Infection (infectious mononucleosis, HIV, HTLV, hepatitis, Lyme disease)	"Post-Lyme" fibromyalgia/CFS condition Post-Lyme disease: the presence of objective evidence of inflammation or organ system dysfunction (vs fibromyalgia patients lack)
Hypothyroidism	Abnormal thyroid function tests
Hyperparathyroidism	Hypercalcemia
Cushing's syndrome	Characteristic facial and skin features, muscle weakness more than pain
Adrenal insufficiency	Not typically associated with chronic, widespread pain
Neuropathies	Clinical and electrical evidence of neuropathy

Abx, antibiotic; CRP, C-reactive protein; ESR, erythrocyte sedimentation rate; HTLV, human T-cell lymphotropic virus; RA, rheumatoid arthritis.

Treatment
- Education of chronic but generally nonprogressive nature of FM
- Identify and treat other coexisting disorders (especially treatable) (eg, depression, restless legs syndrome, sleep apnea, regional musculoskeletal disorders, etc)
- Oral medication
  - Initial: low dose of a tricyclic antidepressants (TCA) (amitriptyline 25 mg or nortriptyline 10–25 mg) qhs or cyclobenzaprine 5 mg tid
  - If (+) more problems with sleep: amitriptyline 25 mg initially (to 199 mg qhs [1st])
    - Pregabalin 75 mg qhs (2nd) upto 150 mg bid, gabapentin 200 to 3,600 mg/d (alternative, cheaper)
  - If (+) more exhaustion: duloxetine 30 mg qd or milnacipran q 12.5 mg a.m. initially
  - Combination: serotonin–norepinephrine reuptake inhibitors (SNRI) q a.m. + anticonvulsant q p.m.
  - Nonsteroidal anti-inflammatory drugs: not effective, not recommended as first-line. May have synergistic effect in combination with central nervous system active drugs
  - Problems: high noncompliance, ~50%
- Low-impact aerobic activities
  - Walking, biking, swimming, or water aerobic exercises
- Cognitive behavioral therapy: most effective if combined with an ongoing exercise program
- For nonresponders
  - To confirm the diagnosis and provide additional advice on management
  - Multidisciplinary therapy may be most useful in such patients

POLYMYALGIA RHEUMATICA (PMR)

Introduction (13)
- Incidence: <2 (Japan) to 113 (Norway)/100,000
  - Female > male by 2 to 3 times
  - Age: >50 YO, prevalence: $700/10^5$, >50 years, average age at diagnosis: >70 years
- Associated with giant cell (temporal) arteritis (GCA)
  - Prevalence of PMR > GCA by 2 to 3 times
  - PMR occurs in ~50% of patients with GCA and 15% to 30% of patients with PMR eventually develop GCA
- Etiology: unknown
  - Both environmental and genetic factors
    - HLA-DR4, similar sequence polymorphism within the hypervariable region of the HLA-DRB1 increased (similarity between PMR and GCA)
    - A cyclical pattern in incidence and seasonal variation
- Prognosis
  - Self-limited course over months to years
  - No evidence of increased mortality associated with PMR

History and physical examination
- Subacute or chronic aching pain and morning stiffness in the shoulders, hip girdles, neck, and torso, usually symmetric
  - Shoulder pain (70%–95%), hip/neck pain (50%–70%); worse with movement; may interfere with sleep
  - Morning stiffness ≥30 (to 45) minutes
    - Bilateral aching and morning stiffness (≥2/3: neck or torso, shoulders or proximal regions of the arms, and hips or proximal aspects of the thighs; ≥30 minutes) for ≥1 month
- Joint swelling, pitting edema of hands/wrists and ankles/feet (dorsum), and tenderness
  - Synovitis and bursitis: ~50%, palpable synovitis in more peripheral joints (knees, wrists, and metacarpophalangeal [MCP] joints); mild, nonerosive, and asymmetric

○ Tenosynovitis: can be the presenting symptom (± paresthesia: carpal tunnel syndrome: 10%–15% of PMR patients)
• Mild muscle tenderness (likely from synovial or bursal rather than direct muscle involvement) and subjective weakness (↓ effort because of pain or disuse atrophy; rather than true weakness)
• Decreased range of motion (ROM) of proximal (and peripheral) joints
• Systemic signs and symptoms: ~40%; malaise, fatigue, depression, anorexia, weight loss, and fever (high spiking fever sometimes in GCA, rare in only PMR)

Diagnosis
• Clinical diagnosis with serologic test
  ○ Mandatory criteria
    ▪ Age ≥50 years at disease onset, aching in both shoulders, abnormal CRP, ESR, or both
  ○ Additional criteria (points)
    ▪ Morning stiffness >45 minutes (2), hip pain or reduced ROM (1), negative RA or CCP Ab (2), absence of peripheral synovitis (1) and US findings of bursitis and synovitis in one shoulder (1), both (2); in imaging findings
  ○ Diagnosis mandatory criteria + ≥4 points for additional criteria without US findings (sensitivity: 68% and specificity: 78%) and ≥5 points with ultrasonographic findings (diagnostic sensitivity and specificity, 66% and 81%, respectively)
• Serologic test
  ○ Increased ESR ≥40 mm/hour (78%–93%) and 100 mm/hour (~20%) and CRP
    ▪ ESR: <40 mm/hour in limited disease with fewer systemic symptoms, treatment with glucocorticoids
    ▪ CRP: >5 mg/L in 99%, >22 mg/L in 90%; more sensitive than ESR
  ○ CBC: normocytic anemia, thrombocytosis (as part of a general inflammatory response), usually (−) ANA/RF/anti-CCP Ab, elevated alkaline phosphatase (more common in GCA than PMR alone)
  ○ For differential diagnosis: blood glucose, urinalysis, blood urea nitrogen, creatinine, aminotransferases, ALP, and calcium
• Imaging studies
  ○ Musculoskeletal ultrasound (additional criteria)
    ▪ ≥1 shoulder with subdeltoid bursitis, biceps tenosynovitis, or glenohumeral synovitis, or ≥hip with synovitis or trochanteric bursitis
    ▪ Subdeltoid bursitis, biceps tenosynovitis, or glenohumeral synovitis in both shoulders
    ▪ Effusions within both shoulder bursae (>90%) (14)
  ○ MRI of shoulder: subacromial and subdeltoid bursitis (typically bilateral) in almost all patients with active PMR
  ○ Baseline bone density measurement for steroid induced osteoporosis
• Differential diagnosis
  ○ Giant cell arteritis (concomitant in 15%–30% of those with PMR)
    ▪ New headache, jaw claudication, scalp tenderness, visual change/loss, fever, or cough in addition to symptoms suggestive of PMR, signs of inflammation of temporal arteries
    ▪ Referral for temporal artery biopsy
      – Routine biopsy strongly discouraged (because they seldom develop ischemic complications)
  ○ Other differential diagnosis

Rheumatoid arthritis or other inflammatory arthropathy	Persistent symmetric polyarthritis of the small joints, only partially responsive to low doses of prednisone; considerable overlap between PMR and seronegative RA in elderly Age onset of 40–50 years, asymmetric symptoms, and ESR <40 mm/hr
RS3PE syndrome	Remitting seronegative symmetrical synovitis with pitting edema, usually more prominent distally, needs to R/O paraneoplastic disorder
Bursitis/tendinitis	Tenderness (minimal/mild in PMR), no systemic symptoms, normal labs
Spondyloarthropathy	Enthesitis, dactylitis, anterior uveitis, sacroiliitis on imaging, and the greater prevalence of HLA-B27
CPPD disease	Characteristic crystals in the joint fluid, + chondrocalcinosis on x-ray
Hypothyroidism	Slow relaxation of DTR, low T4, elevated TSH
Fibromyalgia	Often younger than 50 years, normal labs (ESR, CRP)
Multiple myeloma	± Bone pain, ↑ ESR; (+) SPEP/UPEP
Infective endocarditis	Persistent fever, heart murmur, positive blood cultures, and abnormal echocardiography
Inflammatory myopathy (DM/PM)	↑ Muscle enzymes (CPK), abnormal EMG, and muscle biopsy
Vasculitis	ANCA-associated vasculitis: symptoms of URI, pulmonary hemorrhage, renal disease, neuropathy
Others	Parkinson disease (tremor, cogwheel rigidity), hyperparathyroidism (proximal stiffness and aching), drug-induced myopathy (myalgias and aching), depression (somatic symptoms, weight loss)

ANCA, anti-neutrophil cytoplasmic antibody; CPPD, calcium pyrophosphate dihydrate crystal; CRP, C-reactive protein; DTR, deep tendon reflex; EMG, electromyography; ESR, erythrocyte sedimentation rate; PMR, polymyalgia rheumatica; RA, rheumatoid arthritis; SPEP, serum protein electrophoresis; TSH, thyroid-stimulating hormone; UPEP, urine protein electrophoresis; URI, upper respiratory infection.

Treatment (15)
• Initial therapy: prednisone 15 to 20 mg/d for 1 to 2 months
  ○ Dramatic improvement: often after 1st dose; 50% to 70%, ↓ in pain and stiffness within 3 days
  ○ If symptoms not well controlled within 1 week, increase by 5 mg/d each week up to a maximum of 30 mg/d
  ○ If (+) evening or night-time pain or stiffness: use of a divided (twice daily) dose
• Maintain the effective dose for 1 to 2 months, and then taper 20%/month as tolerated (↓ in 2.5 mg decrements every 2–4 weeks) → taper slowly if the dose reaches 10 mg/d) (↓ 1 mg per month)

- Duration for 1 to 2 (3) years typically
  - Some patients require long-term therapy with stable doses less than 5 mg/d
- Relapses are common with tapering
  - Earlier relapse: associated with higher ESR, larger initial doses of prednisone, and rapid tapering
  - ~10% of patients will relapse within 10 years
- Monitor the clinical response closely
  - Clinical response: presence and/or recurrence of symptoms of PMR or GCA
  - Continued and/or recurrent high levels of ESR/CRP: alternative or additional diagnoses (malignancy or GCA)
  - Order: CBC, ESR, CRP-initially, after 2 months of treatment, then every 3 months during glucocorticoid therapy (interleukin-6 [IL-6]: correlates well with disease activity [16])
- Therapy has not been shown to clearly improve prognosis or prevent progression to GCA
- Glucocorticoid sparing therapies; Not proven to be effective
  - Methotrexate (MTX), tumor necrosis factor (TNF) inhibitors, infliximab, etanercept, and the like
  - NSAIDs
    - Associated with drug-related morbidity
    - If with glucocorticoids: gastrointestinal protection should be used
- Physical therapy (PT)
  - ROM in affected joints and gradual strengthening exercise to prevent deconditioning

CHRONIC FATIGUE SYNDROME

Introduction
- Prevalence: 75–267/100,000, peak in 20 to 55 years, female (up to 80%–90%) > male
  - Well under 10% of patients with chronic fatigue have chronic fatigue syndrome (CFS)
  - 70% of patients with FM meet the criteria for CFS
- Etiology and risk factors; unclear
  - Infection: EBV, xenotropic murine leukemia virus-related virus (XMRV), HIV, human herpes virus-6 (HHV-6), enteroviruses, coxsackie B virus, Ross river virus, Borna disease virus, human T-cell lymphotropic virus (HTLV)
    - Often associated with infection (upper respiratory infection [URI], infectious mononucleosis, etc) although none has been proven to cause CFS
  - Immune dysfunction, endocrine-metabolic dysfunction
  - Neurally mediated hypotension
  - Depression and sleep disruption
  - Genetic predisposition
- Course and prognosis
  - Symptomatic improvement in 64% at 1.5 years but complete resolution in only 2% (17)

History and physical examination
- Relatively sudden onset, overwhelming fatigue
  - Typically highly functioning individuals previously
  - Myalgia and fatigue in >90%
  - Neurocognitive and mood disturbances, headaches, and sleep disturbances
  - History predicting persistent symptoms
    - >8 medically unexplained physical symptoms
    - A lifetime history of dysthymic disorder
    - >1.5 years of chronic fatigue
    - <16 years of formal education and age >38 years at presentation
- Normal physical examination unless overlap with other disorders such as FM

Diagnosis
- Clinical diagnosis: diagnosis of exclusion (18)
  - Unexplained, persistent, or relapsing fatigue with new or definite onset
  - Not the result of ongoing exertion and not alleviated by rest
  - Substantial reduction in previous levels of occupational, educational, social, or personal activities
  - ≥4 of the following symptoms for ≥6 consecutive months
    - Self-reported impairment in short-term memory or concentration
    - Sore throat, tender cervical or axillary nodes
    - Muscle pain (throbbing, shooting often burning), multijoint pain (often migratory) without redness or swelling
    - Headaches of a new pattern or severity
    - Unrefreshing sleep and postexertional malaise lasting ≥24 hours
  - Other symptoms: unexplained muscle weakness, abdominal pain with altered bowel habit, mild fever (37.5–38.6°C) or chills
- Normal laboratory finding: CBC, ESR, chemistry, and thyroid-stimulating hormone (TSH)
  - Do not routinely order EBV, CMV, Lyme disease, or ANA (in the setting of low pretest probability, any positive test is likely to be a false positive)
- Normal radiologic test
- Differential diagnosis
  - FM and temporomandibular dysfunction (19)

Treatment (20)
- No highly effective therapy available; cognitive behavioral and graded exercise therapy are beneficial
- Referral to comprehensive center (sleep center, psychology for depression/panic): less fatigue and better physical function (21)
  - Sleep apnea or nocturnal myoclonus are common
- Cognitive behavioral therapy: to alter beliefs and behaviors that might delay recovery
- Graded exercise therapy: may worsen temporarily
  - PT for cardiovascular fitness training, myofascial release and modality (massage) for a few sessions
- Supportive approach with reassurance
  - Patient and family education and validate the diagnosis
- Medications and diet: none has proved successful
  - Low dose of TCA, if not responsive, add selective serotonin reuptake inhibitors (SSRI)
  - Benzodiazepine low dose if repetitive limb movement
  - Analgesic and NSAIDs as needed
  - Trigger point or tender point injection

PAIN RELATED TO CANCER

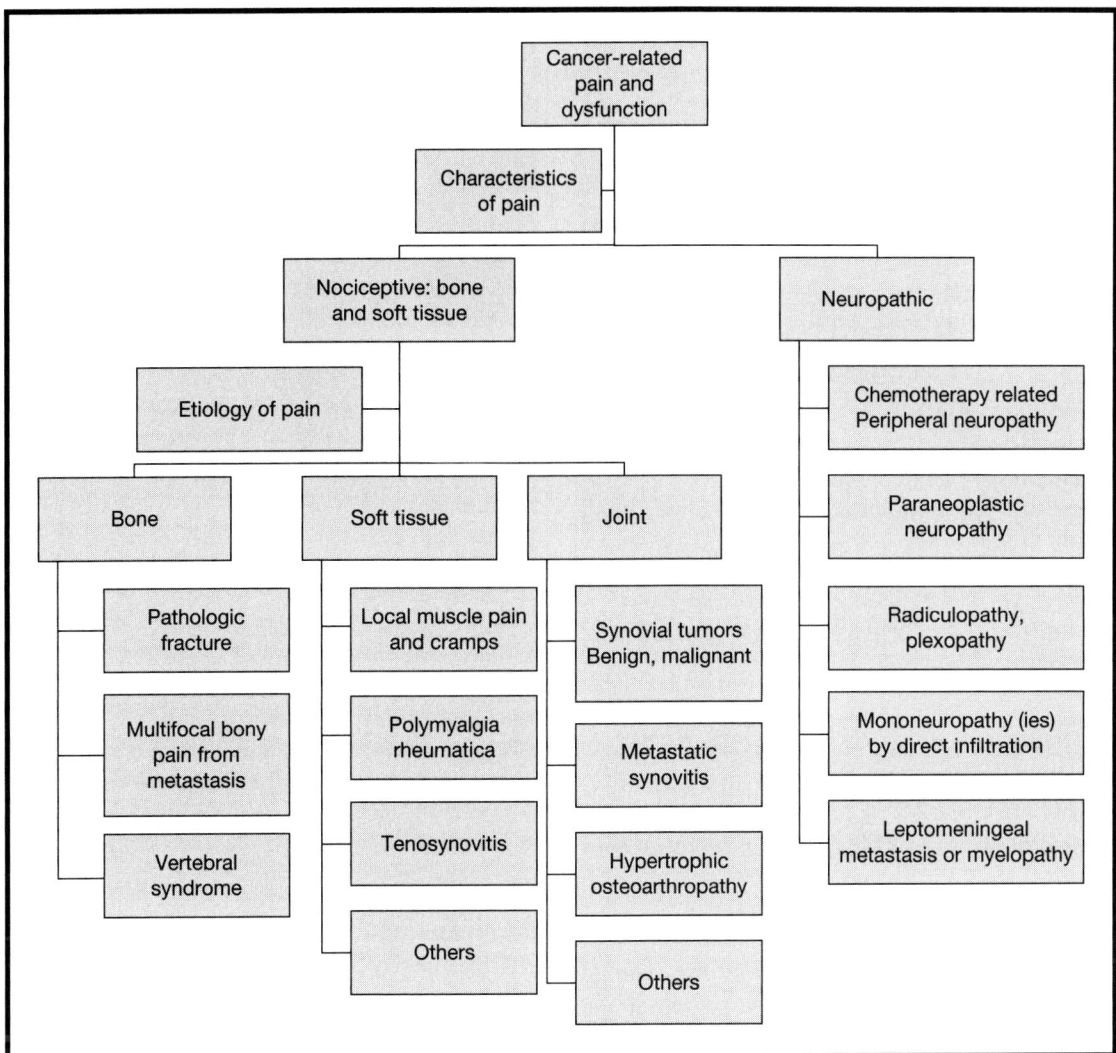

FLOWCHART 11.3
Classification of cancer-related pain.

BONY PAIN RELATED TO TUMOR (22,23)

Pathologic fracture: occurs within a preexisting lesion, sudden onset of limb pain with/without antecedent trauma (Flowchart 11.3)

Multifocal bone pain
• Bone metastases: the most prevalent cause of chronic pain in cancer patients
　○ MC source: solid tumor in the lung, breast, and prostate
　○ The pain due to direct invasion, secondary pathologic fracture, or damage to adjacent structures.
　○ Local field external beam radiation therapy (RT) is a well-recognized and effective palliative modality for painful bone metastases. Pain relief is seen in 80% to 90% of cases.
• Pain mediated by bone marrow expansion by hematologic malignancies with nests of rapidly growing cells in the marrow
• Oncogenic hypophosphatemic osteomalacia
　○ Rare paraneoplastic form of renal phosphate wasting → osteomalacia, multifocal bone pain, and fractures
　○ Associated with mesenchymal neoplasms
　○ Complete tumor removal can lead to rapid correction of the biochemical derangements, remineralization of bone, and symptom improvement

Vertebral syndrome
See Chapters 2 and 6

MUSCLE AND SOFT TISSUE PAIN

Local muscle pain and cramps
• Differential diagnosis of muscular cramps
　○ Radiculopathy or plexopathy or peripheral neuropathy
　○ Paraneoplastic syndrome with electrolytes abnormality
• Sarcoma: painless lump or local muscle pain (common presentation)

Polymyalgia Rheumatica
- Related to myelodysplastic syndrome or atypical presentation with metastatic cancers
  - Earlier onset, asymmetric presentation, ESR <40 or >100 mm/hour, poor or delayed response to low dose glucocorticoid and long-lasting symptoms

Remitting seronegative symmetrical synovitis (tenosynovitis) with pitting edema
- Solid tumor: prostate cancer (MC)
- Hematologic malignancy; >50 years, sudden onset of pitting edema of the hand, high serum level of metalloproteinase 3
  - Hypercalcemia of malignancy: ectopic secretion of parathyroid hormone (PTH)-related peptide (MC)

Others
- Myopathy: cancer cachexia, dermatomyositis, polymyositis, paraneoplastic necrotizing myopathy
- Somatic chest wall pain: common in patients with lung cancer or mesothelioma
  - Direct tumor infiltration of intercostal spaces, or parietal pleura
  - A malignant intercostal neuropathy with mixed nociceptive and neuropathic features.

JOINT DISORDERS/SYNOVITIS (NEOPLASTIC OR PARANEOPLASTIC) (22,24)

- Can be first sign of an occult malignancy or its recurrence

Synovial tumors
- Benign
  - Pigmented villonodular synovitis (PVNS): MC benign tumor of tendon and synovium, knee; MC (up to 80%), infrapatellar fat pad (MC localized form)
    - Giant cell tumor of tendon sheath if originated in the tendon sheath; tendons of hand or wrist (MC involved)
    - MRI; thickened synovium with heterogenous signal intensity with area of high intensity, and gadolinium enhancement.
    - Biopsy with US or CT guidance if MRI is not conclusive
  - Synovial chondromatosis
    - Multiple metastatic cartilaginous nodules under the surface of synovial membrane in joints, tendon, or bursa. Osteochondromatosis if cartilaginous nodules are ossified
    - Pain, synovial effusion ± locking if loose body presents
    - MRI: preferred imaging, can detect chondromas at earlier stages (complete cartilaginous nodules: isointense to the muscle on T1 and high signal enhancement on T2)
  - Hemangioma: rare, adolescent, knee > shoulder and ankle
  - Lipoma arborescens: lipomatous proliferation involving synovium
    - Rare, men in 4th and 5th decades of life. Knee: MC location
- Malignant
  - Synovial sarcoma: young adults, 15 to 40 years, male > female
    - Painless mass more common than pain (15%) and rare constitutional symptoms
    - x-ray: a round or oval radiopacity in the proximity to a large joint, multiple spotty calcifications (characteristic finding in 15%–20%)—often confused with benign lesion
    - Metastatic lesion in 50%; lung, bone, and regional lymph nodes
  - Synovial chondrosarcoma; extremely rare
  - Malignant PVNS; extremely rare, difficult to differentiate from benign aggressive PVNS

Metastatic synovitis
- Solid tumors: rare manifestation, typically monoarthritis of a large joint, such as the knee (MC involved)
  - Bronchogenic adenocarcinoma (MC), less frequently colon, renal, laryngeal, and breast cancer
  - Poor prognosis, chemo and radiation for symptom relief
  - Sanguineous synovial fluid, atypical cells in synovial fluid analysis
- Leukemic arthritis
  - Unexplained joint pain and swelling in leukemic patients (4% in adults and 14% in children with leukemia), asymmetric, oligoarticular, knee (MC involved), improves with treatment of underlying disease

Hypertrophic osteoarthropathy
- A migratory or additive nonerosive, nondeforming, asymmetric polyarthritis of explosive onset, involving more commonly large joints and sparing the wrists and hands, accompanied by constitutional symptoms and elevated markers of inflammation

Paraneoplastic joint disorders
- Polyarthritis: nondeforming, asymmetric polyarthritis of explosive onset involving large joints sparing wrists and hands (when involved → similar to RA), related to solid and hematologic malignancies
- Amyloid arthritis: 0.1% to 0.6% of multiple myeloma, affects shoulders, knees, wrists and MCP, proximal interphalangeal (PIP) joints, subcutaneous nodules
  - Common extra-articular manifestation: macroglossia and submandibular gland involvement
- Polyarthritis and panniculitis (with extensive fat necrosis) and/or bone necrosis, commonly involving ankle, knee, wrist, and MCP joints
  - Pancreatic tumor
- Polyarthritis and palmar fasciitis: ovarian cancer, firm, painful nodules with thickening and erythema of the palmar arch of the hand

NEUROPATHIC PAIN RELATED TO TUMOR

Peripheral neuropathy related to chemotherapy
- Usually subsides over time; however, some patients develop persistent pain
- History and physical examination
- Initial involvement of the feet and distal legs, followed by the hands and arms similar to other axonal neuropathy (dying back phenomenon). The severity of the pain and the presence and degree of neurologic impairment vary widely

- A persistent Raynaud's phenomenon: ~1/3 of patients with testicular tumors treated with regimens containing cisplatin, vincristine, and bleomycin

PARANEOPLASTIC PERIPHERAL NEUROPATHY

Introduction (25)
- Remote effects of malignancy rather than direct invasion usually from autoimmunity
- Epidemiology
  - 0.01% of cancer patients (exception; thymoma and myathenia gravis (MG), small cell lung cancer (SCLC), and myasthenic syndrome)
  - Frequently-related tumors: small cell lung cancer > adenocarcinoma of breast, ovary, and thymoma
  - ~4.5% of patients with unexplained adult onset axonal sensorimotor neuropathy related to malignancy (exact incidence: unknown)
- Common paraneoplastic peripheral neuropathy subtypes
  - Mixed sensory and motor length-dependent axonal neuropathy
    - Commonly related tumors: lung cancer (small cell or non-small cell [SC]), breast cancer, and thymoma
  - Sensory neuropathy, neuronopathy, and ganglionopathy
  - Others: neuromuscular junction disorder, motor neuron disorder, and autonomic ganglionopathy

History and physical examination
- Similar to the peripheral neuropathy (varies depending on phenotypes)
  - Pain with hyperesthesia/paresthesia, weakness (distal to proximal fashion in length dependent neuropathy): relatively rapid progression
  - Pain and numbness: rapidly progressive, upper limb commonly involved and asymmetric, sensory ataxia, + Rhomberg sign, pseudoathetosis, and absent reflex in sensory neuropathy/neuronopathy/ganglionopathy

Diagnosis: clinical diagnosis confirmed with EMG study (for neuromuscular disorder) and serologic study
- Serologic study: autoantibodies (anti-Hu, ANNA-1, CRMP-5 [anti-CV2], amphiphysin, ANNA-2, etc)
- NCS and needle EMG (unable to distinguish it from peripheral neuropathy unrelated to cancer)
- Others: SPEP and UPEP, radiologic survey (for POEMS syndrome; polyneuropathy, organomegaly, endocrinopathy, monoclonal gammopathy, and skin changes)

Treatment
- Work-up for underlying malignancy: referral to oncologist or basic screening for common cancers
- Symptomatic treatment if available (immunotherapy for neuromuscular transmission disease) or referral for treatment of underlying tumor

RADIATION PLEXOPATHY

Introduction
- Declining incidence due to lower dose regimens and better radiation therapy (RT) techniques
- Occurs months to years after RT

History and physical examination
- Weakness and sensory changes. Pain is rarely severe
  - Chronic perineal pain following pelvic RT is often clinically associated with a sacral plexopathy. Burning pain in nature and may extend anteriorly to the vagina or scrotum

Diagnosis
- Clinical diagnosis after the work-up for recurrent tumor

Treatment: symptomatic

LEPTOMENINGEAL METASTASIS

See Chapter 6, Lumbar Spine section, page 268

POLYRADICULOPATHY

Introduction
- Etiology: epidural metastasis (MC), leptomeningeal metastases, or intradural tumor (particularly meningioma, neurofibroma, and ependymoma)
- Mode of epidural metastasis: posterior extension of a tumor from a vertebral body metastasis, or growth into the intervertebral foramen from a paraspinal site

History and physical examination
- Radicular pain: continuous or intermittent, aching or sharp or dysesthetic (eg, burning or electrical-like) in quality ± neurological signs
- Tight band across the chest or abdomen in patients with cancer: a high likelihood of associated epidural tumor/metastasis

Diagnosis
- Clinical suspicion with MRI of cervical, thoracic, lumbar spine with contrast (especially if infiltration of nerve root is suspected) ± cerebrospinal fluid (CSF) examination

Treatment
- Emergency room (admit the patient) and referral to oncology, radiation oncology, and spine surgery

CHRONIC RADIATION MYELOPATHY

Late complication that may develop many years following the completion of RT

Sensory symptoms, including pain, typically precede the development of progressive motor and autonomic dysfunction
- The pain characterized as a burning dysesthesia and localized to the area of spinal cord damage or below this region

The neurological findings may be consistent with a transverse myelopathy, sometimes in a Brown-Sequard pattern

NEUROPATHIC PAIN

CENTRAL POSTSTROKE PAIN SYNDROME (THALAMIC PAIN)

Introduction (26)
- Central poststroke pain (CPSP): ~8 (1–12)% of all stroke patients
  - More common in a patient with sensory deficits (up to 18%)
    - Age, sex, or side of lesion: not consistent predictor
  - Higher incidence after lateral medullary infarct (Wallenberg syndrome) or lesion in the ventroposterior part of the thalamus
    - Any level of somatosensory pathway; spinothalamic tract
  - Onset usually within months of stroke; <1 month (MC), then 1 to 6 months, but can be longer
- Prevalence of chronic pain after stroke: 11% to 55% of patients
  - MC form of chronic post stroke pain: shoulder pain (30%–40%), CPSP, painful spasticity, and tension type headache

History and physical examination
- Spontaneous dysesthesia: MC (up to 85%), 3–6/10 (intensity of pain), fluctuates
  - Aggravated by stress or cold, relieved by rest or distraction
  - Large area (one side of body) more commonly affected than small area (hand or foot)
- Neurological findings depending on location of stroke lesion; no universal nonsensory finding

Diagnosis
- Clinical diagnosis (diagnosis of exclusion): after the other causes of nociceptive, psychogenic, or peripheral neuropathic etiologies ruled out

MANDATORY CRITERIA FOR CPSP	SUPPORTIVE CRITERIA
Pain within an area of the body corresponding to the lesion of the CNS	No primary relation to movement, inflammation, or other local tissue damage
History of a stroke and onset of pain at or after stroke onset	Descriptors such as burning, painful cold, electric shocks, aching, pressing, stinging, and pins and needles, although all pain descriptors can apply
Confirmation of a CNS lesion by imaging or negative or positive sensory signs confined to the area of the body corresponding to the lesion	
Other causes of pain, such as nociceptive or peripheral neuropathic pain, are excluded or considered highly unlikely	Allodynia or dysesthesia to touch or cold

CNS, central nervous system; CPSP, central poststroke pain.

Treatment
- Often trial and error, and psychological management (coping strategies and behavioral therapy)
- Pharmacologic management
  - TCA (amitriptyline), gabapentin, or pregabalin (300–600 mg/d): first line
  - If first line is not effective: serotonin-norepinephrine reuptake inhibitors, lamotrigine, or opioids
  - Transdermal ketamine 50–75 mg/d
  - Referral to pain medicine for IV drug trials: IV morphine, lidocaine, propofol (GABA A receptor agonist)
- Neurostimulation therapy
  - Transcranial magnetic stimulation; modest effect and short lasting, rare adverse effect
  - Referral to neurosurgery for disabling pain despite conservative management: deep brain stimulation for sensory (ventral posterior) thalamus and periventricular gray matter

SPINAL CORD INJURY–RELATED PAIN SYNDROME

Introduction (27)
- Prevalence: up to 70% of individuals with spinal cord injury (SCI) (28)
  - Neuropathic pain: ~40%; pain at level of neurologic level of injury (NLI) sooner than below level (>3 levels of NLI)
  - Nociceptive pain (MC): shoulder pain: 30% to 78%; shoulder impingement syndrome (tendinopathy, bursitis) and rotator cuff tear > hand/wrist (40%–64%) > elbow pathologies
  - Visceral pain: up to 30% in long term (increasing with duration)
- Classification
  - Nociceptive; musculoskeletal, visceral, and others
  - Neuropathic; SCI related (cauda equina or syringomyelia): at level or below level (>3 levels below NLI), at and below or other
  - Other and unknown

History and physical examination
- Neuropathic pain felt at and below injury level, onset usually within 1 year after SCI
  - Usually without any relation to movement or other local tissue damage
  - Characterized by burning, tingling, pins/needles, shooting, squeezing, and freezing
  - Allodynia or hyperalgesia within the pain distribution
- Pain (nociceptive; dull aching) in the shoulder, hand/wrist related (above NLI) to activity ± sensory symptoms in the hand/fingers (from nerve entrapment), and the like
- Physical examination
  - Neurological examination to decide NLI (American Spinal Injury Association [ASIA] classification)
  - Musculoskeletal examination for common pathologies in the upper extremity (rotator cuff syndrome, hand/wrist tendinopathy/carpal tunnel syndrome/arthritis)

Diagnosis
- Clinical diagnosis

CATEGORIES	TYPE	CHARACTERISTICS
Nociceptive	Musculoskeletal	Above, at, or below NLI, in an area of at least some preserved sensation; "dull" or "aching" pain related to movement; tenderness on palpation; response to anti-inflammatory medications; evidence of skeletal pathology Fracture, strain/sprain, shoulder overuse syndrome, muscle spasm/injury
	Visceral pain	Located in the thorax or abdomen; "dull," "aching," or "cramping" related to visceral pathology or dysfunction (eg, infection or obstruction) UTI, ureteric calculus and bowel impaction
	Other nociceptive	Nociceptive pains which do not fit into the musculoskeletal or visceral categories, headache or skin ulcer
Neuropathic	At level of SCI	Located in the segments, including NLI and three levels below the NLI; "burning," "electric," or "shooting"; presence of allodynia and/or hyperalgesia; unilateral or bilateral distribution
	Below level of SCI	Located in segments >3 levels below NLI; diffuse, regional distribution; "burning," "electric," or "shooting"
	At or below	A single pain distribution that is located both at and below NLI
	Others	May be located above, at, or below NLI, but not associated with spinal cord or nerve root lesion; Painful diabetic neuropathy, central poststroke pain
Other pain Unknown pain		Not classified into any of types listed earlier

NLI, neurologic level of injury; SCI, spinal cord injury.

- Imaging study: MRI of spine, CT, and x-ray as necessary
- NCS and EMG for entrapment neuropathy

Treatment
- Pharmacologic treatment (29)
  ○ Pregabalin (150–600 mg/d), gabapentin (1,200–3,600 mg/d) or TCA (amitryptyline; 25–150 mg/d)
    ▪ If not sufficient, may combine lamotrigine 200 to 400 mg/d in incomplete SCI with mechanical allodynia) or consider strong opiod
  ○ Tramadol for predominantly nociceptive/inflammatory pain
- Nonpharmacologic treatment
  ○ Exercise: strengthening/stretching, ergonomics for musculoskeletal pain, cardiovascular and regular physical activity (reducing diffuse and generalized pain)
  ○ Others (with limited evidence): massage, acupuncture, and psychological interventions

COMPLEX REGIONAL PAIN SYNDROME

Introduction (30)
- Epidemiology (31)
  ○ Incidence: 5.5/100,000 person-years (Olmstead county), female > male by ~4 times, median age: 46 years
  ○ Upper limb > lower limb by 2 times, however, the lower limb is more common in children
- Etiology: unclear
  ○ Fracture: MC preceding event, up to 30% in various fracture, sprain, or strain
  ○ Peripheral nerve injury: 1% to 5% of patients with peripheral nerve injury

History and physical examination
- Chronic pain: spontaneous pain, hyperalgesia/hyperesthesia/allodynia (beyond single nerve/root distribution or disproportionate to the inciting event), and/or stiffness/spasm
  ○ Average duration of time to tertiary pain clinic: 30 months, longer in worker's compensation
- Physical examination
  ○ Trophic changes (hypertrophic nails, disturbance of hair growth, atrophic skin), edema, sudomotor abnormalities (dry, warm, erythematous, cold extremity, hyperhidrosis)
  ○ Temperature difference >1°C from site to site (in acute, cold in chronic stage, decreased ROM/contracture, weakness (with pain), tenderness, allodynia ± muscle atrophy (disuse)

Diagnosis
- Clinical diagnosis
  ○ Stages: acute, dystrophic (3–6 months; vasomotor change) and atrophic (>6 months)
  ○ Classification
    ▪ Type I without a specific nerve injury: reflex sympathetic dystrophy
    ▪ Type II with a specific nerve injury: causalgia

DIAGNOSTIC CRITERIA BY INTERNATIONAL ASSOCIATION OF THE STUDY OF PAIN	PROPOSED EXPERIMENTAL REVISION
The presence of initiating noxious event or a cause of immobilization Continuing pain, allodynia, or hyperalgesia with which the pain is disproportionate to any inciting event Evidence of edema, changes in skin blood flow, or abnormal sudomotor activity in the region of pain at some time This diagnosis is precluded by the existence of conditions that would otherwise account for the degree of pain and dysfunction	Continuing pain disproportionate to any inciting event At least one of the following symptoms • Sensory: hyperesthesia • Vasomotor: temperature asymmetry and/or skin color changes or asymmetry • Sudomotor: edema and/or sweating asymmetry • Motor/trophic: decreased ROM, motor dysfunction and/or trophic changes At least one of the following signs • Sensory: hyperalgesia and/or allodynia • Vasomotor; temperature asymmetry and/or skin color changes and asymmetry sudomotor; edema and/or sweating changes and/or asymmetry • Motor/trophic: decreased ROM/motor dysfunction and/or trophic changes

ROM, range of motion.

- Differential diagnosis
  - Extensive: entrapment neuropathy/radiculopathy, neuroma, FM/myofascial pain syndrome, central pain syndrome, postherpetic neuralgia, inflammatory arthropathy, and the like
- Work-up: three phase bone scan (sensitive but lacks specificity), EMG (often unable to tolerate, to evaluate local entrapment syndrome or other peripheral neuropathy), x-ray (patchy osteopenia after 4–8 weeks, in ~40%), autonomic test (abnormal QSART, in ~60%)
  - Diagnostic nerve block (US guided); to address underlying nerve injury or concomitant local entrapment neuropathy

Treatment (32)
- Occupational (or physical) therapy: mirror therapy (33), motor imagery program, desensitization technique, mobilization exercise, flexibility, control edema, isotonic strengthening to progressive resistive strengthening exercise (with increasing weight), modality (electrical stimulation, contrast baths, massage) as tolerated, and manual lymphatic decongestive therapy
- Unna boot application (lower extremity): avoid irritation; control edema, relief pad in the foot with skipped lacing
- Pharmacological treatment (34)
  - Oral prednisone 100 mg qD with 25% reduction q 4Ds, short term (pain, edema, and mobility), not recommended for long term
  - Others: NSAIDs, opioid, bisphosphonate, vitamin C, N-methyl-D-aspartate antagonist (transdermal ketamine)
  - Local anesthetic: topical dimethyl sulfoxide (dimethyl sulfoxide [DMSO] 50% in a grease based cream) for "primarily warm" CRPS
- Injection
  - Sympathetic nerve block for mechanical allodynia, burning pain accompanied by color and temperature changes, advantages without motor nerve block
    - In patients with clinical evidence of vasomotor or sudomotor dysfunction
    - Stellate ganglion block for upper extremity; for sympathetic-mediated symptoms
    - Lumbar sympathetic nerve block (L4–5 vertebral body)
    - Predictor for sympathectomy
  - Referral for pain management for brachial or lumbar plexus block (with indwelling catheter)
    - Works for both sympathetic and nonsympathetic mediated (with concerns of motor block with transient weakness)
  - Peripheral nerve block: median nerve, sciatic nerve, superficial peroneal and saphenous nerve block
  - Acupuncture (35)
- Consider referral for spinal cord stimulator for lower extremity CRPS if failed other treatment

SMALL FIBER NEUROPATHY

Introduction (36)
- Peripheral neuropathy that primarily or exclusively affects small somatic fibers, autonomic fibers, or both (thinly myelinated A-δ fibers and unmyelinated C fibers)
- Unknown epidemiology but underrecognized or often misdiagnosed
- Etiology for somatic small fiber neuropathy (37)
  - Metabolic: impaired glucose intolerance, hyperlipidemia, or hypothyroidism
  - Immune mediated: sarcoidosis, Sjögren syndrome, celiac disease, inflammatory myopathy, paraneoplastic neuropathy
  - Infectious: leprosy, EBV, and the like
  - Toxin and drugs: antiretroviral drugs, metronidazole, nitrofurantoin, alcohol abuse, flecainide, bortezomib, and the like
  - Hereditary: Na(V) 1.7 channel mutations, Fabry disease, erythromelalgia, Ross syndrome, hemochromatosis
  - Idiopathic: idiopathic small fiber neuropathy, burning mouth syndrome
- Prognosis: slowly progressive, spreading proximally over time, neuropathic pain worsened in 30% and resolved spontaneously in ~10%

History and physical examination
- Pain, burning, tingling, or numbness typically affects the limbs in a distal to proximal gradient (length-dependent fashion), worse at night often affecting sleep
  - Non-length-dependent fashion: Sjögren, celiac disease, and paraneoplastic syndrome
  - Frequent autonomic dysfunction: hyper/hypohidrosis, urinary/bowel habit change, gastroparesis, blurry vision,

sicca syndrome, facial flushes, orthostatic intolerance, or sexual dysfunction
- Physical examination
  - Allodynia, hyperalgesia, reduced pinprick and thermal sensation in the affected area. Vibration sensation: mildly reduced at the toes
  - Motor strength, deep tendon reflex, and proprioception (large fibers); usually preserved

Diagnosis (38)
- Clinical diagnosis complemented by skin biopsy (gold standard) and QSART
  - Skin biopsy: 3-mm diameter punch biopsy from the distal leg, distal and proximal thigh
    - Finding: lower or no intraepidermal nerve fiber density (small fibers in the epidermis), normal in early stages
  - QSART: check sweat volume triggered by acetylcholine release by action potential; and other sudomotor testing (thermoregulatory sweat test, silastic skin imprint method, etc)
  - Others: blister biopsy and corneal confocal microscopy (done by ophthalmology) (39)
- Nerve conduction study and needle EMG (to assess large diameter fiber); normal in isolated small fiber neuropathy
  - 13% of those with small fiber neuropathy showed large fiber involvement in 2 years
  - Small fiber neuropathy progressing to mixed fiber neuropathy
    - Differential diagnosis: metabolic (diabetes mellitus [DM], chronic kidney disease), immune-mediated (amyloidosis, vasculitis, SLE, GBS), infectious (HIV, hepatitis C, lyme neuroborreliosis), vitamin B6 overdose, hereditary (familial amyloidosis, Fabry, Tangier disease, Friedreich ataxia, cerebrotendinous xanthomatosis, hereditary sensory autonomic neuropathies)
- Sural nerve biopsy; not indicated generally unless amyloidosis, vasculitis, or another inflammatory process are suspected
- Serologic tests for underlying causes: CBC, metabolic panel, lipid panel, ESR, thyroid function test (TSH, free T4), ANA, nuclear antigen, angiotensin-converting enzyme (ACE) level, serum and urine immunofixation, vitamin B6, and glucose intolerance test (more sensitive than hemoglobin A_{1c} [HgA_{1c}])

Treatment
- Treatment of underlying or other diseases; regular aerobic endurance exercise, weight control, and glucose control
- Wear roomier shoes, education for desensitization/benign neglect, trial of transcutaneous electrical nerve stimulation (TENS; home TENS if effective) for temporary pain control
- Pharmacological management: gabapentin (600–900 tid), pregabalin (75 bid increased to 300 bid), TCA, lidocaine patch, tramadol (50 bid to qid), NSAIDs (less effective than others), and opioids (if not responsive to other medicines)

ERYTHROMELALGIA

Introduction (40)
- Heterogeneous conditions characterized by erythema, edema, and burning pain in the distal extremities
- Prevalence: ~2/100,000 (Norway) and female > male
- Classification and etiology
  - Idiopathic (primary), common in middle age
  - Secondary (extensive)
    - Myeloproliferative disorder (polycythemia in ~60%, thrombocythemia)
    - Small fiber neuropathy and peripheral neuropathies (axonal neuropathy)
    - Diabetes, autoimmune diseases, infectious disorders, mushroom poisoning, medications, and others

History and physical examination (41)
- Intense burning pain, marked erythema, and increased skin temperature in the feet (but can be present in hands, bilateral, gradual onset of intermittent symptoms, worse late in the day)
- Relief of pain with ice water immersion

Diagnosis (41)
- Clinical diagnosis (often difficult to diagnose, symptoms often provoked by immersing in hot water for 10–30 minutes)
- Laboratory work-up; CBC, SPEP, ESR, CRP, PT, partial thromboplastin time (PTT), chemistry, liver function test (LFT) ALP (42)
- Imaging study (R/O spine-mediated pain); normal
- NCS/EMG to evaluate peripheral neuropathy (often large fiber neuropathy coexists, in 39% in one study) and sudomotor function (QSART or skin biopsy for small fiber neuropathy)
- Differential diagnosis
  - CRPS, Raynaud's phenomenon/disease, small fiber neuropathy, peripheral arterial disease, cellulites, spine disorder, and the like

Treatment
- Topical (high-potency capsaicin cream, 10%), gabapentin, aspirin (if related to blood dyscrasia), diltiazem, amitriptyline, sertraline, propranolol 10 mg tid, clonazepam, and the like
- Referral to pain management for sympathetic nerve block (or sympathectomy in recalcitrant case), epidurals, and spinal cord stimulator if refractory
- Workup for associated disorders

REFERENCES

1. Mourão AF, Blyth FM, Branco JC. Generalised musculoskeletal pain syndromes. *Best Pract Res Clin Rheumatol*. 2010;24(6):829–840.
2. Macfarlane GJ. Generalized pain, fibromyalgia and regional pain: an epidemiological view. *Baillieres Best Pract Res Clin Rheumatol*. 1999;13(3):403–414.
3. Kerstman E, Ahn S, Battu S, et al. Neuropathic pain. *Handb Clin Neurol*. 2013;110:175–187.
4. Miller TM, Layzer RB. Muscle cramps. *Muscle Nerve*. 2005;32(4):431–442.
5. Baron R, Binder A, Wasner G. Neuropathic pain: diagnosis, pathophysiological mechanisms, and treatment. *Lancet Neurol*. 2010;9(8):807–819.
6. Ferrari S, Vento S, Monaco S, et al. Human immunodeficiency virus-associated peripheral neuropathies. *Mayo Clin Proc*. 2006;81(2):213–219.
7. Halperin JJ. Lyme disease and the peripheral nervous system. *Muscle Nerve*. 2003;28(2):133–143.

8. Reilly PA. The differential diagnosis of generalized pain. *Baillieres Best Pract Res Clin Rheumatol*. 1999;13(3):391–401.
9. Bromberg MB. An electrodiagnostic approach to the evaluation of peripheral neuropathies. *Phys Med Rehabil Clin N Am*. 2013;24(1):153–168.
10. Clauw DJ. Fibromyalgia: a clinical review. *JAMA*. 2014;311(15):1547–1555.
11. Wolfe F, Clauw DJ, Fitzcharles MA et al. The American College of Rheumatology preliminary diagnostic criteria for fibromyalgia and measurement of symptom severity. *Arthritis Care Res*. 2010;62(5):600–610.
12. Sharma P, Sahni NS, Tibshirani R, et al. Early detection of breast cancer based on gene-expression patterns in peripheral blood cells. *Breast Cancer Res*. 2005;7(5):R634–R644.
13. Weyand CM, Goronzy JJ. Clinical practice. Giant-cell arteritis and polymyalgia rheumatica. *N Engl J Med*. 2014;371(1):50–57.
14. Camellino D, Cimmino MA. Imaging of polymyalgia rheumatica: indications on its pathogenesis, diagnosis and prognosis. *Rheumatology (Oxford)*. 2012;51(1):77–86.
15. Hernández-Rodríguez J, Cid MC, López-Soto A, et al. Treatment of polymyalgia rheumatica: a systematic review. *Arch Intern Med*. 2009;169(20):1839–1850.
16. Weyand CM, Fulbright JW, Evans JM, et al. Corticosteroid requirements in polymyalgia rheumatica. *Arch Intern Med*. 1999;159(6):577–584.
17. Bombardier CH, Buchwald D. Outcome and prognosis of patients with chronic fatigue vs chronic fatigue syndrome. *Arch Intern Med*. 1995;155(19):2105–2110.
18. Fukuda K, Straus SE, Hickie I, et al. The chronic fatigue syndrome: a comprehensive approach to its definition and study. International Chronic Fatigue Syndrome Study Group. *Ann Intern Med*. 1994;121(12):953–959.
19. Aaron LA, Burke MM, Buchwald D. Overlapping conditions among patients with chronic fatigue syndrome, fibromyalgia, and temporomandibular disorder. *Arch Intern Med*. 2000;160(2):221–227.
20. Prins JB, van der Meer JW, Bleijenberg G. Chronic fatigue syndrome. *Lancet*. 2006;367(9507):346–355.
21. White PD, Goldsmith KA, Johnson AL, et al.; PACE trial management group. Comparison of adaptive pacing therapy, cognitive behaviour therapy, graded exercise therapy, and specialist medical care for chronic fatigue syndrome (PACE): a randomised trial. *Lancet*. 2011;377(9768):823–836.
22. Azar L, Khasnis A. Paraneoplastic rheumatologic syndromes. *Curr Opin Rheumatol*. 2013;25(1):44–49.
23. Ashouri JF, Daikh DI. Rheumatic manifestations of cancer. *Rheum Dis Clin North Am*. 2011;37(4):489–505.
24. Marengo MF, Suarez-Almazor ME, Lu H. Neoplastic and paraneoplastic synovitis. *Rheum Dis Clin North Am*. 2011;37(4):551–572.
25. Sharp L, Vernino S. Paraneoplastic neuromuscular disorders. *Muscle Nerve*. 2012;46(6):841–850.
26. Klit H, Finnerup NB, Jensen TS. Central post-stroke pain: clinical characteristics, pathophysiology, and management. *Lancet Neurol*. 2009;8(9):857–868.
27. Finnerup NB. Pain in patients with spinal cord injury. *Pain*. 2013;154 Suppl 1:S71–S76.
28. Cardenas DD, Felix ER. Pain after spinal cord injury: a review of classification, treatment approaches, and treatment assessment. *PM R*. 2009;1(12):1077–1090.
29. Attal N, Mazaltarine G, Perrouin-Verbe B, Albert T; SOFMER French Society for Physical Medicine and Rehabilitation. Chronic neuropathic pain management in spinal cord injury patients. What is the efficacy of pharmacological treatments with a general mode of administration? (oral, transdermal, intravenous). *Ann Phys Rehabil Med*. 2009;52(2):124–141.
30. Bogduk N. Complex regional pain syndrome. *Curr Opin Anaesthesiol*. 2001;14(5):541–546.
31. Allen G, Galer BS, Schwartz L. Epidemiology of complex regional pain syndrome: a retrospective chart review of 134 patients. *Pain*. 1999;80(3):539–544.
32. Shah A, Kirchner JS. Complex regional pain syndrome. *Foot Ankle Clin*. 2011;16(2):351–366.
33. Cacchio A, De Blasis E, De Blasis V, et al. Mirror therapy in complex regional pain syndrome type 1 of the upper limb in stroke patients. *Neurorehabil Neural Repair*. 2009;23(8):792–799.
34. Birklein F, O'Neill D, Schlereth T. Complex regional pain syndrome: An optimistic perspective. *Neurology*. 2015;84(1):89–96.
35. Dowd GS, Hussein R, Khanduja V, Ordman AJ. Complex regional pain syndrome with special emphasis on the knee. *J Bone Joint Surg Br*. 2007;89(3):285–290.
36. Tavee J, Zhou L. Small fiber neuropathy: A burning problem. *Cleve Clin J Med*. 2009;76(5):297–305.
37. Hoeijmakers JG, Faber CG, Lauria G, et al. Small-fibre neuropathies-advances in diagnosis, pathophysiology and management. *Nat Rev Neurol*. 2012;8(7):369–379.
38. Hoitsma E, Reulen JP, de Baets M, et al. Small fiber neuropathy: a common and important clinical disorder. *J Neurol Sci*. 2004;227(1):119–130.
39. Lauria G, Merkies IS, Faber CG. Small fibre neuropathy. *Curr Opin Neurol*. 2012;25(5):542–549.
40. Cohen JS. Erythromelalgia: new theories and new therapies. *J Am Acad Dermatol*. 2000;43(5 Pt 1):841–847.
41. Orstavik K, Mørk C, Kvernebo K, Jørum E. Pain in primary erythromelalgia—a neuropathic component? *Pain*. 2004;110(3):531–538.
42. Norton JV, Zager E, Grady JF. Erythromelalgia: diagnosis and classification. *J Foot Ankle Surg*. 1999;38(3):238–241.

Index

abdominal muscle strain, 284
acetaminophen, 178
acetic acids, 59
Achilles (noninsertional) tendinopathy, 411
Achilles tendon tear, 411–412
AC joint sprain and injury, 146–147
ACL injury, 351–352
AC osteoarthritis, 147–148
active piriformis test, 257
acupuncture, 102, 110, 114, 453–454
   MSK pain, 75
   neck pain, 102
adhesive capsulitis, 148–149
Adson maneuver, 135
Adson test, 98
African palliative outcome scale (APCA), 4
alfentanil, 64
amyloid arthropathy, 154
ankle and foot pain
   in athletes, 383
   causes of severe (disabling) pain, 387
   classification of, 384
   diagnostic studies, 399
      CT scan, 401
      MRI, 401
      plain radiographs, 399–400
      point-of-care US, 400–401
   differential diagnosis
      of ankle equinus, 387–388
      of ankle instability, 388
      of MSK forefoot pain, 386
      of MSK hindfoot and ankle pain, 385
      of MSK midfoot pain, 386
      of pes planus, 387
      of snapping ankle, 388
   lateralization of foot (medial) pain, 426
   lateralization of pain, 388
   musculoskeletal (MSK) causes of, 383
   neuropathic causes of, 386
   physical examination, 395–397
      palpation, 396
      special tests, 397–399
   surface anatomy of foot and ankle, 383
   treatment
      ankle arthrodesis, 406
      ankle arthroscopy, 406
      foot inserts, 403–404
      injections, 402
      medications, 402
      orthoses, 404–405
      physical therapy for therapeutic exercise, 401–402
      shoes, 405–406
      surgery, 406
      taping, 402–403
   at work, 383
ankle arthritis, 415–416
ankle foot instability, 32
ankle impingement syndrome, 408–409
ankle joint, 388–389
ankle ligaments, 390
ankle sprain, 407–408
ankylosing spondylitis, 109, 279–280
anterior and posterior drawer tests, 134
anterior femoral cutaneous neuralgia, 320
anterior interosseous neuropathy, 225
anterior slide test, 134
anterior tarsal tunnel syndrome (deep peroneal nerve entrapment neuropathy), 433–434
anticonvulsants, for greater occipital neuralgia, 105
apophyseal injuries, 314
apophysitis, 23
appendicular skeleton, 21
Appley grind test, 339
apprehension test, 134, 339
arachnoiditis, 269
arterial endofibrosis, 378
arthropathy, 36, 431
   age and, 24
   amyloid, 154
   in Caucasians, 24
   Charcot foot, 420–421
   classification based on underlying pathology, 24
   cuff-tear, 138
   facet, 270–271, 321
   foot, 395
   GH joint, 140
   inflammatory, 138, 147, 153, 219, 310, 322, 331, 347–348, 416, 422–423, 425
   laboratory investigation for, 56
   neuropathic, 406, 416
   in premenopausal women, 24
   presentation of joint pathology, 24
   rotator cuff, 124, 139, 144, 149
avascular necrosis of hip, 312
avulsion fracture, 314
axial skeleton
   anatomy, 20
   pain-sensitive structures in the spine area, 21
axillary artery occlusion
   diagnosis, 161
   history and physical examination, 161
   treatment, 161

Babinski sign, 12
back, anatomy and biomechanics of
   arachnoid, 248
   biomechanics
      degenerative spine cascade, 254
      disc loads, 254
      facet joint, 254
      kinematics, 253–254
      low back in adolescent, 254
      lumbopelvic, 255–256
      mechanism for radiculopathy or myelopathy, 254
      of sacroiliac joint, 255
      sagittal and coronal balance, 254
      stability of spine, 254–255
   of chest wall and thoracic spine, 248–249
   dura mater, 248
   lumbar root and LS plexus, 250
   meninges, 248
   muscles
      buttock, 253
      extrinsic, 253
      paraspinal, 252–253
   nerve innervation of the spine structure, 250
   nerves
      cutaneous, 252
      motor branches, 252
   pia meter, 248
   ribs, 249
   sacroiliac joint, 249–250
   sacroiliac ligament, 250
   somatic nociception, 250
   spine complex, 247
      bony and soft-tissue anatomy with innervation in the lumbar spine, 248
      intervertebral disc, 247
      vertebra, 247
      vertebral canal, 247
   sympathetic nociception, 250
   thoracic spinal nerves and intercostal nerve, 249

back, anatomy and biomechanics of (cont.)
    thoracic spine, 248–249
    ventral root, 250
back pain
    diagnostic studies, 259
        CT scan, 260
        EMG, 262–263
        MRI, 260–262
        plain radiographs, 259–260
        serologic test, 262
    differential diagnosis, 242
        based on mode of onset, 243
        of severe back spasm, 244
        of spine deformity, 244
    epidemiology, 241–242
    lower (LBP), 241–242
        unusual causes of, 243
    in pediatric population, 241
    physical examination
        for bowel/bladder dysfunction/saddle anesthesia, 256
        neurological examination, 256
        palpation, 256
        provocative tests, 256–258
        Waddell's sign for psychological (nonorganic) factors in back pain, 258
    referral pattern from myofascial trigger point and painful facet joint, 243
    sports with higher rates of LBP, 241–242
    treatment
        bracing (orthoses), 263–264
        facet injection and medial branch block, 264
        functional scale for outcome measurement, 263
        lumbar epidural steroid injection (fluoroscopic guided), 264
        nonoperative management, 263
        oral medication, 263
        surgery, 264
        therapeutic exercise, 263
        US-guided lumbar spine procedure, 264
    work-related factors for lumbar disc disease, 241
ballotable patellar test, 338
Baxter's neuropathy, 432
Beatty test, 257
Bennett lesion
    diagnosis, 152
        MRI, 152
        X-ray, 152
    epidemiology, 152
    etiology, 152
    history and physical examination, 152
bicep long-head tendon disorder
    biomechanics and pathophysiology, 144
    diagnosis, 145
        MRI, 145
        X-ray, 145
    history and physical examination, 144–145
    incidence, 144
    nonoperative management, 145
biceps crease interval test, 176
biceps long-head tear and rupture, 145

biceps long-head tendon instability/subluxation, 145–146
biceps squeeze test, 176
bicipitoradial bursitis, 183
bilateral limb swelling, 9
biomechanics (introduction and clinical application), 28–29
    abnormal, 29
bipartite patella, 347
bone, 21
    aging effect on, 24
    cortical and cancellous, 20
    healing, 21
    pediatric bony injury, 22–23
    subchondral, 24
    tumors, 33, 233–234, 276, 282
bone density (BMD), 40
border nerve syndrome, 320–321
Boxer's knuckle, 200
brachial amyotrophy (Parsonage Turner Syndrome), 158–159
Bragard's sign, 256
bursa, 20
    major/anatomic bursae, 126
    minor/adventitial bursae, 127
    scapulothoracic, 127
    subacromial subdeltoid, 126–127
    subcoracoid, 126
bursitis, treatment of, 76
bursopathy, 123
buttock pain, 246–247

calcaneal fracture, 419
calcaneal gait (heel walking), 31–32
calcific tendinopathy, 143–144
    calcific stage, 144
    post-calcific stage, 144
    pre-calcific stage, 144
calcium pyrophosphate dihydrate crystal deposition (CPPD) disease, 348
cancer pain, 441, 449
capitellum fracture, 189
capsaicin cream, 59–60, 178
cardiovascular history/stroke, 8
carpal boss, 233
carpal fracture, 235
carpal tunnel syndrome (CTS), 197, 224–225
carpal (wrist) instability, 230–231
cauda equina syndrome (CES), 266–267
central poststroke pain syndrome (thalamic pain), 452
central slip extensor injury, 224
cervical cord neurapraxia, 107
cervical facet pathology
    common changes of facet degeneration, 110
    degenerative changes, 109
    diagnosis, 109
        intra-articular facet joint injection and diagnostic medial branch block, 109
        X-ray and MRI, 109
    history and physical examination, 109
    neurological examination and provocative tests, 109
    pain referral pattern from cervical facet joint injection, 109
    treatment, 110

cervical myelopathy, 98, 106–107
cervical radiculopathy, 27, 98, 103–104
cervical spine disorder in Down syndrome, 111–112
    common orthopedic manifestations, 111
cervical strain/sprain, 114
chair apprehension signs, 176
Charcot foot (neuroarthropathy), 420–422
chest wall pain, differential diagnosis, 244, 245
chiari malformation, 108
chondroitin sulfate, 59
chondromalacia patella, 347
chordoma, 277–278
chronic exertional compartment syndrome (CECS), 373–374
chronic fatigue syndrome, 448
chronic venous insufficiency (CVI), 379
clavicle fracture, 157
claw toe, 427
CL injury other than thumb, 223
clunk test, 135
CMC grind test, 212
CMC osteoarthritis (trapeziometacarpal), 227
coccygodynia, 285–286
codeine, 64
Coleman's block test, 397, 398
complex regional pain syndrome, 453–454
compression fracture (osteoporotic), 273–275
compression test for interdigital neuritis, 398
coronary artery disease, 122
coronoid fractures, 187
costochondritis, 245
costovertebral joint subluxation, 282
COX-2 inhibitors, 59
Cozen test, 176
crank test, 134
crescent sign, 151
cross arm adduction test, 135
cross leg test, 397
cruciate ligament injury, 351
crystal induced arthritis, 153–154
cuboid subluxation, 430
cystic adventitial disease, 378

deep fascia, 20
deep vein thrombosis, 378–379
degenerative arthritis, 24
degenerative disc disease, 110–111, 271
    possible mechanisms of pain, 110
de Quervain's tenosynovitis/tendinopathy, 218
desipramine, 62
diabetes mellitus (DM), 8
diabetic radiculopathy, 267
diabetic thoracic radiculoneuropathy, 283
dial test, 339
diaphragm irritation and pneumonia, 122
diclofenac, 178
diffuse idiopathic skeletal hyperostosis, 279
diffuse pain syndrome, 441
discogenic thoracic radiculopathy, 283
discoid meniscus, 350–351

distal biceps tendinopathy/tear, 182–183
distal clavicle osteolysis, 148
distal radial (colles) fracture, 234–235
distal radioulnar instability, 232
dragging gait, 12
drawer sign, 398
drop arm test, 133
drop head syndrome, 109
dual-energy X-ray absorptiometry (DEXA), 40
duloxetine, 62
Dupuytren's disease, 222

ECU tendonitis/tenosynovitis/subluxation, 219
effort thrombosis, 379–380
    Paget-Schroetter syndrome, 160–161
elbow
    biomechanics
        fall on outstretched hand, 175
        function in ADL, 174
        kinetic and kinematics, 174
        overhead throwing, 174–175
        stability, 174
    bone, 170
        distal humerus, 170
        tendon attachment site, 170
    epicondyle, 171
    joint
        radiocapitellar and radioulnar, 170
        ulnohumeral (coronoid-trochlear), 170
    joint innervation, 171
    ligament
        lateral ulnar collateral ligament, 171
        medial (ulnar) collateral, 171
    muscle, 172–173
    nerve innervation, 171, 172
    nerves, 171–172
elbow instability, 169
elbow pain
    in athletes, 167
    diagnostic workup and management of, 177
    differential diagnosis, 167, 168
    epicondylitis, 167
    fractures, 186–189
    imaging study
        CT scan, 178
        MRI/MRA, 178
        plain radiographs, 177
        point-of-care ultrasonography, 177–178
    lateral elbow, 167
    medial elbow, 167
    MSK and neuropathic causes of, 167
    neuropathy, 189–194
        entrapment neuropathies at, 190–191
    nonoperative management, 178
        education, 178
        injections, 179
        medications, 178
        orthotics, 178
        physical or occupational therapy, 178
    pathologies and characteristics, 169
    physical examination
        carrying angle, 175
        ecchymosis, 175
        palpation, 175
        range of motion, 175
        special tests, 176
        swelling, 175
    surgery, 179
    ulnar neuropathy at elbow, 167
    at work, 167
elliptical exercise (EE), 33
Ely test, 305, 338
empty can test, 133
enchondroma, 234
enolic acids, 59
entrapment neuropathy, 27
epidermoid inclusion cyst, 234
epidural liposis, 269
epimysial fascia, 20
equinus (ankle), 31
extensor tendon tear/rupture, 219–220
extensor tenosynovitis or tendinopathy, 219
extracorporeal shockwave therapy (ESWT), 76

Fabella syndrome, 360
FABER (Patrick) test, 305
facet arthropathy, 270–271
facet joint injury, 97
FADIR (FAIR) test, 258, 305
fascia
    deep, 20
    epimysial, 20
    superficial, 20
fascial pain, 20. *See also* myofascial pain
FCR tendinopathy/partial tear/tenosynovitis, 220
FCU tendinopathy, 220–221
femoral neck stress fracture, 312–313
femoral N stretch test, 257
femoral shaft stress fracture, 313
femoroacetabular impingement, 311–312
fenamic acids, 59
fentanyl, 64
FHL tendon dysfunction, 415
fibromyalgia, 445–446
finger deformities, 203
Finkelstein test, 212
first rib fracture, 158
flexor pollicis longus tendinopathy/tenosynovitis, 220
flexor tendon tear, 221
fluctuation test, 338
foot. *See also* ankle and foot pain
    big-toe innervation, 392
    biomechanics
        ankle joint, 394
        arches of the foot, 394–395
        compensation mechanism, 394
        foot alignment and deformity, 394–395
        in gait, 394
        midfoot and forefoot, 394
        neutrally aligned feet, 395
        pes cavus (high arch foot), 395
        pes planus (flat foot), 395
        subtalar joint, 394
    joint
        ankle, 388–389
        midtarsal, 389–390
        1st MTP, 390
        subtalar, 389
        TMT (tarsometatarsal), 390
    ligaments, 390
    muscles, 392–393
    nerve innervation, 391–393
    retinaculum, 390–391
foot and ankle pain. *See* ankle and foot pain
foot drop/slap from ankle dorsiflexion weakness, 32
foot orthosis, 402
foot pathologies, 31–32
Fortin finger test, 257
fractures, 21
    avulsion, 314
    calcaneal, 419
    capitellum, 189
    carpal, 235
    clavicle, 157
    complications of, 21–22
    coronoid, 187
    diagnosis, 113
    distal radial (colles), 234–235
    elbow/forearm, 186
    epidemiology of spine fracture, 112
    etiology of spine fracture, 112
    first rib, 158
    Galeazzi's, 187
    hook of hamate, 236
    injury classification of cervical spine fracture, 112
    IP fracture-dislocations, 234
    Jones, 427–428
    MC site for fracture, 234
    metacarpal, 236–237
    metatarsal neck, 237
    Monteggia's, 188
    nightstick, 188
    olecranon, 188
    patellar sleeve (avulsion), 357–358
    pathologic, 22
    pediatric distal radial, 235
    proximal humeral, 156–157
    radial head and neck, 187
    rib, 245
    scaphoid, 235–236
    stress (fatigue), 22
        femoral neck, 312–313
        femoral shaft, 313
        metatarsal (March fracture), 425–426
        pubic ramus, 313
        of tibia, 374–375
        treatment of, 77–78
    supracondylar, 188–189
    talus, 419
    toe, 429
    treatments, 77–78
    triquetral, 236
Freiberg maneuver, 257
Freiberg's disease, 23, 426
functional weakness, 12

gabapentin, 62, 101, 104, 105, 159, 263, 267, 271, 274, 283, 289, 380
    greater occipital neuralgia, 105
Gaenslen's test, 257

gait
　clinical implication of spatiotemporal parameters of, 31
　cycle, 29
　dysfunction, 31–33
　　with ankle and foot pathologies, 31–32
　　characteristics, 31
　　with hip flexion contracture, 31
　　with knee flexion contracture, 31
　　knee instability, 31
　　scissoring gait, 31
　　swing phase problem, 32
　　Trendelenburg gait, 31
　　underlying causes, 31
　excessive pronation and supination during, 32
　Inman's six determinants of, 31
Galeazzi's fracture, 187
Gamekeeper's (Skier's) thumb, 222
ganglion cyst, 232–233
generalized musculoskeletal pain, 442–448
giant cell tumor of tendon sheath, 233–234
Gillet test, 257
glomus tumor, 234
glucosamine, 59
gluteal aponeurotic tear, 288
gluteal compartment syndrome, 290
gluteal tendinopathy/tear, 316–317
glycerol trinitrate, 60
gonalgia paresthetica, 360–361
gout, 423–424
greater occipital neuralgia, 105–106
groin pain
　differential diagnosis, 300
　　for groin mass, 300
　extrinsic causes of, 299
groin region, 300. *See also* hip, anatomy of

hallux limitus and rigidus, 422–423
hallux valgus, 422
hammer toe, 427
Hawkins Kennedy tests (Hawkins' test), 11, 133, 139
heel rise test, 398
hemangioma, 278
hepatobiliary disease, 122
herpes zoster radiculopathy, 267
Hilton's law, 24
hip, anatomy and biomechanics of
　biomechanics
　　center of gravity (COG), 304
　　hip stability, 304
　　joint motion in activities of daily living (ADL), 303–304
　　joint movement, 303
　　kinematics and kinetics, 303–304
　femur
　　blood supply to, 301
　　neck of, 300
　　proximal, 301
　joint
　　acetabulum, 300
　　alignment of, 301
　　capsuloligamentous tension at, 300
　　labrum, 300
　ligament
　　anterior, 301
　　posterior, 301
　muscles, 302–303, 304
　nerves
　　cutaneous, 302
　　femoral, 302
　　obturator, 302
　　sciatic, 302
hip adductor muscle injury, 318–319
hip adductor (Ober test), 10
hip dislocation, 315
hip pain
　in athletes, 295
　in children, 295
　diagnostic studies, 306
　　plain radiographs, 307
　　point-of-care ultrasonography, 307–308
　differential diagnosis, 295
　　based on the location, 299
　　for hip instability, 300
　　of medial groin pain, 300
　　of musculoskeletal, 296
　　of neuropathic, 296
　　traumatic instability, 300
　hip OA, 295
　nerve innervation in the groin area, 298
　pathologies, 298–299
　physical examination, 304–306
　　palpation, 305
　　range of motion (position), 305
　　tests, 305–306
　prevalence, 295
　related to occupational factor, 295
　risk factors, 295
　surface anatomy of hip and groin, 295, 297
　treatment
　　arthroscopy, 308–309
　　assistive devices, 308
　　home exercise program, 308
　　injections, 308
　　nonoperative, 308
　　patient education, 308
　　perioperative rehabilitation, 309
　　physical therapy, 308
　　surgery, 308–309
hip pointer, 314
HIV radiculopathy, 268
Hoffa's fat pad impingement syndrome, 358–359
Hoffman reflex test, 12, 98
hook of hamate fracture, 236
Hook test, 176
Hoover's sign, 12
hydrocodone, 64
hydromorphone, 64
hydromyelia, 108
hyperekplexia, 244
hyperkyphosis, 244, 273
hyperlordosis, 244
hypermobile first-ray syndrome, 424–425
hypertrophic osteoarthropathy, 450
hypothenar hammer syndrome, 237–238

iliolumbar ligament sprain, 281
iliopsoas tendinobursitis, 317–318
impingement syndrome (shoulder), 136
　external impingement, 139
　internal impingement, 139
　structural diagnosis, 139
indentation test (of knee joint effusion), 338
infrapatellar bursitis, 358
insertional Achilles tendinopathy, 412
intercostal muscle strain, 283
intercostal neuritis, 283
internal impingement syndrome (shoulder), 141–142
intersection syndrome, 218
intervertebral disc injury, 97
intoe gait, 32
ischiofemoral impingement, 287–288
ischiogluteal bursitis, 288
isolated neck extensor myopathy, 109

Jendrassik maneuver, 12
Jersey finger, 223
Jogger's Foot (medial plantar nerve), 432–433
joints
　aging effect on, 24
　anatomy, 23–24
　ankle, 388–389
　approach to painful, 25
　cartilaginous, 24
　constraint and stability, 24
　diarthrodial, 23–24
　elbow
　　radiocapitellar and radioulnar, 170
　　ulnohumeral (coronoid-trochlear), 170
　fibrous, 24
　1st MTP, 390
　hip
　　acetabulum, 300
　　alignment of, 301
　　capsuloligamentous tension at, 300
　　labrum, 300
　innervation of, 24
　involvement, classification based on number, 24
　knee
　　femoro-tibial, 332
　　patellofemoral, 331–332
　　proximal tibiofibular, 332
　midtarsal, 389–390
　shoulder, 124–125
　subtalar, 389
　TMT, 390
　wrist and hand
　　distal radioulnar joint, 201
　　IP, 201
　　MCP, 201
　　midcarpal (intercarpal) joint, 201
　　radiocarpal joint (wrist), 201
　　trapezio-1st carpometacarpal (CMC) joint, 201
joint swelling, 9
Jones fracture, 427–428
J sign, 339, 346, 355

Kim test for posteroinferior labral lesion, 135
kinematics, 28
kinetics, 28–29
Kleinman shear test, 212

Klippel-Feil anomaly, 112
knee, anatomy and biomechanics of
    arcuate ligament complex, 334
    biomechanics
        anterior cruciate ligament, 336
        kinematics and kinetics, 334–336
        knee joint in a closed kinetic chain, 335–336
        in knee OA, 336
        knee stability, 336–337
        patellofemoral joint, 334–335
        "screw home" motion, 335
        tibiofemoral joint, 335
        tibiofibular joint, 335
    blood supply, 332
    extra-articular structures, 333
    inferior lateral genicular artery, 332
    inferior medial genicular artery, 332
    joint
        femoro-tibial, 332
        patellofemoral, 331–332
        proximal tibiofibular, 332
    ligaments, 332
        anterior cruciate (ACL), 332
        cruciate, 332
        PCL, 332–333
    meniscus, 333
    middle genicular artery, 332
    nerve innervation of, 334
    popliteal artery, 332
    popliteus muscle, 334
    synovial membrane and fluid, 332
knee instability, 31
knee pain
    in athletes, 327
    bony and soft tissue anatomy, 329
    diagnostic studies, 340
        CT scan, 342
        MRI, 341–342
        plain radiographs, 340–341
        point of care ultrasound examination, 341
    differential diagnosis of, 328–329
        neuropathic, 330
        painful knee snapping, 331
        subjective knee instability, 331
    epidemiology of, 327
    knee OA, 327
    knee swelling without significant trauma, 331
    MSK (musculoskeletal) causes of, 327
    physical examination, 337
        palpation, 337
        range of motion, 337
        special tests, 337–339
    referred pain pattern, 330
    related to occupation, 327
    risk factors for, 327
    surface anatomy of the knee, 327
    treatment
        education for aerobic endurance exercise, 342
        injection, 342–343
        orthoses, 343
        physical therapy, 342
        surgery, 343
        total knee arthroplasty, 343–344

Kohler's disease, 23, 420
Kümmell's disease, 275

labral tear of hip, 310–311
Lachman test, 338
lateral antebrachial cutaneous neuropathy, 194
lateral collateral ligament, 356
lateral epicondylitis, 179–180
lateral femoral cutaneous nerve, 319–320
lateral squeeze test, 398
lateral sural cutaneous neuropathy, 376–377
LCL sprain, 180
leg, anatomy of
    bones
        fibular, 369
        tibia, 369
    muscles, 370
leg pain
    anterior, 368
    in athletes, 367
    claudication, 369
    diagnostic studies, 372
        CT scan, 372
        MRI, 371
        plain radiographs, 371
        point-of-care ultrasound (US), 372
    differential diagnosis, 367
        of calf pain and cramps, 368
        of common tibial deformity, 369
        of leg swelling, 368–369
        of significant atrophy and hypertrophy, 369
    epidemiology, 367
    neurological examination, 371
    physical examination, 371
        palpation, 371
    posterior, 368
    treatment, 372–373
    vascular study, 372
leptomeningeal metastasis/meningeal carcinomatosis, 268
leukemia, 315
levorphanol, 63
Lhermitte's sign, 98
Lichtman's test, 212
lidocaine or lidocaine creams/patches, 59, 63, 106, 178
ligaments
    anatomy, 12–13
    clinical diagnosis, 16
    collagen in, 15
    elbow
        lateral ulnar collateral ligament, 171
        medial (ulnar) collateral, 171
    healing of, 16
    hip
        anterior, 301
        posterior, 301
    injuries, treatment of, 76
    knee, 332
    liscfranc, 390
    pathologies, 16
        abnormality in motor function after injury, 16
    sensorimotor control of joint movement, and, 16

shoulder, 124–125
spring, 390
syndesmosis, 390
wrist and hand
    collateral, 202, 203
    digital cutaneous, 204
    extrinsic, 201
    fingers, 202–204
    intrinsic, 201–202
    retinacular, 202
    transverse retinacular, 203
    triangular fibrocartilage complex, 202
    volar plates, 202
limb advancement problem, 32
limb clearance problem, 32
lisfranc (TMT) joint injury, 430–431
little league elbow, 181
little league shoulder, 155–156
load and shift test, 134
Ludington test, 134
lumbar spinal stenosis, 269–270
lumbosacral radiculopathy with disc disease, 265–266
lunate-triquetral Ballottement test (Reagan test), 212
lunotriquetral sprain and instability, 231
lyme arthritis, 154–155
lyme radiculopathy, 267–268

Mallet finger, 223
Matles test, 398
Maudsley test, 176
MCL bursitis (Voschell's bursitis), 355
MCL sprain or injury, 354–355
McMurray test, 339
medial antebrachial cutaneous neuropathy, 194
medial epicondylitis, 180–181
medial gastrocnemius tear, 375
medial hallucal neuropathy, 435
medial neuropathy at elbow, 193
medial patellofemoral ligament dysfunction, 355–356
medial tibial stress syndrome, 373
Medrol Dosepak. See methylprednisone (Medrol Dosepak)
meniscal injury, 350
meperidine, 64
metacarpal fractures, 236–237
metastasis (to shoulder), 122
metastatic cervical spine tumor, 114
metastatic synovitis, 450
metatarsal neck fracture (Boxer's fracture), 237
metatarsal rise test, 398
metatarsal stress fracture (March fracture), 425–426
methadone, 63–64
methylprednisone (Medrol Dosepak), 138, 216, 263, 402
midcarpal instability, 231
midfoot arthritis, 429
milking maneuver, 176
Mill's test, 176
Milwaukee shoulder, 149, 153
modified Schober Index, 258
Monteggia's fracture, 188

Morale Lavallée lesion, 317
morphine, 63–64
Morton's interdigital neuralgia, 433
motor neuron disease, 109
movements, physiologic diversity of, 29
moving valgus stress test, 176
Mulder's click, 398
multidirectional instability (of shoulder), 151
multiple myeloma, 277
muscle and soft tissue pain, 449–450
muscle relaxants
   ankle and foot pain, 402
   back pain, 247, 263, 271
   greater occipital neuralgia, 105
   myofascial pain syndrome, 115
   neck pain, 101
   shoulder pain, 138
   wrist and hand pain, 216
muscles
   back
      buttock, 253
      extrinsic, 253
      paraspinal, 252–253
   compartmental anatomy, 16
   elbow, 172–173
   hip, 302–303, 304
   injury/injuries
      ankle and foot, 392–393
      chronic exertional compartment syndrome, 19
      classification of, 16
      delayed onset muscular soreness, 19
      inflammatory myopathy, 19
      leg, 370
      muscle trauma, 19
      muscular dystrophy, 19
      myoadenylate deaminase, 19
      myopathies, 19
      myotonic dystrophy and fascioscapulohumeral dystrophy, 19
      neuromyotonia, 19
      pain sensation of, 16
      referred pain, 19–20
      rhabdomyolysis, 19
      vitamin deficiency, 19
   piriformis, 286
   shoulder, 127–129
   skeletal, 16
   wrist and hand, 206–208
musculoskeletal (MSK) disorders, imaging, 33–34
   advanced, 36
   chronic pain in joints, 33
   CT imaging, 37
      common artifacts, 37
      myelogram, 37
   dual-energy X-ray absorptiometry, 40
   guidelines for, 34
   MRI imaging, 37–39
      characteristics of benign tumor versus malignancy, 39
      common artifacts, 39
      contraindications and adverse effects, 37
      determinants of signal intensity (brightness), 37
      findings in common MSK pathologies, 39
      indications, 37
      principle, 37
      sequences commonly used in the evaluation of MSK pathologies, 38
      spin echo images, 37
      tumor findings, 39–40
   neurological symptoms/signs, 33
   radiographs, 33–35
      plain radiographs, 33–34
      stress radiographs, 35
   suspicion for diseases with significant morbidity, 33
   trauma, 33
   ultrasound, 40–56
   X-ray findings in, 36
musculoskeletal (MSK) problems. See also treatment for MSK pain
   chief complaints, 1–4
      chronic neuropathic pathologies, 3
      diffuse pain, 3
      pain distribution from sclerotome, dermatome, and peripheral nerves, 2
      referred pain, 3
      regional/local pain, 2
      severity of pain, 4
      valid (well-accepted) causes of pain, 4
   common pain generator encountered in a musculoskeletal clinic, 13
   common versus uncommon etiologies (diagnosis), 4
   differential diagnosis, 9
   etiologies, 4
   locations of common musculoskeletal injuries based on age, 14
   neurological impairment
      impaired function, 5–6
      sensory dysfunction, 5
      weakness, 4–5
   patient education for MSK disorders
      education and lifestyle modification, 57
      exercise, 57
      exercise and arthritis, 57
      for recovery and expected outcome, 57
   pharmacologic management for MSK pain, 57–64
      aspiration, 65
      capsaicin cream, 59–60
      chondroitin sulfate, 59
      common indications for injections, 64
      dry needling/fenestration, 65
      fluoroscopy-guided steroid injections, 69
      glucosamine, 59
      glycerol trinitrate, 60
      image-guided injections, 65
      injections, 64–67
      lidocaine or lidocaine creams/patches, 59
      for muscle cramps, 60
      muscle (skeletal) relaxant, 60
      neuropathic pain medication, 60–63
      NSAIDs, 58–59
      opioid(s) analgesics, 58, 64
      platelet rich plasma injections, 67
      prolotherapy, 67
      skin preparation for injections, 65
      steroid injections, 66
      topical analgesics, 59–60
      viscosupplementation, 66–67
      WHO analgesic ladder, 2002, 58
   PQRST pain assessment method, 1–4
   relevant histories for MSK disorders
      cancer, 8
      cardiovascular history/stroke, 8
      diabetes mellitus, 8
      occupational risk factors, 8
      pediatric MSK issues, 8
      related to specific sport/recreational activity, 6–7
      relationship between OA and sports/recreational activity, 7–8
   review of system, 8–9
      bowel/bladder dysfunction/saddle anesthesia, 9
      CNS aspects, 8
      constitutional, 8
      gastrointestinal (GI) and renal, 8–9
      HEENT, 8
      respiratory and cardiovascular, 8
   swelling
      bilateral limb swelling, 9
      joint swelling, 9
      unilateral limb swelling, 9
   treatment for MSK pain
      acupuncture, 75
      Alexander technique, 75
      cardiovascular endurance training, 72
      common problems and limitations of therapy, 70
      cryoneuroablation (cryoanalgesia), 69
      diagnostic nerve block with anesthetic, 68
      education for biomechanics and home exercise program, 71
      for elderly, 72
      Feldenkrais, 75
      flexibility exercise, 70
      fluoroscopy-guided steroid injection, 69
      manual therapy, 70–71
      modalities, 73, 75
      nerve sclerosing therapy, 68
      for obese patients, 72
      occupational therapy (OT), 69–70
      for patients with MSK pathologies, 72–73
      peripheral nerve stimulation, 69
      pharmacologic management, 57–64
      physical therapy (PT), 69–70
      pilates, 75
      during pregnancy, 73
      principle of, 58
      prolotherapy, 67
      spinal cord stimulation, 69
      stabilization exercise, 71
      stem cell therapy, 67
      strengthening exercise, 71–72
      tai chi, 75
      US-guided nerve block, 69
      water exercise therapy, 75
      yoga, 75
musculoskeletal (MSK) structure, anatomy of, 121
myasthenia gravis, 109
myofascial LBP, 280–281

myofascial pain syndrome, 20, 64–65, 71, 84, 86, 105, 115, 122, 137–138, 253, 286–287, 289, 373
  definition, 115
  diagnosis, 20, 115
  history and physical examination, 115
  mimicking positive sensory symptoms, 85
  of neck, 122
  of neck (paraspinal/suboccipital) muscles (referred pain), 122
  in the neck-shoulder girdle, 83
  pain patterns, 86
  prevalence, 115
  referral pattern, 299
  of rhomboids, 284
  of scapular stabilizer muscle (trapezius, rhomboids, levator scapular etc) with referred pain, 122
  treatment, 115
    manual, 115
    nonpharmacologic, 115
    pharmacologic, 115
myopathy, 109
myositis ossificans, 186, 321

nalbuphine, 64
navicular osteonecrosis (Müller-Weiss disease), 420
navicular stress fracture, 420
neck, anatomy of, 88, 95
  anterior, 92–93
  carotid artery, 96
  deep cervical fascia, 95
  investing layer, 95
  ligament
    anterior longitudinal ligament (ALL), 90
    atlanto-occipital membrane, 90
    flavum, 90
    posterior longitudinal ligament (PLL), 90
    supraspinous, 90
    transverse, 90
  movements, 92–96
  muscle
    anterior and anterolateral cervical, 92
    posterior cervical, 92
    suboccipital, 94
  nerve
    cervical plexus and brachial plexus, 91
    innervation of the spine structure, 90
    spinal, 90–92
  posterior, 93–94
  regional anatomy
    C1 (atlas) and C2 (axis), 87
    cervical spinal canal and spinal cord, 90
    facet joint orientation, 89
    spine complex (bone and joint), 87–90
    subaxial cervical spine, 87–90
    triangle of, divided by sternocleidomastoid (SCM) muscle, 87
  vertebral artery, 95–96
neck, biomechanics
  cervical spine ROM, 96
  degenerative changes, 96–97
  spinal musculature, role of, 96
neck, imaging of
  CT scan, 101
  MRI imaging, 100
  plain radiographs, 98
    indications with history of trauma, 99
    lateral view, 98
  point-of-care ultrasound, 100
neck, physical examination of
  atrophy of muscles, 97
  bony structure, 97
  motor and sensory examination of upper extremity, 97–98
  muscle and other soft tissue, 97
  position of head in relation to the line of gravity (plumb line), 97
  provocative test
    for cervical myelopathy, 98
    for cervical radiculopathy, 98
    for thoracic outlet syndrome, 98
  range of motion (ROM), 97
neck distraction test (for radiculopathy), 98
neck pain
  in athletes, 83
  diagnostic approach and management for, 99
  differential diagnosis, 83–87
    of nontraumatic, 84
  extrinsic causes of, 85
  indications of plain radiographs, 100
  neurological symptoms associated
    cervicogenic headache, 86
    motor symptoms, 85–86
    multiple joint pain (polyarthralgia) with neck pain, 86
    otolaryngologic sensations, 86
    pseudoangina pectoris or breast pain, 86
    sensory symptoms, 85
    swallowing difficulty, 86
  risk factors for, 83
  spinal cord injury (SCI), 83
  treatment
    acupuncture, 102
    alternative therapy, 102
    common office-based procedures, 101–102
    education for nonspecific neck pain, 101
    interventional procedure with fluoroscopic guidance, 102
    nonoperative management, 101–102
    oral medication for nonspecific neck pain, 101
    physical therapy, 101
    surgical management, 102–103
  unusual causes of, 84
  at work, 83
Neer's test, 133, 139
nerve innervation
  elbow, 171, 172
  foot, 391–393
  hip
    cutaneous, 302
    femoral, 302
    obturator, 302
    sciatic, 302
  knee, 334
  shoulder, 126
  spine structure, 250
  wrist and hand, 204–205
nerve tumor, 268–269
nervous system
  anatomy, physiology, and clinical implication, 26–27
  ascending pathway, 26
  central (brain and spinal cord) and peripheral, 26
  descending pathway, 27
  differential diagnosis and localization, 28
  EMG/NCS analysis, 28
neurolysis, 68
neuropathic pain
  central poststroke pain syndrome (thalamic pain), 452
  classification of
    entrapment neuropathy, 27
    radiculopathy, 27
    traumatic nerve injury, 27
  complex regional pain syndrome, 453–454
  conditions, 441
  diagnostic studies, 444
  examination for, 443–444
  related to tumor, 450
  small fiber neuropathy, 454–455
  spinal cord injury-related pain syndrome, 452–453
neuropathy, treatment of, 76–77
  modification of aggravating factor, 77
  systematic/diffuse, 77
Newton's law, 29
nightstick fracture, 188
noble compression test, 306
nonsteroidal anti-inflammatory drug (NSAID)
  back pain, 263, 272
  calcific tendinopathy, 144
  cervical facet pathology, 110
  elbow pain, 178
  FCR tendinopathy/partial tear/tenosynovitis, 220
  femoroacetabular impingement, 312
  gluteal tendinopathy/tear, 317
  greater occipital neuralgia, 105
  lateral epicondylitis, 180
  myofascial pain syndrome, 115
  osteitis pubis, 314
  rotator cuff arthropathy, 149
  shoulder osteoarthritis, 150
  shoulder pain, 138
  spondylolisthesis, 272
  subacromial impingement syndrome, 140
  subcoracoid impingement syndrome, 141
  Tietze's syndrome, 282
  wrist and hand pain, 216
nortriptyline, 62
  greater occipital neuralgia, 105

Ober test, 10, 306, 338
O'Brien test, 134
obturator internus syndrome, 287
obturator neuropathy, 320
olecranon bursitis, 183–184
olecranon fracture, 188
opioid medications, 9, 58, 63–64, 452, 454–455
  ankle and foot pain, 402
  back pain, 263, 267
  hip and thigh pain, 310
  leg pain, 373, 380
  neck pain, 110
  neuropathy and vascular dysfunction, 159
  shoulder pain, 138
  wrist and hand pain, 216
orthoses (bracing)
  ankle and foot pain, 404–405
  definition, 75
  elbow pain, 178
  knee pain, 343
  problems using orthotics, 75
  shoulder pain, 138
  spine, 256
  wrist and hand pain, 216–217
Osgood-Schlatter disease, 359
Os Peroneum syndrome, 418–419
ossification of PLL, 107–108
Osteitis Condensans Ilii, 285
osteitis pubis, 313–314
osteoarthritis (OA), 184, 295, 327
  ankle, 415–416
  CMC (trapeziometacarpal), 227
  elbow, 184
  of hip, 309–310
  knee, 344–345
  shoulder, 149–150
  of wrist, 227–228
osteochondritis dissecans, 348–349
  of the elbow (capitellum), 184–185
  of talus, 417
osteochondroses, 23
osteonecrosis, 23
  of the femoral head (avascular necrosis), 312
  of the humeral head, 155
  of the knee, 349
oxycodone, 63–64
oxymorphone, 64

pace maneuver test, 257
Paget's disease, 280
painful accessory navicular, 418
painful Os trigonum, 418
paraneoplastic joint disorders, 450
paraneoplastic peripheral neuropathy, 451
Parkinson's disease, 109
patellar glide test, 339
patellar instability, 347
patellar sleeve (avulsion) fracture, 357–358
patellar tilt test, 339
patella tendinopathy and tear, 357
patellofemoral grind test (Clarke sign), 339
patellofemoral syndrome, 345–347
pathologic fractures, 22
Paxinos test, 135
PCL injury, 352

pectoralis muscle strain and tear, 146
pediatric bony injuries, 22–23
  growth-related problems, 22–23
  overuse injuries, 23
  pediatric distal radial fracture, 235
  presentation
    greenstick fracture, 23
    Salter–Harris epiphyseal fracture, 23
    supracondylar fracture, 23
    torus (buckle) fracture, 23
pediatric hip pathology
  diagnostic workup, 322
  history and physical examinations, 322
  individual conditions, 323
pediatric tumors, 315
peripheral arterial disease, 377
peripheral neuropathy, 109
peripheral neuropathy related to chemotherapy, 450–451
peroneal neuropathy, 361–362
peroneal tendon dysfunction, 414–415
pes anserine tendinobursitis, 354
physical therapy (PT), 434, 448, 454
  for adhesive capsulitis, 149
  for ankle and foot pain, 401–402, 408, 410–411
  for back pain, 271–272, 274, 275, 279–281, 288
  for buttock pain, 285
  for cervical strain/sprain, 114
  for hip and thigh pain, 308, 310
  for knee pain, 342, 345–347, 357
  for musculoskeletal problem, 69–70, 76
  for neck pain, 101, 104–106, 108, 110–111, 114
  for nonspecific TOS, 160
  for rheumatoid arthritis, 111
pinch test, 398
piriformis syndrome, 257–258, 286–287
pisotriquetral grind test, 212
pivot shift test, 338
plantar fasciitis, 409–410
plantar fibromatosis, 410–411
plantaris tendon and soleus muscle tear, 375
plica of knee, 353
plica syndrome, 353–354
point-of-care ultrasonography, 45–55
  ankle and foot pain, 400–401
  basic interpretation
    echogenicity (brightness), 41
  basic manual for, 41
  bony evaluation, 44
  challenges in MSK US, 41
  common indications for, 40
  common US findings in MSK disorders, 42–43
  common US image artifacts, 42
  definition, 40
  elbow pain, 177–178
  hip pain, 307–308
  knee pain, 341
  leg pain, 372
  limitations, 41
  muscle evaluation, 44
  peripheral nerve disorder evaluation, 44
  practical tips for scanning and guidance, 55

  role in diagnostic injection, 55
  shoulder pain, 136
  technologies to improve image quality
    beam steering, 56
    elastography, 56
    matrix (array) probe, 55
    spatial compounding image, 55
    using harmonic waves, 55
  US evaluation
    of joint effusion, 43
    of soft tissue mass, 43–44
  wrist and hand pain, 214–215
polymyalgia rheumatica, 446–448, 450
popliteal artery aneurysm, 360
popliteal artery entrapment syndrome, 377–378
popliteal cyst (Baker), 359–360
popliteus tendinopathy, 356
posterior antebrachial cutaneous neuropathy, 193
posterior femoral cutaneous neuropathy, 321
posterior hip impingement test, 306
posterior impingement of the elbow, 185
posterior sag sign, 338
posterolateral corner (PLC) injury, 352–353
posterolateral rotatory-instability test (pivot shift), 176
postlaminectomy, 109
posttraumatic kyphosis, 109
PQRST pain assessment method, 1–4
pregabalin, 63
  greater occipital neuralgia, 105
prepatellar bursitis, 358
propionic acids, 59
propoxyphene, 64
proximal hamstring tendinopathy or tear, 287
proximal humeral fracture, 156–157
proximal tibiofibular sprain and instability, 349–350
pseudogout, 348
PT arthritis/instability, 228
pubic ramus stress fracture, 313
pyrazolidinediones, 59

quadriceps tendinopathy and tear, 356–357
quadrilateral space syndrome, 162

radial tunnel and supinator syndrome, 192–193
radiation plexopathy, 451
radiculopathy, 27
radiculoplexus neuropathy, 267
rectus femoris tendon disorder, 318
relocation test, 134
resisted wrist flexion and pronation, 176
restless leg syndrome, 380
retinacular cyst, 221–222
retrocalcaneal bursitis, 412–413
rheumatoid arthritis, 111, 185–186, 416–417
  cervical spine involvement, 111
  elbow, 185–186
  for foot and ankle, 416–417

of knee, 347–348
prevalence, 111
in shoulder, 152–153
of wrist and hand, 228–230
rib fracture, 245
Roller Wringer effect, 130
Roo's test, 98, 135
rotator cuff arthropathy, 149
rotator cuff tendinopathy and tear, 142–143
running, 32–33

salicylates, 59
Salter–Harris epiphyseal fracture, 23
saphenous mononeuropathy, 435–436
saphenous neuropathy, 360–361
scaphoid fracture, 235–236
scapular fracture, 157
Scheuermann's disease, 275
sciatic neuropathy, 288–289
scissoring gait, 31
scoliosis, 272–273
seated flexion test, 257
seated piriformis test, 258
2nd MTP joint disorder and subluxation, 425
septic arthritis of the GH joint, 154
serratus anterior strain, 284
sesamoid disorders of the hallux, 424
sesamoid pathology, 13
Sever's disease, 412
shoulder
    anatomy, 121–122
        acromioclavicular joint, 124
        acromioclavicular ligament, 124
        bony landmarks, 124
        bursa, 126–127
        glenohumeral joint, 124
        glenohumeral ligament, 124
        glenoid cavity of the scapular and glenohumeral stabilizers, 125
        humerus, 124
        impingement zone, 125
        labrum, 124
        muscle, 127–129
        nerve innervation, 126
        rotator cuff interval, 125–126
        scapula, 124
        sternoclavicular joint, 124–125
        subacromial/coracoacromial arch space, 125–126
    biomechanics of
        GH and scapulothoracic joint motion, 129
        scapular plane and angle of torsion, 130
        scapular protraction and abduction, 130
        scapulothoracic movement, 127
        shoulder stability, 131–132
        six phases of the baseball pitch, 131
        subacromial impingement, 130
        suprascapular nerve traction with scapula position, 130
        throwing, 131
shoulder abduction test, 98
shoulder-hand syndrome (complex regional pain syndrome), 8

shoulder impingement syndrome, 8
shoulder instability, 150–151
shoulder osteoarthritis, 149–150
shoulder pain
    in athletes
        prevalence, 119
        risk (predisposing) factors, 119
        SICK scapula syndrome, 119
        tendon overuse, 119
    diagnostic studies
        AP with stress, 136
        CT scan, 137
        MRA, 137
        MRI, 136–137
        plain radiographs, 135–136
    differential diagnosis of sensory symptoms, 122
    extrinsic causes of, 122
    motor symptoms, 122–123
    musculoskeletal (MSK) causes of, 119
        anatomic structure, 121
        differential diagnosis, 120
    neurological symptoms, 122–123
    neuropathic causes of, 122
        axillary neuropathy, 122
        suprascapular neuropathy, 122
    physical examination
        acromioclavicular joint, 135
        Apley "Scratch test," 133
        atrophy, 132
        biceps tendon, 134
        bony landmarks on sitting with forearm neutral, 132
        GH internal rotation deficit, 133
        GH joint movement, 133
        glenohumeral instability test, 134
        normal scapulothoracic motion, 133
        palpation, 132
        range of motion, 132–133
        scapular positioning, 132
        strength of rotator cuff muscles, 133
        subacromial impingement test, 133
    prevalence, 119
    shoulder instability, 123–124
    snapping shoulder, 123
    surface anatomy of, 119, 120
    treatment, 137
        hemiarthroplasty, 138
        injections, 138
        medications, 138
        physical and occupational therapy and education, 137–138
        reverse arthroplasty, 138
        rotator cuff repair, 138
        shoulder arthroplasty, 138
        surgery, 138
    at work, 119
SICK scapula syndrome, 119
SI joint dysfunction, 284–285
Silfverskiold test for gastrocnemius tightness, 11
Sinding–Larsen–Johansson disease, 359
sinus-tarsi syndrome, 409
skeletal muscles, 29
SLAP (superior labral anteroposterior) lesion, 151–152
slipping rib syndrome, 245

slump test, 257
small fiber neuropathy, 454–455
snapping elbow, 169
snapping shoulder, 123
spinal cord injury-related pain syndrome, 452–453
spondylolisthesis, 271–272
spondylosis, 106
spontaneous osteonecrosis of the knee, 349
sport hernia, 319
Spurling test, 98
squeeze test, 397
stair climbing, 33
standing flexion test, 257
statin myopathy, 380
Stener's lesion, 222
sternoclavicular osteoarthritis, 156
sternoclavicular sprain/injury, 156
stiffness, 169–170
Stinger syndrome (Burner), 159
Stork test, 258
straight leg raise test (SLR), 256
    cross, 257
stress (fatigue) fractures, 22
subacromial impingement syndrome, 139–140
    comparison of open and arthroscopic acromioplasty, 140
    structural pathologies underlying, 139
subcoracoid impingement syndrome, 140–141
subtalar arthritis, 416
subtalar sprain and instability, 409
sufentanil, 64
sulcus sign, 134
sulphonamides, 59
superficial fascia, 20
superficial peroneal nerve entrapment syndrome, 434
superficial peroneal neuropathy, 376
superficial radial neuropathy, 226
superior cluneal nerve entrapment syndrome, 289
superior gluteal arterial disease, 289–290
supraclavicular nerve entrapment syndrome, 106
supracondylar fracture, 188–189
suprascapular neuropathy, 161–162
sural mononeuropathy, 435
syringomyelia, 108

Tailor's bunion (Bunionette deformity), 427
talus fracture, 419
Tarlov cyst, 278
tarsal coalition, 417–418
tarsal tunnel syndrome (tibial nerve), 431
tendinopathy, treatment of, 76
tendinopathy (wrist and hand), in sport, 197
tendinosis, 14
tendon
    aging, 14
    anatomy, 12–13
        gross (macroscopic) anatomic characteristics, 12
        characteristics and clinical implications, 13–14
        characteristics of tendinosis, 14

tendon (cont.)
  common site for tendon-muscle injury, 14
  epidemiology of sports related tendon injury, 15
  and ligament stress-strain relationship curve, 14
  neuronal response to tendon injury, 14
  pathologies
    classification, 14
    predisposing conditions for tendinopathy, tear, or rupture, 15
    tendon healing, 15
tensor fascia lata tendinopathy and tear, 317
TFCC grind test, 212
TFCC lesion, 231–232
TFCC snap test, 212
therapy for patients with neuromuscular disease, 73
Thessaly test, 339
Thomas test, 305, 338
Thompson test, 398
thoracic outlet syndrome, 98, 135
  diagnosis, 159
    X-ray, 160
  epidemiology, 159
  history and physical examination, 159
  location of compression in, 160
  treatment, 160
thoracic radiculopathy, 27
tibialis anterior tendinopathy and tear, 414
tibial neuropathy, 376
Tietze's syndrome, 245
toe fracture, 429
TP tendon dysfunction, 413–414
tramadol, 63
transient osteoporosis, 321–322
transient synovitis or irritable hip, 323
traumatic nerve injury, 27
Trendelenburg gait, 31
triangular fibrous cartilage complex injury, 230
triangular sign (for shoulder instability), 151
triceps tendinopathy and tear, 183
tricyclic antidepressant (TCA), 60–61, 446, 448, 452, 455
  back pain, 263, 267, 271, 274, 283
  buttock pain, 289
  greater occipital neuralgia, 105
  myofascial pain syndrome, 115
  neck pain, 101, 104, 105, 115
  neuropathic pain, 452–453
trigger fingers, 221
triquetral fracture, 236
triquetral impingement, 232
trochanteric bursitis, 315–316
Tromner sign, 98
tumors, 233–234
  bone, 282
  bony pain related to, 449
  lesions, 315

pediatric, 315
of the spine, 275–277
synovial, 450
turf toe, 424

ulnar collateral ligament injury, 181–182
ulnar neuropathy, 189–192
  at elbow, 167
  at wrist, 225–226
ulnar styloid triquetral impaction test, 212
unilateral limb swelling, 9
upper and lower extremities, compartmental anatomy of, 17–18
US-guided lumbar spine procedure, 264
US-guided needle lavage for calcific tendinopathy, 144
US-guided nerve block
  greater occipital neuralgia, 106
  lateral femoral cutaneous nerve block, 308
  for MSK pain, 69
  posterior interosseous nerve block, 216
  saphenous nerve block, 343
  superficial peroneal nerve block, 376
  suprascapular nerve block, 149

valgus extension overload syndrome (posteromedial impingement), 182
valgus stress test, 176, 339
Valleix's phenomenon, 10
varus stress test, 176, 339
venlafaxine, 62
vertebral osteomyelitis, 278–279
visual analogue scale, 4
volar plate injury, 224

Watson's test, 212
whiplash-associated injury, 97, 110
widespread pain, 441
Wright maneuver, 135
Wright's hyperabduction, 98
wrist and hand, anatomy and biomechanics
  biomechanics of
    forearm movement and radioulnar joint, 208
    hand functions, 209
    proximal carpal movements, 208–209
    ROM during activities of daily living (ADL), 208
    wrist stability, 209
  bone
    distal carpal row, 201
    proximal carpal row, 200–201
  joints
    distal radioulnar joint, 201
    IP, 201
    MCP, 201
    midcarpal (intercarpal) joint, 201
    radiocarpal joint (wrist), 201
    trapezio-1st carpometacarpal (CMC) joint, 201

ligaments
  collateral, 202, 203
  digital cutaneous, 204
  extrinsic, 201
  of fingers, 202–204
  intrinsic, 201–202
  retinacular, 202
  transverse retinacular, 203
  triangular fibrocartilage complex, 202
  volar plates, 202
muscle
  hand intrinsic, 207–208
  wrist extensor compartment, 206
  wrist flexor, 206–207
nerve innervation, 204–205
  anterior interosseous, 205
  lateral antebrachial cutaneous, 205
  median, 204
  posterior interosseous, 205
  superficial radial, 204
  ulnar, 204
  ulnar nerve main trunk, 205
wrist and hand pain
  diagnosis
    CT scan, 215
    EMG, 215
    MRI, 215
    plain radiographs, 214
    point-of-care ultrasound, 214–215
  differential diagnosis of, 198
    dorsal-middle snapping, 200
    of finger/wrist drop, 200
    surface anatomy with surface landmark, 197, 198
    ulnar side snapping, 200
  neuropathic causes of, 199
  orthoses, 216–217
  physical examination
    finger, 209–210
    inspection of the position of the hand, 209
    palpation, 210–213
    radial side, 209
    special tests of the hand, 213
    special tests of the wrist, 211–212
    thumb movements, 211
    wrist ROM, 210
  prevalence, 197
  in sports, 197
  tests for median and ulnar neuropathy, 213
  treatment
    common injections, 216
    medications, 216
    nonoperative management, 216
    surgery, 217–218
  vascular test, 213
  at work, 197

Yergason test, 134